Geriatric Rehabilitation
From Bedside to Curbside

REHABILITATION SCIENCE IN PRACTICE SERIES

Series Editors

Marcia J. Scherer, Ph.D.

President
Institute for Matching Person and
Technology
Professor
Physical Medicine & Rehabilitation
University of Rochester Medical Center

Dave Muller, Ph.D.

Visiting Professor
University of Suffolk
Past and Founding Chair of
Chamber of Commerce
Editor-in-Chief
Disability and Rehabilitation
Director
Ipswich Central Ltd.

Published Titles

Ambient Assisted Living, *Nuno M. Garcia and Joel J.P.C. Rodrigues*

Assistive Technology Assessment Handbook, edited by *Stefano Federici and Marcia J. Scherer*

Assistive Technology for Blindness and Low Vision, *Roberto Manduchi and Sri Kurniawan*

Computer Access for People with Disabilities: A Human Factors Approach, *Richard C. Simpson*

Computer Systems Experiences of Users with and Without Disabilities: An Evaluation Guide for Professionals, *Simone Borsci, Maria Laura Mele, Masaaki Kurosu, and Stefano Federici*

Devices for Mobility and Manipulation for People with Reduced Abilities, *Teodiano Bastos-Filho, Dinesh Kumar, and Sridhar Poosapadi Arjunan*

Geriatric Rehabilitation: From Bedside to Curbside, edited by *K. Rao Poduri, MD, FAAPMR*

Human-Computer Interface Technologies for the Motor Impaired, edited by *Dinesh K. Kumar and Sridhar Poosapadi Arjunan*

Multiple Sclerosis Rehabilitation: From Impairment to Participation, edited by *Marcia Finlayson*

Neuroprosthetics: Principles and Applications, *Justin Sanchez*

Paediatric Rehabilitation Engineering: From Disability to Possibility, edited by *Tom Chau and Lillian Fairley*

Quality of Life Technology Handbook, *Richard Schultz*

Rehabilitation: A Post-critical Approach, *Barbara E. Gibson*

Rehabilitation Goal Setting: Theory, Practice and Evidence, edited by *Richard J. Siegert and William M. Levack*

Rethinking Rehabilitation: Theory and Practice, edited by *Kathryn McPherson, Barbara E. Gibson, and Alain Leplège*

Robotic Assistive Technologies: Principles and Practice, edited by *Pedro Encarnção and Albert M. Cook*

Wheelchair Skills Assessment and Training, *R. Lee Kirby*

The discussion of *Geriatric Rehabilitation: From Bedside to Curbside* presented in this multiauthored book provides a comprehensive and up-to-date presentation of the many issues facing older adults and should be read by every physician who treats elderly patients. The chapters are written from the perspective of practicing clinicians, who are internationally recognized experts in the field. Edited by Dr. K. Rao Poduri, the chairperson of physical medicine and rehabilitation at the University of Rochester School of Medicine and Dentistry, this book will be useful to the clinician in daily practice. The field of geriatrics will benefit from this unique resource, which can serve as both a textbook for students and a handy guide for clinicians.

Bradford C. Berk, MD, PhD
Distinguished University Professor in Medicine,
Pathology, and Pharmacology and Physiology
University of Rochester School of Medicine and Dentistry
Director, Rochester Neurorestorative Institute
University of Rochester Medical Center
Rochester, New York

It is with great enthusiasm and delight that I recommend the new book, *Geriatric Rehabilitation: From Bedside to Curbside*, edited by K. Rao Poduri, MD, professor, and chair from the Department of PM&R at the University of Rochester. The 33 chapters of this important new textbook cover the range of physiologic and pathologic changes seen with aging and in the older adult, and provide rehabilitation-specific interventions for management. It is a well-written and informative book that will quickly become a "must have" for the everyday clinician who takes care of older adults. I have known Dr. Poduri for nearly 20 years and am not surprised at the quality and attention to detail contained in this book. It is both an academic reference and a practical resource.

David Cifu, MD
Herman J. Flax, MD, Professor and Chairman
Department of Physical Medicine and Rehabilitation
Virginia Commonwealth University School of Medicine
Richmond, Virginia
Senior TBI Specialist
U.S. Department of Veterans Affairs

Geriatric Rehabilitation
From Bedside to Curbside

K. Rao Poduri

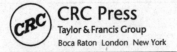

CRC Press
Taylor & Francis Group
Boca Raton London New York

CRC Press is an imprint of the
Taylor & Francis Group, an **informa** business

CRC Press
Taylor & Francis Group
6000 Broken Sound Parkway NW, Suite 300
Boca Raton, FL 33487-2742

First issued in paperback 2019

© 2017 by Taylor & Francis Group, LLC
CRC Press is an imprint of Taylor & Francis Group, an Informa business

No claim to original U.S. Government works

ISBN-13: 978-1-4822-1122-1 (hbk)
ISBN-13: 978-0-367-86880-2 (pbk)

Library of Congress Cataloging-in-Publication Data

Names: Poduri, K. Rao, author.
Title: Geriatric rehabilitation : from bedside to curbside / K. Rao Poduri.
Description: Boca Raton, FL : CRC Press/Taylor & Francis Group, 2017.
Identifiers: LCCN 2016030569| ISBN 9781482211221 (hardback) | ISBN 9781482211238 (ebook)
Subjects: LCSH: Older people–Rehabilitation.
Classification: LCC RC952.5 .P63 2017 | DDC 618.97/703–dc23
LC record available at https://lccn.loc.gov/2016030569

Visit the Taylor & Francis Web site at
http://www.taylorandfrancis.com

and the CRC Press Web site at
http://www.crcpress.com

This book is dedicated to my patients, who inspired me to undertake this project, and to my family for their support during its preparation.

Contents

SECTION I   Basics of Aging

SECTION II   Geriatric Syndromes

SECTION III   Systemic Disorders in Geriatric Rehabilitation

SECTION IV Health Maintenance, Caregiving, and Postacute Rehabilitation: Bedside to Curbside

Foreword

Most potential readers of *Geriatric Rehabilitation: From Bedside to Curbside* will probably already be aware of the demographic impact of the aging of the baby boomer generation. We know that 10,000 Americans for example are turning to 65 years of age every day. From the perspective of healthcare, what is less well appreciated is that the earliest of these boomers are turning 75 and 85 years of age, a trend that will persist for decades ahead. These individuals with increasing longevity, better healthcare, education, and expectations of healthcare present new and even radical challenges to healthcare providers. Geriatricians, physicians who specialize in the care of older adults, are aware that the goals of geriatric healthcare are focused on preservation and improvement of functionality and quality of life, even at the realization that less rather than more conventional medical care is often the prudent choice. The concept of *frailty* is one of the key concepts in good care of older adults. Every medical decision must be based on the prevention of muscle loss, sarcopenia, and potential adverse drug reactions. From the perspective of physiatrists, physicians who specialize in physical medicine and rehabilitation increasingly are being asked to focus less on rehabilitation following acute trauma and more on the improvement of quality of life in patients at 80, 90, or 100 years of age.

This book, carefully edited by Dr. K. Rao Poduri, fills an important educational niche in melding these two specialties so important to the care of older adults. It draws on a distinguished group of authors, most of whom are associated with the University of Rochester School of Medicine and Dentistry in Rochester, New York. Most importantly, these elite authors are the frontline providers of care to older adults. In 33 chapters, this book presents the full spectrum of the unique care needs of older patients who need the combined skills of physical medicine and geriatrics. In the first section, the basics of aging are presented with an emphasis on demographics, health assessment, and the role of function, psychosocial assessment, and principles of exercise in older adults. The second section explores the "geriatric syndromes" that are the key concepts in care. Topics covered include frailty, delirium, incontinence, falls and gait disorders, and pressure ulcers. The three unique features of geriatric care, namely, pain, polypharmacy, and sleep disorders, are also included. Even the placement of these two sections in the front part of this book telegraphs the message that these key care issues are the major determinants of good care. Section III explores some of the key systemic disease states that distinguish the care of older adults from younger patients. These include dysphagia, vision impairment, arthritis, osteoporosis, and diabetes mellitus. Additional topics are cardiovascular and respiratory disorders, cerebrovascular states, cancer, spinal cord damage, Parkinson's disease, and aging with developmental disabilities. The fourth section completes the spectrum of care with chapters on rehabilitation settings, complementary and alternative approaches, assistive technology, ethics, palliative care and end of life, and economics. The final chapter gives a perspective of global geriatric rehabilitation.

Why is this book important? First, the care of our older patients in rehabilitation settings demands the broad understanding of the key differences in strategies to care for older adults. It is unusual that such a broad perspective can be found in a single text. Moreover, these chapters are written by professionals active in the field with real-world experience and expertise. This book is also informative to assist healthcare providers to adapt to the many changes in reimbursement strategies for rehabilitation services. For example, in the United States, Medicare, the federal health insurance program for people who are 65 or older, certain younger people with disabilities, and people with end-stage renal disease, is poised to reward high value care and penalize care not up to quality benchmarks. Various forms of "bundling of payment" for episodes of care defined as the totality of care, which includes an acute hospitalization and all postacute care services over 30 or 90 days are being implemented. Hospitals are already being financially penalized for higher rates of 30-day readmissions following an acute hospitalization. Interestingly, many, if not most, of these readmissions are not related to the initial diagnosis of the first admission but rather to deconditioned frailty states potentially amenable to more targeted rehabilitation services.

There are initiatives to eliminate "silos" of postacute care from the current ones, such as hospital-based rehabilitation, skilled nursing facility care, long-term care hospitals, and home-based care. Benchmarks related to quality measures emphasizing functionality will be the major determinant of reimbursement across the current venues of care with different payment systems. It will be essential that all professionals involved in geriatric and rehabilitation have the expertise to provide some of the unique skills essential to successfully meet quality standards and benchmarks.

Finally, the combined skills embraced in rehabilitation and geriatrics are presenting unprecedented opportunities for both fields to make substantive and even groundbreaking improvements in the lives of millions of older adults who entrust their lives to us. Rarely in one's medical career are such opportunities so evident and achievable. This book provides an easily accessible means of acquiring and improving these new skills.

William J. Hall, MD, MACP
Fine Professor of Geriatrics and Internal Medicine
University of Rochester School of Medicine and Dentistry
Rochester, New York

Acknowledgments

In contributing to this book as an editor, I have inevitably sought out the literature in geriatrics. The wealth of fascinating and inspiring material published on this subject was immensely helpful for my involvement in this production. The information and the up-to-date reports from the Centers for Disease Control (CDC) and the World Health Organization (WHO) enabled me to accurately provide the information needed.

I would like to thank my husband, SRS Rao Poduri, PhD for his helpful suggestions. Special thanks to Patricia DiGiorgio, MS and Cathy Flanagan, RN, MBA for their technical support.

Editor

K. Rao Poduri, MD, FAAPMR, is a professor and the chair of physical medicine and rehabilitation and neurology at the University of Rochester School of Medicine and Dentistry in Rochester, New York. She is the medical director of physical medicine and rehabilitation services at Strong Memorial Hospital at the University of Rochester Medical Center and is the director of the Physical Medicine and Rehabilitation Residency Program. She graduated from Karnataka Medical College, Hubli, India. After 3 years of internal medicine training, Dr. Poduri did residency training in physical medicine and rehabilitation (PM&R) at Strong Memorial Hospital at the University of Rochester. She is fellowship trained in geriatric rehabilitation at the Monroe Community Hospital, an affiliate of the University of Rochester. She is a diplomat of the American Board of Physical Medicine and Rehabilitation, American Academy of Pain Management and Spinal Cord Injury Medicine.

Dr. Poduri joined the faculty in 1981 at the University of Rochester Medical Center. She served as the medical director of the Rochester Rehabilitation Center from 1985 to 1998 and director of the prosthetic clinic at Strong Memorial Hospital from 1989 to 2004. In addition to her medical practice, she teaches medical students, residents, and Fellows at the University of Rochester School of Medicine and Dentistry. Dr. Poduri has been in charge of quality assurance since 1986 and has been the director of quality council for PM&R since 2004. She was a member of the quality assurance committee at the American Academy of Physical Medicine and Rehabilitation (AAPM&R) from 1989 to 1992. She has presented several papers at the annual meetings of AAPM&R, National Stroke Association, and the American Geriatric Society. Her presentation on shoulder pain in stroke patients took her to Germany in 1993. Her research work presentations and publications are in the areas of stroke, brain injury, spinal cord injury, amputations, hypertension, and inpatient rehabilitation outcomes. She had lectured extensively on spinal cord injuries and hypertension in the United States, Canada, and India.

She has authored many journal articles and book chapters and is active in research and has presented many research studies at national and international meetings. She was invited to present her research to her peers in Canada, Germany, India, and United States. She is on the editorial boards of the *AAPM&R's Knowledge NOW, Journal of the Jawaharlal Nehru Medical College Scientific Society, Internet Journal of Medical Update: International Advisory/Reviewers' Committee, Journal Disability and Rehabilitation,* and the *HSOA Journal of Physical Medicine, Rehabilitation and Disabilities.* She is a reviewer for the journals *Archives of Physical Medicine and Rehabilitation, Journal of Neurology,* and *American Journal of Physical Medicine and Rehabilitation.*

Dr. Poduri is a member of many prestigious physical medicine and rehabilitation associations where she holds major leadership positions: American Academy of Physical Medicine and Rehabilitation: served as the chair of the Geriatric Forum at the AAPMR, current chair of General and Medical Rehabilitation Council at AAPMR, and she was the AAPM&R liaison for the American Academy of Neurology to serve as the subject matter expert for AAN's multiple sclerosis Quality Measurement Set Development work group. She served as a subject matter expert for the Quality Tool Box (QTB) on Osteoporosis and Exercise for AAPMR. Dr. Poduri served as a member of the technical expert panel for the development of cross-setting function and quality measures for the Center for Medicaid and Medicare Services (CMS). At the Association of Academic Physiatrists, she is a member of the education committee. In the American Spinal Injury Association, she serves as the chair of by-laws committee and was a member of the autonomic standards committee. Dr. Poduri is a member of International Society of Physical and Rehabilitation Medicine.

Contributors

Bilal Ahmed, MD, FRCP (Edin), FACP, is a professor of clinical medicine at the University of Rochester School of Medicine and Dentistry in Rochester, New York. He received training in internal medicine, geriatrics, and pulmonary medicine in the United Kingdom. He is boarded in internal medicine and palliative care medicine. Dr. Ahmed is on the clinical faculty at Highland Hospital of Rochester, which is a major inpatient geriatric center for the University of Rochester. His major interests are delivering bedside teaching seminars for medical students, internal medicine and family medicine residents, as well as the clinical faculty. He has received more than 35 teaching awards for innovative bedside teaching. His major interests are in the cognitive thought process that drives the medical decision-making process. He has written a book chapter in *Practice of Geriatrics* in (2006) and has numerous other publications, abstracts, and posters to his credit. Dr. Ahmed is a member of the National Board of Medical Examiners (NBME).

Egan Allen, MD, FACP, is an assistant professor of clinical medicine and geriatric hospitalist in the Department of Medicine, Division of Geriatrics, Highland Hospital, University of Rochester School of Medicine and Dentistry, Rochester, New York. Dr. Allen is a board-certified internist and palliative care physician active as a geriatric hospitalist at Highland Hospital, an affiliate of Strong Memorial Hospital in Rochester, New York. He teaches medical students, residents, and fellows in programs in association with the University of Rochester School of Medicine and Dentistry. From 2006 to the present, he has been a part of the Geriatric Fracture Center at Highland Hospital, which specializes in fractures sustained by geriatric patients. He has been the medical director of a neurobehavioral unit at the Highlands at Brighton, a skilled nursing facility in Rochester, New York, since 2008. Dr. Allen earned an MD in 1993 at the University of Rochester School of Medicine and Dentistry and completed a 3-year internal medicine residency in 1996, followed by a chief medical resident position in 1997. He has been a peer reviewer for articles in the geriatric fracture literature, a lecturer in the fields of geriatrics and internal medicine, and a clinical informaticist, working alongside technical personnel in the electronic health record field.

B. Allyn Behling-Rosa, DO, is a physiatrist at the North Shore Osteopathic LLC, Melville, New York, Department of Medicine, Division of Palliative and Hospice Medicine, Northwell Health, Manhasset, New York. She recently completed her residency at Northwell Health's Department of Physical Medicine and Rehabilitation as chief resident. While still a PGY-4, she started a private integrated osteopathic medicine and physical medicine and rehabilitation practice on Long Island, New York. She is also employed part-time by Northwell Health as a teaching associate and palliative medicine fellow in Manhasset, New York. When time permits, she volunteers to lecture for medical students at the Hofstra-Northwell School of Medicine on behalf of the Department of Physical Medicine and Rehabilitation, and is invited to lecture biannually at the regional scleroderma and pulmonary rehabilitation support group. Prior to her undergraduate medical education, she assisted with protocol design, development, and execution of complementary and alternative medicine studies for the University of Michigan Complementary and Alternative Medicine Research Center (CAMRC), as well as coordinated various other studies within the Departments of Endocrinology, Rheumatology, Cardiology, and Cardiac Surgery.

David Berbrayer, MD, is an associate professor in the Division of Physical Medicine and Rehabilitation of the Department of Medicine, University of Toronto. He is a specialist in physical medicine and rehabilitation certified by the Royal College of Physicians and Surgeons of Canada and the American Board of Medical Specialties. Dr. Berbrayer completed a master teacher program at the University of Toronto and is a Harvard Macy graduate. Dr. Berbrayer is the director of outpatient services of physical medicine and rehabilitation at Sunnybrook Health Sciences Centre and the past vice president and chief of staff at Lyndhurst, the Spinal Cord Centre. He is an active consultant at Holland Bloorview Kids Rehab and past president of the staff. He is currently chairman of the section of physical medicine and rehabilitation of the Ontario Medical Association. Dr. Berbrayer is the education chair and pediatric chair of the Canadian Association of Physical Medicine and Rehabilitation, past chair of continuing education of the Canadian Association of Physical Medicine and Rehabilitation. Dr. Berbrayer is an active member of the education committee of the Association of Academic Physiatrists (AAP) and previous chair of the membership committee of AAP. Dr. Berbrayer is a member of the performance metrics committee of AAPM&R and part of the evidence-based committee of AAPM&R. He is a member of the transitions committee of AACPDM and a member of the task force of the American Congress—Geriatrics and also Stroke Sig. Dr. Berbrayer has published numerous peer-reviewed abstracts and continues to review articles for numerous PM&R journals. He has worked with respirology and neurology in the area of sleep medicine pathology and has also lectured on fall prevention and treatment.

Rachel A. Biemiller, MD, earned her medical degree in Augusta, Georgia, at the Medical College of Georgia in 2009. Afterward, she completed her neurology residency in 2013 at the University of Rochester, Rochester, New York. She then was accepted to receive the National Institutes of Health Experimental Therapeutics fellowship at the University of Rochester, where she received further training in the treatment of movement disorders and education in clinical trial design. In 2015, she accepted a position in La Crosse, Wisconsin, in the Gundersen health system.

Kathleen M. Bishop, PhD, is a gerontologist with a specialty in aging with intellectual and developmental disabilities (IDD). She has worked in the IDD field for 40 years, beginning as a preschool special education teacher, an ICF program manager, and then as the assistant director of staff development and training at a large state-run facility for people with IDD. She earned a PhD at Syracuse University in 1998 so she could focus on older adults with IDD. She directed the Program on Aging and Developmental Disabilities at the Strong Center for Developmental Disabilities, University of Rochester (UR) School of Medicine and Dentistry, and with the Finger Lakes Geriatric Education Center also at UR. She has taught gerontology courses at Utica College and New Mexico State University as well as consult for a number of organizations, including the Arc of Oneida/Lewis Counties, on healthy aging in adults with IDD. Dr. Bishop is an active member of the National Task Force on Dementia and ID, cochairing the training committee. After the development of a national curriculum, Dr. Bishop has trained a 2-day course on dementia-capable care and ID across the country and has mentored hundreds of caregivers in a 3-day course on dementia-capable care, which includes a focus on healthcare advocacy for adults with IDD. Additionally, she often presents at conferences and forums in New York State, nationally, and internationally.

Yvonne J. Braver, MD, FACP, is currently the program director in internal medicine and director of ambulatory clinics for Brandon Regional Hospital, Brandon, Florida. She established the first residency program at Brandon Regional Hospital in 2015. Dr. Yvonne went to the University of Florida for her undergraduate education, completed medical school and residency in primary care internal medicine at Emory University. Dr. Yvonne served as the program director for primary care internal medicine and an associate program director in internal medicine at the Cleveland Clinic for more than 10 years.

Philippines G. Cabahug, MD, is a faculty instructor of physical medicine and rehabilitation at the Johns Hopkins School of Medicine and the director of musculoskeletal ultrasound (MSK-US) at the International Center for Spinal Cord Injury, Kennedy Krieger Institute. Dr. Cabahug earned a baccalaureate degree in physical therapy at the University of the Philippines in 1994 and a medical degree at St. Luke's-WHQ Memorial, Philippines, in 2000. She completed a physical medicine and rehabilitation residency at the Philippine General Hospital in 2005. In 2004, she was awarded a UN scholarship to pursue a postgraduate diploma in gerontology and geriatrics at the University of Malta. She completed her second PM&R residency in 2012 and a fellowship in spinal cord injury medicine at the Johns Hopkins Hospital in 2013. Currently, Dr. Cabahug runs two MSK-US clinics at Kennedy Krieger Institute, including a musculoskeletal diagnostic clinic and an ultrasound-guided intrathecal pump access clinic. Dr. Cabahug is actively involved in medical education as the director of the Spinal Cord Injury Medicine Fellowship Program at Kennedy Krieger Institute and the Johns Hopkins School of Medicine. In addition to this role, she also instructs medical students, PM&R residents, and fellows in the fields of spinal cord injury and MSK-US.

Thomas V. Caprio, MD, MPH, MSHPE, CMD, HMDC, FACP, AGSF, is an associate professor of medicine/geriatrics, dentistry, clinical nursing, and public health sciences at the University of Rochester Medical Center in Rochester, New York. He serves as the director of the geriatric medicine fellowship training program, the director of the University of Rochester geriatric assessment clinic, and the director of the Finger Lakes Geriatric Education Center. Dr. Caprio is the medical director for the Visiting Nurse Service Home Care and Hospice and cares for patients in home care, nursing home, and inpatient clinical settings. He is past president for the National Association of Geriatric Education Centers and the National Association for Geriatric Education as well as the past president of the State Society on Aging of New York. He currently oversees the federally funded Finger Lakes Geriatric Workforce Enhancement Program, which provides education and training related to geriatrics and dementia care for healthcare professionals, rural primary care providers, academic health professions faculty, and family caregivers.

Sara J. Cuccurullo, MD, is a professor and the chair of the Department of Physical Medicine and Rehabilitation at Rutgers Robert Wood Johnson Medical School and medical director and vice president of the JFK Johnson Rehabilitation Institute, where she has been the Physical Medicine and Rehabilitation Medicine Residency Program director since 1998. She also serves as a clinician of the JFK Medical Center Consult Service. Dr. Cuccurullo has published three editions of a major textbook *Physical Medicine and Rehabilitation Board Review* (Demos Publishing) and has authored over 24 book chapters and has also authored and coauthored multiple articles and over 60 abstracts on academic medicine, with a major focus on competency assessment of residents. She is president of the National Residency and Fellowship Program Council for PM&R. Dr. Cuccurullo is the co principal investigator on the *Stroke Recovery Research Program Study—Outcomes Trial/Functional Outcomes Trial.* She earned a medical degree at SUNY Downstate.

Richard A. Demme, MD, FACP, is an associate professor of medical humanities and bioethics at the University of Rochester Medical Center (URMC), Rochester, New York. He has been board certified in nephrology for over 20 years. His clinical practice has focused on kidney transplant and dialysis patients. He is the codirector of the Division of Medical Humanities and Bioethics, and the bioethics program director at the URMC. Dr. Demme also serves as the director of the Clinical Ethics Consult Service and chair of the Strong Memorial Hospital Ethics Committee. He has a particular interest in improvement and expansion of advance directives and also writes about allocation of scarce resources and other ethical issues in transplantation.

Matthew Dounel, MD, MPH, FACPM, FAAPMR, is an adjunct assistant professor of preventive medicine at Emory University School of Medicine and voluntary physician at Lenox Hill Hospital located in New York. He completed his residency in preventive medicine at Emory University School of Medicine and subsequently completed his residency in physical medicine and rehabilitation at SUNY Downstate Medical Center. Dr. Dounel recieved master of public health from Mailman School of Public Health at Columbia University. He completed a fellowship in cardiac rehabilitation at Montefiore Medical Center. He is a diplomat of the American Board of Physical Medicine and Rehabilitation and American Board of Preventive Medicine.

Jennifer Anne Fleeman, PsyD, is a licensed psychologist and neuropsychologist in the Department of Physical Medicine and Rehabilitation, University of Rochester Medical Center, Rochester, New York (2007–2015), and director of the Integrative Cognitive Rehabilitation Program (ICRP). She has specialized in the fields of neuropsychology and rehabilitation psychology, providing neuropsychological evaluations and individual psychotherapy for adult and geriatric populations. She was the principal investigator for a grant provided through the Craig H. Neilsen Foundation ("Optimizing Quality of Life for Individuals with Spinal Cord Injury"). She also assisted in the development of a psychosocial rating scale for use with an inpatient rehabilitation population to identify psychosocial issues and interventions to optimize participation and functional outcomes in rehabilitation. Through the ICRP, she worked with an interdisciplinary treatment team, including neuropsychologists, speech-language pathologists, and occupational therapists, to develop a cognitive rehabilitation model focused on a compensatory approach to optimizing daily functioning.

Talya K. Fleming, MD, is an adult physiatrist in the Department of Physical Medicine and Rehabilitation, JFK Johnson Rehabilitation Institute, and the director of the Aftercare Program, Edison, New Jersey, and the director of the Aftercare Program at JFK Johnson Rehabilitation Institute. She oversees the postacute care treatment of patients while guiding them through the rehabilitation continuum. She has been invited to present at various organizations regarding program development and the integration of patients within the rehabilitation continuum to improve patient care. Her clinical interests combine the impact of exercise in the older adult and improving health outcomes, including bone health. She is currently a coprincipal investigator for a clinical research trial comparing medical and functional outcomes of stroke survivors. Dr. Fleming completed her residency training at JFK Johnson Rehabilitation Institute, where she was a chief resident during her final year. As an attending physiatrist of the Aftercare Program, she manages geriatric patients while undergoing neurologic, orthopedic, and cardiopulmonary rehabilitation. She currently maintains board certification in physical medicine and rehabilitation and is a clinical assistant professor at Rutgers Robert Wood Johnson Medical School.

Lindsey Garner, PharmD, MBA, completed her doctor of pharmacy and master of business administration at Drake University in Des Moines, Iowa. As a graduate student, she specialized in drug information, geriatrics, administration, and psychiatry. She is completing a post graduate year-1 residency at the Minneapolis Veterans Affairs Medical Center with plans to pursue a specialty post graduate year-2 residency in geriatrics or psychiatric pharmacy.

Susan Garstang, MD, is a clinical associate professor of physical medicine and rehabilitation (PM&R) at Rutgers–New Jersey Medical School (NJMS). She graduated from PM&R residency in 1998, and following a fellowship in spinal cord injury, she joined an academic practice at the University of Texas Southwestern Medical Center. She became residency program director in 2001 at UT Southwestern and continued in this role until 2014 at Rutgers–New Jersey Medical School. Dr. Garstang is currently associate chief of staff for education at the Veterans Administration, New Jersey. In this role, she is responsible for administrative and accreditation aspects of all medical trainees at the Veterans Administration, including medical students, residents, and fellows. She served two terms as vice chair of the Graduate Medical Education Committee at Rutgers–New Jersey Medical School. She currently serves the Accreditation Council for Graduate Medical Education as a member of the review committee for PM&R. She has been involved in both undergraduate and graduate medical education for most of her academic career.

Diya Goorah, MD, is a physical medicine and rehabilitation resident at SUNY Upstate University Hospital. She attended medical school at St. George's University in Grenada. She completed her undergraduate training at the University of Georgia. She has a particular interest in musculoskeletal and pain medicine.

Holly B. Hindman, MD, MPH, is an ophthalmologist at The Eye Care Center based in Canandaigua, New York. Until 2016, she worked as an associate professor of ophthalmology at the Flaum Eye Institute at the University of Rochester School of Medicine and Dentistry, Rochester, New York, where she also had a secondary appointment in the Center for Visual Science. She completed her undergraduate studies at Stanford University, her medical degree at Harvard Medical School, and her residency in ophthalmology at the Wilmer Eye Institute at Johns Hopkins University. She returned to her hometown of Rochester, New York, for her fellowship training in cornea and external disease at the University of Rochester, where she also completed a master's in public health. She provides medical and surgical treatments for cataract and corneal diseases with expertise on the impact of corneal disease processes on ocular optics and visual function.

Katarzyna Iwan, MD, is a fourth-year resident in the Department of Physical Medicine and Rehabilitation at the University of Rochester Medical Center in Rochester, New York. Dr. Iwan has a distinct interest and experience in the areas of musculoskeletal and pain medicine. She has presented grand rounds and several case reports at the American Academy of Physical Medicine and Rehabilitation (AAPMR), the Association of Academic Physiatrists (AAP), and the American Academy of Pain Management (AAPM) annual assemblies on these topics. Dr. Iwan is proficient in diagnostic and interventional ultrasound applications in physiatry. She will be starting an Accreditation Council for Graduate Medical Education–accredited fellowship in pain management at the University of Rochester Medical Center, Department of Anesthesiology.

Rashmi Khadilkar, MD, completed her medical education, internal medicine residency, and rheumatology fellowship at Temple University in Philadelphia, Pennsylvania. After 5 years as an attending rheumatologist, she completed fellowships in hospice and palliative medicine and geriatric medicine at the University of Rochester. She is board certified in internal medicine, rheumatology, hospice and palliative medicine, and geriatric medicine. Dr. Khadilkar has been involved in medical trainee education throughout her career and has a special interest in community education. She has given lectures and webinars for organizations including the American College of Rheumatology Fellowship Program Directors, Arthritis Foundation, Lupus Foundation, and University of Rochester. She is a recipient of the American Medical Directors Association Foundation Futures Program Scholarship Grant and the Hearst Foundation Hospice and Palliative Medicine Fellowship Grant. She is currently a senior instructor of medicine in the Division of Palliative Care, Highland Hospital, and an associate medical director at Visiting Nurse Hospice, both affiliated with the University of Rochester Medical Center in Rochester, New York.

Susan Maltser, DO, is a physiatrist in the Department of Physical Medicine and Rehabilitation at Northwell Health and an assistant professor of PM&R at the Hofstra Northwell School of Medicine. Dr. Maltser completed her training at the Rusk Institute of Rehabilitation Medicine at NYU Langone Medical Center. She is currently the division chief of cancer rehabilitation at her institution. She spent several years working with geriatric patients in a subacute rehab facility bridging the gap between geriatrics and rehab medicine. She has presented at several national meetings on the topic of cancer rehabilitation.

Kristin Meyer, PharmD, CGP, CACP, FASCP, is an associate professor of pharmacy practice at Drake University College of Pharmacy and Health Sciences and a consultant to the Iowa Veterans Home (IVH). Dr. Meyer precepts third- and fourth-year pharmacy students in specialty geriatrics practice experiences at IVH in addition to various classroom-teaching duties. She is a graduate of Drake University and completed a geriatric specialty pharmacy residency at the Central Arkansas Veterans Healthcare System and University of Arkansas in Little Rock. Her main areas of interest and expertise are Alzheimer's, Parkinson's, and anticoagulation management. Dr. Meyer enjoys being active in the leadership and advocacy efforts of the Iowa Pharmacy Association, the American Society of Consultant Pharmacists, and the American Association of Colleges of Pharmacy.

Armando Miciano, MD, FAAPMR, trained in internal medicine at Baylor College of Medicine in Houston, Texas, and physical medicine and rehabilitation at the National Rehabilitation Hospital Washington, DC. Dr. Miciano is the medical director at the Nevada Rehabilitation Institute in Las Vegas, Nevada, where he subspecializes in geriatric rehabilitation focusing on sleep disorders due to comorbidities. He has presented several scientific abstracts on functional outcomes using performance-based assessments and patient-reported outcomes.

Susanne U. Miedlich, MD, is an endocrinologist at the Division of Endocrinology, Department of Medicine, University of Rochester Medical Center (URMC) in Rochester, New York. Dr. Miedlich is originally from Leipzig, Germany, where she studied medicine at Leipzig University. She completed a residency in internal medicine and worked as a physician–scientist pursuing endocrine research in the Department of Endocrinology and Nephrology. Dr. Miedlich moved to the United States where she continued her basic research on G-protein coupled receptors as well as steroid receptors. She then completed a residency in internal medicine at Wayne State University, Detroit, Michigan, followed by a fellowship in endocrinology at URMC. Since 2014, she has been on faculty in the Division of Endocrinology at URMC, where she sees and teaches patients, fellows, residents, and medical students in endocrinology. She has a special interest in obesity, especially in the growing population of both young and old diabetic patients. Her work has been published in 13 peer-reviewed journals.

Maya Modzelewska, MD, is a pain fellow in the Department of Anesthesia at the University of Rochester Medical Center in Rochester, New York. She completed her residency in physical medicine and rehabilitation at the University of Rochester, where she developed a special interest in musculoskeletal and cancer pain management.

Mary Anne M. Morgan, MD, is an associate professor of medicine at the University of Rochester, where she completed an internal medicine residency and a fellowship in pulmonary and critical care medicine. A graduate of Stanford University (BA) and the University of California, San Francisco (MD), she is boarded in internal medicine, pulmonary medicine, and critical care medicine, and she has a combination of inpatient and outpatient practice specializing in intensive care and pulmonary medicine, with particular interest in the areas of septic shock, sarcoidosis, and lymphangiomyomatosis. She participates in medical education on a variety of levels and is the associate program director for the fellowship in pulmonary and critical care medicine.

Huma Naqvi, MD, has been an attending physiatrist and assistant professor in the Department of Physical Medicine and Rehabilitation at Montefiore Medical Center University Hospital for Albert Einstein College of Medicine Bronx, New York, since 2002, after finishing her residency from the same institution. She has been working as the director of geriatric rehabilitation since 2007. Dr. Naqvi is certified in wound care and acupuncture for pain management in the elderly. She is a recipient of a Global Health Initiative Grant for the neurorehabilitation of Iraqi children with neurodisabilities. She has started a certification course for Iraqi physicians and therapists on rehabilitation techniques and interventions. She has lectured at several international conferences on various geriatric topics.

Jean L. Nickels, MD, is an associate professor in the Department of Physical Medicine and Rehabilitation (PM&R) at the University of Rochester Medical Center (URMC) in Rochester, New York. She earned a medical degree from the Medical College of Wisconsin and completed her residency in physical medicine and rehabilitation at the University of Rochester. Dr. Nickels has served as the medical director of outpatient services in the Department of PM&R at URMC. She enjoys working with geriatric stroke and teaches medical students and residents. Dr. Nickels has served as vice chair of education for the General Rehab Council of the American Academy of Physical Medicine and Rehabilitation. She is currently the associate medical director of the acute rehabilitation unit at Strong Memorial Hospital in Rochester, New York.

Jeffrey B. Palmer, MD, is a professor of physical medicine and rehabilitation, otolaryngogy-head and neck surgery, and functional anatomy/evolution at the Johns Hopkins University School of Medicine and a distinguished professor at Fujita Health University in Nagoya, Japan. Dr. Palmer earned bachelor's and medical degrees at New York University and completed a residency in physical medicine and rehabilitation at the University of Washington. Dr. Palmer has been at Johns Hopkins since 1983, reaching the rank of professor of PM&R in 2002. From 2004 to 2014, he served as chair of the Department of PM&R. His publications include 77 peer-refereed scientific papers, 35 book chapters, and two books. He is a coauthor of *Spinal Cord Injury: A Guide for Living*, a book for people with SCI and their families. Dr. Palmer is the editor-in-chief of *Current Physical Medicine and Rehabilitation Reports*. Dr. Palmer is a fellow of the American Congress of Rehabilitation Medicine, and he received the Distinguished Academician Award from the Association of Academic Physiatrists. He is an honorary member of the Japanese Society for Dysphagia Rehabilitation and the Japanese Association of Rehabilitation Medicine.

Jennifer H. Paul, MD, is a physiatrist and assistant professor in the Departments of Physical Medicine and Rehabilitation and Orthopaedics at the University of Rochester Medical Center, Rochester, New York. She was trained in rehabilitation medicine at the University of Colorado in Denver. She lectures to residents and medical students and has particular interest and experience in arthritis, brain injuries, strokes, spinal cord injuries, and several other neurological and musculoskeletal conditions. In her academic practice, she provides care to patients in outpatient clinics in rehabilitation and orthopaedics.

Annie Philip, MBBS, is an associate professor in the Department of Anesthesiology and Physical Medicine and Rehabilitation. She is the fellowship director of the University of Rochester Pain Management Fellowship Program. She works at the multidisciplinary tertiary pain clinic at the University of Rochester, Department of Anesthesiology, and provides care for pain patients in the acute care setting in the hospital and, also in the outpatient department, caring for pain patients of all ages, including older adults.

Timothy E. Quill, MD, is the Thomas and Georgia Gosnell Distinguished Professor in Palliative Care at the University of Rochester Medical Center (URMC), where he is also a professor of medicine, psychiatry, medical humanities, and nursing. He was the founding director of the URMC Palliative Care Division and a past president of the American Academy of Hospice and Palliative Medicine. Dr. Quill has published and lectured widely about various aspects of the doctor–patient relationship, with a special focus on end-of-life decision making, including delivering bad news, nonabandonment, discussing palliative care earlier, and exploring last-resort options. He is the author of several books on end-of-life care and over 150 peer-reviewed articles. He was the lead physician plaintiff in the New York State legal case challenging the law prohibiting physician-assisted death that was heard in 1997 by the U.S. Supreme Court (*Quill v. Vacco*). Dr. Quill is a fellow in the American Academy of Hospice and Palliative Medicine, a fellow in the American College of Physicians, an ABMS certified palliative care consultant, and a past board member of the American Academy of Hospice and Palliative Medicine.

Rajeev S. Ramchandran, MD, MBA, is an associate professor in the Department of Ophthalmology, Flaum Eye Institute at the University of Rochester Medical Center (URMC), Rochester, New York.

He earned a medical degree at the University of Rochester School of Medicine and Dentistry with distinction in research. He completed his ophthalmology residency at the Duke Eye Center and fellowship in vitreoretinal surgery from the URMC. Dr. Ramchandran is the cofounder of the University of Rochester Telehealth Consortium, and he studies the implementation and value of teleophthalmology enabled remote diagnostic ocular imaging services for early detection and awareness of eye disease in at-risk populations. His work is funded by local health foundations, the National Institutes of Health and the Centers for Disease Control.

Dr. Ramchandran is the director of the Flaum Eye Institute's population eye health initiative, and he is developing a vision health system of western New York, which incorporates screening, education, and care in a vertically integrated community engagement model.

Claudia Ramirez, MD, is a physiatrist and recent graduate of the University of Rochester Medical Center Physical Medicine and Rehabilitation Residency Program. She is completing an Accreditation Council for Graduate Medical Education–accredited pain fellowship at Virginia Commonwealth University, where she continues to expand her training on the management of musculoskeletal disorders. In the past, she has contributed to multiple orthopedic-focused research projects at the University of Pittsburgh Medical Center. She is interested in working with the geriatric population addressing musculoskeletal disorders.

Albert C. Recio, MD, RPT, PTRP, is an assistant professor of physical medicine and rehabilitation at the Johns Hopkins School of Medicine and the medical director of the Aquatherapy Program at the International Center for Spinal Cord Injury at Kennedy Krieger Institute. Dr. Recio is board certified in physical medicine and rehabilitation and spinal cord injury medicine and a licensed physical therapist. Dr. Recio earned his medical degree in 1997 at the Perpetual Help College of Medicine in Biñan, Laguna. He undertook his internship training at the Perpetual Help Medical Center from 1997 to 1998. At Jackson Park Hospital in Chicago, Illinois, from 2002 to 2003, he completed his general internship. While at the Harvard Medical School/Spaulding Rehabilitation Hospital in Boston, Massachusetts, from 2003 to 2006, he completed his residency in physical medicine and rehabilitation. From there, he did a year-long clinical fellowship in spinal cord injury medicine at the University of Washington/Veterans Administration–Puget Sound Health Care System in Seattle, Washington, in 2007. In an effort to provide patients with chronic spinal cord injuries or paralysisgreater independence, his research evaluates the ability of activity-based restorative therapies (ABRT) to help patients recover neurological sensation and physical movement. His fields of interest also include electrical stimulation in the treatment of recalcitrant pressure wounds and the use of functional electrical stimulation to activate nerves innervating extremities affected by paralysis resulting from spinal cord injury.

Michael Reed, RPh, B-Pharm, is a clinical pharmacist in the Department of Pharmacy, Emory University Hospital and Emory Rehabilitation Hospital in Partnership with Select Medical, Atlanta, Georgia. He has worked with geriatric, brain injury, and spinal cord patients for over 25 years. As a clinical pharmacist, he has consulted with physiatrists and physical medicine and rehabilitation residents in the areas of polypharmacy, pharmacokinetics, and anticoagulation. He serves on the Pharmacy and Therapeutics Committee of the Emory Rehabilitation Hospital and was a contributor to *Rational Prescribing Initiative in an Acute Rehabilitation Hospital: Update on a Three Year Quality Improvement Project.*

Irene Hegeman Richard, MD, is a professor of neurology with a secondary appointment in the Department of Psychiatry at the University of Rochester. Dr. Richard specializes in movement disorders and is actively engaged in clinical care of patients with Parkinson's disease (PD) and related conditions. She is dedicated to teaching medical students, residents, and fellows and serves as director of the Movement Disorders Fellowship Program. Dr. Richard conducts clinical research aimed at understanding and developing effective treatments for neurological and psychiatric aspects of movement disorders, with a particular emphasis on depression and anxiety in PD. After graduating from the Yale University School of Medicine in 1991, she completed a neurology residency (1995) and fellowship training at the University of Rochester. She then joined and has remained a member of the faculty. She has received numerous research grants, has many publications in peer-reviewed journals, and has lectured extensively locally, regionally, and at the national level. Her research career began with the study of mood fluctuations in PD, with support from career development awards from the National Institutes of Health (NIH) and the National Alliance for Research on Schizophrenia and Depression (NARSAD). From there, she obtained a clinical trial planning grant followed by an R-01 from NIH to lead a multicenter clinical trial of antidepressants in PD, demonstrating the efficacy and tolerability of two currently available medications (published in *Neurology*, 2012). She has had ongoing collaborations with an international group of colleagues to further understand the phenomenology and optimize evaluation of anxiety in PD that was recently awarded a grant from the Michael J. Fox Foundation to study its treatment. In addition, she has served as a site investigator in numerous multicenter clinical trials in patients with PD. She has served for a number of years as a medical and scientific advisor for the Michael J. Fox Foundation for Parkinson's research and was the recipient of the 2011 Langston Award for her contributions in this regard. In addition to conducting her own research, she has served as a mentor, collaborator, consultant, and reviewer within her area of expertise.

Corey Romesser, MD, is an assistant professor of clinical medicine, Division of Geriatrics, the University of Rochester School of Medicine and Dentistry, Rochester, New York. Dr. Romesser is board certified in internal medicine, geriatrics, and hospice and palliative medicine. He is the director of geriatric inpatient services at Highland Hospital in Rochester, where he works as a geriatric hospitalist and consultant as well as the palliative care consultant service. He is the medical director for the Acute Care for Elders unit and the Hospital Elder Life program. In addition to hospital work, he sees patients at the Highlands at Brighton nursing home, where he attends patients on subacute rehabilitation, long-term care, and dementia units. He participates in a variety of medical student, resident, and fellow education, and in his clinical practice has an interest in delirium.

Roger P. Rossi, DO, is a clinical professor of physical medicine and rehabilitation at Rutgers Robert Wood Johnson School of Medicine and the director of Medical Student Education at the JFK Johnson Rehabilitation Institute in Edison, New Jersey. Dr. Rossi completed his residency in physical medicine and rehabilitation at New York University, the Rusk Institute of Rehabilitation, where he served as chief resident. Dr. Rossi serves as the director of postacute rehabilitation services and the director of the JFK Johnson Parkinson's disease and movement disorders program. He is board certified in physical medicine and rehabilitation and sports medicine. In addition to general rehabilitation, he holds special interests in the areas of neurodegenerative disease, Parkinson's disease, multiple sclerosis, muscular dystrophy, as well as sports medicine and musculoskeletal medicine. Dr. Rossi is a fellow in the American Academy of Medical Acupuncture and has completed certification training in acupuncture at UCLA-Berkeley and Harvard Medical School. Dr. Rossi served as the first physiatrist on the National Parkinson's Disease Centers Review Board, and he has been involved in the areas of Parkinson disease education and program development for various healthcare settings. He has served on the New Jersey Board of Acupuncture for more than 23 years, serving as past president. Dr. Rossi remains involved at the community level as well, serving as a commissioner on his town's local environmental protection committee and the Committee for Individuals with Disability.

He has authored several textbook chapters on various rehabilitation topics as well as numerous articles on topics in physical medicine and rehabilitation and lifestyle medicine.

Sara Z. Salim, MD, is a physiatrist and assistant professor in the Department of Physical Medicine and Rehabilitation at the University of Rochester and Strong Memorial Hospital in Rochester,

New York, where she is a staff physician in the inpatient and outpatient rehabilitation units. She completed an internship in internal medicine at the State University of New York at Buffalo and completed her residency in physical medicine and rehabilitation at UMDNJ/Kessler Institute for Rehabilitation in Newark, New Jersey. Her interests include inpatient and outpatient rehabilitation, ultrasound-guided injections, and spasticity management with Botox.

Deepthi S. Saxena, MD, CPE, FAAPMR, is a physiatrist and the president of Avant-Garde Medicine. Dr. Saxena provides physician and consultant services in postacute care and utilization review. She earned her medical degree at the Deccan College of Medical Sciences in Hyderabad, India, and completed her residency training at Marianjoy Rehabilitation Hospital in Wheaton, Illinois. She is an instructor in PM&R at the Touro University Nevada, College of Osteopathic Medicine, and an adjunct clinical assistant professor in the Department of Internal Medicine at the University of Nevada School of Medicine (UNSOM) (Las Vegas). Dr. Saxena is the chair-elect for the Medical Rehabilitation Council of the American Academy of Physical Medicine and Rehabilitation (AAPM&R) and an editorial board leader of Knowledge Now. She is pursuing an executive MBA at the University of Chicago, Booth School of Business. Dr. Saxena has written book chapters on medical rehabilitation, geriatric rehabilitation, and quality of delivery of rehabilitative care.

Marcia J. Scherer, PhD, MPH, is a rehabilitation psychologist and founding president of the Institute for Matching Person and Technology. She is also a professor of physical medicine and rehabilitation at the University of Rochester Medical Center, where she earned both PhD and MPH degrees. She is the PM&R Department's research director. She is a past member of the National Advisory Board on Medical Rehabilitation Research, National Institutes of Health, and she is the editor of the journal *Disability and Rehabilitation: Assistive Technology.* She is the coeditor of the *Rehabilitation Science in Practice Series* for CRC Press. Dr. Scherer is a fellow of the American Psychological Association, American Congress of Rehabilitation Medicine, and the Rehabilitation Engineering and Assistive Technology Society of North America (RESNA). Dr. Scherer has authored, edited, or coedited nine books and has published over 70 articles in peer-reviewed journals as well as over 25 book chapters on disability and technology. Her research has been cited more than 3000 times by others.

Sandhya Seshadri, PhD, MA, MS, CCC-SLP, is an adjunct assistant professor in the University of Rochester's School of Nursing and speech-language pathologist at the University of Rochester Medical Center. Dr. Seshadri's clinical practice has focused on adult neurogenic communication and swallowing disorders in acute-care settings. Her research interests include the health and well-being of community-dwelling older adults and geriatric communication and swallowing disorders. She is a coresearcher on studies related to geriatric health conducted at the University of Rochester. She has presented research work at national and international conferences.

Margie Hodges Shaw, JD, PhD, is an assistant professor in the Division of Medical Humanities and Bioethics at the University of Rochester School of Medicine and Dentistry, Rochester, New York. She is the director of the Law and Bioethics Pathways Program and director of the Law and Bioethics Theme at the University of Rochester Medical School. She is a member of the clinical consult team and a member of the ethics committee at the University of Rochester Strong Memorial Hospital. She earned a JD at Cornell Law School in 1991. From 2004 to 2011, she earned a master's in philosophy and a PhD in education. Her dissertation is titled "Coaching as a Form of Instruction and a Component of Medical Ethics Education." From 2010 to 2011, she held a fellowship in clinical ethics at the University of Rochester Strong Memorial Hospital. Her research interests include the intersection between clinical bioethics decision making, interprofessional clinical conferencing, and frameworks and pedagogy in adult education.

Silvia Sörensen, PhD, is an associate professor of counseling and human development at the University of Rochester's Warner School of Education and Human Development, Department of Ophthalmology, Department of Psychiatry, and Center for Community Health. She is a researcher in gerontology and an educator in human development and related fields, with interests in facilitating well-being among vulnerable older adults and their families. Dr. Sörensen is a cofounder of the Aging Well Initiative community collaboration with faith-based organizations, and she has a particular interest in empowering underserved groups in order to reduce health disparities. She is the director of the Laboratory for Aging, Population Health, Disparities, and Intervention Research (LAPHDIR) in which new research and community health projects are hatched with the help of a community health-project advisory board. Her specific areas of research include successful aging through preparation for future care, family caregiver stress and coping, interventions with caregivers, interventions with vision-impaired older adults, future thinking among older adults, as well as health literacy and patient education for diabetes prevention.

Dale C. Strasser, MD, earned a BA at Vanderbilt University (1976), an MD at Northwestern University Medical School (1984). He had an integrated PM&R residency (1988), a fellowship in arthritis rehabilitation at the Rehabilitation Institute of Chicago (1998), and a fellowship in geriatric medicine in the Department of Internal Medicine at Northwestern University Medical School (1990). He is currently a professor in the Department of Rehabilitation at Emory University School of Medicine, Atlanta, Georgia. Dr. Strasser was instrumental in opening one of the few acute inpatient rehabilitation units in the United States targeting the needs of the frail elderly. He worked with Veterans Administration-based geriatricians as a core investigator with the Birmingham/Atlanta Geriatric Research, Education, and Clinical Centers (GRECC) for 10 years, and his research interests include geriatric rehabilitation, specifically polypharmacy and the rehabilitation needs of the older adult and rehabilitation team effectiveness. His Veterans Administration Rehab R&D-sponsored research, known as the "VA Rehab Teams Project," is considered a landmark work linking rehabilitation team functioning to patient outcomes. Dr. Strasser's involvement on national committees includes the American Academy of Physical Medicine and Rehabilitation, the AAPM&R representative on several committees with the American Geriatrics Society, the American Association of Neurology/American Psychiatric Association (quality indicators for dementia care), and the American College of Surgeons (geriatric trauma). He has authored 30 peer-reviewed manuscripts, 10 book chapters, and done numerous national and international professional presentations and workshops.

Nicole Strong, DO, is a third-year physical medicine and rehabilitation resident at the University of Rochester Medical Center. She attended medical school at Midwestern University, earning a degree in 2013. Her interest in musculoskeletal medicine stems from her background in kinesiology. She has held various leadership positions in the field of PM&R, through the American Osteopathic College of Physical Medicine and Rehabilitation (AOCPMR), and continues to actively pursue leadership and research challenges during residency.

Bernard Sussman, MD, is a professor of clinical medicine and medical humanities at the University of Rochester, Rochester, New York. For over 30 years, he practiced primary care internal medicine in Rochester. During that time, he also served as a consultant in clinical ethics and palliative care. Since 2012, he has practiced and taught at the University of Rochester Medical Center as a member of the Palliative Care Division, Division of Medical Humanities and Bioethics, and the General Medicine Division. As a bioethics faculty member, he teaches undergraduates, master's students, medical students, medical residents, and fellows.

Rajbala Thakur, MD, is a professor in the Department of Anesthesiology and Physical Medicine and Rehabilitation, palliative care consultant, medical director of Anesthesiology Clinical Research Center, University of Rochester Medical Center, Rochester, New York. She is an anesthesiologist who has been working with chronic/acute pain and palliative care patients for over 20 years. Dr. Thakur has been the principal or subinvestigator on many clinical trials exploring different treatment options for malignant and nonmalignant pain conditions. She coauthored and established inpatient and outpatient policies for Ketamine infusion therapy with the University of Rochester Medical Center. She has published articles in pain journals and presented abstracts/posters at the American Academy of Pain Medicine. She teaches pain fellows and residents. She also is a consultant for the Acute Pain Service Program at the GMCH, India.

Tina Thornhill, PharmD, FASCP, CGP, is an associate professor of pharmacy practice and vice chair for professional education at Campbell University College of Pharmacy and Health Sciences. Dr. Thornhill earned her doctor of pharmacy degree and completed a specialty residency in geriatrics and long-term care at Campbell University in 1991 and 1992, respectively. She worked as a clinical pharmacy specialist in geriatrics for the Veterans Administration before joining the faculty at Campbell University in 1996. She served as a pharmacy preceptor in geriatric medicine for over 19 years at Wake Forest Baptist Medical Center, where she spent the last 12 years as the clinical pharmacist for the Acute Inpatient Rehabilitation and Acquired Brain Injury Units. She has presented at the state and national level and published articles and book chapters on various geriatric-related topics. Dr. Thornhill served on the examination development committee for the Commission for Certification in Geriatric Pharmacy. She teaches in the areas of geriatrics, neurology, and rheumatology to pharmacy, nurse practitioner, and physician assistant students.

Kristen Thornton, MD, CWSP, FAAFP, AGSF, currently serves as an assistant professor of family medicine and medicine at the University of Rochester School of Medicine and Dentistry, Rochester, New York. She is a graduate of Dartmouth Medical School, completed her internship at the Mayo Clinic, and her residency, chief residency, and geriatric medicine fellowship at the University of Rochester. She is board certified in family medicine, geriatric medicine, and hospice and palliative medicine. She is also a certified wound specialist physician (CWSP). Dr. Thornton provides outpatient family medicine care, outpatient geriatric medicine and palliative medicine consults, home visits, and long-term care. She is a codirector of the "Aging Well" at the University of Rochester School of Medicine and is active in geriatric medicine education of medical students, residents, and fellows. She is a fellow of both the American Academy of Family Physicians and American Geriatrics Society.

Brian Tucker, MBBS, is a private practitioner in general medicine and earned his medical degree at Karnatak Medical College, Hubli, India. He was trained in anti-rabies program, medical termination of pregnancy, and essential new-born care. He held many positions at various institutions in India, such as medical officer in Indian Railways and V.M. Salgaocar Mining Co., residential medical officer at Republic Nursing Home, Bangalore, and company medical officer and plantation medical officer at Mahavir Plantations, Highforest T.E. Anamalais, S.I. Plantation, Chandan Tea Co., Mount Stuart T.E., Anamalais, S.I., Parry Agro Industries Ltd., and senior medical officer at Mac Cloud Rossel Tea Company in Assam, India. His publications include HIV–AIDS and the Surgeon, an educational production for general practitioners, and Ageing Gracefully, to address the senior members of the society. He lectured extensively on HIV–AIDS in several prestigious institutions in India. In 1991, he was awarded a life membership in the Indian Society of Health Administrators.

Dr. Tucker organizes and participates in medical camps for the underprivileged in several parts of India. An avid sportsman, he has a passion for cricket, tennis, and golf, and he is a winner of many trophies at the state level in different parts of India.

Krishna J. Urs, MD, is a clinical assistant professor of physical medicine and rehabilitation at Rutgers Robert Wood Johnson Medical School/JFK Johnson Rehabilitation Institute. He has been in practice for the past 10 years. During this time, he has been significantly involved in resident training. He earned a medical degree at the Chicago Medical School. He completed his residency in physical medicine and rehabilitation and fellowship training in brain injury medicine at the JFK Johnson Rehabilitation Institute, where he served as chief resident. Currently, he is the director of Rehabilitation Consult Services at JFK Medical Center. In addition, he is the director of quality improvement and safety for the residency program in physical medicine and rehabilitation. His area of particular interest and experience are stroke and traumatic brain injury. He is board certified in physical medicine and rehabilitation as well as brain injury medicine.

Christopher J. Williams, MD, is chief resident physician at Emory University School of Medicine, Department of Rehabilitation Medicine, Atlanta, Georgia. He is currently in his postgraduate year four of training and has been working in the inpatient rehabilitation setting for the last 3 years. He has an interest in quality improvement, team dynamics, polypharmacy, and regenerative medicine. He is the coinvestigator of Reducing Geriatric Polypharmacy by Promoting Rational Prescribing Practices: Report on a 3-year Quality Improvement Initiative in an Acute Inpatient Rehabilitation Hospital.

Steven D. Wittlin, MD, is a professor of medicine at the University of Rochester School of Medicine and Dentistry, Rochester, New York. He is the clinical director of endocrinology and director of Diabetes Services at the University of Rochester Medical Center/Strong Memorial Hospital, where he has worked since 1993. He served previously as chief of endocrinology and assistant chairman of medicine at Booth Memorial Medical Center. He attended medical school at the Sackler School of Medicine in Tel Aviv. His endocrine training was at New York University, where he worked in the laboratory of Marvin C. Gershengorn. He has published in the areas of general endocrinology, diabetes and cardiovascular disease, assessment of glycemic control, glucose homeostasis, hypoglycemia, and insulin pump therapy.

Hilary Yehling, MD, is a practicing internal medicine and pediatrics primary care physician who specializes in adult and pediatric palliative care at the Elliot Health System in the Manchester, New Hampshire, area. She graduated from Rochester Institute of Technology (BS), SUNY at Buffalo School of Medicine (MD), and completed internal medicine and pediatrics residency and fellowship in palliative care at the University of Rochester. She is boarded in internal medicine, pediatrics, and hospice and palliative medicine.

Mikhail Zhukalin, DO, is a pain medicine fellow at Northwestern University and the Rehabilitation Institute of Chicago. He completed his residency in physical medicine and rehabilitation at Emory University, Atlanta, Georgia. He has been involved with the issue of polypharmacy, especially as it pertains to the geriatric and other vulnerable populations, since his first year of residency training. He created a computer-based medication assessment tool, which became the foundation for the 3-year quality improvement project at Emory Rehabilitation Hospital, with significant reduction in potentially inappropriate medications and anticholinergic burden at discharge in patients 65 years and older. Dr. Zhukalin's interests include promoting rational medication prescribing practices, medical student and resident education, utilizing multidisciplinary and team-based approaches to solve complex medical problems, and developing tools to foster interspecialty communication and continuity of care.

Geriatric Rehabilitation: Introduction

K. Rao Poduri

Geriatrics is a fascinating area of medicine with its intricacies of care that affect the older adults and their health. Health is not the absence of disease for the older adults and maintaining their functional independence is of utmost value at the time of unprecedented challenges in the world. Population is growing at a rapid rate due to a shift in controlling the disease and death rates from leading causes such as infections and communicable diseases all across the globe http://www.nia. nih.gov/research/publication/global-health-and-aging/preface. For the first time in the history of mankind, people can expect to live beyond 65 all the way up to 95 years and beyond. However, the consequences of living longer carry with them many challenges and opportunities for maintaining health, providing the healthcare, and the related costs. Life expectancy is at its highest throughout the world with population aging at an exponential rate.[1] As we discuss about older adults, it is helpful to define older adults.

There is no universally defined or recognized classification of the older population as a group and chronological age is the most universally accepted categorization. In the past, old age was arbitrarily referred to the people older than 65 years of age.

Maddox[2] and Dililierti[3] described the following definitions to appropriately classify geriatric population: Young old 60+ years, Old -old, 75+ years, the oldest -old 85+ years and centurions. Throughout this book, the terms elderly and older adults are used interchangeably referring to the geriatric population. The American Geriatric Society (AGS) prefers referring to the geriatric population as the older adults.

Just 50 years ago, childhood (under the age of 15) mortality was at 45% as compared to 22% for people over the age of 65 and older,[4] in the world's population. The death rates varied for children in different countries; 62% in Africa and Asia, 48% in Latin America, and 54% in the Caribbean while the death rates in the developed countries were at 20%. More interestingly the death rate for older adults (65 and older) has been at 50% or higher.[5]

According to the United Nations, the growth of older adults will rise from 8% in 1950 to 21% in 2050[4] and by then for the first time in history they will outnumber the young. In the developed countries, there is a 50% growth in the number of older adults from 2006 to 2030 compared to 140% in the developing countries for which they will be unprepared. In the United States alone, there were 3-million older adults (4% of the population) in 1900 and the number escalated to 36.8 million (35%) in 2005 of the people 65 years and older comprising one in eight Americans. It is projected that by 2030, one in five Americans will be in this category. By middle of the next century, this number will grow to 82 million and far more than in other developed counties such as Japan, Italy, Germany, Sweden, and United Kingdom. Of note, the 85-years and older age group is the fastest-growing segment of the U.S. population which is expected to grow from 2% to 5% in the next 50 years.[6,7] During the second half of the twentieth century, life expectancy has been rising all across the world due to the decline in fertility and mortality rates and a 20-year increase in the average life span.[8,9]

Increasing life expectancy does not guarantee more years of life in good health. It is associated with increased morbidity and more years spent with disability and dependency. The causes of death and disability are no longer from infectious diseases but instead from noncommunicable diseases. In 2008, 85% of people over 60 years and older died from noncommunicable diseases around the world and the number was higher than 92% in the developed countries. The consequences of living longer include disability from underlying diseases that affect physical, cognitive, and sensory functions. These are described by Bernard Isaacs as the Four Giants of Geriatrics[10] and they include

1. Immobility
2. Instability
3. Incontinence
4. Intellectual impairment

The etiology of these giants is multifactorial and in the older adults, at least one if not more chronic conditions exists creating disability and dependence in physical and cognitive domains.

Besides frailty and age-related decline, common conditions that are responsible for the above four giants, include strokes, spinal cord injuries and other neurological conditions, cardiopulmonary diseases, falls and hip fractures, arthritis and joint replacements, and dementia to name a few. Many of these conditions can be improved with rehabilitation to a level that can improve the quality of life. As the life expectancy is on the rise, keeping the older adults healthy longer, avoiding, or delaying disability with rehabilitative efforts will reduce dependency to a level that is gratifying to the older adults and care givers.

Several measures of disability and limitations in this population have shown improvements in the last decade. Multiple chronic diseases are increasingly prevalent among the older U.S. adults, whereas the prevalence of impairment and disability, while substantial, remain stable.[11]

The older adults lose their mobility due to frailty, multicomorbidity, and become dependent in physical and cognitive functions. These older adults may require longer length of stays in the hospital and have potential for long-term care placement in facilities or community care with services at home or in assisted livings settings. It behooves on us to make every effort to prevent complications of the diseases, minimize secondary complications, and maximize functional gains to maintain independence through rehabilitation. Achieving therapeutic gains may be difficult but still rehabilitation is justified.

The rehabilitation of this population spans from providing care during acute hospitalization to the continuum of care in the community. Rehabilitation is a relatively young specialty which is becoming known throughout the world; more developed, and sophisticated in the West while being still to be recognized as a needed service for older adults. With the advent of modern medical care with its technological and pharmaceutical advances, people are living longer worldwide. The aging population is the beneficiary of rehabilitation in the healthcare continuum. Some of the descriptors such as chronological, physiological, biological, and emotional states are used to identify and explain the disease processes of this particular population. Based on animal models, Beltrán-Sánchez et al.[12] present the empirical evidence which suggests that delayed aging process could result in increased life expectancy. By improving the health of older adults and delaying the aging process, a possibility exists for these age groups to live without disability. Disease and disability carry a huge burden for older adults, care givers, and the society. Functional decline is noted more commonly in the geriatric population. It is questionable if years of life added to an individual will be without a disability. Rehabilitation then plays an important role in improving the function of the older adults and reduces disability. Rehabilitation is defined as restoration of function which is impaired as a result of a disease process with comorbidities and the aging process. In the older adults, there is a high incidence of disability and dependence due to many factors which can be improved to an extent with rehabilitation to optimize the quality of life. Geriatric population utilizes a large proportion of healthcare services. Rehabilitation is an important part of geriatric healthcare. It involves assessing older adults and their needs and functional status design to treatments for various conditions. It is in the context of postacute care that rehabilitation plays a major role in the health, well-being, and functional restoration of older adults at various settings.

The major focus of geriatric healthcare is on functional independence but *not* on disease eradication.

Rehabilitation is a multispecialty and multidisciplinary effort to improve the quality and safety of care provided to hospitalized older adults followed by the postacute care continuum throughout the life span of the individual's life. The concept of the postacute care continuum offers many opportunities and challenges and requires thoughtful evaluation. The integration of care across many settings including acute hospital, acute rehabilitation units in the hospital or freestanding sites, and subacute rehabilitation facilities, in home and at the outpatient settings, calls for new creativity. The care coordination should address the older adults' conditions, diseases, comorbidities, biopsychosocial issues, finances, and community resources. Rehabilitation is provided in different settings, each with their own guidelines, intensity, outcomes and variable costs, and the major determinant is the funding source.

There are four levels of postacute care/rehabilitation that can be provided to this population in the United States which may also be available in some of the countries in the Western Hemisphere.

1. Acute—in a hospital or freestanding rehabilitation care which is highly regulated by the Federal government with a set of rules. Typically in the acute rehabilitation setting with availability of physiatrists (physicians trained in physical medicine and rehabilitation and nursing care 24/7 and physical, occupational, and speech therapies 3 hours per day if they are admitted with a set of diagnostic conditions). They are expected to have medical complexity with comorbidities yet stable enough to participate in 3 hours of therapies a day and make functional gains in a reasonable period of time. The patients should be able to endure the intensity of therapies, which in frail older patients poses a problem. Costs are higher for acute rehabilitation compared to any other setting due to the multidisciplinary approach of provision of care with high intensity and duration of therapies. The programs provide coordinated care with the physiatrist leading the interdisciplinary team. Cost containment has changed the landscape of rehabilitation in the recent years and has led to the growth of subacute rehabilitation facilities.

2. The next level of rehabilitation care is at subacute level provided in a less acute setting such as nursing homes. The difference being the availability of physician supervision with access 24 hours a day on emergency basis with 24-hour nursing care. In this setting, patients are expected to receive 1–2 hours/day of therapies. The coordination of care is not a requisite and length of stay may not be short.

    Post-acute care of older adults with nonhospital-based services has grown exponentially in the last few decades entirely based on economic factors. It is also impacting the type of patients with high acuity of medical conditions being cared for at these units.[13]

3. The next two levels: therapies are provided at home or in the community. The nursing care needs are intermittent and with periodic checkups, physical, occupational, and speech therapies are all provided in the patient's home setting with availability of family support.

4. Finally, therapies are provided in the outpatient facilities geared toward and focusing on functional recovery in mobility and self-care. The goal of rehabilitation is emphasized for improving a person's independence and quality of life. Reasonable expectation of functional improvements is required for continuation of therapies.

The physicians should be knowledgeable of the range of services provided at each level and their benefits and disadvantages in order to appropriately direct the patients to meet their needs and make the timely recommendations.

Hence, the title of this book is *Geriatric Rehabilitation: From Bedside to Curbside*. The various chapters describe the nuances of how different conditions influence the function of older adults along with biological, physiological, and patho-physical, biopsychosocial factors. The authors describe how rehabilitation is provided to this specific population. Although some of the chapters focused in this book are entirely on older adults in the United States, in many instances, they may also be applied to the global geriatric population. This book conveys a message to the medical students and physicians in various specialties to be cognizant of the special needs of aging population and address them in the most appropriate setting. To guide the clinician, the four major sections of this book explain and emphasize various conditions in a comprehensive and evidence-based manner.

Each chapter focuses on individual conditions or diseases, their impact on the physical functioning of the patients, and their rehabilitative management.

REFERENCES

1. World report on ageing and health by World Health Organization (WHO) 2015.
2. Maddox GL, editor. *The Encyclopedia of Aging: a Comprehensive in Gerontology and Geriatrics*. 3rd ed. New York: Springer; 2001. p 435–8.
3. Dililierti W, Eccles M. *Thesaurus of Aging Terminology: Ageline Database on Middle Age and Aging*. 5th ed. Washington (DC): Research Information Center, American Association of Retired Persons; 1994. p 102–3.
4. Department of Social and Economic Affairs, Population Division. World population is ageing 1950–2050, United Nations; 2001 available at https://www.un.org/esa/population/publications/worldageing19502050/pdf/preface_web.pdf
5. United Nations Department of Economic and Social Affairs Population Division. World population is ageing 2013, ST/ESA/SER. A 348.
6. Federal Interagency Forum on Aging Related Statistics. *Older Americans 2000: Key Indicators of Wellbeing*. Washington DC: U.S. Government Printing Office; 2000.
7. U.S. Census Bureau. Available at: http://www.census.gov. Accessed February 2016.
8. Kinsella K, Wan H. U.S. Census Bureau, International Population Reports, p95/09-1, *An Aging World*: 2008, U.S. Government Printing Office, Washington, DC, 2009.
9. Centers for Disease Control and Prevention (CDC). Trends in aging: United States and worldwide. *MMWR Morb Mortal Wkly Rep*. 2003 Feb 14; 52 (6):101–4, 106.
10. Barton A, Mulley G. History of the development of geriatric medicine in the UK. *Postgrad Med J*. 2003 Apr; 79(930):229–34; quiz 233-4. See comment in PubMed Commons below.
11. Hung WW, Ross JS, Boockvar KS, Siu AL. Recent trends in chronic disease, impairment and disability among older adults in the United States. *BMC Geriatrics BMC Series* 2011.
12. Beltrán-Sánchez H, Soneji S, Crimmins EM. Past, present, and future of healthy life expectancy. *Cold Spring Harb Perspect Med*. 2015 Nov 2; 5(11):1–11.
13. Shaughnassey PW, Kramer AM. The increased needs of patients in nursing homes and patients receiving home health care. *N Engl J Med*. 1990: 322(1):21–27.

Section I

Basics of Aging

1 Demographics, Biology, and Physiology

K. Rao Poduri

CONTENTS

1.1 DEMOGRAPHICS

Worldwide, there is an unprecedented increase in the population of older adults. According to the United Nations, this rate of growth of the aging population in the developed countries is expected to rise to 50% as compared to 140% in developing countries from 2006 to 2030. As life expectancy is escalating to new heights all around the world, the aging population is not only surviving longer but also carrying the burden of disease and disability and consuming a lot of resources. Chronic health problems are common in this population. Older adults have high prevalence of comorbid conditions. The prevalence of multimorbidity is significantly high with aging population.[1,2] More than 45% of adults, living in the community are reported as having one or more chronic conditions in the United States.[2] Having two or more chronic conditions is a high risk for functional dependency.[3] Poor health, chronic disease, and comorbidities accompany advanced age and declining functional status for basic mobility and self-care. Correlation between economic deprivation[4,5] and the incidence of comorbidities and multimorbidity tends to be high. The period of disability before death poses both societal and economic impact. On an average, persons 65 and older visit a physician more frequently than their younger counterparts. They are hospitalized twice as often as younger persons and stay 50% longer. Avoidable admissions and preventable complications in the hospital setting are higher for individuals with chronic conditions.[6]

The growth of the aging population carries a special significance because of its implications for disability and its impact on those who provide preventative or restorative care. Disability may be physical, emotional, or social.

- Physical disability
  - Sensory and motor performance
  - Mobility and activities of daily living (ADL)
  - Community skills

- Emotional disability
  - Anxiety
  - Unhappiness
  - Dissatisfaction

- Social disability
  - Social interaction
  - Isolation from family and friends

The etiology for the above disabilities is multifactorial and can be classified as age related and disease related.[7,8] Biological, psychological, and social factors certainly play a role.

Biological causes that are age related include cardiac and pulmonary function, muscle strength, vital capacity, orthostatic changes, peripheral resistance, vital capacity, minute volume, and aerobic capacity. Psychological factors include beliefs about self, recovery, and rehabilitation in addition to delayed learning pace needing more repetitions. In the social arena, less frequent referrals to needed rehabilitative care, negative views of ageism,[9] financial barriers, and self-ageism all impact the older adults in coping with disability and obtaining rehabilitation. On the other hand, disease-related causes under biological category encompass multiple diseases (comorbidities), polypharmacy, disease-to-disease interactions, subclinical organ dysfunction, deconditioning, and contractures from immobility. The psychological factors are depression, lack of motivation, cognitive deficits, and atypical presentations. In addition, the social factors include lack of services and resources, inaccessibility to buildings, restricted reimbursement, and financial difficulties.

1.2 BIOLOGY OF AGING

Aging is defined[10] as a progressive decline and deterioration of functional properties at the cellular, tissue, and organ levels that lead to loss or decreased ability to adapt to internal or external stimuli and increased vulnerability to disease and mortality. The changes that occur with age in the cellular and molecular level are unique to the specific cells, tissues, and organs. Other changes occur across organ systems and have common effect on the functional capacity of the older adult. The onset of aging along with the rate and extent of progression is very individualized and differs from individual to individual. Depending on the functional capacity, the biological age is the metric for the biology of aging, and not the chronological age.

There are evolutionary, genetic, physiologic, and other theories of aging. In this book, emphasis is given to physiologic theory that describes various changes that occur to the cellular, molecular, and organ systems. They are common to a disease condition and to all ages in general. Age-related changes occur in the skin, muscles, nerves, bones, eyes, ears, endocrine, digestive, cardiovascular, pulmonary, urinary, and immune systems. Some of the changes are summarized below:

Skin. There is a decrease in moisture content, epidermal appendages, and melanocytes; hair turns gray due to the decrease in the melanocytes. The remaining melanocytes produce less melanin. Reduced elastin combined with increased collagen cross-links results in loss of elasticity of the skin. Capillaries are decreased resulting in the loss of blood supply followed by diminished sensitivity to touch, pain, and temperature, and this predisposes to pressure sores. Color of the nails becomes yellow and they become brittle with the formation of longitudinal ridges.

Muscles. Loss of muscle tissue results in the reduction of lean body mass; lypofuscin and fat get deposited in the muscles. It may result in an increase of body fat up to 30% of the body weight. The higher relative composition of body fat prolongs the half-life of lipid-soluble drugs. Hence, this factor should be considered when fat-soluble drugs are prescribed for older adults.

These changes coupled with the normal changes in the nervous system from advanced age result in loss of muscle tone and contractibility, strength, and endurance.

Bones. They become thinner and brittle, especially in females after menopause. Loss of fluid in the intervertebral discs and mineral content of the vertebrae results in shortening of the spine and trunk. These changes in addition to the flattening of the arches of the feet result in the loss of height. Other skeletal changes include the anterior thrust of the head, cervical spine extension, thoracic kyphosis, and straightened lumbar spine. Hips and knees are more flexed and ankle dorsiflexion is diminished. The above structural and postural changes result in flexing of the knees and the center of gravity shifts behind the hips.[11] The functional effect of these changes will require the use of aides for gait such as canes and walkers. Reflexes are diminished with an increase in reaction time. The gait becomes slower with shorter step length. The ability to stand on one leg and balance gets difficult and walking becomes unsteady.

Nervous system. Decline in the sensory and motor nerves resulting in decrease in strength and contractibility of the muscles. The axons lose their speed causing delays in starting of a motion. A speed of motor activities is compromised. Fine motor control is reduced due to the diminished capacity of the neurons to grow branches in the axons and dendrites. Neuronal cell membranes, blood vessels, and myelin reduce the blood flow causing slower action potentials and contraction of the muscle cell, which explains the decreased muscle strength during quick movements. Decreased visual acuity, vibratory, and proprioceptive loss with diminished vestibular and cerebellar function result in gait abnormalities.[11] The decrease in muscle strength in older adults is more prominent in proximal muscles and in the lower limbs than the upper limbs. This explains the reason for the difficulty of the older adults rising up from a low chair or a toilet seat. They do better with chairs having firm seats and arm rests, with their hips and knees at 90° angle and feet flat on the floor. There is a gradual decline in cognitive function due to decreased central processing and short-term memory.

Eyes. The eyes need double the illumination for every 13 years to see and maintain recognition in dim light. Pupil diameter decreases and accommodation is diminished due to the onset of fibrosis in the iris in later age. New central epithelial cells form in front of the lens making it large and rigid. These changes result in presbyopia and cataract formation. The chapter on vision impairment describes in detail these changes and their consequences later in this book.

Ears. Conductive deafness for low-frequency sounds is common due to the thickening of the tympanic membrane, and loss of elasticity in addition to inefficient function of the ossicular articulation. Sensory neural deafness for high-frequency sounds occurs due to the loss or atrophy of the hair cells in the organ of corti, and changes in spiral ganglion from the loss of cochlear neurons and restricted blood supply to the cochlea. Narrowing of the auditory canal also contributes to the loss of hearing.

Endocrine system. The changes in endocrine system for each gland differ with age. The thyroid gland may show changes with nodule formation and fibrosis with decrease in T4 production. Since the rate of clearance of T4 is slow, the serum thyroxin level remains normal. In parathyroid gland, there is an increase in fat deposition. In women after the age of 40, the level increases while its metabolism decreases affecting bone mineral homeostasis. The pituitary gland changes are minimal with advanced age. Growth hormone declines affecting the lean body mass to fat ratio. In the pineal gland, a reduction in diurnal melatonin rhythm, which is responsible for sleep, affects the sleep rhythm in older adults.

Cardiac function decreases from systematic vasoconstriction as a result of the increase in norepinephrine secretion. The adrenal glands respond to aging with a decrease in aldosterone secretion that can explain the orthostatic hypotension experienced by this population. Pancreas responds with very little change as people age. The thymus gland produces decreased thymosin in older adults affecting the immune system and contributing to increased risk for infection and cancer. Testosterone decreases with age resulting in the above-mentioned changes in the bone, skin, and muscles. In older women, decrease in estrogen and progesterone results in altered bone mineral density and increased low density lipoprotein levels.

Immune system. There is a slow decline in immune function and the older adults show decreased primary and secondary responses. The T cell function decreases and the immune response to an exposure to pathogens is reduced. With decreased function, the B cells are unable to fight the newly introduced antigens. Autoimmune antibodies are increased and abnormal antibodies are produced by B cells with age. Decreased thymus production due to the atrophy of the thymus gland with age compromises the immune system by reducing the T lymphocytes production and cytokines required for the maturation and growth of the B cells. The hematopoietic stem cells lose their ability to self-renew and result in the loss of immune function, predisposing the older adults to infections.

Temperature control. As an example of system-wide failure to maintain and regulate function, older adults lose thermoregulation resulting in hypo and hyperthermia when they are exposed to cold or hot temperatures. Loss of the sweat glands, thinning of the skin, decreased blood flow to the surface of the skin and reduction of the muscle mass are all responsible for the decrease in the functional capacity and the inability to maintain body temperature. The febrile response to infection is also altered leading to missed diagnosis and treatment of the older adults.

Digestive system. Decreased production of saliva can make the older adults susceptible to infection in the mouth and their digestive system may be affected in several ways. Difficulty in swallowing due to the increased spontaneous contractions of the esophagus occurs in older adults along with herniation and diverticulae. Delayed gastric emptying following a fatty meal are the common symptoms. In the small intestines, increased incidence of diverticular formation, decreased fat absorption due to delayed gastric emptying and decreased lipase production are the related changes. Absorption of Vitamin B12, iron, and calcium are decreased with age. Decreased transit time, constipation, and the formation of diverticula result from the atrophy of mucosal layers of the large intestine and the increase of the connective tissue. Constipation for the older adults is a problem from the gastro-intestinal (GI) system but it is also due to decreased mobility.

Genito-urinary system. Many age-related changes occur in the kidneys; there is a decline in the concentrating ability, glomerular filtration rate, kidney size and weight, functional glomeruli, and bladder capacity. At the bladder level in males, benign prostrate hypertrophy interferes with emptying. Changes that occur due to lymphocyte infiltration, trabaculae, prolapse, and urethral mucosal atrophy may predispose the older adults to urinary tract infections and associated incontinence.

Cardio-pulmonary system. With age, cardiac reserve, heart rate with exercise and baroreceptor sensitivity decrease. Increased systolic and diastolic arterial blood pressure predispose to strokes and myocardial infarctions. Maximal oxygen consumption decreases due to decreases in heart rate, cardiac output, and the muscle extraction of oxygen from blood. Similarly, many changes in pulmonary function occur due to age. They include decreased vital capacity, increased residual volume, decreased forced expiratory volume, and forced vital capacity. Chest wall compliance decreases and mucus glands in the bronchi are increased.

These changes in the heart and lung diminish the exercise tolerance in older adults. However, the changes in cardio-pulmonary system and the functional deficits are mainly due to disease and not due to age itself.

1.3 PHYSIOLOGY

Physiological changes of aging are summarized in Table 1.1.

TABLE 1.1
Physiological Changes of Aging

Body System	Change	Consequences
Nervous	↓ Number of neurons	↓ Muscle innervation
	↓ Action potential speed	↓ Fine motor control
	↓ Axon/dendrite branches	
Muscle	Fibers shrink	Tissue atrophies
	↓ Type II (fast twitch) fibers	↓ Tone and contractility
	↑ Lipofuscin and fat deposits	↓ Strength
Skin	↓ Thickness	Loss of elasticity
	↑ Collagen cross-links	
Skeletal	↓ Bone density	Movement slows and may become limited
	Joints become stiffer, less flexible	
Cardiovascular		
Heart	↑ Left ventricular wall thickness	Stressed heart is less able to respond
	↑ Lipofuscin and fat deposits	
Vasculature	↑ Stiffness	
	↓ Responsiveness to agents	
Pulmonary	↓ Elastin fibers	↓ Effort dependent and independent respiration (quiet and forced breathing)
	↑ Collagen cross-links	↓ Exercise tolerance and pulmonary reserve
	↓ Elastic recoil of the lung	
	↑ Residual volume	
	↓ Vital capacity, forced expiratory volume, and forced vital capacity	
Eyes	↑ Lipid infiltrates/deposits	↓ Transparency of the cornea
	↑ Thickening of the lens	Difficulty in focusing on near objects
	↓ Pupil diameter	↓ Accommodation and dark adaptation
Ears	↑ Thickening of tympanic membrane	↑ Conductive deafness (low-frequency range)
	↓ Elasticity and efficiency of ossicular articulation	↑ Sensorineural hearing loss (high-frequency sounds)
	↑ Organ atrophy	
	↓ Cochlear neurons	
	↓ Number of neurons in the utricle, saccule, and ampullae	↓ Detection of gravity, changes in speed, and rotation
	↓ In size and number of otoliths	
Digestive	↑ Dysphagia	
	↑ Achlorhydria	
	Altered intestinal absorption	↓ Iron absorption
	↑ Lipofuscin and fat deposition in pancreas	↓ B_{12} and calcium absorption
	↑ Mucosal cell atrophy	↑ Incidence of diverticula, transit time, and constipation
Urinary	↓ Kidney size, weight, and number of functional glomeruli	↓ Ability to resorb glucose
	↓ Number and length of functional renal tubules	↓ Concentrating ability of kidney
	↓ Glomerular filtration rate	
	↓ Renal blood flow	
Immune	↓ Primary and secondary response	↓ Immune functioning
	↑ Autoimmune antibodies	

(Continued)

TABLE 1.1   (*Continued*)
Physiological Changes of Aging

Body System	Change	Consequences
	↓ T-cell function, fewer naïve, and more memory T cells	↓ Response to new pathogens
	Atrophy of thymus	↓ T lymphocytes, natural killer cells, cytokines needed for growth, and maturation of B cells
Endocrine	↑ Atrophy of certain glands (e.g., pituitary, thyroid, and thymus)	Changes in target organ response, organ system homeostasis, response to stress, and functional capacity
	↓ Growth hormone, dehydroepiandrosterone, testosterone, and estrogen	
	↑ Parathyroid hormone, atrial natriuretic peptide, norepinephrine, baseline cortisol, and erythropoietin	

Source: Fedarko NS, McNabney MK. *Geriatrics Review Syllabus: A Core Curriculum in Geriatric Medicine*, 9th edn. New York, American Geriatrics Society, 2016. Reprinted with permission. Also available: http://geriatricscareonline.org/

REFERENCES

1. Fortin M, Bravo G, Hudon C, Vanasse A, Lapointe L. Prevalence of multimorbidity among adults seen in family practice. *Ann Fam Med* 2005; 3:223–228.
2. Hoffman C, Rice D, Sung HY. Persons with chronic conditions, their prevalence and costs. *JAMA* 1996; 276(18):1473–1479.
3. Koller D, Schön G, Schäfer I, Glaeske G, van den Bussche H, Hansen H. Multimorbidity and long-term care dependency—A five-year follow-up. *BMC Geriatr* 2014; 14:70, May 28.
4. Barnett K, Mercer SW, Norbury M, Watt G, Wyke S, Guthrie, B. Epidemiology of multimorbidity and its implications for health care, research, and medical education: A cross-sectional study. *Lancet* 2012; 380:37–43.
5. McLean G, Gunn J, Wyke S, Guthrie B, Watt GC, Blane DN, Mercer SW. The influence of socioeconomic deprivation on multimorbidity at different ages: A cross-sectional study. *Br J Gen Pract* 2014; 64(624):e440–e447, July.
6. Wolff JL, Starfield B, Anderson G. Prevalence, expenditures, and complications of multiple chronic conditions in the elderly. *Arch Intern Med* 2002; 162(20):2269–2276.
7. Brummel-Smith K. Rehabilitation. In Cassel CK (ed.), *Geriatric Medicine*. New York, Springer-Verlag, 1990, p. 129.
8. Ham RJ, Sloane PD (eds). *Primary Care Geriatrics: A Case-Based Approach*. St. Louis, Missouri, CV Mosby, 1992, p. 142.
9. Butler RN. A disease called ageism. *J Am Geriatr Soc* 1990; 38(2):178–180, February.
10. Holliday R. Aging: The reality: The multiple and irreversible causes of aging. *J Gerontol A Biol Sci Med Sci* 2004; 59(6):B568–B572.
11. Steinberg FU. Gait disorders in the aged. *J Am Geriatr Soc* 1972; 20:537–540.
12. Fedarko NS, McNabney MK. Biology. In Medina-Walpole A, Pacala JT, Potter JF, (eds), *Geriatrics Review Syllabus: A Core Curriculum in Geriatric Medicine*, 9th edn. New York, American Geriatrics Society, 2016. Also available: http://geriatricscareonline.org/.

2 Geriatric Assessment and the Physical Examination of the Older Adult

Bilal Ahmed and Yvonne J. Braver

CONTENTS

2.1 INTRODUCTION

Physical examination is an integral component in the assessment, diagnosis, and management of disease. The objective clues gathered while doing a physical examination of the elderly patient can provide information of more than just the presence or absence of disease. The patient's general appearance for instance can provide an estimation of care, nutritional status, alertness, and evidence of discomfort. The elderly often do not volunteer this information and might not be able to express an accurate description of their ailments.

It is uncommon for the elderly to present with a discrete set of symptoms that can be translated to an easily recognizable diagnosis. Many elderly patients misinterpret their dysfunction as normal signs of aging. A combination of frailty and other psychosocial factors interact with their symptomatology, as well as their ability to clearly state the reasons for which they might seek care.

Multiple comorbidities are also the rule rather than an exception in geriatrics and a problem-based approach is not very well adapted to care for the elderly, given the complexity of the presentation. Although the patient is the primary source of information, coexistent cognitive and sensory impairment often interferes with accurate data gathering.

All of this is often complicated by communication barriers. These include depression, memory loss, hearing and visual impairment, inadequate description of the chief complaint, and cultural differences. These factors make it all the more important to carry out a thorough physical examination to focus and narrow the disease spectrum for these patients.

Physical examination is not an isolated exercise in the geriatric population and should complement a comprehensive geriatric assessment, which includes the patient's past medical history, mental status examination, social history, living arrangements, medication history, impediments to compliance as well as a complete review of systems. A large majority issues identified are connected with concern worsening cognition, frailty, immobility, incontinence, or falls.

Another important caveat to remember in assessing the older adult is the fact that the patient's presentation may be symptomatic of a completely unrelated pathology. A classic example would be delirium presenting as symptoms of a urinary tract infection.

Geriatric assessment is a multidimensional diagnostic instrument that is designed to collect information on a variety of factors and should ideally consist of an interdisciplinary approach.

A multidisciplinary approach is also crucial to determine the patient's mental health, social and environmental circumstances as well as their functional ability. This approach also helps in the development of treatment plans, coordination of management, and evaluation of long-term care needs.

The aim of the comprehensive geriatric assessment is to paint a more complete picture of the patient's medical problems as well as functional and psychosocial issues. The constraints of time can make it difficult to coordinate and assess all these facets in a patient's presentation when confronted with multiple concerns. A approach would be to perform a continuous assessment over several visits.

2.1.1 SUMMARY

- Geriatric assessment is a multidimensional and multidisciplinary exercise, which includes known medical domains, such as functional capacity and quality of life.
- Attention to nutrition, vision, hearing, incontinence, and balance is vital.
- The elderly accrue a vast number of symptoms and pathology over time and often have complex and interlinked comorbidities.
- Assessment of the functional status is of primary importance in the elderly.
- Attention to polypharmacy, noncompliance with medications, and drug interactions is crucial in geriatric assessment.
- Social history and nutritional history are also often-neglected facets in geriatric patients.

2.2 SYSTEMATIC APPROACH TO GERIATRIC CLINICAL ASSESSMENT

Collecting clinical data in the elderly can be a daunting task. Impediments to documenting an accurate history include factors such as cognitive impairment, visual and auditory handicaps, as well as difficulties in assessing the primary reason for presentation on account of multiple coexisting comorbidities.

An effective history might require the presence of family members or other caregivers. The availability of a documented list of previous diagnoses as well as a medication list can be extremely helpful. The physical examination itself can be time consuming on account of the patient's decreased mobility, frailty, and the changing physiologic nature of the human organ systems.

We will now go through a stepwise approach of gathering data for a comprehensive geriatric assessment.

2.3 SOURCES OF INFORMATION

The clinical decision-making process is an interesting iterative exercise, which relies heavily on observation, data gathering, as well as physical examination. An objective history in the elderly can often be difficult to gather on account of cognitive impairment and memory issues. But a history gathered from caregivers and family members can often be biased on account of their review and interpretation of the patient's situation. It is important to note the identity of the historian and if it is a caregiver, their objectivity. Due respect should be paid to confidentiality as well as to patient's cultural and social background. If the patient's responses to questions point to cognitive impairment, the mental status examination precedes the rest of the data gathering process.

2.4 GETTING STARTED

- The interview and the physical examination should be conducted in a quiet room.
- Backlighting should preferably be avoided.
- Interruptions should be minimized.
- The elderly prefer honorific titles such as "Mr." and "Mrs."
- Due respect should be accorded to the patient.
- The physician should speak clearly and slowly.
- The patient and the physician should preferably be at the same level and position.
- The interviewer should be cognizant of the possibility of hearing and visual impairment.
- A notepad to write questions in large print should be accessible if a speech amplifier is not available.
- Introducing oneself, a kind and empathic attitude, and eye contact can go a long way in establishing initial rapport with the patient.

2.4.1   Why Is Geriatric History Taking Different? Key Issues to Keep in Mind

* The extensive list of complaints that the elderly usually present with can make it very hard to identify the primary issue at the time of presentation. Some patients might present to physicians after being told to do so by their spouse or children.
* The elderly often misinterpret many of the complaints as a part and parcel of the aging process.
* Many of the presenting symptoms in the elderly are complexly interlinked.
* This facet of the geriatric practice often makes the complete examination of individual systems difficult.
* It is best to start with an objective assessment of cognitive status.
* This can be followed by assessment of mobility and balance.
* The functional status in the elderly has a significant influence on their well-being and presentation.
* Realistically, most of the geriatric assessments are performed under constraints of time and resources. The focus of data gathering and physical examination should be directed at the presenting complaints. This approach can work well in relatively high-functioning elders.
* However, most of these assessments take place over multiple visits. Soliciting information from a multidisciplinary team can be crucial for a comprehensive geriatric assessment.
* An interventional treatment strategy based on input from social work, nutrition, physical and occupational therapy and sometimes speech therapy as well as other specialties such as psychiatry, ophthalmology, and audiology would be desirable in ideal circumstances.
* Some practices also rely on assessment instruments in which the patients are asked to complete questionnaires and perform specific tasks prior to visiting their caregivers.
* This information can provide a useful insight into the patient's activities of daily living as well as their cognitive ability.

2.4.2   Simplifying the Assessment Tools/Prescreening

Administrating a previsit to questionnaire as mentioned above can improve the validity of data gathered in the patient's first visit.

Some aspects of this questionnaire can include

* Mobility around the house
* Ability to perform functional tasks
* History of falls
* Sources of social support
* The patient and hearing difficulties
* Advanced directives and durable power of attorney

2.5   PHYSICAL EXAMINATION

The examination of the elderly necessitates a multidisciplinary approach. The goal of this information gathering is to obtain a perspective of an individual's overall functional ability. This includes a patient's ability to function in their environment and their ability to overcome physical and cognitive challenges.

The information gathered from the history obtained from the patient and caregivers, physical examination, and psychosocial as well as functional capabilities is used to formulate a care plan. This concerns the patient as well as a constellation of required services.

These interventions might include the need for rehabilitative services, arranging for home visits, meals, physical therapy, and determination for long-term care requirements, and also understanding how to best use the available healthcare resources.

Geriatric physical examination has overarching similarities to an adult physical examination. The following list is given as an outline but gives an idea of information that needs to be gathered in the assessment of the elderly:

- History of the present illness and its functional impact on the patient's activities
- Past medical history
- A complete review of systems
- Personal and social functional ability
- Recent relevant life changes
- Patient's situation in reference to availability of healthcare providers and family members and their geographic proximity
- Caregiver network
- Living environment and its relevance to patient's functional abilities
- Emotional health and substance abuse
- Status of services being provided such as *Meals on Wheels*
- Rehabilitative status
- Advanced directives and documentation concerning healthcare proxy

In addition to the special areas of focus discussed above, the elderly have other variables that can have a significant impact on their well-being and functional capabilities. Physical examination is not an isolated exercise and forms a part of a continuum of an assessment.

We have now obtained the history and review of systems. The next steps are to collect a comprehensive record of the patient's pharmacotherapy. Where possible, it is useful to ask the patient or the family to bring with them the medications that they are taking. The examination routine described here is to both serve as an aid to a quick overview of the patient's functional status and act as a template in a thorough and efficient assessment of physical abnormalities.

2.5.1 General Observation

Observational clues to the general well-being of the elderly can be very helpful.

- The patient's appearance can provide clues about their hygiene, nutritional status, recall, and ability to interact appropriately.
- Important inferences can be drawn from the patient's reaction to the environment, posture and motor activity, as well as their facial expression.
- The patient's height and weight should be measured and recorded at every visit.

Check the blood pressure, pulse, and orthostatics. Orthostatics in the elderly are preferably checked after a few minutes of postural change.

2.5.2 Examination of the Face

A careful observation can provide a wealth of information and might provide clues that point to

- Parkinson's disease
- Cushing's syndrome
- Sign of hypo- or hyperthyroidism
- Horner's syndrome

- VIIth nerve palsy
- Parotid gland enlargement
- Systemic sclerosis
- Cachexia/malnutrition
- Poor dentition/dentures

A helpful hint is to divide the parts of the face into their constituents and ask yourself the question, "Is this normal?"

2.5.3 ASSESSING HYDRATION STATUS

The assessment of volume status in the elderly requires good clinical skills and a history of prior events. The most helpful sign of volume depletion is acute weight loss. Physical examination-based assessment of fluid status in the elderly is somewhat less specific. Skin turgor is best tested on the inner aspect of the thigh or the sternum. Examination of the mouth for dryness of the tongue and mucous membranes could be helpful but can be ordered by certain medications. Reduced turgor of the eyes and muscle weakness also point to dehydration. Postural hypotension and tachycardia can be indicative of hypovolemia.

2.5.4 HEAD, EYES, EAR, NOSE, AND THROAT (HEENT) EXAMINATION

2.5.4.1 Examination of the Oral Cavity

This examination is carried out with adequate lighting, and other necessary equipment might include tongue depressor and gauze sponge.

Sialadenitis is a painful infection that is usually caused by bacteria. It is more common among elderly adults with salivary gland stones. The opening of the parotid salivary gland duct, also called the Stensen's duct, is seen in the punctate soft tissue next to the maxillary second molar tooth.

The buccal mucosa is examined for hyperplastic reaction from chronic irritation from dentures or broken teeth. The tongue might have white spots consistent with oral candidiasis. A smooth and glossy tongue might indicate vitamin B12 deficiency. Dental hygiene can result in dental plaques and gingival inflammation.

2.5.4.2 Neck

Osteoarthritis and cervical spondylosis often impair the elderly patient's neck mobility. Caution is recommended in hyperextending the neck of people with rheumatoid arthritis due to the involvement of the odontoid process. Wasting of the interosseous muscles of the hand can provide an indirect clue about cervical myelopathy malnutrition or diabetic neuropathy.

2.5.4.3 Carotid Auscultation

Auscultation of the carotid arteries should take place in a quiet room. The patient should preferably be in a sitting or supine position. Start with palpating the carotid arteries. The stethoscope bell should form a seal over the carotid pulse. It is helpful to ask the patient to hold their breath during the auscultation as it eliminates interference from respiratory sounds. Cardiac and thoracic vascular sounds could also be transmitted to the carotid arteries and the best method to locate the origin of a murmur is to slowly move the stethoscope down the carotid. Cardiac murmurs will increase in intensity as the stethoscope moves toward the precordium.

2.5.4.4 Jugular Vein Pressure

Jugular vein pressure (JVP) examination is an integral part of the examination and yields gratifying results with clinical implications. It is an important marker of intravascular fluid status and can guide us in our clinical decision-making process.

The jugular vein lies behind the anterior belly of the sternocleidomastoid muscle and the waveform seen on the neck is transmitted through the overlying tissue. The JVP can however be hard to assess. A well-lit room and the patient positioned at a 45° angle can be very helpful. Past light shown tangentially across the neck can help to accentuate the jugular venous pulsations. It is helpful to palpate either the carotid pulse or the radial pulses during the JVP examination. The carotid impulse coincides with palpated radial artery pulsation. The jugular venous pulse tends to the sinuous compared to the carotid pulse, which is a single up-and-down pulsation. The jugular venous pulse can also be obliterated by applying pressure just above the clavicle. Once the top of the jugular venous column is identified, the vertical distance from the top of this column to the manubrium sternum is measured and 5 cm is added to this to obtain the JVP height.

The hepatojugular reflux can confirm that the pulsations originate in the jugular venous pulse. The pressure to the right upper quadrant has to be sustained and the height of the column should have a demonstrable sustained rise, immediately after the hepatic pressure is applied.

2.5.4.5 Thyroid Gland

A multinodular goiter is a common finding in the elderly. If a goiter is suspected, palpate the gland with the right index and middle fingers below the thyroid cartilage. The two lobes of the thyroid gland are then palpated laterally. The patient can be asked to swallow while the thyroid gland is palpated. The neck should be slightly flexed while the gland is being palpated.

2.5.4.6 Lymph Nodes

Careful assessment for lymph node enlargement is an essential part of geriatric physical examination. The important nodes to remember are the supraclavicular nodes of the anterior cervical chain and the axillary lymph nodes. Detection of an enlarged left sided lymph node is always a cause for concern as it can signify an occult abdominal malignancy.

2.5.4.7 Head

The elderly often have some temporal subcutaneous fat atrophy. Significant atrophy can point to malnutrition. Palpate the temporal arteries if there is a recent history of headaches or visual changes. The temporal artery is palpated for tenderness or absence of pulsation. On account of its exposure to solar radiation, the head and the forehead are the most common sites for actinic damage. Dermatologic examination to look for actinic keratosis or other malignancies such as basal cell cancer, malignant melanoma, and squamous cell cancer is indicated.

2.5.4.8 Ears

Presbycusis is very common in the elderly. Hearing aids can facilitate the retention of cerumen. Refer to Section 2.5.14. Otoliths of the semicircular canals and the consequent positional vertigo are common causes of dizziness in the elderly.

Approximately 25%–50% of dizziness in the elderly can be secondary to benign positional vertigo. In a recent study, about 9% of urban-dwelling elders were found to have Benign paroxysmal positional vertigo (BPPV) (Oghalai et al., 2000). BPPV is diagnosed by performing the Dix–Hallpike maneuver. This is performed with the patient sitting upright on the examination table. The patient's head is then rotated on one side by 45°. The clinician then facilitates the patient to lie backward with the head turned and at approximately 20° of extension. Having the head hang at the edge of the bed is a helpful maneuver. Remember to ask the patient to keep their eyes open to observe the nystagmus.

The test is considered positive if rotational nystagmus is observed. There can be 5–10 seconds latency before the nystagmus manifests itself. This test is contraindicated in patients with cervical radiculopathies, vertebral column instability, and carotid and vertebral vascular disease.

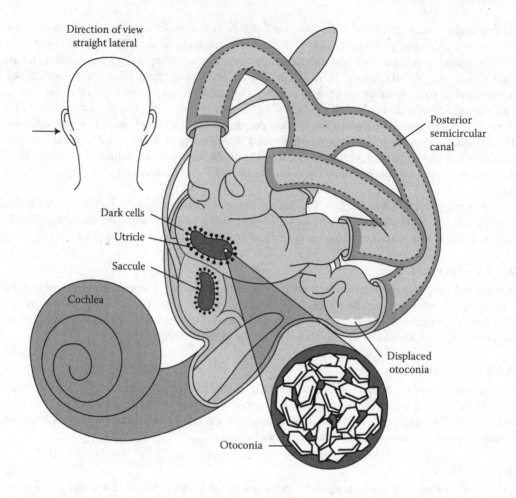

Direction of view straight lateral

Posterior semicircular canal

Dark cells

Utricle

Saccule

Cochlea

Displaced otoconia

Otoconia

DIX-Hallpike manueuver

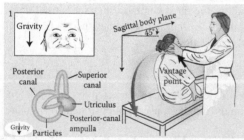

The examiner stands at the patient's head, 45° to the right, to align the right posterior semicircular canal with the sagittal plane of the body.

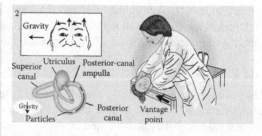

The examiner moves the patient, whose eyes are open, from the seated to the supine, right-ear-down position and then extends the patient's neck slightly so that the chin is pointed slightly upward. The latency, duration, and direction of nystagmus, if present, and the latency and duration of vertigo, if present, should be noted. Inset: The arrows over the eyes depict the direction of nystagmus in patients with typicaI BPPV. The presumed location in the labyrinth of the free-floating debris thought to cause the disorder is also shown.

Source: epomedicine.com.

2.5.4.9 Eyes

The incidence of cataracts, glaucoma, macular degeneration, and retinopathy rises with aging. Visual acuity can consequently be affected and has a significant impact on activities of daily living. Annual eye examinations are best conducted by optometrists or ophthalmologists. Visual acuity screening with a Snellen's chart should be conducted annually on office visits. The important objective findings to look for are

- Cataracts
- Arcus senilis (this is common and clinically not significant)
- Dry eyes
- Entropion and ectropion
- Macular degeneration screening

The easiest way of assessing macular function in an office setting is using an Amsler grid. It consists of a piece of paper on which a 10 cm × 10 cm grid box is printed with a black dot in the center. The patient is asked to cover one eye and fix their gaze on the central dot. The patient is asked if they can see the four corners of the box. They are then told to comment on any distortions or missing areas within the box. If able to, the patient can draw the areas of distortion on and this provides a record of disease progression. This should be repeated for the fellow eye. This gives a reasonable indication of macular function. This simple tool can be used by the patient who can self-test at home and report early if changes are detected. Straight lines in the pattern appear wavy, or some of the lines are missing.

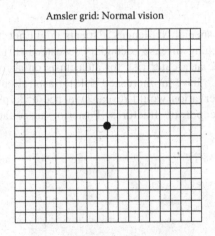

Amsler grid: Normal vision

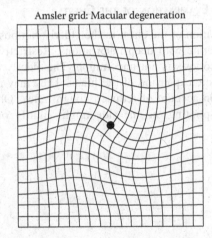

Amsler grid: Macular degeneration

1. Do the test with each eye separately by covering the eye that is not being tested.
2. Hold the test grid directly in front of the patient about 14 inches from your face, and ask them to look at the dot in the center of the grid, *not at the lines*.
3. While looking at the dot, all the lines, both vertical and horizontal, should appear straight and unbroken.

2.5.5 Dermatologic Examination

The incidence of aging-related dermatologic disorders is increasing. The physiologic changes that occur with aging include thinning of the epidermis, loss of strength and stratum corneum's ability to retain water, decreased wound healing, decreased number of apocrine sweat glands, and impaired immune responsiveness.

Excessive UV exposure produces photo damage in all layers of the skin. Photo damage is the most common change in the Caucasian skin and commonly presents as actinic keratoses and solar lentigines. The presence of these conditions can predict a higher risk of sunlight-induced skin cancer.

2.5.5.1   Common Dermatologic Conditions Seen in the Office

2.5.5.1.1   Solar or Traumatic Purpura (Senile Purpura)

These are ecchymotic, purpuric patches on the forearms, arms, or legs (Figure 2.1). These usually follow minor trauma and are more common in people taking aspirin and blood thinners. No treatment is required for these.

2.5.5.1.2   Seborrheic Keratosis

These are probably the most common benign skin growths in the elderly. These are hyperkeratotic plaques that appear to be stuck onto the skin surface (Figure 2.2). They tend to congregate on the trunk. The cause is unknown but there might be a genetic predisposition. Therapy is usually not necessary unless they are inflamed.

2.5.5.1.3   Stasis Dermatitis

This affects approximately 7% of older adults. This worsens with standing and progresses throughout the day. Over time, this develops into a dermatitis, which could be scaly red and edematous (Figure 2.3). This can also often mimic cellulitis and is a common cause for prescription of inappropriate antibiotics. Varicose veins are also common as are decubitus ulcers secondary to pressure and friction in sedentary patients.

2.5.6   Examination of the Chest

Examination of the chest in the elderly can pose special challenges. Patients might not be able to cooperate with deep inspirations. Restrictive lung disease secondary to osteoarthritis and kyphoscoliosis is not uncommon. The elderly are at greater risk for atelectasis on account of incomplete expansion of the lungs. They may also have an increased risk for aspiration pneumonia on account of reduced cough reflex. Observation would reveal evidence of kyphoscoliosis. Splinting on one side might signify osteoporotic fractures. Posterior auscultation is

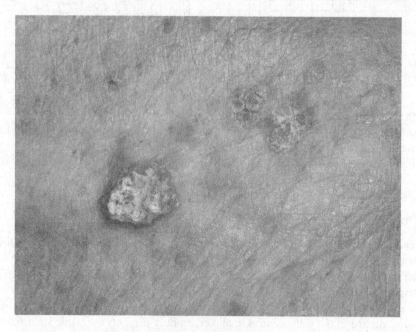

FIGURE 2.1   Actinic keratosis. (From *Global Dermatology*.)

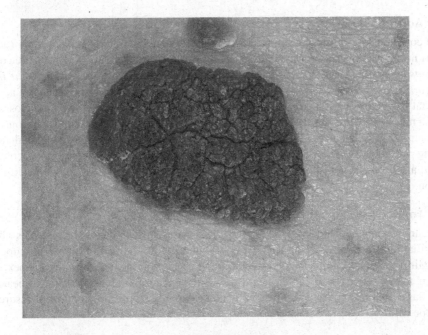

FIGURE 2.2 Seborrheic keratosis. (University of Maryland.)

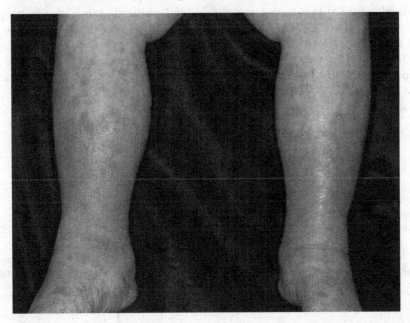

FIGURE 2.3 Stasis dermatitis. (VisualDx.)

recommended as it has the greatest yield. Reduced air entry and basal crackles can be present even in the absence of pathology.

2.5.7 EXAMINATION OF THE HEART

Examination of the jugular venous pulse as well as the carotid pulses has been described above. It is recommended to auscultate an area specific to the corresponding valves. Common findings in the elderly include the following.

2.5.7.1   Aortic Stenosis

The most commonly heard murmur in the elderly is aortic stenosis. Calcification of the aortic well is part of the normal aging process. The intensity of the murmur has no relation to the degree of stenosis. *The most important predictive factor for the cross-sectional valve area tends to be the intensity of the second heart sound.* The softer the sound, the more severe the stenosis. This is on account of the fact that the heart sounds are produced by valve closure. A heavily calcified valve closes gradually with a much less force and the associated intensity of the second heart sound. Late onset of the systolic murmur can also be predictive of the severity of the aortic valve cross-sectional area. The slow rising plateau pulse (Pulsus parvus et tardus) is not very helpful in the elderly on account of the associated arteriosclerosis leading to poor transmission of pulse pressure to the peripheral arterial circulation.

2.5.7.2   Fourth Heart Sound

Fourth heart sound is not uncommon due to a reduced ventricular compliance. It is absent in atrial fibrillation. It is low in frequency and is best heard with the bell of the stethoscope placed lightly against the chest wall. Though often soft and most prominent at the cardiac apex, the left ventricular fourth heart sound can be heard over other precordial areas. The fourth heart sound typically has a dull or thudding quality, and it can be suppressed by applying firm pressure on the stethoscope bell.

2.5.7.3   Ankle/Brachial Index

Ankle/brachial index (ABI) is an undervalued and underutilized examination technique that is often performed incorrectly. ABI is a noninvasive clinical test that can be applied to diagnose peripheral arterial disease (PAD) and also to provide important prognostic information about future cardiovascular events. Although ABI has been employed in clinical practice for some time, it is poorly understood and often incorrectly performed. It is extremely important that we understand all aspects of this crucial test, as it is now being recommended as part of a patient's routine health risk assessment.

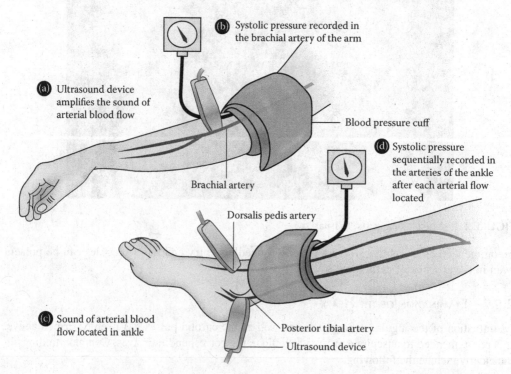

(a) Ultrasound device amplifies the sound of arterial blood flow

(b) Systolic pressure recorded in the brachial artery of the arm

Blood pressure cuff

Brachial artery

(d) Systolic pressure sequentially recorded in the arteries of the ankle after each arterial flow located

Dorsalis pedis artery

(c) Sound of arterial blood flow located in ankle

Posterior tibial artery

Ultrasound device

ABI is calculated by measuring the systolic blood pressure from both the brachial arteries and diastolic blood pressure from both the dorsalis pedis and posterior tibial arteries. The equipment required for this is blood pressure cuff, stethoscope, hand-held Doppler, and ultrasound gel. It is best to begin with the right arm, followed by the right leg, then the left leg, and finally the left arm. The patient should be in the supine position. The cuff is inflated to about 20 mmHg above the expected systolic pressure. The transducer is placed in the antecubital fossa over the brachial artery. A notation is made of the pressure at which the Doppler signal appears. The ankle pressure is then measured by placing the ultrasound gel over the dorsalis pedis and posterior tibial arteries. The cuff can be placed proximal to the malleoli. ABI is calculated by taking the higher pressure of two arteries at the ankle, divided by the brachial artery systolic pressure for each leg. In normal individuals, they should be at a minimal gradient.

$$ABI = \frac{\text{ankle systolic pressure}}{\text{arm systolic pressure}}$$

2.5.7.3.1 Interpretation of the ABI

ABI	Interpretation	Action
>1.2	Atherosclerosis from peripheral vascular disease	Monitor
0.9–1.2	Acceptable	None
0.8–0.9	Mild arterial disease	Manage risk factors
0.5–0.8	Moderate arterial disease	Vascular surgery referral
<0.5	Severe arterial disease	Urgent vascular surgery referral

2.5.7.4 Peripheral Edema

Edema of the lower extremity is very common in the elderly patients. This can occur in the absence of heart disease. The common cause of lower extremity edema is venous stasis. There could be a diurnal pattern to this as a venous stasis edema improves overnight. Long-standing edema leeds to hemosiderin deposits in the subcutaneous tissues and this can often be confused with cellulitis and can lead to inappropriate antibiotic use. Long-standing venous stasis can also lead to stasis ulcers.

2.5.8 EXAMINATION OF THE ABDOMEN

The examination of the abdomen in the elderly can pose special challenges. The patient's dignity should be foremost while conducting this examination. Draping the groin and the sheath is recommended. The patient might not be able to lie flat on account of kyphoscoliosis or congestive heart failure, or the patient may be wheelchair bound.

The general appearance as well as the rest of the examination can provide a multitude of clues. Organ enlargement might be visible to the naked eye. Ascites is suggested by fullness in the flanks. Examination for hernias is best done by asking the patient to raise the head off the bed. Midline, incisional, and groin hernias are common in the elderly. Be cognizant of heparin or insulin injection sites with associated ecchymosis and erythema. A bruise around the umbilicus (Cullen's) or in the femoral area (Grey Turner) signifies a retroperitoneal bleed.

Auscultation of the abdomen is done with the diaphragm the stethoscope. It is best done just lateral to the umbilicus. High-pitched bowel sounds can indicate an ileus or a small bowel obstruction. Abdominal palpation is performed with one's hands and inquiring about any tender areas that are either avoided or examined at the end of the session. Liver edge is best palpated with the ulnar edge of the hand. Gentle pressure is applied downward as the patient breathes in. A mass in the left or the right lower quadrant should be followed up to exclude the possibility of inflammatory bowel disease, diverticulitis, or colon cancer. Spleen is palpated by asking the patient to roll on to the right side. The hand is placed along the left costal margin and the patient is asked to exhale the soft and hard to palpate. Abdominal ascites can be clinically apparent. Shifting dullness continues to be a very helpful sign. Percussion is started in the midline and the pleximeter (finger on the abdomen) is slowly moved to the flank. Percussion is stopped where the dullness is appreciated and the patient is asked to roll over to the other side. Percussion is recommenced after about 30 seconds. The return of a tympanitic note signifies free fluid, which gravitates to the dependent area of the abdomen.

2.5.8.1 Rectal Exam

The patient has to be informed that they will experience a sensation of pressure. The first part of the anal reflex is contraction. After about 5 seconds, the sphincter relaxes and the fingers can then be advanced into the anal orifice. Once the finger is inserted, each quadrant is examined, starting at the 12 o'clock position. The prostate gland is felt anteriorly and its size symmetry, nodularity, and consistency are noted.

2.5.9 NEUROLOGICAL EXAMINATION

Comprehensive neurological examination[1] is a daunting task for a busy practitioner. This quick general overview can provide a relatively good overall assessment. Language assessment is a significant part of the dominant hemisphere. Language is composed of fluency, comprehension, and repetition. Fluency can be assessed during history taking and it would be evident if the patient is having trouble coming up with appropriate words. Comprehension is tested by giving a three-step command. This could be: Take the right thumb, touch your left ear, and stick out your tongue. If the patient can perform this function, it would suggest intact receptive language and also give an idea about the right hand's motor function and proprioception. Repetition is tested by asking the patient a simple phrase. These simple steps will help differentiate between receptive and expressive dysphasia and give significant clues about the mental status of the patient.

2.5.9.1 Cranial Nerves

Testing the cranial nerves individually is a significant time commitment. The highest-yield cranial nerve examination involves information about the pupils, extraocular movements, facial strength, and visual fields. The best way to examine the patient's fields is the "confrontation" method. The examiner's face should be about 3 feet from the patient. Ask the patient to look at your nose. The examiner's hand should be halfway between themselves and the patient. The patient is asked to point to the hand that is wiggling. The intent is to compare the examiner's peripheral field of vision with that of the patient. Asking the patient to show their teeth and raise their eyebrows is a quick test of the seventh nerve. The third, fourth, and sixth nerves as can be tested by moving the finger in the shape of the letter "H" and asking the patient to follow the finger as it moves.

2.5.9.2 Motor Exam

A quick and easy way to test the motor system includes testing for pronator drift and fast finger movements and toe taps. This is then followed by testing one muscle group in each of the four extremities. Testing the hand grip is a poor assessment of motor strength as the strong flexor muscles are the last to exhibit weakness. It would be helpful to spend time distinguishing between upper and lower motor weakness by testing the reflexes.

2.5.9.3 Sensory Exam

This is notoriously difficult to perform and replicate as well as interpret. As far as the sensory exam is concerned, peripheral neuropathy is the commonest entity in the elderly. If the sensations in the toe are intact, continuing with the sensory examination is not necessary.

2.5.9.3.1 Romberg's Test

Romberg's test can be informative and valuable. The patient is asked to stand up and then bring their feet completely together. The patient is then asked to close their eyes. The Romberg's test is positive only if the patient falls after closing their eyes.

2.5.9.4   Reflexes

The symmetry of reflexes is more important than individual reflexes. Elderly people often do not have an ankle reflex.

2.5.9.5   Coordination

The best way to test coordination is to have the patient walk.

2.5.9.6   Delirium

Delirium is a common clinical syndrome. It is characterized by inattention and acute cognitive dysfunction. Among elderly patients, one of the most prominent risk factors for delirium is dementia, with two-thirds of all cases of delirium in this age group occurring in patients with dementia. There might be any number of modifiable risk factors leading to delirium as well. These include sensory impairment, immobilization (catheters or restraints), pain, polypharmacy, sleep deprivation, and so on.

A quick assessment tool that is commonly used is the confusion assessment method (CAM). This provides a brief, validated diagnostic algorithm that is currently in widespread use for the identification of delirium. The CAM algorithm relies on the presence of acute onset of symptoms and a fluctuating course, inattention, and either disorganized thinking or an altered level of consciousness.

2.5.9.6.1   Short CAM Version   The short CAM version is easier to administer by the bedside.[2]

2.5.9.6.1.1   Feature 1: Acute Onset and Fluctuating Course   This feature is usually obtained from a family member or nurse and is shown by positive responses to the following questions:

1. *Is there evidence of an acute change in mental status from the patient's baseline?*
2. *Did the (abnormal) behavior fluctuate during the day, that is, tend to come and go, or increase or decrease in severity?*

2.5.9.6.1.2   Feature 2: Inattention   This feature is usually obtained by interacting with the patient, but may also be reported by family members or staff and is shown by a positive response to the following question:

3. *Did the patient have difficulty focusing attention, for example, being easily distractible or having difficulty keeping track of what was being said?*

2.5.9.6.1.3   Feature 3: Disorganized Thinking   This feature is usually obtained by interacting with the patient, but may also be reported by family members or staff and is shown by a positive response to the following question:

4. *Was the patient's thinking disorganized or incoherent, such as rambling or irrelevant conversation, unclear or illogical flow of ideas, or unpredictable switching from subject to subject?*

2.5.9.6.1.4   Feature 4: Altered Level of Consciousness   This feature is obtained by observing the patient and is shown by any answer other than "alert" to the following question:

5. *Overall, how would you rate this patient's level of consciousness?*
   Alert (normal)
   Vigilant (hyperalert)
   Lethargic (drowsy, easily aroused)
   Stupor (difficult to arouse)
   Coma (unarousable)

2.5.9.6.2   Scoring the Test (Please Tick as Appropriate)

	Positive	Negative
Feature 1		
Feature 2		
Feature 3		
Feature 4		

2.5.9.6.3   Interpreting the CAM

Rate each symptom of delirium listed in the short CAM instrument as: Absent (0), Mild (1), and Marked (2). Acute onset or fluctuation is rated as absent or present. Summarize these scores into a composite that ranges from 0 to 7 (higher scores indicate more severe delirium).

2.5.10   MUSCULOSKELETAL SYSTEM EXAMINATION

Loss of muscle mass (sarcopenia) accompanies the normal process of aging. This can be easily discernible in the interosseous muscles. A quick review of muscle strength can be done by asking the patient to touch the back of their head with both hands. Elderly people might appear weak during the testing of muscle strength. The patients might have increased muscle tone and this too is a normal finding in the elderly. Cogwheel rigidity would however be abnormal.

Joints should be examined for tenderness, swelling, subluxation, crepitus, warmth, and redness. Heberden's nodes (bony overgrowths at the distal interphalangeal joints) or Bouchard nodes (bony overgrowths at the proximal interphalangeal joints) signify osteoarthritis. Rheumatoid arthritis is bilaterally symmetrical and is often accompanied by ulnar deviation of the fingers. Active and passive range of joint motion should be determined. The presence of contractures should be noted. Variable resistance to passive manipulation of the extremities sometimes occurs with aging.

Comprehensive geriatric assessment is a multidisciplinary exercise and aims to identify medical, psychosocial, and functional limitations of a frail older person in order to develop a coordinated plan. In addition to the system-based examination discussed above, some aspects that are unique to the examination of the elderly will now be discussed.

These include

- Functional status
- Nutrition
- Vision
- Hearing

2.5.11   FUNCTIONAL STATUS

This refers to a person's ability to perform tasks that are required for daily living. The two key aspects of functional ability are

- *Activities of daily living (ADLs).* The person performs these activities on a daily basis and include
  - Eating, dressing, and bathing
  - Transferring between bed in a chair
  - Using the toilet and controlling bladder or bowel functions
- *Instrumental activities of daily living (IADLs).* These activities are needed to live independently and include
  - Doing housework, preparing meals, managing finances, and using the telephone
  - Taking medications properly

Physicians can acquire useful functional information by simply observing older patients as they complete tasks such as buttoning and unbuttoning a shirt, writing a sentence, and climbing up and down from the examination table.

The commonly used instruments in assessing ADL and IADL include the Katz ADL scale (Table 2.1) and the Lawton IADL scale (Table 2.2). Another valuable and relatively quick office assessment of the person's functional status is the Timed Get Up and Go test. The Timed Get Up and Go test is a measurement of mobility. It includes a number of tasks such as standing up from a seating position, walking, turning, stopping, and sitting down, which are all important tasks needed for a person to be independently mobile. For the test, the person is asked to stand up from a standard chair and walk a distance of approximately 10 feet (measure as 3 meters), turn around and walk back to the chair, and sit down again. The individual uses his/her usual footwear and can use any assistive walking device they normally use, such as a cane. The person is seated with his/her back to the chair, their arms resting on the arm rests, and any walking aid they may use should be in hand. Timing, using either a wristwatch with a second hand or a stopwatch, begins when the individual starts to rise from the chair and ends when he/she is once again seated in the chair.

The normal time required to finish the test is between 7 and 10 seconds. Individuals, who cannot complete the task in that time probably have some mobility problems, especially if they take more than 20 seconds. This information should be documented as a baseline and repeated if any change in mobility occurs or at least yearly.

TABLE 2.1

Katz Index of Independence in Activities of Daily Living

Activities Points (1 or 0)	Independence (1 Point) NO Supervision, Direction or Personal Assistance	Dependence (0 Points) WITH Supervision, Direction, Personal Assistance or Total Care
BATHING Points: _____	(1 POINT) Bathes self completely or needs help in bathing only a single part of the body such as the back, genital area, or disabled extremity	(0 POINTS) Need help with bathing more than one part of the body, getting in or out of the tub or shower. Requires total bathing
DRESSING Points: _____	(1 POINT) Get clothes from closets and drawers and puts on clothes and outer garments complete with fasteners. May have help tying shoes	(0 POINTS) Needs help with dressing self or needs to be completely dressed
TOILETING Points: _____	(1 POINT) Goes to toilet, gets on and off, arranges clothes, cleans genital area without help	(0 POINTS) Needs help transferring to the toilet, cleaning self or uses bedpan or commode
TRANSFERRING Points: _____	(1 POINT) Moves in and out of bed or chair unassisted. Mechanical transfer aids are acceptable	(0 POINTS) Needs help in moving from bed to chair or requires a complete transfer
CONTINENCE Points: _____	(1 POINT) Exercises complete self-control over urination and defecation	(0 POINTS) Is partially or totally incontinent of bowel or bladder
FEEDING Points: _____	(1 POINT) Gets food from plate into mouth without help. Preparation of food may be done by another person.	(0 POINTS) Needs partial or total help with feeding or requires parenteral feeding

Total Points: _____

Score of 6 = High, patient is independent.

Score of 0 = Low, patient is very dependent.

TABLE 2.2
Instrumental Activities of Daily Living (IADL)

A. Ability to Use Telephone	Score
1. Operates telephone on own initiative; looks up and dials numbers, etc.	1
2. Dials a few well-known numbers	1
3. Answers telephone but does not dial	1
4. Does not use telephone at all	0

B. Shopping	Score
1. Takes care of all shopping needs independently	1
2. Shops independently for small purchases	0
3. Needs to be accompanied on any shopping trip	0
4. Completely unable to shop	0

C. Food Preparation	Score
1. Plans, prepares, and serves adequate meals independently	1
2. Prepares adequate meals if supplied with ingredients	0
3. Heats and serves prepared meals, or prepares meals but does not maintain adequate diet	0
4. Needs to have meals prepared and served	0

D. Housekeeping	Score
1. Maintains house alone or with occasional assistance (e.g., "heavy work domestic help")	1
2. Performs light daily tasks such as dishwashing, bed making	1
3. Performs light daily tasks but cannot maintain acceptable level of cleanliness	1
4. Needs help with all home maintenance tasks	1
5. Does not participate in any housekeeping tasks	0

E. Laundry	Score
1. Does personal laundry completely	1
2. Launders small items; rinses stockings, etc.	1
3. All laundry must be done by others	0

F. Mode of Transportation	Score
1. Travels independently on public transportation or drives own car	1
2. Arranges own travel via taxi, but does not otherwise use public transportation	1
3. Travels on public transportation when assisted or accompanied by another	1
4. Travel limited to taxi or automobile with assistance of another	0
5. Does not travel at all	0

G. Responsibility for Own Medications	Score
1. Is responsible for taking medication in correct dosages at correct time	1
2. Takes responsibility if medication is prepared in advance in separate dosages	0
3. Is not capable of dispensing own medication	0

H. Ability to Handle Finances	Score
1. Manages financial matters independently (budgets, writes checks, pays rent and bills, goes to bank), collects and keeps track of income	1
2. Manages day-to-day purchases, but needs help with banking, major purchases, etc.	0
3. Incapable of handling money	

Instructions: Circle the scoring point for the statement that most closely corresponds to the patient's current functional ability for each task. The examiner should complete the scale based on information about the patient from the patient him-/herself, informants (such as the patient's family member or other caregiver), and recent records.

Scoring: The patient receives a score of 1 for each item labeled A–H if his or her competence is rated at some minimal level or higher. Add the total points circled for A–H. The total score may range from 0 to 8. A lower score indicates a higher level of dependence.

Source: Cromwell DA, Eagar K, Poulos RG. The performance of instrumental activities of daily living scale in screening for cognitive impairment in elderly community residents. *J Clin Epidemiol.* 2003;56(2):131–137; Lawton MP. The functional assessment of elderly people. *J Am Geriatr Soc.* 1971;19(6):465–481; Lawton MP, Brody EM. Assessment of older people: Self-maintaining and instrumental activities of daily living. *Gerontologist.* 1969;9(3):179–186; Polisher Research Institute. Instrumental Activities of Daily Living Scale (IADL). Available at: http://www.abramsoncenter.org/PRI/documents/IADL.pdf. Accessed February 15, 2005.

2.5.12   NUTRITIONAL STATUS

It is surprisingly difficult to determine whether an elderly patient is malnourished. The methods used to assess nutritional status in younger patients have not been validated in elderly persons. Skeletal height decreases with aging and as the body mass decreases the proportion of adipose tissue increases. The standard height and weight charts and a body mass index (BMI) nomograms can be unreliable in older adults.[3]

Poor nutrition in the elderly can often reflect a medical illness. It can also point to depression, functional losses, and financial hardship. This information is not often volunteered by the elderly. A key element of assessing the elderly is inspection, and malnutrition can be very evident on inspection. It is important to measure and document the patient's height, weight, and BMI. BMI of less than 20 kg per square meter or unintentional weight loss of more than 10 pounds will require further history and investigation.

Poor nutrition in the elderly can also be symptomatic of a number of concomitant factors. These include alcohol and drug misuse, dental problems, medical problems, poor vision, dementia, medication side effects, social isolation, functional dependencies, depression and other psychiatric disorders, environmental factors, poverty, limited access to or intake of food, food attitudes and cultural preferences, and elder abuse.

Weight loss in the elderly has been associated with increased mortality and morbidity. Loss of more than 4% per year is an independent predictor of mortality.[4] Physical examination might be misleading in the detection of early malnutrition as some of the loss of muscle may be an age-related process. However, changes in nail, hair, and tongue, and cheilosis in the angle of the mouth can point to specific nutrient deficiencies:

Hair: Easily plucked, thin; protein or biotin deficiency

Mouth: Tongue fissuring (niacin), decreased taste/smell (zinc)

The most widely used screening tool for detecting nutritional deficits is the Mini Nutritional Assessment (MNA®). The MNA is a simple, low-cost, and noninvasive method that can be done at the bedside.[5]

MNA scores allow one to screen the elderly and identify those who have an adequate nutritional status, as well as those who are at risk of malnutrition. As is evident from the MNA table, the scoring system consists of both anthropometric as well as global indicators such as reduced fluid intake, weight loss of more than 3 kg of body weight, and reduced mobility.

Another population-specific tool to subjectively assess nutritional status is the subjective global assessment (SGA) scale. The SGA was developed to assess hospitalized individuals, investigating the recent weight loss, changes in food consumption, loss of functional capacity, and disease-associated stress found on physical examination.[6]

2.5.12.1   Clinical Examination to Assess Nutritional Status

Start your assessment by asking questions about appetite and intake. Assessing taste changes, dentition, dysphagia, feeding independence, and vitamin/mineral supplements can be very helpful. Enquire about eating patterns. These can include daily and weekend intake, diet restrictions, ethnicity, eating away from home, and fad diets. Obtain diet intake from 24-hour recall and food-frequency questionnaire. Food diary can help where recall is an issue. This helps in identifying the physical signs of malnutrition. Keep in mind that signs do not appear unless severe deficiencies exist.

Examine patients for temporal wasting, cheilosis (usual appearance is a roughly triangular area of erythema, edema (swelling), and maceration at either corner of the mouth), loss of subcutaneous fat, and edema. Most of the signs and symptoms described above indicate two or more deficiencies. The SGA scale requires a physical assessment of

- Loss of subcutaneous fat (triceps, chest)
- Muscle wasting (quadriceps, deltoids)

- Ankle edema
- Sacral edema
- Ascites

Mini Nutritional Assessment
MNA®

**Nestlé
NutritionInstitute**

Last name: First name:

Sex: Age: Weight, kg: Height, cm: Date:

Complete the screen by filling in the boxes with the appropriate numbers. Total the numbers for the final screening score.

Screening

A Has food intake declined over the past 3 months due to loss of appetite, digestive problems, chewing or swallowing difficulties?
0 = severe decrease in food intake
1 = moderate decrease in food intake
2 = no decrease in food intake   ☐

B Weight loss during the last 3 months
0 = weight loss greater than 3 kg (6.6 lbs)
1 = does not know
2 = weight loss between 1 and 3 kg (2.2 and 6.6 lbs)
3 = no weight loss   ☐

C Mobility
0 = bed or chair bound
1 = able to get out of bed / chair but does not go out
2 = goes out   ☐

D Has suffered psychological stress or acute disease in the past 3 months?
0 = yes   2 = no   ☐

E Neuropsychological problems
0 = severe dementia or depression
1 = mild dementia
2 = no psychological problems   ☐

F1 Body Mass Index (BMI) (weight in kg) / (height in m²)
0 = BMI less than 19
1 = BMI 19 to less than 21
2 = BMI 21 to less than 23
3 = BMI 23 or greater   ☐

IF BMI IS NOT AVAILABLE, REPLACE QUESTION F1 WITH QUESTION F2.
DO NOT ANSWER QUESTION F2 IF QUESTION F1 IS ALREADY COMPLETED.

F2 Calf circumference (CC) in cm
0 = CC less than 31
3 = CC 31 or greater   ☐

Screening score (max. 14 points)

12-14 points: Normal nutritional status
8-11 points: At risk of malnutrition
0-7 points: Malnourished   ☐ ☐

Ref. 1.Vellas B, Villars H, Abellan G, et al. Overview of the MNA® - Its History and Challenges. J Nutr Health Aging 2006;10:456-465. 2.Rubenstein LZ, Harker JO, Salva A, Guigoz Y, Vellas B. Screening for Undernutrition in Geriatric Practice: Developing the Short-Form Mini 3.Nutritional Assessment (MNA-SF). J. Geront 2001;56A: M366-377. 4.Guigoz Y. The Mini-Nutritional Assessment (MNA®) Review of the Literature - What does it tell us? J Nutr Health Aging 2006; 10:466-487. 5.Kaiser MJ, Bauer JM, Ramsch C, et al. Validation of the Mini Nutritional Assessment Short-Form (MNA®-SF): A practical tool for identification of nutritional status. J Nutr Health Aging 2009; 13:782-788. ® Société des Produits Nestlé, S.A., Vevey, Switzerland, Trademark Owners © Nestlé, 1994, Revision 2009. N67200 12/99 10M
For more information: www.mna-elderly.com

MNA®

2.5.12.2   SGA Scoring Guidelines

The clinician rates each medical history and physical examination parameter as A, B, or C on the SGA scoring sheet. On the basis of all of these parameter ratings, the clinical observer assigns an overall SGA classification, which corresponds to his or her subjective opinion of the patient's nutritional status. SGA is not a numerical scoring system. Therefore, it is inappropriate just to add the number of A, B, and C ratings to arrive at the overall SGA classification.

The clinician should examine the form to obtain a general feel for the patient's status. If there seem to be more checks on the right-hand side of the form (more B and C ratings), the patient is more likely to be malnourished. If the ratings seem to be on the left-hand side, the patient is likely to be nourished. The severely malnourished (C) rating is given whenever a patient has physical signs of malnutrition, such as severe loss of subcutaneous fat, severe muscle wasting, or edema, in the presence of a medical history suggestive of risk, such as continuing weight loss with a net loss of 10% or more, or a decline in dietary intake: GI symptoms and functional impairments usually exist in these patients. Severely malnourished patients will rank in the moderate to severe category in most sections of the SGA form.

When weight loss is 5%–10% with no subsequent gain, in conjunction with mild subcutaneous fat or muscle loss and a reduction in dietary intake, the patient is assigned the mildly/moderately malnourished (B) rating. These patients may or may not exhibit functional impairments or GI symptoms. The B rating is expected to be the most ambiguous of all the SGA classifications. These patients may have a ranking in all three categories. In general, if the severely malnourished (C) or well-nourished (A) rating is not clearly indicated, assign the patient to the moderately malnourished classification.

If there is no physical signs of malnutrition, no significant weight loss, no dietary difficulties, no nutritionally related functional impairments, or no GI symptoms that might predispose to malnutrition, the patient should be assigned to the well-nourished (A) category.

If the patient has recently gained weight, and other indicators, such as appetite, show improvement, the patient may be assigned the A rating, despite previous loss of fat and muscle, which may still be physically apparent. On the other hand, obese patients can be moderately or severely malnourished based upon their poor medical history and signs of muscle loss. Even patients with a normal appearance could be classified as mildly or moderately malnourished because of a poor medical history.[7]

2.5.13   VISION

Assessment of the visual acuity in the elderly is best carried out by asking specific questions, which include

- Difficulty of driving, including glare and night vision problems
- Sudden or recent onset of visual loss that might be central, partial, or complete
- Inability to read or watch television
- Diplopia or eye pain
- Lifestyle restrictions necessitated by decrease in visual acuity

Visual impairment is a major risk factor associated with falls and associated hip fractures in the elderly. In a screening study of the senior citizens in the community, the visual acuity was measured with a standard Snellen's chart. Nearly 72% had impaired vision. There was a significant association between visual impairment and female sex, history of diabetes or glaucoma, cataract, and infrequent eye examination.[8]

Common disorders associated with visual impairment in the elderly include cataracts, macular degeneration, glaucoma, diabetic retinopathy, hypertensive retinopathy, temporal arteritis, and retinal detachment.

The implications of vision change in the elderly include impact on safety, inability to read medication labels, difficulty navigating stairs of curbs, difficulty driving, and falls. Visual acuity should be examined in all elderly patients. This initial screening test can be done with a Snellen's chart in the office.

Visual fields should be examined and the best way in the primary care setting is to do confrontational visual field test; however, this only works when the patient can cooperate with instructions as it is a comparison of the patient's with the examiner's own the visual fields.

The provider sits directly opposite the patient at a distance of about 3 feet. The patient is asked to cover one eye and the provider covers the contralateral eye. So that both the covered eyes are opposite to each other. In the elderly, it might be easier to say, "cover one eye with your hand" and then follow their cue. This is on account of the fact that the elderly can often confuse instructions, especially ones pertaining to the left and right side of the body. The patient is asked to indicate when the examiner's finger is visible at the edge of the visual field. This is done in all the quadrants and is then repeated for the other eye. It is important to keep reminding the patient to look into the examiner's eye.

Low intraocular pressure can manifest itself as a soft eyeball over the closed lids. Very hard eyeball can indicate high intraocular pressures. Tonometers can be used if available. Checking for the light reflex can unmask abnormal pupillary reactions, indicating an optic nerve pathology or previous history of iridocyclitis.

2.5.14　Hearing

Hearing loss affects one-third of the people above 65 years of age, two-thirds of those older than 70 years, and three-fourths of those 80 years of age or older.[9] The most common type of hearing loss is presbycusis. Hearing loss is initially for high-frequency sounds but progresses to lower frequencies. Patients often have an inability to hear a significant proportion of the consonant sounds, which makes speech unintelligible. Understanding is more difficult in crowded rooms.

Start by taking a history of any changes in hearing. An important question to ask is if the patient has difficulty understanding higher-pitched frequencies such as a child speaking. Difficulty in understanding telephone conversations and when more than one person is speaking can also point to hearing loss.

The examination is commenced by doing an otoscopic examination. Cerumen impaction is common and its removal can often lead to improvement in hearing. A whisper test is done by standing about 6 inches behind the patient and whispering 10 words. A 256 Hz tuning fork can be placed on the base of the mastoid process and then transferred to the external auditory meatus. Air conduction is normally louder than bone conduction. If this is not so, the patient probably has presbycusis. The patient can be referred for formal audiological testing. Hearing aids can often be prohibitively expensive and this has to be a consideration while making referrals for formal consults to audiology.[10]

The physical examination of the elderly differs from standard medical evaluation. The caregiver has to be cognizant of challenges posed by physical limitations and multiple disorders. A comprehensive interview and examination can avert delays in diagnoses and avoid morbidity. Early detection of pathology requires an open mind and keen observation. Paying attention to facets of the examination described above can lead to early recognition of disease entities and improve quality of life.

REFERENCES

1. Gesensway D. The high-yield neuro exam. *Today's Hospitalist*. January 2012.
2. Inouye SK, van Dyck CH, Alessi CA et al. Clarifying confusion: The confusion assessment method. A new method for detection of delirium. *Ann Intern Med* 1990; 113:941–948.

3. Rueben DB, Greendale GA, Harrison GG. Nutrition screening in older persons. *J Am Geriatr Soc* 1995; 43:415–425.
4. Wallace JI, Schwartz RS, LaCroix AZ, Uhlmann RF, Pearlman RA. Involuntary weight loss in older outpatients: incidence and clinical significance. *Format: Abstract J Am Geriatr Soc* 1995; 43(4):329–337.
5. Guigoz Y, Garry JP. Mini nutritional assessment: A practical assessment tool for grading the nutritional state of elderly patients. *Facts Res Gerontol* 1994; (Suppl 2):15–59.
6. Makhija S, Baker J. The subjective global assessment: A review of its use in clinical practice. *Nutr Clin Pract* 2008, 23(4):405–409.
7. Baxter Healthcare Corporation, Renal Division, 1620 Waukegan Road (Society of Hospital Medicine Clinical Toolbox for Geriatric Care).
8. Wun YT, Lam CC, Shum WK. Impaired vision in the elderly: A preventable condition. *Fam Pract* 1997; 14:289–292.
9. Wilson PS, Fleming DM, Donaldson I. Prevalence of hearing loss among people aged 65 and over: Screening and hearing aid provision. *Br J Gen Pract* 1993; 43:406–409.
10. Fleming KC, Evans JM, Weber DC, Chutka, DS. Practical functional assessment of elderly persons: A primary care approach. Mayo Foundation for Medical Education, 1995.
11. Cromwell DA, Eagar K, Poulos RG. The performance of instrumental activities of daily living scale in screening for cognitive impairment in elderly community residents. *J Clin Epidemiol.* 2003;56(2):131–137.
12. Lawton MP. The functional assessment of elderly people. *J Am Geriatr Soc.* 1971;19(6):465–481.
13. Lawton MP, Brody EM. Assessment of older people: Self-maintaining and instrumental activities of daily living. *Gerontologist.* 1969;9(3):179–186.
14. Polisher Research Institute. Instrumental Activities of Daily Living Scale (IADL). Available at: http://www.abramsoncenter.org/PRI/documents/IADL.pdf. Accessed February 15, 2005.

3 Psychosocial Assessment

Jennifer Anne Fleeman

CONTENTS

3.1 THE BIOPSYCHOSOCIAL MODEL IN GERIATRIC REHABILITATION

Within the current healthcare environment, an integrative and multidisciplinary approach to rehabilitation is imperative. Although not by any means a new concept in medicine, the development of the biopsychosocial model[1] helped to define and add to a greater understanding of this important concept. The biopsychosocial model emphasizes the importance of understanding human health, illness, and functioning by considering the complex interplay between biological, psychological, and social factors. Within this model, clinical conditions are viewed as comprising psychological and social components, which will impact a patient's understanding of the condition, will guide their health-related behavior, and can affect the clinical course of that condition.[2]

The biopsychosocial model has natural applications within geriatric rehabilitation, particularly given the additional factors that one must consider with the older adult. The older adult population demonstrates unique psychosocial aspects of aging that must be considered for optimizing treatment and the resulting well-being and functional status in this population. These concepts will be further explored in this chapter.

As an example of the application of the biopsychosocial model, social and psychological factors may have contributed to the development of the clinical condition. Further, a person's unique history and characteristics are a significant factor in how the patient understands their diagnosis and prognosis. Social and psychological factors have a prominent role in the person's response to their diagnosis and the subsequent involvement in health-related behaviors, in turn impacting functional recovery and overall clinical course. There is an ever-growing body of empirical literature that suggests that a patient's perceptions of health, as well as psychosocial factors, influence the likelihood that the patient will engage in health-promoting behaviors or adhere to treatment recommendations.[3] The literature indicates that the outcomes of healthcare for the older adult population are dependent on a combination of their physical health status, interventions to address their medical needs, and attention to psychosocial factors.[3]

3.2 THEORIES OF ADJUSTMENT AND COPING

There are numerous theoretical frameworks used to describe coping and adjustment following illness and injury, particularly as it relates to the individual's psychological and physical health. Commonly cited theories include Lazarus and Folkman's Transactional Model of Stress and Coping,[4] the Self-Regulation Model,[5] and the Self-Determination Theory.[6] These theories have been applied in various settings, including applications to describe emotional adjustment and coping following injury/illness. Lazarus and Folkman's theory has been widely studied within this context; therefore, a general overview of this theory will be provided here.

As part of Lazarus and Folkman's theory,[4] stressful experiences are construed as person–environment transactions. Stress emerges when the relationship between the person and the environment is appraised as exceeding his or her resources and as threatening their well-being. In addition to demographics and biological factors, adjustment to illness/injury is mediated by several coping processes. These coping processes include cognitive appraisal, coping strategies, and coping resources, which interact to help determine outcomes of adjustment. In terms of cognitive appraisal, the individual evaluates a stressor's potential for threat, controllability, and challenge. The individual then responds to the stressor by utilizing coping strategies and coping resources. Examples of coping strategies include emotion-, problem-, and meaning-focused approaches. Coping resources can include internal resources (e.g., personality, optimism, and hope) and external resources (e.g., social support system). These appraisals, coping strategies, and coping resources can be modified by both internal and external factors throughout one's adjustment to a stressor.

In regards to the coping strategies outlined in Lazarus and Folkman's theory,[4] an emotion-focused approach is characterized by the individual directing attention toward dealing with the distress associated with the stressor (by approach or avoidance). Within a problem-focused approach, the individual focuses on dealing with the problem that is causing the distress, including strategies such as analyzing the problem, seeking information, developing a plan to resolve or change the stressor, and engaging in problem-solving action. A meaning-focused approach can be characterized by the individual creating, rebuilding, or reinstating meaning within the context of the stressful event. Rebuilding of meaning can include finding reasons for why something has happened and looking for the positive aspects of the event (e.g., positive reframing).

The concept of self-efficacy is an important component of Lazarus and Folkman's theory of cognitive appraisal.[4] Self-efficacy has also become a prominent theme within the research field related to social-cognitive models of health behavior.[7,8] Self-efficacy has been defined as the extent or strength of one's belief in one's own ability to complete tasks and to reach goals.[9] Within this theory, people with a higher level of self-efficacy are more likely to view difficult tasks as something to be mastered rather than something to be avoided. This theory naturally has implications with regard to behaviors affecting health. Choices affecting health are seen as being dependent on self-efficacy. Self-efficacy beliefs can influence how an individual will set their health goals, whether health behavior change will be initiated, how much effort will be expended, and how long the health behavior will be sustained in the face of obstacles.[10,11] Self-efficacy has been found to be associated with patient adherence and satisfaction.[12] The role of self-efficacy has also been examined within the context of clinician–patient relationships and engagement in treatment. This will be discussed later in this chapter.

3.3 ADJUSTMENT AND COPING RESPONSES

There is a wide spectrum of emotional responses to illness/injury, with one's coping and adjustment playing a significant role in the response. Some individuals will demonstrate signs of the normal grieving process following the onset of an injury or illness that impacts their functioning. Within the rehabilitation setting, it is also common to observe the presence of frustration, anxiety, and emotional liability related to the physiological impact of neurological conditions as well as one's response to the impact of these conditions (e.g., frustration due to aphasia). It is important for the rehabilitation clinician to monitor the grieving process and any other emotional or behavioral responses to help guard against any worsening of symptoms of depression or anxiety. Providing active interventions to address depressive and anxiety symptoms early on in the process can help to avoid prolongation of this process and guard against a worsening of these symptoms.

According to the DSM-5,[13] responses to a significant loss (which can include medical illness or disability) may include symptoms that resemble a depressive episode (e.g., feelings of intense sadness, rumination about the loss, insomnia, poor appetite, and weight loss). While these symptoms may be considered appropriate or understandable due to the loss, the presence of a major depressive episode or adjustment disorder should also be considered. Differential diagnosis can be challenging, but should take into account clinical judgment based on the individual's history and the cultural norms for the expression of distress in the context of loss. In differentiating between grief and a major depressive episode, an additional point to consider is the predominant affect and thoughts that the individual experiences; grief and loss are characterized by feelings of emptiness and loss while a major depressive episode is characterized by persistent depressed mood and the inability to anticipate happiness or pleasure. Additional information about differential diagnosis is available in the DSM-5.[13]

Along the spectrum of responses to illness/injury, some individuals will experience symptoms of an adjustment disorder, which can include any combination of depressed mood, anxiety, or behavioral changes in response to a stressor. To meet DSM-5 criteria[13] for an adjustment disorder, the symptoms must have a clinically significant impact on functioning (as defined by either marked distress that is out of proportion to the severity of the stressor or significant impairment in social, occupational, or other important areas of functioning).

When depressive symptoms persist, worsen, and/or significantly impact functioning, a major depressive episode must also be considered and treated promptly. The diagnostic criteria for a major depressive disorder and differential diagnosis are discussed in detail within the DSM-5.[13] To summarize, a certain number of symptoms (five or more) must be present during the same 2-week period, and the symptoms must not be attributable to other conditions or causes (as detailed in the DSM-5). The symptoms outlined in the DSM-5 include depressed mood, loss of interest or pleasure, significant changes in appetite or weight loss/gain, insomnia or hypersomnia, psychomotor agitation or retardation, fatigue, feelings of worthlessness or guilt, problems with concentration, and/or recurrent thoughts of death or suicidal ideation. In addition, to meet criteria, the symptoms must cause clinically significant distress or impairment in social, occupational, or other areas of functioning.

Anxiety is also a common response to illness/injury and can have a significant impact on one's functioning. A person can experience anxiety related to the diagnosis or prognosis itself as well as its implications for changing various aspects of their lives. Within the rehabilitation setting, it is also commonly observed that individuals can experience anxiety associated with pain, fear of falling, meeting the requirements of therapies, and discharge planning. These symptoms are common experiences when an individual copes with illness/injury and may not be at a level to warrant diagnosis (i.e., they could be judged as being appropriate or understandable based on the loss, as described above). However, when the symptoms of anxiety cause clinically significant distress or impairment in functioning, the presence of an adjustment disorder or other anxiety disorder should be considered. In addition, some individuals within the rehabilitation setting experience symptoms of acute stress disorder or posttraumatic stress disorder (PTSD), with a variety of traumatic events that could trigger this response (e.g., a traumatic accident causing injury, the trauma of being in the ICU, etc.). Symptoms that might indicate such a response include intrusive memories, dreams, or flashbacks about the event, intense psychological distress or physiological reactions upon exposure to cues that resemble the traumatic event, avoidance of stimuli associated with the traumatic event, negative alterations in cognitions and mood associated with the event, and alterations in arousal and reactivity.[13]

In addition to new-onset psychiatric diagnoses that can occur in association with injury/illness in individuals with no prior psychiatric history, some individuals already have a premorbid psychological disorder that can be exacerbated by the additional stressor of injury/illness. Pre-existing psychological disorders also need to be considered in relation to the potential impact on adjustment and health-related behaviors. Another consideration is that the individual may have been experiencing a subsyndromal or undiagnosed psychological disorder that became evident within the context of their adjustment to the stressors related to their medical condition.

One's ability to adjust to and cope with illness/injury has been widely studied. Studies indicate that perseverative negative cognitive processes (e.g., worry, suppression, and avoidance of undesirable thoughts), have been linked to persistence of depression.[14] Further, depression has been found to be significantly related to functional recovery.[15] Positive psychological variables present during the rehabilitation stay may help to predict positive functional outcomes after discharge within rehabilitation populations. For example, Kortte et al.[16] found that hope accounted for a statistically significant amount of the variance in the prediction of functional role participation at 3 months postdischarge, underscoring the importance of incorporating interventions that enhance hope and build on the individual's psychological strengths. Although empirical investigation into the concept of hope following illness and disability is still limited, there are studies that have similarly demonstrated that hope is an important mediating factor in the coping process contributing to optimal recovery.[17]

The role of coping and emotional functioning has also been examined in specific patient populations commonly treated within the rehabilitation field. Van Leeuwen et al.[18] conducted a systematic literature review within the spinal cord injury (SCI) population in regards to the associations between psychological factors and quality of life ratings. In their review, they found that locus of control, sense of coherence, self-worth, hope, purpose in life, and positive affect were consistently associated with greater quality of life; negative affect was consistently associated with lower quality of life.[18] Peter et al.[19] similarly conducted a systematic literature review of psychological resources in the SCI population, with self-efficacy and self-esteem consistently associated with positive adjustment indicators, including better mental health.

Other studies have also investigated coping and adjustment as it relates to outcomes, with findings indicating that appraisals and coping are significantly related to functional outcome, psychological adjustment, and quality of life.[20,21] The presence of hope and positive affect were associated with greater life satisfaction during the initial acute rehabilitation period as well as at 3 months after discharge for individuals with SCI.[22] Social support was found to be associated with life satisfaction after SCI for at least up to 1 year after inpatient rehabilitation.[23] Increases in life satisfaction were also found in persons with SCI for at least up to 5 years after discharge from inpatient rehabilitation when associated with factors such as high functional status, low pain, good social skills, and high self-efficacy.[24] In contrast, individuals with SCI who utilized emotion-focused coping styles reported greater ratings of depression during acute rehabilitation, and physical setbacks were more likely to contribute to negative mood.[25] Similarly, the use of disengagement coping skills helped to predict levels of depression and PTSD in individuals with SCI.[26]

Within the stroke population, Skidmore et al.[27] found that cognitive impairment (e.g., executive dysfunction) and depressive symptoms correlated significantly with participation during stroke rehabilitation. Similarly, Ostir et al.[28] found that positive emotion ratings at discharge from inpatient rehabilitation were significantly associated with higher overall functional status and cognitive status at 3 months postdischarge. Depression, which is common following stroke, has been associated with increased morbidity and mortality.[29] The presence of preinjury factors in predicting life satisfaction following traumatic brain injury (TBI) has also been examined. For example, Davis et al.[30] demonstrated that preinjury functioning (e.g., education and employment) and preinjury condition (e.g., psychiatric and substance use problems, learning problems, prior TBI) each contributed significantly to variance in life satisfaction following TBI.

3.4 STRESSORS AND THEIR IMPACT ON COPING AND OUTCOME WITHIN THE OLDER ADULT POPULATION

Adjustment to stressors in one's life depends on multiple variables. Naturally, relevant examples of stressors in the rehabilitation population include illnesses, injuries, and changes to functional status. Given the increased incidence of diseases in older adults, there is an associated increase in the number and frequency of stressors as the individual ages. For the older adult, this can include a combination of chronic and acute stressors, all playing a role in the individual's response to illness, treatment adherence, and clinical course.

There are certain common stressors in the older adult population that should be considered, given their impact on physical and emotional functioning as well as adherence and health-related behaviors. Examples of these common stressors include changes in social roles and relationships, changes in family structure, loss within the support system, caregiving roles, retirement, financial changes, decreased level of functioning, decreased independence, changes in social opportunities, social isolation, etc. Frequently, these factors contribute to existential issues regarding the meaning of one's life, their mortality, and the role of illness in their lives. Subsequently, the individual might engage in revisions of their self-definition, life goals, and values. With loss within the support system and/or changes in the nature of social relationships, there is often less support available to assist the older adult with the process of coping and adjusting to stressors. This can become problematic, particularly given research findings that indicate that social support serves as a strong external coping resource. The role of social support is discussed further in this chapter.

Within the acute rehabilitation setting, an additional layer of stressors can become apparent. Not only is the individual adjusting to an acute medical issue, but they are also adjusting to changes in functional status, independence, identity, and goals for the future. These can be further compounded by pain, poor sleep, and decreased energy. In addition, the individual is in an unfamiliar environment away from home and may have less access to their usual social supports while in the hospital. They may also be experiencing distress related to medical procedures and events that occurred earlier in their hospital stay. Individuals within the acute rehabilitation setting also face the additional stressor of discharge planning and decision-making surrounding this important step in the recovery process.

After discharge from the acute rehabilitation setting, the individual often continues to experience the impact of stressors that were first encountered during their rehabilitation stay. They also face the additional adjustment to the transition back home, moving in with a family member or friend, or transferring to a subacute rehabilitation setting. There is also an adjustment to changes in the social environment and social roles upon transition to the community. Changes in level of functioning can impact the nature of social roles (e.g., social supports taking on responsibilities that the individual used to have and/or providing additional assistance for the individual). In addition, those in the social support system may have different levels of understanding or expectations of the individual's level of functioning.

When returning to the community from acute or subacute rehabilitation, there is a decrease in the level of medical supervision and decreased frequency of restorative therapies. Without the high level of structure inherent in one's daily schedule during acute rehabilitation, there is the potential for decreased involvement in restorative therapies, thereby impacting functional improvement and recovery. Medication adherence is another potential factor that becomes highlighted for community-dwelling older adults. Falls are also common in older adults, with prevalence increasing with age.[31] Falls can result in declines in health status, in the ability to undertake activities of living, and in lifestyle and quality of life, contributing to additional stressors.

If the older adult lives alone, there are fewer external resources available to help motivate them to participate in restorative therapies and to adhere to treatment recommendations. Thus, this motivation must arise internally. The presence of psychosocial factors and stressors may impact this internal motivation. When the older adult lives alone, there is also the potential for increased social isolation, as they may not be able to drive, may have fewer visitors, and no longer have the daily interactions with the acute rehabilitation treatment team. As discussed below, social isolation is a risk factor for declines in physical and emotional status.

3.5   SOCIAL/INTERPERSONAL FACTORS AND THE ROLE OF SOCIAL SUPPORT

The older adult understands health and illness through frameworks based on generational factors, social and cultural contexts, and personal beliefs and values. There are an infinite number of ways in which different individuals view illness and treatment based on these factors. It is important to consider these individual and social factors in the treatment of illness. The role of social support has been widely researched from perspectives including social support as a protective factor, social isolation as a risk factor, and social support as it relates to adjustment/coping.

Considering the social network as a system, the advent of an acute medical event or diagnosis can have a significant impact on existing social relationships. There is a complex interplay within this social system, including the impact of how each of the individuals within the social system cope with a medical event, how this impacts each of the relationships within the system, and how the social system responds as a whole to the medical event. Ideally, the introduction of a stressor such as a medical event contributes to cohesion within the social structure. Unfortunately, the result can also be that of increased conflict within the system, particularly when all members do not agree on the best course of action or if they have differing views and expectations surrounding the medical event. The individual diagnosed with the medical condition rarely adjusts to this stressor in isolation; rather, there is a ripple effect within the social context.

The role of social support has been studied in various diagnostic populations, with a common theme emerging: the presence of social support is positively related to physical and mental health.[32–38] Social isolation has consistently been found to be a prevalent health problem among community-dwelling older adults, leading to numerous health conditions and affective disorders. Particularly given the increasing older adult population, social isolation will continue to be a prominent focus in regards to its impact on the health, well-being, and quality of life of older adults. In a systematic literature review, Nicholson[39] found that there is extensive evidence demonstrating numerous negative health outcomes and potential risk factors related to social isolation.

Investigators have also examined the mechanisms through which social isolation and loneliness affect health, including health-related behavioral and biological factors. As investigated by Shankar et al.,[40] loneliness and social isolation may affect health through their effects on health behaviors (e.g., greater risk of multiple health-risk behaviors) as well as through biological processes associated with the development of cardiovascular disease (e.g., social isolation being positively associated with blood pressure, C-reactive protein, and fibrinogen levels). Both social isolation and loneliness have been found to be associated with increased mortality in the older adult population.[41] Holwerda et al.[42] also investigated the increased risk of mortality associated with social isolation in older adults, finding that at 10 years follow up, feelings of loneliness were found to be a major risk factor for increasing mortality in older men.

Regarding the nature and quality of relationships, Seeman[43] found through literature review that social relationships have the potential for both health-promoting and health-damaging effects in older adults. Protective effects have been documented with respect to mental and physical health outcomes and better recovery after disease onset. On the contrary, there is also a growing awareness of the potential for negative health effects from social relationships characterized by more negative patterns, with increased risks for depression. There is also literature that supports biological pathways related to the impact of social interactions, with more negative social interactions being associated with certain physiological profiles (e.g., elevated stress hormones, increased cardiovascular activity, and depressed immune function).[43]

In regards to the role of marital quality in physical health in the geriatric population, it has been found that higher levels of negative spousal behaviors uniquely contributed to more physical symptoms, chronic health problems, and physical disability.[44] Caregivers providing care to chronically ill family members have been found to be at risk for caregiver burden as well as at increased risk, compared to their noncaregiving peers, for health problems, depression, and poor quality of life.[45,46] Heavy caregiving burden has been associated with various health effects, hospitalization, and mortality among community-dwelling dependent older adults.[47-50] These findings lead to the conclusion that the reduction of caregiver burden and improvement of caregiver well-being may not only prevent the deterioration of caregiver health but also reduce adverse health outcomes for care recipients.

3.6 PSYCHOLOGICAL AND COGNITIVE FACTORS IMPACTING FUNCTIONING

In terms of additional psychological factors, the older adult may have pre-existing psychological disorders or substance abuse issues that can impact the course of their medical diagnoses as well as their understanding of and response to medical conditions. There is a relatively high prevalence rate for depression and other mental health disorders in the older adult population. The American Association for Geriatric Psychiatry[51] has estimated that 20% of adults aged 55 and older have a mental health disorder (e.g., mood disorder, anxiety, or cognitive impairment) that is not part of normal aging. According to the Geriatric Mental Health Foundation (GMHF),[52] an estimated 15%–20% of adults older than 65 in the United States have experienced depression. The GMHF also estimates that approximately 25% of those with chronic illness are affected by depression, most commonly observed in patients with ischemic heart disease, stroke, cancer, chronic lung disease, arthritis, Alzheimer disease, and Parkinson disease.

Depression, even including subsyndromal depression, has been associated with increased use of health services and increased healthcare costs in addition to poor functional and health outcomes, including functional impairment, medical comorbidity, and the complication of chronic conditions such as heart disease, diabetes, and stroke.[53-57] Depression has also been tied to higher mortality from suicide and cardiac disease.[54,58] Another point to consider is that increased cognitive impairment is a common symptom of depression for the older adult, sometimes to the extent that it can mimic dementia. Older adults with symptoms of generalized anxiety disorder have been found to have increased functional disability, greater healthcare utilization, and lower health-related quality of life.[59] Clearly, the presence of difficulties with adjustment and emotional functioning can have a significant impact on the individual's participation in rehabilitation activities and subsequent outcomes.

Decreased cognitive functioning is another factor that can have implications in terms of an individual's ability to understand medical issues and to follow recommended treatment. For example, cognitive impairments can impact the individual's ability to understand the diagnosis and prognosis and can impact medical decision-making. Cognitive impairments may impact the individual's insight into their medical conditions and the importance of adhering to treatment recommendations. Cognitive factors can also impact the patient's ability to remember the details of the treatment recommendations given to them and to remember to follow through with these recommendations. Cognitive impairment can also impact their ability to engage in self-care activities. Even in the absence of dementia or cognitive impairments related to other conditions, there are some normal age-related cognitive changes that can impact these areas of functioning. Within the acute rehabilitation setting, studies have shown cognitive dysfunction to be associated with a poorer rehabilitation

outcome compared to cognitively intact individuals.[60] Studies have also demonstrated a longer rehabilitation length of stay, increased risk of adverse incidents, and increased mortality in individuals
with impaired cognition.[61] Clearly, difficulties with memory can impact the older adult's ability
to remember to consistently take their medication, with obvious potential consequences. In those
needing medication support, lack of medication assistance was associated with higher risk of hospitalization in community-dwelling disabled elderly adults.[62]

Within the acute rehabilitation setting, symptoms of delirium or dementia can impact the individual's participation in therapies as well as other areas of day-to-day functioning. Various symptoms are common within these conditions. Although not an exhaustive list, the following symptoms
should be identified and appropriate interventions provided: anxiety, depression, apathy, sleep disturbance, appetite changes, irritability, mood liability, disinhibition, wandering, verbal or physical
aggression, delusions/hallucinations, decreased insight, resistance to care, fluctuation in symptoms,
etc. In these situations, it is important to identify any environmental precipitants (e.g., changes in
room or roommate, changes in routine, overstimulation, etc.) and attempt to avoid or modify them.
Reorientation and the provision of structured routines and activities are also helpful within this
context. Formal behavioral interventions, such as those provided by psychologists, can also be very
helpful in this regard.

3.7 PSYCHOSOCIAL FACTORS AND HEALTH BEHAVIORS

Consistent with the biopsychosocial model, the rehabilitation process involves multiple biological,
psychological, and social factors that influence how well a person benefits from medical rehabilitation. There is ample evidence in the literature supporting the concept that patients must be actively
involved or engaged in the rehabilitation process to maximize the functional benefits of rehabilitation.[63] Adherence to and avoidance of treatment recommendations play an important role in rehabilitation outcomes.[64]

Meta-analytic studies have continued to identify a number of stable and consistent factors that
affect patient adherence.[33,65–67] Results of many studies have also found that successful attempts to
improve patient adherence and subsequent outcome depend upon many factors, some of which are
potentially modifiable. Examples of potentially modifiable factors include patients' understanding
of the recommended interventions, effective communication between health professionals and their
patients, trust in the therapeutic relationship,[68] illness beliefs,[69] patient attitudes/perceptions of the
effectiveness of treatment, spiritual and religious beliefs,[70,71] social support, and medical comorbidity.[72] Additional factors impacting adherence can also include pain and energy level.

In a meta-analysis of available literature on health beliefs, disease severity, and patient adherence, Di Matteo et al.[73] found that adherence is significantly positively correlated with the patients'
beliefs in the severity of the disease to be prevented or treated. Results suggested that the objective
severity and subjective awareness of the severity of the patients' disease conditions can predict
adherence; patients who are most severely ill are at greater risk for nonadherence to treatment.

In a review of the literature regarding health outcomes related to medication adherence among
seniors,[74] evidence suggested that polypharmacy and poor patient–healthcare provider relationships
may be major determinants of nonadherence among older persons. They noted that available data
provided some support for increased health risks associated with nonadherence. Similarly, Vik
et al.[75] examined the risk for hospitalization and/or mortality associated with medication nonadherence in older, at-risk adults residing in the community. They found that nonadherent clients showed
an increased but nonsignificant risk for an adverse health outcome during follow up. They found that
nonadherence was more often associated with depressive symptoms, a high drug regimen complexity, residence in a private home (vs. assisted-living setting), and absence of assistance with medication administration. Additional factors that have been found to be associated with medication
nonadherence in the older adult population include inadequate or marginal health literacy, comorbid
conditions, and the presence of cognitive, vision, and/or hearing impairment.[76]

Psychological factors also play a role in adherence and outcome. Level of engagement in recovery at 3 months has been found to be negatively correlated with depression and positively correlated with level of functioning.[77] Depression has been found to be a risk factor for noncompliance with medical treatment.[67] As noted previously, social support plays a significant role in a patient's adjustment to stressors as well as adherence and health-related behavior. In a meta-analysis of the literature related to social support and patient adherence to medical treatment,[33] adherence was found to be significantly higher in patients from cohesive families and significantly lower in patients from families in conflict. Further, marital status and living with another person increased adherence modestly.[33]

Healthcare availability and access can also contribute significantly to an individual's adherence to treatment recommendations, disease management, and outcome. As an example, financial difficulties can impact the individual's ability to meet basic needs important for health (e.g., paying for food, medical bills, and copayments for medications). In addition, decreased access to preventive services, delayed diagnosis, and poor monitoring and control of chronic disease can contribute to serious health consequences and increased mortality.[78,79]

3.8 THE REHABILITATION CLINICIAN'S ROLE IN PSYCHOSOCIAL ASSESSMENT

3.8.1 The Clinician–Patient Relationship

The role of the clinician–patient relationship cannot be underestimated. The nature of the relationship itself can impact the quality of information that the clinician is able to gather during the assessment process and can also have significant bearing on the success of the clinician's interventions. Further, the clinician–patient relationship can have an important effect on the patient's adherence and subsequent health outcomes.[33,80,81]

As previously noted, there is a growing body of evidence to suggest that the outcomes of healthcare for older adults are dependent upon care for the patients' psychosocial needs. Optimizing patient adherence to treatment recommendations depends on several key factors, among which include clear and effective communication between clinicians and their patients, nurturance of trust in the therapeutic relationship, and mutual collaboration.[3,68,82] Adherence can be optimized by the clinician's ability to assess and treat the individual within the context of their beliefs, cultural context, social supports, and emotional health.[68] Several meta-analyses of relevant literature indicate that there is a significant positive correlation between patient adherence and both physician communication and physician–patient collaboration.[82,83] Fuertes et al.[12] also investigated dimensions of the physician–patient relationship (working alliance) in relation to patient's adherence and satisfaction. Results demonstrated moderate to strong relationships between the physician–patient relationship and beliefs about the usefulness of treatment, adherence self-efficacy (beliefs about being able to adhere to treatment), adherence to their treatment plan, and patient realization of benefit.

Several characteristics that contribute to effective clinician–patient relationships as well as empirical support for these methods in optimizing adherence and health outcomes have been investigated.[3,68] One component of effective communication deals with information delivery, including the clinician's ability to successfully convey information in a clear and comprehensible format. This typically includes communicating information about the diagnosis, options for treatment, and strengths and weaknesses of those treatment options. It is an important skill for the clinician to be able to gauge the appropriate amount of this information to be given to each individual patient (avoiding the possibility of overwhelming them with too much information vs. contributing to distress or confusion with too little information). Additional characteristics of the effective clinician–patient relationship include the concept of a partnership, mutual cooperation, and a patient-centered approach that takes into account the individual's personal values, preferences, and choice in their treatment. The goal is for the clinician and patient to form a therapeutic alliance within which both partners actively work together in joint decision-making to improve the patient's health.[3]

Empathy, trust, integrity, and respect are other crucial characteristics of the effective clinician–patient relationship. The concept of empathy in medicine can be tied back to the biopsychosocial model of integrative care. Empathy requires trying to understand another's experience of the world and conveying this understanding to them through both verbal and nonverbal feedback. Verbal feedback can include active listening/reflection, words of supportiveness, expressions of understanding, or encouragement for the patient to tell their story of the experience of illness/injury. Nonverbal feedback can occur by listening with attentiveness, facing the patient, making eye contact, not interrupting or rushing the patient, and having a closer interactional distance than in more formal interactions.[3]

Motivational interviewing (MI)[84–87] involves communication that elicits behavior change by helping the patient to explore and resolve ambivalence about change, thereby facilitating and engaging the patient's intrinsic motivation to work toward a change in behavior. Active components of the MI approach include a relational component, focused on empathy and rapport, and a technical component, focused on evoking and reinforcing the patient's communication about change. This approach does not impose change (which might be inconsistent with the person's own values, beliefs, etc.) but instead supports change in a manner that is congruent with these values and beliefs.

MI techniques, characterized by nonconfrontation, collaboration, and self-efficacy, have been widely applied to address health behavior change and treatment adherence in health settings.[88] Within the context of a neurorehabilitation program, Medley and Powell[88] provided a review of potential positive contributions of MI techniques in three areas, including setting the stage for therapeutic alliance and case formulation, facilitating acceptance of deficits and realistic goal-setting, and promoting engagement in clinical interventions.

3.8.2 PSYCHOSOCIAL ASSESSMENT THROUGH INTERVIEW, RECORD REVIEW, AND COLLABORATION

Given the significant contribution of psychosocial factors within the older adult population, the important role for rehabilitation practitioners is to assess for the presence and impact of stressors as well as the individual's coping/adjustment to these stressors. There are various methods for assessing these factors.[89] These methods should be aimed at identifying both strengths and weaknesses in the individual's coping process.

One component of psychosocial assessment occurs within the context of the clinician–patient relationship. Important information can be gathered during discussion with the patient, collateral interviews with family or other members of their social network, and through behavioral observations. Information provided by discussion with other members of the treatment team can provide crucial information in determining the effect of emotional functioning on rehabilitation participation.

A sign that the individual is engaging in problematic coping processes is the presence of adjustment difficulties. When these difficulties become apparent, it is important for the clinician to assess the individual's adjustment status and coping processes. Assessing for the presence of depression, anxiety, and other psychological symptoms is an important part of the discussion between the clinician and patient. Diagnostic criteria are outlined within the DSM-5,[13] which can assist with knowing the right questions to ask to assess for the presence of these symptoms within the interview and while gathering background information. Common symptoms of depression and anxiety were reviewed within Section 3.3 Adjustment and Coping Responses of this chapter.

Suicide risk assessment is also a critical component to assessment of emotional functioning, particularly when it becomes evident that an individual is having difficulty coping with stressors and exhibiting difficulties with emotional functioning. Symptoms of depression, comments about suicide or self-harm, statements of not-wanting to live, or the presence of hopelessness should trigger an evaluation of suicidality. Assessing for the presence of suicidal ideation, a plan, and intention to follow through with the plan are key components of the suicide risk assessment. An assessment of suicidal ideation involves exploration of the person's thoughts about harming or killing themselves.

Further, one must assess for whether or not the person has a plan and if so, the lethality of that plan. In addition, assessing for the individual's access to firearms, medications, etc. is an important aspect of suicide risk assessment. Another significant component of the suicide assessment is determining whether the person has an intent to carry out the plan for suicide. One must also consider supports available and the individual's belief systems that may serve as protective factors to minimize the risk for suicide. A mental health professional should also be consulted to further evaluate risk for suicide.

Consultation with a mental health professional is an important component of psychosocial assessment and the provision of recommendations for interventions. Mental health professionals (e.g., psychiatrists, psychologists/neuropsychologists, psychiatric nurse practitioners, mental health counselors, and clinical social workers) have specialized training in the identification and treatment of psychological conditions, and they should be consulted when there is question about the individual's emotional functioning or risk for suicide. In addition to the screening measures that the clinician can utilize (discussed below), the mental health professional is able to provide a more comprehensive and detailed assessment of the individual's emotional functioning. They also serve a crucial role in providing interventions to assist in minimizing psychological symptoms.

3.8.3 SCREENING MEASURES FOR EMOTIONAL FUNCTIONING, COGNITIVE FUNCTIONING, AND REHABILITATION ENGAGEMENT

In addition to the clinical interview, the presence and severity of depression, anxiety, and other psychological conditions can also be more formally assessed through various screening measures. It is important to note that while screening identifies the likelihood that the individual may have depression, anxiety, or other psychological symptoms, it is not in itself a diagnosis. There are many screening measures available to assess emotional functioning, cognitive functioning, and rehabilitation engagement. Although by no means an exhaustive list, some of the commonly used screening measures appropriate for the older adult rehabilitation population are briefly described here

- *The 9 Item Patient Health Questionnaire (PHQ-9)*[90]: a multiple-choice self-report inventory that includes nine items covering the diagnostic criteria for major depressive disorder. This measure can be used for screening of depressive symptoms and for serial assessment to evaluate response to treatment interventions.
- *Beck Depression Inventory—2nd edition (BDI-II)*[91]: a 21-question multiple-choice self-report inventory used to identify symptoms of depression.
- *Beck Depression Inventory—Fast Screen for Medical patients (BDI-Fast Screen)*[92]: a version of the BDI-II designed specifically for medical patients. This is a 7-item self-report instrument used to identify symptoms of depression, while excluding symptoms that might be related to medical problems.
- *Beck Anxiety Inventory (BAI)*[93]: a 21-item self-report inventory used to assess anxiety levels.
- *Geriatric Depression Scale (GDS)*[94]: a 30-item self-report assessment used to identify symptoms of depression in the elderly. This measure minimizes somatic and sleep-related questions, given that these symptoms can be affected by physical illness and do not necessarily represent symptoms of depression.
- *Hospital Anxiety and Depression Scale (HADS)*[95]: a 14-item scale used to determine the levels of anxiety and depression in people with physical health problems. The HADS is designed to avoid reliance on aspects of depression and anxiety that are also common somatic symptoms of illness.
- *Brief Symptom Inventory (BSI)*[96]: a 53-item, self-report scale assessing various symptoms, including symptom scales of somatization, obsessive–compulsive, interpersonal sensitivity, depression, anxiety, hostility, phobic anxiety, paranoid ideation, and psychoticism.

- *The Center for Epidemiologic Studies Depression Scale—Revised (CESD-R)*[97,98]: a 20-item scale that measures symptoms of depression in nine different groups (including sadness, loss of interest, appetite, sleep, thinking/concentration, guilt, fatigue, movement, and suicidal ideation).
- *The Hopkins Rehabilitation Engagement Rating Scale (HRERS)*[77]: a 5-item clinician-rated measure developed to quantify engagement in acute rehabilitation services.
- *The Mini-Mental State Examination (MMSE)*[99]: a brief 30-point test that is used to screen for cognitive impairment, to estimate the severity of cognitive impairment at a given point in time, to follow the course of cognitive changes in an individual over time, and to document an individual's response to treatment.
- *Montreal Cognitive Assessment (MoCA)*[100]: a brief 30-point cognitive screening measure that assesses several cognitive domains, including orientation, attention, memory recall, language, visuospatial abilities, and executive functions.

3.9   ROLE OF THE REHABILITATION CLINICIAN IN ADDRESSING PSYCHOSOCIAL FACTORS

Following psychosocial assessment, the rehabilitation clinician's role is to identify relevant interventions to address psychosocial issues. The choice of intervention approaches should be devised based on the information gathered through the psychosocial assessment process. Although there is substantial overlap in interventions available within different settings (e.g., acute rehabilitation, subacute rehabilitation, and community settings), there are also interventions that are most relevant within each of these settings. In addition, there are universal interventions that should be provided to each individual, regardless of psychosocial status, in addition to more specific interventions provided based on the presence of particular psychosocial factors.[101,102]

3.9.1   UNIVERSAL PSYCHOSOCIAL INTERVENTIONS

There are many psychosocial interventions available regardless of the rehabilitation setting. As discussed previously in this chapter, the nature of the clinician–patient relationship itself is an important intervention within the psychosocial realm. MI is also an intervention, as are the approaches to promote an effective clinician–patient relationship that were described earlier. Providing support to one's patient is critical, regardless of the setting. Individuals who have difficulty coping with illness/injury will likely require additional support from the clinician and other members of their treatment team. Important elements of this additional support include the concept of reflective listening and acknowledgement of the individual's thoughts and feelings related to the stressors that they are facing. Psychoeducation is also an important component of psychosocial intervention. Providing the individual with additional information about symptoms of their illness/injury, the process of recovery, prognosis, etc. can help to ease some of the inherent anxiety that is present with the unknown. Psychoeducation can also be a helpful tool in terms of providing information about common emotional responses to injury/illness (e.g., stages of grief, common feelings of sadness, anger, anxiety within the context of stressors, etc.) as well as some of the physiologically based emotional responses in neurological conditions (e.g., emotional liability after stroke or TBI). This education can help to provide some sense of "normalization" of their experiences.

Providing practical interventions to assist with adherence to treatment recommendations is also an important universal intervention. This can include simplifying complex treatment regimens, reviewing the most important details, encouraging the patient to ask questions as they arise, and putting treatment recommendations/interventions in writing (e.g., list of medications and medication changes, exercise regimen, referral sources and upcoming appointments, etc.). In addition, providing practical compensatory strategies for remembering important tasks can also enhance adherence (e.g., recommending the use of pillboxes, calendars, and reminder calls for appointments).

The clinician's ability to collaborate with other professionals and to assist in identifying available resources are important components of psychosocial intervention, regardless of the setting. Availability of particular referral sources and resources have the tendency to vary, depending on the setting. The importance of continued monitoring and follow up cannot be understated, underscoring the importance of continuity of care ranging from one rehabilitation setting to another as the patient progresses through the stages of recovery.

3.9.2 Psychosocial Interventions in Acute and Subacute Rehabilitation

In addition to the universal interventions described above, certain interventions may be available for the individual within the acute and subacute rehabilitation settings. Additional support and interactions with members of the rehabilitation treatment team can go a long way in assisting an individual to cope with changes associated with an illness/injury. The treatment team members can also assist in promoting participation in enjoyable activities outside of the patient's room and can facilitate increased visits from individuals within the patient's support system.

Referrals and consultations for additional services within the acute and subacute rehabilitation setting are also important components in optimizing emotional well-being. Recreational therapy is an extremely beneficial intervention to provide additional access to enjoyable activities and opportunities for socialization/decreased isolation. Depending on the individual's faith and spirituality, chaplain services may also be available to provide additional spiritual support. When pain, end-of-life, and/or existential issues are impacting the individual, palliative care services may also be available to assist in addressing these factors. When cognitive deficits are present, consultation with a speech-language pathologist and/or neuropsychologist is common within the acute rehabilitation setting. If behavioral concerns are present, a psychologist can be consulted to assist with implementation of a behavioral plan. Environmental modifications are also helpful to address behavioral concerns. Additional services that may be available in the acute or subacute rehabilitation setting include support groups (general support groups and support groups for specific medical conditions), peer support visitors, music therapy, massage therapy, pet therapy, etc.

As noted previously, consultation with a mental health professional is also an important piece to assist the individual in the coping process while facing the impact of illness/injury during the rehabilitation process. The clinician should be attuned to possible barriers to such a referral, however, including the finding that many older adults and society itself may have a stigma against mental illness and mental health treatment. If this barrier is present, it is even more important for the clinician to discuss these viewpoints and to provide additional education on psychological symptoms and the role of mental health interventions in helping to treat them.

In terms of utilization of mental health interventions, both medications and psychotherapy can be effective in isolation. However, extensive literature over the years has supported the finding that psychotherapy combined with psychotropic medication is associated with greater and longer-lasting improvement in psychiatric symptoms. There are several commonly used interventions in psychotherapy that are utilized in the treatment of individuals with medical conditions. Examples include cognitive-behavioral, interpersonal, and problem-solving therapy approaches. Additional modalities include life review/reminiscence, supportive approaches, behavioral interventions, relaxation techniques, etc.

Planning and coordinating follow-up care after discharge from the acute/subacute rehabilitation setting is also imperative, including follow-up mental healthcare if the individual has struggled with coping and emotional adjustment during his/her rehabilitation stay. As a starting point, the rehabilitation clinician should provide information to the patient's primary care provider in the community regarding the presence and severity of psychological symptoms that were present during rehabilitation. The primary care provider can then assist in the ongoing monitoring and treatment of residual symptoms. The rehabilitation clinician should also be sure to address psychosocial factors and psychological symptoms during their hospital follow-up visits with the patient. When appropriate, referral to outpatient mental health services should also be a part of the discharge planning process when an individual transitions from acute or subacute rehabilitation to the community setting.

When there is any question regarding suicide risk, a suicide risk assessment should be completed. If suicidal ideation, plan, and/or intent are present, consultation with a mental health professional for a more formal evaluation is indicated. The mental health professional will assist in determining suicide risk and the need for inpatient psychiatric treatment. If suicidal ideation is present in the absence of plan or intent, the individual may not require inpatient psychiatric treatment, but outpatient psychiatric treatment would be highly indicated. Regardless, the individual should be provided with a suicide hotline phone number in preparation for discharge.

The rehabilitation clinician can also assist in connecting patients to community resources. These can include community resources such as support groups and diagnosis-specific organizations for additional resources and support. Additional community resources are discussed below.

3.9.3 Psychosocial Interventions in the Community Setting

Within the community setting, the rehabilitation clinician plays an important role in coordinating appropriate services to help address psychosocial factors. This can include referral for mental health treatment as well as providing the patient with a suicide hotline phone number, as appropriate. Referral to a neurologist, geriatrician, and/or neuropsychologist can also assist with additional diagnosis and treatment for a variety of conditions.

The rehabilitation clinician in the community can also provide information to assist the patient in connecting to various community resources. There are many community resources available to assist individuals with various medical conditions. The clinician can play an important role in minimizing barriers and identifying resources to ensure access and availability of preventative services and medical care for the diagnosis and ongoing management of health conditions. Diagnosis-specific organizations can provide a wealth of information for the patient about their medical condition, additional resources, support groups, online support venues, etc. Often, these associations provide links to local associations within the individual's community. There are also local resources available through aging and older adult services agencies, respite services, day programs, fall prevention initiatives, etc. A list of organizations/associations, including those available for diagnoses commonly treated in the rehabilitation setting, is included at the end of this chapter.

3.10 CONCLUSION

Within the biopsychosocial model,[1] human health, illness, and functioning are understood by considering the complex interplay between biological, psychological, and social factors. The combination of these factors can influence how the individual copes with illness/injury, how they implement health behavior change and adhere to treatment recommendations, and can impact the clinical course and outcome of the condition. From a psychological standpoint, some individuals will demonstrate signs of the normal grieving process following the onset of illness/injury, while others may experience symptoms of an adjustment disorder, depressive disorder, or anxiety disorder. Pre-existing psychological symptoms may also be exacerbated by the onset of stressors associated with the illness/injury. Cognitive deficits can also impact the understanding of the illness/injury, adherence to treatment, and resulting outcomes. There are also many social factors that can impact coping, health behavior, and clinical outcome within the context of illness/injury. These include generational factors, access to services, stressors common in the geriatric population, the person's social and cultural context, their beliefs and values, and the quality of social support systems available to them.

The rehabilitation clinician plays a crucial role in the assessment and provision of interventions based on the biopsychosocial factors noted above. Important components of psychosocial assessment include the clinician–patient relationship, discussion with the patient, and discussion with individuals who are familiar with the patient. There are also many screening measures available to assess emotional functioning, cognitive functioning, and rehabilitation engagement. The interventions recommended by the rehabilitation clinician should take into account the biopsychosocial factors unique to the individual. Universal interventions, regardless of the rehabilitation or community setting, include the clinician–patient relationship itself, psychoeducation, practical interventions to assist with treatment adherence, and collaboration with other professionals. Coordination of follow-up services within the community is also an important intervention allowing the clinician to promote access to community resources, preventative services, and ongoing medical care for management of health conditions.

ADDITIONAL RESOURCES/ASSOCIATIONS

- Alzheimer's Association—www.alz.org
- American Association for Geriatric Psychiatry—www.aagponline.org
- American Cancer Society—www.cancer.org
- American Diabetes Association—www.diabetes.org
- American Geriatrics Society (AGS)—www.americangeriatrics.org
- Arthritis Foundation—www.arthritis.org
- Brain Injury Association of America—www.biausa.org
- Center for Mental Health Services, US Substance Abuse and Mental Health Services Administration—www.samhsa.gov
- Family Caregiver Alliance/National Center on Caregiving—www.caregiver.org
- Institute on Aging—www.ioaging.org
- Mental Health America—www.mentalhealthamerica.net
- National Alliance on Mental Illness—www.nami.org
- National Amputation Foundation—www.nationalamputation.org
- National Institutes of Health—Senior Health—www.nihseniorhealth.gov
- National Institute of Mental Health—nimh.nih.gov
- National Multiple Sclerosis Society—www.nationalmssociety.org
- National Spinal Cord Injury Association—www.spinalcord.org
- National Stroke Association—www.stroke.org
- National Suicide Prevention Lifeline—1-800-273-8255
- Positive Aging Resource Center—www.positiveaging.org
- The Portal of Geriatrics Online Education (POGOe)—www.pogoe.org

REFERENCES

1. Engel GL. The need for a new medical model: A challenge for biomedicine. *Science* 1977;196:129–136.
2. Engel GL. The clinical application of the biopsychosocial model. *American Journal of Psychiatry* 1980;137:535–544.
3. Williams SL, Haskard KB, DiMatteo MR. The therapeutic effects of the physician–older patient relationship: Effective communication with vulnerable older patients. *Clinical Interventions in Aging* 2007;2(3):453–467.
4. Lazarus RS, Folkman S. *Stress, Appraisal and Coping.* New York: Springer Publishing; 1984.
5. Leventhal H, Nereenz, DR, Steele DJ. Illness perceptions and coping with health threat. In: Baum A, Taylor SE, Singer JE (eds.). *Handbook of Psychology and Health, Volume IV: Social Psychological Aspects of Health.* Hillsdale, New Jersey: Erlbaum; 1984, 219–252.
6. Deci EL, Ryan RM. *Intrinsic Motivation and Self-Determination in Human Behavior.* New York: Plenum; 1985.
7. Schwarzer, R (ed.). *Self-Efficacy: Thought Control of Action.* Washington, DC: Hemisphere Publishing Corp.; 1992.

8. Armitage CJ, Conner M. Social cognition models and health behaviour: A structured review. *Psychology and Health* 2000;15:173–189.

9. Bandura A. Self-efficacy: Toward a unifying theory of behavioral change. *Psychological Review* 1977;84(2):191–215.

10. Luszczynska A, Schwarzer R. Social cognitive theory. In: M. Conner, P. Norman (eds.). *Predicting Health Behavior*, 2nd edn. Revised. Buckingham, England: Open University Press; 2005, 127–169.

11. Conner M, Norman P (eds.). *Predicting Health Behavior*, 2nd edn. Revised. Buckingham, England: Open University Press; 2005.

12. Fuertes JN, Mislowack A, Bennett J, Paul L, Gilbert TC, Fontan G, Boylan LS. The physician–patient working alliance. *Patient Education and Counseling* 2007;66(1):29–36.

13. American Psychiatric Association. *Diagnostic and Statistical Manual of Mental Disorders*, 5th edn. Arlington, Virginia: American Psychiatric Publishing; 2013.

14. Dickens C, Coventry P, Khara A, Bower P, Mansell W, Bakerly ND. Perseverative negative cognitive processes are associated with depression in people with long-term conditions. *Chronic Illness* 2012;8(2):102–111.

15. Cully JA, Gfeller JD, Heise RA, Ross MJ, Teal CR, Kunik ME. Geriatric depression, medical diagnosis, and functional recovery during acute rehabilitation. *Archives of Physical Medicine and Rehabilitation* 2005;86(12):2256–2260.

16. Kortte KB, Stevenson JE, Hosey MM, Castillo R, Wegener ST. Hope predicts positive functional role outcomes in acute rehabilitation populations. *Rehabilitation Psychology* 2012;57(3):248–255.

17. Popovich JM, Fox PG, Burns KR. "Hope" in the recovery from stroke in the U.S. *The International Journal of Psychiatric Nursing Research* 2003;8(2):905–920.

18. van Leeuwen CM, Kraaijeveld S, Lindeman E, Post MW. Associations between psychological factors and quality of life ratings in persons with spinal cord injury: A systematic review. *Spinal Cord* 2012;50(3):174–187.

19. Peter C, Möller R, Cieza A, Geyh S. Psychological resources in spinal cord injury: A systematic literature review. *Spinal Cord* 2012;50(3):188–201.

20. Kennedy P, Lude P, Elfström ML, Smithson E. Appraisals, coping, and adjustment pre and post SCI rehabilitation: A 2-year follow-up study. *Spinal Cord* 2012;50(2):112–118.

21. Kennedy P, Evans M, Sandhu N. Psychological adjustment to spinal cord injury: The contribution of coping, hope, and cognitive appraisals. *Psychology, Health and Medicine* 2009;14(1):17–33.

22. Kortte K, Gilbert M, Gorman P, Wegener ST. Positive psychological variables in the prediction of life satisfaction after spinal cord injury. *Rehabilitation Psychology* 2010;55(1):40–47.

23. van Leeuwen CM, Post MW, van Asbeck FW, van der Woude LH, de Groot S, Lindeman E. Social support and life satisfaction in spinal cord injury during and up to one year after inpatient rehabilitation. *Journal of Rehabilitation Medicine* 2010;42(3):265–271.

24. van Leeuwen CM, Post MW, van Asbeck FW, Bongers-Janssen HM, van der Woude LH, de Groot S, Lindeman E. Life satisfaction in people with spinal cord injury during first five years after discharge from inpatient rehabilitation. *Disability and Rehabilitation* 2012;34(1):76–83.

25. Moore AD, Bombardier CH, Brown PB, Patterson DR. Coping and emotional attributions following spinal cord injury. *International Journal of Rehabilitation Research* 1994;17(1):39–48.

26. Livneh H, Martz E. The impact of perceptions of health control and coping modes on negative affect among individuals with spinal cord injuries. *Journal of Clinical Psychology in Medical Settings* 2011;18(3):243–256.

27. Skidmore ER, Whyte EM, Holm MB, Becker JT, Butters MA, Dew MA, Munin MC, Lenze EJ. Cognitive and affective predictors of rehabilitation participation after stroke. *Archives of Physical Medicine and Rehabilitation* 2010;91(2):203–207.

28. Ostir GV, Berges IM, Ottenbacher ME, Clow A, Ottenbacher KJ. Associations between positive emotion and recovery of functional status following stroke. *Psychosomatic Medicine* 2008;70(4):404–409.

29. Roger PR, Johnson-Greene D. Comparison of assessment measures for post-stroke depression. *The Clinical Neuropsychologist* 2009;23(5):780–793.

30. Davis LC, Sherer M, Sander AM, Bogner JA, Corrigan JD, Dijkers MP, Hanks RA, Bergquist TF, Seel RT. Preinjury predictors of life satisfaction at 1 year after traumatic brain injury. *Archives of Physical Medicine and Rehabilitation* 2012;93(8):1324–1330.

31. Roe B, Howell F, Riniotis K, Beech R, Crome P, Ong BN. Older people and falls: Health status, quality of life, lifestyle, care networks, prevention and views on service use following a recent fall. *Journal of Clinical Nursing* 2009;18(16):2261–2272.

32. DiMatteo MR, Martin LR. *Health Psychology*. Boston, Massachusetts: Allyn and Bacon; 2002.

33. DiMatteo MR. Social support and patient adherence to medical treatment: A meta-analysis. *Health Psychology* 2004;23(2):207–218.

34. Sayers SL, Riegel B, Pawlowski S, Coyne JC, Samaha FF. Social support and self-care of patients with heart failure. *Annals of Behavioral Medicine* 2008;35:70–79.

35. Luttik ML, Jaarsma T, Moser D, Sanderman R, van Veldhuisen DJ. The importance and impact of social support on outcomes in patients with heart failure: An overview of the literature. *The Journal of Cardiovascular Nursing* 2005;20(3):162–169.

36. Müller R, Peter C, Cieza A, Geyh S. The role of social support and social skills in people with spinal cord injury: A systematic review of the literature. *Spinal Cord* 2012;50(2):94–106.

37. Blais MC, Boisvert JM. Psychological and marital adjustment in couples following a traumatic brain injury (TBI): A critical review. *Brain Injury* 2005;19(14):1223–1235.

38. Blais MC, Boisvert JM. Psychological adjustment and marital satisfaction following head injury. Which critical personal characteristics should both partners develop? *Brain Injury* 2007;21(4): 357–372.

39. Nicholson NR. A review of social isolation: An important but underassessed condition in older adults. *The Journal of Primary Prevention* 2012;33(2–3):137–152.

40. Shankar A, McMunn A, Banks J, Steptoe A. Loneliness, social isolation, and behavioral and biological health indicators in older adults. *Health Psychology* 2011;30(4):377–385.

41. Steptoe A, Shankar A, Demakakos P, Wardle J. Social isolation, loneliness, and all-cause mortality in older men and women. *Proceedings of the National Academy of Sciences of the United States of America* 2013;110(15):5797–5801.

42. Holwerda TJ, Beekman AT, Deeg DJ, Stek ML, van Tilburg TG, Visser PJ, Schmand B, Jonker C, Schoevers RA. Increased risk of mortality associated with social isolation in older men: Only when feeling lonely? Results from the Amsterdam Study of the Elderly (AMSTEL). *Psychological Medicine* 2012;42(4):843–853.

43. Seeman TE. Health promoting effects of friends and family on health outcomes in older adults. *American Journal of Health Promotion* 2000;14(6):362–370.

44. Bookwala J. The role of marital quality in physical health during the mature years. *Journal of Aging and Health* 2005;17(1):85–104.

45. Chang HY, Chiou CJ, Chen NS. Impact of mental health and caregiver burden on family caregivers' physical health. *Archives of Gerontology and Geriatrics* 2010;50(3):267–271.

46. Saban KL, Sherwood PR, DeVon HA, Hynes DM. Measures of psychological stress and physical health in family caregivers of stroke survivors: A literature review. *The Journal of Neuroscience Nursing* 2010;42(3):128–138.

47. Kuzuya M, Enoki H, Hasegawa J, Izawa S, Hirakawa Y, Shimokata H, Akihisa I. Impact of caregiver burden on adverse health outcomes in community-dwelling dependent older care recipients. *The American Journal of Geriatric Psychiatry* 2011;19(4):382–391.

48. Schulz R, Beach SR. Caregiving as a risk factor for mortality: The Caregiver Health Effects Study. *The Journal of the American Medical Association* 1999;282(23):2215–2219.

49. Bobinac A, van Exel N, Rutten FF, Brouwer WB. Health effects in significant others: Separating family and care-giving effects. *Medical Decision Making* 2011;31(2):292–298.

50. Chappell NL, Reid RC. Burden and well-being among caregivers: Examining the distinction. *The Gerontologist* 2002;42(6):772–780.

51. American Association for Geriatric Psychiatry. Geriatrics and mental health—The facts, 2008. www.aagponline.org.

52. Geriatric Mental Health Foundation. Depression in late life: Not a natural part of aging, 2008. www.gmhfonline.org.

53. Lyness JM, King DA, Cox C, Yoediono Z, Caine ED. The importance of subsyndromal depression in older primary care patients: Prevalence and associated functional disability. *Journal of the American Geriatrics Society* 1999;47(6):647–652.

54. Frederick JT, Steinman LE, Prohaska T, Satariano WA, Bruce M, Bryant L, Ciechanowski P et al. Community-based treatment of late life depression: An expert panel-informed literature review. *American Journal of Preventative Medicine* 2007;33(3):222–249.

55. Katon WJ, Lin E, Russo J, Unützer J. Increased medical costs of a population-based sample of depressed elderly patients. *Archives of General Psychiatry* 2003;60(9):897–903.

56. Snowden M, Steinman L, Frederick J. Treating depression in older adults: Challenges to implementing the recommendations of an expert panel. *Preventing Chronic Disease* 2008;5(1):A26.

57. Unützer J, Patrick DL, Simon G, Grembowski D, Walker E, Rutter C, Katon W. Depressive symptoms and the cost of health services in HMO patients aged 65 years and older: A 4-year prospective study. *The Journal of the American Medical Association* 1997;277(20):1618–1623.

58. Snowden M, Steinman L, Frederick J, Wilson N. Screening for depression in older adults: Recommended instruments and considerations for community-based practice. *Clinical Geriatrics* 2009;17(9):26–32.

59. Porensky EK, Dew MA, Karp JF, Skidmore E, Rollman BL, Shear MK, Lenze EJ. The burden of late-life generalized anxiety disorder: Effects on disability, health-related quality of life, and healthcare utilization. *The American Journal of Geriatric Psychiatry* 2009;17(6):473–482.

60. Diamond PT, Felsenthal G, Macciocchi SN, Butler DH, Lally-Cassady D. Effect of cognitive impairment on rehabilitation outcome. *American Journal of Physical Medicine and Rehabilitation* 1996;75(1):40–43.

61. Poynter L, Kwan J, Sayer AA, Vassallo M. Does cognitive impairment affect rehabilitation outcome? *Journal of the American Geriatrics Society* 2011;59(11):2108–2111.

62. Kuzuya M, Hirakawa Y, Suzuki Y, Iwata M, Enoki H, Hasegawa J, Iguchi A. Association between unmet needs for medication support and all-cause hospitalization in community-dwelling disabled elderly people. *Journal of the American Geriatrics Society* 2008;56(5):881–886.

63. Lequerica AH, Kortte K. Therapeutic engagement: A proposed model of engagement in medical rehabilitation. *American Journal of Physical Medicine and Rehabilitation* 2010;89(5):415–422.

64. Kortte KB, Veiel L, Batten SV, Wegener ST. Measuring avoidance in medical rehabilitation. *Rehabilitation Psychology* 2009;54(1):91–98.

65. DiMatteo MR. Variations in patients' adherence to medical recommendations: A quantitative review of 50 years of research. *Medical Care* 2004;42(3):200–209.

66. DiMatteo MR, Giordani PJ, Lepper HS, Croqhan TW. Patient adherence and medical treatment outcomes: A meta-analysis. *Medical Care* 2002;40(9):794–811.

67. DiMatteo MR, Lepper HS, Croghan TW. Depression is a risk factor for noncompliance with medical treatment: A meta-analysis of the effects of anxiety and depression on patient adherence. *Archives of Internal Medicine* 2000;160(14):2101–2107.

68. Martin, LR, Williams SL, Haskard KB, DiMatteo MR. The challenge of patient adherence. *Therapeutics and Clinical Risk Management* 2005;1(3):189–199.

69. Stafford L, Jackson HJ, Berk M. Illness beliefs about heart disease and adherence to secondary prevention regimens. *Psychosomatic Medicine* 2008;70(8):942–948.

70. Maggi L, Ferrara PE, Aprile I, Ronconi G, Specchia A, Nigito C, Amabile E, Rabini A, Piazzini DB, Bertolini C. Role of spiritual beliefs on disability and health-related quality of life in acute inpatient rehabilitation unit. *European Journal of Physical and Rehabilitation Medicine* 2012;48(3):467–473.

71. Lucchetti G, Lucchetti AG, Badan-Neto AM, Peres PT, Moreira-Almeida A, Gomes C, Koenig HG. Religiousness affects mental health, pain and quality of life in older people in an outpatient rehabilitation setting. *Journal of Rehabilitation Medicine* 2011;43(4):316–322.

72. Zivin K, Kales HC. Adherence to depression treatment in older adults: a narrative review. *Drugs and Aging* 2008;25(7):559–571.

73. DiMatteo MR, Haskard KB, Williams SL. Health beliefs, disease severity, and patient adherence: A meta-analysis. *Medical Care* 2007;45(6):521–528.

74. Vik SA, Maxwell CJ, Hogan DB. Measurement, correlates, and health outcomes of medication adherence among seniors. *The Annals of Pharmacotherapy* 2004;38(2):303–312.

75. Vik SA, Hogan DB, Patten SB, Johnson JA, Romonko-Slack L, Maxwell CJ. Medication nonadherence and subsequent risk of hospitalisation and mortality among older adults. *Drugs and Aging* 2006;23(4):345–356.

76. MacLaughlin EJ, Raehl CL, Treadway AK, Sterling TL, Zoller DP, Bond CA. Assessing medication adherence in the elderly: Which tools to use in clinical practice? *Drugs and Aging* 2005;22(3):231–255.

77. Kortte KB, Falk LD, Castillo RC, Johnson-Greene D, Wegener ST. The Hopkins Rehabilitation Engagement Rating Scale: Development and psychometric properties. *Archives of Physical Medicine and Rehabilitation* 2007;88(7):877–884.

78. Chen, H, Landefeld SC. The hidden poor: Care of the elderly. In: King WM (ed.). *Medical Management of Vulnerable and Underserved Patients.* New York: McGraw-Hill; 2007, 199–209.

79. Sudano JJ, Baker DW. Explaining US racial/ethnic disparities in health declines and mortality in late middle age: The roles of socioeconomic status, health behaviors, and health insurance. *Social Science and Medicine* 2006;62(4):909–922.

80. Stewart MA. What is a successful doctor–patient interview? A study of interactions and outcomes. *Social Science and Medicine* 1984;19(2):167–175.

81. Stewart MA. Effective physician–patient communication and health outcomes: A review. *Canadian Medical Association Journal* 1995;152(9):1423–1433.

82. Zolnierek KB, DiMatteo MR. Physician communication and patient adherence to treatment: A meta-analysis. *Medical Care* 2009;47(8):826–834.

83. Arbuthnott A, Sharpe D. The effect of physician–patient collaboration on patient adherence in non-psychiatric medicine. *Patient Education and Counseling* 2009;77(1):60–67.

84. Miller WR. Motivational interviewing with problem drinkers. *Behavioural Psychotherapy* 1983;11(2):147–172.

85. Miller, WR, Zweben, A, DiClemente, CC, Rychtarik, RG. *Motivational Enhancement Therapy Manual: A Clinical Research Guide for Therapists Treating Individuals with Alcohol Abuse and Dependence.* Project MATCH Monograph Series V.2. Rockville, Maryland: National Institute on Alcohol Abuse and Alcoholism (NIAAA); 1992.

86. Miller WR, Rose GS. Toward a theory of motivational interviewing. *The American Psychologist* 2009;64(6):527–537.

87. Miller WR, Rollnick, S. *Motivational Interviewing: Preparing People for Change*, 2nd edn. New York: Guilford Press; 2002.

88. Medley AR, Powell T. Motivational interviewing to promote self-awareness and engagement in rehabilitation following acquired brain injury: A conceptual review. *Neuropsychological Rehabilitation* 2010;20(4):481–508.

89. Heinemann AW. Measures of coping and reaction to disability. In Cushman LC, Scherer MJ (eds.). *Psychological Assessment in Medical Rehabilitation.* Washington, DC: APA Books; 1995, pp. 39–100.

90. Kroenke K, Spitzer RL, Williams JB. The PHQ-9: Validity of a brief depression severity measure. *Journal of General Internal Medicine* 2001;16(9):606–613.

91. Beck AT, Steer, RA, Brown GK. *Manual for the Beck Depression Inventory-II.* San Antonio, Texas: Psychological Corporation; 1996.

92. Beck AT, Steer RA, Brown GK. *Manual for the BDI-Fast Screen for Medical Patients.* San Antonio, Texas: Psychological Corporation; 2000.

93. Beck AT, Steer RA. *Beck Anxiety Inventory Manual.* San Antonio, Texas: Psychological Corporation; 1993.

94. Yesavage JA, Brink TL, Rose TL, Lum, O, Huang V, Adey M, Leirer VO. Development and validation of a geriatric depression screening scale: A preliminary report. *Journal of Psychiatric Research* 1982–1983;17(1):37–49.

95. Zigmond AS, Smith RP. The hospital anxiety and depression scale. *Acta Psychiatrica Scandinavica* 1983;67(6):361–370.

96. Derogatis L, Melisaratos N. The brief symptom inventory: An introductory report. *Psychological Medicine* 1983;13(3):595–605.

97. Radloff LS. The CES-D scale: A self-report depression scale for research in the general population. *Applied Psychological Measurement* 1977;1(3):385–401.

98. Eaton WW, Muntaner C, Smith C, Tien A, Ybarra M. Center for Epidemiologic Studies Depression Scale: Review and revision (CESD and CESD-R). In: Maruish ME (ed.). *The Use of Psychological Testing for Treatment Planning and Outcomes Assessment*, 3rd edn. Mahwah, New Jersey: Lawrence Erlbaum; 2004, 363–377.

99. Folstein MF, Folstein SE, McHugh PR. "Mini-mental state". A practical method for grading the cognitive state of patients for the clinician. *Journal of Psychiatric Research* 1975;12(3):189–198.

100. Nasreddine ZS, Phillips NA, Bédirian V, Charbonneau S, Whitehead V, Collin I, Cummings JL, Chertkow H. The Montreal Cognitive Assessment, MoCA: A brief screening tool for mild cognitive impairment. *Journal of the American Geriatrics Society* 2005;53(4):695–699.

101. Scherer MJ 2010. Rehabilitation psychology. In IB. Weiner and WE. Craighead (eds.). *The Concise Corsini Encyclopedia of Psychology*, 4th edn., Vol. 4. Hoboken, New Jersey: John Wiley & Sons, Inc. 1444–1447.

102. Frank RG, Rosenthal M, Caplan B (eds.). *Handbook of Rehabilitation Psychology*, 2nd edn., Washington, DC: APA Books.

4 Functional Assessment and Measures

Deepthi S. Saxena

CONTENTS

4.1 INTRODUCTION

The number of persons 65 years of age and older continues to increase dramatically in the United States to an estimated 70 million by 2030. The elderly comprise the fastest growing segment of our population who also require the highest proportion of medical care amongst all age groups.[1] When impaired older persons become ill, they are at a high risk of functional deterioration that leads to institutionalization.[2] Today, we must provide good quality at a lesser cost as it is linked to reimbursement, with indicators such as length of stay (LOS) and readmissions in acute care hospitals. Prolonged hospitalization is possible only in postacute care (PAC) settings. However, due to the intensity of regulation in PAC settings, patients who continue to be functionally impaired after acute hospitalization may not qualify for PAC services to meet all their medical, rehabilitative, and social needs.[2] Therefore, prevention is imperative. Both primary and secondary prevention are becoming increasingly important for older individuals. Due to increased longevity and complex comorbidities, a multidisciplinary approach is needed to provide comprehensive medical and social assessment as well as treatment, often with an emphasis on rehabilitation. Since a multidisciplinary approach entails multiple providers to communicate with a common language that ties in disease with disability, it is imperative to use an organized approach with objective measurements to target key areas of functional status, with a comprehensive geriatric assessment (CGA). A CGA is not simply a diagnostic tool because it also includes the efficacious management of the older adult.

4.2 SECTION A: COMPREHENSIVE GERIATRIC ASSESSMENT

A CGA evaluates the physical, psychosocial, and environmental factors that impact the well-being of older adults, over the age of 65 years.

An emerging new paradigm is geriatric assessment units, which favorably affect health status, functional activities, and discharge to more independent living. However, there have been few randomized trials to evaluate the effectiveness of such units. Studies have found that treatment in the geriatric assessment units reduced subsequent mortality and institutionalization, lowering healthcare costs per year of life.[2] The challenge with these settings is that a long-term measurement component outside of these settings at inpatient consultation and in the outpatient clinics is needed to identify patients at risk. A randomized control trial (RCT) has shown that the benefits of an inpatient CGA on mortality and physical function may be greatest when there is moderate illness and moderate functional impairment.[2] Given the multiple medically complex conditions in the elderly, simple screening instruments stratify risk for common conditions, but they may not be effective in reducing healthcare utilization or costs, unless a CGA is conducted to evaluate patients with risk for imminent morbidity or mortality.[3] The CGA leads to preventive care and proactive medical management, which is needed in addition to disease-specific intervention.[4] According to the summary statement of a National Institute on Aging Consensus, the most effective forms of assessment are those that target at-risk patients and that combine assessment with intensive treatment and rehabilitation.[5] Therefore, this chapter focuses on the CGA, which is the functional assessment of the older adult, which can be used by all practitioners working in multidisciplinary teams. This chapter emphasizes on assessment and measurement tools that are available easily, particularly on public domains, and can be administered with time efficiency and at little or no cost.

4.2.1 COMPONENTS OF THE CGA

The most important components of the CGA,[3] that is, the functional assessment of the older adult, are the following:

1. Functional status
2. Injury prevention (gait and falls)
3. Polypharmacy
4. Sensory perception (dizziness, visual, and hearing deficits)
5. Mental status (cognition and mood)
6. Nutrition
7. Pressure sores
8. Continence
9. Pain
10. Sexuality
11. Immunizations
12. Frailty assessment
13. Social issues (elder abuse and advance directives)

Geriatric syndromes comprise a spectrum of disease and disability states in geriatric health, which occur from the accumulated effect of multiple disorders superimposed on age-related changes. Falls, sensory deficits, malnutrition, incontinence, pressure sores, immune deficiencies, sexual dysfunction, impaired cognition and mood, and elder abuse are among a long list of geriatric syndromes, which are related to, but are not specific to disease states. Therefore, another goal of this chapter is to encourage a systematic assessment of various areas of potential risk to create a database, in the context of both disease and disability, which is unique to the concerns of the elderly. Multiple visits can be used to perform the entire assessment, as all information is difficult to gather in one patient encounter, in acute care hospital, outpatient, acute inpatient rehabilitation hospital (or unit), subacute rehabilitation, and in other PAC settings.

4.3   SECTION B: FUNCTIONAL ASSESSMENT AND MEASUREMENT TOOLS

4.3.1   FUNCTIONAL STATUS

Functional status refers to the individual's ability to move and perform activities of daily living (ADLs) and mobility. This assessment determines whether the patient is independent in their activities or if they require supportive assistance. The *level of supportive assistance* that is needed is determined by asking the patient and/or caregiver about the patient's ability to perform the ADLs and mobility. Having the patient complete a structured series of activities, such as the performance test of activities of daily living (PADL), provides similar information without any reporting bias.

An older adult's functional status can be assessed at three levels:

1. *Basic activities of daily living (BADLs)*: BADLs refer to self-care tasks and include bathing, dressing, toileting, continence, grooming, feeding, and transferring.
2. *Instrumental or intermediate activities of daily living (IADLs)*: IADLs include tasks that are required for independent living, such as housework including laundry and meal preparation, medication self-administration, grocery shopping, public transportation or driving, communication device use such as telephone and Internet, and financial management.
3. *Advanced activities of daily living (AADLs)*: AADLs vary between individuals and include participation in family, society, local community, recreational, or occupational endeavors.

Older adults are vulnerable to functional decline leading to disability, due to their decreased physiological reserves and decreased compensatory strategies when there is illness or injury. Hospitalization contributes to this decrease due to the hazards of immobilization.

Several assessment instruments are used to assess the patient's functional status in different settings, which are referred to in Section C under performance measures/metrics, with rehabilitation measurement tools covered in Chapter 27, measurement in acute and subacute inpatient rehabilitation.

The functional independence measure (FIM) instrument scale used in inpatient rehabilitation facilities (IRF), that is, in acute rehabilitation assesses physical and cognitive disability. This scale focuses the level of disability indicating the burden of care.

Items are scored on the level of assistance required for an individual to perform ADLs. The scale includes 18 items, of which 13 items are physical domains based on the Barthel Index and five items are cognition items. Each item is scored from 1 to 7 based on the level of independence, where 1 represents total dependence and 7 indicates complete independence. The scale can be administered by a physician, nurse, therapist, or a layperson. Possible scores range from 18 to 126, with higher scores indicating more independence. Alternatively, 13 physical items could be scored separately from five cognitive items.

4.3.2   INJURY PREVENTION

Falls are associated with reduced overall functioning and early admission to long-term care (LTC) facilities, and lead to greater morbidity and mortality in the older population. Geriatric patients are at a higher risk of falling due to postural hypotension, balance and gait impairment, polypharmacy, impaired cognitive ability, and mental health issues. These should be evaluated within the context of the individual's social situation, not by screening every patient, but by screening those with any *change* in physical or mental function. The May 2001 Guideline for the Prevention of Falls in Older Persons aims at assessment of fall risk and the management of older adults who have fallen or are at risk of falling. It was a joint endeavor of the American Geriatrics Society (AGS), the British Geriatrics Society (BGS), and the American Academy of Orthopedic Surgeons (AAOS). According to the update published in 2010,[6,7] a fall is defined as "an event whereby an individual unexpectedly comes to rest on the ground or another lower level without known loss of consciousness." The guideline recommends that all older persons who are under the care of a health professional or caregivers should be asked at least once a year about

1. Falls (the number of falls)
2. Frequency of falling
3. Gait or balance impairment

Any positive answer to the screening questions puts the person screened in a high-risk group needing further evaluation. A multifactorial fall risk assessment should be performed for community-dwelling older persons who report recurrent (two or more) falls, report difficulties with gait or balance and/or seek medical attention, or present to the emergency department because of a fall. Multifactorial fall risk assessment is the assessment of known predisposing factors within the person and in the environment that increase the risk of falling. *Intervention domains or categories* for fall prevention include medication, exercise, vision, postural hypotension, heart rate and rhythm, vitamin D, footwear, and home environment to name a few. A *multifactorial fall risk assessment* is important because falls are responsible for a significant number of accidental deaths and traumatic injuries among the elderly. One-third of patients with confirmed falls may not recall falling. A *single intervention* is in one of the preceding categories, such as a balance and strength exercise program, medication adjustment, vision improvement, or home/environmental modification. A *multifactorial intervention* is made up of a subset of interventions to address the specific risk factors identified through a multifactorial fall risk assessment. *Multicomponent interventions* are a set of interventions (population method) addressing more than one intervention domain or category offered to all participants in a program. The algorithm for the Guideline for the Prevention of Falls in Older Persons (AGS, BGS, and AAOS) is recommended for use in the clinical setting for assessment and intervention to reduce falls among community-residing older persons (>65 years).[6,7]

The U.S. Preventive Services Task Force (USPSTF) in the second edition of its *Guide to Clinical Prevention Services*[9] recommended fall prevention as an assessment category unique to patients 65 years of age and older as the annual incidence of falls in persons over 65 years of age who live independently is approximately 25%, rising to 50% in those over 80 years of age.[8,9] Therefore, a comprehensive risk assessment for falls incorporates a review of all potential intrinsic and extrinsic factors, as well as a focused physical examination. Intrinsic factors that contribute to falls include age-related changes in postural control, gait, and visual ability, and the presence of acute and chronic diseases that affect sensory input, the central nervous system, and musculoskeletal system, including strength, balance, gait, and coordination.

4.3.2.1 Medications

Medications that increase the risk of falling include the following categories[6]:

1. Sedative, hypnotic, and anxiolytic drugs (especially long-acting benzodiazepines)
2. Tricyclic antidepressants (TCADs)
3. Major tranquilizers (phenothiazines and butyrophenones)
4. Antihypertensive drugs

5. Cardiac medications
6. Corticosteroids
7. Nonsteroidal anti-inflammatory drugs (NSAIDs)
8. Anticholinergic drugs
9. Hypoglycemic agents
10. Any medication that is likely to affect balance

4.3.2.2 Osteoporosis

Patients with osteoporosis may present with a pathologic fracture preceding the fall. Therefore, *screening should be directed at risk assessment for osteoporosis.*

The American Academy of Physical Medicine and Rehabilitation (AAPM&R) recommends the use of a Quality Tool Box (QTB)[10] for specific health conditions to bring together a variety of already existing resources on a particular condition in one centralized location. The QTB identifies core constructs based on the International Classification of Functioning, Disability and Health (ICF) Framework. These core constructs, as per the ICF Framework, help assess the patient in physical, social, and environmental contexts as they are classified into

1. Risk
2. Symptom quality
3. Activity limitation/participation restrictions
4. Quality of life (QOL)

The *International Classification of Functioning, Disability and Health (ICF), endorsed by 191 Nations, including the Unites States* is published by the World Health Organization (WHO) to provide a standard language and framework for Health and Disability.[11] The ICF is a description of health and health-related states as domains that describe changes in body function and structure. This includes what a person with a health condition *can do* in a standard environment (level of capacity), and what they *actually do* in their usual environment (level of performance). These domains are classified from body, individual, and societal perspectives into two lists: a list of body functions and structure and a list of domains of activity and participation. In the ICF, the term functioning refers to all body functions, activities, and participation. Impairments are problems in body functions and structure such as significant deviation or loss. Disability is similarly an umbrella term for impairments, activity limitations, and participation restrictions. ICF also lists environmental factors that interact with all these components. Activity is the execution of a task or action. *Participation* is the involvement in a life situation. Activity limitations are difficulties in executing activities and occur in the personal sphere. Participation restrictions are problems in involvement in the societal or environmental spheres. The commonly used measurement tools today identify the ICF domain that they address.

The commonly referenced and recommended, easily available, and easy to use practical measurement tools referenced by guidelines, consensus panels, and professional societies are available at rehabmeasures.org.[12] Measurement tools pertinent to the CGA are as follows:

1. *Timed up and go test (TUG)*: The TUG takes less than 3 minutes to administer, is free, and assesses the ICF domain activity, as a dual-task (up and go) dynamic measure for identifying individuals who are at risk for falls (reference will be helpful).[13–15]
2. *The Berg balance scale*: It assesses the ICF domain activity with a 14-item objective measure designed to assess static balance and fall risk. This takes 10–15 minutes to administer, is free except for the cost of the equipment such as a stopwatch, step stool, and chair with arm rests in adult populations (reference will be helpful).[16–18]
3. *Tinetti performance-oriented mobility assessment*: It measures an older adult's gait and balance abilities including fall risk (reference will be helpful). This takes 10–15 minutes to administer, is free, and assesses the ICF domain activity.[19]

4. *Dynamic gait index (DGI)*: It measures an individual's ability to modify balance while walking in the presence of external demands. The DGI takes less than 10 minutes to administer, is free, and assesses the ICF domain activity (reference will be helpful).[20,21]

5. *Functional gait assessment (FGA)*: It assesses postural stability during various walking tasks (reference will be helpful). The FGA takes less than 10 minutes to administer, is free, and assesses the ICF domain activity.[22–24]

6. *Four step square test (FFST)*: The FFST takes less than 5 minutes to administer, is free, and assesses the ICF domain activity. It is a test of dynamic balance that clinically assesses the person's ability to step over objects forward, sideways, and backwards (reference will be helpful).[25–27]

7. *Tinetti falls efficacy scale (TFES)*: It assesses the perception of balance and stability during ADLs; and the fear of falling in the elderly population (reference will be helpful). The TFES takes 10–15 minutes to administer, is free, and assesses the ICF domains of activity and participation.[28,29]

8. *Functional reach test (FRT)*: It assesses the patient's stability by measuring the maximum distance an individual can reach forward while standing in a fixed position (reference will be helpful). The modified version of the FRT requires the individual to sit in a fixed position. The FRT takes 5 minutes or less to administer, is free, and assesses the ICF domain of activity.[30]

4.3.3 POLYPHARMACY

Twenty percent of Medicare beneficiaries have five or more chronic conditions and 50% receive five or more medications.[31] This is of particular concern in the elderly because it sets the stage for drug–drug interactions and adverse effects in the context of age-related changes and multiple medically complex comorbidities, which are common in this population. This is worsened by other factors such as the geriatric syndromes of decreased sensory perception, decreased nutrition, and cognitive impairments. While overprescribing is a concern, undertreatment with appropriate medication is also an issue, as in the case of managing pain. There is often confusion on the part of providers and caregivers as to whether changes in clinical status, particularly cognition are due to pain medication, such as narcotics versus the pain itself. Therefore, appropriate management of the elderly entails judicious and also adequate use of appropriate and necessary medications. Several indices are used as assessment tools or instruments to avoid polypharmacy and they are as follows:

1. Beers criteria[32–34] are used to improve the awareness of and clinical outcomes for older adults with polypharmacy and at risk of adverse drug events (ADEs). They are explicit, and therefore have simple application and wide dissemination, and can be easily integrated into an electronic health record (EHR). EHRs are equipped to send providers instant feedback with suggested alternatives when a drug on the list of drugs to avoid or use-with-caution is prescribed in a particular care setting. Implicit criteria may include factors such as therapeutic duplication and drug–drug interactions. Beers criteria are not suitable for all situations, and must be applied properly. They should not be used in a punitive manner or to make financial decisions about Medicare Part D drugs, because these situations do not consider the individual or the clinician's best judgment, particularly with certain populations, such as individuals near the end of life. Judicious application of the criteria allows closer monitoring of medications, real-time e-prescribing and interventions to decrease ADEs in the elderly, leading to better patient outcomes.

2. Medication Appropriateness Index gives implicit criteria, to guide the tailoring of medications to the individual patient, but this can be relatively difficult and time consuming to implement compared with Beer's criteria.[32–34]

3. The Screening Tool of Older Persons potentially inappropriate Prescriptions and Screening Tool to Alert doctors to the Right Treatment (STOPP/START criteria)[35] version 2 is a screening tool with a broader application. This was created by a consensus panel of experts in the field of pharmacotherapy of older people, which was selected from 14 European, including two from the Netherlands. They are crucial to improving the health of older adults as they are organized according to the physiological systems and include clinical stopping rules. As they cover some areas that the AGS Beers criteria do not, in spite of an overlap with the Beers, they are to be used in a complementary manner.

Studies[36,37] have found that a small number of medications are responsible for most ADEs in older adults. In a recent study[38], four medications or medication classes (anticoagulants, insulin, oral antiplatelet agents, and oral hypoglycemic agents) were associated with most ADEs.

4. FORTA (Fit FOR The Aged)[39,40] which has a consensus validation from a panel of geriatricians, rates medications into four categories based on the individual patient's indication for the medication. These are the following:
   a. Clear benefit
   b. Proven but limited efficacy or some safety concerns
   c. Questionable efficacy or safety profile—consider alternative
   d. Clearly avoid and find alternative[39,40]
5. Assessing Care of Vulnerable Elders (ACOVE) project recommends the documentation of the indication for a new drug therapy, current medication lists, patient education on the risk profile of new medication, monitoring response to therapy, and periodical reviewing of the ongoing need to continue medication management.[41]

4.3.4 SENSORY PERCEPTION

4.3.4.1 Dizziness

Dizziness refers to various abnormal sensations of body orientation in space, which are difficult to describe. Dizziness is multifactorial, with medications contributing to other causes.[42,43] The prevalence of dizziness in the community is more than 30% among the elderly, compared with 1.8% in young adults. It has four subtypes

1. Vertigo is an episodic spinning or rotational sensation from a vestibular disorder.
2. Disequilibrium is a feeling of imbalance or unsteadiness from visual, proprioceptive compromise, with or without a vestibular component.
3. Presyncope results from cardiovascular causes such as orthostatic hypotension.
4. Atypical dizziness, the most common type of dizziness, has features and etiologies of more than one of the above. Another etiology is medications, such as antianxiety drugs, antidepressants, anticonvulsants, antipsychotics, antihypertensives, and anticholinergics.

Studies[42–44] on diagnosing dizziness have been conducted in highly selected homogeneous groups of patients only.

Measurement tools include the following:

1. *Head impulse test (HIT/head thrust test [HTT])*[42]: The HIT is done with the examiner abruptly accelerating and then decelerating the head, moving the head rapidly at high speed and then stopping. A positive test result is diagnostic of peripheral vestibular dysfunction and a negative test result is diagnostic of central peripheral dysfunction. The HIT takes 1 minute to administer, is free, and assesses the ICF domains body structure and body function.

2. *Dix–Hallpike maneuver*[45]: This test takes less than 5 minutes, is free, and assesses the ICF domain body structure. It is used to diagnose benign paroxysmal positional vertigo (BPPV) of the posterior semicircular canal.[45]
3. *Dizziness handicap inventory (DHI/DHI-S)*[46]: It is a 25-item self-assessment inventory designed to evaluate the self-perceived handicapping effects imposed by dizziness. This takes 10 minutes to administer, is copyrighted by the American Medical Association (AMA), available on multiple sites, and assesses the ICF domains body structure, body function, and participation.
4. Clinical test of sensory interaction and balance (CTSIB); modified clinical test of sensory interaction and balance (mCTSIB).[47,48]

The mCTSIB takes less than 10 minutes to administer, is free, and assesses the ICF domain activity by evaluating the patient's balance under a variety of conditions to infer the source of instability. The mCTSIB provides the clinician with a means to quantify postural control under various sensory conditions. The CTSIB additionally uses the visual conflict dome, takes 20–30 minutes to administer, and measures the ICF domains of body function and activity.

4.3.4.2 Hearing

Hearing loss in the older adult affects physical, social, and cognitive health. Risk factors for hearing loss include increasing age, history of exposure to loud noises or ototoxic agents, including occupational exposures, previous recurrent inner ear infections, genetic factors, and certain systemic diseases, such as diabetes. In all, 20%–40% of older adults over 50 years and 80% of elderly over 80 years have hearing loss. However, only 20% of them are screened routinely and only 32% of persons with moderate to marked hearing loss use a hearing aid.[3] The most common type of hearing loss in the elderly is presbycusis, which is a progressive high-frequency hearing loss, which also decreases the ability to interpret speech, leading to inability to communicate, and subsequent social isolation and depression.

The USPSTF concludes that the current evidence is insufficient to assess the balance of benefits and harms of screening for hearing loss in asymptomatic adults aged 50 years or older. However, persons seeking evaluation for perceived hearing problems or for cognitive or affective symptoms that may be related to hearing loss should be assessed for objective hearing impairment and treated when indicated.[49]

Measurement tools:

The USPSTF recommends the following screening tests for hearing:

1. Whispered voice test
2. Finger rub test
3. Watch tick test
4. Single-item screening (e.g., asking "Do you have difficulty with your hearing?")
5. Multiple-item patient questionnaire (Hearing Handicap Inventory for the Elderly-Screening [HHIE-S])
6. Handheld audiometer

The reference standard for establishing hearing impairment is pure tone audiometry, which can be combined with questionnaires such as the HHIE-S version to improve screening effectiveness.[3]

4.3.4.3 Vision

Prevalence of vision impairment increases with age and ranges from 1% in persons aged 65–69 years to 17% in persons older than 80 years,[3] with uncorrected refractive errors, cataracts, and age-related macular degeneration being the most common causes. In a 2009 update, USPSTF defined impaired visual acuity as best-corrected vision worse than 20/40 but better than 20/200, the threshold for legal blindness.[50]

Since older adults may not perceive sensory deficits as a problem and may not modify activity to adapt to sensory deficits, they are at an increased risk of falls. Vision remains a subjective measurement. The USPSTF is in the process of updating its recommendations on screening elderly for vision, and is open to comments to date. As per the 2009 update, the recommendation is for a visual acuity test (Snellen eye chart) as the usual method for screening for visual acuity impairment in the primary care setting. The conclusion is that screening questions are not as accurate as visual acuity testing for identifying visual acuity impairment.

4.3.5 Mental Status (Cognition and Mood)

The main cognitive disorders in the elderly are dementia, depression, and delirium.

Dementia is chronic and progressive. It is characterized by the gradual onset of impaired memory and deficits in two or more areas of cognition, such as anomia, agnosia, or apraxia, with no alteration of consciousness and no underlying medical cause to explain the deficits.

Amnestic mild cognitive impairment (MCI) is an early stage of Alzheimer's dementia (AD) in which there is limited anterograde long-term memory impairment, with preserved function. In AD, memory impairment occurs first, followed by decline in language and visuospatial skills relatively early in the disease. Deficits in executive function and behavioral or neuropsychiatric symptoms, such as apathy, isolation, agitation, psychosis, and wandering are indicative of advanced AD.[51]

Depression as opposed to dementia, has a relatively rapid onset, may or may not be associated with decreased cognition and generally has time-limited duration. It significantly increases both morbidity and mortality.

Delirium is characterized by acute onset of increased confusion and fluctuating course, with disorganized thinking, inattention, and altered level of consciousness.

Delirium can lead to long-term cognitive impairment. Delirium being fatal, the safest clinical approach is to consider all confusion as delirium until proven otherwise.

Delirium and dementia are each a risk factor to the other. There is thought[52] that delirium may unmask previous dementia or initiate a process of cognitive decline. It is difficult to diagnose delirium from Lewy-body dementia because of common features such as hallucinations and a fluctuating course.[52] Cognitive assessments should include history and a search for delirium precipitants such as medical disease including infections and drug interactions because precipitants to delirium may be occult or atypical.[53]

Measurement tools:

1. *Mini-mental state examination (MMSE)*[54]: MMSE-1 is freely available on the Internet. The current version of the MMSE (MMSE-2) is owned by Psychological Assessment Resources (PAR). MMSE provides a quantitative assessment of cognitive impairment and is used to record cognitive changes over time.
2. *Clock drawing test (CDT)*[55]: CDT takes 1–2 minutes to administer, is free, addresses the ICF domain of body function, and assesses visuospatial and praxis abilities (may reflect both attention and executive dysfunction).
3. *Montreal Cognitive Assessment (MOCA)*[56]: It is a rapid screen of cognitive abilities designed to detect mild cognitive dysfunction.
4. *Geriatric depression scale (GDS)*[57]: The GDS takes 5–10 minutes to administer and is free. It avoids issues related to physical symptoms and asks questions requiring only a "yes" or "no" answer. It assesses depression and suicide ideation in elderly individuals.
5. *Patient health questionnaire (PHQ-9)*[58]: The PHQ-9 takes 1–3 minutes to administer, is free, and assesses the presence and intensity of depressive symptoms. The PHQ 9 was designed to diagnose both the presence of depressive symptoms as well as to characterize the severity of depression.

6. *Yale depression screen*[3]: This is a one-question screen, which asks, "Do you often feel sad or depressed?" It is an effective screening tool when time is limited. An assessment for suicide risk is important in geriatric patients who appear depressed. The best way to accomplish this is to ask direct, but nonthreatening questions by beginning with asking patients if they are concerned that they are becoming a burden to their family and if they have ever felt that their family might be better off without them. This is followed by questions about active suicidal ideation.

7. *Hospital anxiety and depression scale (HADS)*[59] The HADS takes 2–6 minutes to administer, requires no training, and is not free. It is a two-dimension scale developed to identify depression and anxiety among physically ill patients. A validation study suggests that the HADS should be used only for screening and not as a case identifier of depression or other psychiatric disorders.

8. *Cornell scale for depression in dementia*: An alternative to patient testing for dementia is a structured family report using the Informant Questionnaire on Cognitive Decline in the Elderly (IQCDE),[60] which, unlike the MMSE, is not affected by a patient's educational level or premorbid intelligence. Combining these tools can increase the sensitivity of the screening process and identify additional patients in the early stages of dementia.

9. A shortened version of the mini-mental state (MMSE) that includes only the recall of three words and the orientation to month, year, and address is a valid and time-efficient assessment tool.[61]

4.3.6 NUTRITION

Nutritional problems occur in the elderly due to physiological changes and the presence of medical disease, including psychiatric disorders, use of medications, social, and environmental factors.[62,63] Medications cause anorexia or can reduce nutrient availability in older adults.

Physiological factors leading to anorexia include the following:

1. Age-related decrease in taste and smell sensitivity
2. Delayed gastric emptying
3. Early satiety
4. Impairment in the regulation of food intake

As defined by the Omnibus Budget Reconciliation Act (OBRA) of 1987, nursing home residents in the United States are considered to have meaningful weight loss if they lost 5% of usual body weight in 30 days or 10% in 6 months.[62,63]

Lean body mass, that is, muscle mass, is inversely related to mortality risk in older adults. It is best to avoid therapeutic diets unless there is evidence as basis for their clinical value. Appetite stimulants have not been shown to improve long-term survival and their adverse effects must be considered before prescribing them. Malnutrition in older adults spans a wide range, from undernutrition to overnutrition. Age-related changes in physiology, metabolism, and function can alter older adults' nutritional requirements, and therefore their recommended daily intake (RDI). Owing of this, nutritional screening, assessment, and interventions are required to improve the health, well-being, QOL, and independence in older adults.

Serum albumin is used as a risk indicator and prognosticator to determine malnutrition; however, hypoalbuminemia is not sensitive or specific to malnutrition as albumin is an acute-phase reactant. Serum prealbumin is a more sensitive indicator of short-term changes in nutrition, than albumin because it has a shorter half-life and is present in the body in smaller amounts.

Measurement tools:

1. *Simplified nutrition assessment questionnaire (SNAQ)*[64]: This is a four-item screening tool. The SNAQ (pronounced snack) takes less than 2 minutes to administer. This test is to detect and treat malnutrition in hospitalized patients.
2. *Seniors in the community: risk evaluation for eating and nutrition (SCREEN II)*: This is a valid and reliable 17-item tool for nutritional risk assessment of seniors in the community.[65]
3. *Malnutrition universal screening tool (MUST)*[66]: MUST assesses body mass index (BMI), weight loss in 3–6 months, and acute disease. It is administered in community settings, and is easier to use than the mini nutritional assessment (MNA).
4. *DETERMINE*[67,68]: DETERMINE is a nine-item checklist, which is developed by the USA Nutrition Screening Initiative (NSI). It is general and nonspecific and has a high false positive rate. The RENAL DETERMINE helps assess nutritional risk among renal patients. DETERMINE is a screening tool, which also helps increase nutritional risk awareness. DETERMINE is a mnemonic for the questions the tool asks:

   Disease, eating poorly, tooth loss/mouth pain, economic hardship, reduced social contact, multiple medications, involuntary weight loss/gain, needs assistance in self-care and elder years > age 80 years.
5. *MNA*[69–71]: The MNA is a global assessment and subjective perception of health. It is a valid tool, which is clinician administered, takes 10–15 minutes to use, and has a role in the community, hospital, and LTC settings.

4.3.7 CONTINENCE

The prevalence of incontinence is 11%–34% in elderly men and 17%–55% in elderly women.[3] Overall prevalence is 15%–30% in adults greater than and equal to 65 years old. Fortunately, this is frequently reversible without which there are significant social and emotional consequences, which paradoxically is the reason relatively few patients volunteer to seek treatment. Types of incontinence are the following:

1. Urge incontinence, which occurs with urgency to void, seen commonly in men and women.
2. Stress incontinence where leakage is associated with coughing, sneezing, laughing, and physical activity; second most common form in women and occurs in men after prostatectomy.
3. Mixed incontinence where leakage occurs with both urgency and activity; common in women.
4. Urinary incontinence from incomplete emptying is associated with increased postvoiding residual (PVR, generally 200 mL) and intermittent small dribbling. It is a relatively uncommon condition compared with the other types. A combination of both urge incontinence and increased PVR occurs in detrusor hyperactivity with impaired contractility (DHIC) in the frail elderly without bladder outlet obstruction.

Urinary incontinence leads to poor QOL, increased caregiver burden, sexual dysfunction due to coital incontinence, and infections leading to greater morbidity with an increased risk of falls.[72]

The first step in screening for urinary incontinence is to ask if the individual is experiencing any problems. Two simple questions are (a) if the individual ever loses urine without wanting to and (b) if urine was lost on at least six separate days. A positive screen is when the answer is yes to both the questions, which needs further evaluation. Next question to ask is if urine is lost when the person coughs, exercises, lifts, sneezes, or laughs.[73] Since urinary incontinence needs a multifactorial management and can have a multifactorial etiology, cognitive function, fluid intake, mobility, medication side effects and previous urologic surgeries must all be considered during its assessment. The physical examination should focus on the lower genitourinary tract in women and the prostate gland in men with a rectal examination for fecal impaction, and a urinalysis to screen for infection or glycosuria.[3]

Measurement tool:

1. International consultation on incontinence questionnaire-short form (ICIQ-SF)[74,75]

The ICIQ-SF takes less than 5 minutes to administer, is free, and assesses the ICF domain body function. It is a subjective measure of severity of urinary loss and QOL for those with urinary incontinence. It has been used in primary stress urinary incontinence in women (primary stress urinary incontinence [SUI] describes someone who has not had a surgical procedure for their incontinence), and in men undergoing a perineal sling procedure for stress urinary incontinence after treatment for prostate cancer.

4.3.8 PRESSURE SORES

Pressure ulcers, which affect one million adults in the United States, are caused due to pressure and shear forces leading to tissue compression between a bony prominence and an external surface over time. Pressure ulcers are an important national health issue in LTC, are a primary marker of quality in this setting, and are monitored throughout the continuum of care. Centers for Medicare and Medicaid Services (CMS) currently do not pay for hospital-acquired stage III and IV pressure ulcers. As they are debilitating to the elderly and cause the loss of independent living due to the care that they entail, clinicians are expected to be aggressive in their prevention and treatment.

Measurement tools:

1. *Pressure ulcer scale for healing (PUSH)*[76,77]: The PUSH tool takes 20–30 minutes to administer, is free, assesses the ICF domain body structure, and measures the change in pressure ulcer status over time, including size, the amount of exudate, and tissue type.
2. *Braden scale (pressure ulcer)*[78]: The Braden scale takes 20–30 minutes to administer, is free, addresses the ICF domain body structure, and assesses the likelihood of the individual developing pressure ulcers.

4.3.9 PAIN

Older adults are likely to minimize pain. They may not report pain due to language or cognitive impairments. Persistent pain is often undertreated because of provider's hesitation to administer adequate analgesics due to the fear of causing or worsening the patient's cognition. Pain-related behaviors that are important clues to the presence of pain are resistance to giving a history, withdrawal, and inappropriate, combative, abusive, and disruptive behaviors.[79–81]

Measurement tools:

1. *West Haven-Yale Multidimensional Pain Inventory*[82]: This is recommended for use with behavioral and psychophysiological strategies, assesses chronic pain in individuals, takes 31–60 minutes to administer, is free of cost, and requires no training to administer.
2. *McGill pain questionnaire*[83]: This is a self-reported measure of pain, takes 30 minutes to administer, is free, requires no training, and assesses the ICF domain of body function.

4.3.10 IMMUNIZATIONS

A 1990 report[84] indicated that fewer than 30% of adults had received updated tetanus–diphtheria (Td), influenza, and pneumococcal immunizations. The poor compliance rate was determined to be due to patients' concerns about adverse reactions to immunizations and physicians' overlooking the need for immunizations. However, recently, the rates of immunization have improved, with data from the Centers for Disease Control and Prevention (CDC) that the 1997 rates for influenza and pneumococcal vaccinations were 65.5% and 45.5%, respectively. The USPSTF recommendation is for an annual influenza vaccination in the fall for all elderly patients, and at least one pneumococcal vaccination in the lifetime of patients over 65 years, with high-risk patients receiving a second pneumococcal vaccine in 6 years. The Td toxoid vaccine is recommended to be given every 10 years, and again after 5 years if the patient suffers a wound.

4.3.11   SEXUALITY

The estimated proportions of men and women 60 years and over who are sexually active are 73.8% for married men and 55.8% for married women; among unmarried men and women, the proportions are 31.1% and 5.3%, respectively.[3,85] The levels decrease significantly with age in both genders. Of these, 35.3% of married men are estimated to have erectile impotence. Decreased mobility and lack of sexual activity are interrelated in both genders. Impotency is associated with a history of myocardial infarction, urinary incontinence, and use of sedatives. Other problems that cause a decline in sexual function in older adults are arthritis, diabetes, fatigue, fear of precipitating a myocardial infarction, alcohol, prescription drugs, and over-the-counter medications. The physician must initiate discussions about sexuality with open and direct questions. The elderly must be treated as normal sexual persons. Problems in enjoying sexual relations are not to be considered to be due to normal aging.

Measurement tool: Sexual interest and satisfaction scale (SIS)[85]—The SIS measures sexual adjustment after spinal cord injury (SCI). The SIS is designed to assess sexuality and sexual function before and after the injury in two domains: interest and satisfaction. It takes 5 minutes or less to administer, requires no training, is free, and assesses the ICF domain function.

4.3.12   FRAILTY ASSESSMENT

Frailty is a clinical syndrome, which is at the core of geriatric rehabilitation because it predisposes elderly to stressors. Frailty occurs due to altered genetic and cellular processes, which result in dysregulation of physiological mechanisms leading to disease at a critical threshold. Frailty is diagnosed when three of more of the following criteria are met:

1. Weight loss of greater than 10 pounds in 1 year
2. Slowed gait (tested as time to walk 15 feet based on gender and height)
3. Exhaustion (self-reported)
4. Low activity level (expenditure <270 kcal per week)
5. Weakness, measured by grip strength with a hand dynamometer

Measurement tool: Fatigue severity scale[86]—This is a nine-item scale, which has been studied in the elderly. It measures the severity of fatigue and its effect on a person's activities and lifestyle in patients with a variety of disorders. It takes 5 minutes or less to administer, requires no training, is free of cost, and measures the ICF domains activity and participation.

4.3.13   SOCIAL ISSUES (ELDER ABUSE AND ADVANCE DIRECTIVES)

Multiple social aspects, sedatives, living arrangements, finances, and activities influence functional ability, and therefore independent living in the elderly. This information is important to obtain during geriatric assessment from the patient and caregivers to determine the availability of support systems, and to make support accessible to them. Care must be provided with the patients' and the caregivers' goals in mind. Advance directives, living will, and durable power of attorney must be discussed at geriatric assessment. USPSTF recommends training family members of geriatric patients in cardiopulmonary resuscitation.

Measurement tools:

1. *WHO Quality of Life-BREF (WHOQOL-BREF)*[87]: WHOQOL-BREF assesses QOL within the context of an individual's culture, value systems, personal goals, standards, and concerns. It takes 6–30 minutes to administer, requires no training, is free of cost, and measures the ICF domains, activity, participation, and environment.
2. *London handicap scale (LHS)*[88]: The LHS measures health status in patients with chronic, multiple, or progressive diseases, including evaluation of interventions deployed in their treatment. It takes 5 minutes or less to administer, requires no training, is free of cost, and measures the ICF domain participation.
3. *Participation measure for postacute care (PM-PAC)*[89]: The PM-PAC assesses participation outcomes in outpatient or in home-care settings based on the ICF classification scheme. It takes 15 minutes to administer, requires no training, is free of cost, and measures the ICF domain participation.
4. *Medical Outcomes Study Short Form 36 (SF 36)*[90]: It is used commonly to assess QOL, includes 36 items in eight domains: physical function, role limitations due to physical and emotional health, bodily pain, social functioning, mental health, vitality, and general health perceptions. It has been tested extensively in community-living adults and hospitalized patients. But because it is insensitive to important changes in clinical status, it is not recommended for the frail elderly.
   The SF-36 takes 10 minutes to administer, is available for purchase at SF-36.org, and measures the ICF domains of body function, activity, and participation.
5. One recent study indicated that short-term memory and orientation are the domains most closely associated with ADL dependence; therefore, making the short form of the MMSE an effective tool with testing only the recall of three words and the orientation to month, year, and address.[3,61]

The FIM in acute inpatient rehabilitation and the MDS 3.0 in subacute rehabilitation are among the PAC measurement tools[91], which measure the individual's function as it relates to ADLs, mobility, and social and environmental factors. These are covered in Chapter 27.

4.4   SECTION C: PERFORMANCE MEASURES/METRICS

The required performance measures of a provider or a healthcare system are compared against local and national benchmarks. Performance is measured as a ratio. For example, a metric can capture the percentage of patients who were screened for falls in comparison to the number of patients who were eligible or needed fall screening. *Safety* is achieved by reducing errors to provide patients with "freedom from accidental injury." *Error* is the failure of a planned action to be completed as intended or the use of a wrong plan. Reliability means consistency of processes. Transparency supports safety by making the reliability of organizations visible by offering comparisons through public reporting of performance measures.

Since performance metrics transform healthcare quality by measuring the outcomes of quality improvement methods with data-driven processes, they entail collaborative involvement of multiple stakeholders including patients, provider organizations, payers, consumer representatives, and communities. Current metrics necessitate a multidisciplinary approach with physicians, nurses, therapists, nutritionists, pharmacists, case managers, and all categories of clinicians and nonclinicians in organizations.

Performance measurement started in 1998 with the Joint Commission's (JCH) ORYX initiative (A proprietary methodology that enables standardized outcome and performance measurement for healthcare organizations; established by the Joint Commission on Accreditation of Healthcare Organizations [JCAHO].), the first national program to measure hospital quality. Subsequent to this, a study of 4000 hospitals from 2004 to 2008, published in the *Journal of Hospital Medicine* in 2011, showed that JCH accredited hospitals outperformed nonaccredited hospitals in nationally standardized quality measures like heart failure and pneumonia. However, interpretation of this data led to the question as to whether accreditation signifies higher and improved quality or if it also increases the value of care provided. That performance measurement increases value of care is now an important consideration because developing these measures is a complex and expensive process.

Current thought is that "accountability" measures achieve the goal of maximizing health benefits to patients, improving quality, and also the value of care, because they must be vetted with strict criteria[92,93]:

1. *Research*: There must be randomized controlled trials and more than one study providing scientific evidence to demonstrate that a given process of care improves healthcare outcomes (either directly or by reducing the risk of adverse outcomes).
2. *Proximity*: The process being measured must be connected to the outcome it impacts.
3. *Accuracy*: The measure should be able to assess whether an evidence-based process is effectively delivered for improvement to occur.
4. *Adverse effects*: The measure should minimize or eliminate unintended adverse effects.

Though outcomes are central to assessing quality, we have more process measures today.

Modern day health delivery systems take into account patient safety, care coordination, high reliability, and team management. When these newer variables are taken into account, measures of quality[94] are as follows:

1. Evidence-based medicine (structure)
2. Process improvement and decision support (process)
3. Outcomes management (outcome)
4. Access
5. Patient experience

The Annual National Healthcare Quality Report (NHQR) released in May of 2014[95] reported that 70% of recommended care has wide variations amongst different states. Several important dimensions of quality are not currently being measured. These dimensions pertaining to rehabilitation medicine that need measure development include, but are not limited to, pain reduction and functional improvement in patients undergoing orthopedic surgery and functional decline in multiple sclerosis patients. The NHQR report found that over 4 years, while the quality of hospital care is improving, the quality of ambulatory care is slow to improve. Therefore, developing new measures, which add value and maximize patient benefits is critical, even as older measures with lesser utility and accountability are being discontinued.

Today, higher cost of care is also associated with poorer quality of care. However, it is imperative to be aware that improvement in value cannot be done by cost containment alone. A cultural change involving innovation and accountability is critical to improving value in healthcare delivery, which is possible with performance measurement because of the transparency involved in reporting measures. The principles of performance measurement are in the lines of Six Sigma's cycle of define, measure, analyze, improve, and control (DMAIC), known to other industries.[96] DMAIC and Lean Management principles are used best with a cultural change across healthcare in order to share organized information for patient safety.

Measure development: Measure development is an expensive process because measures have an intricate life cycle. It needs financial, human, technological, and educational environments over long time lines to reduce variation in care delivery between different states and locally within states.

For example, the life cycle of a measure by the National Quality Forum which sets priorities for performance measurement is as follows[97]:

1. Researching and accumulating evidence-based data on disease prevalence
2. Using assessment tools to study disease severity

3. Creating local initiatives to measure quality improvement with newer processes, by measure testing various practice settings (e.g., testing ambulatory measures in solo to large-sized practices)
4. Making changes leading to improvement locally
5. Public reporting on local performance
6. Endorsing the measure as a National Consensus Standard
7. Retooling the measure for use in EHRs
8. Inclusion in CMS's Meaningful Use program so that the measure adoption is widespread and leads to improvement in patient care.

As measures are complex and expensive to develop, the current focus is explicitly on measures maximizing health benefits to patients, which includes replacing poorly performing measures with better ones for use in national transparency and payment programs. Measures are tested by different agencies before they are vetted.

The AMA, JCAHO, and the National Committee for Quality Assurance (NCQA) have a consensus on what a performance measure must achieve. According to their consensus, the measure must address a topic of high priority which is also financially important, demonstrate improvement, and improve patient outcomes; while having well-defined specifications, documented reliability and validity, and allowing risk while being feasible, confidential, and publicly available.

The AMA's Physician's Consortium for Process Improvement (PCPI) is one of several agencies which test measures. It tests the six areas of needs assessment, feasibility and implementation, reliability, validity, unintended consequences, and applications.

A challenge in the use of measures which are all publicly reported is that they are collected in databases or registries linked to EHRs across providers, but they must be reported with transparency while still preserving patient privacy. This becomes more complex when there are multiple stakeholders and cross-cutting measures; therefore, entailing training and monitoring of providers.[98]

Performance measures are used as follows:

1. *Improve hospital performance*: Many measures are robust, with excellent evidence basis to link process, performance, and patient outcomes. This has resulted in improved performance of hospitals. For example, in 2009, a total of 98.3% of eligible patients with acute myocardial infarction received a beta-blocker at hospital discharge, as compared with 87.3% of such patients in 2002.[99]
2. *Link quality to reimbursement*: Performance metrics are used to incentivize providers, individuals, organizations, and health plans to improve quality through accountability, to achieve the Institute of Medicine (IOM) six aims[99] of safety, timeliness, effectiveness, equity, efficiency, and patient centeredness.
3. *Align providers to the National Quality Strategy's (NQS) six priorities*:
   a. Safer care by reducing harm in the delivery of care
   b. Engaging each person and family in their own care
   c. Promoting effective communication and coordination of care
   d. Promoting the most effective prevention and treatment of the leading causes of mortality, starting with cardiovascular disease
   e. Promoting wide use of best practices to enable healthy living in communities
   f. Developing and spreading new healthcare delivery models for affordable quality care for individuals, families, employers, and governments
4. *Identify priorities*: Highly vetted accountability measures have transformed passive payers and consumers into buyers of efficient high-quality healthcare, that is, value-based purchasing (VBP). Value equates quality or outcomes/cost of episode of care (not individual services).[100] Measuring value in the context of improvement with performance metrics allows decisions on which healthcare services need more spending and which ones need reduction.

5. *Identify priorities with risk adjustment*[101]: Providers and organizations serve patients with risk factors which are patient characteristics, such as age, gender, race, admitting diagnoses, socioeconomic status, education, social support, substance use, comorbidities, communities, etc., which create a statistically significant level of variance. The problem with this variance is that it is an impediment to make valid comparisons between providers and organizations. Risk-adjusted measures use a large reference population to compute the weight of each risk factor that affects any given outcome, with statistical testing comparing specific predicted versus actually observed differences in performance and outcomes to determine if these variations are random or significant. Such a specific level of standardization helps in identifying priorities in performance improvement.

6. *Provide evidence-based data, which all clinicians relate to*: This aligns multidisciplinary teams when they jointly review evidence-based data that performance metrics provide to meet a common goal of improving clinical processes.

7. *Provide decision support*: Performance metrics gathered over time become clinical intelligence, which is particularly important in the management of chronic diseases. The future of a national network of such intelligence can be envisioned, because of enterprise resource planning (ERP) which integrates databases. When linked, databases make it possible to share information across points of care, to individuals, organizations, populations, and currently local healthcare networks.[102]

8. Support pay-for-performance initiatives and accreditation in health plans by becoming a source for purchasers and payers to enforce quality while containing healthcare expenditure with VBP. Payers such as Medicare, WellPoint, and Aetna do differential reimbursement and determine accreditation of providers to their plans based on measurement and comparison.

9. *Support patient safety*: Health plan accreditation standards are used to ensure that they are performing on par with industry standards in quality by measuring their performance. Consumers use this data to compare plans and shop, while other purchasers like employers and state and federal regulators use this data for pay-for-performance. Agencies such as the NCQA, Utilization Review Accreditation Commission (URAC), and the Joint Commission (JC) rank insurance plans by using tools such as the Medicare Health Outcomes Survey (HOS) in which all managed care organizations holding Medicare Advantage contracts are required to enroll in. Health Effectiveness Data Information Set (HEDIS) and the Agency for Healthcare Research and Quality's (AHRQ) Consumer Assessment of Health Providers and Systems (CAHPS) are such tools. The Leapfrog group advocates for quality and safety in hospitals with transparency in pricing and reports on several performance measures, which compare hospitals with various indicators, including prevention of medication errors, appropriate ICU staffing, steps to avoid harm, managing serious errors, safety-focused scheduling, and hospital-acquired conditions. The peer-reviewed Hospital Safety Score methodology grades hospitals as A, B, C, D, or F based on how safe they are for patients by measuring infections, injuries, and medical and medication errors that frequently cause harm or death during a hospital stay. Performance metrics data from the CMS is available through its Hospital Compare website at www.hospitalcompare.hhs.gov.

Public reporting by CMS on nursing homes and measuring the performance of Home and Community-Based Services (HCBS) with linked financial incentives have been steps toward improving healthcare quality in the long-term and PAC arenas.

Physician performance metrics are gathered through Physician Quality Reporting System (PQRS), which are tied to financial incentives and penalties. The public reporting of performance metrics is a driver of healthcare quality because it encourages transparency and accountability. By tying in reimbursement to quality, the healthcare industry has made performance measurement the answer to making determinations on the delivery of healthcare today.

REFERENCES

1. Devons CA. Comprehensive geriatric assessment: Making the most of the aging years. *Current Opinion in Clinical Nutrition and Metabolic Care*. 2002;5(1):19.
2. Applegate WB, Miller ST, Graney MJ, Elam JT, Burns R, and Akins DE. A randomized, controlled trial of a geriatric assessment unit in a community rehabilitation hospital. *New England Journal of Medicine*. 1990;322:1572–1578.
3. Miller KE, Zylstra RG, and Standridge JB. The geriatric patient: A systematic approach to maintaining health. *American Family Physician*. 2000;61(4):1089–1104.
4. Reuben DB, Maly RC et al. Physician implementation of and patient adherence to recommendations from comprehensive geriatric assessment. *American Journal of Medicine*. 1996;100:444–451.
5. David SF, Brown AS et al. National Institutes of Health Consensus Development Conference statement: Geriatric assessment methods for clinical decision-making. *Journal of the American Geriatric Society*. 1988;36:342–347.
6. American Geriatrics Society (AGS)/British Geriatrics Society (BGS) Clinical Practice Guideline. Prevention of Falls in Older Persons, 2010. Available at http://geriatricscareonline.org/FullText/CL014/CL014_BOOK003.
7. Thomas JG. Fall Prevention in the Elderly. American Academy of Physical Medicine and Rehabilitation (AAPM&R) Knowledge Now. November 2011. Available at http://me.aapmr.org/kn/article.html?id=77.
8. Fuller GF. Falls in the elderly. *American Family Physician*. 2000;61(7):2159–2168.
9. US Preventive Services Task Force. Guide to Clinical Preventive Services: Report of the U.S. Preventive Services Task Force. 2nd edn. Baltimore, Maryland: Williams & Wilkins, 1996.
10. http://www.aapmr.org/research/evidence-based/Documents/QTB_OSTEO_6.02.pdf
11. Towards a Common Language for Functioning, Disability and Health, ICF. World Health Organization, Geneva, 2002. Available at http://www.who.int/classifications/icf/training/icfbeginnersguide.pdf.
12. http://www.rehabmeasure.org.
13. Lundin-Olsson L, Nyberg L et al. Attention, frailty, and falls: The effect of a manual task on basic mobility. *Journal of the American Geriatric Society*. 1998;46(6):758–761.
14. Maranhao-Filho PA, Maranhao ET et al. Rethinking the neurological examination II: Dynamic balance assessment. *Arq Neuropsiquiatr* 2001;69(6):959–963.
15. Rockwood K, Awalt E et al. Feasibility and measurement properties of the functional reach and the timed up and go tests in the Canadian study of health and aging. *Journals of Gerontology. Series A, Biological Sciences and Medical Sciences* 2000;55(2):M70–73.
16. Berg K, Wood-Dauphinee S et al. The Balance Scale: reliability assessment with elderly residents and patients with an acute stroke. *Scandanavian Journal of Rehabilitation Medicine* 1995;27(1):27–36.
17. Berg KO, Maki BE et al. Clinical and laboratory measures of postural balance in an elderly population. *Archives of Physical Medicine Rehabilitation* 1992;73(11):1073–1080.
18. Berg KO, Wood-Dauphinee SL et al. Measuring balance in the elderly: validation of an instrument. *Canadian Journal Public Health* 1992;83 Supplement 2:S7– S11.
19. Tinetti ME. Performance-oriented assessment of mobility problems in elderly patients. *Journal of the American Geriatric Society* 1986;34(2):119–126.
20. Chiu YP, Fritz SL et al. Use of item response analysis to investigate measurement properties and clinical validity of data for the dynamic gait index. *Physical Therapy* 2006;86(6):778–787.
21. Jonsdottir J and Cattaneo D. Reliability and validity of the dynamic gait index in persons with chronic stroke. *Archives of Physical Medicine and Rehabilitation* 2007;88(11):1410–1415.
22. Leddy AL, Crowner BE et al. Functional gait assessment and balance evaluation system test: Reliability, validity, sensitivity, and specificity for identifying individuals with Parkinson disease who fall. *Phys Ther* 2011;91(1):102–113.
23. Wrisley DM and Kumar NA. Functional gait assessment: Concurrent, discriminative, and predictive validity in community-dwelling older adults. *Physical Therapy* 2010;90(5):761–773.
24. Wrisley DM, Marchetti GF et al. Reliability, internal consistency, and validity of data obtained with the functional gait assessment. *Physical Therapy* 2004;84(10):906–918.
25. Dite W and Temple VA. A clinical test of stepping and change of direction to identify multiple falling older adults. *Arch Phys Med Rehabil* 2002;83(11):1566–1571.
26. Duncan RP and Earhart GM. Four square step test performance in people with parkinson disease. *Journal of Neurologic Physical Therapy* 2013;37(1):2–8.
27. Whitney SL, Marchetti GF et al. The reliability and validity of the four square step test for people with balance deficits secondary to a vestibular disorder. *Arch Phys Med Rehabil* 2007;88(1):99–104.

28. Huang TT and Wang WS. Comparison of three established measures of fear of falling in community-dwelling older adults: Psychometric testing. *International Journal of Nursing Studies* 2009;46(10):1313–1319.

29. Jorstad EC, Hauer K et al. Measuring the psychological outcomes of falling: A systematic review. *Journal of the American Geriatrics Society* 2005;53(3):501–510.

30. Rockwood K, Awalt E et al. Feasibility and measurement properties of the functional reach and the timed up and go tests in the Canadian study of health and aging. *Journals of Gerontology. Series A, Biological Sciences and Medical Sciences* 2000;55(2):M70–73.

31. Tinetti ME, Bogardus ST Jr, Agostini JV. Potential pitfalls of disease-specific guidelines for patients with multiple conditions. *New England Journal of Medicine* 2004;351(27):2870.

32. American Geriatrics Society Updated Beers Criteria for Potentially Inappropriate Medication Use in Older Adults. The American Geriatrics Society Updated 2012 Beers Criteria Update Expert Panel.

33. Fick D, Selma T. American geriatrics society beers criteria: New Year, new criteria, new perspective. *JAGS.* 2012;60(4):614–615.

34. Geller AI, Strasser D. Polypharmacy. American Academy of Physical Medicine and Rehabilitation (AAPM&R) Knowledge Now, December 2012. Available at http://me.aapmr.org/kn/article.html?id=93.

35. Knol W, Verduijn MM, Lelie-van der Zande AC, van Marum RJ, Brouwers JR van der Cammen TJ, Petrovic M, Jansen PA. Detecting inappropriate medication in older people: The revised STOPP/START criteria. *Ned Tijdschr Geneeskd.* 2015;159:A8904. [Article in Dutch]

36. Donna M and Semla TP 2012. American Geriatrics Society Beers Criteria: New Year, New Criteria, New Perspective.

37. Hamilton H, Gallagher P, Ryan C et al. Potentially inappropriate medications defined by STOPP criteria and the risk of adverse drug events in older hospitalized patients. *Archives of Internal Medicine* 2011;171:1013–1019.

38. Budnitz DS, Lovegrove MC, Shehab N, Richards CL. Emergency hospitalizations for adverse drug events in older americans. *N Engl J Med* 2011;365:2002-2012. doi: 10.1056/NEJMsa1103053.

39. Wehling M. Multimorbidity and polypharmacy: How to reduce the harmful drug load and yet add needed drugs in the elderly? Proposal of a new drug classification: Fit for the aged. *Journal of the American Geriatric Society* 2009;57(3):560–561.

40. Kuhn-Thiel AM, Weib C, Wehling M. Consensus validation of the FORTA (fit for the aged) list: A clinical tool for increasing the appropriateness of pharmacotherapy in the elderly. *Drugs Aging.* 2014;31(2):131–140.

41. Shrank WH, Polinski JM, Avorn J. Quality indicators for medication use in vulnerable elders. *Journal of the American Geriatric Society* 2007;55(Suppl 2):S373.

42. Dros J, Maarsingh OR, van der Horst HE, Bindels PJ, ter Riet G, and van Weert HC. Tests used to evaluate dizziness in primary care. *CMAJ.* 2010;182(13):E621–E631.

43. Sloane PD, Coeytaux RR et al. Dizziness: State of the science. *Annals of Internal Medicine* 2001;134(9 Pt 2):823–832.

44. Dros J, Maarsingh OR, van der Horst HE, Bindels PJ, ter Riet G, and van Weert HC. Tests used to evaluate dizziness in primary care. *CMAJ.* 2010;182(13):E621–E631.

45. Noda K, Ikusaka M et al. Predictors for benign paroxysmal positional vertigo with positive dix–hallpike test. *International Journal of General Medicine* 2011;4:809–814.

46. Gamiz MJ and Lopez-Escamez JA. Health-related quality of life in patients over sixty years old with benign paroxysmal positional vertigo. *Gerontology* 2004;50(2):82–86.

47. Suttanon P, Hill KD et al. Retest reliability of balance and mobility measurements in people with mild to moderate Alzheimer's disease. *International Psychogeriatrics* 2011;23(7):1152–1159.

48. Whitney SL and Wrisley DM. The influence of footwear on timed balance scores of the modified clinical test of sensory interaction and balance. *Archives of Physical Medicine and Rehabilitation* 2004;85(3):439–443.

49. http://www.uspreventiveservicestaskforce.org/Page/Document/RecommendationStatementFinal/hearing-loss-in-older-adults-screening#consider

50. http://www.uspreventiveservicestaskforce.org/Page/Document/RecommendationStatementFinal/impaired-visual-acuity-in-older-adults-screening1#consider

51. Kelley BJ and Petersen RC. Alzheimer's disease and mild cognitive impairment. *Neurological Clinics* 2007;25:577–609.

52. Fick DM, Agostini JV, and Inouye SK. Delirium superimposed on dementia: A systematic review. *Journal of the American Geriatrics Society* 2002;50:1723–1732.

53. Saxena DS. Dementia and Delirium. American Academy of Physical Medicine and Rehabilitation (AAPM R) Knowledge Now. 2013. Available at http://me.aapmr.org/kn/article.html?id=74

54. Tombaugh TN and McIntyre NJ. The mini-mental state examination: A comprehensive review. *Journal of the American Geriatrics Society.* 1992;40:922–935.

55. Adunsky A, Fleissig Y et al. Clock drawing task, mini-mental state examination and cognitive-functional independence measure: Relation to functional outcome of stroke patients. *Archives of Gerontological Geriatrics* 2002;35(2):153–160.

56. Nasreddine ZS, Phillips NA et al. The montreal cognitive assessment, MoCA: A brief screening tool for mild cognitive impairment. *Journal of the American Geriatrics Society* 2005;53(4):695–699.

57. Cheng ST, Yu EC et al. The geriatric depression scale as a screening tool for depression and suicide ideation: A replication and extension. *American Journal of Geriatric Psychiatry* 2010;18(3):256–265.

58. Gilbody S, Richards D et al. Screening for depression in medical settings with the patient health questionnaire (PHQ): A diagnostic meta-analysis. *Journal of General Internal Medicine* 2007;22(11):1596–1602.

59. Spinhoven P, Ormel J, Sloekers PP, Kempen GI, Speckens AE, and Van Hemert AM. A validation study of the hospital anxiety and depression scale (HADS) in different groups of dutch subjects. *Psychological Medicine* 1997;27(2):363–370.

60. Jorm AF and Jacomb PA. The informant questionnaire on cognitive decline in the elderly (IQCODE): Socio-demographic correlates, reliability, validity and some norms. *Psychological Medicine* 1989;19:1015–1020.

61. History Gill TM, Williams CS, Richardson ED, Berkman LF, and Tinetti ME. A predictive model for ADL dependence in community-living older adults based on a reduced set of cognitive status items. *Journal of the American Geriatrics Society* 1997;45:441–445.

62. Wilson MMG, Thomas DR, Rubenstein LZ, Chibnall JT, Anderson S, Baxi A, Diebold MR, and Morley JE. Appetite assessment: Simple appetite questionnaire predicts weight loss in community-dwelling adults and nursing home residents. *American Journal of Clinical Nutrition* 2005;82(5):1074–1081.

63. Morley JE and Thomas DR. *Geriatric Nutrition.* Boca Raton, FL: CRC Press, Taylor & Francis Group, 2007.

64. Kruizenqa HM, Seidell JC, de Vet HC, Wierdsma NJ, and Bokhorst-de van der Schueren MA. Development and validation of a hospital screening tool for malnutrition: The short nutritional assessment questionnaire (SNAQ). *Clinical Nutrition* 2005;24:75–82.

65. Keller HH1, Goy R, Kane SL. Validity and reliability of SCREEN II (seniors in the community: Risk evaluation for eating and nutrition, version II). *European Journal of Clinical Nutrition* 2005;59(10):1149–57.

66. Elia M. The MUST Report. *Nutritional Screening of Adults: A Multidisciplinary Responsibility.* Malnutrition Advisory Group (MAG). Redditch: BAPEN, 2003.

67. Report of Nutrition Screening I: Toward a Common View. Washington DC: Nutrition Screening Initiative; 1991. The Nutrition Screening Initiative, a project of the American Academy of Family Physicians, the American Dietetic Association, and the National Council on the Aging, Inc.

68. Posner BM, Jette AM, Smith KW, and Miller DR. Nutrition and health risks in the elderly: The nutrition screening initiative. *American Journal of Public Health* 1993;83(7):972–978. doi: 10.2105/AJPH.83.7.972.

69. MNA (actual tool). Available at http://www.mna-elderly.com/forms/mini/mna_mini_english.pdf

70. Rubenstein LZ, Harker JO, Salva A, Guigoz Y, and Vellas B. Screening for undernutrition in geriatric practice: Developing the Short-Form Mini Nutritional Assessment (MNA-SF). *Journals of Gerontology* 2001;56A:M366–M377.

71. Kaiser MJ, Bauer JM et al. Validation of the mini nutritional assessment short-form (MNA®-SF): A practical tool for identification of nutritional status. *Journal of Nutrition Health and Aging* 2009;13:782–788.

72. Brown JS, Vittinghoff E, Wyman JF, Stone KL, Nevitt MC, Ensrud KE, and Grady D. Urinary incontinence: Does it increase risk for falls and fractures? Study of Osteoporotic Fractures Research Group. *Journal of the American Geriatrics Society* 2000;48(7):721–725.

73. Goode PS, Burgio KL, and Richter HE. Incontinence in older women. *Journal of the American Medical Association (JAMA)* 2010;303(21):2172–2181.

74. Avery K, Donovan J et al. ICIQ: A brief and robust measure for evaluating the symptoms and impact of urinary incontinence. *Neurourological Urodynamics* 2004;23(4):322–330.

75. Ku JH, Jeong IG, Lim DJ, Byun SS, Paick JS, and Oh SJ. Voiding diary for the evaluation of urinary incontinence and lower urinary tract symptoms: Prospective assessment of patient compliance and burden. *Neurourological Urodynamics* 2004;23(4):331–335.

76. Berlowitz DR, Ratliff C et al. The PUSH tool: A survey to determine its perceived usefulness. *Advanced Skin Wound Care* 2005;18(9):480–483.

77. de Gouveia Santos VL, Sellmer D et al. Inter rater reliability of Pressure Ulcer Scale for Healing (PUSH) in patients with chronic leg ulcers. *Revista Latino-Americana de Enfermagem* 2007;15(3):391–396.

78. Bergquist S and Frantz R. Braden scale: Validity in community-based older adults receiving home health care. *Applied Nursing Research* 2001;14(1):36–43.

79. Miller KE, Zylstra RG, and Standridge JB. The geriatric patient: A systematic approach to maintaining health. *American Family Physician* 2000;61(4):1089–104.

80. American Geriatrics Society (AGS) Panel. The pharmacological management of persistent pain in older persons uideline. *JAGS.* 2009;57:1331–1346.(2009)

81. Saxena DS. History. In Geriatrics: RMQR (*Rehabilitation Medicine Quick Reference*). Buschbacher R, Means K, Kortebein P (eds). New York: Springer Publishing, 2012.

82. Kerns RD, Turk DC et al. The west haven-yale multidimensional pain inventory (WHYMPI). *Pain* 1985;23(4):345–356.

83. Dworkin RH, Turk DC et al. Development and initial validation of an expanded and revised version of the short-form McGill pain Questionnaire (SF-MPQ-2). *Pain* 2009;144(1–2):35–42.

84. Reese S, Owen P et al. Influenza and pneumococcal vaccination levels among adults aged > or = 65 years—United States, 1997. *Morbidity and Mortality Weekly Report (MMWR).* 1998;47:797–802.

85. Diokno AC, Brown MB, and Herzog AR. Sexual function in the elderly. *Archives of Internal Medicine* 1990;150:197–200.

86. Herlofson K and Larsen JP. The influence of fatigue on health-related quality of life in patients with parkinson's disease. *Acta Neurologica Scandinavica* 2003;107(1):1–6.

87. Bonomi A, Patrick D et al. Validation of the United States' version of the World Health Organization Quality of Life (WHOQOL) instrument. *Journal of Clinical Epidemiology* 2000;53(1):1–12.

88. Ackerley SJ, Gordon HJ et al. Assessment of quality of life and participation within an outpatient Rehabilitation setting. *Disability Rehabilitation* 2009;31(11):906–913.

89. Gandek B, Sinclair SJ et al. Development and initial psychometric evaluation of the participation measure for post-acute care (PM-PAC). *American Journal of Physical Medicine and Rehabilitation.* 2007;86(1):57–71.

90. McNaughton HK, Weatherall M et al. Functional measures across neurologic disease states: Analysis of factors in common. *Archives of Physical Medicine and Rehabilitation* 2005;86(11):2184–2188.

91. Granger CV, Hamilton BB et al. Advances in functional assessment for medical rehabilitation. *Topics in Geriatric Rehabilitation* 1986;1(3):59–74.

92. Saxena DS. Performance *Metrics. Braddom's Physical Medicine and Rehabilitations*, 5th edition. Philadelphia, PA: Elsevier, 2015.

93. Chassin MR, Loeb JM, Schmaltz SP and Wachter RM. Accountability measures—using measurement to promote quality improvement. *The New England Journal of Medicine* 2010;363:683–688. doi: 10.1056/NEJMsb1002320.

94. Granger CV (Chief Editor), Cailliet R. *Quality and Outcome Measures for Rehabilitation Programs.* Buffalo, NY: Medscape, 2015.

95. http://www.ahrq.gov/research/findings/nhqrdr/nhqdr14/index.html

96. Chassin M. Is health care ready for Six Sigma? *Milbank Quarterly* 1998;76(4):565–591.

97. National Quality Forum, Field Guide to NQF Resources. Available at http://www.qualityforum.org/Field_Guide/Infographics.aspx

98. Aspden P, Corrigan JM, Wolcott J, Erickson SM (Eds). *Committee on Data Standards for Patient Safety: Achieving a New Standard for Care*, 550 pages, Washington, DC: The National Academies Press, 2004. ISBN: 030909776.

99. Institute of Medicine. *Crossing the quality chasm: A new health system for the 21st Century.* Washington, DC: National Academies Press, 2001.

100. Porter ME. What is value in healthcare. New England Journal of Medicine 2010;363:2477–2481. doi: 10.1056/NEJMp1011024.

101. Mainz J. Methodology matters, defining and classifying clinical indicators for quality improvement, The National Indicator Project and University of Aarhus, Denmark. *International Journal for Quality in Health Care* 2003;15(6):523–530.

102. Diamond CC, F Mostasshari, Shirky C. Collecting and sharing data for population health: A new paradigm. *Health Affairs* 2009;28(2):454-466.

5 Pharmacology in Geriatric Rehabilitation

Kristin Meyer, Tina Thornhill, and Lindsey Garner

CONTENTS

5.1 INTRODUCTION

Geriatrics encompasses all aspects of aging including physiological, psychological, functional, social, and economical sequelae of advancing age. It is vitally important for the clinician to appreciate that *all* aspects of geriatrics can be impacted by medications. The safe and effective use of medications is a challenging balance for the healthcare practitioner, but is particularly more difficult when working with older adult patients. A disproportionate amount of medication use is seen in older adults when compared to their younger counterparts often leaving the physiatrist to unravel the complicated medication history. Moreover, trying to discern whether a new or long-standing symptom is a sign of a true physiological condition or whether it is a medication side effect becomes daunting. While evidence-based medicine is important, outcomes pertaining to senior care (e.g., function, independence, and cognitive impairment) are difficult to assess and measure in clinical research requiring the clinician to utilize general knowledge and expertise when prescribing many drugs in this population.

5.2 PHARMACOKINETICS

Pharmacokinetics, simply stated, is what the body does to the drug. Pharmacokinetics encompasses absorption, distribution, metabolism, and excretion (ADME), all of which are affected to varying extents by the normal aging process and various disease states commonly associated with advanced age. Changes in kidney function are frequently highlighted as being significant in older adults, but it is also important to consider changes in liver and gastrointestinal (GI) functions, as these can affect the results of certain medication choices. Age-related alterations in pharmacokinetics and the resultant potential effects on drug disposition are summarized in Table 5.1 and further discussed.

5.2.1 ABSORPTION

Of the four pharmacokinetic parameters, absorption seems to be the least affected by aging. Changes in the GI tract that occur with aging include reduction in blood flow, decreased gut motility, delayed gastric emptying, and decreased gastric acid production. There is some evidence that

TABLE 5.1
Pharmacokinetic Changes in the Elderly

Process	Pharmacokinetic Change	Effect on Drug Disposition
Absorption (oral)	Reduced intestinal blood flow	Altered absorption of drugs relying on gastric acidity for
	Decreased gut motility	dissolution may have
	Delayed gastric emptying	Increased absorption of some high hepatic extraction ratio
	Decreased gastric acid production	drugs
	Reduced first-pass metabolism	Decreased absorption of drugs from prodrugs
Distribution	Decreased albumin	Increased (free) serum levels of highly protein-bound drugs
	Increased alpha 1-glycoprotein	Decreased (free) serum levels of alpha 1-glycoprotein-bound
	Decreased total body water	drugs
	Increased adipose tissue	Decreased volume of distribution of hydrophilic drugs
	Decreased muscle mass	Increased volume of distribution of lipophilic drugs
		Increased permeability of blood–brain barrier
Metabolism	Reduced liver size	Decreased metabolism of some drugs
	Decreased liver blood flow	Increased bioavailability of high hepatic extraction ratio drugs
Excretion	Decreased kidney size	Decreased elimination of renally eliminated drugs
	Fibrosis and tubular atrophy	

Source: Sera LC, McPherson ML. *Clin Geriatr Med* 2012; 28:273–86.

the active diffusion of some nutrients, such as iron, calcium, and vitamin B_{12} is diminished, but further research has not found significant changes in absorption of drugs due to aging (2).

First-pass metabolism is an absorption phenomenon affected by age-related changes in the liver. Reductions in liver size and hepatic blood flow result in decreased first-pass metabolism of certain drugs (e.g., morphine, propranolol, and diazepam). A hepatic extraction ratio is the measure of how well the liver can eliminate drug from circulation. Drugs with high hepatic extraction ratios, such as propranolol and amitriptyline, may have an increased amount of drug available for absorption; while prodrugs that require this process for conversion to their active forms (e.g., codeine and primidone) may have a reduced serum level (3).

When discussing drug absorption, age-related changes can alter drugs absorbed via skin, muscle, subcutaneous layer, lungs, and oral mucosa. With advancing age there is a reduction in tissue blood flow, which can decrease the rate of subcutaneous and intramuscular drug absorption. Transdermal drug delivery avoids concerns with first-pass metabolism; however, aging skin can alter topical drug penetration (1). Age-related changes include drying of the stratum corneum, changes in sebaceous gland activity, lipid composition in the surface layers, and flattening of the dermoepidermal junction with a decrease in the number of dermal capillary loops (4). More hydrophilic compounds (e.g., acetylsalicylic acid) may be better absorbed, whereas more lipophilic compounds (e.g., fentanyl, testosterone, and estradiol) may be less absorbed (4). In a study of transdermal fentanyl in older postoperative patients, the time it took for plasma drug levels to double after application was twice as long as in younger patients, but there was no difference in total absorption or in elimination between the groups (5).

Inhaled drugs may have decreased absorption because of reductions in chest wall compliance, ventilation-perfusion matching, and alveolar surface tension (6). According to the Centers for Disease Control, more than 15 million Americans report that they have been diagnosed with chronic obstructive pulmonary disorder (COPD), which included emphysema, chronic bronchitis, and sometimes asthma (7). Advancing age is a risk factor for COPD, and as such, it is important to consider the dosage form used when administering inhaled medications. Dry powder inhalers can also be problematic due to a reduced inspiratory force to activate the inhaler. Metered-dose inhalers can be difficult for older adults to appropriately self-administer if they have conditions associated with aging such as osteoarthritis or Parkinson's disease. For these reasons, nebulizer solutions and the newer Respimat® inhalers would be more ideal for older adult patients.

5.2.2 DISTRIBUTION

A drug's volume of distribution (Vd) as well as its protein binding can be affected by aging. Vd is a term used to describe the ratio of total drug in the body to the amount of drug in the plasma. Changes in body composition that may alter Vd in the older adults include a decrease in total body water and an increase in adipose tissue. The Vd of hydrophilic drugs (e.g., alcohol) decreases with aging with a consequent increase in drug concentration; whereas the opposite is true for lipophilic drugs, such as amiodarone, haloperidol, and diazepam. The plasma half-life of a drug (the amount of time it takes for one-half the drug to be eliminated) is directly related to its Vd; if the Vd increases, as with lipophilic agents, the drug is retained longer in the body. Decreased muscle mass frequently occurring in older patients may also affect Vd. Drugs that are active in muscle tissue, such as digoxin, may have a decreased Vd and increased plasma concentrations potentially leading to digoxin toxicity (1).

There are primarily two proteins involved in drug binding: alpha-1-acid glycoprotein and albumin. Alpha-1-acid glycoprotein binds basic drugs, but has not been demonstrated to be affected by the aging process (8). Albumin binds acidic drugs such as naproxen, phenytoin, and warfarin. The aging process can result in a 20% decrease in serum albumin levels; causing an increase in the drug's free fraction and subsequent toxicity (1). This can be an issue of clinical significance for the older adult receiving phenytoin or warfarin, for example. If the older adult has hypoalbuminemia attributable to the aging process or exacerbated by comorbid disease, a lower dose of the medication would theoretically be necessary to produce the same clinical result. If a serum phenytoin level is warranted, it is important to evaluate a serum albumin level, or preferably, obtaining a free phenytoin level to depict a more accurate concentration.

5.2.3 METABOLISM

The liver is the primary route by which drug metabolism occurs, converting drugs into more water-soluble compounds so that they may be eliminated from the body.

With advancing age, liver size is reduced by as much as 35% and blood flow can be reduced more than 40% (1). The clinical impact of this change is most significant on drugs with high extraction ratios. Propranolol and verapamil are examples of drugs that may have decreased metabolism; consequently, if using these medications in the geriatric rehabilitation patient, initiating therapy with a lower dose (e.g., at least half of the usually recommended dose) is warranted (9).

Metabolic enzyme reactions via the cytochrome P450 system occur by either phase I or phase II reactions. Although it has been established that phase II reactions appear unchanged with aging, it remains unclear what the significance of aging is on phase I reactions (1). Studies have shown no difference in enzyme activity in older subjects, yet there appear to be age-dependent differences in metabolic clearance of many drugs including some benzodiazepines, theophylline, imipramine, propranolol, and indomethacin (9). These decreases are more likely caused by reduced hepatic blood flow than specific alterations in liver enzymes. Polypharmacy, which frequently occurs in older patients, may play a role in changes in metabolism as well. Not only are some medications substrates for phase I enzymes but can also either inhibit or induce their activity, thus affecting the metabolism of other medications the patient takes (1). If adding a medication that may inhibit or induce a CYP 450 enzyme, consider whether it induces or inhibits an enzymatic reaction. Inhibition will happen immediately, while induction of a CYP enzyme requires days or weeks to see the full effect.

5.2.4 EXCRETION

Although drugs may be eliminated via urine, feces, bile, or lungs, the primary focus of a discussion of age-related changes in pharmacokinetics centers around renal elimination. A decrease in excretion of renally eliminated drugs is the most important consideration of all ADME parameters when caring for the geriatric patient. The kidney decreases in size by 20%–30% between age 30 and 80 years, with fibrosis and tubular atrophy also occurring (10). These changes contribute as much as a 50% decrease in glomerular filtration rate (GFR) from age 25 to 85 years (11). A GFR of 30–60 mL/min, suggestive of stage 3 kidney disease, has been observed in 15%–30% in older adults; although many likely lack a formal diagnosis of chronic kidney disease (12).

Renal function is commonly monitored using serum creatinine values. In older adults, because of the age-related decline in muscle mass, serum creatinine may over-represent renal function. A more accurate assessment of renal function can be made by collecting a 24-hour urine; however, this is rarely realistic to execute, especially in rehabilitation. When estimating creatinine clearance, it is best to use the Cockcroft–Gault equation. The evaluation of several different kidney function estimation equations (e.g., Wright, Jelliffe, and Modification of Diet in Renal Disease) have been researched and found to be somewhat inconclusive because, unsurprisingly, each formula has its strengths and limitations (13). However, the Cockcroft–Gault equation is most commonly used by drug manufacturers as the basis for determining dose adjustments in renal impairment. A list of selected medications requiring dosage adjustment in renal impairment and potential toxicity can be found in Table 5.2. A variety of drugs have recommended dose reductions based on GFR. Since GFR is almost always an estimate, it is vital to consider individual sensitivity to medications and the risk versus benefit of using a more aggressive dose in geriatric patients with decreased renal function.

TABLE 5.2
Selected Medications Requiring Dose Adjustment in Renal Impairment

Drug/Drug Class	Potential Toxicity
Antibiotics	
Aminoglycosides and vancomycin	Ototoxicity and nephrotoxicity
Carbapenems	Seizures
Fluoroquinolones	CNS stimulation
Penicillins	CNS stimulation and seizures
Sulfonamides	Crystalluria
Antiviral Agents	
Acyclovir, famciclovir, and valacyclovir	Seizures, confusion, and nephrotoxicity
Cardiovascular Agents	
ACE-I (except fosinopril)	Nephrotoxicity
Apixaban, dabigatran, edoxaban, rivaroxaban, enoxaparin and fondaparinux	Bleeding
Atenolol	Bradycardia and hypotension
Digoxin	Heart block, confusion, and nausea
Spironolactone	Hyperkalemia
Triamterene	Hyperkalemia and hyponatremia
CNS Agents	
Amantadine	Confusion and hallucinations
Duloxetine	Nausea and diarrhea
Gabapentin, levetiracetam, and tramadol	Somnolence and confusion
Lithium	Sedation, confusion, tremors, and seizures
Meperidine	Confusion and seizures
Pregabalin	Confusion, blurred vision, and ataxia
Others	
Allopurinol	Nephrotoxicity and exfoliative dermatitis
Colchicine	GI, neuromuscular, and bone marrow toxicity
Glyburide	Hypoglycemia
H-2 antagonists	Confusion
Probenecid	Loss of effectiveness

Source: Hutchison LC, O'Brien C. *J Pharm Pract* 2007; 20:4–12; American Geriatrics Society 2015 Updated Beers Criteria Update Expert Panel. American Geriatrics Society 2015 Updated Beers Criteria for Potentially Inappropriate Medication Use in Older Adults; *J Am Geriatr Soc,* 2015; 63:2227–46, http://onlinelibrary.wiley.com/doi/10.1111/jgs.13702/pdf; Accessed October 21, 2015.

5.3 PHARMACODYNAMICS

Pharmacodynamics is the study of the drug's effects on the body. The pharmacodynamic changes of aging with regard to medication therapy are less well defined compared to pharmacokinetics. In general, aging patients demonstrate an increased sensitivity to drugs by mechanisms that are not all entirely understood. Increased sensitivity to warfarin, sedative-hypnotics, narcotic analgesics, and anticholinergic medications has been reported in older adults (8,14). Select changes in specific body systems are discussed below.

5.3.1 Cardiovascular System

There are several physiological changes with aging that may affect an older adult's response to antihypertensive medications. Diminished baroreceptor sensitivity results in an increased response to calcium-channel blockers, the lack of rebound tachycardia when withdrawn, and an increased risk of orthostatic hypotension (OH) (1). A decrease in the number and sensitivity of beta receptors results in reduced effectiveness of beta-blockers (16). Lastly, impaired renal function is the primary cause for the reduced response to diuretics, making it more common for older adult patients to require two diuretics that act at different sites in the kidney for the desired diuresis (1). Diuretics are commonly prescribed to decrease lower extremity edema in older adults. Since there is a reduced response to diuresis in these patients, mechanical (e.g., the use of pressure stockings) means may be more appropriate in most patients.

5.3.2 Fluids and Electrolytes

The aging patient has a reduced reserve capacity to respond to environmental stressors and there are a number of factors that further contribute to this vulnerability. Decreased creatinine clearance and thirst response, impaired renal response to salt intake, and sometimes even the reluctance to take in enough fluid for fear of incontinent symptoms can put the patient at greater risk for adverse drug effects such as hyponatremia, syndrome of inappropriate antidiuretic hormone, hyperkalemia, and dehydration (14,17).

5.3.3 Central Nervous System

The changes occurring in the aging brain may be most important when discussing pharmacodynamics, yet possibly still the least understood. As with other systems, there seems to be a phenomenon of decreased reserve, which predisposes the older adult to adverse drug events related to medications affecting various neurotransmitter systems (14). Possibly the most clinically significant example of pharmacodynamic change is the response of the older adult to benzodiazepines. Changes in gamma-aminobutyric acid (GABA) receptors have been proposed as the cause for the increased response to benzodiazepines, given that the increases in responses seen in these patients are beyond what can be accounted for by pharmacokinetics (18–20). Patients receiving benzodiazepines should be monitored for ataxia, sedation, and cognitive impairment (14). Antipsychotics, another drug class to which aging patients have demonstrated a pharmacodynamically altered response, can result in greater susceptibility to sedation, anticholinergic effects, OH, and arrhythmias (21). Decreases in the number of dopaminergic neurons in the substantia nigra put the elderly patient at increased risk for extrapyramidal side effects (EPS) (22).

5.4 ADVERSE DRUG EVENTS

During acute rehabilitation, the clinician uses a variety of therapies, including drug therapy, to facilitate functional recovery. It is commonplace to use narcotics for pain management, antiplatelet therapy for secondary stroke prevention, and antiepileptic agents for seizure prophylaxis; however, while making medical decisions often in very complex patients, it is important to recognize that many pharmacological agents used in rehabilitation can negatively affect function. A study by Hilmer et al. (23) found that in community-dwelling seniors, anticholinergic and sedative medications are associated with poorer function. There is a paucity of scientific data evaluating the impact of medications in seniors undergoing inpatient or outpatient rehabilitation; however, the astute clinician can anticipate possible functional adverse effects when considering the drug's pharmacology, its pharmacokinetic and pharmacodynamic properties, along with age-related changes in physiological function.

Figure 5.1 illustrates contributors to both physical and psychological function while also considering the influence of age-related changes and pharmacological therapy. It is important to note

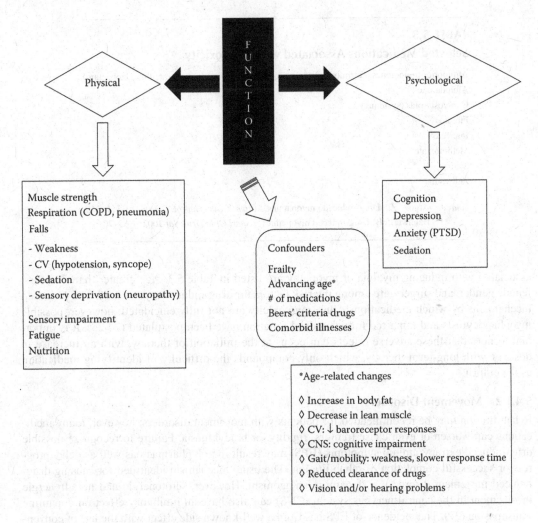

FIGURE 5.1 Medications and function.

that the physiatrist must consider physiological age in addition to chronological age while treating patients in rehabilitation. People in their fourth or fifth decade may not be viewed as "geriatric" based on their chronological age. Physiologically, however, their health may be more aligned with that of a 65- or 70-year-old, making drug selection as important as it is in an older adult patient.

The reasons why persons are referred to rehabilitation are frequently due to amputation, multiple trauma, spinal cord injury, orthopedic disorders, and neurological conditions, including brain injury. Whether the older adult patient has experienced a traumatic event or had premorbid weakness, consideration must be given to the potential impact of medications on function. Moreover, as many older adults have multiple comorbidities and frequently take multiple medications, it is also important to consider the indirect impact medication side effects may have on function.

5.4.1 Adverse Effects on Physical Function

5.4.1.1 Myotoxicity

Muscle strength can be weakened by drugs that cause myalgia, myositis, myopathy, and life-threatening rhabdomyolysis. These adverse effects may not be easily recognizable in a geriatric patient because of age-related weakness and the high incidence of frailty. Medications frequently

TABLE 5.3

Selected Medications Associated with Myotoxicity

Antibiotics (quinolones, cotrimoxazole, isoniazid, minocycline, and piperacillin–tazobactam)

Amiodarone

Corticosteroids (systemic)

Fibrates

Interferon

Methotrexate

Statins

Zidovudine

Source: Argov Z. Drug-induced myopathies. *Curr Opin Neurol* 2000; 13:541–545;
Bannwarth B. Drug-induced myopathies. *Expert Opin Drug Saf* 2002; 1:65–70.

associated with inducing myalgia or myopathy are listed in Table 5.3. Age greater than 70 years, female gender, and surgery are among the risk factors for drug-induced myotoxicity. The proposed mechanisms by which medications cause myotoxicity are not fully elucidated; however, possible myophagocytosis and impaired mitochondrial function have been postulated (24,25). It is important to note that these adverse effects can occur at the initiation of therapy, with an increase in dose, or with long-term therapy, which only compounds the difficulty of identifying medication as the culprit.

5.4.1.2 Movement Disorders

Rehabilitation may be recommended for patients with movement disorders; however, many medications can worsen or even cause tremors, rigidity, or bradykinesia. Failure to recognize possible drug-induced extrapyramidal symptoms (EPS) may result in polypharmacy as well as delay progress or successful completion of rehabilitation. The usual mechanism identified for causing drug-induced movement disorders is dopamine antagonism. However, serotonergic and noradrenergic involvement in the central nervous system (CNS) can also have an inhibitory effect on dopamine transmission (27). The incidence of EPS has been a well-known side effect with the use of conventional (typical) antipsychotics (e.g., haloperidol); this is why the newer (atypical) neuroleptics are more frequently used. Clozapine, quetiapine, and iloperidone appear to have the lowest risk of EPS; while risperidone and paliperidone appear to have the highest risk of dose-dependent EPS (28). The incidence of EPS is as high as 30%–40% in patients receiving the antiemetics promethazine, droperidol, or prochlorperazine and in those receiving the gastric motility agent metoclopramide. Although with lower frequency, EPS, especially in patients with underlying movement disorders, has also been reported with the use of selective serotonin reuptake inhibitors (SSRIs) and tricyclic antidepressants (TCAs) (28). Advancing age and female gender are additional risk factors for drug-induced EPS.

5.4.1.3 Respiratory Disorders

Patients with respiratory disorders (e.g., COPD, pneumonia) are frequently referred to rehabilitation due to deconditioning. Symptoms as subtle as nonproductive cough, exertional dyspnea, and diminished lung capacity can be easily overlooked in someone with known respiratory illness; however, these symptoms could also represent pulmonary toxicity due to medications. A list of agents associated with respiratory toxicity is in Table 5.4. Seniors unable to get a good, deep breath will find exercise, including attempting simple activities of daily living (ADLs), difficult to perform. Sleep disrupted cough and shortness of breath, for example, can adversely impact a senior's reserve to complete a more intensive therapy schedule. Unless the clinician is aware of the possibility of

TABLE 5.4
Selected Medications Associated with Pulmonary Toxicity

ACE inhibitors
Amiodarone
Aspirin
Bleomycin
Bromocriptine
Cyclophosphamide
Methotrexate
Nitrofurantoin
NSAIDs
Methotrexate
Psyllium

Source: Trewet, CB. *Drug-Induced Diseases*, 2nd ed., Chapter 21. Bethesda,
MD: ASHP; 2010; Leader WG, Mohundro BL. *Drug-Induced
Diseases*, 2nd ed., Chapter 22. Bethesda, MD: ASHP; 2010.

drug-induced respiratory disease, the senior patient may be viewed as "intolerant" of therapy simply because it appears as if the underlying condition precludes their participation and success in the program.

5.4.1.4 Hypotension

OH, a potentially disabling problem resulting in falls, fractures, and syncope, is another condition frequently encountered in the rehabilitation patient. Although the incidence of OH in healthy elderly is rare, 68% of elderly discharged from the hospital and 50% of patients with cerebrovascular accident admitted to an inpatient rehabilitation unit experienced OH (31,32). Autonomic dysfunction, dehydration, blood loss, or overly aggressive treatment of hypertension are frequent causes of OH. Table 5.5 lists medications associated with OH. Many of the causative agents are antihypertensive drugs that are initiated in acute care when a patient presents with hypertensive urgency or emergency. In the acute setting, intravenous fluids (IVFs) are often administered to maintain metabolic

TABLE 5.5
Selected Medication Inducing Hypotension

ACE inhibitors	Diuretics
ARBs	Dopamine agonists
Antiparkinsonian agents	Nitrates
Antipsychotics	Opiates
Alpha-agonists	Phosphodiesterase inhibitors
Alpha-blockers	Trazodone
Beta-blockers	TCAs
Calcium-channel blockers	Vancomycin

Source: Gupta V, Lipsitz LA. *Am J Med* 2007; 120:841–847; Lipsitz
LA. *NEJM* 1989; 321:952–957; Tinetti ME et al. *J Am
Geriatr Soc* 1995; 43:1214–1241.

stability, but following admission to rehabilitation or when the patient is discharged to home, IVFs are discontinued. In 1–2 weeks after hypertension treatment begins, the drugs reach their full clinical effect causing the physiologically frail elderly patient to experience orthostasis, weakness, and/or a fall.

5.4.1.5 Renal Impairment

The older adult is at risk for having or developing renal impairment as a result of dehydration, physiological aging, and medication use. Maintaining good hydration can be difficult in these patients due to age-related changes in thirst drive, dysphagia, depression, and altered mental status (AMS). Furthermore, as previously mentioned, serum creatinine may not be a reliable marker for evaluating renal function in a senior patient. It is also important to note that in the presence of reduced creatinine clearance, many medications may require dosage reduction. Failure to properly dose medications may result in accumulation and eventual drug toxicity. Medications implicated in drug-induced kidney injury are listed in Table 5.6.

5.4.1.6 Hepatic Impairment

Liver injury can occur as a result of trauma, alcohol consumption, hepatitis, and/or medications. Frequently, the rehab clinician is forced to interpret transaminitis and attempt to differentiate the cause(s). In older adults, 20% of the cases of jaundice and 25% of fulminant hepatic failure are due to medications making the etiology important to define (38). The two biggest culprits of drug-induced liver impairment are acetaminophen and HMG-CoA reductase inhibitors (statins). The incidence of acetaminophen-induced hepatotoxicity is rare, but will be higher if greater than 4 g/day are repeatedly consumed. Additional risk factors for acetaminophen-induced hepatotoxicity are hypovolemia, severe renal impairment, alcoholism, hepatic impairment, and chronic malnutrition (39). Acetaminophen is readily available and is frequently combined with narcotic analgesics and cough and cold medications making unintentional overdose possible. Although consumption of maximum recommended doses of acetaminophen (4 g) in patients with chronic, stable liver disease did not cause any clinically relevant adverse effects, the manufacturer recommends a dose of ≤3 g/day be consumed, especially in the elderly (40).

TABLE 5.6

Selected Medications Worsening Renal Function

ACE inhibitors

ARBs

Aminoglycosides

COX-2 inhibitors

Cyclosporine

Diuretics

Indinavir

NSAIDs

Radiocontrast media

Sulfonamides

Tacrolimus

Vancomycin

Source: Hricik DE, Dunn MJ. *J Am Soc Nephrol* 1990; 1:845–858; Scwartz J et al. *Clin Pharmacol Ther* 202; 72:50–61.

5.4.1.7 Hypertension

Many of the medications used in the care of patients undergoing rehabilitation have been associated with causing hypertension. Whether the patient has a history of hypertension or not, it is important to recognize this usually unwanted side effect. Those with renal impairment or pre-existing hypertension are at highest risk (41). In the presence of possible drug-induced hypertension, it is important to reevaluate the need for the medication before treating the side effect of a medication with another medication. Sympathomimetic drugs (e.g., dextroamphetamine, methylphenidate, and pseudoephedrine), as CNS stimulants, cause dose-related increases in blood pressure. Corticosteroids causing sodium retention can also result in dose-related fluid retention and increased blood pressure. Nonsteroidal anti-inflammatory drugs (NSAIDs) and cyclooxygenase-2 (COX-2) inhibitors (e.g., ibuprofen and celecoxib) through prostaglandin inhibition also cause sodium and water retention. Serotonin/norepinephrine reuptake inhibitors (SNRIs) (e.g., venlafaxine, duloxetine) by increasing the levels of norepinephrine can result in the potentiation of noradrenergic neurotransmission. Immunosuppressants (e.g., cyclosporine and tacrolimus) increase prostaglandin synthesis and thereby reduce water and sodium excretion (42).

Evaluating the older adult patient for possible drug-induced problems in rehabilitation takes an astute eye and time to perform a thorough drug regimen review. Obtaining an accurate medication history is paramount, but not always easy to accomplish. If a possible adverse event is reported, it is important to carefully listen to what other team members are reporting—especially with regard to function and cognition.

5.4.2 Adverse Effects on Cognition

While medications can directly negatively impact function, there are additional medication side effects that can indirectly affect function. These adverse effects are also very important for the physiatrist to consider in caring for the older adult patient.

5.4.2.1 Seizures

Whether the older adult patient in rehabilitation has a history of seizures or is now at risk due to a traumatic event, it is important to recognize that certain medications can lower seizure threshold. Although the incidence of drug-induced seizures is rare, known risk factors include a history of seizures or epilepsy, malignancy, compromised blood–brain barrier, not properly adjusting the dose of hepatically or renally eliminated medications, and concomitant use of CNS stimulants (43). The clinician must also remember that seizures may result due to toxicity of many of the antiepileptic medications (e.g., phenytoin, phenobarbital, and carbamazepine) and when suspected, serum drug level monitoring is recommended. Table 5.7 lists medications associated with drug-induced seizures. The risks and benefits of using these medications in an older adult patient with known risk factors for seizures should be carefully weighed. It is also important to remember that overdose is a major contributory factor to drug-induced seizures.

5.4.2.2 Altered Mental Status

One of the biggest challenges in geriatric rehabilitation is accurately differentiating between premorbid cognitive status and current cognitive status. The importance of accurately identifying contributor(s) of AMS may make the difference between admission to an acute inpatient rehabilitation unit and skilled nursing facility for therapy. Cognitive status can be negatively impacted by traumatic brain injury (e.g., fall, surgery, and stroke), delirium (e.g., postop, infection, and stool impaction), unrecognized or undertreated depression, metabolic abnormalities (e.g., dehydration, hyponatremia, and hypoglycemia), sensory deprivation, and medications. Nearly all medications can be psychoactive in the elderly; therefore, it is crucial to perform a thorough review of medications given on a scheduled

---

TABLE 5.7

Selected Medications Lowering Seizure Threshold

Antipsychotics
Bupropion
Carbapenems
Cyclosporine
Fluoroquinolones
Meperidine
Theophylline
Tramadol

Source: Stimmel GI, Dopheide JA. *CNS Drugs* 1996; 5:37–50.

TABLE 5.8

Selected Medications Altering Mental Status

ANTICHOLINERGICS

Amantadine	Meclizine
Amitriptyline	Olanzapine
Benztropine	Oxybutynin
Cimetidine	Paroxetine
Cyclobenzaprine	Prochlorperazine
Cyproheptadine	Promethazine
Darifenacin	Ranitidine
Dicyclomine	Scopolamine
Diphenhydramine	Solifenacin
Diphenoxylate atropine	Tolterodine
Doxepin	Triphexyphenidyl
Hydroxyzine	Trospium
Hyoscyamine	Fluoroquinolones
Benzodiazepines	NSAIDs
Corticosteroids	Opiates
Digoxin	

Source: American Geriatrics Society 2015 *J Am Geriatr Soc* 2015;63, 2227–46, http://onlinelibrary.wiley.com/doi/10.1111/jgs.13702/pdf; Accessed October 21, 2015; Ancelin ML et al. *BMJ* 2006; 332:455; Larson EB et al. *Ann Intern Med* 1987; 107:169–173.

---

basis as well as those given only as needed. It is also important to consider possible drug interactions, alcohol and medication withdrawal as the offender. Medications with anticholinergic activity are the most offending agents associated with AMS in geriatric patients (45). Pharmacodynamic changes with advancing age, as discussed earlier, make the elderly more sensitive to the effects of anticholinergic agents. In addition to confusion, anticholinergic medications can also lead to unwanted urinary retention and constipation, which can be detrimental in most patients, but particularly in the older adults and in those with a spinal cord injury. Table 5.8 lists medications associated with AMS.

5.4.2.3 Depression

With advancing age, chronic comorbidities, physical decline, and a devastating life event, such as an ischemic stroke, depression can be difficult to recognize as a clinical phenomenon. Many medications have been implicated in worsening or causing depression. The highest incidence appears to be with gonadotropin-releasing hormone agonists (e.g., leuprorelin and triptorelin) and primidone, but interferon, tamoxifen, corticosteroids, topiramate, levetiracetam, and vigabatrin are causative agents as well (48). There is limited data regarding the prevention of drug-induced depression; however, if the drug is suspected, the benefits of continued treatment should be weighed against the risks of discontinuation. If the medication cannot be discontinued, then antidepressant therapy with a SSRI, for example, should be initiated. If a stimulant is used, the clinician must be cognizant of precipitating anxiety or insomnia. Medications with stimulating effects should be administered early in the day to help prevent insomnia. Treatment of these side effects can result in polypharmacy and should be avoided.

5.4.2.4 Anxiety and Insomnia

In the presence of anxiety or insomnia, it is important for the clinician to evaluate untreated or poorly treated depression in addition to other possible causes, such as medications. Stimulants such as caffeine, amphetamines, bupropion, modafinil, pseudoephedrine, and SSRIs have been associated with causing or worsening anxiety and causing insomnia especially if taken late in the day. Paradoxical reactions have been associated with antipsychotics, benzodiazepines, and hypnotics. When this occurs it is easy for the clinician to misinterpret behavior and increase the dose of the medication. If unwanted behaviors persist despite an increase in dose, the medication should be discontinued to evaluate for possible drug-induced causes. It is important to note that medication withdrawal (e.g., narcotics, gabapentin, and benzodiazepines) can also result in anxiety-like symptoms (49).

5.4.3 Adverse Effects on Appetite

It is estimated that 20% of community-dwelling elderly and as many as 65% of hospitalized elderly are malnourished (50). Loss of appetite is usually multifactorial, but proper nutrition is vitally important for overall health and well-being. Factors such as depression, cognitive impairment, nausea, and feelings of futility can dramatically reduce oral intake in seniors. Also when the diet is undesired by the patient (e.g., pureed and cardiac prudent) intake is also difficult. When nutrition is significantly compromised, clinicians have to consider alternatives to oral feeding, such as nasogastric or percutaneous endoscopic gastrostomy tubes. Drug-induced xerostomia and lowered taste sensation is frequently associated with anticholinergic medications. Dry mouth can also negatively affect mastication and swallowing. Dysgeusia has been related to recent anesthesia, antihypertensive medications, antibiotics, and opiate analgesics (51,52). An evaluation of the patient's medication list may also reveal possible drug-induced causes of failure to thrive.

5.5 DRUG INTERACTIONS

Although drug–drug interactions and drug–disease interactions are common in older adults, there is little published data regarding important clinical implications of such interactions (53). Older age, female gender, polypharmacy, and multimorbidity have been identified as significant risk factors for hospital admission due to drug interactions (54,55). Another consideration is the contribution of geriatric syndromes such as frailty, falls, cognitive impairment, immobility, and urinary incontinence on the risk of clinically significant outcomes from drug interactions or the impact of drug interactions on older patients falling victim to these syndromes (53). This remains an area where additional research is needed to shape clinical guidelines for safe medication use.

The majority of drug interactions occur when the action of one drug alters the ADME of another drug. The most frequently cited medications associated with drug interactions are warfarin, NSAIDs, diuretics, and angiotensin-converting enzyme (ACE)-inhibitors (56). If the clinician understands how two drugs may potentially interact, monitoring and avoidance of serious clinical consequences are possible. For example, NSAIDs (e.g., ibuprofen and celecoxib) can competitively inhibit the antiplatelet effect of low-dose aspirin (81–325 mg daily). Acute renal failure can occur when a patient takes an ACE-inhibitor or angiotensin receptor blockers (ARB) along with a diuretic (e.g., hydrochlorothiazide or chlorthalidone) and NSAID; frequently referred to as the "triple whammy." The GFR is reduced by the ACEI/ARB due to its vasodilation of the efferent arteriole coupled with the diuretic that causes vascular volume depletion and the NSAID that causes vasodilation of the afferent arteriole (57,58).

5.6 PRINCIPLES AND PRESCRIBING OPTIMIZATION

5.6.1 TOOLS TO ASSIST IN PRESCRIBING FOR THE OLDER ADULTS

Given the complexity of geriatric care, three tools have been developed to assist with identifying and preventing the use of potentially inappropriate medications. The American Geriatric Society Beers' Criteria is the national standard for quality indicators and geriatric clinical care. These evidence-based criterion were updated in 2015 and now include medications requiring dosage adjustment in renal impairment and select drug–drug interactions known to cause harm in seniors (15). It is important to remember that the Beers Criteria are meant to guide clinicians in selecting medications for senior patients. The Quality of Evidence and Recommendations are based on the general elderly population and may not apply to a specific patient in a special population such as traumatic brain injury.

The STOPP/START criteria, updated in 2014, are standards developed to identify potentially inappropriate prescribing in seniors as well as to identify medication that is clinically indicated, but omitted (59). STOPP, or Screening Tool to Older Person's Prescriptions, identified potentially inappropriate medication similar to Beers' criteria. For example, the use of amitriptyline, a highly anticholinergic medication, would be relatively contraindicated in a senior with known urinary retention or with a history of glaucoma. If treatment was aimed at neuropathic pain, then a safer alternative such as gabapentin may be recommended. Another example would be the use of a benzodiazepine, such as lorazepam, for anxiety. Given its pharmacokinetic property of high lipophilicity combined with the increase in adipose tissue and decline in lean body mass with advancing age, the sedative effects may be more significant in a senior patient. Moreover, the use of benzodiazepines can adversely affect functional outcomes; therefore, the STOPP criteria would suggest considering a safer alternative for anxiety such as a SSRI (60).

Conversely, START, or Screening Tool to Alert to Right Treatment, helps identify when a medication is indicated, but omitted. Reasons why clinically indicated medications are often left out of an elderly patient's treatment plan include insufficient data in patients of old age, the desire to avoid polypharmacy, or the patient's desire for palliative care rather than preventative measures (59). For example, in a patient with a history of atrial fibrillation not receiving anticoagulation despite no contraindications, START would prompt the prescriber to evaluate why warfarin had not been initiated. In the setting of rehabilitation this could be of great benefit as the patient frequently has multiple prescribers and sometimes complicated histories. While there has been no evidence showing the application of the STOPP/START criteria decreases morbidity or mortality, it may warrant implementation in an effort to prevent untoward reactions while attempting to maximize pharmaceutical care.

5.6.2 MEDICATIONS GIVEN VIA TUBES

Patients with functioning GI tracts unable to tolerate oral feedings for extended periods of time will require nutrition administered via a tube, such as a nasogastric tube (NG-tube) or percutaneous endoscopic gastrostomy tube (PEG-tube). When long-term enteral feedings are needed, the use of a PEG-tube is preferred. In the rehabilitation setting, consideration for medication administration through the tube must be made. The method by which the feeding occurs (e.g., continuous, bolus, or nocturnal), possible medication–nutrient interactions, and the formulation of the medication available must be taken into account.

Ideally, patients should be transitioned to bolus or nocturnal tube feedings for easier rehabilitation participation and to reduce caregiver burden. These methods of nutrition administration also help to minimize drug–nutrient interactions, if the enteral formula is not given directly with the medication, and the tube is flushed with a bolus of water before and after each feeding. It is important to consider the formulations available when prescribing medications to patients unable to safely swallow. When available, liquid preparations (e.g., elixirs or suspensions) are preferred (61). Some syrups, especially those with a pH ≤ 4, may cause clumping if given with the enteral feeding possibly resulting in a clogged tube (61). It is noteworthy that many liquid preparations contain sorbitol, an artificial sweetener added to improve palatability. If given in excessive quantities (>10–20 g/day), GI upset, especially diarrhea, can result. If diarrhea persists in a patient receiving medications via a tube, it is always important to evaluate the total daily dose of sorbitol received and to evaluate possible concomitant laxative use. Solid dosage forms (e.g., nonenteric coated, compressible tablets) rarely undergo any significant pharmacokinetic changes with crushing. Caution, however, must be taken when a solid formulation is prescribed containing beads, pellets, or granules that are extended-release. Based on the manufacturer's recommendation, these products may be opened and the contents sprinkled into the tube followed by water flushes. Extended-release products should never be crushed. It is important to note when a patient is receiving a long-acting preparation, a change to an immediate-release formulation will likely result in a change in dosage frequency. Formulations that should not be given via a tube include those with enteric-coating and products designed for buccal or sublingual absorption.

The serum concentrations of warfarin, phenytoin, and fluoroquinolones can be significantly altered if not administered properly when patients are receiving these medications via a tube (62). Whether the medication binds to a portion of the enteral feeding (e.g., protein and divalent cations) or simply adheres to the tube, thus reducing systemic absorption, it is imperative to closely monitor these medications and their clinical effects.

In time, patients often regain their ability to safely swallow allowing for medications to be given by the oral route. When this occurs, careful consideration should be made when switching from liquid to solid dosage forms and accounting for possible drug–nutrient interactions. Prescribers are encouraged to consult a pharmacist or the manufacturer before prescribing medications requiring tube administration or when therapeutic drug monitoring is warranted.

5.6.3 Evidence-Based Medicine in Geriatric Patients

Although evidence-based and expert consensus clinical practice guidelines have improved clinical care, the applicability to the patient requires clinical judgment by the clinician. Moreover, the clinician must weigh the possible benefits to the patient's quality of life (63). When it comes to the geriatric patient, an approach of conservative prescribing is best. Examples of this behavior on the part of clinician would include a preference for nondrug therapies, vigilance for monitoring for medication adverse effects, skepticism about new drugs to the market until they have proven themselves to be safe and effective for the elderly, and shared decision-making with patients about treatment plans (64).

5.6.4 Medication Discontinuation

Unnecessary medication use is a common problem in rehab medicine. Patients with chronic medical conditions may continue to take the same medication(s) for years without assessment of necessity or new medications may be initiated during a hospitalization and continued indefinitely when they were intended for short-term use only. Some commonly identified unnecessary medications at transitions of care are proton-pump inhibitors, CNS medications and vitamin and mineral supplements (65). In rehabilitation, careful consideration for the continued use of opioid analgesics, muscle relaxants, and NSAIDs should be given; medications deemed unnecessary can be safely discontinued utilizing a systematic approach (66).

5.6.5   HELPFUL RESOURCES

With over 100,000 mobile health apps available, it is difficult for providers and patients to know which are useful and which to avoid (67). For a healthcare provider, a desirable app is one that both simplifies the job while simultaneously improving efficiency and quality of patient care. The American Geriatric Society promotes the following three apps for any healthcare professional working with geriatric patients. These apps work with both Apple and Android devices and are free or cost less than $20.00 (USD) per year (68).

Geriatrics at Your Fingertips

- Contains specialized, up-to-date evaluation and management strategies for common geriatric conditions
- Offers in-app purchases ($20.00 USD for annual subscription)

Multimorbidity GEMS

- Developed by a grant from the American Geriatrics Society and the Agency for Healthcare Research and Quality (AHRQ)
- Helps guide the clinician through an approach to managing senior patients with multiple comorbidities

iGeriatrics

- Combines clinical information offered by the AGS
- Offers in-app purchases ($5.99 USD for annual subscription)

For senior patients, a desirable medical app is easy to use and understand, but is also trustworthy and reliable. The following apps will work with both Apple and Android devices.

Good Rx or www.goodrx.com

- Provides cost of medications, manufacturer coupons, and pill identification
- Price: Free

MyMedSchedule Mobile

- Provides medication schedule and reminder program, has picture of the medications
- Provides a picture of the medication along with schedule of administration
- Price: Free

Drugs.com

- Provides drug information, pill identification, and drug interaction checker
- Allows input on own personal medication records
- Price: Free

Websites offering suggestions and opportunities for patients and prescribers seeking assistance with medication costs include www.benefitscheckup.org, www.rxassist.org, and www.rxhome.com. It is always worthwhile looking at the manufacturer's website for patient assistance programs, especially if the medication is not generically available.

REFERENCES

1. Sera LC, McPherson ML. Pharmacokinetics and pharmacodynamic changes associated with aging and implications for drug therapy. *Clin Geriatr Med* 2012; 28:273–86.
2. Russell RM. Changes in gastrointestinal function attributed to aging. *Am J Clin Nutr* 1992; 55:1203S–7S.
3. Davies RO, Gomez HJ, Irwin JD et al. An overview of the pharmacology of enalapril. *Br J Clin Pharmacol* 1984;18:215S–29.
4. Cusack BJ. Pharmacokinetics in older persons. *Am J Geriatr Pharmacother* 2004; 2:274–302.
5. Thompson JP, Bower S, Liddle AM et al. Perioperative pharmacokinetics of transdermal fentanyl in elderly and young patients. *J Clin Pharmacol* 1995; 35:31–36.
6. Allen S. Are inhaled systemic therapies a viable option for the treatment of the elderly patient? *Drugs Aging* 2008; 25:89–94.
7. Centers for Disease Control and Prevention. Chronic obstructive pulmonary disease among adults—United States, 2011. *MMWR* 2012; 61:938–943.
8. Bressler R, Bahl JJ. Principles of drug therapy for the elderly patient. *Mayo Clin Proc* 2003; 78:1564–1577.
9. Turnheim K. Drug dosage in the elderly: Is it rational? *Drugs and Aging* 1998; 13:357–379.
10. McLean AJ, Le Couter DG. Aging biology and geriatric clinical pharmacology. *Pharmacol Rev* 2004; 56:163–84.
11. Lee JK, Mendoza DM, Mohler M, Lee EM. Geriatrics. In: Chisholm-Burns MA, Wells BG, Schwinghammer TL, Malone PM, Kolesar JM, DiPiro JT. eds. *Pharmacotherapy Principles and Practice*, 3rd ed. New York: McGraw-Hill; 2013. http://ppp.mhmedical.com.cowles-proxy.drake.edu/content.aspx?bookid=1450&Sectionid=81142870. Accessed November 01, 2015.
12. Aymanns C, Keller F, Maus S, Hartmann B, Czock D. Review on pharmacokinetics and pharmacodynamics and the aging kidney. *Clin J Am Soc Nephrol* 2010; 5:314–27.
13. Ainsworth NL, Marshall A, Hatcher H, Whitehead L, Whitfield GA, Earl HM. Evaluation of glomerular filtration rate estimation by Cockcroft-Gault, Jelliffe, Wright and Modification of Diet in Renal Disease (MDRD) formulae in oncology patients. *Ann Oncol* 2012; 23:1845–53.
14. Hutchison LC, O'Brien C. Changes in pharmacokinetics in and pharmacodynamics in the elderly patient. *J Pharm Pract* 2007; 20:4–12.
15. American Geriatrics Society 2015 Updated Beers Criteria Update Expert Panel. American Geriatrics Society 2015 updated beers criteria for potentially inappropriate medication use in older adults; *J Am Geriatr Soc* 2015;63: 2227–46, http://onlinelibrary.wiley.com/doi/10.1111/jgs.13702/pdf; Accessed October 21, 2015.
16. Schutzer W, Mader S. Age-related changes in vascular adrenergic signaling: Clinical and mechanistic implications. *Ageing Res Rev* 2004; 2:169–190.
17. Allison, SP. Fluid and electrolytes in the elderly. *Curr Opin Clin Nutr Metab Care* 2004; 7:27–33.
18. Rissman RA, Nocera R, Fuller LM et al. Age-related alterations in GABAA receptor subunits in the nonhuman primate hippocampus. *Brain Res* 2006; 1073–1074:120–30.
19. Greenblatt D, Harmatz J, vonMoltke L et al. Age and gender effects on the pharmacokinetics and pharmacodynamics of triazolam, a cytochrome P450 3A substrate. *Clin Pharmacol Ther* 2004; 76:467–469.
20. Platten HP, Schweizer E, Dilger K et al. Pharmacokinetics and pharmacodynamic action of midazolam in young and elderly patients undergoing tooth extraction. *Clin Pharmacol Ther* 1998; 63:552–60.
21. Mangoni AA, Jackson SHD. Age-related changes in pharmacodynamics: basic principles and practical applications. *Br J Clin Pharmacol* 2003; 1:6–14.
22. Zubenko G. Sutherland T. Geriatric psychopharmacology: Why does age matter? *Harv Rev Psychiatry* 2000; 7:311–333.
23. Hilmer SN, Mager DE, Simonsick EM et al. A drug burden index to define functional burden of medications in older people. *Arch Intern Med* 2007;167:781–787.
24. Argov Z. Drug-induced myopathies. *Curr Opin Neurol*. 2000; 13:541–545.
25. Williams C. Myopathy In: Tisdale JE, Miller DA, eds. *Drug-Induced Diseases*, 2nd ed., Chapter 53. Bethesda, MD: ASHP; 2010.

26. Bannwarth B. Drug-induced myopathies. *Expert Opin Drug Saf* 2002; 1:65–70.
27. Sanders-Bush E, Hazelwood L. 5-Hydroxytryptamine (Serotonin) and dopamine. In: Brunton LL, Chabner BA, Knollmann BC, eds. *Goodman and Gilman's The Pharmacological Basis of Therapeutics*, 12th ed., Chapter 13. New York: McGraw-Hill; 2011. http://accessmedicine.mhmedical.com.proxy.campbell.edu/content.aspx?bookid=374&Sectionid=41266219. Accessed October 17, 2015.)
28. Chen JJ, Swope DM. Movement disorders In: Tisdale JE, Miller DA, eds. *Drug-Induced Diseases*, 2nd ed., Chapter 12. Bethesda, MD: ASHP; 2010.
29. Trewet, CB. Interstitial lunch disease/pulmonary fibrosis. In: Tisdale JE, Miller DA, eds. *Drug-Induced Diseases*, 2nd ed., Chapter 21. Bethesda, MD: ASHP; 2010.
30. Leader WG, Mohundro BL. Asthma and bronchospasm. In: Tisdale JE, Miller DA, eds., Chapter 22. *Drug-Induced Diseases*, 2nd ed., Bethesda, MD: ASHP; 2010.
31. Weiss A, Grossman E, Beloosesky Y, Grinblat J. Orthostatic hypotension in acute geriatric ward. Is it a consistent finding? *Arch Int Med* 2002; 162: 2369–2374.
32. Kong KH, Chuo AM. Incidence and outcome of orthostatic hypotension in stroke patients undergoing rehabilitation. *Phys Med Rehab* 2003; 84:559–562.
33. Gupta V, Lipsitz LA. Orthostatic hypotension in the elderly: Diagnosis and treatment. *Am J Med* 2007; 120:841–847.
34. Lipsitz LA. Orthostatic hypotension in the elderly. *NEJM* 1989; 321:952–957.
35. Tinetti ME, Doucette J, Claus E et al. Risk factors for serious injury during falls by older persons in the community. *J Am Geriatr Soc* 1995; 43:1214–1241.
36. Hricik DE, Dunn MJ. ACE-inhibitor induced renal failure: Causes, consequences, and diagnostic uses. *J Am Soc Nephrol* 1990; 1:845–858.
37. Scwartz J, Vandomael K, Malice MP et al. Comparison of rofecoxib, celecoxib and naproxen on renal function in elderly subjects receiving a normal salt diet. *Clin Pharmacol Ther* 202; 72:50–61.
38. Eastwood HOH. Causes of jaundice in the elderly: A survey of diagnosis and investigation. *Gerontol Clin* 1971; 13:69.
39. Acetaminophen. Micromedex 2.0. Truven Health Analytics, Inc. Greenwood Village, CO. Available at: http://www.micromedexsolutions.com. Accessed October 28, 2015.
40. Kuffner EK, Dart RC, Bogdan GM et al. Effect of maximal daily doses of acetaminophen on the liver of alcohol patients. *Arch Intern Med* 2001; 161:2245–2252.
41. Grossman E, Messerli FH. Drug-induced hypertension: An unappreciated cause of secondary hypertension. *Am J Med* 2012; 125:14–22.
42. Saseen JJ. Hypertension. In: Tisdale JE, Miller DA, eds. *Drug-Induced Diseases*, 2nd ed., Chapter 27. Bethesda, MD: ASHP; 2010.
43. Welty TE. Seizures In: Tisdale JE, Miller DA, eds. *Drug-Induced Diseases*, 2nd ed., Chapter 10. Bethesda, MD: ASHP; 2010.
44. Stimmel GI, Dopheide JA. Psychotropic drug-induced reductions in seizure threshold: Incidence and consequences. *CNS Drugs* 1996; 5:37–50.
45. Rudolph JL, Salow MJ, Angelini MC et al. The anticholinergic risk scale and anticholinergic adverse effects in older persons. *Arch Intern Med* 2008; 168:508–513.
46. Ancelin ML, Artero S, Portet F et al. Non-degenerative mild cognitive impairment in elderly people and use of anticholinergic drugs: Longitudinal cohort study. *BMJ* 2006; 332:455.
47. Larson EB, Kukull WA, Buchner D et al. Adverse drug reactions associated with global cognitive impairment in elderly persons. *Ann Intern Med* 1987; 107:169–173.
48. Botts S, Ryan M. Depression In: Tisdale JE, Miller DA, eds. *Drug-Induced Diseases*, 2nd ed., Chapter 18. Bethesda, MD: ASHP; 2010.
49. Dopheide JA. Anxiety In: Tisdale JE, Miller DA, eds. *Drug-Induced Diseases*, 2nd ed., Chapter 19. Bethesda, MD: ASHP; 2010.
50. Wells JL, Dumbrell AC. Nutrition and aging: Assessment and treatment of compromised nutritional status in frail elderly patients. *Clin interv Aging* 2006:1:67–79.
51. Ackerman BH, Kasbekar N. Disturbances of taste and smell induced by drugs. *Pharmacotherapy* 1997; 17:482–496.
52. Roberston RG, Montagnini M. Geriatric failure to thrive. *Am Fam Phys* 204; 70:343–50.
53. Gnjidic D, Johnell K. Clinical implications from drug–drug and drug–disease interactions in older people. *Clin Exp Pharmacol Physiol* 2013; 40:320–5.
54. Brewer L, Williams, D. Drug interactions that matter. *Clin Pharmacol.* 2012; 40:371–375.
55. Reimche L, Forster AJ, Van walraven C. Incidence and contributors to potential drug–drug interactions in hospitalized patients. *J Clin Pharmacol.* 2011; 51:1043–50.

56. Braverman SE Howard RS, Bryant et al. Potential drug interactions in a physical medicine and rehabilitation clinic. *Am J Phys Med Rehabil* 1996; 75:44–49.
57. Bakris GL, Weir MR. Angiotensin-converting enzyme inhibitor-associated elevations in serum creatinine: Is this a cause for concern? *Arch Intern Med* 2000; 160:685–93.
58. National Kidney Foundation. K/DOQI Clinical Practice Guidelines on Hypertension and Antihypertensive Agents in Chronic Kidney Disease. http://www2.kidney.org/professionals/KDOQI/guidelines_bp/guide_12.htm (Accessed October 28, 2015).
59. OMahony D, OSullivan D, Byrne S et al. STOPP/START criteria for potentially inappropriate prescribing in older people: Version 2. *Age Ageing* 2014; 44(2):213–8.
60. Puustinen J, Nurminen J, Kukola M et al. Associations between use of benzodiazepines or related drugs and health, physical abilities and cognitive function: A non-randomized clinical study in the elderly. *Drugs Aging* 2007; 24:1045–59.
61. Williams NT. Medication administration through enteral feeding tubes. *Am J Health Syst Pharm* 2008; 65:2347–2357.
62. Thomson FC, Naysmith MR, Lindsay A. Managing drug therapy in patients receiving enteral and parenteral nutrition. *Hospital Pharmacist* 2000; 7:155–64.
63. Boyd CM, Darer J et al. Clinical practice guidelines and quality of care for older patient with multiple comorbid diseases: Implications for pay for performance. *JAMA* 2005; 294:716–724.
64. Schiff GD, Galanter WL, Duhig J et al. Principles of conservative prescribing. *Arch Intern Med* 2011; 171:1433–1440.
65. Steinman MA, Hanlon JT. Managing medications in clinically complex elders: There's got to be a happy medium. *JAMA* 2010; 304:1592–1601.
66. Garfunkel D, Mangin D. Feasibility study of a systematic approach for discontinuation of multiple medications in older adults: Addressing polypharmacy. *Arch Intern Med* 2010; 18:1648–1654.
67. http://research2guidance.com/ Accessed October 18, 2015.
68. http://www.americangeriatrics.org/publications/shop_publications/smartphone_products/Accessed October 18, 2015.

6 Exercise in the Older Adult

Susan Garstang

CONTENTS

6.1 INTRODUCTION

By the year 2030, 70 million people (20% of the population) will be older than 65 years, with those 85 years and older being the fastest growing segment of our population. It is estimated that up to 45% of adults between 65 years and 74 years, and 51% of adults over 75 years have no leisure-time physical activity.[1] Current evidence clearly shows that increasing physical activity can be beneficial in the management of common health conditions in the older adult, and may in fact reverse some of the usual age-related decline in physiological processes seen with normal aging.[2] This chapter reviews the physiology of normal aging in both sedentary and active older adult populations, and discusses the deleterious effects of physical inactivity. The benefits of participation in various types of exercise will be covered, including aerobic (endurance) exercise, resistive exercise, and exercise aimed at balance and flexibility. Considerations for recommending and prescribing exercise will be discussed, including ways to assess fitness prior to beginning an exercise program, and contraindications to exercise. Recommendations and exercise prescriptions for different conditions common in the elderly will be reviewed, including osteoarthritis, cardiovascular disease (CVD), diabetes, respiratory disease, stroke, and osteoporosis. Suggestions for lifestyle modification to promote physical activity, as well as ways to overcome barriers to exercise and improve adherence to an exercise program will also be provided.

There are physiological changes that are associated with aging that are considered to be very similar to those seen with physical inactivity. Many of these changes, such as reduced aerobic capacity, changes in body composition, bone loss, skeletal muscle atrophy, and muscle weakness, are often reversible with exercise. The Department of Health and Human Services published for the first time in 2008 Physical Activity Guidelines for Americans.[3] These guidelines recommend 150 minutes per week of physical activity for health benefits. Note that additional benefits occur as the amount of physical activity increases through higher intensity, greater frequency, and/or longer duration. However, these guidelines stress that if an older adult cannot do 150 minutes of moderate intensity aerobic activity per week because of chronic conditions, they should be as physically active as their abilities and conditions allow.[4] Even 10 minutes a day of exercise has been shown to be more beneficial than being sedentary.

Regular participation in physical activity has a variety of benefits in the older adult, including the following:

- Minimizing the physiological changes associated with typical aging
- Contributing to psychological health and well-being
- Increasing longevity and decreasing the risk of many common chronic diseases
- Functioning as a primary or adjunctive treatment for certain chronic diseases
- Preventing and treating complications of disability[5]

6.2   BENEFITS OF REGULAR PHYSICAL ACTIVITY IN OLDER ADULTS

The benefits of regular physical activity in older adults are extensive. Regular physical activity has been shown to reduce the risk of both development and worsening of many different chronic diseases thought by some to be a part of "normal" aging.[6] Clinical practice guidelines identify a substantial therapeutic role for physical activity in coronary heart disease,[7–9] hypertension (HTN),[9–11] peripheral vascular disease,[12] type 2 diabetes,[13] obesity,[14] elevated cholesterol,[9,15] osteoporosis,[16,17] osteoarthritis,[18,19] claudication,[20] colon cancer,[21,22] breast cancer,[23,24] and chronic obstructive pulmonary disease.[25] Clinical practice guidelines identify a role for physical activity in the management of depression and anxiety disorders,[26] dementia,[27] pain,[28] congestive heart failure,[29] stroke,[30] back pain,[31] and constipation.[32] Of particular importance to older adults, there is substantial evidence that physical activity reduces risk of falls and injuries from falls,[33] prevents or mitigates functional limitations,[34–37] and is an effective therapy for many chronic diseases. There is also some evidence that physical activity prevents or delays cognitive impairment,[38–40] disability,[35,41–43] and improves sleep (Table 6.1).[44,45]

6.3   DEFINITIONS

Physical activity: Body movement that is produced by the contraction of skeletal muscles that increases energy expenditure.

TABLE 6.1

Health Benefits of Physical Activity in Adults

Strong evidence

Decreased risk of early death, heart disease, stroke, type 2 diabetes mellitus, high
   blood pressure, adverse blood lipid profile, and metabolic syndrome

Decreased risk of colon and breast cancer

Prevention of weight gain

Weight loss, when combined with healthy diet

Improved cardiorespiratory and muscular fitness

Fall prevention

Reduced depression and anxiety

Improved cognitive function

Moderate-to-strong evidence

Improved functional health

Reduced abdominal obesity

Moderate evidence

Weight maintenance after weight loss

Decreased risk of hip fracture

Increased bone density

Improved sleep quality

Decreased risk of lung and endometrial cancers

Source: US Department of Health and Human Services, Office of Disease
        Prevention and Health Promotion. 2008. *Physical Activity Guidelines for
        Americans.* Washington, DC: US Department of Health and Human
        Services.

Exercise: Planned, structured, and repetitive movement to improve or maintain one or more components of physical fitness.

Resistive exercise training (RET): Exercise that causes muscles to work or hold against an applied force or weight which may also be referred to as strength training (ST).

Aerobic exercise training (AET): Exercises in which the body's large muscles move in a rhythmic manner for sustained periods.

Metabolic equivalent of task (MET): A physiological measure expressing the energy cost of physical activities. MET is the ratio of metabolic rate during a specific activity to a reference metabolic rate (3.5 mL O_2/kg/min). 1 MET is considered the resting metabolic rate.

Flexibility exercise: Activities designed to preserve or extend the range of motion (ROM) around a joint.

Balance training: Refers to a combination of activities designed to increase lower body strength and reduce the likelihood of falling.

Physical fitness: A state of well-being with a low risk of premature health problems and energy to participate in a variety of physical activities, which results from participation in exercise and the performance of physical activity; includes the summation of cardiorespiratory endurance, muscle power, flexibility, and body composition.

Lifestyle modification: Using opportunities in a person's daily routine (e.g., carry groceries or climbing stairs) to increase energy expenditure, and substitute activity for leisure time.

Older adult: In most cases, "old age" guidelines apply to individuals aged 65 years or older, but they can also be relevant for adults aged 50–64 years with clinically significant chronic conditions or functional limitations that affect movement ability, fitness, or physical activity.

6.4   PHYSIOLOGY OF NORMAL AGING

Many physiological changes have been found to occur as part of normal aging. There is a decrease in maximal aerobic capacity and maximal heart rate, and an increase in heart rate and blood pressure response to submaximal exercise. There is a decrease in tissue elasticity, muscle strength, muscle power, and endurance. Motor coordination and neural reaction time also decrease. Oxidative and glycolytic capacity decline with a reduction in mitochondrial volume. Gait parameters including step length, cadence, speed, and stability also decrease. Attention span, memory, cognitive processing speed, and accuracy decrease. Rapid eye movement (REM) and slow wave sleep duration decrease. Heat and cold intolerance increases, and temperature regulatory capacity decreases.

Most cardiovascular functions also decrease, including maximal cardiac output, stroke volume, endothelial reactivity, skeletal blood flow, and capillary density. Arterial distensibility and vascular sensitivity also decrease, as does glomerular filtration rate (GFR). Baroreflex function becomes more impaired, and postural hypotension can be exacerbated. Pulmonary function also decreases with aging, including a decline in vital capacity and peak flow rates.

There are also effects on the nutritional status of the body, including decreased metabolic rate and total energy expenditure. Total body water, potassium, calcium, and nitrogen also decrease, as do protein synthesis rates, amino acid uptake into skeletal muscle, nitrogen retention, and protein turnover. Appetite also decreases, and dehydration is more common as thirst decreases while the number of nephrons decreases, and the kidneys become less sensitive to the effects of antidiuretic hormone. Metabolic changes are also part of normal aging. Glycogen storage capacity, glycogen synthase, GLUT-4 transporter protein content, and translocation to the cell membrane all decrease. With aging, lipoprotein lipase activity decreases, while total cholesterol and low density lipoprotein (LDL)-C increase. High density lipoprotein (HDL)-C decreases, so does insulin-like growth factor (IGF)-1 and growth hormone.

Body composition also changes with aging. There is an increase in adipose mass and a decline in fat-free mass (FFM). Adipose tissue deposition patterns shift, increasing both visceral and truncal adiposity. There is a decrease in muscle mass (sarcopenia) and type 2 (fast twitch) muscle fiber types. There is an increase in intramuscular fat and connective tissue, with a decline in muscle quality. There is also decreased bone mass and density, with an increase in bony fragility.

6.5   SUCCESSFUL AGING AND THE ROLE OF PHYSICAL ACTIVITY AND EXERCISE IN CHRONIC DISEASE PREVENTION AND TREATMENT

Age is a primary risk factor for developing chronic diseases such as CVD, type 2 diabetes, obesity, as well as degenerative musculoskeletal conditions such as osteoporosis, arthritis, and sarcopenia. Fortunately, despite the long list of systems that are adversely affected by aging, increased physical activity or exercise can either slow the decline seen with aging, or even improve the health of these systems. Studies have shown a statistically significant decrease in the relative risk of cardiovascular and all-cause mortality among persons who are highly fit/active, as compared with those who are normally fit/active or low fit/sedentary.[46]

Regular physical activity increases average life expectancy through its influence on chronic disease development (via reduction of secondary aging effects). A graded, inverse relationship between total physical activity and mortality has been identified. Physical activity, even when initiated later in life, can lessen morbidity and improve mortality rates, while postponing the onset of disability. This concept has been termed "disability threshold"; which is when the person goes from independent to disabled. This can be modified in a positive way with muscle strengthening and increased mass, and can also be affected by environmental changes such as home modifications or assistive devices. These changes can influence the age at which a person becomes disabled (Figure 6.1).

In an analysis of more than 10,000 older adults in the Established Populations for Epidemiologic Studies of the Elderly, there was an almost twofold increased likelihood of dying without disability

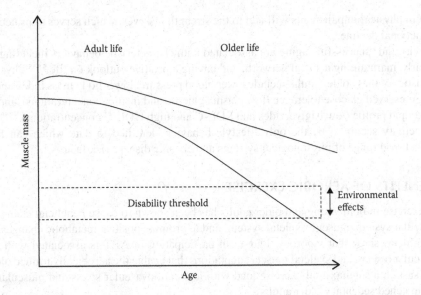

FIGURE 6.1 How the disability threshold changes with age, muscle mass, and environment.

among those most physically active compared with those who were sedentary.[47] The largest increment in mortality benefit is seen when comparing sedentary adults with those in the next highest
physical activity level.[46] The DHHS report "Physical Activity Guidelines Advisory Committee
Report" provides a comprehensive summary of the evidence linking lower levels of physical activity
with a higher risk of developing and dying from a variety of different conditions.[3]

Physical activity can also limit the impact of secondary aging through restoration of functional
capacity in older adults who have previously been sedentary. However, helping older adults benefit
from increased physical activity can be difficult. Older adult populations not only have a reduction
in overall amounts of physical activity, but also the intensity of physical activity may be less. The
most popular activities in older adults tend to be of lower intensity such as walking, gardening, golf,
and low-impact aerobic activities, compared to activities such as running, sports, and high-impact
aerobic activities preferred by younger adults.

Healthy sedentary older adults have the same physiological responses to submaximal aerobic
exercise as do younger adults, although not always to the same degree. This response includes the
control of arterial blood pressure and vital organ perfusion, augmentation of oxygen and substrate
delivery and utilization within the active muscle, maintenance of arterial blood homeostasis, and
dissipation of heat.[48] Healthy older adults are also able to demonstrate normal cardiovascular and
neuromuscular responses to RET. Thus, the normal age-associated changes in physiologic function should not preclude participation in physical activity. Although absolute improvements tend to
be less in older adults versus their younger counterparts, there are similar relative increases from
baseline in VO$_2$max, submaximal metabolic responses, and exercise tolerance with AET and limb
muscle strength, endurance, and muscle size in response to RET.[49–51] However, older adults may
take longer to achieve these improvements with exercise, and often have reduced exercise tolerance
with heat or cold stress. In addition, cessation of AET in older adults leads to rapid loss of cardiovascular and metabolic fitness, just as it does in younger populations.

It is important to note that improvement in physiological parameters does not always translate
into functional gains. Studies have demonstrated that endurance exercise alone with minimal resistance training is less likely to have a significant effect on function, but does improve cardiovascular
health. There is also a threshold of strength where frail adults can have a marked improvement in
function with minimal change in strength, whereas healthy older adults may not have as much of
a benefit with the same percent increase in strength.[52,53] Above the functional threshold, additional

reduction in physical impairments will add to the strength reserves, which serves to protect against future functional decline.

Longevity and "successful" aging are associated with characteristic behaviors including exercising regularly, maintaining a social network, and having a positive outlook on life.[54,55] Physiological characteristics of these older adults include lower blood pressure, lower body mass index and central adiposity, preserved glucose tolerance (low plasma glucose and insulin concentrations), and a favorable blood lipid profile (low triglycerides and LDL-C and high HDL-C concentrations).[55,56] Regular physical activity seems to be the only lifestyle behavior identified to date which can favorably influence a broad range of physiological systems and chronic disease risk factors.[4]

6.6   BENEFITS OF AEROBIC EXERCISE

Aerobic exercise in both young and older adults has been shown to cause beneficial changes in the cardiovascular system, musculoskeletal system, and to promote positive metabolic changes. Studies of older athletes show that vigorous, long-term participation in AET is associated with elevated cardiovascular reserve and skeletal muscle adaptations that enable the aerobically trained older individual to sustain a submaximal exercise load with less cardiovascular stress and muscular fatigue than age-matched sedentary older adults.

Aerobic exercise capacity can be increased in healthy middle-aged and older adults by regular aerobic exercise with an intensity of at least 60% of pretraining VO_2max, at least 3 days per week, for at least 16 weeks.[57] This regimen can produce an average increase in VO_2max of 15%–20% as compared with nonexercise controls. Larger improvements in VO_2max can occur with longer durations of training (20–30 weeks), but intensities greater than 70% of VO_2max do not necessarily result in further increases. Significant increases in VO_2max with training can also occur in older adults over 75 years of age. Men and women in their 60s and 70s can increase their VO_2max with AET, but with different mechanisms per gender; older men have increases in maximal cardiac output and systemic A-VO_2 differences, whereas older women primarily show increases in A-VO_2 difference alone.[58]

Interestingly, studies of families and twin pairs have found a significant genetic influence on baseline physiological function and the exercise-induced changes in aerobic fitness, skeletal muscle properties, and cardiovascular risk factors.[47,59] The influence of genetics on the training response to exercise probably explains some of the differences between responders and nonresponders to different training stimuli.

Cardiovascular adaptations are typically seen after 3 or more months of moderate-intensity AET (≥60% of VO_2max); these include lower heart rate at rest[57] and with submaximal exercise,[60] smaller rises in systolic, diastolic, and mean blood pressures during submaximal exercise,[51] and improved vasodilator and O_2 uptake capacity in trained muscles.[61–63] In addition, there are cardioprotective effects, including reductions in atherogenic risk factors (reduced triglycerides and increased HDL-C), reductions in large elastic artery stiffness,[64] improved endothelial and baroreflex function,[65,66] and increased vagal tone.[66]

Aerobic exercise can positively influence body composition. Studies show that moderate-intensity AET without dietary modification is effective in reducing total body fat, as well as slowing the age-related accumulation of central body fat. AET can result in fat loss from the intra-abdominal (visceral) region by more than 20%.[67] Average losses in overweight older adults during 2–9 months of AET ranged from 1% to 4% of total body weight, with the magnitude of total fat loss related to the total number of exercise sessions. In contrast to its effects on body fat, most studies report no significant effect of AET on FFM. A metaanalysis identified significant increases in total FFM in only eight of 36 studies that involved AET, and these increases were generally less than 1 kg.[68] This is probably due to the fact that AET does not generally improve muscle strength or size.

The metabolic effects of aerobic exercise can also be pronounced. Moderate AET, independent of dietary changes, can induce multiple changes that enhance the body's ability to maintain glycemic control at rest, to clear atherogenic lipids triglycerides (TG) from the circulation, and to preferentially use fat as a muscular fuel during submaximal exercise.[56,69-71] Note that the effects of AET on metabolic parameters seem to depend on the intensity of AET, with higher-intensity AET increasing the glucose transporter (GLUT-4) content in the muscles, which results in greater improvements in whole-body insulin action and glycemic control.[72]

6.7   BENEFITS OF RESISTIVE EXERCISE

RET or progressive resistance training refers to the use of muscles to generate force that moves or resists a given weight. Weight resistance can be created using elastic bands, weighted cuffs, free weights, weight machines, or even the patient's own body weight (e.g., mini-squats). RET maintains or improves muscle strength, power, and endurance; these factors then translate into other functional and health benefits. The benefits of RET may also be in part due to a modification of the adverse effects of chronic diseases due to metabolic changes.[73,74] Women who regularly participate in strengthening exercises for as little as 30 minutes a week have a similar risk reduction (23%) in CVD as those who engage in brisk walking for 30 minutes or more each day (18%).[75]

Muscle strength is basically the ability to generate force. Studies have shown that impaired strength is associated with functional impairment and disability in older adults.[53,76-78] Thus, it is not surprising that evidence shows that RET may be an optimal way to improve or maintain function in older adults.[5,79] Older adults can increase their strength with RET from 25% to 100% depending on the study and outcome variable.[80] This strength may translate to functional gains such as sit to stand, but may not affect other variables such as walking speed or distance. Some studies show similar strength gains between younger and older athletes, while others find that strength gains are less in the older adult.[81-83] The effects of age on strength gains may also be influenced by gender, duration of the training period, genetic factors, and specific muscle groups trained.[84-87]

Muscle power is the force of the muscle contraction multiplied by its velocity. The loss of muscle power, which accelerates later in life, is strongly associated with functional decline.[88,89] Studies have shown that functional performance in older adults is associated more with muscle power than muscle strength.[90-93] In addition, the loss of muscle power that occurs with aging happens at a greater rate than the loss of strength; this is thought due to a disproportionate reduction in the size of type II fibers.[86,94-97] Fortunately, RET in older adults has been shown to substantially increase muscle power. Muscle power can be improved in older adults with resistive exercise with a high-velocity component.

RET in older adults has been shown to increase muscle quality, which is muscular performance (strength and/or power) per unit of muscle volume. Studies on the effects of RET on muscle quality in older adults show that increases in strength and power with RET are greater than would be expected based on changes in muscle mass alone.[84,98-100] The primary contributors to increased muscle quality after RET are thought to be increased motor-unit recruitment although other changes such as decreased activation of antagonistic muscle groups, alterations in muscle architecture and tendon stiffness, and selective hypertrophy of type II muscle fiber areas may also influence muscle quality.[82,83,88,101] Note that the hypertrophic response is diminished in older adults. The adaptations seen after RET in older adults seem similar between older men and women.

Muscle endurance, which is the ability to repeatedly produce muscular force and power over an extended period of time, may also be a determinant of functional status. However, RET's effects on muscular endurance are relatively understudied. Increases in muscular strength, secondary to neurological, metabolic, and/or hypertrophic adaptations, are likely to translate into increased muscular endurance in several ways. These adaptations include reduced motor-unit activation required for submaximal tasks, reduced coactivation of antagonistic muscles, increased high-energy phosphate (e.g., adenosine triphosphate [ATP]) availability, and increased mitochondrial density and oxidative capacity.[4] Marked improvements of 34%–200% in muscular endurance have been reported after RET using moderate- to higher-intensity protocols.[81,102]

Body composition can also be positively influenced by RET. Compared with age-matched AET athletes, RET athletes have more total muscle mass, higher bone mineral density (BMD), and higher muscle strength and power.[103,104] Most studies report an increase in FFM with RET, with similar increases from baseline in older men and women. Increases in FFM can be attributed to increases in muscle cross-sectional areas and volumes.[105,106] A recent review of 20 studies found that older adults demonstrate hypertrophy of muscle tissue of between 10% and 62% after RET, depending on the intensity and duration of RET.[107] Moderate- or high-intensity RET can also decrease total body fat mass, with losses between 1.6% and 3.4%.[4] Older RET-trained athletes tend to have higher muscle mass, and are 30%–50% stronger than their sedentary peers.[103]

The evidence for RET as a countermeasure for abdominal obesity is less clear. One study reported significant reductions in intraabdominal fat in older women with RET.[106] Another study found a 10% reduction in visceral fat and an 11% reduction in subcutaneous abdominal fat with RET in older men with type 2 diabetes, despite a 16% increase in energy intake after only two exercise sessions per week for 16 weeks.[108] This study had no dietary controls, and thus subjects may have been also attempting dietary modifications. After participating in a 25-week RET program, women lost significant visceral fat in response to exercise, but men did not. Both groups had similar total fat loss. Fat infiltration into muscle increases with age but this may be partially reversed with RET.[109,110] In addition, cessation of RET in trained older persons increases muscle fat infiltration, while resumption of exercise decreases it.[110]

Studies on the effects of RET on basal metabolic rate (BMR) in the older adult are inconsistent, with some studies showing increases of 7%–9% in BMR, and others demonstrating no differences with 12–26 weeks of training.[111–113] RET may be able to alter the preferred fuel source used under resting conditions, with RET favoring the use of fat as fuel by increasing lipid oxidation and decreasing carbohydrate and amino acid oxidation at rest.[112–114] RET can also increase HDL-C by 8%–21%, decrease LDL-C by 13%–23%, and reduce triglyceride levels by 11%–18%.[115–117] There is some evidence of the effects of RET on a variety of hormones, including possibly increasing IGF-1 or decreasing cortisol, without clear conclusions. There is no consistent evidence of an increase in total or free testosterone with RET.[4]

Physical inactivity is one of the behavioral risk factors thought to influence the development of metabolic syndrome.[118] The metabolic syndrome is a cluster of interrelated risk factors for the development of atherosclerotic CVD, diabetes, and HTN. Muscular strength has been found to be inversely related to metabolic syndrome and all-cause mortality.[119,120] An increased risk of metabolic syndrome, independent of abdominal fat, was strongly associated with high insulin levels, low muscle mass, and low strength in middle-aged and older adults.[121]

RET improves insulin sensitivity and glucose uptake; some studies attribute this to an increased FFM, while others point to qualitative changes in muscle.[122–126] The improved insulin action may be due to increased protein content of glucose transport protein 4 insulin receptor (GLUT-4), protein kinase B, and glycogen synthase.[127–129]

Postmenopausal women have an increase in the risk of metabolic syndrome, thought to be due to increased hepatic lipogenesis in conjunction with intraabdominal fat, both of which are linked to insulin resistance.[130,131] ST may improve insulin sensitivity by reducing hepatic lipogenesis. Given that fat deposition depends on the balance between lipogenesis and fatty acid oxidation, these results also suggest a possible mechanism for ST reducing intraabdominal fat.

The literature on the effects of RET on dyslipidemia is not as clear. There is some evidence for the role of RET in reducing triglycerides, but no consistent evidence for lowering other lipids. In a metaanalysis by Kelley and colleagues, RET reduced total cholesterol by 2.7%, LDL-C by 4.6%, triglycerides by 6.4%, and total cholesterol/HDL-C increased by 1.4% (with no significant overall changes for HDL-C).[132,133] Other reviews support the concept that pharmacological interventions (such as statins) or AET may be more effective for improving lipids and lipoproteins in adults.[134–136] Note that in one study significant reductions were observed in triglycerides and LDL-C levels, and increase in HDL-C levels compared with a nonexercise control group after 11 weeks of RET in 70- to 87-year-old women.[115]

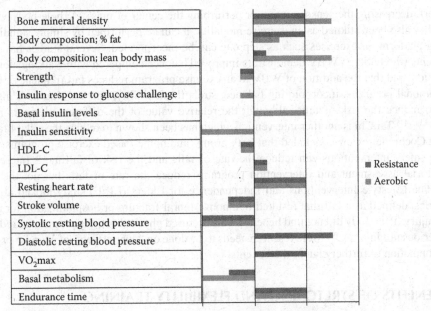

Bone mineral density
Body composition; % fat
Body composition; lean body mass
Strength
Insulin response to glucose challenge
Basal insulin levels
Insulin sensitivity
HDL-C
LDL-C
Resting heart rate
Stroke volume
Systolic resting blood pressure
Diastolic resting blood pressure
VO$_2$max
Basal metabolism
Endurance time

■ Resistance
■ Aerobic

Decreases   No change   Increases

FIGURE 6.2 Comparison of AET and RET on different physiological conditions. (Modified from Pollock, M. L. et al. AHA Science Advisory. Resistance exercise in individuals with and without cardiovascular disease: Benefits, rationale, safety, and prescription: An advisory from the Committee on Exercise, Rehabilitation, and Prevention, Council on Clinical Cardiology, American Heart Association; Position paper endorsed by the American College of Sports Medicine. *Circulation* 101(7):828–833.)

RET can produce small reductions in exercise and resting blood pressure; again the significance of these changes is not clear. In a study of older men and women with pre-HTN (systolic blood pressure [SBP] 120–139/diastolic blood pressure [DBP] 80–89), a heavy-resistance, high-volume RET program significantly reduced resting blood pressure for up to 48 hours following an ST session and were sufficient to shift diastolic BP in men from the prehypertensive category to the normal range. There may also be a role for genotype influencing these reductions. Older men and women with specific genotypes within their angiotensin II type 1 receptor and angiotensinogen genes experience a greater reduction in their resting blood pressure (BP) in response to RET than those with other genotypes at these loci.[137] In the American College of Sports Medicine (ACSM) position stand on exercise and HTN, it was concluded that RET reduces both SBP and DBP in subjects with normal BP, pre-HTN, or HTN.[11] Note that the absolute magnitude of these changes tends to be small, 3.2–6.0 mmHg systolic BP and 3.5–4.7 mmHg diastolic BP (Figure 6.2).

6.8 BENEFITS OF BALANCE TRAINING

Several studies have examined relationships among age, exercise, and balance, with the most research being conducted in populations at risk for falling. Several large cohort studies show that higher levels of physical activity, particularly walking, are associated with a 30%–50% reduction in the risk of osteoporotic fractures.[138] However, it is not clear whether the risk of fracture is reduced due to improved balance, or if balance training alone helps to prevent these fractures. Balance training activities such as lower body strengthening and walking over difficult terrain have been shown to significantly improve balance in many studies, and are thus recommended as part of an exercise intervention to prevent falls.[138–141] Balance regimens should include one to two sets of four to 10 different exercises involving dynamic positions; difficulty should be progressed by decreasing the base of support, decreasing the sensory input, or perturbing the center of mass.[5] Whole-body vibration (WBV) has also been studied as an exercise modality; it can be performed by simply standing on a vibrating platform, or exercises such as stepping can be incorporated. Several studies have shown that patients who undergo WBV demonstrate improved balance compared with walking alone as an intervention, and that the addition of WBV to an exercise program reduces fall frequency.[142]

Multimodal programs incorporating balance, strength, flexibility, and walking have also been shown to reduce the risk of falls, although the relative value of the different elements remains unclear.[53,143–145] Tai Chi is another intervention which has been shown to reduce the risk of fall.[146,147] A recent Cochrane review concluded that both group- and home-based exercise programs, as well as home safety interventions can reduce the rate of falls and the risk of falling.[138] Interestingly, multifactorial assessment and intervention programs reduce the rate of falls but not the risk of falling. The Lifestyle Interventions and Independence for Elders (LIFE) study looked at serious fall injuries, defined as a fall that resulted in a nonvertebral fracture or hospitalization for another serious injury. This study did not find benefit for a structured physical activity program to reduce the risk of serious fall injuries.[148] More research needs to be done on "dose effects" of exercise programs in this population to further clarify the benefits.

6.9 BENEFITS OF STRETCHING AND FLEXIBILITY TRAINING

Stretching exercises have been shown to increase tendon flexibility, and to improve joint ROM and function. However, there is no consensus about how much (frequency or duration) or what types of ROM exercises (static vs. dynamic) are the safest and most effective for older adults. It is recommended that both aerobic and resistance training programs should be complemented by the stretching program that exercises the major muscle or tendon groups at least 2–3 days per week.[8] Singh et al. recommend flexibility training 1–7 days each week, for all major muscle groups with a sustained (20 seconds) stretch of each muscle group.[5] A suggested technique is proprioceptive neuromuscular facilitation, which involves stretching as far as possible, relaxing, and then attempting to stretch further; at maximal stretch the position is held for 20 seconds.

6.10 BENEFITS OF EXERCISE ON SPECIFIC CONDITIONS

6.10.1 IMPROVED BONE HEALTH WITH EXERCISE

Several metaanalyses have concluded that RET and AET both have positive effects on BMD in both premenopausal and postmenopausal women.[149–152] Most studies show a 1%–2% increase with RET, that is higher intensity, progressive, and novel loading, as well as with higher strain rates, although other studies have shown only preservation of BMD over the course of the study.[153–155] Higher-intensity bone loading activities such as stair climbing, brisk walking or walking with weighted vests, or jogging have more effect on BMD in postmenopausal women over a short-term period.[156] Interestingly, WBV can be more effective than walking, and similar to ST for improving bone mass in postmenopausal women.[142] Note that low-intensity weight-bearing activities such as walking (3–5 days a week) for up to a year have minimal effects on BMD in postmenopausal women (0%–2% increase in hip and spine BMD).[156] However, these activities may counteract the age-related loss of BMD and may also lower hip fracture risk. Research on the effectiveness of exercise for bone health in older men is still emerging, but one prospective study found that middle-aged and older men who ran nine or more times per month exhibited lower rates of lumbar bone loss than men who jogged less frequently.[150,157]

6.10.2 IMPROVED PSYCHOLOGICAL WELL-BEING AND QUALITY OF LIFE WITH EXERCISE

Regular physical activity is associated with significant improvements in overall psychological well-being. Both physical fitness and participation in AET are associated with a decreased risk for clinical depression and anxiety. Both higher physical fitness and participation in AET are associated with a decreased risk for clinical depression or anxiety, as well as improvements in overall well-being, and quality of life (QOL), with response rates ranging from 25% to 88%.[158-163] Moderate- and high-intensity tasks seem more likely to improve depression and overall QOL. Most well-controlled exercise training studies result in significant improvements in both physical fitness and self-efficacy for physical activity in older adults.[114] In addition, physical self-efficacy is not only an important outcome measure as a result of participation in activity, but it may also be an important predictor of sustained behavioral change in sedentary populations.[164] Exercise and physical activity have been proposed to impact psychological well-being and health-related QOL through their moderating and mediating effects on constructs such as self-concept and self-esteem.[4]

Physical activity has been shown to be positively associated with most domains of QOL. In a group of older adults who increase their physical activity over the 4-year period, there were increases in physical self-esteem and positive affect, but only positive affect directly influenced improvements in QOL. These findings lend support to the position that physical activity effects on QOL are in part mediated by intermediate psychological outcomes and that physical activity can have long-term effects on well-being.[165] Healthy older adults who regularly participated in physical activity of at least moderate intensity for more than 1 hour per week had higher health-related quality of life (HRQL) measures in both physical and mental domains than those who were physically less active. Therefore, incorporating more physical activity into the lifestyles of sedentary or slightly active older individuals may improve their HRQL.[166]

6.10.3 IMPROVED FUNCTIONING AND DAILY LIFE ACTIVITIES WITH EXERCISE

The effects of exercise on functional abilities are poorly understood, and do not seem to be linear. RET has been shown to favorably impact walking speed, rising from a chair, and balance activities, but more information is needed to understand the precise nature of the relationship between exercise and functional performance.[4] While some studies demonstrate improvements across a variety of functional tasks, other studies suggest functional performance adaptations are more specific, resulting in changes in one functional measure (e.g., walking) but not others (e.g., chair rise or stair climb performance).[73,167-170] There does seem to be a relationship between maintaining cardiovascular fitness levels and the likelihood of becoming functionally dependent in an 8-year follow-up study of older adults.[171] Task-specific training has also been shown to improve function, including tasks such as bed mobility, transfers, and general mobility.[167,172,173] The nature and strength of the relationship between physical activity and functional performance are likely to vary as a function of the specific physical activity functional measures selected.

6.10.4 IMPROVED COGNITIVE FUNCTION WITH EXERCISE

Participation in regular physical activity has been linked to a reduced risk of dementia or cognitive decline in older adults.[174,175] Increases in walking speed and distance have been shown to be related to delayed onset of cognitive impairment.[176,177] The converse has also been shown to be true; decreases in physical mobility (i.e., walking speed, chair stands) and strength are linked to the hastening of cognitive decline.[35,178] However, the causative relationship between physical activity and cognitive status has not been clearly identified, nor has the type of activity been defined. The LIFE study looked at 1635 community-living adults aged 70–89 years who could walk at least 400 m but were at risk for mobility disability.[179] A physical activity program that included walking, resistance training, and flexibility exercises as compared with an education program did not result in changes in global or domain-specific cognitive function. Notably, in a subset of participants over the age of 80 years and those with poorer baseline physical performance, there were improvements in executive functioning.

Studies have shown an inverse relationship between muscular strength and prevalence of Alzheimer's disease (AD), with several studies showing that the incidence of AD was significantly associated with grip strength independent of muscle mass.[180–182] In a study looking at total body strength (assessed in 11 muscle groups), each one unit increase in baseline strength was linked to a 43% decrease in the risk of AD, even when adjusted for other variables such as body mass index (BMI) physical activity, and vascular risk factors, among others.[183] Muscle strength was also associated with a reduced risk of mild cognitive impairment, and an improved working memory with RET (especially when a heavy resistance training load is used).[184] Some hypothesize that the causal association is the IGF-1 (insulin-like growth factor) which increases with exercise, and has been shown to induce neurogenesis in the hippocampus.[185]

6.10.5 STROKE PREVENTION WITH EXERCISE

Physical activity improves stroke risk factors such as HTN, hyperlipidemia, obesity, and diabetes mellitus (DM), and may reduce stroke risk itself. Data from clinical trials show clearly that exercise reduces BP, improves endothelial function, reduces insulin resistance, improves lipid metabolism, and may help reduce weight. Epidemiological research strongly suggests that, on average, high levels of leisure-time physical activity and moderate levels of occupational physical activity are associated with a 10%–30% reduction in the incidence of stroke and coronary heart disease (CHD) in both men and women.

Stroke survivors are often deconditioned and predisposed to a sedentary lifestyle that adversely impacts performance of activities of daily living, increases the risk for falls, and may contribute to a heightened risk for recurrent stroke and other CVDs. With regard to the effectiveness of exercise for secondary prevention of stroke, there are several studies that have shown that aerobic exercise and ST improve cardiovascular fitness after stroke.[186] Exercise training improves functional capacity, the ability to perform activities of daily living, and QOL, and it reduces the risk for subsequent cardiovascular events. Physical activity goals and exercise prescription for stroke survivors need to be customized for the individual to maximize long-term adherence.

For patients with ischemic stroke or transient ischemaic attack (TIA) who are capable of engaging in physical activity, at least three to four sessions (30–40 minutes) per week of moderate- to vigorous-intensity aerobic physical exercise are reasonable to reduce stroke risk factors. For patients who are able and willing to initiate increased physical activity, referral to a comprehensive, behaviorally oriented program is reasonable. For individuals with disability after ischemic stroke, supervision by a health-care professional such as a physical therapist or cardiac rehabilitation professional, at least on initiation of an exercise regimen, is recommended.[187]

6.10.6 CANCER PREVENTION AND MANAGEMENT WITH EXERCISE

Many studies have demonstrated the effects of exercise on both primary and secondary prevention of colon cancer.[188] It is known that physically active individuals have a lower risk of colorectal cancer.[22,189] Exercise appears to have a dose–response in the reduction of colon cancer; this benefit is demonstrated with greater than 4 hours of exercise per week. In the US Nurses' Health Study, there was a 24% reduced risk of colon cancer overall with exercise when comparing the most active to the least active women.[190] Women who expended more than 21 MET-hours per week on leisure-time physical activity had a relative risk of colon cancer of 0.54 in comparison with women who expended less than 2 MET-hours per week.[191] These levels are equivalent to brisk walking for 5–6 hours per week in the most active and 0.5 hours per week in the least active. The significant inverse association between leisure-time physical activity and incidence of colon cancer in women in this study is consistent with what has been found in men. Several mechanisms have been proposed for the role of physical activity in reducing colon cancer risk including reduced insulin resistance and hyperinsulinemia, anti-inflammatory action, direct immune action, decreased intestinal transit time, and/or higher vitamin D levels.

Obesity is also associated with an increased risk of colon cancer. Women who had a body mass index greater than 29 kg/m^2 had a relative risk of colon cancer of 1.45 in comparison with women who had a body mass index of less than 21 kg/m^2.[190] It is interesting to note that increased body fatness in childhood and adolescence, independent of adult obesity, has been shown to be a possible risk factor for colorectal cancer in women, with a weaker association in men.[192]

Once a person develops colon cancer the benefits of exercise appear to continue both by increasing QOL and reducing cancer-specific and overall mortality.[21] Patients with a diagnosis of stage III colon cancer who engaged in at least 18 MET-hours per week of physical activity showed a better outcome, with 47% having significant improvement in disease-free survival. Recreational physical activity after the diagnosis of stage I–III colorectal cancer also reduces the risk of cancer-specific and overall mortality. Both low- and moderate-intensity aerobic exercise programs can be equally effective in improving physiologic and psychologic functions in cancer survivors. There is recent evidence that QOL, cancer-specific mortality, and overall mortality are improved with exercise after colon cancer is diagnosed. Thus, aerobic exercise is a valuable addition to the cancer rehabilitation plan.

There is also a beneficial role of exercise in breast cancer prevention and treatment. There is strong evidence for an inverse association between physical activity and postmenopausal breast cancer, with risk reductions ranging from 20% to 80%.[193] However, the evidence is stronger for postmenopausal breast cancer than for premenopausal cancer. For pre- and postmenopausal breast cancer combined, physical activity is associated with a 15%–20% decreased risk.[193] Evidence of a dose–response relationship also exists. Women who engaged in regular strenuous physical activity in their 30s, between 30 and 60 minutes per day moderate to vigorous intensity exercise, have a 14%–18% decreased risk of postmenopausal breast cancer.[24,194] Even brisk walking 1.25–2.5 hours per week decreases the risk of breast cancer. There appears to be a 6% decrease in breast cancer risk for each additional hour of physical activity per week, assuming sustained activity over time.[193] The protective effects of exercise were most pronounced in those with a BMI <24, but also were observed for women with BMI 24.1–28.4.[194]

The associations between physical activity and breast cancer risk are strongest for activity sustained over a lifetime or done after menopause, and for moderate to strenuous physical activity that is done regularly. This effect is stronger in postmenopausal women, women who are parous, women of normal weight, and those without a family history of breast cancer.[195] In one review, the odds ratio (OR) of breast cancer among women who, on average, spent 3.8 or more hours per week participating in physical exercise activities was 0.42 relative to those who were inactive. The effect was stronger among women who had a full-term pregnancy (OR of 0.28 for parous and 0.73 for nulliparous women).[196] Risk factors for breast cancer may include adiposity, sex hormones, insulin resistance, adipokines, and chronic inflammation.

There is also evidence of the benefits of exercise in breast cancer patients and survivors. Increasing physical activity after breast cancer diagnosis may reduce the risk of death from this disease.[197] The greatest benefit occurred in women who walked the equivalent of 3–5 hours per week at an average pace. In a systematic review and metaanalysis of exercise in the breast cancer population, exercise was found to lead to statistically significant improvements in QOL and physical functioning, and reduced symptoms of fatigue in breast cancer patients and survivors.[198]

6.11 SCREENING OLDER ADULTS FOR SAFE PARTICIPATION IN AN EXERCISE PROGRAM

Screening examinations of older adults for safe participation in an exercise program should generally include (1) screening individuals for safe participation in exercise; (2) identifying medical problems that would require modification of the exercise prescription, and (3) identifying the impairments and conditions to be targeted by the exercise program.[38] The medical history and physical examination should address all pertinent systems, including neurologic, musculoskeletal, pulmonary, and cardiac.

The history should include questions regarding vision (retinal disease, diplopia, cataracts, glaucoma, and hemianopsia), cognitive status (dementia or delirium), psychiatric status (anxiety or depression), cardiovascular status (abdominal aortic aneurysm [AAA], orthostatic hypotension, and HTN), peripheral vascular disease, hydration status, and pulmonary conditions (chronic obstructive pulmonary disease [COPD], bronchitis, or asthma), neurologic (stroke, neuropathy, weakness, and movement disorders), endocrine conditions such as diabetes or hypothyroidism, hernias, hemorrhoids, arthritis, or other joint impairments, stress incontinence, and osteoporosis.

The goals of exercise and a functional history should also be obtained. Particular importance should be placed on a history of falls or impaired balance, vertigo or dizziness, insufficiency fractures or osteoporosis, and prior exercise preferences, successes, and challenges.

Physical examination should include assessment of cognitive status, including orientation, attention, and short-term memory, assessment of pulses and circulatory status, auscultation of heart and lungs, abdominal examination including inspection for hernias, auscultation for bruits, and a screening neuromusculoskeletal examination looking at strength, coordination, sensory impairment, and assessment of balance and mobility skills.

Findings that require further assessment or modification of the exercise program include previously undiagnosed heart murmur (especially if consistent with aortic stenosis), resting tachycardia, bradycardia, or other arrhythmia (rate controlled), orthostasis, undiagnosed vascular murmur or bruit (carotid or abdominal), pericardial rub, enlarged aorta or AAA, and symptomatic or undiagnosed hernia. Joint laxity, strength impairment, or evidence of reduced ROM, impaired flexibility, contracture, or sensory loss are other findings that may require modification of the exercise program, but do not preclude participation in exercise.

Additional tests should include a resting electrocardiogram looking for ischemic changes or rhythm disturbances (atrial fibrillation or flutter, bradycardia, and tachycardia). The ACSM does recommend cardiac stress testing for men greater than and equal to 45 years and women greater than or equal to 55 years who plan to exercise at greater than or equal to 60% of VO_2max.[199] In addition, those with known coronary artery disease or cardiac symptoms, two or more coronary artery disease risk factors, diabetes, or known or major signs/symptoms of pulmonary or metabolic disease should also undergo cardiac stress testing.[200]

The ACSM and American Heart Association (AHA) also recommend a screening exercise tolerance test for all older adults for whom moderate to vigorous exercise is considered.[7,199] In most older adults, moderate activity corresponds to 2.5–5.5 METs, equivalent to level walking at 2.0–4.5 miles per hour (mph). In situations where obtaining a screening exercise tolerance test is not feasible, it is reasonable to monitor older persons with no overt cardiac disease for signs and symptoms of cardiovascular abnormalities during the initial stages of an exercise program. Further evaluation should be obtained if the person develops symptoms including angina, decrease in SBP more than 20 mmHg, increase in SBP to more than 250 mmHg or DBP to more than 120 mmHg, or increases in heart rate to greater than or equal to 90% of age-predicted maximum.

Note that the usual formula for age-predicted maximal heart rate, $HR_{max} = 220 - age$, may underestimate maximal heart rate in older adults. A study looking at a broader age distribution showed that this formula often underestimated the maximal heart rate in older subjects and a revised formula fitted to the data resulted in this formula: $HR_{max} = 208 - 0.7(age)$.[201] Another look at this showed good correlation to stress testing results using $HR_{max} = 207 - 0.7(age)$ with a p-value of <0.001 (Table 6.2).[202]

Contraindications to resistance training are similar to the above, and include unstable angina, uncontrolled HTN (SBP ≥160 mmHg and/or diastolic BP ≥ 100 mmHg), uncontrolled dysrhythmias, a recent history of congestive heart failure that has not been evaluated and effectively

---

TABLE 6.2

Contraindications to Participation in an Aerobic Exercise Program

Unstable angina or severe left main coronary disease

End-stage congestive heart failure

Severe valvular heart disease

Malignant or unstable arrhythmias

Elevated resting blood pressure (SBP > 200 mmHg, DBP > 110 mmHg)

Large or expanding abdominal aortic aneurysm

Known cerebral aneurysm or recent intracranial bleed

Uncontrolled or end-stage systemic disease

Acute retinal hemorrhage or recent ophthalmologic surgery

Acute or unstable musculoskeletal injury/condition

Severe dementia or behavioral disturbance

Source: Abbott, R. D et al. 2004. *JAMA* 292(12):1447–1453.

---

treated, severe stenotic or regurgitant valvular disease, and hypertrophic cardiomyopathy.[203] As patients with myocardial ischemia or poor LV function may develop wall-motion abnormalities or serious ventricular arrhythmias during resistance training exertion, moderate to good LV function and cardiorespiratory fitness (>5–6 METs) without angina symptoms or ischemic ST-segment depression have been suggested as additional prerequisites for participation in traditional resistance training.

In addition, for older persons with cardiovascular concerns, resistance training, as opposed to endurance training, may be the initially chosen mode of exercise. Consensus is growing that resistance training may actually reduce the risk for cardiovascular events in comparison to aerobic exercise.

6.12 OVERCOMING BARRIERS TO EXERCISE IN THE OLDER ADULT

There are multiple common barriers to exercise in the older adult. For each of these, there are strategies to reduce or overcome the barrier. One of the most common problems in the older adult is low self-efficacy. Self-efficacy is the confidence in one's ability to carry out a planned behavior. Low self-efficacy has been shown to be correlated with difficulty climbing stairs, impaired balance, increased risk of falls, and functional decline in the elderly. Older adults may also be reluctant to start exercise as they feel it is "too late" or that they are "too old"; this is also associated with fear of injury or discomfort caused by exercise. They may also lack motivation, have depression or cognitive issues that limit their desire to participate in activities, or simply may lack knowledge of the benefits of exercise. Unsurprisingly, habit is the single best predictor of inactivity across all age groups.

Adherence to an exercise program is better in older adults with fewer functional limitations, better overall functional performance, a stronger sense of self-efficacy, and a history of fewer falls.[204] Factors influencing exercise participation include beliefs about exercise, perception of benefits of exercise, past experience with exercise, goals of exercising, personality, and minimizing unpleasant sensations with exercise. A useful way to conceptualize introducing exercise into a routine is to think of it as incorporating physical activity into the daily routine. This avoids sometimes negative connotations "exercise" may have.

Environmental factors or logistical issues may also make exercising more difficult to achieve. These include lack of access to equipment, trouble with transportation, lack of resources such as money for a gym membership, or limited access to technology (like a computer or video player).

And finally, having a mobility impairment that makes transfers, standing, or walking difficult may present what seems like an insurmountable challenge to exercise.

The following are suggestions for some of the common barriers to exercise:[205]

Self-efficacy	Start with exercises that are easily accomplished; provide frequent encouragement; incorporate increased activity into daily tasks; and advance the exercise program gradually.
Attitude	Promote positive personal benefits of exercise and identify enjoyable activities (such as walking in the mall).
Discomfort	Vary intensity and range of exercise; employ cross-training; start slowly; and avoid overdoing.
Disability	Specialized exercises; consider a personal trainer or a physical therapist to design an appropriate program.
Poor balance/ataxia	Assistive devices can increase safety as well as increase exercise intensity. Exercises can be performed from a sitting position. Aquatic therapy can be prescribed.
Fear of injury/falls	Balance and ST initially; use of appropriate clothing, equipment, and supervision; start slowly.
Habitual inactivity	Incorporate into daily routine; repeat encouragement; and promote active lifestyle (such as exercising in front of the television).
Subjective norms	Identify and recruit others who will support interests and education of patient and influential family/friends.
Fixed income	Walking and other simple exercises; use of household items (such as canned goods instead of weights); and promote active lifestyle.
Environmental factors	Walk in the mall (in inclement or overly warm weather); use senior centers; and promote active lifestyle.
Cognitive decline	Incorporate physical activity into daily routine; keep exercises simple and provide clear written instruction with pictures.
Illness/fatigue	Use a range of exercises/intensities that patients can match to their varying energy level. Encourage small amounts of activity as better than no activity.

Instead of focusing on the need to "exercise," a better strategy may be to implement some of these suggestions for promoting physical activity in older adults.

- Reduce sedentary behavior and incorporate activity into daily life
- Increase moderate activity and give less emphasis to the attainment of high levels of activity
- Take a gradual or stepwise approach
- Perform muscle-strengthening activity as well as other recommended types of activity
- Encourage any amount of physical activity as preferable to no activity
- Emphasize both individual activity and community-based activity with others
- Use risk management strategies to prevent injury (such as removing fall hazards or ensuring supervision when a new activity is started)

6.13   WRITING THE EXERCISE PRESCRIPTION

Patients are five to six times more likely to participate in an exercise program when it is recommended by a physician. A successful exercise prescription should be concise, have measurable targets, be realistic for the patient given prior limitations, and address compliance expectations and possible barriers. The exercise prescription should include frequency, intensity, type, time (duration), and progression. A combination of aerobic and resistive exercise, as well as exercise for flexibility and balance ideally should be included; this allows for reduced risk of injury, optimization of health outcomes, and improved adherence.[205]

Aerobic training should start gradually and include low-impact activities such as walking, bicycle riding, dancing, golf (without a cart), yard work, swimming, or housework. Participants should be taught a perceived exertion scale (like the Borg rating of perceived exertion [RPE] scale), or

---

TABLE 6.3

Activities Requiring Moderate Intensity Exercise

Walking briskly (3–4 mph)

Cycling leisurely (≤10 mph)

Swimming with moderate effort

Doubles tennis

Golf—using a pull cart

Fishing—stand and cast

Canoeing leisurely (2–4 mph)

Mowing lawn with power mower

Home repair, painting

Source: Nied, R. J. and B. Franklin. 2002. *American Family Physician* 65(3):419–426.

Note: Moderate intensity is defined as 3–6 METs, or 4–7 kcal/min and slightly lower (2.5–5.5 METs) for older adults.

---

follow simple instructions such as the "talk test" where they should be able to have a conversation while exercising. This prevents overexertion, especially when starting an exercise program.

Older adults starting resistance training should start slowly and gradually. Resistive bands/tubing or light weights (2 lb hand weights or even canned goods), or simple exercises such as rising from a chair repeatedly and/or without using the arms, should be suggested to start. While adults younger than 50 years often do 8–12 repetitions, cardiac patients and those over 50–60 years should do 10–15 repetitions at a lower relative resistance. Training regimens can be increased gradually to avoid fatigue or pain, and to help the participant continue to make gains. Activities that strengthen muscles include calisthenics, carrying groceries, pilates, exercises with bands or weights, yard work/gardening, and heavier chores (such as scrubbing the floor or vacuuming). Note that for higher weight, weight machines may be safer than free weights, especially for those with poor vision, impaired balance, musculoskeletal pains, to avoid dropping the weights and causing potential injuries (Table 6.3).[8]

For frail patients, chair- and bed-based exercises should be used initially. They should also be considered as a starting point for lower functioning patients. A good way to assess what is needed is to have the patient rise from a chair, stand with eyes closed, open their eyes, and then walk across the room. If standing on the chair is difficult, or requires use of the arms, strengthening exercise should be prescribed first.[42] If standing balance is impaired, balance exercises are also indicated. Only if these first two tests are performed easily should aerobic exercise be prescribed before balance exercise.

The activities and intensity levels chosen should depend on the patient's overall health, goals for exercise, energy level, and the routine should vary to maintain interest and promote continued gains. At a minimum, 150 minutes a week of moderate-intensity aerobic activity plus muscle-strengthening activities on 2 days each week should be performed to achieve important health benefits. These benefits will increase with an increase in the activity to 300 minutes per week of moderate-intensity aerobic activity. If the intensity of the aerobic exercise is vigorous, less time per week will be needed to obtain the same beneficial effects.[206]

To support behavior change, physicians should use the five A's (assess, advise, agree, assist, and arrange) when prescribing exercise. The first step is to assess beliefs, behaviors, and knowledge about exercise and its benefits. Physicians should also assess the patient's current fitness level and willingness to begin an exercise program. Patients can complete an activity readiness questionnaire (e.g., the PAR-Q from the Canadian Society for Exercise Physiology, available at http://www.csep.ca/forms.asp), which can be reviewed with the physician prior to initial exercise prescription.[207] Next, physicians should advise their patients about the specific health risks they face, and the benefits of change. Goals for the exercise program should be agreed upon by the patient and the physician, and be based on their interest and confidence in changing their behavior. Long-term exercise compliance is facilitated by the presence of a support network within the family and community, thus assessment of support should occur during the visit as well.[207]

Other techniques to improve adherence include making sure exercise programs incorporate social activities or solitude (depending on patient preference), and giving written instructions including benefits of exercise, illustrations, and guidelines of specific exercises. Additional things to consider include exercise history, cultural norms, instructional needs, health literacy, habitual activities, readiness and motivation for exercise, self-discipline (locus of control) or need for external input, and logistics.[205] Finally, the physician should arrange specifics for follow-up, including suggesting patient journals for completion, and support via phone and during follow-up visits to encourage continued participation. An exercise prescription should be reviewed and adjusted periodically to maintain the desired effect. The ideal prescription is a product of patient–physician shared decision-making, with realistic goals based on specific activities clearly defined.

6.14 SPECIAL CONSIDERATIONS FOR INITIATION OF PHYSICAL ACTIVITY IN OLDER ADULTS[206]

Older adults are often inactive at baseline, thus it is appropriate to start with a light-intensity activity that lasts less than 10 minutes. The duration and intensity of the activity can be slowly progressed as the patient becomes more comfortable with activity, and the numbers of days a week can also be increased. A good beginning activity is walking at a comfortable pace; vigorous activity should initially be avoided to avoid injury and allow confidence to develop. Functional limitations should be taken into account when designing the exercise program, including impairments such as poor balance or limited flexibility. If one of the goals of exercise is weight loss, dietary changes may also need to be implemented for the physical activity to lead to weight loss. If there is a break in the exercise routine due to injury or illness, the intensity and duration should be started at a lower level and gradually increased again. Generally, older or less fit adults need a longer warm-up and cool down period than an active younger adult; this should also be built into the exercise program.

The key practices for promoting physical activity in older adults, with a focus on those with chronic disease or low fitness and those with low levels of physical activity, include (a) a multidimensional activity program that includes endurance, strength, balance, and flexibility training; (b) including principles of behavior change including social support, self-efficacy, active choices, health contracts, assurances of safety, and positive reinforcement enhance adherence; (c) managing risk and avoiding injury by beginning at low intensity but gradually increasing to moderate physical activity, and (d) monitoring intensity to aid in progression and motivation.[206]

Exercise programs should be progressed based on the functional and fitness status of the participant. In addition, different types of exercise can be progressed through different stages of intensity. For aerobic exercise, the ways of progressing include increasing the length of the exercise session, increasing the number of days per week exercising, increasing the intensity slightly over the course of the exercise session, or adding brief bursts during each session. For resistive exercise, when 15 low-intensity weight repetitions are too easy (Borg RPE scale 12–14), increase weight by 10% and reduce the repetitions. Then gradually work up the number of repetitions again. For flexibility training, the participant can add new stretches, progress from static to dynamic moves, or reduce reliance on balance support.

6.15   EXERCISE RECOMMENDATIONS FOR SPECIFIC DISEASES

6.15.1   OSTEOARTHRITIS

Recommendations:

   RET: two to three times weekly at 13–17 on the Borg scale, two to three sets of eight to 10
      repetitions; greater strength gains will be achieved at higher Borg scale ratings.
   AET: two to three times weekly at 11–13 on the Borg scale, progress up to 30–40 minutes.

   Special considerations: When starting aerobic exercise, if uncomfortable or difficult, start with
10 minutes of cardiovascular exercise and increase by 5 minutes per sessions until the goal of 30
minutes is met. For aerobic exercise, use low-impact exercises such as walking, bicycling, or aquatic
exercise. Emphasize functional activities such as sit to stand and stair climbing. If resistive exercise
is painful, start with two to three repetitions and work up as tolerated. For flexibility training, do
ROM of affected joints only within pain-free range[207].
   Contraindications: Avoid vigorous, repetitive activities that use unstable joints, limit activity
during active joint flares for inflammatory arthritis, plan exercise sessions during time of day when
pain is less (e.g., not in the morning if morning stiffness present), and cease activity if joints become
painful or swollen, or lose ROM.

6.15.2   DIABETES

Recommendations:

   RET: two to three times weekly at 13–17 on the Borg scale, two to three sets of eight to 10
      repetitions; greater strength gains will be achieved at higher Borg scale ratings. Use major
      muscle groups; can also use higher repetitions (15–20) with lower intensity (40%–60% of
      one rep max).
   AET: (e.g., walking, biking, and aquatic exercise) two to three times weekly at 11–13 on the
      Borg scale, progress up to 30–40 minutes.

   Special considerations: Aim to expend at least 1000 kcal per week (equivalent to walking
10 miles). For weight loss, aim for 2000 kcal per week. Have patients screened for cardiovascular,
renal, and nervous system abnormalities (including neuropathy and retinopathy) before starting an
exercise program[207].
   Contraindications: Watch for acute hyperglycemia during intense RET, and for postexercise
hypoglycemia in patients on insulin or oral hypoglycemic agents. Patients with peripheral neuropathy may have gait and balance impairment, and will need attention to appropriate footwear.
With autonomic neuropathy emphasize the Borg progressive resistive exercise (PRE) in addition to
heart rate (HR) and BP response to exercise. Polyuria may contribute to dehydration and compromised thermoregulation.

6.15.3   RESPIRATORY/PULMONARY DISEASE

Recommendations:[208]
   Train both upper and lower extremities separately at 60% exercise-tested maximal work
capacity, which is roughly equivalent to 11–13 on the Borg scale.
   Upper-body exercises include arm ergometry, canoeing, swimming, and low-resistance high-repeti-
tion weight lifting. Shoulder girdle, arm, and inspiratory muscles should be targeted for strengthening.
   Lower-body exercises include walking or stationary bicycling, and stair climbing.

Note that RET at higher resistance does not have proven benefit.

Perform exercise three to six times weekly progressing to 30–60 minutes per session.

Special considerations: Initial sessions should be monitored by a professional. Teach patients to self-monitor dyspnea and heart rate. While the minimum frequency goal is exercising 3–5 days per week, those with impaired functional capacity should exercise daily for at least 10 minutes[207].

Contraindications: Oxygen saturations between 88% and 92% are acceptable, consider supplemental oxygen as needed if saturations decline during exercise[25].

6.15.4 OSTEOPOROSIS

Recommendations:

RET: two to three times weekly at 13–17 on the Borg scale, two to three sets of eight to 10 repetitions.

Note greater strength gains will be achieved at higher Borg scale ratings. Specific attention to spinal extensors is important.

AET: only strenuous aerobic exercise, including combinations of fast walking, stair climbing, jogging, or calisthenics have been shown to be beneficial.[208]

Special considerations: Focus should be on balance and function (such as chair stands and stair climbing). Aerobic activities should be weight bearing, at least 4 days a week. Painful activities should be avoided[207].

Contraindications: Avoid high-impact activities and explosive movements, if there is a significant risk factor for fracture. Limit exercises that involve extremes of trunk flexion and twisting.

6.15.5 STROKE

Recommendations:

RET: two to three times weekly at 13–17 on the Borg scale; two to three sets of eight to 10 repetitions. Greater strength gains will be achieved at higher Borg scale ratings.

AET: treadmill walking at normal gait speed or slightly faster, more impaired subjects may benefit from supported treadmill walking, two to three times weekly, progress to 30–40 minutes, 11–13 on the Borg scale.

Task-specific training: perform functional tasks such as rising from chair, climbing stairs, and squatting. Progress to two to three sets of eight to 10 repetitions[208].

Special considerations: If HTN is present, focus on aerobic activities that use large muscle groups, and aim to exercise daily for at least 30 minutes. Intensities of 40%–70% of a one repetition maximum can be equally effective as higher intensities. Use lower repetitions and more repetitions for RET[207].

Contraindications: Note that beta-blockers may attenuate heart rate response and reduce exercise capacity.

6.15.6 CARDIOVASCULAR DISEASE

Recommendations:

RET: two to three times weekly at 13–17 on the Borg scale, two to three sets of eight to 10 repetitions; greater strength gains will be achieved at higher Borg scale ratings.

AET: (e.g., walking, biking, and aquatic exercise) two to three times weekly at 11–13 on the Borg scale, progress up to 30–40 minutes[208].

Special considerations: If HTN is present, focus on aerobic activities that use large muscle groups, and aim to exercise daily for at least 30 minutes. Intensities of 40%–70% of one rep max can be equally effective at higher intensities. Use lower repetitions and more repetitions for RET[207].

Contraindications: Note that beta-blockers may attenuate heart rate response and reduce exercise capacity.

6.15.7   FALLS, POOR BALANCE, AND MOBILITY PROBLEMS

Recommendations:

RET: two to three times weekly at 13–17 on the Borg scale, two to three sets of eight to 10 repetitions.
Note greater strength gains will be achieved at higher Borg scale ratings.
AET: (e.g., walking, biking, and aquatic exercise) two to three times weekly at 11–13 on the Borg scale, progress up to 30–40 minutes.
Dynamic exercises: Tai Chi and high-velocity training exercises with a concentric component performed as quickly as possible to augment muscle power. Examples: repeated performance of leg exercises on exercise machines or common functional tasks such as chair rise or climbing a step.[208]

6.16 SUMMARY OF PHYSICAL ACTIVITY RECOMMENDATIONS FOR OLDER ADULTS BASED ON THE ACSM/AHA POSITION STATEMENT

1. To promote and maintain health, older adults should maintain a physically active lifestyle.
2. Older adults should perform moderate-intensity aerobic (endurance) physical activity for a minimum of 30 minutes on 5 days each week or vigorous intensity aerobic activity for a minimum of 20 minutes on 3 days each week.
   a. Moderate-intensity aerobic activity involves a moderate level of effort relative to an individual's aerobic fitness. On a 10-point scale, where sitting is 0 and all-out effort is 10, moderate-intensity activity is a 5 or 6 and produces noticeable increases in heart rate and breathing. For example, given the heterogeneity of fitness levels in older adults, for some older adults a moderate-intensity walk is a slow walk, and for others it is a brisk walk.
   b. Vigorous intensity activity is a 7 or 8 and produces large increases in heart rate and breathing.
3. Combinations of moderate- and vigorous-intensity activity can be performed to meet this recommendation. These moderate- or vigorous-intensity activities are in addition to the light-intensity activities frequently performed during daily life (e.g., self-care, washing dishes) or moderate-intensity activities lasting 10 minutes or less (e.g., taking out trash, walking to parking lot at store or office).
4. In addition, to promote and maintain health and physical independence, at least twice each week older adults should perform muscle-strengthening activities using the major muscles of the body that maintain or increase muscular strength and endurance. It is recommended that eight to 10 exercises be performed on at least 2 nonconsecutive days or per week using the major muscle groups.
   a. To maximize strength development, a resistance (weight) should be used that allows 10–15 repetitions for each exercise. The level of effort for muscle-strengthening activities should be moderate to high. On a 10-point scale, where no movement is 0, and

maximal effort of a muscle group is 10, moderate-intensity effort is a 5 or 6 and high-intensity effort is a 7 or 8.

5. Participation in aerobic and muscle-strengthening activities above minimum recommended amounts provides additional health benefits and results in higher levels of physical fitness.

   a. Older adults should exceed the minimum recommended amounts of physical activity if they have no conditions that preclude higher amounts of physical activity, and they wish to do one or more of the following: (a) improve their personal fitness, (b) improve management of an existing disease where it is known that higher levels of physical activity have greater therapeutic benefits for the disease, and/or (c) further reduce their risk for premature chronic health conditions and mortality related to physical activity.

   b. In addition, to further promote and maintain skeletal health, older adults should engage in extra muscle-strengthening activity and higher-impact weight-bearing activities as tolerated.

   c. To help prevent unhealthy weight gain, some older adults may need to exceed minimum recommended amounts of physical activity to the point that is individually effective in achieving energy balance, while considering diet and other factors that affect body weight.

6. To maintain the flexibility necessary for regular physical activity and daily life, older adults should perform activities that maintain or increase flexibility on at least 2 days each week for at least 10 minutes each day.

7. To reduce risk of injury from falls, community-dwelling older adults with substantial risk of falls should perform activities that maintain or improve balance.

8. Older adults with one or more medical conditions for which physical activity is therapeutic should perform physical activity in a manner that effectively and safely treats the condition. When chronic conditions preclude activity at minimum recommended levels for prevention, older adults should engage in regular physical activity according to their abilities and conditions so as to avoid sedentary behaviors.

9. Older adults should have a plan for obtaining sufficient physical activity that addresses each recommended type of activity. In addition to specifying each type of activity, care should be taken to identify, how, when, and where each activity will be performed. Those with chronic conditions for which activity is therapeutic should have a single plan that integrates prevention and treatment. For older adults who are not active at recommended levels, plans should include a gradual (or stepwise) approach to increase physical activity over time using multiple bouts of physical activity ($\geq$10 minutes) as opposed to continuous bouts when appropriate. Many months of activity at less than recommended levels are appropriate for some older adults (e.g., those with low fitness) as they increase activity in a stepwise manner. Older adults should also be encouraged to self-monitor their physical activity on a regular basis and to reevaluate plans as their abilities improve or as their health status changes.

6.17   RESOURCES FOR PATIENT EDUCATION

CDC Physical Activity for Everyone: http://www.cdc.gov/physicalactivity/everyone/guidelines/olderadults.html

- Lists CDC guidelines for all types of physical activity, with definitions and explanations for each item.

Go4Life from the National Institute on Aging at the NIH: https://go4life.nia.nih.gov/
- Has videos and pictures of exercises, as well as worksheets for goal setting and to track progress.

Silver Sneakers: http://www.silversneakers.com/
- Describes Silver Sneakers program (exercise program at local health clubs aimed at older adults) with locations of program and how to determine eligibility.

Arthritis Foundation: http://www.arthritis.org/resources/
- Comprehensive website about the Arthritis Foundation and resources; information for a wide variety of arthritis. Has patient information, links to resources, and provides a "support/discussion community."

NIH Exercise and Physical Activity Guide: https://www.nia.nih.gov/health/publication/exercise-physical-activity
- Downloadable comprehensive guide to help older adults become more active; includes basic introductory information, goal-setting worksheets, and clear pictures with descriptions of simple exercises.

Sit and be Fit: http://www.sitandbefit.org/
- Program on public television public broadcasting service (PBS); website has links to videos of the program, a channel guide to find the program on TV, and an online blog with tips for exercising.

VHA National Center for Health Promotion and Disease Prevention: MOVE program handouts: http://www.move.va.gov/handouts.asp?physical
- MOVE is program for veterans, but website provides helpful handouts and worksheets for patients; includes information not only about exercise/physical activity, but also behavior and nutrition.

6.18 LIST OF PERTINENT GUIDELINES AND POSITION PAPERS (IN REVERSE CHRONOLOGIC ORDER)

Physical Activity and Exercise Recommendations for Stroke Survivors: A Statement for Healthcare Professionals from the American Heart Association/American Stroke Association (2014).

Guidelines for the Prevention of Stroke in Patients with Stroke and Transient Ischemic Attack: A Guideline for Healthcare Professionals from the American Heart Association/American Stroke Association (2014).

Exercise and Type 2 Diabetes: American College of Sports Medicine and the American Diabetes Association Joint Position Statement of (2010).

Clinical Practice Guideline on the Treatment of Osteoarthritis of the Knee. American Academy of Orthopedic Surgeons (2010).

Exercise and Physical Activity for Older Adults. American College of Sports Medicine Position Stand (2009).

Exercise Training for Type 2 Diabetes Mellitus: Impact on Cardiovascular Risk. American Heart Association (2009).

Department of Health and Human Services (DHHS) Physical Activity Guidelines for Americans (2008).

Physical Activity and Public Health in Older Adults: Recommendation from the American College of Sports Medicine and the American Heart Association (2007).

Bone Health and Osteoporosis: A Report of the Surgeon General (2004).

Physical Activity and Exercise Recommendations for Stroke Survivors: American Heart Association (2004).

Exercise and Hypertension: Position Stand, American College of Sports Medicine (2004).

Exercise and Physical Activity in the Prevention and Treatment of Atherosclerotic Cardiovascular Disease: American Heart Association (2003).

Third Report of the National Cholesterol Education Program (NCEP) Expert Panel on Detection, Evaluation, and Treatment of the High Blood Cholesterol in Adults (Adult Treatment Panel III) (2001).

Resistance Exercise in Individuals with and without Cardiovascular Disease: Benefits, Rationale, Safety, and Prescription. An Advisory from the Committee on Exercise, Rehabilitation, and Prevention, Council on Clinical Cardiology, American Health Association (2000).

REFERENCES

1. US Department of Health and Human Services. 2011. *Healthy People 2020.* Washington, DC: US Department of Health and Human Services; 2010.
2. Nelson, M. E., W. J. Rejeski, S. N. Blair, P. W. Duncan, J. O. Judge, A. C. King, C. A. Macera, and C. Castaneda-Sceppa. 2007. Physical activity and public health in older adults: Recommendation from the American College of Sports Medicine and the American Heart Association. *Medicine and Science in Sports and Exercise* 39(8):1435–1445.
3. US Department of Health and Human Services, Office of Disease Prevention and Health Promotion. 2008. *Physical Activity Guidelines for Americans.* Washington, DC: US Department of Health and Human Services.
4. American College of Sports Medicine, W. J. Chodzko-Zajko, D. N. Proctor, M. A. Fiatarone Singh, C. T. Minson, C. R. Nigg, G. J. Salem, and J. S. Skinner. 2009. American College of Sports Medicine position stand: Exercise and physical activity for older adults. *Medicine and Science in Sports and Exercise* 41(7):1510–1530, doi:10.1249/MSS.0b013e3181a0c95c.
5. Singh, M. A. 2002. Exercise comes of age: Rationale and recommendations for a geriatric exercise prescription. *The Journals of Gerontology, Series A: Biological Sciences and Medical Sciences* 57(5): M262–M282.
6. Haskell, W. L., I.-M. Lee, R. R. Pate, K. E. Powell, S. N. Blair, B. A. Franklin, C. A. Macera, G. W. Heath, P. D. Thompson, and A. Bauman. 2007. Physical activity and public health: Updated recommendation for adults from the American College of Sports Medicine and the American Heart Association. *Circulation* 116(9):1081.
7. Fletcher, G. F., G. J. Balady, E. A. Amsterdam, B. Chaitman, R. Eckel, J. Fleg, V. F. Froelicher et al. 2001. Exercise standards for testing and training: A statement for healthcare professionals from the American Heart Association. *Circulation* 104(14):1694–1740.
8. Pollock, M. L., B. A. Franklin, G. J. Balady, B. L. Chaitman, J. L. Fleg, B. Fletcher, M. Limacher et al. 2000. AHA Science Advisory. Resistance exercise in individuals with and without cardiovascular disease: Benefits, rationale, safety, and prescription: An advisory from the Committee on Exercise, Rehabilitation, and Prevention, Council on Clinical Cardiology, American Heart Association; Position paper endorsed by the American College of Sports Medicine. *Circulation* 101(7):828–833.
9. Thompson, P. D., D. Buchner, I. L. Pina, G. J. Balady, M. A. Williams, B. H. Marcus, K. Berra et al. 2003. Exercise and physical activity in the prevention and treatment of atherosclerotic cardiovascular disease: A statement from the Council on Clinical Cardiology (Subcommittee on Exercise, Rehabilitation, and Prevention) and the Council on Nutrition, Physical Activity, and Metabolism (Subcommittee on Physical Activity). *Circulation* 107(24):3109–3116, doi:10.1161/01.CIR.0000075572.40158.77.
10. Chobanian, A. V., G. L. Bakris, H. R. Black, W. C. Cushman, L. A. Green, J. L. Izzo Jr, D. W. Jones, B. J. Materson, S. Oparil, and J. T. Wright Jr. 2003. The Seventh Report of the Joint National Committee on Prevention, Detection, Evaluation, and Treatment of High Blood Pressure: The JNC 7 Report. *JAMA* 289(19):2560–2571.
11. Pescatello, L. S., B. A. Franklin, R. Fagard, W. B. Farquhar, G. A. Kelley, and C. A. Ray. 2004. Exercise and hypertension: American College of Sports Medicine position stand. *Medicine and Science in Sports and Exercise* 36(3):533–553.
12. McDermott, M. M., K. Liu, L. Ferrucci, M. H. Criqui, P. Greenland, J. M. Guralnik, L. Tian, J. R. Schneider, W. H. Pearce, and J. Tan. 2006. Physical performance in peripheral arterial disease: A slower rate of decline in patients who walk more. *Annals of Internal Medicine* 144(1):10–20.

13. Sigal, R. J., G. P. Kenny, D. H. Wasserman, and C. Castaneda-Sceppa. 2004. Physical activity/exercise and type 2 diabetes. *Diabetes Care* 27(10):2518–2539, doi:27/10/2518 [pii].

14. US Preventive Services Task Force. 2003. Screening for obesity in adults: Recommendations and rationale. *Annals of Internal Medicine* 139(11):930.

15. Geliebter, A., M. M. Maher, L. Gerace, B. Gutin, S. B. Heymsfield, and S. A. Hashim. 1997. Effects of strength or aerobic training on body composition, resting metabolic rate, and peak oxygen consumption in obese dieting subjects. *The American Journal of Clinical Nutrition* 66(3):557–563.

16. Going, S., T. Lohman, L. Houtkooper, L. Metcalfe, H. Flint-Wagner, R. Blew, V. Stanford, E. Cussler, J. Martin, and P. Teixeira. 2003. Effects of exercise on bone mineral density in calcium-replete postmenopausal women with and without hormone replacement therapy. *Osteoporosis International* 14(8):637–643.

17. US Department of Health and Human Services. 2004. *Bone Health and Osteoporosis: A Report of the Surgeon General*. Rockville, Maryland: US Department of Health and Human Services, Office of the Surgeon General 87.

18. Gamble, R., J. Wyeth-Ayerst, E. L. Johnson, W.-A. Searle, and S. Beecham. 2000. Recommendations for the medical management of osteoarthritis of the hip and knee. *Arthritis and Rheumatism* 43(9):1905–1915.

19. Katz, P., M. O'Grady, G. Davis, C. H. Rojas-Fernandez, B. Ferrell, R. Levy, D. C. Neiman, M. A. Young, S. Radcliff, and B. B. Reitt. 2001. Exercise prescription for older adults with osteoarthritis pain: Consensus practice recommendations—A supplement to the AGS clinical practice guidelines on the management of chronic pain in older adults. *Journal of the American Geriatrics Society* 49(6):808–823.

20. Stewart, K. J., W. R. Hiatt, J. G. Regensteiner, and A. T. Hirsch. 2002. Exercise training for claudication. *New England Journal of Medicine* 347(24):1941–1951.

21. Meyerhardt, J. A., E. L. Giovannucci, M. D. Holmes, A. T. Chan, J. A. Chan, G. A. Colditz, and C. S. Fuchs. 2006. Physical activity and survival after colorectal cancer diagnosis. *Journal of Clinical Oncology: Official Journal of the American Society of Clinical Oncology* 24(22):3527–3534, doi:JCO.2006.06.0855 [pii].

22. Slattery, M. L. 2004. Physical activity and colorectal cancer. *Sports Medicine* 34(4):239–252.

23. Holmes, M. D., W. Y. Chen, D. Feskanich, C. H. Kroenke, and G. A. Colditz. 2005. Physical activity and survival after breast cancer diagnosis. *JAMA* 293(20):2479–2486.

24. Lee, I. M. 2003. Physical activity and cancer prevention—Data from epidemiologic studies. *Medicine and Science in Sports and Exercise* 35(11):1823–1827, doi:10.1249/01.MSS.0000093620.27893.23.

25. Pauwels, R. A., A. S. Buist, P. M. A. Calverley, C. R. Jenkins, and S. S. Hurd. 2012. Global strategy for the diagnosis, management, and prevention of chronic obstructive pulmonary disease. *American Journal of Respiratory and Critical Care Medicine* 163(5): 1256–1276.

26. Brosse, A. L., E. S. Sheets, H. S. Lett, and J. A. Blumenthal. 2002. Exercise and the treatment of clinical depression in adults. *Sports Medicine* 32(12):741–760.

27. Doody, R. S., J. C. Stevens, C. Beck, R. M. Dubinsky, J. A. Kaye, L. Gwyther, R. C. Mohs et al. 2001. Practice parameter: Management of dementia (an evidence-based review). Report of the Quality Standards Subcommittee of the American Academy of Neurology. *Neurology* 56(9):1154–1166.

28. AGS Panel on Persistent Pain in Older Persons. 2002. The management of persistent pain in older persons. *Journal of the American Geriatrics Society* 50(6 Suppl):S205–S224, doi:jgs5071 [pii].

29. Remme, W. J., K. Swedberg, and Task Force for the Diagnosis and Treatment of Chronic Heart Failure, European Society of Cardiology. 2001. Guidelines for the diagnosis and treatment of chronic heart failure. *European Heart Journal* 22(17):1527–1560, doi:10.1053/euhj.2001.2783.

30. Gordon, N. F., M. Gulanick, F. Costa, G. Fletcher, B. A. Franklin, E. J. Roth, T. Shephard et al. 2004. Physical activity and exercise recommendations for stroke survivors: An American Heart Association scientific statement from the Council on Clinical Cardiology, Subcommittee on Exercise, Cardiac Rehabilitation, and Prevention; the Council on Cardiovascular Nursing; the Council on Nutrition, Physical Activity, and Metabolism; and the Stroke Council. *Stroke: A Journal of Cerebral Circulation* 35(5):1230–1240, doi:10.1161/01.STR.0000127303.19261.19.

31. Hagen, K. B., G. Hilde, G. Jamtvedt, and M. F. Winnem. 2002. The cochrane review of advice to stay active as a single treatment for low back pain and sciatica. *Spine* 27(16):1736–1741, doi:00007632-200208150-00010 [pii].

32. Bharucha, A. E., J. H. Pemberton, and G. R. Locke 3rd. 2013. American Gastroenterological Association technical review on constipation. *Gastroenterology* 144(1):218–238, doi:10.1053/j.gastro.2012.10.028.

33. Orthopaedic Surgeons Panel on Falls Prevention. 2001. Guideline for the prevention of falls in older persons. *Journal of the American Geriatrics Society* 49(5):664–672.

34. Kesaniemi, Y. K., E. Danforth Jr, M. D. Jensen, P. G. Kopelman, P. Lefebvre, and B. A. Reeder. 2001. Dose–response issues concerning physical activity and health: An evidence-based symposium. *Medicine and Science in Sports and Exercise* 33(6 Suppl):S351–S358.

35. Keysor, J. J. 2003. Does late-life physical activity or exercise prevent or minimize disablement? A critical review of the scientific evidence. *American Journal of Preventive Medicine* 25(3):129–136.

36. Nelson, M. E., J. E. Layne, M. J. Bernstein, A. Nuernberger, C. Castaneda, D. Kaliton, J. Hausdorff et al. 2004. The effects of multidimensional home-based exercise on functional performance in elderly people. *The Journals of Gerontology, Series A: Biological Sciences and Medical Sciences* 59(2):154–160.

37. Pahor, M. 2006. Effects of a physical activity intervention on measures of physical performance: Results of the lifestyle interventions and independence for elders pilot (LIFE-P) study. *The Journals of Gerontology, Series A: Biological Sciences and Medical Sciences* 61(11): 1157–1165.

38. Abbott, R. D., L. R. White, G. W. Ross, K. H. Masaki, J. D. Curb, and H. Petrovitch. 2004. Walking and dementia in physically capable elderly men. *JAMA* 292(12):1447–1453.

39. Larson, E. B., L. Wang, J. D. Bowen, W. C. McCormick, L. Teri, P. Crane, and W. Kukull. 2006. Exercise is associated with reduced risk for incident dementia among persons 65 years of age and older. *Annals of Internal Medicine* 144(2):73–81.

40. Weuve, J., J. H. Kang, J. E. Manson, M. M. B. Breteler, J. H. Ware, and F. Grodstein. 2004. Physical activity, including walking, and cognitive function in older women. *JAMA* 292(12):1454–1461.

41. Penninx, B. W. J. H., S. P. Messier, W. J. Rejeski, J. D. Williamson, M. DiBari, C. Cavazzini, W. B. Applegate, and M. Pahor. 2001. Physical exercise and the prevention of disability in activities of daily living in older persons with osteoarthritis. *Archives of Internal Medicine* 161(19):2309–2316.

42. Singh, M. A. F. 2002. Exercise to prevent and treat functional disability. *Clinics in Geriatric Medicine* 18(3):431–462.

43. Tseng, B. S., D. R. Marsh, M. T. Hamilton, and F. W. Booth. 1995. Strength and aerobic training attenuate muscle wasting and improve resistance to the development of disability with aging. *The Journals of Gerontology, Series A: Biological Sciences and Medical Sciences* 50(Spec No):113–119.

44. King, A. C., R. F. Oman, G. S. Brassington, D. L. Bliwise, and W. L. Haskell. 1997. Moderate-intensity exercise and self-rated quality of sleep in older adults: A randomized controlled trial. *JAMA* 277(1):32–37.

45. Singh, N. A., K. M. Clements, and M. A. Fiatarone. 1997. A randomized controlled trial of the effect of exercise on sleep. *Sleep* 20(2):95–101.

46. Blair, S. N. and M. Wei. 2000. Sedentary habits, health, and function in older women and men. *American Journal of Health Promotion* 15(1):1–8.

47. Bouchard, C. and T. Rankinen. 2001. Individual differences in response to regular physical activity. *Medicine and Science in Sports and Exercise* 33(6 Suppl):S446–S451; discussion S452–S453.

48. Seals, D. R., J. A. Taylor, A. V. Ng, and M. D. Esler. 1994. Exercise and aging: Autonomic control of the circulation. *Medicine and Science in Sports and Exercise* 26(5):568–576.

49. Huang, G., C. A. Gibson, Z. V. Tran, and W. H. Osness. 2005. Controlled endurance exercise training and VO$_2$max changes in older adults: A meta-analysis. *Preventive Cardiology* 8(4):217–225.

50. Lemmer, J. T., D. E. Hurlbut, G. F. Martel, B. L. Tracy, F. M. Ivey, E. J. Metter, J. L. Fozard, J. L. Fleg, and B. F. Hurley. 2000. Age and gender responses to strength training and detraining. *Medicine and Science in Sports and Exercise* 32(8):1505–1512.

51. Seals, D. R., B. F. Hurley, J. Schultz, and J. M. Hagberg. 1984. Endurance training in older men and women II. Blood lactate response to submaximal exercise. *Journal of Applied Physiology: Respiratory, Environmental and Exercise Physiology* 57(4):1030–1033.

52. Camacho, T. C., R. E. Roberts, N. B. Lazarus, G. A. Kaplan, and R. D. Cohen. 1991. Physical activity and depression: Evidence from the Alameda County Study. *American Journal of Epidemiology* 134(2):220–231.

53. Campbell, A. J., M. C. Robertson, M. M. Gardner, R. N. Norton, M. W. Tilyard, and D. M. Buchner. 1997. Randomised controlled trial of a general practice programme of home based exercise to prevent falls in elderly women. *BMJ (Clinical Research Ed.)* 315(7115):1065–1069.

54. Seeman, T. E., L. F. Berkman, P. A. Charpentier, D. G. Blazer, M. S. Albert, and M. E. Tinetti. 1995. Behavioral and psychosocial predictors of physical performance: MacArthur studies of successful aging. *The Journals of Gerontology, Series A: Biological Sciences and Medical Sciences* 50(4):M177–M183.

55. Spirduso, W. W., K. L. Francis, and P. G. MacRae. 2005. *Physical Dimensions of Aging.* Champaign, Illinois: Human Kinetics.

56. Holloszy, J. O. 2000. The biology of aging. *Mayo Clinic Proceedings* 75(Suppl):S3–S8; discussion S8–S9.

57. Huang, G., X. Shi, J. A. Davis-Brezette, and W. H. Osness. 2005. Resting heart rate changes after endurance training in older adults: A meta-analysis. *Medicine and Science in Sports and Exercise* 37(8):1381–1386, doi:00005768-200508000-00018 [pii].

58. Adams, K. J., A. M. Swank, J. M. Berning, P. G. Sevene-Adams, K. L. Barnard, and J. Shimp-Bowerman. 2001. Progressive strength training in sedentary, older African American women. *Medicine and Science in Sports and Exercise* 33(9):1567–1576.

59. Rico-Sanz, J., T. Rankinen, D. R. Joanisse, A. S. Leon, J. S. Skinner, J. H. Wilmore, D. C. Rao, C. Bouchard, and HERITAGE Family Study. 2003. Familial resemblance for muscle phenotypes in the HERITAGE family study. *Medicine and Science in Sports and Exercise* 35(8):1360–1366, doi:10.1249/01.MSS.0000079031.22755.63.

60. Hagberg, J. M., J. E. Graves, M. Limacher, D. R. Woods, S. H. Leggett, C. Cononie, J. J. Gruber, and M. L. Pollock. 1989. Cardiovascular responses of 70- to 79-yr-old men and women to exercise training. *Journal of Applied Physiology (Bethesda, Md.: 1985)* 66(6):2589–2594.

61. Jubrias, S. A., P. C. Esselman, L. B. Price, M. E. Cress, and K. E. Conley. 2001. Large energetic adaptations of elderly muscle to resistance and endurance training. *Journal of Applied Physiology (Bethesda, Md.: 1985)* 90(5):1663–1670.

62. Martin, W. H. 3rd, W. M. Kohrt, M. T. Malley, E. Korte, and S. Stoltz. 1990. Exercise training enhances leg vasodilatory capacity of 65-yr-old men and women. *Journal of Applied Physiology (Bethesda, Md.: 1985)* 69(5):1804–1809.

63. Wray, D. W., A. Uberoi, L. Lawrenson, and R. S. Richardson. 2006. Evidence of preserved endothelial function and vascular plasticity with age. *American Journal of Physiology: Heart and Circulatory Physiology* 290(3):H1271–H1277, doi:00883.2005 [pii].

64. Tanaka, H., F. A. Dinenno, K. D. Monahan, C. M. Clevenger, C. A. DeSouza, and D. R. Seals. 2000. Aging, habitual exercise, and dynamic arterial compliance. *Circulation* 102(11):1270–1275.

65. DeSouza, C. A., L. F. Shapiro, C. M. Clevenger, F. A. Dinenno, K. D. Monahan, H. Tanaka, and D. R. Seals. 2000. Regular aerobic exercise prevents and restores age-related declines in endothelium-dependent vasodilation in healthy men. *Circulation* 102(12):1351–1357.

66. Okazaki, K., K. Iwasaki, A. Prasad, M. D. Palmer, E. R. Martini, Q. Fu, A. Arbab-Zadeh, R. Zhang, and B. D. Levine. 2005. Dose–response relationship of endurance training for autonomic circulatory control in healthy seniors. *Journal of Applied Physiology (Bethesda, Md.: 1985)* 99(3):1041–1049, doi:00085.2005 [pii].

67. Hurley, B. F. and J. M. Hagberg. 1998. Optimizing health in older persons: Aerobic or strength training? *Exercise and Sport Sciences Reviews* 26(1):61–90.

68. Toth, M. J., T. Beckett, and E. T. Poehlman. 1999. Physical activity and the progressive change in body composition with aging: Current evidence and research issues. *Medicine and Science in Sports and Exercise* 31(11 Suppl):S590–S596.

69. Katsanos, C. S. 2006. Prescribing aerobic exercise for the regulation of postprandial lipid metabolism. *Sports Medicine* 36(7):547–560.

70. Kirwan, J. P., W. M. Kohrt, D. M. Wojta, R. E. Bourey, and J. O. Holloszy. 1993. Endurance exercise training reduces glucose-stimulated insulin levels in 60- to 70-year-old men and women. *Journal of Gerontology* 48(3):M84–M90.

71. Sial, S., A. R. Coggan, R. C. Hickner, and S. Klein. 1998. Training-induced alterations in fat and carbohydrate metabolism during exercise in elderly subjects. *The American Journal of Physiology* 274(5 Pt 1):E785–E790.

72. DiPietro, L., J. Dziura, C. W. Yeckel, and P. D. Neufer. 2006. Exercise and improved insulin sensitivity in older women: Evidence of the enduring benefits of higher intensity training. *Journal of Applied Physiology (Bethesda, Md.: 1985)* 100(1):142–149, doi: 00474.2005 [pii].

73. Bean, J. F., S. Herman, D. K. Kiely, I. C. Frey, S. G. Leveille, R. A. Fielding, and W. R. Frontera. 2004. Increased velocity exercise specific to task (InVEST) training: A pilot study exploring effects on leg power, balance, and mobility in community-dwelling older omen. *Journal of the American Geriatrics Society* 52(5):799–804.

74. Borst, S. E., K. R. Vincent, D. T. Lowenthal, and R. W. Braith. 2002. Effects of resistance training on insulin-like growth factor and its binding proteins in men and women aged 60 to 85. *Journal of the American Geriatrics Society* 50(5):884–888.

75. Asikainen, T.-M., K. Kukkonen-Harjula, and S. Miilunpalo. 2004. Exercise for health for early postmenopausal women. *Sports Medicine* 34(11):753–778.

76. Brown, M., D. R. Sinacore, and H. H. Host. 1995. The relationship of strength to function in the older adult. *The Journals of Gerontology, Series A: Biological Sciences and Medical Sciences* 50(Spec No):55–59.

77. Jette, A. M., S. F. Assmann, D. Rooks, B. A. Harris, and S. Crawford. 1998. Interrelationships among disablement concepts. *The Journals of Gerontology, Series A: Biological Sciences and Medical Sciences* 53(5):M395–M404.

78. Rantanen, T., J. M. Guralnik, L. Ferrucci, B. W. J. H. Penninx, S. Leveille, S. Sipilä, and L. P. Fried. 2001. Coimpairments as predictors of severe walking disability in older women. *Journal of the American Geriatrics Society* 49(1):21–27.

79. McCartney, N., A. L. Hicks, J. Martin, and C. E. Webber. 1995. Long-term resistance training in the elderly: Effects on dynamic strength, exercise capacity, muscle, and bone. *The Journals of Gerontology, Series A: Biological Sciences and Medical Sciences* 50(2):B97–B104.

80. Fahlman, M. M., N. McNevin, D. Boardley, A. Morgan, and R. Topp. 2011. Effects of resistance training on functional ability in elderly individuals. *American Journal of Health Promotion* 25(4):237–243.

81. Grimby, G., A. Aniansson, M. Hedberg, G. B. Henning, U. Grangard, and H. Kvist. 1992. Training can improve muscle strength and endurance in 78- to 84-yr-old men. *Journal of Applied Physiology (Bethesda, Md.: 1985)* 73(6):2517–2523.

82. Häkkinen, K., W. J. Kraemer, R. U. Newton, and M. Alen. 2001. Changes in electromyographic activity, muscle fibre and force production characteristics during heavy resistance/power strength training in middle-aged and older men and women. *Acta Physiologica Scandinavica* 171(1):51–62.

83. Hakkinen, K., R. U. Newton, S. E. Gordon, M. McCormick, J. S. Volek, B. C. Nindl, L. A. Gotshalk et al. 1998. Changes in muscle morphology, electromyographic activity, and force production characteristics during progressive strength training in young and older men. *The Journals of Gerontology, Series A: Biological Sciences and Medical Sciences* 53(6):B415–B423.

84. Ivey, F. M., S. M. Roth, R. E. Ferrell, B. L. Tracy, J. T. Lemmer, D. E. Hurlbut, G. F. Martel et al. 2000. Effects of age, gender, and myostatin genotype on the hypertrophic response to heavy resistance strength training. *The Journals of Gerontology, Series A: Biological Sciences and Medical Sciences* 55(11):M641–M648.

85. Ivey, F. M., B. L. Tracy, J. T. Lemmer, M. NessAiver, E. J. Metter, J. L. Fozard, and B. F. Hurley. 2000. Effects of strength training and detraining on muscle quality: Age and gender comparisons. *The Journals of Gerontology, Series A: Biological Sciences and Medical Sciences* 55(3):B152–B157; discussion B158–B159.

86. Izquierdo, M., K. Hakkinen, J. Ibanez, M. Garrues, A. Anton, A. Zuniga, J. L. Larrion, and E. M. Gorostiaga. 2001. Effects of strength training on muscle power and serum hormones in middle-aged and older men. *Journal of Applied Physiology (Bethesda, Md.: 1985)* 90(4):1497–1507.

87. Welle, S., K. Bhatt, B. Shah, and C. A. Thornton. 2002. Insulin-like growth factor-1 and myostatin mRNA expression in muscle: Comparison between 62–77 and 21–31 yr old men. *Experimental Gerontology* 37(6):833–839.

88. Connelly, D. M. and A. A. Vandervoort. 2000. Effects of isokinetic strength training on concentric and eccentric torque development in the ankle dorsiflexors of older adults. *The Journals of Gerontology, Series A: Biological Sciences and Medical Sciences* 55(10):B465–B472.

89. Bean, J. F., D. K. Kiely, S. Herman, S. G. Leveille, K. Mizer, W. R. Frontera, and R. A. Fielding. 2002. The relationship between leg power and physical performance in mobility-limited older people. *Journal of the American Geriatrics Society* 50(3):461–467.

90. Earles, D. R., J. O. Judge, and O. T. Gunnarsson. 1997. Power as a predictor of functional ability in community dwelling older persons. *Medicine and Science in Sports and Exercise* 29(5):11.

91. Evans, W. J. 2000. Exercise strategies should be designed to increase muscle power. *The Journals of Gerontology, Series A: Biological Sciences and Medical Sciences* 55(6):M309–M310.

92. Foldvari, M., M. Clark, L. C. Laviolette, M. A. Bernstein, D. Kaliton, C. Castaneda, C. T. Pu, J. M. Hausdorff, R. A. Fielding, and M. A. Singh. 2000. Association of muscle power with functional status in community-dwelling elderly women. *The Journals of Gerontology, Series A: Biological Sciences and Medical Sciences* 55(4):M192–M199.

93. Skelton, D. A., A. Young, C. A. Greig, and K. E. Malbut. 1995. Effects of resistance training on strength, power, and selected functional abilities of women aged 75 and older. *Journal of the American Geriatrics Society* 43(10):1081–1087.

94. Hakkinen, K., W. J. Kraemer, M. Kallinen, V. Linnamo, U. M. Pastinen, and R. U. Newton. 1996. Bilateral and unilateral neuromuscular function and muscle cross-sectional area in middle-aged and elderly men and women. *The Journals of Gerontology, Series A: Biological Sciences and Medical Sciences* 51(1):B21–B29.

95. Izquierdo, M., E. Gorostiaga, M. Garrues, A. Anton, J. L. Larrion, and K. Haekkinen. 1999. Maximal strength and power characteristics in isometric and dynamic actions of the upper and lower extremities in middle-aged and older men. *Acta Physiologica Scandinavica* 167:57–68.

96. Klein, C. S., G. D. Marsh, R. J. Petrella, and C. L. Rice. 2003. Muscle fiber number in the biceps brachii muscle of young and old men. *Muscle and Nerve* 28(1):62–68.

97. Lexell, J., D. Y. Downham, Y. Larsson, E. Bruhn, and B. Morsing. 1995. Heavy-resistance training in older Scandinavian men and women: Short- and long-term effects on arm and leg muscles. *Scandinavian Journal of Medicine and Science in Sports* 5(6):329–341.

98. Bamman, M. M., V. J. Hill, G. R. Adams, F. Haddad, C. J. Wetzstein, B. A. Gower, A. Ahmed, and G. R. Hunter. 2003. Gender differences in resistance-training-induced myofiber hypertrophy among older adults. *The Journals of Gerontology, Series A: Biological Sciences and Medical Sciences* 58(2):B108–B116.

99. Frontera, W. R., C. N. Meredith, K. P. O'Reilly, H. G. Knuttgen, and W. J. Evans. 1988. Strength conditioning in older men: Skeletal muscle hypertrophy and improved function. *Journal of Applied Physiology (Bethesda, Md.: 1985)* 64(3):1038–1044.

100. Tracy, B. L., F. M. Ivey, D. Hurlbut, G. F. Martel, J. T. Lemmer, E. L. Siegel, E. J. Metter, J. L. Fozard, J. L. Fleg, and B. F. Hurley. 1999. Muscle quality. II. Effects of strength training in 65- to 75-yr-old men and women. *Journal of Applied Physiology (Bethesda, Md.: 1985)* 86(1):195–201.

101. Macaluso, A., G. De Vito, F. Felici, and M. A. Nimmo. 2000. Electromyogram changes during sustained contraction after resistance training in women in their 3rd and 8th decades. *European Journal of Applied Physiology* 82(5–6):418–424.

102. Vincent, K. R., R. W. Braith, R. A. Feldman, P. M. Magyari, R. B. Cutler, S. A. Persin, S. L. Lennon, A. H. Gabr, and D. T. Lowenthal. 2002. Resistance exercise and physical performance in adults aged 60 to 83. *Journal of the American Geriatrics Society* 50(6):1100–1107.

103. Klitgaard, H., M. Mantoni, S. Schiaffino, S. Ausoni, L. Gorza, C. Laurent-Winter, P. Schnohr, and B. Saltin. 1990. Function, morphology and protein expression of ageing skeletal muscle: A cross-sectional study of elderly men with different training backgrounds. *Acta Physiologica Scandinavica* 140(1):41–54.

104. Suominen, H. 2006. Muscle training for bone strength. *Aging Clinical and Experimental Research* 18(2):85–93.

105. Roth, S. M., F. M. Ivey, G. F. Martel, J. T. Lemmer, D. E. Hurlbut, E. L. Siegel, E. Jeffrey Metter, J. L. Fleg, J. L. Fozard, and M. C. Kostek. 2001. Muscle size responses to strength training in young and older men and women. *Journal of the American Geriatrics Society* 49(11):1428–1433.

106. Treuth, M. S., G. R. Hunter, T. Kekes-Szabo, R. L. Weinsier, M. I. Goran, and L. Berland. 1995. Reduction in intra-abdominal adipose tissue after strength training in older women. *Journal of Applied Physiology (Bethesda, Md.: 1985)* 78(4):1425–1431.

107. Hunter, G. R., J. P. McCarthy, and M. M. Bamman. 2004. Effects of resistance training on older adults. *Sports Medicine* 34(5):329–348.

108. Ibanez, J., M. Izquierdo, I. Arguelles, L. Forga, J. L. Larrion, M. Garcia-Unciti, F. Idoate, and E. M. Gorostiaga. 2005. Twice-weekly progressive resistance training decreases abdominal fat and improves insulin sensitivity in older men with type 2 diabetes. *Diabetes Care* 28(3):662–667, doi:28/3/662 [pii].

109. Borkan, G. A., D. E. Hults, S. G. Gerzof, and A. H. Robbins. 1985. Comparison of body composition in middle-aged and elderly males using computed tomography. *American Journal of Physical Anthropology* 66(3):289–295.

110. Taaffe, D. R., T. R. Henwood, M. A. Nalls, D. G. Walker, T. F. Lang, and T. B. Harris. 2009. Alterations in muscle attenuation following detraining and retraining in resistance-trained older adults. *Gerontology* 55(2):217–223, doi:10.1159/000182084.

111. Campbell, W. W., M. C. Crim, V. R. Young, and W. J. Evans. 1994. Increased energy requirements and changes in body composition with resistance training in older adults. *The American Journal of Clinical Nutrition* 60(2):167–175.

112. Hunter, G. R., C. J. Wetzstein, D. A. Fields, A. Brown, and M. M. Bamman. 2000. Resistance training increases total energy expenditure and free-living physical activity in older adults. *Journal of Applied Physiology (Bethesda, Md.: 1985)* 89(3):977–984.

113. Treuth, M. S., G. R. Hunter, R. L. Weinsier, and S. H. Kell. 1995. Energy expenditure and substrate utilization in older women after strength training: 24-H calorimeter results. *Journal of Applied Physiology (Bethesda, Md.: 1985)* 78(6):2140–2146.

114. Mcauley, E. and J. Katula. 1998. Physical activity interventions in the elderly: Influence on physical health and psychological function. *Annual Review of Gerontology and Geriatrics* 18(1):111–154.

115. Fahlman, M. M., D. Boardley, C. P. Lambert, and M. G. Flynn. 2002. Effects of endurance training and resistance training on plasma lipoprotein profiles in elderly women. *The Journals of Gerontology, Series A: Biological Sciences and Medical Sciences* 57(2):B54–B60.

116. Hagerman, F. C., S. J. Walsh, R. S. Staron, R. S. Hikida, R. M. Gilders, T. F. Murray, K. Toma, and K. E. Ragg. 2000. Effects of high-intensity resistance training on untrained older men. I. Strength, cardiovascular, and metabolic responses. *The Journals of Gerontology, Series A: Biological Sciences and Medical Sciences* 55(7):B336–B346.

117. Joseph, L. J. O., S. L. Davey, W. J. Evans, and W. W. Campbell. 1999. Differential effect of resistance training on the body composition and lipoprotein-lipid profile in older men and women. *Metabolism* 48(11):1474–1480.

118. Libby, P. 2005. Prevention and treatment of atherosclerosis. *Harrisons Principles of Internal Medicine* 16(2):1430.

119. Jurca, R., M. J. Lamonte, C. E. Barlow, J. B. Kampert, T. S. Church, and S. N. Blair. 2005. Association of muscular strength with incidence of metabolic syndrome in men. *Medicine and Science in Sports and Exercise* 37(11):1849.

120. Jurca, R., M. J. Lamonte, T. S. Church, C. P. Earnest, S. J. Fitzgerald, C. E. Barlow, A. N. Jordan, J. B. Kampert, and S. N. Blair. 2004. Associations of muscle strength and aerobic fitness with metabolic syndrome in men. *Medicine and Science in Sports and Exercise* 36:1301–1307.

121. Atlantis, E., S. A. Martin, M. T. Haren, A. W. Taylor, and G. A. Wittert. 2009. Inverse associations between muscle mass, strength, and the metabolic syndrome. *Metabolism* 58(7):1013–1022.

122. Close, G. L., A. Kayani, A. Vasilaki, and A. McArdle. 2005. Skeletal muscle damage with exercise and aging. *Sports Medicine* 35(5):413–427.

123. Miller, J. P., R. E. Pratley, A. P. Goldberg, P. Gordon, M. Rubin, M. S. Treuth, A. S. Ryan, and B. F. Hurley. 1994. Strength training increases insulin action in healthy 50- to 65-yr-old men. *Journal of Applied Physiology (Bethesda, Md.: 1985)* 77(3):1122–1127.

124. Misra, A., N. K. Alappan, N. K. Vikram, K. Goel, N. Gupta, K. Mittal, S. Bhatt, and K. Luthra. 2008. Effect of supervised progressive resistance-exercise training protocol on insulin sensitivity, glycemia, lipids, and body composition in Asian Indians with type 2 diabetes. *Diabetes Care* 31(7):1282–1287, doi:10.2337/dc07-2316.

125. Smutok, M. A., C. Reece, P. F. Kokkinos, C. M. Farmer, P. K. Dawson, J. DeVane, J. Patterson, A. P. Goldberg, and B. F. Hurley. 1994. Effects of exercise training modality on glucose tolerance in men with abnormal glucose regulation. *International Journal of Sports Medicine* 15(6):283–289, doi:10.1055/s-2007-1021061.

126. Tresierras, M. A. and G. J. Balady. 2009. Resistance training in the treatment of diabetes and obesity: Mechanisms and outcomes. *Journal of Cardiopulmonary Rehabilitation and Prevention* 29(2):67–75, doi:10.1097/HCR.0b013e318199ff69.

127. Holten, M. K., M. Zacho, M. Gaster, C. Juel, J. F. Wojtaszewski, and F. Dela. 2004. Strength training increases insulin-mediated glucose uptake, GLUT4 content, and insulin signaling in skeletal muscle in patients with type 2 diabetes. *Diabetes* 53(2):294–305.

128. Khaw, K. T., N. Wareham, R. Luben, S. Bingham, S. Oakes, A. Welch, and N. Day. 2001. Glycated haemoglobin, diabetes, and mortality in men in Norfolk cohort of European prospective investigation of cancer and nutrition (EPIC-Norfolk). *BMJ (Clinical Research Ed.)* 322(7277):15–18.

129. Manley, S. 2003. Haemoglobin A1c—A marker for complications of type 2 diabetes: The experience from the UK Prospective Diabetes Study (UKPDS). *Clinical Chemistry and Laboratory Medicine* 41(9):1182–1190.

130. Kotronen, A. and H. Yki-Jarvinen. 2008. Fatty liver: A novel component of the metabolic syndrome. *Arteriosclerosis, Thrombosis, and Vascular Biology* 28(1): 27–38, doi: ATVBAHA.107.147538 [pii].

131. Samuel, V. T., Z. X. Liu, X. Qu, B. D. Elder, S. Bilz, D. Befroy, A. J. Romanelli, and G. I. Shulman. 2004. Mechanism of hepatic insulin resistance in non-alcoholic fatty liver disease. *The Journal of Biological Chemistry* 279(31):32345–32353, doi:10.1074/jbc.M313478200.

132. Kelley, G. A. and K. S. Kelley. 2009. Impact of progressive resistance training on lipids and lipoproteins in adults: A meta-analysis of randomized controlled trials. *Preventive Medicine* 48(1):9–19.

133. Kelley G. A. and K. S. Kelley. 2009. Impact of progressive resistance training on lipids and lipoproteins in adults: Another look at a meta-analysis using prediction intervals. *Preventive Medicine* 49(6):473–475.

134. Braith, R. W. and K. J. Stewart. 2006. Resistance exercise training: Its role in the prevention of cardio-vascular disease. *Circulation* 113(22):2642–2650, doi:113/22/2642 [pii].

135. Hurley, B. F. and S. M. Roth. 2000. Strength training in the elderly. *Sports Medicine* 30(4):249–268.

136. Williams, M. A., W. L. Haskell, P. A. Ades, E. A. Amsterdam, V. Bittner, B. A. Franklin, M. Gulanick et al. 2007. Resistance exercise in individuals with and without cardiovascular disease: 2007 Update: A scientific statement from the American Heart Association Council on Clinical Cardiology and Council on Nutrition, Physical Activity, and Metabolism. *Circulation* 116(5):572–584, doi:CIRCULATIONAHA.107.185214 [pii].

137. Hurley, B. F., E. D. Hanson, and A. K. Sheaff. 2011. Strength training as a countermeasure to aging muscle and chronic disease. *Sports Medicine* 41(4):289–306.

138. Gillespie, L. D., M. C. Robertson, W. J. Gillespie, C. Sherrington, S. Gates, L. M. Clemson, and S. E. Lamb. 2012. Interventions for preventing falls in older people living in the community. *Cochrane Database of Systematic Reviews* 9(11).

139. Booth, F. W., S. H. Weeden, and B. S. Tseng. 1994. Effect of aging on human skeletal muscle and motor function. *Medicine and Science in Sports and Exercise* 26(5):556–560.

140. Patla, A. E., J. S. Frank, and D. A. Winter. 1992. Balance control in the elderly: Implications for clinical assessment and rehabilitation. *Canadian Journal of Public Health; Revue Canadienne De Sante Publique* 83(Suppl 2):S29–S33.

141. Said, C. M., P. A. Goldie, A. E. Patla, E. Culham, W. A. Sparrow, and M. E. Morris. 2008. Balance during obstacle crossing following stroke. *Gait and Posture* 27(1):23–30.

142. Gómez-Cabello, A., I. Ara, A. González-Agüero, J. A. Casajús, and G. Vicente-Rodriguez. 2012. Effects of training on bone mass in older adults. *Sports Medicine* 42(4):301–325.

143. Campbell, A. J., M. C. Robertson, M. M. Gardner, R. N. Norton, and D. M. Buchner. 1999. Psychotropic medication withdrawal and a home-based exercise program to prevent falls: A randomized, controlled trial. *Journal of the American Geriatrics Society* 47(7):850–853.

144. Campbell, A. J., M. C. Robertson, M. M. Gardner, R. N. Norton, and D. M. Buchner. 1999. Falls prevention over 2 years: A randomized controlled trial in women 80 years and older. *Age and Ageing* 28(6):513–518.

145. Norton, R., G. Galgali, A. J. Campbell, I. R. Reid, E. Robinson, M. Butler, and H. Gray. 2001. Is physical activity protective against hip fracture in frail older people? *Age and Ageing* 30(3):262–264.

146. Li, F., P. Harmer, K. J. Fisher, E. McAuley, N. Chaumeton, E. Eckstrom, and N. L. Wilson. 2005. Tai chi and fall reductions in older adults: A randomized controlled trial. *The Journals of Gerontology, Series A: Biological Sciences and Medical Sciences* 60(2):187–194, doi:60/2/187 [pii].

147. Wolf, S. L., R. W. Sattin, M. Kutner, M. O'Grady, A. I. Greenspan, and R. J. Gregor. 2003. Intense tai chi exercise training and fall occurrences in older, transitionally frail adults: A randomized, controlled trial. *Journal of the American Geriatrics Society* 51(12):1693–1701.

148. Gill, T. M., M. Pahor, J. M. Guralnik, M. M. McDermott, A. C. King, T. W. Buford, E. S. Strotmeyer et al. 2016. Effect of structured physical activity on prevention of serious fall injuries in adults aged 70–89: Randomized clinical trial (LIFE Study). *BMJ (Clinical Research Ed.)* 352:i245, doi:10.1136/bmj.i245.

149. Kelley, G. A. 1998. Exercise and regional bone mineral density in postmenopausal women. *American Journal of Physical Medicine and Rehabilitation* 77(1):76–87.

150. Kelley, G. A., K. S. Kelley, and Z. V. Tran. 2000. Exercise and bone mineral density in men: A meta-analysis. *Journal of Applied Physiology (Bethesda, Md.: 1985)* 88(5):1730–1736.

151. Wallace, R. B. 2000. Bone health in nursing home residents. *JAMA* 284(8):1018–1019.

152. Wolff, I., J. J. Van Croonenborg, H. C. G. Kemper, P. J. Kostense, and J. W. R. Twisk. 1999. The effect of exercise training programs on bone mass: A meta-analysis of published controlled trials in pre- and postmenopausal women. *Osteoporosis International* 9(1):1–12.

153. Rhodes, E. C., A. D. Martin, J. E. Taunton, M. Donnelly, J. Warren, and J. Elliot. 2000. Effects of one year of resistance training on the relation between muscular strength and bone density in elderly women. *British Journal of Sports Medicine* 34(1):18–22.

154. Stewart, K. J., A. C. Bacher, P. S. Hees, M. Tayback, P. Ouyang, and S. Jan de Beur. 2005. Exercise effects on bone mineral density: Relationships to changes in fitness and fatness. *American Journal of Preventive Medicine* 28(5):453–460.

155. Vincent, K. R. and R. W. Braith. 2002. Resistance exercise and bone turnover in elderly men and women. *Medicine and Science in Sports and Exercise* 34(1):17–23.

156. Bloomfield, S. A., K. D. Little, M. E. Nelson, and V. R. Yingling. 2004. Position stand. *Medicine and Science in Sports and Exercise* 195(9131/04):3611–1985.

157. Michel, B. A., N. E. Lane, A. Bjorkengren, D. A. Bloch, and J. F. Fries. 1992. Impact of running on lumbar bone density: A 5-year longitudinal study. *The Journal of Rheumatology* 19(11):1759–1763.

158. Greist, J. H., M. H. Klein, R. R. Eischens, J. Faris, A. S. Gurman, and W. P. Morgan. 1979. Running as treatment for depression. *Comprehensive Psychiatry* 20(1):41–54.

159. Martinsen, E. W. 2008. Physical activity in the prevention and treatment of anxiety and depression. *Nordic Journal of Psychiatry* 62(suppl 47):25–29.

160. Martinsen, E. W., A. Medhus, and L. Sandvik. 1985. Effects of aerobic exercise on depression: A controlled study. *British Medical Journal (Clinical Research ed.)* 291(6488):109.

161. Mather, A. S., C. Rodriguez, M. F. Guthrie, A. M. McHarg, I. C. Reid, and M. E. McMurdo. 2002. Effects of exercise on depressive symptoms in older adults with poorly responsive depressive disorder: Randomised controlled trial. *The British Journal of Psychiatry: The Journal of Mental Science* 180:411–415.

162. Singh, N. A., K. M. Clements, and M. A. Fiatarone. 1997. A randomized controlled trial of progressive resistance training in depressed elders. *The Journals of Gerontology, Series A: Biological Sciences and Medical Sciences* 52(1):M27–M35.

163. Singh, N. A., K. M. Clements, and M. A. Singh. 2001. The efficacy of exercise as a long-term antidepressant in elderly subjects: A randomized, controlled trial. *The Journals of Gerontology, Series A: Biological Sciences and Medical Sciences* 56(8):M497–504.

164. Dunn, A. L., M. H. Trivedi, J. B. Kampert, C. G. Clark, and H. O. Chambliss. 2005. Exercise treatment for depression: Efficacy and dose response. *American Journal of Preventive Medicine* 28(1):1–8.

165. Elavsky, S., E. McAuley, R. W. Motl, J. F. Konopack, D. X. Marquez, L. Hu, G. J. Jerome, and E. Diener. 2005. Physical activity enhances long-term quality of life in older adults: Efficacy, esteem, and affective influences. *Annals of Behavioral Medicine* 30(2):138–145.

166. Acree, L. S., J. Longfors, A. S. Fjeldstad, C. Fjeldstad, B. Schank, K. J. Nickel, P. S. Montgomery, and A. W. Gardner. 2006. Physical activity is related to quality of life in older adults. *Health and Quality of Life Outcomes* 4(1):1.

167. Bean, J., S. Herman, D. K. Kiely, D. Callahan, K. Mizer, W. R. Frontera, and R. A. Fielding. 2002. Weighted stair climbing in mobility-limited older people: A pilot study. *Journal of the American Geriatrics Society* 50(4):663–670.

168. Henwood, T. R. and D. R. Taaffe. 2005. Improved physical performance in older adults undertaking a short-term programme of high-velocity resistance training. *Gerontology* 51(2):108–115, doi: 82195 [pii].

169. Holviala, J. H., J. M. Sallinen, W. J. Kraemer, M. J. Alen, and K. K. Hakkinen. 2006. Effects of strength training on muscle strength characteristics, functional capabilities, and balance in middle-aged and older women. *Journal of Strength and Conditioning Research/National Strength and Conditioning Association* 20(2):336–344, doi: R-17885 [pii].

170. Schlicht, J., D. N. Camaione, and S. V. Owen. 2001. Effect of intense strength training on standing balance, walking speed, and sit-to-stand performance in older adults. *The Journals of Gerontology, Series A: Biological Sciences and Medical Sciences* 56(5):M281–M286.

171. Paterson, D. H., D. Govindasamy, M. Vidmar, D. A. Cunningham, and J. J. Koval. 2004. Longitudinal study of determinants of dependence in an elderly population. *Journal of the American Geriatrics Society* 52(10):1632–1638.

172. Alexander, N. B., A. T. Galecki, M. L. Grenier, L. V. Nyquist, M. R. Hofmeyer, J. C. Grunawalt, J. L. Medell, and D. Fry-Welch. 2001. Task-specific resistance training to improve the ability of activities of daily living-impaired older adults to rise from a bed and from a chair. *Journal of the American Geriatrics Society* 49(11):1418–1427.

173. Schnelle, J. F., P. G. MacRae, J. G. Ouslander, S. F. Simmons, and M. Nitta. 1995. Functional incidental training, mobility performance, and incontinence care with nursing home residents. *Journal of the American Geriatrics Society* 43(12):1356–1362.

174. Laurin, D., R. Verreault, J. Lindsay, K. MacPherson, and K. Rockwood. 2001. Physical activity and risk of cognitive impairment and dementia in elderly persons. *Archives of Neurology* 58(3):498–504.

175. Yaffe, K., D. Barnes, M. Nevitt, L.-Y. Lui, and K. Covinsky. 2001. A prospective study of physical activity and cognitive decline in elderly women: Women who walk. *Archives of Internal Medicine* 161(14):1703–1708.

176. Fiatarone, M. A., E. C. Marks, N. D. Ryan, C. N. Meredith, L. A. Lipsitz, and W. J. Evans. 1990. High-intensity strength training in nonagenarians: Effects on skeletal muscle. *JAMA* 263(22):3029–3034.

177. Marquis, S., M. M. Moore, D. B. Howieson, G. Sexton, H. Payami, J. A. Kaye, and R. Camicioli. 2002. Independent predictors of cognitive decline in healthy elderly persons. *Archives of Neurology* 59(4):601–606.

178. Tabbarah, M., E. M. Crimmins, and T. E. Seeman. 2002. The relationship between cognitive and physical performance: MacArthur studies of successful aging. *The Journals of Gerontology, Series A: Biological Sciences and Medical Sciences* 57(4):M228–M235.

179. Sink, K. M., M. A. Espeland, C. M. Castro, T. Church, R. Cohen, J. A. Dodson, J. Guralnik, H. C. Hendrie, J. Jennings, and J. Katula. 2015. Effect of a 24-month physical activity intervention vs health education on cognitive outcomes in sedentary older adults: The LIFE randomized trial. *JAMA* 314(8): 781–790.

180. Alfaro-Acha, A., S. Al Snih, M. A. Raji, Y. F. Kuo, K. S. Markides, and K. J. Ottenbacher. 2006. Handgrip strength and cognitive decline in older Mexican Americans. *The Journals of Gerontology, Series A: Biological Sciences and Medical Sciences* 61(8):859–865, doi: 61/8/859 [pii].

181. Buchman, A. S., R. S. Wilson, J. L. Bienias, R. C. Shah, D. A. Evans, and D. A. Bennett. 2005. Change in body mass index and risk of incident Alzheimer disease. *Neurology* 65(6):892–897, doi: 65/6/892 [pii].

182. Gustafson, D., E. Rothenberg, K. Blennow, B. Steen, and I. Skoog. 2003. An 18-year follow-up of overweight and risk of Alzheimer disease. *Archives of Internal Medicine* 163(13):1524–1528.

183. Boyle, P. A., A. S. Buchman, R. S. Wilson, S. E. Leurgans, and D. A. Bennett. 2009. Association of muscle strength with the risk of Alzheimer disease and the rate of cognitive decline in community-dwelling older persons. *Archives of Neurology* 66(11):1339–1344.

184. Lachman, M. E., S. D. Neupert, R. Bertrand, and A. M. Jette. 2006. The effects of strength training on memory in older adults. *Journal of Aging and Physical Activity* 14(1):59.

185. Chang, Y.-K., C.-Y. Pan, F.-T. Chen, C.-L. Tsai, and C.-C. Huang. 2012. Effect of resistance exercise training on cognitive function in healthy older adults: A review. *Journal of Aging and Physical Activity* 20(4):497–517.

186. Billinger, S. A., R. Arena, J. Bernhardt, J. J. Eng, B. A. Franklin, C. M. Johnson, M. MacKay-Lyons et al. 2014. Physical activity and exercise recommendations for stroke survivors: A statement for healthcare professionals from the American Heart Association/American Stroke Association. *Stroke; A Journal of Cerebral Circulation* 45(8):2532–2553, doi: 10.1161/STR.0000000000000022.

187. Kernan, W. N., B. Ovbiagele, H. R. Black, D. M. Bravata, M. I. Chimowitz, M. D. Ezekowitz, M. C. Fang et al. 2014. Guidelines for the prevention of stroke in patients with stroke and transient ischemic attack: A guideline for healthcare professionals from the American Heart Association/American Stroke Association. *Stroke: A Journal of Cerebral Circulation* 45(7):2160–2236, doi: 10.1161/STR.0000000000000024.

188. Trojian, T. H., K. Mody, and P. Chain. 2007. Exercise and colon cancer: Primary and secondary prevention. *Current Sports Medicine Reports* 6(2):120–124.

189. Li, T., S. Wei, Y. Shi, S. Pang, Q. Qin, J. Yin, Y. Deng et al. 2016. The dose-response effect of physical activity on cancer mortality: Findings from 71 prospective cohort studies. *British Journal of Sports Medicine* 50(6):339–345, doi: 10.1136/bjsports-2015–094927.

190. Wolin, K. Y., Y. Yan, G. A. Colditz, and I. M. Lee. 2009. Physical activity and colon cancer prevention: A meta-analysis. *British Journal of Cancer* 100(4):611–616.

191. Martinez, M. E., E. Giovannucci, D. Spiegelman, D. J. Hunter, W. C. Willett, and G. A. Colditz. 1997. Leisure-time physical activity, body size, and colon cancer in women. Nurses' Health Study Research Group. *Journal of the National Cancer Institute* 89(13):948–955.

192. Zhang, X., K. Wu, E. L. Giovannucci, J. Ma, G. A. Colditz, C. S. Fuchs, W. C. Willett et al. 2015. Early life body fatness and risk of colorectal cancer in U.S. women and men-results from two large cohort studies. *Cancer Epidemiology, Biomarkers and Prevention: A Publication of the American Association for Cancer Research, Cosponsored by the American Society of Preventive Oncology* 24(4):690–697, doi: 10.1158/1055-9965.EPI-14-0909-T.

193. Monninkhof, E. M., S. G. Elias, F. A. Vlems, I. van der Tweel, A. J. Schuit, D. W. Voskuil, F. E. van Leeuwen, and TFPAC. 2007. Physical activity and breast cancer: A systematic review. *Epidemiology (Cambridge, Mass.)* 18(1):137–157, doi: 10.1097/01.ede.0000251167.75581.98.

194. McTiernan, A., C. Kooperberg, E. White, S. Wilcox, R. Coates, L. L. Adams-Campbell, N. Woods, and J. Ockene. 2003. Recreational physical activity and the risk of breast cancer in postmenopausal women: The Women's Health Initiative Cohort Study. *JAMA* 290(10):1331–1336.

195. Lynch, B. M., H. K. Neilson, and C. M. Friedenreich. 2010. Physical activity and breast cancer prevention. In *Physical Activity and Cancer*, 13–42, Berlin Heidelberg: Springer.

196. Bernstein, L., B. E. Henderson, R. Hanisch, J. Sullivan-Halley, and R. K. Ross. 1994. Physical exercise and reduced risk of breast cancer in young women. *Journal of the National Cancer Institute* 86(18):1403–1408.

197. Holmes, M. D., W. Y. Chen, D. Feskanich, C. H. Kroenke, and G. A. Colditz. 2005. Physical activity and survival after breast cancer diagnosis. *JAMA* 293(20):2479–2486.

198. McNeely, M. L., K. L. Campbell, B. H. Rowe, T. P. Klassen, J. R. Mackey, and K. S. Courneya. 2006. Effects of exercise on breast cancer patients and survivors: A systematic review and meta-analysis. *CMAJ: Canadian Medical Association Journal; Journal De L'Association Medicale Canadienne* 175(1):34–41, doi: 175/1/34 [pii].

199. American College of Sports Medicine. 2013. *ACSM's Guidelines for Exercise Testing and Prescription.* China: Lippincott Williams & Wilkins.

200. Gill, T. M., L. DiPietro, and H. M. Krumholz. 2000. Role of exercise stress testing and safety monitoring for older persons starting an exercise program. *JAMA* 284(3):342–349.

201. Tanaka, H., K. D. Monahan, and D. R. Seals. 2001. Age-predicted maximal heart rate revisited. *Journal of the American College of Cardiology* 37(1):153–156.
202. Gellish, R. L., B. R. Goslin, R. E. Olson, A. McDonald, G. D. Russi, and V. K. Moudgil. 2007. Longitudinal modeling of the relationship between age and maximal heart rate. *Medicine and Science in Sports and Exercise* 39(5):822–829, doi: 10.1097/mss.0b013e31803349c6.
203. Pollock, M. L., Franklin, B. A., Balady, G. J., Chaitman, B. L., Fleg, J. L., Fletcher, B., Limacher, M. et al. 2000. AHA Science Advisory. Resistance exercise in individuals with and without cardiovascular disease: Benefits, rationale, safety, and prescription: An advisory from the Committee on Exercise, Rehabilitation, and Prevention, Council on Clinical Cardiology, American Heart Association; Position paper endorsed by the American College of Sports Medicine. *Circulation* 101(7):828–833.
204. Resnick, B. and A. M. Spellbring. 2000. Understanding what motivates older adults to exercise. *Journal of Gerontological Nursing* 26(3):34–42.
205. Nied, R. J. and B. Franklin. 2002. Promoting and prescribing exercise for the elderly. *American Family Physician* 65(3):419–426.
206. Elsawy, B. and K. E. Higgins. 2010. Physical activity guidelines for older adults. *American Family Physician* 81(1):55–59.
207. Mcdermott, A. Y. and H. Mernitz. 2006. Exercise and older patients: Prescribing guidelines. *American Family Physician* 74(3):437–444.
208. Bean, J. F., A. Vora, and W. R. Frontera. 2004. Benefits of exercise for community-dwelling older adults. *Archives of Physical Medicine and Rehabilitation* 85:31–42.

Section II

Geriatric Syndromes

7 Frailty

Egan Allen

CONTENTS

7.1 INTRODUCTION

Loosely applied, the term "frailty" could be explained of as something that a physician "knows it when she sees it." A frail patient may appear overly thin and "weak"; he or she may give the general impression that reserves are low, risks for complications high, and recovery will likely be protracted if recovery from an acute illness is possible at all. A particular patient may be very old or appear much older than the stated age. However, appearances of frailty may not actually mean the patient is frail. Not all thin and older patients are frail. Some very thin patients recover quicker than expected; some very old patients do better than expected. This begs the need for a more systematic use of the term "frailty." Although there is not a single accepted definition of frailty, attempts made to define it share many criteria that help make the application of the term more relevant and useful.

Aging brings with it an accumulation of deficits across multiple systems that take their tolls on a human body over time. Frailty is a threshold past which those tolls incur a net negative in terms of a wide variety of outcomes. Some patients reach this threshold as a result of a string of acute events; others may gradually reach it without these acute punctuations. However a patient becomes clinically frail, it is a clinically important diagnosis to make; accurate prognostication and the laying out of reasonable diagnostic and/or treatment options may depend on it. Specifically, falls, disability, hospitalization, and death are all outcomes that occur with higher frequency in frail patients. A physician might be operating under the assumption that his or her patient is "feeble," "fragile," or "weak" without explicitly diagnosing frailty. However, as in many clinical situations when diagnostic clarity is not achieved, if a physician is not explicit about frailty he or she risks being inconsistent and making inappropriate recommendations to the patient and his family. Being explicit about frailty provides an important basis upon which to construct the work-up and treatment of a patient.

The frail patient may not do well with the "usual" treatments in a particular acute condition; risks can often outweigh benefits. Compounding this, the frail patient may also have multiple chronic medical problems, might take several medications, can endorse a variety of symptoms, and exhibit a variety of impairments in function. Despite the association with aging and the latter complexities, frailty should be considered a distinct entity. Doing so, the approach to an acute condition in a frail patient typically leads to the thoughtful modification of a "standard" set of treatment options for that condition. In turn, this can alter the diagnostic work-up considered. These are some of the most vulnerable patients and applying the "less is more" dictum is usually appropriate, especially in its final stage, when frailty becomes "failure to thrive" (FTT). Symptom-based approaches, under the auspices of a palliative care approach, may become more appropriate at this stage.

Medical decision-making in frail patient brings psychosocial factors to the fore. Making difficult decisions requires the involvement of the healthcare agent, family, and other supports. Reviewing advance directives (ADs) and having goals of care discussions become increasingly important. Framing these discussions while explicitly using the diagnosis of frailty can center what may already be a challenging plan of care.

What follows is a discussion of what we know about defining frailty, its prevalence, pathophysiology, and utility in predicting outcomes. Furthermore, the discussion will focus on what we know about preventing frailty and the systems of care that are optimally suited to frail patients.

7.1.1 DEFINING FRAILTY

There is no universally accepted definition of frailty [1]. That fact might seem to prevent substantive discussion about the subject before it is even started: If one cannot agree about what frailty is then how can one meaningfully speak about it, let alone use it productively in a particular clinical context? That does not mean that serious attempts to define frailty are lacking. Multiple indices and tools exist to define and/or measure frailty. These share in common several features that together serve to preserve the term *frailty's* usefulness.

There are some valid reasons why a precise definition of frailty does not exist. First, frailty represents a spectrum of illness and/or physical state. One cannot simply state exactly when frailty begins or, for that matter, advances to FTT (the end stage of frailty). Second, the biopsychosocial factors that together culminate in frailty are multiple, complex, usually chronic, and, if considered individually, often carry their own respective and variable clinical trajectories.

There is broad agreement that frailty involves decline in some key patient characteristics. A frail patient has impaired function, is physically weak, and has a low physiologic reserve. Acute conditions and invasive investigations and treatments have a more profound impact on frail patients as a result: Recovery is slowed, if possible at all, and negative outcomes are more likely and of greater magnitude when they do occur. A conference regarding frailty sponsored by the American Geriatrics Society and the National Institute on Aging in 2004 yielded the following definition:

> "[Frailty is] a state of increased vulnerability to stressors due to age-related declines in physiologic reserve across neuromuscular, metabolic and immune systems" [2].

The term, "phenotype," is used by some in the literature to encompass specific patient criteria; therefore, it is an operationally useful definition of frailty. To develop a phenotype Fried et al. defined frailty by selecting criteria that predicted poor outcomes (falls, worsening mobility, disability, hospitalization, and death). Fried et al. found that frailty could be operationally defined as a clinical syndrome in which three or more of the following criteria were present [3]:

1. Unintentional weight loss (10 lbs or more than 5% of body weight in past year)
2. Self-reported exhaustion
3. Weakness (grip strength in lowest 20th percentile)
4. Slow walking speed (15 ft; lowest 20th percentile)
5. Low physical activity (kcals spent per week: males expending <383 kcals and females <270 kcals)

Furthermore, the group found that patients were at risk if they met two of these criteria and were also at higher risk of developing the poor outcomes as given above. Patients meeting no criteria were nonfrail. The Fried Frailty Phenotype, given the fact that it used data from the Cardiovascular Health Study [4], is also referred to as the Cardiovascular Health Study (CHS) index.

Frailty is usually discussed in the context of the geriatric patient. The above five criteria have been in use in Europe (Survey of Health, Ageing and Retirement in Europe [SHARE]). Accordingly, a comparison of the 5-item SHARE-FI criteria (SHARE Frailty Instrument: weakness, exhaustion, weight loss, slowness, and low activity) [5] were compared to a modified version of the comprehensive geriatric assessment (CGA) tool, which consists of a lengthy list of criteria [6]. It was found that the simpler phenotype approach (SHARE-FI) was simpler to use and about as accurate.

The Study of Osteoporotic Fractures (SOF) index used a reduced set of criteria than the CHS and is more clinically performable [7]. A patient is defined as frail if they meet two of three of the following:

1. Weight loss of 5% over the past year
2. Inability to rise from a chair five times in succession (without use of arms)
3. Responding, "no," to the question: "Do you feel full of energy?"

Still other studies incorporate additional factors into the definition: nutritional measurements, deficit accumulation, cognitive function, and absolute weight [1,8,9].

Frailty has been shown to be an independent entity from other factors that are often considered part of frailty. Comorbidities and old age have been shown to be independent risks for frailty, and disability is thought to be an independent outcome. Poor or declining cognitive function, on the other hand, has been variously incorporated into the defining criteria for frailty by some groups and has also been shown to be a separate factor by others. In one study frailty was shown to be a risk factor for cognitive impairment [10]. Poor cognitive function and frailty together compound the risk for poor outcomes [11]. Some factors that might be related to frailty need more research. The association of mood disorders with frailty, for example, is not thoroughly understood.

Among the multitude of sets of criteria for defining frailty are those that can be used in clinical settings and those that lend themselves to research settings. In a 2011 review of the literature it was found that among 22 sources reviewed the screening tools, indices, criteria, and so on often were used to fit the particular requirements of the study at hand and were not always aimed at standardizing the definition [6]. The criteria used in each respective set can range from the three in the SOF index to 70 in the Rockwood frailty index [9]. When compared together the various instruments used to define frailty have been shown to identify separate but overlapping groups of patients on a large scale [12]. Not surprisingly, conclusions such as "need more study" and "a consensus is needed" are frequently arrived at.

7.1.2 Transitions

Frailty is understood as a disorder that can exist in different states. Patients can transition between nonfrail, prefrail, and frail states. Typically, once a patient has become frail it is very uncommon to transition back to nonfrail. Furthermore, frailty progresses to FTT and, ultimately, to death [16]. The idea that a patient can dynamically change frailty states (more important, including less frail states) has prompted interest in the concept of treating patients to reduce their frail state [13].

It is important to differentiate disability from frailty [14]. Disability can contribute to frailty, and vice versa, but the two conditions are not the same. Disability is defined as impaired ability to perform activities of daily living (ADLs) and/or instrumental activities of daily living (IADLs) or difficulty with mobility. However, disability does not occur across multiple organ systems as does frailty [15]. Among disabled older patients only 28% are frail; nearly 75% of frail older patients can complete ADLs and 40% do not have difficulty performing IADLs [3].

The various indices used (albeit, often in specialized research contexts) do share common categories of criteria: weight loss, objective evidence of generalized weakness and/or reduced function, and a subjective (chronic) feeling of exhaustion. And these general traits, when combined, are associated with a variety of poor outcomes in several clinical contexts (medical and surgical).

The differential for frailty includes multiple conditions that can present with weight loss, weakness, and decreased mobility [13]. These conditions may be treatable, or are at the very least significantly different, and should therefore be excluded, from frailty. Example conditions include congestive heart failure (with cachexia), cancer, neurologic wasting diseases, Parkinsonism, polymyalgia rheumatic, inflammatory arthritis, and infection. Usually, the presentation of conditions such as these should be obvious, except for perhaps occult malignancy; nonetheless, frailty is a diagnosis of exclusion.

7.1.3 EPIDEMIOLOGY

How common is frailty? Because most of the published work on frailty comes from varying definitions of it and therefore on specific study populations (from which the indices discussed above were developed and utilized), we do not have a definitive sense of prevalence in the general population. However, several studies have yielded useful measurements from which we can establish a reasonably good idea about its incidence and prevalence. In the CHS, frailty existed in about 7% of the patients; in the SOF it was about 11%. In their 80s approximately 20% of patients develop frailty [16]. A Canadian study found that among community-dwelling adults living in one of 10 provinces (aged 65–102) 22.7% were frail and among those 85 or older nearly 40% were frail [17]. Up to about 30% of 90-year-olds were found to be frail in another study [14]. Thus, frailty increases with age. Furthermore, the 4-year incidence of frailty in older patients is 7% [3]. This fact has potentially profound implications given that the baby-boom generation began cresting the 65-year-old threshold in 2011; 40 million Americans were 65 or older in 2011 and 50 million Americans will be in 2019.

Frailty is more common in women than in men [18] and more common in African Americans and Asians than in Hispanics or Caucasians [19]. Interestingly in the latter study single men were more likely to be frail than married men. Frailty is associated with lower income as well [3].

7.2 ETIOLOGY

The causes of frailty are complex. To date no definitive or singular physiologic mechanism has been identified. Multiple clinical factors have been associated with the development of frailty, and some have described a genotype consisting of environmental, medication, age, and disease-related factors rendering patients prone to develop frailty [20]. Other experts have posited specific intrinsic factors, chiefly sarcopenia, and related metabolic pathogenic factors, atherosclerosis, cognitive impairment, and malnutrition that interact to form the underpinnings of frailty [21].

A "frailty spiral" that incorporates several disease- and aging-related factors is a helpful construct when contemplating how the frail state is arrived to [14] (see Figure 7.1).

At the molecular and cellular level multiple abnormal physiologic systems are likely operating. The systems involved include immune and inflammatory, endocrine, vascular, and other metabolic systems. Within the immune and inflammatory systems some biomarkers have been shown to correlate with frailty. Specifically, interleukin-6 and c-reactive protein (IL-6 and CRP) can be elevated; the latter leads to the elevation of the former [22]. Also, researchers have noted elevation in components related to clotting: fibrinogen, d-dimer, and factor VIII [23].

Within the endocrine system, glucose (postprandial and fasting) and insulin have been found to be higher than normal in frail patients; these abnormal levels in turn have been associated with sarcopenia. Leptin resistance, seen with hyperinsulinemia (often found in obese patients), is associated with cognitive impairment. In turn, cognitive decline can lead to decreased oral intake and nutritional deficiency [24]. Dehydroepiandrosterone sulfate (DHEA-S) is a precursor to testosterone

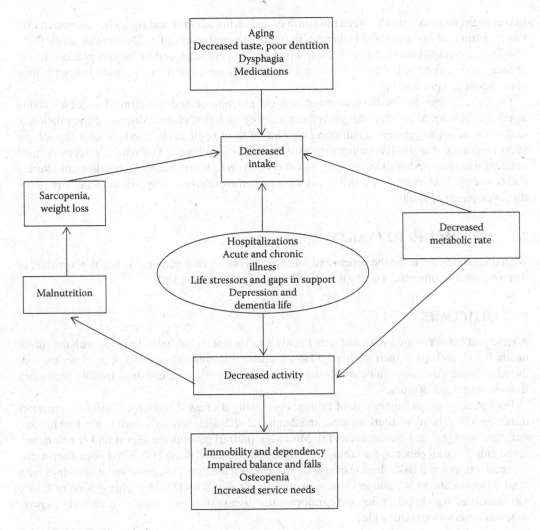

FIGURE 7.1 Frailty spiral.

and influences muscles mass and attenuates inflammation [25]. DHEA-S has been shown to be low in frail patients [26]. However, low testosterone is not associated directly with frailty [27]. Indirectly, we know that low testosterone is associated with decreased muscle strength and physical activity, factors that may compound or contribute to frailty. Growth hormone regulates cell growth and development. Insulin-like growth factor stimulates the release of growth hormone and has been found to be low in frail patients [26]. Furthermore, growth hormone itself has been found to decrease with age [28]. Cortisol, which is a stress steroid and is anti-immune and impacts muscle mass, has higher late-afternoon levels in frail patients [29].

Although not usually framed by researchers as a direct cause of frailty, some have regarded atherosclerosis as an important etiologic factor via indirect pathways [21]; namely, peripheral vascular disease can lead to immobility and diminished muscle perfusion (hence, compounding sarcopenia). Cerebrovascular disease can lead to vascular dementia and subsequent nutritional decline. Coronary atherosclerosis can lead to congestive heart failure leading to decreased activity and, in advanced cases, cardiac cachexia.

Many other biologic factors are thought be a part of the etiologic picture of frailty. Malnutrition contributes to frailty [30]. A multitude of chronic diseases can lead to malnutrition via cachexia, and aging itself is associated with anorexia and subsequent risk for inadequate nutritional intake.

Interestingly, no association between lipid profiles and serum albumin and frailty has been seen [31]. Low vitamin D levels strongly correlated with frailty in a study focused on Dutch older adults [32].

It is important to note that it is not clear whether the above neuroendocrine factors cause frailty or codevelop as a part of frailty. This is important to understand as will be discussed below in terms of treatment and prevention.

Frailty's etiology is best thought about as a culmination of multiple clinical variables acting together over time. Molecular changes related to aging, genetics, chronic disease, dysregulation of multiple systems, and impaired nutrition either manifest through and/or combine with physiologic stress responses that involve endocrine and inflammatory pathways. Ultimately, sarcopenia (and resultant weakness, exhaustion, wasting, and slowness) and a low resilience to equilibrium-altering events emerge. Factors like cognitive impairment and atherosclerosis serve to accelerate or magnify the development of frailty.

7.3 APPROACHES TO FRAILTY

What does frailty mean for the patient and for those caring for frail patients? Is frailty reversible? Is it preventable? In other words, why does the diagnosis of frailty matter?

7.4 OUTCOMES

A variety of outcomes are associated with frailty. Studies that include (and designed with the subset in mind) frail patients in their study populations utilize differing definitions discussed above, and, therefore, some outcomes can be within a narrow niche; however, one can draw useful conclusions from the aggregate of studies.

Frail patients are at higher risk of falling, developing decreased mobility, declining in performance of ADLs, being institutionalized, and death (1.2–2.5-fold increase), when controlled for age, race, sex, smoking, and comorbidities [3]. Moreover, prefrail patients are also at higher risk (albeit not as much as frail patients) for falling, institutionalization, and death [14]. It has been shown that frail patients mount a less robust response to influenza vaccination [33], have worse outcomes with renal transplantation [34], and in some general surgical situations [35]. A higher degree of frailty was associated with hypertension and cardiovascular disease in older Midwestern adults in a cross-sectional observational study [36].

7.5 TREATMENT

Reversing or treating frailty is problematic. There may be some possibility in reversing the prefrail stage, but once full frailty (and also in the failure-to-thrive stage) is established it is generally considered irreversible [16,37]. Treating frail patients involves treating chronic conditions that contribute to frailty and avoiding or mitigating factors that cause sarcopenia. Exercise has been shown to help in patients who are not at the end-stages of frailty. Between 30 and 60 min of exercise 3 times per week has been shown to improve some frailty markers when the period of exercise ranges from 3 to 6 months. Furthermore, programs involving stretching, resistance training, and tai-chi have been shown to benefit [14]. Exercise activity has even been shown to be beneficial in a program involving as little as 2 days per week [38].

There is hope that research into nutritional factors in the older adults might eventually apply to frail patients [14]. Weight loss with exercise, more than either individually, in obese patients improved frailty markers [39]. It should be noted that medications such as megestrol acetate and dronabinol have not been shown to be very effective in increasing appetite in patients cared for in skilled nursing facilities [37]. Furthermore, these drugs have significant side effects.

Targeting the inflammatory and endocrine pathophysiologic factors directly has not yielded much in the way of effective treatments. The following have been studied and have yet to show positive outcomes: growth hormone (and growth hormone-releasing factor) and DHEA-S [40]. Testosterone has been shown to increase muscle mass but may have potentially negative outcomes given its link to changes in the prostate gland [41] and elevated cholesterol [42]. Low vitamin D (25(OH)D) levels were found in frail patients in one study [32]; further investigation into vitamin D replacement and sarcopenia and frailty may prove helpful.

7.6   PREVENTION

Prevention measures should be applied generally. In the broader geriatric population, exercise is probably the best measure that can be utilized besides treating and optimizing other chronic conditions. The benefits that have been shown in older patients with exercise include increased mobility, enhanced performance of ADLs, improved gait, decreased falls, improved bone mineral density, and increased general well-being [43–46]. Although no prospective study exists, it is not unreasonable to infer from this that exercise imparts some preventive benefit in the development of frailty; there seems little in the way of negatives.

If frailty (fully established frailty) cannot be prevented or reversed then the negative outcomes that go along with it should be ideally managed within a framework of comprehensive care. The model systems of care that have evolved over the past few decades for use in treating older patients with challenges across wide spectrums of disease and disability apply to frail patients as well.

7.7   COMPREHENSIVE GERIATRIC ASSESSMENT, PACE, AND ACE

The CGA is an evaluation of an older patient with complex medical problems incorporating elements considered "usual" in a standard medical evaluation but with additional emphasis on function, quality of life, and expertise from many disciplines. The range of issues assessed in the CGA include physical (pain, mobility/ADLs, falls, incontinence, sensory deficits, general health), mental (cognitive and affective), social (including network of support), financial, environmental, and spiritual. The purpose of the CGA is to identify specific areas where the appropriate resource can be applied to either reverse or mitigate challenges in the many areas assessed. It takes a team to do this and typically involves one or more medical providers, nurses, pharmacists, a social worker, an occupational therapist, and a physical therapist. Ideally it helps to identify patients who are most likely to benefit from comprehensive management: not too well and not too ill. Management can take the form of both outpatient- and inpatient-based care programs. These are conducted with the hope that positive outcomes can be achieved: decreased hospitalization, decreased nursing home admission, and mortality. Maintaining patients' level of independence and at their baselines for as long as possible is the goal. Quality of life can be as important as, or more important than, quantity of life for many patients.

The program for all-inclusive care for the elderly (PACE) is a long-term comprehensive management model that aims to decrease hospitalizations and nursing home care in older patients [47]. Beginning in the 1990s in San Francisco, California, the program has been replicated across the country. In 1997, it became a permanent Medicare program due to its success [48]. Patients are followed across the continuum of care: outpatient clinics, day centers, home environments, and, if necessary, hospitals and nursing homes; the latter two settings attempting to be minimized but not program-ending for patients—patients are followed until the end of their lives.

In a hospital setting, where frail patients are especially vulnerable to bad outcomes, an analogous model of care, called Acute Care for Elders (ACE), can be utilized [49]. Hospitals that have ACE units aim to treat acutely ill or injured older patients across a variety of medical and surgical problems utilizing multiple services to minimize iatrogenic complications and functional decline or improve function if decline has occurred. The following benefits have been observed employing components of the ACE model: decreases in falls, delirium, functional decline, hospital length of stay, discharge to a nursing home, and costs [50].

7.8 POSTACUTE CARE REHABILITATION AND FRAILTY

We know that applying the CGA to nonrobust older patients (and by extension, to frail patients) in home and hospital settings has a positive impact. Unfortunately, outcomes for frail patients in postacute care rehabilitation settings must be inferred from knowledge in frail patients in other settings. More research is needed. Patients with cognitive impairment, which can commonly coexist with frailty, have been shown to have worse outcomes in postacute care rehabilitation programs [51]. Patients who have frailty have less reserve and are more likely to do worse with polypharmacy, invasive procedures, and repeated trips to the hospital. In clinical practice, the frail patient who was sick enough to be admitted to the hospital is the type of patient who faces a worse prognosis in general after an acute stay—including in long-term care settings, skilled nursing rehabilitation programs, and at home. Setting expectations in terms of what patients and families can potentially achieve in a rehabilitation program is important; hopefully, future studies can help guide providers in their discussions with them. We *can* say that frail patients have been shown to have the generally higher risk of falling, developing decreased mobility, declining in performance of ADLs, being institutionalized, and death. Any transition in care, including one to a skilled rehabilitation program, is an opportunity to discuss openly with patients and families the reality of what frailty is and the impact it likely will have.

7.9 FRAILTY AND ADVANCE DIRECTIVES

Advance directives (AD) are formal ways to document a patient's wishes, at a time when he or she has decision-making capacity, pertaining to medical interventions that might be considered at a future time when the patient no longer has decision-making capacity. Designation of a surrogate decision-maker (by the patient when she or he has decision-making capacity) in the event of the patient losing capacity is typically part of the process. The types of decisions that are typically documented pertain to life-threatening illnesses. Specific life-sustaining interventions that are commonly listed for consideration include cardiopulmonary resuscitation (CPR), mechanical ventilation, artificial hydration and nutrition, and intravenous antibiotics. In relevant clinical scenarios, the withholding of any or all of these interventions carry a high risk of death; hence, the need for ADs. A Do Not Resuscitate (DNR) order is placed when a patient's AD states that no CPR is to be attempted under any circumstance. A Do Not Intubate (DNI) order is placed when a patient's AD states that no mechanical ventilation is to be utilized in any circumstance.

A patient admitted to the hospital who suffers a cardiac arrest and undergoes an attempt to be resuscitated is faced with a poor prognosis. In general, such a patient faces an 82% chance of not surviving until discharge. Furthermore, about one-half of these survivors will leave the hospital with moderate-to-severe neurologic deficits [52]. Although there is no specific literature on patients with frailty who undergo resuscitation it has been shown that patients with significant severity of illness markers present at the time they suffer a cardiac arrest do even worse. Patients who are admitted from a skilled nursing facility; have combination of chronic liver, kidney, or lung disease; and advanced age (>75 years); are not neurologically intact on admission; and are presenting other acute clinical factors can have as little as <1% chance of surviving with little or no neurologic injury until discharge [53]. It is not unreasonable to extrapolate that frail patients, who have many of these characteristics, will frequently be among the groups who will do poorly after attempted resuscitation. A diagnosis of frailty should prompt the physician to ensure that a patient's ADs are current and that the patient and/or his or her surrogate decision-maker understand the risks of CPR so that the appropriateness of a DNR order is considered.

7.10 REFLECTIONS

It is important to reiterate that aging is not synonymous with frailty. It is a subset of older patients who develop it. Exercise, maximizing nutritional status, and optimizing chronic conditions are the best measures to mitigate frailty's impact; pharmacologic agents do not presently play a role in treating frailty as a specific entity. The presence of weight loss, low activity, a subjective report of exhaustion, objective weakness, and slowness in a patient may suggest frailty. Once a patient becomes frail, a comprehensive care plan is ideal. It takes a village, so to speak, to optimally care for the frail older patient.

Frail patients are in a declining trajectory that can be accelerated if they are approached in the same way as nonfrail patients are approached. The dictum "less is more" usually applies. In clinical practice, it is the frail patient who is more likely to suffer from cascades of unintended consequences and complications. The nursing home resident whose family states "has been declining over the past few months" is sent to the emergency department for evaluation of altered mental status who then is diagnosed with pneumonia and dehydration. The patient is started on antibiotics and intravenous fluids. His or her sleep cycle is disrupted and mental status worsens further. He or she is lethargic during most of the daylight hours and unable to participate with even minimal physical therapy or simple transfers. Now essentially bed-bound, his or her skin becomes rapidly at risk for breakdown given her low activity, poor nutritional status, low circulating blood volume, and cachectic bony frame. Abdominal cramping develops and a CT scan of the abdomen and pelvis are ordered with intravenous contrast. Later, diarrhea begins and *Clostridium difficile* colitis is diagnosed. Unfortunately, the patient's renal function declines rapidly due to the intravenous contrast given during the prior CT scan. Furthermore, the CT scan also reports the incidental finding of a lesion suspicious for malignancy in one of the kidneys. Several days of severe illness has deconditioned the patient significantly by this time and the patient has developed a stage 2 decubitus ulcer. If this patient survives the acute hospital stay and returns to his or her skilled nursing facility he or she will likely be described by family as "never the same since that last hospitalization" and by the nursing home staff as having a "new and weaker baseline." This is the kind of patient where goals of care discussions with patient and family have great importance. Questions like, "Do we pursue a work-up of the renal lesion?" "Does 'full code', as an advance directive, make the most sense?" "Do we avoid sending back to the hospital for a similar acute condition?" "Is hospice, or a palliative-centric care plan a consideration now?" For a practicing geriatrician caring for hospitalized patients, this type of scenario is common. Thoughtful, deliberate, and cautious approaches to frail patients are a necessity.

REFERENCES

1. Sternberg SA, Wershof Schwartz A, Karunananthan S et al. The identification of frailty: A systematic literature review. *J Am Geriatr Soc* 2011; 59:2129.
2. Walston J, Hadley EC, Ferrucci L et al. Research agenda for frailty in older adults: Toward a better understanding of physiology and etiology: Summary from the American Geriatrics Society/National Institute on Aging Research Conference on Frailty in Older Adults. *J Am Geriatr Soc* 2006; 54:991.
3. Fried LP, Tangen CM, Walston J et al. Frailty in older adults: Evidence for a phenotype. *J Gerontol A: Biol Sci Med Sci* 2001; 56:M146.
4. Kiely DK, Cupples LA, Lipsitz LA. Validation and comparison of two frailty indexes: The MOBILIZE Boston Study. *J Am Geriatr Soc* 2009; 57:1532.
5. Romero-Ortuno R, Walsh CD, Lawlor BA et al. A frailty instrument for primary care: Findings from the Survey of Health, Ageing and Retirement in Europe (SHARE). *BMC Geriatr* 2010; 10:57.
6. Romero-Ortuno R. The frailty instrument for primary care of the Survey of Health, Ageing and Retirement in Europe predicts mortality similarly to a frailty index based on comprehensive geriatric assessment. *Geriatr Gerontol Int* 2013; 13:497–504.
7. Ensrud KE, Ewing SK, Taylor BC et al. Comparison of 2 frailty indexes for prediction of falls, disability, fractures, and death in older women. *Arch Intern Med* 2008; 168:382.
8. Chin A, Paw MJ, Dekker JM et al. How to select a frail elderly population? A comparison of three working definitions. *J Clin Epidemiol* 1999; 52:1015.
9. Rockwood K, Andrew M, Mitnitski A. A comparison of two approaches to measuring frailty in elderly people. *J Gerontol A: Biol Sci Med Sci* 2007; 62:738.

10. Boyle PA, Buchman AS, Wilson RS et al. Physical frailty is associated with incident mild cognitive impairment in community-based older persons. *J Am Geriatr Soc* 2010; 58:248.

11. Avila-Funes JA, Amieva H, Barberger-Gateau P et al. Cognitive impairment improves the predictive validity of the phenotype of frailty for adverse health outcomes: The three-city study. *J Am Geriatr Soc* 2009; 57:453.

12. Cigolle CT, Ofstedal MB, Tian Z et al. Comparing models of frailty: The Health and Retirement Study. *J Am Geriatr Soc* 2009; 57:830.

13. Gill TM, Gahbauer EA, Han L et al. Transitions between frailty states among community-living older persons. *Arch Intern Med* 2006; 166:418.

14. Ahmed N, Mandel R, Fain MJ. Frailty: An emerging geriatric Syndrome. *Am J Med* 2007; 120:748.

15. Fried LP, Ferruci L, Anderson G et al. Untangling the concepts of disability, frailty, and comorbidity: Implications for improved targeting and care. *J Gerontol A: Biol Sci Med Sci* 2004; 59(3):255.

16. Fried LP, Darer J, Walston J, Frailty, in Cassel C, Leipzig R, Cohen H et al., eds. *Geriatric Medicine: An Evidence-Based Approach.* 4th edition. New York: Springer-Verlag; 2003:1067.

17. Song X, Mitnitski A, Rockwood K. Prevalence and 10-year outcomes of frailty in older adults in relation to deficit accumulation. *J Am Geriatr Soc* 2010; 58:681.

18. Walston J, Fried LP. Frailty and the older man. *Med Clin North Am* 1999; 83:1173.

19. Cawthon PM, Marshall LM, Michael Y et al. Frailty in older men: Prevalence, progression, and relationship with mortality. *J Am Geriatr Soc* 2007; 55:1216.

20. Wilson JF. Frailty—and its dangerous effects—might be preventable. *Ann Intern Med* 2004; 141:489.

21. Morley J, Perry HM, Miller DK. Editorial: Something about frailty. *J Gerontol A: Biol Sci Med Sci* 2002; 57:M698.

22. Leng S, Chaves P, Koenig K et al. Serum interleukin-6 and hemoglobin as physiological correlates in the geriatric syndrome of frailty: A pilot study. *J Am Geriatr Soc* 2002; 50:1268.

23. Walston J, McBurnie MA, Newman A et al. Frailty and activation of the inflammation and coagulation systems with and without clinical comorbidities: Results from the Cardiovascular Health Study. *Arch Intern Med* 2002; 162:2333.

24. Morley J, Kim MJ, Haren MT. Frailty and hormones. *Rev Endocr Metab Disord* 2005; 6:101.

25. Schmidt M, Naumann H, Weidler C et al. Inflammation and sex hormone metabolism. *Ann N Y Acad Sci* 2006; 1069:236.

26. Leng S, Cappola AR, Anderson RE et al. Serum levels of IGF-1 and DHEAS-S and their relationship with IL-6 in the geriatric syndrome of frailty. *Aging Clin Esp Res* 2004; 16:153.

27. Mohr BA, Bhasin S, Kupelian V et al. Testosterone, sex hormone-binding globulin, and frailty in older men. *J Am Geriatr Soc* 2007; 55:548.

28. Lanfranco F, Gianotti L, Giordano R et al. Ageing, growth hormone and physical performance. *J Endocrinol Invest* 2003; 26:861.

29. Varadhan R, Walston J, Cappola AR et al. Higher levels and blunted diurnal variation of cortisol in frail older women. *J Gerontol A: Biol Sci Med Sci* 2008; 63:190.

30. Morley JE. Decreased food intake with aging. *J Gerontol Biol Sci Med Sci* 2001; 56A(special issue ii):81.

31. Jones KM, Song X, Rockwood K. Operationalizing a frailty index from a standardized comprehensive geriatric assessment. *J Am Geriatr Soc* 2004; 52:1929.

32. Puts MT, Visser M, Twisk JW et al. Endocrine and inflammatory markers as predictors of frailty. *Clin Endocrinol (Oxf)* 2005; 63:403.

33. Yao X, Hamilton RG, Weng NP et al. Frailty is associated with impairment of vaccine-induced antibody response and increase in post-vaccination influenza infection in community-dwelling older adults. *Vaccine* 2011; 29:5015.

34. Garonzik-Wang JM, Govindan P, Grinnan JW et al. Frailty and delayed graft function in kidney transplant recipients. *Arch Surg* 2012; 147:190.

35. Makary MA, Segev DL, Pronovost PJ et al. Frailty as a predictor of surgical outcomes in older patients. *J Am Coll Surg* 2010; 210:901.

36. Klein BE, Klein R, Knudtson MD et al. Frailty, morbidity and survival. *Arch Gerontol Geriatr* 2005; 41:141.

37. Robertson RG. Geriatric failure to thrive. *Am Fam Physician* 2004; 70:343.

38. Hunter GR, McCarthy JP, Bamman MM. Effects of resistance training on older adults. *Sports Med* 2004; 34:329.

39. Villareal DT, Chode S, Parimi N et al. Weight loss, exercise, or both and physical function in obese older adults. *N Engl J Med* 2011; 364:1218.

40. Lamberts SW. The somatopause: to treat or not to treat? *Horm Res* 2000; 53(Suppl 3):42.

41. Tenover JS. Androgen replacement therapy to reverse and/or prevent age-associated sarcopenia in men. *Baillieres Clin Endocrinol Metab* 1998; 12:419.

42. Lamberts SW, van den Beld AW, van der Lely AJ. The endocrinology of aging. *Science* 1997; 278:419.

43. Daley MJ, Spinks WL. Exercise, mobility and aging. *Sports Med* 2000; 29:1.

44. Spirduso WW, Cronin DL. Exercise dose-response effects on quality of life and independent living in older adults. *Med Sci Sports Exerc* 2001; 33:S598.

45. Keysor JJ. Does late-life physical activity or exercise prevent or minimize disablement? A critical review of the scientific evidence. *Am J Prev Med* 2003; 25:129.

46. Province MA, Hadley EC, Hornbrook MC et al. The effects of exercise on falls in elderly patients. A preplanned meta-analysis of the FICSIT Trials. Frailty and injuries: Cooperative studies of intervention techniques. *JAMA* 1995; 273:1341.

47. Eng C, Pedulla J, Eleazer GP et al. Program of All-inclusive Care for the Elderly (PACE): An innovative model of integrated geriatric care and financing. *J Am Geriatr Soc* 1997; 45:223.

48. Mukamel DB, Peterson DR, Temkin-Greener H et al. Program characteristics and enrollees' outcomes in the Program of All-Inclusive Care for the Elderly (PACE). *Milbank Q* 2007; 85:499.

49. Counsell SR, Holder CM, Liebenauer LL et al. Effects of a multicomponent intervention on functional outcomes and process of care in hospitalized older patients: A randomized controlled trial of Acute Care for Elders (ACE) in a community hospital. *J Am Geriatr Soc* 2000; 48:1572.

50. Fox MT, Persaud M et al. Effectiveness of acute geriatric care using Acute Care for Elders components: A systematic review and meta-analysis. *J Am Geriatr Soc* 2012; 60:12.

51. Landi F, Bernebei R, Cocchi A. Predictors of rehabilitation outcomes in frail patients treated in a geriatric hospital. *J Am Geriatr Soc* 2002; 50(4):679.

52. Peberdy MA, Kaye W, Ornato JP et al. Cardiopulmonary resuscitation of adults in the hospital: A report of 14720 cardiac arrests from the National Registry of Cardiopulmonary Resuscitation. *Resuscitation* 2003;58(3):297–308.

53. Ebell MH, Jang W, Shen Y et al. Development and validation of the good outcome following attempted resuscitation (GO-FAR) score to predict neurologically intact survival after in-hospital cardiopulmonary resuscitation. *JAMA Intern Med* 2013; 173(20):1872–1878.

8 Delirium

Corey Romesser

CONTENTS

8.1 INTRODUCTION

Delirium is a common condition encountered in the care of older adults. Delirium is an acute mental status change that is characterized by a disorder of attention and cognitive function that is typically a consequence of a medical condition. By definition, delirium develops over a short period of time (hours to days) and tends to fluctuate during its course. Although most often associated with hospitalization and in ICUs, delirium is present wherever there are sick patients. Recognition and diagnosis of delirium can be elusive and treatment options are limited. Patients at most risk are those with underlying predisposing conditions as well as those with more severe acute illnesses.

The prevalence of delirium ranges from 14% to 24% on hospital admission, and the incidence of delirium arising during hospitalization is 6%–56% among general hospital populations [1]. Rates are higher for older adults as well as patients with more severe illness. The rate of delirium is highest in patients in intensive care units, which can range from 70% to 87% [2]. The consequences of delirium are significant in many respects. Delirium is associated with increased hospital length of stay, increased hospital costs, increased morbidity and mortality, persistent functional decline, high rates of nursing home placement, and an increase in incidences of falls [3]. In-hospital mortality rates in patients with delirium range from 22% to 76% [4], and there is a 62% increase risk of mortality at 1 year in those who experience delirium during a hospital stay [5]. The costs related to delirium are estimated to be about US$143 billion to US152 billion per year [6]. Delirium commonly persists after discharge [7] and can have significant effects on recovery and long-term outcomes [8].

Delirium has been described in medicine going back to the time of Hippocrates. Over time, it has been referred to by many names, which can contribute to confusion by providers in terms of diagnosis and importance. Acute confusional state, altered mental status, acute brain failure, ICU psychosis, organic brain syndrome, toxic or acute encephalopathy, organic psychosis, and acute cerebral insufficiency are just some of the terms that have been used. Despite differences in terminology, there are many other reasons that delirium is insufficiently diagnosed, and this is more pronounced in older adults. Coexisting dementia combined with lack of understanding of baseline mental status by healthcare providers may lead to assumptions that symptoms related to delirium are normal. Many older adults present with the so-called quiet delirium, which can be more subtle. There can also be a tendency to "normalize" some of the symptoms of delirium in an older patient as well.

Delirium is associated with worsening outcomes, and so prevention is vitally important. Once delirium occurs, prompt recognition, evaluation, and treatment are critical. Delirium is associated with a 3-fold increased risk of death up to 6 months after hospital discharge [9].

8.2   DIAGNOSIS

The diagnosis of delirium is a clinical one, a conclusion based on careful observation of several key features. Diagnosis is overlooked for many reasons, so it is crucial to be aware of the criteria and clinical presentations.

The American Psychiatric Association's *Diagnostic and Statistical Manual of Mental Disorders* (4th edition, *DSM-IV*) lists four key features that characterize delirium [10].

- Disturbance of consciousness with reduced ability to focus, sustain, or shift attention
- A change in cognition of the development of a perceptual disturbance that is not better accounted for by a preexisting, established, or evolving dementia
- The disturbance develops over a short period of time and tends to fluctuate during the course of the day
- There is evidence from the history, physical examination, or laboratory findings that the disturbance is caused by a medical condition, substance intoxication, or medication side effect

Additional features that may be present include the following:

- Psychomotor behavioral disturbances such as hypoactivity, hyperactivity with increased sympathetic activity, and impairment in sleep duration and architecture
- Variable emotional disturbances, including fear, depression, euphoria, or perplexity

Several diagnostic and rating scales exist for diagnosing or screening for delirium. The Delirium Rating Scale—Revised 98 (DRS-R98) and the Confusion Assessment Method (CAM) are both commonly used in the literature. In clinical practice, the CAM is most often used, as it is fairly simple and accurate. It has also been modified for use in ICU patients (CAM-ICU). The CAM is a diagnostic algorithm that has been validated for the clinical diagnosis of delirium and has demonstrated a sensitivity of 94%–100% and specificity of 90%–95%. The CAM algorithm requires that a patient meet both of the first criteria and then either criteria 3 or 4 [11].

1. Acute onset and fluctuating course
2. Inattention
3. Disorganized thinking
4. Altered level of consciousness

When evaluating patients for suspected delirium, or just doing routine screening, it is helpful to use a short test to evaluate attention. There are several tests that can be done quickly as part of any bedside exam. These can be done as quick screening evaluations or as part of a more formal delirium assessment. Asking a patient to recite the days of the week or months of the year backwards is one test. Another is using a digit span test. This involves asking a patient to recall a series of numbers immediately after recitation. The sequence increases in number until the patient is unable to correctly recall the full series. Correct recitation of five to nine digits is considered normal. Vigilance A testing can also be used. This involves the provider reciting a series of letters and asking the patient to raise their hand whenever the letter A is used.

8.3 CLINICAL CHARACTERISTICS

Delirium is commonly missed in clinical practice, and so familiarity of the key features is extremely important. Delirium is often a marker for more severe underlying disease, and many consider the development of delirium to be a medical emergency. Recognition requires knowledge of the various characteristics that often occur in a patient with delirium. It also requires accurate assessment with knowledge of a patient's baseline cognitive status.

8.3.1 ACUTE ONSET/FLUCTUATIONS

Delirium is by definition an acute syndrome. Symptoms often develop and progress over a matter of a few minutes to several hours or days. The symptoms must represent a change from baseline mental status. There is typically a fluctuation in symptoms that occur over the course of the condition, and these changes may also occur over hours or days. Fluctuations can be wild and abrupt. Swings in attention and arousal occur unpredictably and irregularly, but many times there may be an identifiable pattern. Typically, worsening occurs at night and may be labeled as "sun-downing." The unpredictability of the fluctuations can make recognition difficult as the patient may be more lucid when seen by a healthcare provider but be quite altered a few hours later. For this reason it is often important to elicit additional information from patient's families or caregivers. Patients with underlying cognitive impairment may also have fluctuations in mental status but in a more usual, predictable pattern. Knowledge of this underlying pattern is vital to determining when there is an acute change that may be due to the development of delirium.

8.3.2 ATTENTION DEFICIT

Disturbance of attention is the true hallmark of delirium. Attention must be distinguished from arousal (which is discussed later), and the level of disturbance can have a wide range. In a delirious patient, there is distractibility with impaired ability to maintain or appropriately shift attention. In some patients there is limited ability to focus on any stimuli, whereas others may be hyper-alert and, therefore, extremely distractible. Patients may have difficulty following a conversation or answering questions. Patients may be easily distracted by any outside stimuli.

8.3.3 CONFUSION/DISORGANIZED THINKING

Patients with delirium are unable to maintain coherent or clear thought patterns. Speech may shift from subject to subject and be tangential and at times incoherent. There may be repetitions and perseverations within the speech pattern. Thoughts may be illogical or scant and preservative.

8.3.4 ALTERED LEVEL OF CONSCIOUSNESS AND PSYCHOMOTOR ACTIVITY

Patients with delirium may have lethargy or decreased arousal, while others may be hyperalert or hypervigilant. Patients can also fluctuate between the two. Patients with hyperalertness will still have difficulty maintaining appropriate attention or focus. It is not normal for a patient to fall asleep during a clinical interview and should not be dismissed as sleep deprivation. This level of lethargy is typical in a delirious patient. The altered level of consciousness is often associated with changes in psychomotor activity. Hyperalertness is typically associated with agitation and overactivity. A patient may continuously "pick" at clothing, attempt to remove catheters or IVs, and may frequently attempt to get out of bed.

8.3.5 PERCEPTUAL AND EMOTIONAL DISTURBANCES

Delirious patients commonly have disturbances in perception of time and place. Hallucinations can occur and are most often visual in nature. Hallucinations can be frightening in many patients. Some patients will also have delusional episodes related to disorientation. This may manifest as paranoia or persecutory ideation. Other patients may exhibit emotional lability with periods of fear, crying, or even playful behaviors. Older patients often display symptoms of depression in the setting of delirium.

8.3.6 SLEEP/WAKE CYCLE DISTURBANCES

It is quite common for symptoms of delirium to be more prevalent at nighttime. The term "sundowning" is often used to describe this phenomenon. This often results in an increase in restlessness at night, and many patients may remain awake for much of the night. This then results in daytime drowsiness, and many patients will nap much of the day. This then further exacerbates the nighttime issues and creates a cycle of day/night of sleep/wake reversal.

8.3.7 MEMORY IMPAIRMENT/DISORIENTATION

Disorientation is very common in delirium. Most often a patient will be first disoriented to time, but patients are also frequently disoriented to place and situation. Patients will often "replace" the unfamiliar situation with a more familiar one. Hospitalized patients will report that they are at a relative's home or even in their own bedroom. It is important to be aware of a patient's baseline level of orientation as patients with dementia are also often disoriented. Disorientation due to delirium should represent a change from baseline. Patients may also have impaired recent memory due to decreased registration and attention issues.

8.4 DELIRIUM SUBTYPES

Delirium can have many presentations but is often classified into three categories primarily based on level of arousal and psychomotor activity. There are the hyperactive, hypoactive, and mixed subtypes. Hyperactive delirium more typically involves agitation, restlessness, and hyper vigilance and may include delusions or hallucinations. In contrast, patients with hypoactive delirium have more sedation and lethargy and more psychomotor retardation. The hypoactive form occurs most frequently in older adults. Hyperactive delirium represents about 25% of cases and hypoactive about 50%. The remaining 25% are mixed. The patient with hyperactive delirium is typically easy to identify, and the reverse is true for hypoactive delirium. Hypoactive delirium is sometimes referred to as "quiet delirium." It is these patients, with hypoactive delirium, who are often at greater risk due to lack of identification that may lead to lack of work-up and appropriate treatment.

8.5 PREDISPOSING AND PRECIPITATING FACTORS

The development of delirium typically involves the interplay of multiple factors. There are several risk factors that have been identified that can help predict a patient's inherent risk of developing delirium. In a sense, every patient has their own threshold for when delirium might occur. There are then precipitating factors that are usually an acute change/noxious insult that have the effect of lowering the threshold that leads to an episode of delirium. It is the combination of the underlying risk (vulnerable patient) and the precipitating factors (noxious insult) that leads to the development of delirium.

Typically a patient with more risk factors will be more likely to develop delirium with a more minor precipitating factor, and a patient with fewer risk factors will require a more severe precipitating event or multiple factors at one time. An example of this would be a frail older adult with dementia and multiple medical comorbidities who is exposed to relatively benign insult, like a sedative medication. Conversely, an otherwise healthy adult with no cognitive impairment can develop delirium in the setting of a severe infection requiring ICU care and mechanical ventilation. Table 8.1 includes several risk factors associated with delirium. Within this list, visual impairment, severe illness, cognitive impairment, and dehydration are independent risk factors that predispose to delirium [1].

There are literally hundreds of causes or provocative factors that can be the precipitating event that leads to the development of delirium in an older patient. Oftentimes, there are multiple conditions present in patient. Table 8.2 contains a list of some of the most common conditions.

Medications are a leading cause of delirium, especially in older adults. Older patients are often on multiple medications and are typically more at risk for adverse effects from medications. Both intoxication and withdrawal may lead to delirium. In patients who develop delirium, evaluation of medication lists for new or stopped medications is advised. Medications are often additive in effect, especially those with anticholinergic effects. Many over-the-counter cold medications, antihistamines, neuroleptics, and antidepressants have anticholinergic effects. Other medications associated with delirium include narcotic analgesics, sedative-hypnotics, especially longer-acting benzodiazepines, antiparkinsonian drugs, as well as corticosteroids. Withdrawal from several medications can lead to delirium. This includes barbiturates, benzodiazepines, amphetamines, as well as alcohol. Withdrawal from alcohol is always an important consideration as delirium tremens can be severe and life threatening. Withdrawal from antidepressants/SSRIs can lead to a discontinuation syndrome that can sometimes lead to delirium as well.

Infections, both obvious and occult, can lead to delirium. Just about any infection can lead to delirium, both systemic and CNS related. Urinary tract infections, pneumonia, and septicemia are common causes, but consideration for encephalitis or meningoencephalitis should be considered. Immunocompromised patients are at greater risk of infection and prompt work-up should always be considered.

TABLE 8.1
Risk Factors

Age >70
Dementia/cognitive impairment
Depression
Past cerebrovascular accident (CVA)
Alcohol abuse
Psychoactive medications
Multiple medical comorbidities
Dehydration
Impaired activities of daily living (ADLs)/functional dependence
Malnutrition
Polypharmacy
Vision impairment
Hearing impairment
Severe or terminal illness

TABLE 8.2

Causes of Delirium

Drugs
  Anticholinergic
  Sedative hypnotics
  Narcotic analgesics
  Alcohol or drug withdrawal
Acute illnesses
  Dehydration
  Metabolic disorders (hypoxemia, hypoglycemia, hyper- or
    hyponatremia, hyper- or hypocalcemia)
  Infections
  Myocardial infarction
  Congestive heart failure
  Stroke
  Seizure/postictal
  Shock
  Hypoxia
  Malignancy
  Pain
Environmental
  Sleep deprivation
  Indwelling bladder catheters
Surgery/anesthesia
Urinary retention
Constipation/obstipation

Primary central nervous system disorders are a potential, but less frequent, cause of delirium. The frequency of delirium associated with at TIA is quite low, but delirium can occur with strokes. Hypertensive encephalopathy, CNS vasculitis, temporal arteritis, subdural hematomas, and migraine can also lead to delirium.

There are several environmental factors that should be considered as contributing to dementia. Sleep deprivation is a very important one. Interference of sleep/wake cycles can occur in hospitalized patients due to interruptions at night and poor sleep environment. A noisy, unfamiliar hospital unit may be enough to precipitate delirium in a vulnerable patient. This sensory overload may be a factor in producing "ICU psychosis."

8.6 PATHOPHYSIOLOGY

The pathophysiology of delirium is incompletely understood. There are several theories described in the literature, and it is unlikely that a single mechanism is fully responsible. It is likely that the condition of delirium represents a final common pathway of many pathophysiologic disturbances with multiple "causes."

Disturbance in the balance of neurotransmitters is one of the more widely accepted explanations. Acetylcholine and dopamine are the most often implicated neurotransmitters, but others, including serotonin and norepinephrine, may be involved.

There is extensive evidence to support the concept of cholinergic deficiency in delirium [12]. Patients with anticholinergic poisoning have long been described as "mad as a hatter" in medical lexicon, administration of anticholinergic drugs can induce delirium [13], and physostigmine has been shown in case studies to reverse delirium [14]. Other studies have demonstrated increased serum anticholinergic activity in patients with delirium [15,16].

Dopamine excess is another possible contributor to delirium. Dopamineric drugs like levodopa are often responsible for the development of delirium. Also, dopamine antagonists are often effective in treating the symptoms of delirium (see Section 8.8). Other suggested contributors to delirium are systemic inflammatory conditions including cytokines, including interleukin-1, -2, -6 (ILS-1, -2, -6) and tumor necrosis factor alpha [17]. These cytokines can increase permeability of the blood–brain barrier and alter neurotransmission. Given the multiple causes and heterogeneous presentation of delirium, it is likely that there are several pathogenic mechanisms that result in the development of delirium.

8.7 PATIENT EVALUATION

Evaluation of a delirious patient involves two important aspects: First, one must recognize the condition exists, and second, one must diligently evaluate for the underlying medical illness or illnesses that have caused the delirium. A thorough understanding of a patient's baseline mental status must be obtained, as the changes associated with delirium may be subtle and are often attributed to other factors (fatigue, dementia, and age). Understanding of the risk factors, causes, and presenting signs as described above can increase recognition. Once diagnosed, a thorough evaluation for potential causes should be undertaken.

Patient history is often the most important part of the evaluation. Caregivers or family members are often needed to provide additional details to establish baseline abilities as well as when changes were first noted. History of medication changes and careful review of all medications, including over-the-counter medications, is imperative. If history cannot be obtained, it is recommended that the patient be assumed to be delirious until proven otherwise. History should include identification of underlying risk factors as well as symptoms of potential causes. It is important to consider psychosocial changes as well, as this can also contribute to the development of delirium. Examples of this may be a change in living situation or loss of a family member or caregiver.

Physical exam should be focused evaluation of mental status as well as identification of systemic or neurologic illnesses. Due to the numerous causes of delirium, exam should be comprehensive and thorough. Vital signs may reveal fever from an infectious illness or hypoxia due to CHF, pneumonia, or COPD. Careful evaluation for signs of infection or dehydration should be performed. Neurologic exam should include evaluation for meningismus or head trauma along with any evidence for new focal deficits that may suggest a new ischemic event. Patients with delirium may exhibit asterixis or myoclonus.

Essential laboratory testing includes electrolytes, blood urea nitrogen, creatinine, glucose, thyroid function testing, urinalysis, as well as complete cell count to evaluate for evidence of infection or anemia. In many instances drug levels and toxicology screening are appropriate. In patients with respiratory symptoms or chronic pulmonary conditions an arterial blood gas can be helpful. Liver function testing and ammonia levels can be considered for patients when there is concern for hepatic dysfunction. Electrocardiogram should be done in older adults as delirium may be the only present symptom of myocardial infarction.

Imaging is typically a bit more selective in working up delirium. Chest x-rays to evaluate for pneumonia, congestive heart failure, and so on are worth consideration. Abdominal x-rays may be helpful in identifying occult obstipation or ileus, and ultrasound of the bladder (bladder scan) may be helpful to evaluate for urinary retention. Computed topography of the brain is not universally needed. It is always appropriate in a patient with any new, unexplained focal deficits, but not every patient with delirium requires a CT scan and such imaging is unhelpful when used routinely [18]. Acute stroke may present as delirium, but this is less likely in a patient without additional physical findings suggestive of an acute infarct. In patients with recent known or suspected trauma, brain imaging is appropriate to evaluate for intracranial hemorrhage. It is important to remember that older patients may have some brain atrophy, and so a slowly developing subdural hematoma may not present clinically until several weeks after initial trauma.

Lumbar puncture is not required in most cases [19], but should be considered in cases when cause is uncertain or there is concern for meningitis or encephalitis. CT or MRI should be done first, especially if signs of increased ICP, trauma, or space occupying lesion. EEG testing is also a consideration in patients where seizure or postictal state is considered or when cause is uncertain.

8.8 MANAGEMENT

Management/treatment of delirium can be difficult and involves the use of multiple strategies. Since there are so many possible causes of the condition, the treatment can be equally complex and multifaceted. The mainstays of therapy involve four components. First and foremost is to identify and treat the underlying condition(s). Second is to avoid additional insults that can prolong or worsen the condition. Third, we must provide supportive and restorative care that will allow the patient time to recover safely. Finally, treatment may need to be initiated to manage harmful or dangerous behaviors that may be present and may interfere with the first three components of management. Treatment can be both nonpharmacologic and pharmacologic. It is important to note that there are no proven treatments or models of care that successfully reduce the duration of delirium once it has developed.

Delirium can be caused by literally hundreds of illnesses, and it is important to evaluate patients carefully to identify a cause. Oftentimes, there are multiple "causes," and a complete investigation is warranted before determining the exact cause or cause. Once identified, appropriate treatment and management of that condition should be promptly initiated. Management of fluid and electrolyte disturbances, treatment of infections, correction of metabolic disorders, as well as removal of offending medications and treatment of withdrawal of alcohol or sedatives are typical in the treatment of delirium. Management of these conditions is beyond the scope of this chapter, but mentioning of alcohol withdrawal is particularly important due to its potential morbidity and mortality when not recognized and treated promptly.

In any delirious patient, it is possible to make the situation worse by prescribing inappropriate medications or by failing to provide a suitable environment and, therefore, inadvertently worsen or prolong delirium. Avoiding medications that can exacerbate delirium is extremely important. Providing an environment with natural lighting and reduced stimulation can be helpful. Limiting the use of "tethers" can also be effective. Telemetry monitoring, Foley catheters, and even IV lines can contribute to worsening delirium symptoms. Of particular importance is the management of pain. Untreated pain and inadequate analgesia in the perioperative setting are strong risk factors for delirium [20], and use of nursing protocols to better manage pain in hip fracture patients has demonstrated a reduction in severity and duration but not incidence of delirium [21]. However, use of opioid analgesics for pain management may themselves precipitate or prolong delirium [22]. Therefore, there must be careful balance of risks and benefits in pain management of patients at high risk for delirium. In my experience, the undertreatment of pain is more often the culprit for delirium than the use of opioids.

Delirium can take days, weeks, or even longer to resolve. During this time, patients are at risk for complications related to their confusion and immobility that can lead to functional decline. For this reason it is important to focus on maintaining adequate hydration and nutrition as well as attempting to maintain mobility and preventing skin breakdown. Providing adequate pain relief and monitoring for the development of aspiration issues should be done to prevent the patient from developing additional issues that could further worsen or prolong a delirious episode. Patients should be provided with their own, or replacements of, vision or hearing aids to limit sensory deprivation. Increasing activity levels and maximizing mobility during the day can be helpful in many ways including reestablishing a day/night sleep cycle. A calm environment with supportive caregivers and family are helpful. Good illumination, preferably natural light during the day, with quiet and calm, and a dark room for sleep, all will help in patient recovery. Attempts at limiting interruptions of sleep by appropriate timing of vital signs and medications is appropriate. Limiting changing of rooms and caregivers is also helpful. Attention to bowel and bladder function is also important.

Managing disruptive behaviors or agitation in delirium is often the most challenging aspect of care. These behaviors may create a situation that leads to additional patient or even staff harm. Patients may wander or attempt to get out of bed without assistance when they are physically unsafe to do so. They may pull out intravenous catheters, urinary catheters, or feeding tubes. In these situations, physical restraints may be used, but the use of restraints is generally discouraged. Restraints can increase agitation as well as increase risk for injuries, aspiration, and pressure ulcers. One study noted a 3-fold increase of persistent delirium at the time of discharge in patients who had been restrained [23]. In patients who demonstrate behaviors that create an unsafe situation, alternatives include use of medications, as discussed below, or the use of constant observation. Observation by medical staff or family members may be enough to limit the risk of harm. Use of family members can be helpful in managing some behaviors. It offers an opportunity to educate caregivers and can form a partnership in dealing with a potentially frightening condition. Family members can provide frequent reassurance and reorientation along with touch from familiar persons, which may be calming to the patient.

Treatment of disruptive behaviors related to delirium with medications is difficult, and the available data to guide treatment are unfortunately limited. Patients with delirium are vulnerable, and use of any medication can often result in an unintended worsening of the condition. In addition, many of the medications used for this purpose have risk for additional side effects, particularly in older adults. However, there are times when the risk of harm from the behavioral symptoms outweighs the risks of the medication. It is important to weigh this risk/benefit ratio carefully and cautiously.

Medications that have been studied include typical antipsychotics, atypical antipsychotics, benzodiazepines, and cholinesterase inhibitors. Most of the studies have been small and underpowered, and very few are placebo controlled. While many studies have shown improvement in delirium symptoms, it is difficult to know if this was due to natural course of the disease or truly related to drug effects. Currently, there are no medications that are specifically indicated for treatment of delirium, and so all use is considered "off-label." Therefore, any decision to use medications should be carefully considered with appropriate safeguards put in place.

The medication that is most often used or recommended is haloperidol. Despite this recommendation, the data on its efficacy are still quite limited. Most authors recommend use of low-dose haloperidol in older adults, usually 0.25–0.5 mg as a starting dose with slow titration upward [24]. Haloperidol can be given orally or parenterally. Oral dosing is associated with increased risk of extrapyramidal side effects, but IV has higher risk of cardiac complications. When using haloperidol for delirium, it is important to check an EKG prior to use and to continue monitoring for signs of ischemia or QT prolongation. Haloperidol is not recommended for patients with underlying parkinsonism. A study done in hip fracture patients using low dose, scheduled haloperidol did demonstrate safety in a short duration of therapy [25].

The newer, atypical antipsychotic agents have also been used. These agents typically have fewer side effects than haloperidol, but there is still a relative lack of evidence. A recent review article with two RCTs, five open-label studies, and one retrospective cohort showed quetiapine resolves symptoms of delirium more quickly than placebo and has efficacy equal to that of haloperidol [26]. A meta-analysis of three small studies that compared haloperidol with risperidone and olanzepine showed that the three agents were similarly effective [27].

Benzodiazepines are indicated for use in patients with delirium related to sedative medication or alcohol withdrawal. However, use of benzodiazepines can increase the risk for developing delirium [28] and has not shown benefit compared to neuroleptic use [29]; therefore, its use is limited to patients with withdrawal-related delirium only. Use of cholinesterase inhibitors is also discouraged, as a trial using rivastigmine compared to placebo in hospitalized patients with delirium was stopped early due to higher mortality in the rivastigmine group [30].

The use of medication to manage patients with delirium is often necessary but should be used as a last resort. It is important that medication be used only with a goal to decrease risk of harm or injury to the patient or caregivers or to allow for additional management. Medication should not be used to decrease annoying behaviors or for simple sedation. It is recommended that medications be used on a short-term basis as prolonged use increases risk of complications, particularly with antipsychotics [31].

8.9 PREVENTION

A lack of effective, proven interventions for treatment of delirium has led to the increased focus on prevention strategies. These efforts focus on managing modifiable risk factors and have demonstrated a reduction in the development of delirium. The most effective prevention programs involve multiple interventions. There are several nonpharmacologic interventions that are typically recommended by experts. However, additional study is needed to determine the individual effectiveness of these recommendations:

- Avoidance of immobility and sensory deprivation
- Provision of glasses, assistive hearing devices, appropriate orienting stimuli (clocks, calendars, and natural lighting)
- Regular review of medications and minimization of psychoactive medications and discontinuation of unnecessary drugs
- The use of staff or family members who can provide interpersonal contact with use of reorientation strategies and encouragement for increasing activity and increased oral intake
- Use of restraints as well as unneeded "tethers" such as urinary catheters or telemetry monitors should be avoided
- Allowance for uninterrupted sleep with appropriate night-time lighting and noise should be provided for
- Natural lighting and encouragement for activity during daytime can also be helpful

One landmark study utilized a multicomponent intervention with standardized protocols to screen and control for six risk factors [32]. This study looked at 852 hospitalized patients aged 70 years or older. The risk factors were cognitive impairment, sleep deprivation, immobility, visual impairment, hearing impairment, and dehydration. Interventions were targeted to these risk factors in an attempt to reduce the development of delirium during the hospital stay. The interventions included orientation and cognitive stimulation for patients with cognitive impairment, nonpharmacologic sleep protocols for insomnia, early mobilization, visual and hearing aids, and early volume repletion.

This program resulted in a reduction of delirium from 15% to 9.9%. There was no effect on the severity of delirium when it did occur [32]. This intervention has led to the development of a program that has been replicated in other hospitals with similar reductions in delirium [33]. A modified version of this program effectively reduced the rates of delirium in older surgical patients who have undergone abdominal procedures [34].

Despite several trials, the current available evidence does not support the use of medications to prevent delirium. A 2013 systemic review and meta-analysis including six studies evaluated the effects of neuroleptic medications in surgical patients. The study concluded that such treatment reduced the incidence of delirium but not the severity or duration and did not reduce the associated adverse events [35]. However, one well-done study looked at low-dose haloperidol (0.5 mg tid) given routinely to hip surgery patients starting pre-op and continued until 3 days post-op. This study showed no reduction in delirium rates, but it did show a positive effect on severity and duration of delirium (5.4 days vs. 11.8 days) [25].

8.10 CLINICAL OUTCOMES

The duration and prognosis of delirium is quite variable. In general, the condition may only last for a day or two, but it often lasts much longer with some studies demonstrating delirium symptoms up to 12 months after diagnosis [7]. Delirium is often a marker for severe illness but is also independently associated with poor outcomes. It is associated with increased mortality and institutional placement, independent of age, sex, comorbid illness or illness severity, and presence of dementia at baseline [36].

About 40% of patients with delirium during hospitalization who survive to discharge will die within 1 year [1], and there is a 62% increase of mortality compared to patients without delirium [5]. Patients admitted to postacute care with delirium had a cumulative 1-year mortality of 39% and patients with persistent delirium after discharge were 2.9 times more likely to die compared to those whose delirium was resolved [37]. Pooled results from several studies estimated 1- and 6-month mortality to be 14% and 22%, respectively [38].

Delirium can have significant effects on short- and long-term functional outcomes. A recent study of 343 medical inpatients with delirium demonstrated a poor functional recovery in 69% of patients with 13% having a functional decline at 103 days after discharge [39]. Another prospective study of delirious hospitalized patients demonstrated the loss of almost one activity of daily living (ADL) at 3 months after discharge [40]. There is also an increased risk of falls in patients with delirium at 13 months after a delirium episode [3]. These issues are often interrelated to the need for higher level of care.

Many studies have demonstrated increased rates of institutional placement in patients who have an episode of delirium. In one study of 433 patients aged 70 years and older it was demonstrated that there was an increased rate of nursing home placement or death in patients who had delirium during a hospitalization compared to those who didn't. The rates were even higher when comparing patients whose delirium persisted at discharge versus patients in whom the delirium resolved prior to discharge (83% vs. 67.7%) [8]. Similarly, in a study that evaluated outcomes of delirium in poststroke patients, the presence of delirium at admission to the rehabilitation department was an independent risk factor for institutionalization or in-hospital death [41].

8.11 DELIRIUM AND COGNITIVE IMPAIRMENT

The relationship between dementia and delirium is an important part of any discussion of delirium. Cognitive impairment as risk factor for delirium has long been clear. Dementia is the single largest risk factor in the development of delirium, with about two-third of patients with delirium having underlying dementia [42]. However, what is perhaps more interesting is the role delirium plays in the progression of cognitive impairment. In clinical practice, an episode of delirium is often the impetus that leads to the work-up and diagnosis of dementia. This is often due to the lack of identification of a preexisting cognitive disorder, but there may be more to that. There is some evolving evidence that the two conditions are more interrelated and the pathologic processes that cause delirium may also contribute to dementia or at least its progression [43]. While it is not clear that delirium itself causes dementia, there is an associated decline in cognitive functional abilities in patients with dementia who experience delirium [44]. Delirium contributes to worsening functional and cognitive status in patients with dementia with acceleration in the rate of cognitive decline [45]. This new decline may be what leads to the "uncovering" of dementia in a patient who experienced an episode of delirium. A relatively common clinical scenario is for a patient who has experienced delirium to "never return to baseline" and to continue on a steeper rate of decline than seen previously.

8.12 DELIRIUM AND POSTACUTE CARE/REHABILITATION

After an acute hospitalization, many older people are unable to return to their homes due to ongoing physical or cognitive limitations or impairments. Postacute care facilities, including rehabilitation hospitals and skilled nursing facilities (SNF), are frequently used for these patients. As has been discussed, delirium can persist for several weeks or even months and so will often persist at the time of discharge from an acute hospitalization. Unfortunately, there is not a lot of available information on the effects of delirium in the postacute setting as opposed to acute in-hospital environment. Formal assessment for delirium at admission to postacute care is limited and can be challenging, but a few studies have found the rates of delirium to be about 16%–23% [46,47].

Patients who are admitted to postacute facilities with delirium are at increased risk for complications [48] and have worsened functional outcomes [47]. One study showed increased risk for both geriatric syndrome complications (including falls) and medical complications like pneumonia in patients with delirium at admission. In addition, they had increased rates of death at the post-acute facility and were readmitted to the hospital at an increased rate. The patients with delirium were much less likely to be discharged back to the community compared to those with no delirium. Perhaps most concerning is the 6-month mortality rate for patients with delirium was 25% and was only 5.7% for those with no delirium [48]. In patients with delirium superimposed on dementia (DSD), the outcomes are even worse. DSD at admission to postacute care was found to be associated with almost a 15-fold increase in odds of walking dependence, 5-fold increase in risk for institutionalization, and a 2-fold increase in mortality compared to patients without either dementia or delirium [49].

It should be noted, however, that resolution of delirium during postacute care is a marker for improved recovery. In one study, patients whose delirium resolved within 2 weeks without recurrence regained 100% of their prehospital functional level, whereas patients who did not resolve their delirium recovered in less than 50% of the cases [50].

Much of our knowledge about management of delirium comes from inpatient settings. Translating appropriate prevention strategies and management plans to other settings is difficult due to lack of studies. Applying similar, nonpharmacologic approaches for both prevention and management would seem to be appropriate when possible. However, current evidence is not available to support this claim. A delirium abatement program was developed by several experts in an attempt to improve detection and management in postacute admissions. This program consisted of a nurse-driven protocol that focused on initial assessment and correction of common reversible causes of delirium, prevention of complications of delirium, and restoration of function. In a randomized controlled trial of this program, the results were disappointing. There was an increase in detection of delirium, but there was no effect on the persistence of delirium. The study was limited by low percentages of adherence by staff to execute important steps of the intervention [51].

8.13 CONCLUSIONS

Delirium is a complex, geriatric syndrome that is commonly encountered in the care of older adults. Development of delirium is related to underlying risk factors in conjunction with acute precipitating causes—usually acute medical illness or medication issue. Management of delirium involves treatment of underlying causes and the use of both multifaceted nonpharmacologic and pharmacologic interventions. Treatment of delirium once it occurs does not reduce the severity or duration of delirium, and so prevention strategies should be a priority of care in vulnerable patients.

REFERENCES

1. Inouye SK. Delirium in older persons. *New England Journal of Medicine*. March 2006;354:1157–1165.
2. Pisani MA, McNicoll L et al. Cognitive impairment in the intensive care unit. *Clinical Chest Medicine*. Dec 2003;24(4):727–737.
3. DeCrane S, Culp K et al. Twelve-month fall outcomes among delirium subtypes. *Journal for Healthcare Quality*. 2012;34(6):13–20.
4. American Psychiatric Association. Practice guideline for the treatment of patients with delirium. *American Journal of Psychiatry*. 1999;156(suppl):1–20.

5. Leslie DL, Zhang Y et al. Premature death associated with delirium at 1-year follow up. *Archives of Internal Medicine*. July 2005;165:1657–1662.
6. Leslie DL, Inouye SK. The importance of delirium: Economic and societal costs. *The Journal of the American Geriatrics Society*. Nov 2011;59(suppl 2):S241–S243.
7. McCusker J, Cole M et al. The course of delirium in older medical inpatients: A prospective study. *Journal of General Internal Medicine*. 2003;18(9):696.
8. McAvay GJ, Van Ness PH et al. Older adults discharged from the hospital with delirium: 1-Year outcomes. *Journal of the American Geriatrics Society*. Aug 2006;54(8):1245–1250.
9. Ely EW, Shintani A et al. Delirium as a predictor of mortality in mechanically ventilated patients in the intensive care unit. *JAMA*. April 2004;291(14):1753–1762.
10. American Psychiatric Association. *Diagnostic and Statistical Manual of Mental Disorders*. 4th ed. Washington, DC: APA, 1994.
11. Inouye SK, van Dyck CH et al. Clarifying confusion: The Confusion Assessment Method. A new model for detection of delirium. *Annals of Internal Medicine*. Dec 1990;113(12):941–948.
12. Hshieh TT, Fong TG et al. Cholinergic deficiency hypothesis in delirium: A synthesis of current evidence. *Journal of Gerontology, Series A: Biological Sciences and Medical Sciences*. July 2008;63(7):764–772.
13. Han L, McCusker J et al. Use of medications with anticholinergic effect predicts clinical severity of delirium symptoms in older medical inpatients. *Archives of Internal Medicine*. Apr 2001;161(8):1099–1105.
14. Blitt CD, Petty WC. Reversal of lorazepam delirium by physostigmine. *Anesthesia and Analgesia*. 1975;54(5):607–608.
15. Flacker JM, Cummings V et al. The association of serum anticholinergic activity with delirium in elderly medical patients. *American Journal of Geriatric Psychiatry*. 1998;6(1):31–41.
16. Mussi C, Ferrari R et al. Importance of serum anticholinergic activity in the assessment of elderly patients with delirium. *Journal of Geriatric Psychiatry and Neurology*. 1999;12(2):82–86.
17. Cunningham C. Systemic inflammation and delirium: Important co-factors in the progression of dementia. *Biochemical Society Transactions*. 2011;39(4):945–953.
18. Koponen H, Hurri L et al. Acute confusional states in the elderly: A radiological evaluation. *Acta Psychiatrica Scandinavia*. 1987;76:726–731.
19. Warshaw G, Tanzer F. The effectiveness of lumbar puncture in the evaluation of delirium and fever in the hospitalized elderly. *Archives of Family Medicine*. 1993;2:293–297.
20. Lynch EP, Laxo MA et al. The impact of post-operative pain on the development of postoperative delirium. *Anesthesia and Analgesia*. 1998;86:781.
21. Milisen K, Forman MD et al. A nurse-led interdisciplinary intervention program for delirium in elderly hip fracture patients. *Journal of American Geriatrics Society*. 2001;49:53.
22. Gaudreau JD, Gangno P et al. Opioid medications and the longitudinal risk of delirium in hospitalize cancer paints. *Cancer*. 2007;109:2365.
23. Inouye SK, Zhang Y et al. Risk factors for delirium at discharge: Development and validation of a predictive model. *Archives of Internal Medicine*. 2007;167:1406.
24. American Psychiatric Association. Practice guidelines for the treatment of patients with delirium. *American Journal of Psychiatry*. 1999;15(suppl 5):1–20.
25. Kalisvaart KJ, de Johnge JF et al. Haloperidol prophylaxis for elderly hip surgery patients at risk for delirium: A randomized placebo-controlled study. *JAGS*. 2005;53:1658–1666.
26. Hawkins SB, Bucklin M et al. Quetiapine for the treatment of delirium. *Journal of Hospital Medicine*. 2013;8(4):215–220.
27. Lonergan E, Britton AM et al. Antipsychotics for delirium. *Cochrane Database of Systematic Reviews*. 2007;CD005594.
28. Pandharipande P, Shitani A et al. Lorazepam is an independent risk factor for transitioning to delirium in intensive care unit patients. *Anesthesiology* 2006;104:21.
29. Lonergan E, Luxemberg J et al. Benzodiazepines for delirium. *Cochrane Database of Systematic Reviews*. 2009;CD006379.
30. van Eijk MM, Roes KC et al. Effect of rivastigmine as an adjunct to usual care with haloperidol on duration of delirium and mortality in critically ill patients: A multicenter, double-blind, placebo-controlled randomized trial. *Lancet*. 2010;376:1829.
31. Scheider LS, Dagarman KS et al. Risk of death with atypical antipsychotics for dementia: Meta-analysis of randomized controlled trials. *JAMA*. 2005;294:1934.
32. Inouye SK, Bogardus ST et al. A multicomponent intervention to prevent delirium in hospitalized older patients. *NEJM*. 1999;340(9):669–676.

33. Rubin, F. Williams, J et al. Replicating the Hospital Elder Life Program in a community hospital and demonstrating effectiveness using quality improvement methodology. *Journal of the American Geriatrics Society.* 2006;54(6):969–974.

34. Chen CC, Lin MT et al. Modified Hospital Elder Life Program: Effects on abdominal surgery patients. *Journal of American College of Surgeons.* 2011;213(2):245–252.

35. Hirota T, Kishi, T. Prophylactic antipsychotic use for postoperative delirium: A systematic review and meta-analysis. *Journal of Clinical Psychiatry.* Dec 2013;74(12):e1136–e1144.

36. Witlox J, Eurelings LS et al. Delirium in elderly patients and the risk of postdischarge mortality, institutionalization and dementia: A meta-analysis. *JAMA.* 2010;304(4):443.

37. Kiely D, Mercantonio E et al. Persistent delirium predicts greater mortality. *Journal of American Geriatrics Society.* 2009;57(1):55–61.

38. Cole MG, Primeau FJ. Prognosis of delirium in elderly hospital patients. *Canadian Medical Association Journal.* 1993;149(1):41.

39. Dasgupta M, Brymer C. Prognosis of delirium in hospitalized elderly: Worse than we thought. *International Journal of Geriatric Psychiatry.* May 2014:29(5):497–505.

40. Murray AM, Levkoff SE et al. Acute delirium and functional decline in the hospitalized elderly patient. *Journal of Gerontology.* Sept 1993;48(5):M181–M186.

41. Turco R, Bellilli G et al. The effect of poststroke delirium on short-term outcomes of elderly patients undergoing rehabilitation. *Journal of Geriatric Psychiatry and Neurology.* June 2013;26(2):63–68.

42. Fong TG, Tulebeav SR et al. Delirium in older adults: Diagnosis, prevention and treatment. *Nature Reviews Neurology.* April 2009;5(4):210–220.

43. Eikelenboom P, Hoogendijk WJ. Do delirium and Alzheimer's dementia share specific pathogenetic mechanisms? *Dementia and Geriatric Cognitive Disorders.* 1999;10:319–324.

44. Saczynski JS, Marcantonio MD et al. Cognitive trajectories after postoperative delirium. *New England Journal of Medicine.* July 2012;367:30–39.

45. Fong TG, Jones RN et al. Delirium accelerates cognitive decline in Alzheimer disease. *Neurology.* 2009;72:1570–1575.

46. Kiely DK, Bergman MA et al. Delirium among newly admitted post-acute facility patients: Prevalence, symptoms and severity. *Journal of Gerontology, Series A: Biological Sciences and Medical Sciences.* 2003;58A:441–445.

47. Marcantonio ER, Simon SE et al. Delirium symptoms in post-acute care. Prevalent, persistent and associated with poor functional recovery. *Journal of American Geriatric Society.* 2003;51:4–9.

48. Marcantonio ER, Kiely DK et al. Outcomes of older people admitted to postacute facilities with delirium. *Journal of the American Geriatrics Society.* 2005;53:963–969.

49. Morandi A, Davis D et al. Delirium superimposed on dementia strongly predicts worse outcomes in older rehabilitation inpatients. *JAMDA.* 2014;15;349–354.

50. Kiely DK, Jones RN et al. Association between delirium resolution and functional recovery among newly admitted postacute facility patients. *Journal of Gerontology: Medical Sciences.* 2006;61A(2);204–208.

51. Marcantonio ER, Bergmann MA et al. Randomized trial of a delirium abatement program for postacute skilled nursing facilities. *Journal of the American Geriatrics Society.* June 2010;58(6):1019–1026.

9 Urinary Incontinence in Older Adults

Nicole Strong, Sara Z. Salim, Jean L. Nickels,
and K. Rao Poduri

CONTENTS

9.1 INTRODUCTION

Urinary incontinence (UI), defined as involuntary leakage of urine, is a common health problem among older adults.[1] Over 17 million adult Americans are currently believed to be living with UI, which is associated with a significant decrease in psychosocial health and overall quality of life.[1] The prevalence of UI has been shown to consistently increase with age and is overall higher for women. Prevalence varies by source but was recently reported to be 30%–50% of women and 17%–24% of men older than age 60.[2-4] Rates as high as 85% have been reported for those individuals currently living in long-term care facilities.[5]

Notably, 6% of nursing facility admissions have been attributed to UI.[5] The annual cost of UI has been estimated at US$66 billion.[6] Direct costs of UI include those accrued for diagnostic studies, therapeutic procedures, pharmacotherapy, and other available treatment options.[7] Indirect costs include those added due to complications of UI or other resulting disability, including sleep disturbance, mood abnormality, falls, pressure sores, depression, caregiver expense, and nursing facility placement.[7]

The identification and treatment of UI in the geriatric population presents an ongoing challenge due to significant underreporting of symptoms.[8] Many individuals consider UI to be a normal part of aging and do not seek medical evaluation, while others are too embarrassed or ashamed to initiate conversation about UI with medical providers.

9.2 DEFINITIONS

There are six main types of urinary incontinence that are classified by symptomatology and underlying etiology, including urgency urinary incontinence (UUI), stress urinary incontinence (SUI), mixed urinary incontinence (MUI), overflow urinary incontinence (OUI), transient urinary incontinence, and functional urinary incontinence. Overactive bladder (OAB) is a syndrome that often results in incontinence, which will be addressed separately. Neurogenic bladder is not a type of UI but rather a form of bladder dysfunction that may itself result in UI.

Urgency urinary incontinence (UUI) is the sudden imperative need to void during or preceding an incontinent episode.[1,9] UUI prevalence, in the geriatric population, was recently reported as 35% in women and 25.5% in men.[4] Previously, 40%–70% of all UI in older adults was attributed to the UUI variety.[10] This is known to be the most commonly seen form of UI in older adults.[11]

Stress urinary incontinence (SUI) is incontinence that occurs upon increased effort, exertion, coughing, or sneezing.[1,12] It is more commonly seen in women (39.1%) than in men (13.9%).[4,11] The number one cause of SUI in men is iatrogenic following prostate surgery.[9]

Mixed urinary incontinence (MUI) is a combination of SUI and UUI types of urinary incontinence. MUI currently represents over 30% of cases of incontinence in women.[13]

Overflow urinary incontinence (OUI) occurs due to overfilling of the bladder without the necessary muscle contractions to empty.[9] This results in an increased bladder pressure prior to an incontinent episode. The presence of small or large volumes of urine leakage, along with elevated postvoid residual volumes (PVRs) is characteristic of OUI.[9] It is most common in older men due to the high incidence of benign prostatic hyperplasia (BPH).[1]

Transient incontinence is a form of reversible incontinence due to factors outside of the lower urinary tract.[1] A few examples would be infection, change in cognition, or side effects of medications.[1]

Functional incontinence is a subcategory of transient incontinence. It is the involuntary and unpredictable passage of urine due to inability to reach the appropriate place to void in time or due to unwillingness to seek an appropriate place to void.[1,9] It is seen in individuals with decreased mobility, cognitive impairment, difficulty with verbal expression, and during environmental situations when there is lack of easily accessible bathroom facilities.[1]

Overactive bladder (OAB) is characterized by symptoms of urinary urgency (compelling urge to void) with or without the presence of incontinence.[14,15] It is usually accompanied by nocturia (waking up from sleep to void) and frequency of voiding symptoms.[15] OAB is more common than UI, with prevalence rates subjectively reported as "sometimes" being present in 40.4% of men and 46.9% in women aged 65 and older.[14] Progressive worsening of OAB symptoms have been correlated to advancing age.[16]

UUI and OAB are often referred to interchangeably; however, this is not accurate because two-thirds of individuals with OAB do not have UI.[17]

Neurogenic bladder is bladder dysfunction secondary to acquired or traumatic neurologic damage of the central nervous system (CNS), peripheral nervous system (PNS), or both. The presentation of neurogenic bladder is extremely variable and includes urinary retention with or without overflow incontinence, urgency incontinence, and frequency.[18] Neurogenic bladder is most commonly associated with spinal cord injury (SCI), multiple sclerosis (MS), spina bifida, stroke, Parkinson's Disease, and transverse myelitis.[18]

9.3 IMPACT

Urinary incontinence has an overwhelming impact on multiple facets of the geriatric individual's life. Some of the areas most commonly reported and, therefore, studied include physical health, psychological well-being, social balance, and financial condition. When considering that all of these substantial areas have potential to be influenced by the single medical condition of UI, the total impact on quality of life may be recognized.

9.3.1 PHYSICAL HEALTH

People with UI are at higher risk for skin breakdown due to the ammonia content of urine. This can be painful to the individual and requires frequent skin checks and proper hygiene for successful prevention.[12] Urinary tract infections (UTI) are also more common in incontinent individuals, adding to their medical complexity and potentially exacerbating their bladder symptoms.[12]

In addition, studies have demonstrated an impairment of mobility for those with UI.[19,20] Geriatric fall and fracture risk have been reported to increase for those with UI.[21] One study specifically reported a 1.8-fold increased risk of falls and a 2.7-fold increase in high fear of falling among community-dwelling women with urgency and/or UUI.[22] It is speculated that more frequent rushing to the bathroom in an attempt to limit incontinent events and the embarrassment surrounding them may be contributing to this increase in fall risk.[22]

Another physical characteristic associated with UI is its impact on sexual health. Sexual dysfunction is known to increase with age, while sexual frequency often decreases. Despite this, many older adults continue to stay sexually active well into the ninth decade.[23] UI has been noted to have negative implication on sexual function. In fact, one study noted that men with OAB and UUI were less likely to report being sexually active than those with erectile dysfunction.[23] Another study reported that UI had a negative impact on both women's sexual satisfaction and quality of life.[24] Higher volumes of urine lost and nocturnal incontinence have both been independently associated with decreased sexual activity.[24] Furthermore, it was determined that less severe UI was associated with greater sexual satisfaction and less use of self-blame as a coping mechanism.[24] Healthy sexual function requires the synergy of a complex interplay of factors. This includes partner factors, relationship factors, individual factors, life stressors, medical comorbidity, cultural influences, and mental health.[23] It is important that intervention efforts focus both on the individual affected, as well as their partner, in order to optimize results and relationship health.[24]

9.3.2 PSYCHOLOGICAL WELL-BEING

Patients have frequently reported to healthcare workers feelings of shame, self-doubt, embarrassment, depression, anger, and low self-esteem related to their UI.[12,14,25] The need for increased dependence on the caregiver for mobility and hygiene may lead to feelings of being burdensome and a sense of loss of control over function and life in general. Depression scores of older adults with UI are significantly higher than those without UI.[25] Anxiety may also develop due to the individual's concern regarding availability of a bathroom when needed; this may be even more prominent in those with limited mobility when they are in a less familiar environment.[14]

9.3.3 SOCIAL BALANCE

Increased dependence on caregivers may also introduce stress into interpersonal relationships.[12] Sometimes family is not comfortable performing the hygiene tasks required or the individual prefers that family not assist with continence care. This may result in the increased expense that accompanies external assistance and may contribute to the decision for care to be transferred to a nursing facility.[5] As mentioned earlier, anxiety has been frequently reported by individuals with UI and may stem from the constant worry regarding potential of an incontinent episode while outside of the home. The development of anxiety may also contribute to eventual social isolation.[14] This decrease in community and social involvement may then continue the cycle of isolation as further strain is exerted on relationships with family and friends.

9.3.4 FINANCIAL CONDITION

The financial impact of UI is significant when considering both direct and indirect costs. Direct costs include any cost attributed to diagnosing and treating the medical condition itself, including all diagnostic procedures, lab testing, therapy, pharmacology, or other forms of treatment. The indirect costs are those accrued by the individual and caregiver themselves, including incontinence products, laundering costs, bathing, and skin products. Estimated total annual societal cost of UI continues to rise with one of the more recent figures reported at US$66 billion.[6]

9.3.5 QUALITY OF LIFE

Together, all of the discussed components create a very significant impact on an individual's life. Studies have consistently demonstrated a decreased subjective report of quality of life in individuals with incontinence compared to those without, through the use of questionnaires.[24,26] It is difficult for older adults to maintain their identity with the overall loss of control and life changes that come with UI. Healthcare professionals must be sensitive to the underlying, albeit very significant, impact UI has on quality of life when caring for these individuals.

9.4 BASIC ANATOMY/PHYSIOLOGY

The main structures of the urinary system include the upper urinary system composed of the kidneys and ureters as well as the lower urinary tract, made up of the bladder, bladder neck, urethra, and urethral sphincters.[9,27] The kidneys form and concentrate urine. The ureters connect the kidneys to the bladder. The bladder stores urine, while the urethra acts as a conduit for which urine is eliminated.[27] The internal and external urethral sphincters, along with pelvic floor musculature, allow for storage and release of urine.[9,27] During the micturition reflex the urethral sphincters relax while the detrusor muscle of the bladder contracts.[9] The lower urinary tract is made up of smooth muscle and specialized epithelium, called urothelium.[27] The main innervation of the bladder is via extrinsic neurons outside of its wall.[27]

The interstitial cells of the bladder form close contacts with surrounding structures (nerves and other cells).[27] They are functionally innervated and play an intermediary role between the nervous system and cells of the bladder wall.

Urothelial cells of the bladder respond to different chemical and physical stimuli by releasing neuroactive mediators such as ATP, nitric oxide (NO), acetylcholine, and substance P.[27] These mediators have the ability to modulate sensory nerve endings of the urothelium.[27]

9.4.1 INNERVATION

The act of micturition is under both voluntary and involuntary control. There are two main micturition control centers (MCCs): the pontine micturition center (PMC) of the brainstem and pons, and the micturition control center (MCC) located in the cortex of the frontal lobe.[9] The PMC is under involuntary control and serves an excitatory role that is pro-void.[9] This control center coordinates detrusor contraction and sphincter relaxation for successful voiding. The MCC provides tonic inhibition of the PMC at rest to promote storage of urine when it is inappropriate to void.[9]

Micturition will not take place without proper functioning of the autonomic nervous system, made up of the parasympathetic and sympathetic nervous systems. Both systems are responsible for the involuntary functions of the bladder.[9,27]

1. The parasympathetic system releases acetylcholine and causes urine elimination via relaxation of the internal urethral sphincter and contraction of the smooth bladder muscle. The parasympathetic nerves act via muscarinic receptors located in the bladder. The two types are M2 and M3, present in a ratio of 3:1. The M3 receptors are the subgroup responsible for bladder contraction and emptying.[9]
2. The sympathetic system releases norepinephrine and acts on the alpha-1, beta-2, and beta-3 receptors.[28] Contraction of the internal urethral sphincter occurs through the action of alpha-1 receptors. Relaxation of the detrusor occurs through action on the beta-2 and beta-3 receptors. These combined actions ultimately lead to urinary storage.

The bladder receives indirect innervation by the parasympathetic autonomic nerves of the sacral parasympathetic nucleus via the pelvic nerve.[27] It also receives indirect sympathetic innervation from the thoracolumbar spinal cord via the hypogastric, pelvic, and lumbosacral sympathetic chain ganglia.[27] Direct innervation is present through efferent fibers of the parasympathetic postganglionic nerves of the pelvic ganglia.[27] Both the hypogastric and pelvic ganglia also supply the urethra.[27] The external urethral sphincter is directly innervated via motor neurons of the sacral segments of the spinal cord.[9]

Sympathetic preganglionic neurons within the intermediolateral cell column of the dorsal grey commissure of T_{12}–L_2 in the spinal cord activate efferent pathways and promote storage by relaxing the bladder detrusor muscle and contracting the urethral sphincter.[27]

At sacral cord levels S2–S4, a group of parasympathetic preganglionic neurons are located in the sacral parasympathetic nucleus.[27] Activation of these neurons leads to contraction of the detrusor and the bladder empties.[27]

The somatic nervous system voluntarily controls the function of the external urethral sphincter, pelvic floor, and abdominal musculature.[9,27] To release urine, voluntary relaxation of the external urethral sphincter is required. In addition, voluntary contraction of the muscles of the pelvic floor and abdomen may help control the flow of the urine stream.

Onuf's nucleus contains the motor neurons that innervate the striated muscle of the external urethral sphincter via the pudendal nerve.[27] The striated muscle is tonically active during bladder filling; this contraction allows for prevention of urine leakage during bladder filling.[9,27]

9.4.2 Micturition Reflex

Micturition is a two-phase process (filling and emptying) that occurs via involuntary and voluntary reflexes.[9,27] Urine is stored involuntarily due to relaxed detrusor and tonic contraction of urethral sphincter. When the bladder is full, sensory afferents sense bladder wall stretch via proprioceptive receptors.[9] The sacral afferents signal the need to urinate by sending sensory impulses to the PMC.[9,27] Sensory information is also transmitted through the thalamus, hypothalamus, and areas of forebrain.[27] The cortical MCC interprets sensory information and modulates voluntary control of the bladder, thereby preventing inappropriate emptying. When the decision is made that it is appropriate to void, the cortical inhibition is discontinued, and the PMC sends pro-void impulses down the spinal cord to the detrusor muscle.[9] This results in elimination of urine via simultaneous sphincter opening and detrusor contraction.[9] This efferent control over the micturition reflex requires an intact path between the PMC and spinal cord.[27] The ability to start and stop a void and to control the flow rate of a void comes from the complex coordination of sensory and motor components of both autonomic and somatic nervous systems.[27]

9.4.2.1 Anatomical Changes with Age

Much of our understanding of anatomical bladder changes that occur with age is from animal studies. Exact mechanisms of changes are not well understood. Main changes include progressive decrease in sensitivity of bladder, impairment of calcium signaling, increase in bladder collagen content, decreased muscle mass, decreased urothelial thickness, and reduction of the sympathetic innervation.[27] In older humans it has been noted that smooth muscle or detrusor atrophy occurs with vacuolated sarcoplasm and myofilament disorganization. In addition, degenerated neuronal processes and depleted synaptic vesicles have been reported.[27]

9.5 PATHOPHYSIOLOGY

Recognized physiologic changes that occur with aging include decreased bladder capacity, decreased elasticity of bladder, increased frequency of detrusor contractions, decreased ability to postpone micturition (causing more frequent voids), decreased detrusor muscle strength and contractility, incomplete bladder emptying, and decreased urethral closing pressure (may contribute to leakage of urine).[29,30]

The two main theories of etiology believed to cause OAB dysfunction and potentially lead to UI are of neurogenic and myogenic origin.[30] Neurogenic bladder changes occur in the setting of neurologic disease or injury, such as MS, SCI, and stroke. Common causes of dysfunction include decreased suprapontine inhibition of the micturition reflex, damage to axonal paths in spinal cord, increased lower urinary tract afferent nerve input, loss of peripheral inhibition, or enhancement of excitatory neurotransmission in the micturition reflex pathway.[31] The proposed myogenic theory is that in the presence of outlet obstruction, an increase in intravesicular pressure will lead to partial neurologic denervation of bladder smooth muscle.[31] When the smooth muscle degenerates there is an increase in spontaneous action potentials (APs) and ability of APs to propagate from cell to cell. Denervation, therefore, results in "micromotions" of the detrusor smooth muscle that cause increase intravesicular pressure and stimulation of afferent receptors.[31] Afferent nerves will then feedback to the CNS and cause sensations of OAB.[31]

The exact etiology of UUI remains unknown. Essentially, the detrusor muscle develops involuntary overactivity or uninhibited contractions during the filling phase, which forces urine through the urethra.[9,14,29] It is often seen in association with SCI, MS, and stroke.[15] The most common type of detrusor abnormality that results in UUI is detrusor hyperactivity with impaired contractility (DHIC).[30]

SUI occurs with activities such as sneezing that cause an increase in intra-abdominal pressure.[1,9,30,32] The etiology of SUI is either hypermobility of the urethra when normal muscle supports at the urethral junction fail or due to intrinsic sphincter deficits.[29] When either abnormality is present, total bladder pressure may exceed the urethral closing pressure and produce incontinence.[30] Potential causes of urethral hypermobility include multiple vaginal deliveries or vaginal surgery, postmenopausal decrease in estrogen, prostate surgery, neurogenic disease, and age-related changes.[29,30,32] Intrinsic sphincter deficit is a less common cause of SUI.[29] It may be seen with the normal aging process, decreased estrogen, side effects of irradiation, meningomyelocele, prior vaginal surgery, sacral cord lesion, or trauma.[29,33] The number one cause of SUI in men is iatrogenic during surgical treatment of benign prostatic hypertrophy (BPH) or prostate cancer due to damage of the sacral nerves or pelvic musculature.[9] Radical prostatectomy is associated with the highest rates of SUI (approaching 50%),[33] while transurethral resection of the prostate (TURP) has been reported to result in much lower rates of SUI (<0.5%).[9,34]

MUI is a combination of stress and urge incontinence pathologies as described above.[9]

Overflow incontinence is caused by an atonic and over-distended bladder, urethral obstruction, or detrusor sphincter dyssynergia (DSD).[9,29] It occurs when there is incomplete emptying of bladder during voiding effort or due to absent sensation of bladder fullness. The bladder fills to capacity, without the muscle contractions essential to result in a void.[9] A void will only occur in the setting of OUI when urethral pressure is overcome by extremely elevated intravesical bladder pressure, resulting in the release of urine.[9] DSD is seen with neurogenic bladder pathology, when the detrusor and urethral sphincter contract at the same time.[29] Finally, in men, the most common cause of OUI is BPH causing urethral obstruction.[9] Urinary dribbling, difficulty initiating void, weak stream, straining, and nocturia are often reported with overflow incontinence.[1]

Transient UI is the result of external factors that negatively affect the urinary tract.[35] The pneumonic DIAPPERS has been used to list potential causes for transient UI that have been described.[35] It stands for delirium, infection, atrophic urethritis/vaginitis, psychological disorder, pharmacology, excess urine output, restricted mobility, and stool impaction.[35] All of these causes are reversible physical and psychological sources of UI.

Functional UI is also caused by conditions external to the urinary system and is considered to be a form of transient UI.[1,30] Individuals have incontinence due to impaired mobility limiting their ability to make it to the toilet in time.[1] In other cases, change in cognition creates new challenges due to the person's inability to recognize the toilet, its use, or the process of removing clothing in order to void.[1] Some older adults simply develop an unwillingness to go to the toilet.[30]

9.6 RISK FACTORS

Many studies have attempted to identify risk factors of UI in the geriatric population. There has been some variability in the results that is likely attributable to differences in the populations studied (age, location, culture, race, and gender). Modifiable risk factors described are tobacco, alcohol, caffeine, obesity, cognitive impairment, physical inactivity, constipation, and medications.[11,14,19,25,36] Nonmodifiable risk factors mentioned in the literature include age, Caucasian race, menopause, parity, impaired mobility, and asthma.[1,8,19,20,36,37]

Tobacco use is believed to have an irritating effect on the bladder and may contribute to incontinence.[14] A recent study reported that overall risk of need for repeated surgical treatment for patients with SUI was higher among tobacco users.[38] The need for anticholinergic treatment was also significantly associated with tobacco use.[38] It is suspected that caffeine and alcohol are risk factors due to the diuretic effect and potential for increasing urinary frequency. Caffeine is speculated to have a stimulant effect on detrusor muscle activity.[14] In addition, chronic tobacco use may lead to increased intra-abdominal pressure in the setting of frequent upper respiratory infections and cough.[3]

Obesity may increase risk of UI due to extra abdominal weight applying pressure to the bladder.[1] One study demonstrated double the risk of UI in individuals with BMI >30 when compared to those with BMI less than 30.[37] In addition, significant improvement of continence has been demonstrated after weight loss in randomized control trials.[11]

A recent 2014 study of community-dwelling, frail older adults demonstrated partial or total dependence with ambulation or transfers, and cognitive impairment were all independent risk factors for UI.[19] Limited evidence does report bronchial asthma as a potential risk factor of SUI. This observation was proposed to be due to more frequent bursts of increased intra-abdominal pressure due to cough.[37] In the same study, high parity (described as greater than three vaginal deliveries) was associated with twice the risk of severe SUI. Many medications have been proposed to contribute to UI, but evidence remains very limited. Medication classes suspected of contributing to UI include calcium channel blockers, alpha agonists, antagonists, anti-Parkinsonian medications, diuretics, nonsteroidal anti-inflammatory drugs (NSAIDs), and sedatives.[11]

Low socioeconomic status, regardless of healthcare accessibility, was determined to be a risk factor for decreased likelihood of discussing UI with a medical provider.[39] It was proposed that this result may be due to prohibitive copays, rigorous jobs, or family responsibilities that hinder the ability to seek provider assistance.[39] Furthermore, it is suspected that deprioritization of UI may occur when it is present along with other psychosocial difficulties in this population.[39]

9.7 COMORBIDITIES

There are a number of medical conditions found to be associated with UI. Individuals with a diagnosis of dementia were determined to have 3 times the rate of UI compared to those without dementia.[40] Diabetes and hypertension are independent risk factors for UI. Women with diabetes were found to have 2.5 times the risk for UI compared to nondiabetic women,[41] and women aged 60 years or older with hypertension were found to have a significantly higher risk of UI compared to those without hypertension.[42]

Frailty in older adults has also been linked to UI. In one study, UI was suggested to be an indicator of frailty in older adults and determined to be a mortality risk factor.[2]

Prostatic diseases, including benign prostatic hypertrophy and prostate cancer, are associated with UUI in men. When combined with prostatectomy or radiation treatment, there is a higher risk of SUI. The most common cause of SUI in men is prostate surgery, with the two most common surgeries being transurethral resection of the prostate (TURP) and radical prostatectomy. The external urethral sphincter may be damaged in either of these surgeries. Overflow urinary incontinence may also occur in men with prostatic diseases. In OUI, bladder outlet obstruction and impaired detrusor contractility lead to incomplete emptying and overfilling. This results in bedwetting (nocturia) overnight when the pelvic floor muscles relax.[43]

Pelvic organ prolapse is associated with UI in women. As pelvic organs descend and herniate beyond the vaginal walls, bladder and urethral function is affected and can result in SUI in early stages and urinary output obstruction in advanced stages. Risk of pelvic organ prolapse is higher in women with a history of hysterectomy or multiparity.[44]

A number of neurologic conditions can result in UI. Neurogenic bladder is a dysfunction in voiding due to neurologic injury and can affect urine storage and coordinated voluntary voiding. The micturition reflex involves detrusor contraction and urethral sphincter relaxation, the coordination of which allows for normal voiding. This is regulated by the PMC.

Suprapontine lesions result in loss of voluntary inhibition of the micturition reflex. The effect on the bladder is detrusor hyperreflexia. In Parkinson's disease, abnormalities in the midbrain lead to loss of dopamine that results in detrusor hyperreflexia.[45] Similarly, cerebrovascular accidents to the forebrain also lead to dopamine loss and detrusor hyperreflexia. This is particularly true for lesions involving the cingulate gyrus (involved in executive function, learning, and motivation). Detrusor hyperreflexia in turn leads to OAB and urinary urge incontinence.[46] In multiple system atrophy (formerly known as Shy-Drager syndrome) there is dysfunction of oligodendrocytes leading to autonomic nervous system dysfunction. The effects on the micturition reflex include detrusor hyperreflexia with an open bladder neck and synergic (coordinated) sphincter that results in urge incontinence.[45]

Lesions to the spinal cord also result in detrusor hyperreflexia but with a dyssynergic sphincter. There is a loss of coordination between detrusor contraction and sphincter activity, resulting in elevated bladder pressures and incomplete voiding. This leads to urinary retention and can lead to overflow incontinence. In MS the effects on micturition may vary depending on the location of the lesion; however, the most common finding on cystometry is detrusor hyperreflexia, with elevated postmicturition residual volumes.[47]

Lesions to the cauda equina result in detrusor areflexia but with the sphincter retaining a fixed tone. This creates an obstructive pattern and overflow incontinence is possible. A similar pattern may be seen in neurogenic bladder due to other conditions affecting lower motor neurons, including diabetes mellitus, Guillain-Barre syndrome, and poliomyelitis.

Central nervous system shock is the acute phase of most CNS lesions that results in temporary areflexia, including an areflexic bladder, which can last for days to several weeks.[48]

9.8   EVALUATION

A completed medical history and exam are required for accurate diagnosis of UI and to rule out potential reversible causes for the disorder. Referral to a urological specialist may be necessary for more invasive diagnostic testing and to formulate the correct diagnosis. Challenges when taking a patient's history may arise due to impaired memory, inability to describe urinary symptoms, embarrassment regarding urinary condition, or severe cognitive impairment that limits providing history altogether.

Underreporting continues to be a significant challenge when treating these individuals. Unfortunately, many older adults hold the misconception that UI is a normal part of aging and are not aware of the effective treatments that are available.[8,49,50] For this reason they do not raise concerns to medical providers. It is important to proactively initiate conversations regarding lower urinary tract health in order to identify disease early. Worsening of disease progression, increased UTIs, and skin breakdown are all potential complications of unrecognized UI.[8]

One large, six-year study with 829,614 older adults (mean age of 78 years) revealed that only 48%–50% of people who considered themselves to have a "small problem," and 77%–79% people who described themselves as having a "big problem" related to UI had discussed their condition with a physician.[8] In addition, less than 30% of participants with "small problem" and less than 50% of "big problem" participants had received UI treatment each year during the study period.[8]

9.8.1   History

Important aspects of the history may be obtained by asking direct questions as listed below.[12,31,49,51]

- How frequent is incontinence occurring? Establish voiding pattern throughout the day (number, time of day, and triggers).
- What is the severity of incontinence (number of pads or volume)?
- How long has incontinence been present?
- Once you get the urge to void how long can you successfully delay a void?
- Is a feeling of urgency present when you void?
- Do you have incontinence with coughing, sneezing, or exercise/exertion?
- Are you aware when you are incontinent or do you just notice later on that you are wet?
- Is it difficult to initiate a void?
- Is the urine stream continuous or interrupted?
- Please describe all urinary symptoms.
- Please describe associated symptoms, if any.
- Any recent fever, chills, or pain with urination?
- How is incontinence affecting daily activities and quality of life?

- Please describe your home environment (lighting, stairs, and bathroom locations). How far away is your bathroom from your bed?
- How often do you drink fluids? About how much do you drink during the day and what is the timing of your fluid intake?
- Do you have any history of neurologic disease or radiation therapy?
- Are you currently taking any blood pressure or diuretic medication?

Obtaining a full past medical history and surgical history is important, since some comorbidities are associated with higher risk of UI. A medical provider is often able to establish a diagnosis and initial plan for UI with history, examination, and basic testing alone.[52]

9.8.2 PHYSICAL EXAM

A full physical examination is expected as the standard of care when evaluating for UI. Highlights of the exam include a comprehensive abdominal exam to assess for any pelvic or abdominal masses or hernias that may be contributing. Gait should be evaluated along with a neurological examination to also include assessment of speech. Sacral dermatomes need to be evaluated for any sensory or motor changes, including a rectal exam to assess anal tone and contraction.[31,52] The prostate size and character should also be evaluated during the rectal exam for all male patients. Skin around the genitalia must be inspected for any breakdown. Urodynamic testing is only indicated for complex or cases refractory to conservative treatments.[51] Women require a vulvo-vaginal exam to assess for atrophic vaginitis, prolapse, masses, and pelvic floor dysfunction.[31,51] It is recommended that a vaginal exam be completed with a full bladder to check for incontinence and prolapse and then repeated with an empty bladder to more easily assess pelvic organs.[31] When the bladder is full a stress test may be done, in which the patient is asked to cough while the urethral meatus is observed for urinary leakage.[12] A mini-mental examination may also be completed to further evaluate cognitive functioning.

9.8.3 DIAGNOSTIC STUDIES

Diagnostic testing should include a urinalysis on initial visit to check for evidence of UTI. Bladder scan may be completed at the time of the initial visit or after initiation of empiric treatment to obtain a postvoid residual (PVR) measurement.[31,51] A normal PVR is less than 50 mL, while any volume above 200 mL necessitates urological referral.[12] Urodynamic testing is reserved for cases that are very complex, refractory to conservative treatment, have very large PVRs, or have very low uroflow.[31] It is usually not necessary prior to initiating conservative treatment.

The goal of urodynamic studies (UDS) is to further study the storage and voiding function of the bladder and outlet in order to determine whether bladder dysfunction is the cause of the lower urinary tract symptoms (LUTS).[53] It should only be utilized if findings of the study may change management of the patient. Urodynamic testing has many components, and only the most appropriate ones are completed based on the clinician's judgment.[53] During this testing, patients should be sitting or standing rather than lying supine. Reproducing bladder symptoms is often more challenging in the supine position and, therefore, negatively affects the UDS results.

The following are key components of urodynamic studies (UDS).[53]

Uroflowmetry: A noninvasive measure of urine flow rate over time. The hydrostatic pressure from urine accumulation is measured via gravimetric meter. A rate less than 12 mL/s is suggestive, but not diagnostic of obstruction.

Multichannel urodynamics: Includes cystometry (CMG) and electromyography (EMG).

CMG—A measure of the change in bladder pressure during filling and voiding. It is used to evaluate involuntary detrusor contractions, sensation, compliance, and bladder capacity during filling.

EMG—Provides a continuous measure of pelvic floor muscle contraction and a comparison to detrusor contraction through use of patch or needle electrodes. It allows for evaluation of synergy of muscle contractions.

Pressure flow studies (PFS): An invasive measure of urine flow and detrusor pressure. It evaluates bladder contractility and outlet obstruction.

Videourodynamics: Combines genitourinary fluoroscopy with multichannel UDS. It is used when anatomy and function must be further investigated to obtain a definitive diagnosis.

Abdominal leak point pressure (ALPP) and Valsalva leak point (VLP): Interchangeable terms for the lowest abdomen-generated pressure, in absence of detrusor contraction, that causes UI. The patient completes a Valsalva maneuver and cough at different urine volumes.

Detrusor leak point pressure: Lowest detrusor pressure able to cause incontinence. A phasic rise in detrusor pressure during filling is a sign of overactivity that has potential to result in leakage of urine.

Urethral point pressure: The urethral pressure is measured at different anatomical points using a transducer catheter. This is an important part of the SUI evaluation because it provides part of the maximal urethral closure pressure measurement.

9.9   TREATMENT

The treatment of UI in the older adults requires a multidisciplinary and often step-wise approach. The management goal is to decrease incontinent episodes, prevent complications of incontinence, and, if possible, regain continence. More conservative measures should be attempted prior to the addition of pharmacologic or invasive treatment options. In all cases, education is important, and it enables the patient to take an active role in their own care while allowing them to cope with the effects of UI in a healthy way. The management plan does differ depending on the type of UI experienced. However, patients will benefit from behavioral therapy and lifestyle modifications in nearly all cases of UI.

9.9.1   Behavioral Therapy

This treatment approach has a large body of evidence as support. It aims to improve symptoms through education and institution of healthy voiding habits.

Timed voiding: It requires a schedule for voiding be put in place. It is recommended that voids be attempted approximately every 3 hours to avoid incontinent episodes.[1] The schedule may be adjusted based on the individual's symptoms and daily routine.

Bladder-training therapies: These are used to promote complete contraction and emptying of bladder. The two main techniques used are double voiding and bladder inhibition.[1] Double voiding is a technique that encourages increased urinary drainage through position changes. Often, after the initial void, a brief period of standing is completed prior to a second void attempt.[1] Bladder inhibition encourages development of urge control by implementing specific strategies. Some of the strategies include holding body still, slow deep breaths, mental concentration, distraction to reduce awareness, and voluntarily contracting pelvic floor muscles to inhibit detrusor activity.[1,54]

Pelvic floor muscle therapy (PFMT), also known as Kegel exercises, is a broad term used to describe any form of muscle training geared at strengthening the pelvic floor in an attempt to improve stress, urgency, and mixed forms of UI, in both men and women.[1,11] There has been a wealth of investigations of this intervention with overall positive short-term results reported. PFMT does require daily compliance for improvement as well as the ability to perform a proper technique. Biofeedback may be used to improve effectiveness of exercises.[31] Rectal or vaginal sensors are used to provide a visual indication of pelvic muscle activity and strength.[7] Patients are able to gain control of these muscles using biofeedback.[29] It has also been reported that patients in contact with a healthcare professional have increased subjective improvement of UI than those not in contact with a healthcare professional.[55] PFMT is commonly taught by nursing staff, who are able to follow and guide patients throughout their treatment to encourage their compliance with exercises. The current PFMT recommendations are that the patients tighten their pelvic muscles as if holding in a void for approximately 10 seconds, 3 times per day. Improvement is usually noted after 6–12 weeks of treatment.[1]

Attempts are being made to reach out to more individuals who may not have access or may be too embarrassed to seek medical attention for their UI. In 2014, a web-based treatment approach for women with SUI was initiated and evaluated. It was made up of an evidence-based PFMT video treatment program that could be accessed online, from the comfort of home, for a 3-week period. In total, 1053 people from around the world viewed the online program and 34 finished it completely, including the postprogram survey. Over 85% of participants reported improved UI symptoms after the 3-week PFMT program.[56] This result is very positive, not only regarding the effectiveness of PFMT as a conservative treatment option but also in terms of reaching a greater audience with a web-based approach for education and treatment of UI.

Electrical stimulation: An electrical unit is used to apply stimulation to the pelvic musculature via a rectal or vaginal probe. The goal is to inhibit the micturition reflex while strengthening pelvic musculature. This method is very time consuming with improved UI results being equivalent to the less time-consuming PFMT option.[7]

Weighted cones: These are worn vaginally to encourage contraction of pelvic musculature. A cone is inserted into the vagina and pelvic muscles are contracted to keep it in place for 15 minutes twice a day.[52] Slowly, the weight of the cone used is increased as tolerated. Weighted cones are another example of a biofeedback technique.[52] Studies have demonstrated that the use of weighted cones is superior to no treatment at all.[57] In addition, they are equally effective in the treatment of UI when compared to PFMT.[58]

9.9.2 LIFESTYLE ADJUSTMENTS

Initial research investigating the effects of weight loss on improvement of UI symptoms has been very encouraging. One study of overweight women, demonstrated a decrease in frequency for both urge and stress UI events after weight loss.[59] A 2015 study of obese men and women (had either a BMI >40 or BMP >35 with reversible obesity-related comorbidities) confirmed the positive impact of bariatric surgery on UI.[60] After bariatric surgery, 83% of subjects reported significant improvement of their UI symptoms and 33% described complete resolution of UI.[60]

Elimination of potential bladder irritants and substances with diuretic properties is key to improving bladder control and the voiding schedule. These potential irritants include caffeine, tobacco, and alcohol.

Attempting to limit or have a controlled schedule of fluid intake may also be helpful.[50] Currently, there is a dearth of evidence regarding the potential effect of fluid restrictions and fluid intake pattern on UI symptoms in the older adult population. Despite this, it is recommended that caution be exercised with fluid intake changes in the older adult population because they are more vulnerable to dehydration.[50] Those with nocturnal UI may benefit from a decrease of fluid intake after dinner, with appropriate increase in intake during the day, resulting in a safe balance. Starting a bladder diary allows individuals to make effective adjustments more easily to their personal voiding and fluid intake schedules.[50]

The reduction of poly-pharmacy in the older adults is another consideration when managing patients with UI. It is important to educate patients on medication side effects that may contribute to UI and make adjustments to medication regimens when there are alternative pharmacological options. The main medication classes that have been implicated in potential exacerbation of UI are as follows: diuretics, calcium channel blockers, NSAIDs, oral estrogens, alpha-blocking agents, sedative hypnotics, antidepressants, and ACE inhibitors.[61]

A few simple self-care and environmental alterations that may be made to minimize UI episodes are the wearing of nonrestrictive clothing, bed level low to the ground, and having a bedside commode available in the home.[11]

9.9.3 PHARMACOLOGIC

There are many medications that are effective in the treatment of UI. Unfortunately, they all have side effects that the older adult population is more susceptible to.

Anticholinergic medications include oxybutynin chloride, tolterodine tartrate, darifenacin, festerodine, solifenancin, and trospium. Oxybutynin is promoted as the gold standard with which other pharmacologic agents are compared.[7] Many of these medications have both long-acting and short-acting formulations.[7] Oxybutynin now comes in pill, gel, and patch forms. These medications bind to the M2 and M3 receptors of the bladder and decrease the detrusor contraction in intensity and frequency.[7] They are very effective, but significant side effects of dry mouth, dry eye, constipation, urinary retention, tachycardia, blurred vision, and cognitive impairment may be limiting their use.[7] Anticholinergic medication use is contraindicated when comorbidities of dementia, urinary retention, intestinal obstruction, chronic constipation, or uncontrolled narrow-angle glaucoma are present.[11] It is recommended that these medications be started at very low doses and titrated up slowly when used in the older adult population. This allows for close monitoring of tolerance and side effects prior to dose increases.

Alpha-adrenergic blocker medications include tamsulosin, silodosin, doxazosin, and alfuzosin. They act by blocking the alpha-adrenergic receptors (alpha-1 and alpha-2) in the bladder and prostate gland, causing relaxation of the bladder neck smooth muscle and prostatic tissue.[30] This relaxation ultimately results in less resistance to urine flow.[30,52] Silodosin and tamsulosin are third-generation alpha-receptor antagonists and are considered to be uroselective because they strictly target the prostate alpha-1 receptors.[9] Alfuzosin is a second-generation alpha-1 blocker that is also uroselective. Uroselectivity is worth noting because these medications are associated with decreased cardiovascular side effects.[9] A meta-analysis evaluating efficacy of all the alpha-blockers in the treatment of BPH symptoms demonstrated a mean decrease in symptom scores and increase in urinary flow rate.[62] These medications may be used alone or in combination with 5-alpha reductase inhibitors. Alpha-blockers must be used with caution in older adults, as they may induce orthostatic hypotension.[30]

The 5-alpha reductase inhibitors include finasteride and dutasteride. These medications inhibit conversion of testosterone to dihydrotestosterone and therefore aid in reducing prostate hypertrophy.[9] This ultimately reduces obstruction of the urethra by the prostate in BPH. Positive effects may not be noticed for up to 6 months after initiation of treatment.[9]

The only beta-3 adrenergic agonist used in UI treatment, at this time, is mirabegron (Myrbetriq).[1] It is a daily medication that is better tolerated than anticholinergic medications due to its fewer side effects profile.[1] The main side effects that can occur include hypertension and tachycardia. It should not be used in patients with poorly controlled blood pressure, specifically if systolic is above 180 or diastolic is above 110.[1] Mirabegron is typically used as a second- or third-line option when anticholinergic medications are either contraindicated, not effective, or have intolerable side effects.[49]

9.9.4 INVASIVE PROCEDURES AND SURGICAL OPTIONS

9.9.4.1 Bulking Agents

Multiple agents such as collagen, carbon spheres, silicone, calcium hydroxyapatite, and ethyl vinyl alcohol may be used as bulking agents.[63] They are injected near the urinary sphincter and around the bladder neck and urethra with the goal of causing compression.[63] They reduce incontinence by assisting to close the bladder opening by thickening the surrounding tissues.[29] A skin test is required prior to the procedure to rule out a potential allergy to the particular substance being used.[29] Repeat injections are often required every 6–12 months because the body slowly eliminates the bulking agents.[29,64] This procedure is generally well tolerated with few side effects or complications.[51]

9.9.4.2 Botulinum Toxin (Botox)

Treats both hyperactive detrusor muscle and hypersensitive bladder afferent nerves.[31] Botox is usually injected at 20 different sites that are at least 1 cm apart on the detrusor muscle.[65,66] Its effect is case-dependent but usually lasts for 6–9 months.[66] A randomized double-blind, placebo-controlled trial demonstrated the safety and efficacy of botulinum toxin A, when one-third of women participants achieved continence.[66] Of note, symptoms of urgency and incontinence improved more than urinary frequency.[66] The most common adverse events were UTI (31%) and need for self-catheterization (16%).[50,66] It is worth mentioning that this study used a BONT-A dose of 200 units, but later studies determined 100 units to be the optimal dose in terms of both safety and efficacy.[65-67]

A recent 2015 study by Chun-Hou et al. examined the effect of Botox use in the frail older adults.[65] It demonstrated similar results of decreased UUI and increased quality of life as prior studies. However, there was an increased risk of high PVR after Botox and the long-term success rate was lower.[65] The possibility of postprocedure need for straight catheterization regimen, in the vulnerable older adult population, requires careful consideration of risks and benefits before initiation of Botox treatments.

9.9.4.3 Vaginal Devices

A pessary is an intravaginal stiff support ring that may be inserted by a medical provider as a treatment option for UI. The pessary applies pressure to the vagina and nearby urethra.[51] Stress incontinence improves due to manipulated position of the urethra.[51] Patients must be educated on risk of UTI, vaginal infections, vaginal odor, pelvic discomfort, and bleeding.[7] A healthcare professional should regularly follow these individuals, in order to monitor pessary use.[29] Pessaries are typically removed, cleaned, and reinserted every 4–6 weeks.[50]

Disposable urethral inserts also exist as treatment for SUI. These devices are small silicone cylinders that are inserted into the urethra via an insertion probe. A small balloon is inflated after insertion, to hold the device in place. Urethral inserts decrease UI by blocking off the urethra temporarily.[11,68] They should only be worn for short periods of time, for example, while exercising. A prospective study did demonstrate reduction of UI events, decrease of pad weights (a quantitative measure of the amount of urine that leaked into the incontinence pad), and improvement of quality-of-life scores.[68] The main disadvantages associated with urethral inserts are high rate of UTI (31%) and discomfort.[11]

9.9.4.4 Neurosacral Modulation/Sacral Nerve Stimulation (SNM or SNS)

Neurosacral modulation/sacral nerve stimulation is sacral stimulation through an implanted device at approximately the S3 level.[50,52] The sacral nerves innervating the bladder are stimulated first by an external stimulator. If positive effect is noted of at least 50% reduction in symptoms, then a surgeon will implant the device using a minimally invasive technique.[29] Study of this technique has consistently established improvement potential of UI symptoms.[20,52] In one study, a decrease of UI symptoms by 50% or complete resolution was noted in 76% of the patients.[69]

9.9.4.5 Pudendal Nerve Stimulation

This is a neuromodulation technique with same mechanism as neurosacral modulation. However, the electrodes are placed directly onto the pudendal nerve, allowing for more specific stimulation.[63] Lead placement was previously more difficult with this procedure and lead migration was more common, making it less desirable than neurosacral modulation.[63] However, a recent study evaluated a new laparoscopic technique that demonstrated significant improvement of UI and OAB symptoms with no noted lead migration.[70]

9.9.4.6 Percutaneous Tibial Nerve Stimulation

A form of neuromodulation in which projections of the posterior tibial nerve to the sacral plexus are electrically stimulated to target symptoms of urgency, frequency, and UI.[50] Stimulation occurs at the ankle via fine needle insertion.[50] Typically, 30-minute treatments occur weekly for 12 weeks total, followed by treatments as needed.[50] A randomized control trial demonstrated lasting improvements 1 year post-treatment.[71]

9.9.4.7 Surgery

The bladder position may change over time, especially for women following childbirth. Surgical techniques are typically used with the main goal of supporting the bladder in treatment of SUI and diverting the bladder in UUI.[64] Surgery is typically reserved for refractory cases where all other measures have failed and quality of life is significantly affected.

9.9.4.7.1 Retropubic Suspension

Sutures are used to support the bladder neck. The most common type is the Burch procedure, which entails securing urethral support threads to the pelvic ligaments.[29] This procedure is typically completed at the time of an abdominal procedure, such as a hysterectomy.[65]

9.9.4.7.2 Sling Procedure

This technique is completed through a vaginal incision in women and perianal incision in men.[51] Either natural or man-made slings may be used. The classic autologous sling is a strip of the patient's own rectus fascia that is used to cradle the bladder neck.[51] The ends of the strip are either attached to the pubic bone or to the front of the abdominal wall near the pubic bone.[51]

9.9.4.7.3 Mid-Urethral Sling

This procedure is also referred to as transvaginal tape (TVT) or transobturator tape (TOT).[51] These slings are made of synthetic mesh and are applied mid-way along the urethra in order to support it and decrease hypermobility.[51] This is an outpatient surgical procedure, in which specialized needles are used to place the synthetic tape under the urethra.[29,50] Overall, the efficacy rates in older women with SUI have been very good, with 77%–96% reporting significant improvement or cure.[51,50] The mid-urethral sling procedure is typically well tolerated, but complications reported include difficulty emptying bladder, urgency, and local discomfort.[51]

9.9.4.7.4 Adjustable Continence Therapy

This is a balloon device that has been developed for treatment of stress incontinence due to intrinsic sphincter deficiency.[63] It is made up of two balloons that are each attached to an injectable port in the labia majora or scrotum. The port allows for postoperative alteration of balloon pressure to increase compression of urethra for additional effect.[63,72] A prospective study of women demonstrated significant improvement of UI symptoms in 70% of the study subjects, with 68% reporting being dry after the procedures.[72] Adjustable continence therapy was also evaluated prospectively in male subjects after undergoing prostatectomy. Significant improvement of UI symptoms was noted in 92% of subjects.[73] In addition, 2 years after the procedure, median quality-of-life score nearly doubled.[73]

9.9.4.7.5 Artificial Urinary Sphincter

This option has three main working parts: a cuff, a reservoir, and a pump.[51] The cuff is applied around the urethra and when it is filled the urethra is compressed. The cuff is connected to a pump that is placed in the scrotum in men and labia majora in women.[51] When the pump is manually activated the cuff deflates and fluid is pumped from the cuff to a reservoir that is implanted in the abdomen.[51] This option requires dexterity to activate the pump. There is also risk of mechanical failure and implant infection.[51] One study did demonstrate that men over age 80 years were more likely to experience erosion and infection after device placement than younger men.[74]

9.9.4.7.6 Prolapse Repair

Prolapse repair requires a more significant surgery that often follows or accompanies a hysterectomy when prolapsed pelvic organs are contributing to UI. The two main types of prolapse repair are obliterative and reconstructive surgery.[75] Obliterative surgery narrows or closes off a portion of the vaginal canal to provide support for the prolapsed organs.[74] Sexual intercourse is not possible after an obliterative surgery.[75] Reconstructive surgery is the more common option and varies in method depending on the goals of each individual case. The approach may be through the vagina or abdomen, but the ultimate goal is to restore pelvic organs to their original position.[76] Fixation or suspension may be achieved via the patient's own ligaments or using a mesh.[76] New SUI or exacerbation of prior SUI symptoms following a pelvic organ prolapse repair is fairly common, so concomitant incontinence procedure is often done.[76,77] One study compared prolapse repair and concomitant TVT, prolapse repair with TVT completed 3 months later, and prolapse repair alone.[77] Results demonstrated high SUI cure rates of over 89% in both prolapse and TVT repair groups, compared to only 27% in the prolapse-repair-only group.[77]

9.9.4.7.7 Augmentation Cystoplasty (Reconstructive Surgery)

A section of vascularized small bowel is inserted into the bladder to expand its capacity.[14,51,64] This surgery is now able to be performed macroscopically. Augmentation cystoplasty has been shown to be effective, but complications of recurrent UTI and need for intermittent straight catheterization may occur. It is an option for severe cases of refractory urge incontinence only.[51]

9.9.4.7.8 Urinary Diversion

A section of the small intestine is used to connect the ureters to the abdominal wall with definitive stoma formation. The bladder may be left in place or removed. This surgery does cure the UI symptoms, but complications such as stenosis, infections, renal calculi, hernia, and metabolic disturbance may occur.[51]

9.9.4.7.9 Surgical Management of BPH

BPH is the main cause of OUI in older men, due to urethral obstruction.[9] Surgical options are very effective in treating LUTS; however, these procedures have potential to worsen or even cause SUI in some cases.[9] For this reason, surgery is only pursued for those individuals who have severe symptoms, recurrent UTIs, bladder stones, acute urinary retention, complication of renal insufficiency, or hematuria.[9] The surgical gold standard at this time is transurethral resection of the prostate (TURP), which is an inpatient procedure.[9] Other options include transurethral incision of the prostate (TUIP), open prostatectomy, and laser treatments.[9] TUIP is an outpatient procedure, requires only two incisions, and has been determined to be the most effective option.[9,78,79] Open prostatectomy is associated with more complications and longer postoperative hospitalization and recovery; so it is reserved for only those individuals with prostates greater than 75 cm³ in size.[9]

9.9.5 MANAGEMENT BY TYPE OF UI

9.9.5.1 Stress UI

The main first-line treatment options are behavioral and lifestyle. Medications have only demonstrated mild benefit.[1,51] There is some support that topical estrogen may help vaginal atrophy in postmenopausal women, but evidence of improvement of SUI is minimal.[1] Oral estrogen replacement is not supported by current literature.[7] Alpha-agonist medications have shown some benefit due to action on the urethral sphincter; however, their use in SUI is considered to be off-label.[1] Duloxetine (Cymbalta), a serotonin norepinephrine reuptake inhibitor (SNRI), has been shown to improve symptoms of SUI through its effect on the pudendal nerve via neurotransmitters and ultimately by increasing urethral closing pressure.[1,7] It is currently being used in Europe to treat SUI, but is not

FDA-approved for this treatment purpose in the US.[1] In refractory cases, the procedures that have demonstrated effectiveness in treating SUI include the retro pubic suspension, sling, mid-urethral sling, and artificial urinary sphincter as described earlier. For men with UI after prostatectomy, first-line surgical treatment is either a sling procedure (for mild UI) or AUS (for moderate-to-severe UI).[64]

9.9.5.2 Urgency UI

Behavioral and lifestyle modifications are also first-line treatment options. Pharmacologically, both anticholinergic and beta antagonist medication classes have established efficacy in treatment of UUI. Botox is a more invasive third-line treatment option when conservative and pharmacologic measures have not produced significant improvement of symptoms.[30] Neuromodulation modalities (neurosacral modulation, pudendal nerves stimulation, and posterior tibial nerve stimulation) are also more invasive techniques that may be used prior or in addition to botulinum toxin as the next step in management of UUI. Insertion of temporary catheter is not recommended as it can aggravate UUI symptoms. Leakage around the catheter may result from bladder spasms. Finally, augmentation cytoplast and urinary diversion are both viable surgical options for severe and refractory cases.

9.9.5.3 Mixed UI

Again, the first-line treatment is behavior and lifestyle modification. Anticholinergic and beta-3 adrenergic antagonist medications have demonstrated improvement of symptoms, but SUI component often persists.[54] Vaginal estrogen cream may have mild short-term benefits, but no long-term improvement has been reported.[54] Anti-incontinence surgeries, as described previously, may be beneficial for both SUI and UUI components. However, studies have revealed lower overall cure rates for MUI compared to SUI.[54] Surgery must be approached with caution for cases of MUI because it may aggravate preexisting UUI symptoms or contribute to development of storage abnormalities.[54]

9.9.5.4 Overflow UI

This form of incontinence is most often due to benign prostatic hyperplasia (BPH) in men.[9] It may also result from neurogenic bladder secondary to a multitude of etiologies. The ultimate goal of treatment is complete emptying of the bladder at appropriate periodic intervals. Overflow UI is initially treated with conservative measures of both behavioral and lifestyle changes.[9] Fluid management is especially important to prevent excessive bladder overflow during times of high oral intake.[9] If there is no response to conservative measures over a period of months, or if PVRs are exceptionally high, then pharmacologic management is initiated.[52] Depending on the severity of symptoms, an alpha-adrenergic blocker is started independently or along with a 5-alpha reductase inhibitor.[9,52] Historically, bethanecol, a muscarinic agonist medication, has been used for treatment of OUI.[64] Its proposed mechanism of increasing bladder contractility remains understudied. Most available studies of bethanecol have been uncontrolled, so its efficacy in the treatment of UI remains undetermined.[64]

For those with significantly elevated PVRs or overflow incontinence due to neurogenic bladder pathology, initiation of a clean intermittent catheter (CIC) program is the most effective aspect of management.[64] CIC programs are ideal for older adults who are not cognitively impaired and have adequate mobility and dexterity of their hands. Preferably, the bladder should be emptied every 4–5 hours throughout the day.[64] If leakage occurs between catheterizations then frequency of catheterization may be increased, and an anticholinergic medication may be added as supplemental treatment.[64]

Unfortunately, for patients unable to perform independent straight catheterization the responsibility falls on the caregiver. In more challenging cases, for instance, when urine output is high while on essential diuretic medication, CIC may not be a sustainable or effective option. In these situations an indwelling urethral or a suprapubic catheter may be necessary. Both alternatives are considered less satisfactory than CIC to patients and have higher rates of bacteriuria and urethral complications.[64,80] In-dwelling urethral catheters are less comfortable than suprapubic catheters; in addition, they add risk of urethral erosion, epididymitis, orchitis, prostatitis, and urethral stricture.[64]

Urethral catheters also create more sexual challenges than do suprapubic catheters or CIC. Another important consideration for those patients with either form of in-dwelling catheter is the necessity of periodic urologic surveillance due to significantly increased risk for development of squamous cell bladder cancer.[64]

Finally, when overflow UI symptoms continue to be substantial despite conservative and pharmacologic treatment, surgery should be considered.[52] In the case of outflow obstruction in men, the TURP is the most commonly pursued surgical option.[9] Urinary diversion (augmentation cystoplasty) may also be pursued in select cases.

9.9.5.5 Transient UI

Treatment simply entails treating the underlying cause of UI. In the case of infection, UI resolves with resolution of the infection.[1] Current medication list should be reviewed and any new or potentially contributing medications discontinued or adjusted. In the case of functional incontinence, lifestyle modifications such as bedside commode or urinal, timed voiding, assistive devices in readily available areas, and nonrestrictive clothing are key aspects of the treatment plan.[1]

9.10 MANAGEMENT OF URINARY INCONTINENCE IN THE OLDER ADULT ACROSS DIFFERENT SETTINGS

9.10.1 In-Hospital and Inpatient Rehabilitation Units

The prevalence of UI is 35%–42% of hospitalized adult patients and 51% of older adult hospitalized patients.[81] The prevalence is slightly higher in women than men (57% vs. 43%).[81] It did not matter to most patients whether they were approached by the physician or the nurse about their incontinence but of those with a preference, there was a trend toward being approached by the nurse first.[81]

Urinary incontinence in any hospitalized older adults should be addressed. A thorough history should include medications; history of bladder infections and conditions; past abdominal and urological surgeries; urinary symptoms including dysuria, hematuria, hesitation, sensation of full bladder with inability to empty; the frequency and situation of the incontinence; prior self-management strategies for incontinence; prior medical incontinence treatments; history of abdominal or pelvic trauma; and bowel movement patterns.[82] Next, the physical examination should consist of an abdominal exam looking for distention, hard stool, masses, and/or tenderness; a neurological exam looking for brain, spinal cord, or peripheral nerve damage; a rectal examination looking for stool impaction, perianal sensation, and a bulbocavernosus reflex; and in women, a gynecological examination, and in men, prostate examination.[82]

Based on the history and examination the incontinence can be characterized as transient (reversible, associated with an acute medical condition) or established (chronic/long-standing or newly acquired but not anticipated to improve).[82] Transient urinary incontinence can be a mechanical issue due to immobility and lack of access to a toilet. It may also be due to a medical issue such as UTIs, vaginal infections, constipation, atrophic/infectious vaginitis, acute prostatitis, sexually transmitted diseases, irritating skin rashes, underarousal states (coma, delirium), among many other conditions. Diagnostic testing would be guided by the history and physical examination and may include urinalysis and cultures (urinary, vaginal, urethral). Medications must also be reviewed as they can cause incontinence due to frequency/urgency (diuretics), sedation (narcotics, sedatives), or effects on sphincter/detrusor strength (e.g., muscle relaxants). Transient urinary incontinence resolves when the underlying cause is treated and eliminated. In the older adult, isolated bacteruria does not necessarily mean infection and treatment for asymptomatic bacteruria can be deferred; however, pyuria should be treated.[82]

Established incontinence may take several forms. It is important to determine the type of incontinence prior to initiating a medication. A medication to cause urinary retention may help for urge incontinence but would worsen overflow incontinence.

Postvoid residuals can help distinguish between flaccid bladders with overflow and hypertonic bladders. A bladder scan ultrasonically determines residual bladder volume after voiding. Alternatively, this volume can be measured by straight catheterization of the patient after a void. Volumes would normally be less than 30–50 mL within the first 20 minutes after voiding. Volumes larger than this suggest retention and a hypotonic bladder.[82] Urine flowmetry can help to rule out bladder outlet obstruction.[82] A flow of more than 25 mL/s rules out obstruction.[82] Ultrasound can rule out obstructing bladder stones. The presence of hydronephrosis suggests high bladder pressures. Voiding cystourethrograms may be contraindicated in the older adults due to the risks of contrast use in older patients with renal insufficiency. Urodynamic studies to evaluate the detrusor and sphincter response to bladder filling require the skill of a urological consultant. This may not be possible in the hospital setting. It may be useful in evaluating sphincter overactivity as the cause of retention. The use of medications to increase bladder contractions would be contraindicated in these patients. Increased intravesicular pressure would develop with contraction against a closed sphincter and could lead to hydroureter and hydronephrosis.

Treatment in the inpatient setting is multifaceted. If patient is unable to get to the toilet, commodes or bed pans are substituted. Absorbent incontinence bed pads and garments are used. Patient must be checked frequently for incontinence and if present incontinence products are changed promptly and skin is cleansed and dried. Condom catheters can be an option for men, but they are not without drawbacks including poor fit, skin irritation, and balantitis.[82] Prompted or scheduled toileting may also be helpful. For a hypotonic bladder, bethanechol 10–30 mg 3–4 times a day may be tried.[82] For uninhibited bladder contractions many medications are available. Oxybutynin 5 mg 3 times a day is frequently used.[82] Many other anticholinergic agents are also available. Side effects of anticholinergic medications may be more pronounced in the older adults and include dry mouth, blurred vision, constipation, and cognitive deficits.[82,83] Anti-muscarinic agents (e.g., tolterodine) have been shown to be less likely to affect cognition.[83] Baclofen, used in doses of 5–10 mg twice a day, can relax the OAB but side effects include fatigue and weakness of limbs and sphincter muscles. Urology can be consulted for detrusor botulinum toxin injections; however, this is normally done in an outpatient setting. Artificial sphincters may be considered, but risks of surgery in the older adult must be weighed and the sphincter may be difficult for the older adult to manipulate.[82]

9.10.2 SKILLED NURSING REHABILITATION UNITS AND LONG-TERM CARE FACILITIES

Most literature studies regarding UI are limited by their subjects being predominantly women.[83,84] Many factors may contribute to UI in the skilled nursing facility setting. These factors may be cumulative and include

- Limitations in mobility
- Limitations is accessing a toilet
- Limitations in clothing management
- Impaired cognition, especially dementia
- Urinary tract infection
- Skin irritation
- Depression
- Underlying bladder disorders[85]

The prevalence of UI in the nursing home setting may range from 20% to 70% and is reported to be more common in women.[85] The likelihood of UI increases with duration of time in the nursing home, particularly for patient with progressive physical and/or cognitive impairments and for men.[85] Reports of UI care plan documentation in nursing homes varies between studies with one study reporting 81% of those with UI had a reversible cause at onset but only 34% had it addressed and as little as 3% had treatment. However, another study showed nursing facilities had 100%

documentation of bladder status on admission, defined treatment goals in the majority, a documented discussion of UI and treatment in 41%, and had a bladder diary or volume chart in 34%.[85] Only 2% of family members report being included in decisions regarding the UI plan.[85] No studies reported whether or not the nursing home resident was involved in UI treatment plan or goal-setting.[85] This suggests that the resident and family need to be included more in UI treatment plans and goals.

Urinary incontinence has many negative consequences. These may include but are not limited to psychological distress, physical discomfort, pressure sores, incontinence dermatitis, skin and bladder infections, and a higher rate of hospitalization.[85] New or worsening UI is associated with a decline in quality-of-life (QoL) scores.[85]

The first step toward treatment is a review of medications with consideration of decreasing or weaning off medications that may contribute to incontinence.[85] This would include medications that can cloud mentation (such as narcotics, benzodiazepines, and sleep promoting agents), weaken sphincter muscles (muscle relaxants, sedatives), or increase urinary urgency (diuretics). Conflicting bladder medications should also be evaluated as patients may be on a medication to prevent bladder contractions as well as a medication that promotes bladder emptying.[83]

Cost-effectiveness is important in deciding upon an UI treatment plan. Patients with sufficient cognitive abilities may be taught pelvic floor exercises, but data are limited as to the long-term outcomes and cost-effectiveness in the nursing home setting.[83] A physical exercise program has been shown to improve the patient's mobility; however, this does not result in a decrease in UI.[83] However, it may decrease nursing burden for changing clothing, bedding, and incontinence products, thereby increasing nursing staff efficiency. In-dwelling catheters do eliminate incontinence and the direct cost of purchase is cheaper than incontinence products.[83] However, when the indirect costs of staff management, infections, and hospital-related infections are considered, it is not cost-effective to use catheters.[83] The long-term cost-effectiveness of condom catheters has not been effectively studied in the nursing home setting.[83] Scheduled, frequent, prompted toileting has also been studied. Costs of labor are high as two staff members may be needed for patient safety and it is time intensive. Staff time costs are much higher than laundry and incontinence product costs.[83] These studies did not specifically look at indirect costs of any skin health costs. Other studies showed that the degree of immobility and incontinence did not correlate with skin health and integrity.[83] Good skin hygiene showed an improvement in skin condition, a decrease in incidence of stage 1 decubiti, and a decrease in incontinence dermatitis.[83] Studies showed that pH cleansers were healthier for the skin than soap and water.[83] There was a trend for barrier cream plus a pH cleanser to be better than the pH cleanser alone and to decrease nursing time spent with hygiene.[83] Long-term adherence of the nursing staff to the skin hygiene program was not studied.[83] As a result, absorbent pads are the primary treatment plan for UI in most nursing care programs.[85]

9.10.3 HOME

It is not uncommon that older adults will not bring UI to the attention of their physician.[86] Seeking help is related to the duration of symptoms, severity of incontinence, the physical and emotional symptoms associated with the incontinence, and the presence of other physical symptoms, especially obstruction.[86] It is important that the physician ask a screening question regarding incontinence.

As mentioned above, patients may have different kinds of incontinence: stress, urge, overflow, functional, and total. Urge incontinence (also known as detrusor overactivity) is the most common.[82,87] The goal of treatment is to increase the amount of time the urge to void can be suppressed to allow time for the older adult to reach the toilet.[87] The patient is taught pelvic floor–strengthening exercises.[87] This may be combined with biofeedback and electrical stimulation.[87] Routine or prompted voiding every 2 hours is also helpful.[87] Tolderodine 1–2 mg orally twice a day or oxy-butynin 2.5–5 mg nightly to 3 times a day are treatments of choice and can decrease incontinence by 15%–60%.[87] Side effects include dry mouth, blurred vision, constipation, urinary retention, and confusion.[87]

The mainstay of treatment for stress incontinence is pelvic floor–strengthening or Kegel exercises, with or without biofeedback.[87] In women, oral or vaginal estrogen reverses urogenital atrophy and urethritis and may reduce symptoms.[87] Progestin should be given with the estrogen to minimize risk.[87] Estrogens may be prothrombotic and considered carefully in older women with cardiovascular or neurovascular disease. Alpha-adrenergics (e.g., terazosin, tamsulosin, finasteride) should also be used cautiously in older adults with hypertension, cardiac dysrhythmias, and/or angina.[87] Surgical suspension surgeries are successful in eliminating incontinence in 80%–95% of women with stress incontinence.[87] Periurethral bulking injections may be used to narrow the bladder neck.[87] Vaginal inserts that narrow the urethra are now available over the counter, but the evidence base for effectiveness is limited.

Overflow incontinence may be related to prostatic hypertrophy in older men.[87] Alpha-adrenergics may be helpful but as explained above must be used cautiously.[87] Transurethral resection of the prostate may also be of benefit.[87] Patients may require an intermittent catheterization program to empty the bladder regularly and prevent overflow.[87] Not all older patients can manage this and an in-dwelling catheter is needed.[87] In-dwelling catheters increase the risk for infection and must be routinely changed.

REFERENCES

1. Testa A. 2015. Undersstanding urinary I incontinence in adults. *Urol Nurs.* 35(2):82–86.
2. Berardelli M, DeRango F, Morelli F et al. 2013. Urinary incontinence in the elderly and in the oldest of the old: Correlation with frailty and mortality. *Reju Res.* 16(3):206–211.
3. Buttaro TM, Trybulski JA, Bailey PR et al. 2013. *Primary Care: A Collaborative Practice.* 4th ed. Elsevier, St. Louis, MO.
4. Wherberger C, Madershbacher S, Jungwirth S et al. 2012. Lower urinary tract symptoms and urinary incontinence in a geriatric cohort—A population-based analysis. *BJU Int.* 110(10):1516–1521.
5. Morrison A, Levy R. 2006. Fraction of nursing home admission attributable to urinary incontinence. *Value Health.* 9(4):272.
6. Coyne KS, Wein A, Nicholson S. Economic burden of urgency urinary incontinence in the United States: A systematic review. 2014. *J Manag Care Pharm.* 20(2):130–140.
7. Schuessler B, Baessler K. 2003. Pharmacologic treatment of stress urinary incontinence: Expectations for outcome. *Urology.* 62(4 Suppl 1):31–38.
8. Luo X, Chuang CC, Yang E et al. 2015. Prevalence, management and outcomes of medically complex vulnerable elderly patients with urinary incontinence in the United States. *Int J Clin Pract.* 69(12):1517–1524.
9. Miller SW, Miller MS. 2016. Urological disorders in men: Urinary incontinence and benign prostatic hyperplasia. *J Pharm Pract.* 24(4):374–385.
10. Chutka DS, Fleming KC, Evans MP et al. 1996. Urinary incontinence in the elderly population. *Mayo Clinic Proc.* 71(1):93–101.
11. Parker WP, Griebling TL. 2015. Nonsurgical treatment of urinary incontinence in elderly women. *Clin Geriatr Med.* 31(4):471–485.
12. Loh K, Sivalingam N. 2006. Urinary incontinence in the elderly population. *Med J Malaysia.* 61(4):506–511.
13. Chaliha C, Khullar V. 2004. Mixed incontinence. *Urology.* 63(2 Suppl 1):51–57.
14. Sexton C, Coyne K, Thompson C et al. 2011. Prevalence and effect of health-related quality of life of overactive bladder in older Americans: Results from the epidemiology of lower urinary tract symptoms study. *J Am Geriatr Soc.* 59(8):1465–1470.
15. Kraus S, Bavendam T, Brake T et al. 2010. Vulnerable elderly patients and overactive bladder syndrome. *Drugs Aging.* 27(9):697–713.
16. Coyne KS, Sexton CC, Vats V et al. 2011. National community prevalence of over-active bladder in the United States stratified by sex and age. *Urology.* 77(5):1081–1087.
17. Abrams P, Andersson K-E, Birder L et al. 2010. Evaluation and treatment of urinary incontinence, pelvic organ prolapse, and fecal incontinence. *Neurourol Urodyn.* 29(1):213–240.

18. Cameron AP. 2016. Medical management of neurogenic bladder with oral therapy. *Transl Androl Urol.* 5(1):51–62.

19. Hsu A, Conell-Price J, Cenzer IS et al. 2014. Predictors of urinary incontinence in community-dwelling frail older adults with diabetes mellitus in a cross-sectional study. *BMC Geriatrics.* 14:137.

20. Greer JA, Xu R, Propert KJ et al. 2015. Urinary incontinence and disability in community-dwelling women: A cross-sectional study. *Neurol Urodyn.* 34(6):539–543.

21. Brown JS, Vitanghoff E, Wyman JF et al. 2000. Urinary incontinence: Does it increase risk for falls and fractures? Study of osteoporotic fractures research group. *J Am Geriat Soc.* 48(7):721–725.

22. Moon SJ, Kim YT, Lee TY et al. 2011. The influence of an overactive bladder on falling: A study of females aged 40 and older in the community. *Int Neurourol J.* 15(1):41–47.

23. Tannebaum C. 2015. Associations between urinary symptoms and sexual health in older adults. *Clin Geriatr Med.* 31(4):581–590.

24. Senra C, Pereira MG. 2015. Quality of life in women with urinary incontinence. *Rev Assoc Med Bras.* 61(2):178–183.

25. Sahin-Onat S, Unsal-Delialiogu S, Güzel O et al. 2014. Relationship between urinary incontinence and quality of life/depression in elderly patients. *J Clin Gerontol Geriatr.* 5(3):86–90.

26. Kwong PW, Cumming RG, Chan L et al. 2010. Urinary incontinence and quality of life among older community-dwelling Australian men: The CHAMP study. *Age Ageing.* 39(3):349–354.

27. Ranson RN, Saffrey MJ. 2015. Neurogenic mechanisms in bladder and bowel ageing. *Biogerontology* 16(2):265–284.

28. Ruggieri M, Braverman A, Pontari M. 2005. Combined use of alpha-adrenergic and muscarinic antagonists for the treatment of voiding dysfunction. *J Urol.* 174(5):1743–1748.

29. Scemons D. 2013. Urinary incontinence in adults. *Nursing.* 43(11):52–60.

30. Jung HB, Kim HJ, Cho ST. 2015. A current perspective on geriatric lower urinary tract dysfunction. *Korean J Urol.* 56(4):266–275.

31. Wein AJ, Rackley RR. 2006. Overactive bladder: A better understanding of pathophysiology, diagnosis and management. *J Urol.* 175(3 Pt 2):S5–S10.

32. Herbruck LF. 2008. Stress urinary incontinence: Prevention, management, and provider education. *Urol Nurs.* 28(3):200–206.

33. Sanduh JS. 2010. Treatment options for male stress urinary incontinence. *Nat Rev Urol.* 7(4):222–228.

34. Rassweiler J, Teber D, Kunta R et al. 2006. Complications of transurethral resection of the prostate (TURP)-incidence, management, and prevention. *Eur Urol.* 50(5):969–979.

35. Yong YC. 2009. Diagnosis and treatment of geriatric urinary incontinence. *Incont Pelvic Floor Dysfunct.* 3(3):69–72.

36. Jerez-Roig J, Santos MM, Souza DL et al. 2016. Prevalence of urinary incontinence and associated factors in nursing home residents. *Neurourol Urodyn.* 35(1):102–107.

37. El-Hefnawy A, Wadie B. 2011. Severe stress urinary incontinence: Objective analysis of risk factors. *Maturitas.* 68(4):374–377.

38. Sheyn D, James RL, Taylor AK et al. 2015. Tobacco use as a risk factor for reoperation in patients with stress urinary incontinence: A multi-institutional electronic medical record database analysis. *Int Urogynecol J.* 26(9):1379–1384.

39. Duralde ER, Walter LC, Van Den Eeden SK et al. 2015. Bridging the gap: Determinants of undiagnosed or untreated urinary incontinence in women. *Am J Gynecol.* 214(2):266.e1-9. doi: 10.1016/j.ajog.2015.08.072

40. Grant RL, Drennan VM, Rait G et al. 2013. First diagnosis and management of incontinence in older people with and without dementia in primary care: A cohort study using the health improvement network primary care database. *PLoS Med.* 10(8):e1001505.

41. Izci Y, Topsever P, Filiz TM et al. 2009. The association between diabetes mellitus and urinary incontinence in adult women. *Int Urogynecol J Pelvic Floor Dysfunct.* 20(8):947–952.

42. Chang KM, Hsieh CH, Chiang HS et al. 2014. Risk factors for urinary incontinence among women aged 60 or over with hypertension in Taiwan. *J Obstet Gynecol.* 53(2):183–186.

43. Shamliyan TA, Wyman JF, Ping R et al. 2009. Male urinary incontinence: Prevalence, risk factors, and preventive interventions. *Rev Urol.* 11(3):145–165.

44. Rortveit G, Brown JS, Thom DH et al. 2007. Symptomatic pelvic organ prolapse: Prevalence and risk factors in a population-based, racially diverse cohort. *Obstet Gynecol.* 109(6):1396.

45. Sakakibara R, Hattori T, Uchiyama T et al. 2001. Videourodynamic and sphincter motor unit potential analyses in Parkinson's disease and multiple system atrophy. *J Neurol Neurosurg Psychiatry.* 71(5):600–606.

46. Khan Z, Hertanu J, Yang WC et al. 1981. Predictive correlation of urodynamic dysfunction and brain injury after cerebrovascular accident. *J Urol.* 126(1):86–88.

47. Betts CD, D'Mellow MT, Fowler CJ. 1993. Urinary symptoms and the neurological features of bladder dysfunction in multiple sclerosis. *J Neurol Neurosurg Psychiatry.* 56(3):245–250.

48. Bellucci CH, Wöllner J, Gregorini F et al. 2013. Acute spinal cord injury-do ambulatory patients need urodynamic investigations? *J Urol.* 189(4):1369–1373. Epub 2012 Oct 12.

49. Bedoya-Ronga A, Currie I. 2014. Improving the management of urinary incontinence. *Practitioner.* 258(1769):21–24.

50. Goode P, Burgio K, Richter H et al. 2010. Incontinence in older women. *JAMA.* 303(21):2172–2181.

51. Rai J, Parkinson R. 2014. Urinary incontinence in adults. *Renal Urol Surg III.* 32(6):286–291.

52. Iqbal P, Castleden C.1997. Management of urinary incontinence in the elderly. *Gerontology.* 43(3): 151–157.

53. Yared JE, Gormley EA. 2015. The role of urodynamics in elderly patients. *Clin Geriatr Med.* 31(4):567–579.

54. Gomelsky A, Dmochowski RR. 2011. Treatment of mixed urinary incontinence in women. *Curr Opin Obstet Gyn.* 23(5):371–375.

55. Hay-Smith EJ, Herderschee R, Dumoulin C et al. 2011. Comparisons to approaches of pelvic floor muscle training for urinary incontinence in women. *Cochrane Database of Syst Rev.* 12:CD009508. doi: 10.1002/14651858.

56. Barbato KA, Wiebe JW, Cline TW et al. 2014. Web-based treatment for women with stress urinary incontinence. *Urol Nurs.* 34(5):252–257.

57. Herbison P, Plevnik S, Mantle J. 2002. Weighted vaginal cones for urinary incontinence. *Cochran Database Syst Rev.* 1:CD002114.

58. Gameiro MO, Moreira EH, Gameiro FO. 2010. Vaginal weight cone versus assisted pelvic floor muscle training in the treatment of urinary incontinence: A prospective, single-blind, randomized trial. *Int Urogynecol J Pelvic Floor Dysfunct.* 21(4):395–399.

59. Subback LL, Wing R, West DS et al. 2009. Weight loss to treat urinary incontinence in overweight and obese women. *N Engl J Med.* 360(5):481–490.

60. O'Boyle CJ, O'Sullivan OE, Shabana H et al. 2015. The effect of bariatric surgery on urinary incontinence in women. *Obesity Surg.* 26:1–8. doi: 10.1007/s11695-015-1969-z.

61. Kashyap M, Tu LM, Tannenbaum C. 2013. Prevalence of commonly prescribed medications potentially contributing to urinary symptoms in a cohort of older patients seeking care for incontinence. *BMC Geriatrics.* 13:57.

62. Nickel JC, Sander S, Moon TD. 2008. A meta-analysis of the vascular-related safety profile and efficacy of alpha-blockers for symptoms related to benign prostatic hyperplasia. *Int J Clin Pract.* 62(10):1547–1559.

63. Lee C, Chermansky CJ, Damaser MS. 2016. Translational approaches to the treatment of benign urologic conditions in elderly women. *Curr Opin Urol.* 26(2):184–192.

64. MacLachlan LS and Rovner ES. 2015. New treatments for incontinence. *Adv Chronic Kidney Dis.* 22(4):279–288.

65. Liao CH, Kuo HC. 2015. Practical aspects of botulinum toxin—A treatment in patients with overactive bladder syndrome. *Int Neurourol.* 19(4):213–219.

66. Bing M, Uhlman M, Kreder K. 2013. An update in the treatment of male urinary incontinence. *Curr Opin Urol.* 23(6):540–544.

67. Dmochowski R, Chapple C, Nitti VW et al. 2010. Efficacy and safety of onabotulinumtoxinA for idiopathic overactive bladder: A double blind placebo controlled, randomized, dose ranging trial. *J Urol.* 184(6):2416–2422.

68. Sirls LT, Foote JE, Kaufman JM. 2002. Long-term results of the FemSoft urethral insert for the management of female stress urinary incontinence. *Int Urogynecol J Pelvic Floor Dysfunct.* 13(2):88–95.

69. Abrams P, Blaivas JG, Fowler CJ et al. 2003. The role of neuromodulation in the management of urinary urge incontinence. *BJU Int.* 91(4):355–359.

70. Possover M. 2014. A novel implantation technique for pudendal nerve stimulation for treatment of overactive bladder and urgency incontinence. *J Minimal Evasive Gynecol.* 21(5):888–892.

71. MacDiarmid SA, Peters KM, Shobeiri A et al. 2010. Long-term durability of percutaneous tibial nerve stimulation for the treatment of overactive bladder. *J Urol.* 183(1):234–240.

72. Kocjancic E, Civellaro S, Smith JJ 3rd et al. 2008. Adjustable continence therapy for treatment of recurrent female urinary incontinence. *J Endouro.* 22(7):1403–1407.

73. Hubner WA, Schlarp OM. 2005. Treatment of incontinence after prostatectomy using a new minimally invasive device: Adjustable continence therapy. *BJU Int.* 96(4):587–594.

74. Ziegelmann MJ, Linder BJ, Rivera ME et al. 2016. Outcomes of artificial sphincter placement in octogenarians. *Int J Urol.* 23(5):419–423. doi: 10.1111/iju.13062.
75. Kenton K. 2016. Pelvic organ prolapse in women: Obliterative procedures (colpocleiisis). In: *UpToDate*, Post LB (Ed), UpToDate, Waltham, MA (Accessed on March 18, 2016).
76. Nager CW, Tan-kim J. 2016. Pelvic organ prolapse and stress urinary incontinence in women: Combined surgical treatment. In: *UpToDate*, Post LB (Ed), UpToDate, Waltham, MA (Accessed on March 18, 2016).
77. Borstad E, Abdelnoor M, Staff AC et al. 2010. Surgical strategies for women with pelvic organ prolapse and urinary stress incontinence. *Int Urogynecol J.* 21(2):179.
78. Edwards J. 2008. Diagnosis and management of benign prostatic hyperplasia. *Am Fam Physician.* 77(10):1403–1410.
79. Paolone DR. 2010. Benign prostatic hyperplasia. *Clin Geriatr Med.* 26(2):223–239.
80. Esclarin De Ruz A, Garcia Leoni E, Herruzo Cabrera R. 2000. Epidemiology and risk factors for urinary tract infection in patients with spinal cord injury. *J Urol.* 164(4):1285–1289.
81. Zürcher S, Saxer S, Schewendimann R. 2011. Urinary incontinence in hospitalised elderly patients: Do nurses recognize and manage the problem? *Nurs Res Pract.* 2011:671302. doi: 10.1155/2011/671302.
82. Ouslander J. 1981. Urinary incontinence in the elderly. *West J Med.* 145(6):482–491.
83. Zarowitz, B, Allen C, O'Shea T et al. 2015. Challenges in the pharmacological management of nursing home residents with overactive bladder or urinary incontinence. *J Am Geriatr Soc.* 63(11):2298–2307.
84. Flanagan L, Roe B, Jack B et al. 2013. Factors with the management of incontinence and promotion of continence in older people in care homes. *J Adv Nurs.* 70(3):476–496.
85. Roe B, Flanagan L, Jack B et al. 2010. Systematic review of the management of incontinence and promotion of continence in older people in care homes: Descriptive studies with urinary incontinence as primary focus. *J Adv Nurs.* 67(2): 228–250.
86. Teynissen D, van Weel C, Lagro-Janssen T. 2005. Urinary incontinence in older people living in the community: Examining help-seeking behavior. *Br J Gen Pract.* 55(519):776–778.
87. Merkelj I, Quillen J. 2001. Urinary incontinence in the elderly. *South Med J.* 94(10):952–957.

10 Falls and Gait Impairment

Kristen Thornton and Thomas V. Caprio

CONTENTS

10.1 BACKGROUND

Falls and gait impairment are considered geriatric syndromes, as their incidence is greatest among older adults and tends to increase with age. Older adults with disorders of gait and balance are at particularly high risk for falls. Falls are associated with significant morbidity and mortality, and represent one of the greatest threats to maintaining functional independence in older adults. Falls and gait impairment tend to be multifactorial in etiology, demanding a careful and comprehensive approach to clinical assessment and intervention.

A fall is defined as when a person unintentionally comes to rest on the ground or a lower level. The majority of falls are not associated with a loss of consciousness. More than one-third of community-dwelling persons age 65 years or older and one-half of persons over age 80 years will fall each year, and most often, falls are recurrent [1,2]. The incidence of falls differs among community and clinical settings. Hospitalized and institutionalized older adults have a greater incidence of falls compared with community dwellers. The annual incidence of falls in hospitals is 1.4 falls per bed, and in long-term care facilities is estimated at 1.6 falls per bed [3].

Morbidity and mortality related to falls increase with age. Each year, at least 10% of older people will suffer a major injury from a fall, such as a fracture or head injury, and injury from a fall accounts for a significant portion of emergency department visits and is implicated in two-thirds of accidental deaths in older adults [3]. This increased susceptibility to injury is due in part to a higher prevalence of chronic illnesses, such as osteoporosis. Physiologic changes of aging, such as slowed protective reflexes during a fall, may also contribute to higher risk of injury. Falls in community-dwelling older adults are strongly associated with eventual placement in a skilled nursing facility [2].

The inability to get up after a fall can lead to additional morbidity. If a person remains on the floor and is immobilized for an extended period of time, they are at increased risk of developing dehydration, rhabdomyolysis, pressure ulcers, and pneumonia. Additionally, inability to get up after a fall may lead to an increased fear of falling. Such fears may contribute to a person's decline in function as a result of limiting their mobility as an attempt to reduce their risk of another fall [4].

10.2 RISK FACTORS

While some falls have a clearly identifiable etiology, the majority are the result of a combination of multiple intrinsic and extrinsic risk factors. Intrinsic factors include muscle weakness, impaired gait and balance, osteoarthritis, and functional and visual impairments. Cognitive impairment, particularly involving deficits in executive function, is also associated with a higher risk of falls and hip fractures [5]. Extrinsic factors include environmental hazards (e.g., poor lighting and inappropriate footwear) [6].

Environmental hazards and accidents are the leading contributor for falls in older adults. A review of the home environment may help identify potential safety risks. Poor lighting, narrow paths between furniture, clutter, throw rugs, and electrical cords are potential contributors to falls. Safety bars in the bathroom may reduce the risk of slipping on wet floors and assist with bath/shower and toilet transfers. Stable handrails should be available for all stairs and inclines. Additionally, the home environment should be assessed to ensure that it can accommodate the functional needs of the patient. For instance, patients with urge incontinence may benefit from making a toilet or commode more easily accessible or having a raised toilet seat to make it easier to transfer from the commode.

Many acute illnesses, as well as complications of chronic illnesses, contribute to the higher prevalence of gait disorders and falls in the older adult population. Older adults are at even greater risk of falling in the month after discharge from the hospital [7,8]. Conditions that cause fatigue, hemodynamic instability, dyspnea, pain, altered mentation, altered sensory perception, and impaired motor function can contribute to fall risk.

Polypharmacy is an important iatrogenic cause but potentially modifiable risk factor for falls. Both clinician-prescribed and over-the-counter medications can be factors in polypharmacy. The more medications a patient takes, the higher the potential risk of falls [9]. This is due to adverse drug effects, drug–disease, and drug–drug interactions. Medications that affect the central nervous system, particularly anticholinergic and psychotropic medications, are associated with higher fall risk. Antihypertensive medications may increase the risk of orthostatic hypotension, thereby, increasing the risk for unsteadiness, disequilibrium, and syncope.

A history of prior falls is likely the strongest predictor of future falls. The use of assistive devices for ambulation is aimed at mitigating fall risk but the need for such devices by an older adult should be also viewed by a clinician as a higher risk stratification for future falls. Falls may also result from improper use of and assistive device or inappropriate device selection for the type of impairment. Regular straight canes should be utilized for the sole purpose of improving proprioception and should not be used to offset weight. Offset canes and quad canes may be used for very limited weight bearing and should be held in the hand opposite the weaker or painful lower extremity. Three wheeled walkers may be easier to navigate in tight spaces but are unstable and topple easily and therefore generally should not be used. Walkers with brakes require the cognitive function to employ them correctly. Patients utilizing wheelchairs and scooters may be at risk for falls during transfers.

10.3 CLINICAL EVALUATION

Clinicians should ask all older adult patients at least annually whether they have fallen within the previous year and whether they have difficulties with walking or balance (Table 10.1). Those who seek medical attention for injuries from a fall, report multiple falls, report a single fall but have poor gait and balance on assessment, or report difficulty with walking or balance should receive a multifactorial fall risk assessment.

Falls in older adults are frequently multifactorial in origin, and therefore require a systematic clinical approach to their evaluation. A comprehensive history should include information about

---

TABLE 10.1
Screening Patients for Falls

- Ask: Have you fallen in the past year?
- Conduct gait/mobility assessments
- Check use and fit of assistive devices (cane/walker)
- Inspect footwear

TABLE 10.2

Falls History

- Circumstances of fall: sudden loss of consciousness, sudden leg weakness, tripped, position change, head back or far to side, tight collar, cough/urination, postprandial, incontinence, palpitations/angina, dizziness/giddiness
- Major medical problems: cardiac, musculoskeletal, vision, neurologic (including cognitive disorders)
- Medication review: cardiac, diuretic, psychoactive, analgesic, ETOH

TABLE 10.3

Physical Examination

- Vital signs: postural blood pressure to assess for orthostatic changes
- HEENT: vision, hearing, nystagmus
- Neck: ROM, motion-induced vertigo, bruits
- Cardiopulmonary: pulmonary edema, arrhythmia, murmur
- Extremities: arthritis, edema, range of motion, deformities, feet
- Neurological: mental status, gait/balance deficit, weakness, focal findings, tremor, rigidity, peripheral neuropathy
- Gait: direct observation of gait and position change

a patient's activity and environmental setting at the time of the fall, prodromal symptoms, and whether there was loss of consciousness (Table 10.2). In addition to the circumstances surrounding a recent fall, a history of prior falls may help a clinician identify patterns of causation and target therapeutic interventions. Fear of falling, any self-restriction of activity, and personal safety awareness should be explored. A careful medication history should be completed, reviewing all prescription and over-the-counter medications the patient is taking. In addition to obtaining a list of medications, inquiring about how one manages, organizes, and administers medications may provide insight into whether medications are being properly dosed. Particular attention should be paid to antihypertensive medications and drugs affecting the central nervous and cardiovascular system. Obtaining a history regarding use of alcohol and illicit drugs is imperative.

The physical examination after a fall should attempt to identify acute injury, as well as any physical findings indicative of conditions contributing to fall risk. Orthostatic blood pressures may identify a patient with orthostatic hypotension. Close attention should be paid to the cardiovascular, neurologic, and musculoskeletal examination (Table 10.3). Visual acuity should be assessed. At minimum, a basic evaluation of cognitive function should be completed. Gait should be carefully observed, with the patient rising from a seated position in an exam room and walking a distance in the hallway. Footwear should also be evaluated for fit, tread wear on the soles, and heel height. Laboratory studies, cardiac monitoring, echocardiography, neurologic imaging, and other radiologic studies should be judiciously obtained based on history and physical examination findings. Histories or physical exam findings suggestive of seizure activity, syncope, or drop attacks will likely require additional targeted evaluation and testing.

10.4 GAIT AND BALANCE DISORDERS

Gait and balance disorders are significant contributors to risk of falls in older adults. Normal gait is dependent on a complex interplay between the central and peripheral nervous systems, and unhindered musculoskeletal function. Gait disorders affect up to 15% of people age 60 years and older, and 80% or more of those who are age 85 years and older [10]. While disordered gait is not an inevitable consequence of aging, there are some physiologic changes associated with normal aging that increase the risk of falls and gait impairment. Sarcopenia, which involves both the loss of muscle mass and a decrease in muscle strength, accelerates with advancing age. These losses are often more pronounced in the lower extremities compared with the upper extremities. Decline in proprioception and in the vestibular system are commonly seen with aging. Older individuals tend to activate proximal muscles more before distal muscles when confronted with alterations in their support surface, which thereby reduces postural stability [10].

Direct observation of gait is a critical portion of the multifactorial fall risk evaluation. Stance width, gait initiation and fluidity, posture, arm swing, step height, stride length, and velocity should be assessed (Table 10.4). The "Get Up and Go" test is a brief screen that provides the clinician the opportunity to observe a patient's balance, gait speed, and gait pattern. It involves having a patient rise from chair, walk a distance of 3 meters, turn, walk back to the chair, and sit back down again. The times to completion of the test are compared with mean times within an age group. The mean times to completion for ages 60–69, 70–79, and 80–99 years are 8.1, 9.2, and 11.3 s, respectively [11]. Abnormal gait features observed by the clinician during this test may assist in targeting interventions.

The Performance Oriented Mobility Assessment tool (POMA) is a metric that assesses both balance and gait [12]. The tool assesses nine features of balance and seven features of gait using a numerical scale for scoring, which can then stratify individuals in low fall risk, medium fall risk, and high fall risk categories. The Berg Balance test is a useful tool that assigns scores for 14 separate balance-related tasks and allows for a more detailed assessment of postural stability [13]. Included in this assessment are measures of sitting and standing while unsupported, transfers, turning, and forward reach.

Gait speed has been demonstrated to reflect overall health and functional status. Slower gait speeds predict increased fall risk. Additionally, reduced gait speeds are associated with lower rates of survival, particularly over the age of 75 years [14,15]. Walking smoothness, particularly in the context of forward progression, may also provide additional insight into physical function and the quality of one's control during ambulation [16].

There is no clearly accepted standard of what constitutes a normal gait pattern in an older adult [17]. However, there are commonly observed changes in gait with older age. Compared with persons in their twenties, healthy persons in their seventies have a 10%–20% decrease in gait velocity and stride length. Older adults are more likely to demonstrate bent posture and have an increased stance width. There is less force generated at the moment of push off and they tend to spend an increased proportion in the double support phase with both feet on the ground [18]. What has historically been referred to as the "senile gait" pattern (i.e., slow, broad-based, shuffling pattern) is likely a manifestation of underlying disease, particularly cardiovascular disease, parkinsonism, or dementia [18].

Gait disorders may be classified as neurological, nonneurological, or multifactorial in origin. Neurologic causes of abnormal gait include conditions resulting in the upper and lower motor neuron syndromes, sensory and proprioceptive impairments, neurodegenerative conditions, and cognitive dysfunction. Impaired peripheral sensory function may manifest with gait impairment. A deafferentation patterned gait results from impaired proprioception, most commonly from dysfunction

---

TABLE 10.4

Mobility Screen

- Watch the patient walk
- Stand from seated position, arms crossed
- Get up and go test: Get up from chair, walk 10 feet (3 meters), turn, and return/sit down in the chair
  - Most adults can complete in 10 s
  - Most frail older adults can complete in 11–20 s
  - Need for >10 s = ↑ risk of falls
  - Need for >20 s → comprehensive evaluation
- Results are strongly associated with functional independence in ADLs

of the posterior column of the spinal cord or severe sensory peripheral neuropathy. Deafferentation presents as a wide-based, steppage gait (exaggerated hip flexion, knee extension, and foot lifting). They will often display a worsening of their gait stability in darkened environments and may report frequently bumping into objects. They will typically have a positive Romberg sign on physical examination. As a common cause of this pattern in older adults is cervical myelopathy, spinal cord imaging should be considered in evaluation of this gait pattern to rule out cord compression. Additionally, such patients should also have a serum vitamin B12 level and syphilis serology included in their evaluation. Patients with vestibular disorders often display a weaving gait and may lurch toward the side of the affected ear. Patients with visual impairment may demonstrate an uncertain, hesitant, and uncoordinated gait, particularly in low lighting conditions.

The pattern demonstrated in upper motor neuron-associated weakness typically involves impairment in hip flexion, foot and toe dorsiflexion, leg flexion at the knee (hamstrings), and thigh abduction. This results in toes scuffing and inadequately clearing the ground. Patients with this gait pattern may circumduct at the hip to help their toes clear the ground. Those with spasticity, hemiplegia, hemiparesis, paraplegia, and paraparesis may also demonstrate features of this gait pattern. Paraplegia and paraparesis may also result in scissoring during ambulation.

Impaired peripheral motor function may occur due to lower motor neuron lesions, myopathic weakness, pain, or musculoskeletal deformities. A lower motor neuron patterned gait may involve weakened quadriceps, toe, and foot plantar flexion. The hip flexors often remain strong in a lower motor neuron patterned gait and may result in high steppage and foot drop. Myopathic weakness in the limb girdle may present with a waddling gait and abnormal pelvic tilt. An antalgic gait often results from attempting to limit weight bearing on a painful area or surrounding a painful joint. A parkinsonian gait may result from idiopathic Parkinson's disease, or parkinsonism from other neurodegenerative conditions, such as supranuclear palsy, multiple system atrophy, or corticobasal degeneration. Parkinsonism may also be a manifestation of cerebrovascular disease, subcortical dementia, or even dementia with Lewy bodies. Persons with a parkinsonian gait demonstrate a festinating, shuffling, short stride strength, absent or reduced arm swing, and turning "en bloc." In patients with Parkinson's disease, gait impairment may improve with a trial of levodopa therapy. Failure to respond to levodopa therapy may suggest an atypical parkinsonism.

Cerebellar ataxia presents with poor trunk control and coordination. Gait may be observed as stumbling, lurching, or staggering. Step length is frequently reduced and gait is wide-based. Those with a cerebellar ataxia gait pattern will often have other signs of ataxia. Frontal lobe dysfunction can alter gait as a result of impaired motor programming and abnormalities in executive function. It may result in a gait that is cautious due to perceived disequilibrium. Additional features include difficulty initiating gait, shuffling, and en bloc turns. Normal-pressure hydrocephalus often presents with a cautious gait and en bloc turns. Gait abnormalities due to frontal lobe dysfunction share many features with the parkinsonian gait pattern. However, those with frontal lobe dysfunction often lack the other physical signs commonly seen with parkinsonism (rigidity, bradykinesia, and trunk flexion). Gait impairment may also be seen in delirium due to impaired attention. Psychogenic gait disorders often present with bizarre patterns that cannot be attributed to other neurological or organic causes.

10.5 INTERVENTION AND MANAGEMENT

Following a multifactorial evaluation in patients at risk for or experiencing falls, interventions should be targeted at identified contributing factors. Efforts should be made to minimize polypharmacy, with particular attention paid to medications that increase risk of orthostasis, agents that act as central nervous system depressants, and psychotropics. Visual impairment should be addressed with appropriate ophthalmic care. Environments should be modified when possible to reduce fall risk, including appropriate home safety modifications (grab bars, hand rails, and night lights). Patients should be advised on the use of proper footwear, oftentimes this may mean replacing an old or worn-out pair of shoes. Older adults should be advised that walking with shoes of low heel height and high surface contact area may reduce the risk of falls. Persons over the age of 65 years with low serum 25-hydroxyvitamin D levels are at increased risk for loss of muscle mass, strength, and hip fractures [19,20]. There is some evidence that suggests that vitamin D supplementation reduces the risk of falling, but this is by no means definitive. However, vitamin D supplements of at least 800 IU per day should be considered for people with suspected vitamin D deficiency or who are otherwise at increased risk for falls [21].

There is no evidence that restraints, bed or chair alarms reduce the risk of falls in the inpatient or long-term care setting [22,23]. The use of restraints may actually increase a person's risk for injury or falls [24]. While there are a number of hip protectors commercially available, evidence overall is lacking in their effectiveness in reducing hip fractures from falls, particularly as compliance in wearing the protectors is generally low [25].

Exercise programs that target strength, gait, and balance are effective interventions to reduce falls. Tai chi has been demonstrated to reduce fall risk in community-dwelling older adults [26]. Exercise may be performed in groups or as individual (home) exercises, as both are effective in preventing falls. The exercise program should include regular review, progression, and adjustment of the exercise prescription as appropriate [21].

Older adults who are appropriate candidates for anticoagulation have often been denied this treatment if they have a history of falls or are at high risk of falls. However, the risk of intracranial hemorrhage in anticoagulated patients is often overestimated. The risk of a subdural hematoma from falling in patients with atrial fibrillation with an average risk of stroke, a person would have to fall approximately 300 times in a year for the risk of anticoagulation to outweigh its benefits in reducing stroke [27–29].

REFERENCES

1. Tinetti ME. Preventing falls in elderly persons. *NEJM*. 2003; 348:42–49.
2. Tinetti ME, Williams SC. Falls, injuries due to falls, and the risk of admission to a nursing home. *NEJM*. 1997; 337:1279–1284.
3. Rubenstein LZ, Josephson KR. The epidemiology of falls and syncope. *Clin Geriatr Med*. 2002 18:141–158.
4. Tinetti ME, Liu WL, Claus EB. Predictors and prognosis of inability to get up after falls among elderly persons. *JAMA*. 1992; 269:65–70.
5. Muir SW, Gopaul K, Montero Odasso MM. The role of cognitive impairment in fall risk among older adults: A systematic review and meta-analysis. *Age Ageing*. 2012; 41(3):299–308.
6. American Geriatrics Society, British Geriatrics Society, and American Academy of Orthopaedic Surgeons on Falls Prevention. Guidelines for the prevention of falls in older persons. *J Am Geriatr Soc*. 2001; 49:664–672.
7. Mahoney J, Sager M, Dunham NC, Johnson J. Risk of falls after hospital discharge. *J Am Geriatr Soc*. 1994; 42:269–274.
8. Mahoney JE, Palta M, Johnson J et al. Temporal association between hospitalization and rate of falls after discharge. *Arch Intern Med*. 2000; 160(18):2788–2795.
9. Ganz DA, Bao Y, Shekelle PG, Rubenstein LZ. Will my patient fall? *JAMA*. 2007; 297:77–86.
10. Woollacott MH, Shumway-Cook A, Nashner LM. Aging and posture control: Changes in sensory organization and muscular coordination. *Int J Aging Hum Dev*. 1986; 23(2):97–114.
11. Bohannon RW. Reference values for the timed up and go test: A descriptive meta-analysis. *J Geriatr Phys Ther*. 2006; 29:64–68.
12. Tinetti ME. Performance-oriented assessment of mobility problems in elderly patients. *J Am Geriatr Soc*. 1986; 34:119–126.
13. Berg K, Wood-Dauphinee S, Williams JI, Maki, B. Measuring balance in the elderly: Validation of an instrument. *Can J Pub Health*. July/August supplement 1992; 2:S7–11.
14. Studenski S, Perera S, Patel K et al. Gait speed and survival in older adults. *JAMA*. 2011; 305:50–58.
15. Viccaro LJ, Perera S, Studenski SA. Is time up and go better than gait speed in predicting health, function, and falls in older adults? *J Am Geriatr Soc*. 2011; 59:887–892.

16. Lowry KA, VanSwearingen JM, Perera S, Studenski SA, Brach JS. Walking smoothness is associated with self-reported function after accounting for gait speed. *J Gerontol A: Biol Sci Med Sci*. 2013; 68(10):1286–1290.

17. Alexander NB. Gait disorders in older adults. *J Am Geriatr Soc*. 1996; 44(4):434–441.

18. Salzman B. Gait and balance disorders in older adults. *Am Fam Phys*. 2010; 82(1):61–68.

19. Visser M, Deeg DJ, Lips P. Low vitamin D and high parathyroid hormone levels as determinants of loss of muscle strength and muscle mass (sarcopenia): The Longitudinal Aging Study Amsterdam. *J Clin Endocrinol Metab*. 2003; 88(12):5766–5772.

20. Cauley JA, Lacroix AZ, Wu L et al. Serum 25-hydroxyvitamin D concentrations and risk for hip fractures. *Ann Intern Med*. 2008; 149(4):242–250.

21. AGS/BGS Clinical Practice Guideline: Prevention of Falls in Older Persons (Accessed January 2016) http://www.americangeriatrics.org/health_care_professionals/clinical_practice/clinical_guidelines_recommendations/prevention_of_falls_summary_of_recommendations/

22. Capezuti E, Maislin G, Strumpf N, Evans LK. Side rail use and bed-related fall outcomes among nursing home residents. *J Am Geriatr Soc*. 2002; 50(1):90–96.

23. Shorr RI, Chandler AM, Mion LC, Waters TM, Liu M, Daniels MJ, Kessler LA, Miller ST. Effects of an intervention to increase bed alarm use to prevent falls in hospitalized patients: A cluster randomized trial. *Ann Intern Med*. 2012; 157(10):692–699.

24. Tinetti ME, Liu W, Ginter SF. Mechanical restraint use and fall-related injuries among residents of skilled nursing facilities. *Ann Intern Med*. 1992; (95):369–374.

25. Parker MJ, Gillespie WJ, Gillespie LD. Effectiveness of hip protectors for preventing hip fractures in elderly people: Systematic review. *BMJ*. 2006; 332(7541):571–574.

26. Gillespie LD, Robertson MC, Gillespie WJ, Lamb SE, Gates S, Cumming RG, Rowe BH. Interventions for preventing falls in older people living in the community. *Cochrane Database Syst Rev*. 2009; (2):CD007146.

27. Man-Son-Hing M, Laupacis A. Anticoagulant-related bleeding in older persons with atrial fibrillation: Physicians' fears often unfounded. *Arch Intern Med*. 2003; 163(13):1580–1586.

28. Man-Son-Hing M, Nichol G, Lau A, Laupacis A. Choosing antithrombotic therapy for elderly patients with atrial fibrillation who are at risk for falls. *Arch Intern Med*. 1999; 159(7):677–685.

29. Sellers MB, Newby LK. Atrial fibrillation, anticoagulation, fall risk, and outcomes in elderly patients. *Am Heart J*. 2011; 161(2):241–246.

11 Pressure Ulcers in Older Adults

Huma Naqvi

CONTENTS

11.1 DEFINITION

A pressure ulcer is a localized injury to the skin and/or the underlying tissue usually over a bony prominence as a result of pressure or pressure in combination with shear.[1] Pressure ulcers are also called decubitus ulcers, bedsores, or pressure sores. Pressure ulcers vary in severity from reddening of the skin to deep craters with muscle and bone involvement. Pressure ulcers develop fast and are difficult to treat; they usually develop over bony prominences such as heels, ankles, and the sacrum.[1,2] Populations that are at the highest risk for developing pressure ulcers are individuals with medical conditions requiring prolonged confinement to beds or wheelchairs and who have a limited ability to change position. Pressure ulcers need a multidisciplinary approach in order to prevent and treat.

Pressure ulcers are seen in the general practice setting, and are most likely to occur in those over 85 years of age. Preventive strategies within the general practice setting should concentrate on the elderly population.

11.2 EPIDEMIOLOGY

The incidence and prevalence of pressure ulcers vary greatly depending on the clinical setting.[3,4] Hospital incidence rates range from 1% to 30% of patients in the ICUs due to immobility and severe system illnesses. Long-term care facility incidence and prevalence ranges from 3% to 30%, and for individuals at home, the range is 4%–15%.

11.3 SKIN FACTS AND FUNCTIONS

The skin is the largest organ of the body. We lose about 30,000–40,000 dead skin cells every minute, and about 600,000 particles of skin every hour. We shed approximately 1.5 lbs of skin per year and we regrow outer skin cells about every 27 days. Each square inch of human skin consists of 20 feet of blood vessels.

11.3.1 FUNCTIONS OF SKIN

The skin provides us with protection from bacterial invasions and against external elements such as water, chemicals, bacteria, viruses, and ultraviolet radiations. The skin also prevents excessive loss of fluids and electrolytes, while always striving for a homeostatic environment. Our skin produces sebum, a lipid (rich, oily substance) secreted by the sebaceous gland that provides an acidic coating, which retards the growth of microorganisms. Melanin, a pigment produced in the skin that gives human skin, hair, and eyes color, protects against ultraviolet rays. To protect against harmful ultraviolet rays, the skin produces melanin when exposed to the sun. The level of melanin depends on race and amount of sunlight exposure. Other skin functions are to hold the body in shape, sense the environment, and filter basic types of sensations: pain, touch, temperature, and pressure. Our skin retains water in tightly packed cells of the stratum corneous, which provides protection against water loss, maintains body temperature, and maintains thermoregulation by the primary mechanism of circulation and sweating. Blood vessels supply blood to the skin. When the body's temperature increases, vasodilation occurs in order to dissipate heat, and when the body's temperature decreases, vasoconstriction occurs in order to retain heat. When bacteria invade the epidermis, the skin activates an immunological response where the white blood cells in the skin capture and destroy the bacteria. When skin is exposed to ultraviolet radiation from sunlight, the cells in the epidermis convert cholesterol-related steroid to vitamin D, also known as cholecalciferol, which results in the maintenance of calcium and phosphorus levels in the bone and blood.

11.4 ETIOLOGY

Literature reviews show several etiologies of pressure ulcers. The international NPUAP/EPUAP clinical practice guideline states, "pressure ulcers develop as a result of the internal response to external mechanical load."[1] For example, pressure ulcers may develop from pressure-induced capillary closure, cutting blood supply and leading to tissue ischemia, injury, and/or death. Magnetic resonance imaging (MRI) studies have documented cellular distortion and damage from pressure.

External pressure is transmitted from the epidermis inward toward the bone as well as by counterpressure from the bone. As a result, the loaded soft tissues, including skin and deeper tissues (adipose tissue connective tissue and muscle), will deform, resulting in strain and stress within the tissue.[5]

Different body tissues have different tolerances to pressure; muscle is more sensitive to pressure damage than skin.[1,6] Tissue tolerance is compromised further by extrinsic and intrinsic facts. The skin of elderly people is more fragile, thin, less elastic, and drier than the skin of younger people: their cell production is slower, which increases their vulnerability for damage. The basement membrane forms the junction between the dermis and epidermis of skin; during aging, the membrane flattens and diminishes the amount of surface between the layers, which reduces the nutrient transfer and diffusion of bioactive molecules in both directions, thus making the skin less resistant to shearing forces and more prone to skin breakdown.

Based on current data, Stage I pressure ulcers are classified as likely beginning 12–24 hours prior to appearing on the skin. Stage II pressure ulcers likely began 24 hours prior, and Stage III and IV pressure ulcers likely began at least 72 hours prior to appearance. Suspected deep tissue injury pressure ulcers are categorized as purple tissue without epidermal loss and which likely began 48 hours prior to their appearance on skin.

11.5 RISK FACTORS

There are several risk factors for pressure ulcers: sustained pressure, shear and friction forces, moisture, impaired mobility, malnutrition, impaired sensibility, advanced age, and a history of previous pressure ulcers. Risk factors can be stratified into one of two categories: extrinsic and intrinsic. The majority of pressure ulcers can be prevented by using pressure ulcer risk assessment tools to identify at-risk individuals. Once identified, at-risk individuals will benefit from interdisciplinary interventions designed to prevent pressure ulcers, including education, positioning, mobility, nutrition, and management of incontinence (Figure 11.1).

11.5.1 Extrinsic Factors

The most common extrinsic physical factors that cause pressure ulcers are interface (axial) pressure, shearing, friction, and excessive moisture.

11.5.1.1 Shearing

Shearing pressure occurs when the bone and the subcutaneous layer move against the skin block in opposite directions to each other. The capacity to maintain a stable position while sitting or lying is impaired with age.

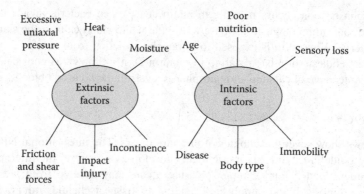

FIGURE 11.1   Factors contributing to pressure ulcers.

Older adults may tend to slide down while sitting on a chair or even from a lying position, caus-ing sheering. In the older adult, shearing also occurs due to reduction in elasticity of the skin, which increases local torsion.

11.5.1.2   Friction

Friction is caused by two forces moving in opposite directions, such as the surface of an external object against the skin. An example is when an elderly agitated person rubs their heels or elbows and causes the formation of intraepidermal blisters. This action may damage the skin and accelerate the formation of pressure ulcers. The effect of friction on developing ulcers is increased fivefold with accompanying moisture access.

11.5.1.3   Moisture

Moisture causes maceration of skin, which facilitates injury to the skin even with light pressure. Moisture can be from urinary or fecal incontinence and other body secretions such as perspirations by fever or a hot environment, fistula drainage, or excessive wound secretions.

11.5.1.4   Pressure

Interface pressure causes a decrease in capillary blood flow and occlusion of blood perfusion to the local territory, causing ischemia.

The average intravascular capillary pressure is 32 mmHg, lying in bed causes a local pressure of 54–94 mmHg on the heels, sacrum, and scapula. A pressure ulcer may result as a product of both the intensity and duration of such pressure.

There is an inverse correlation between the duration of sitting and the intensity of pressure, that is, a pressure ulcer may develop in less sitting time with strong intensity or in response to a longer duration of sitting with low intensity.[7] Therefore, reducing the intensity of the pressure through the use of a pressure-relieving surface is as important as frequently repositioning the patient in order to reduce the duration of pressure on any particular area of the skin.

11.5.2   Intrinsic Factors

Intrinsic factors predispose the aging skin to pressure ulcers. They focus on a patient's pathology, including multiple disease, functional status, skin dryness (xerosis), and skin trauma from various factors:

- Immobility
- Conditions that reduce sensitivity

- Concomitant diseases
- Age
- Poor skin condition
- Poor nutritional status
- Infections
- Urinary and fecal incontinence

11.6 COMMON SITES OF PRESSURE ULCERS

Most pressure ulcers arise in hospitals where the prevalence among in-patients is 3%–14%, although it can be as high as 70% in elderly in-patients with orthopedic problems.[8]

11.7 STAGES OF PRESSURE ULCERS

The National Pressure Ulcer Advisory Panel (NPAUP), a professional organization that promotes the prevention and treatment of pressure ulcers, defines the four stages of pressure ulcers, and guides treatment of pressure ulcers.

The European Pressure Ulcer Advisory Panel (EPUAP) offers similar definitions on the stages of ulcers except for the presence of suspected deep tissue injury and unstageable ulcers.

According to the NPUAP and EPUAP, there are six categories of pressure ulcers.

NPUAP refers to these categories as stages and the EPUAP refers to them as grades according to increasing degrees of skin and tissue damage.

Stage I: Pressure injury
Stage II: Partial thickness skin loss
Stage III: Full thickness skin loss
Stage IV: Full thickness tissue loss
Unstageable: Depth unknown
Suspected deep tissue injury: Depth unknown

Moisture-induced lesions on bony prominences should not be considered pressure ulcers, for example, skin tears, tape burns, perineal dermatitis, or excoriation. The wound should be staged according to its deepest extent.

Stage I ulcers are characterized by intact-skin, nonblanchable redness in a localized area usually over a bony prominence. The area is usually painful, firm or soft, warmer or cooler compared to the adjacent tissue. Skin that is pigmented darkly may not have visible blanching, but its color may appear different from the surrounding area (Figure 11.2).

Stage II ulcers are characterized by partial thickness dermal loss presenting as a shallow open ulcer with a reddish-pink wound bed without slough. The ulcer is generally superficial and may manifest as an abrasion (Figures 11.3 and 11.4).

Stage III ulcers may be identified by full thickness dermal loss and subcutaneous fat may be visible. Exposed bone, tendon, or slough may be present but does not obscure the depth of tissue loss; undermining and tunneling may also be seen (Figure 11.5).

Stage IV ulcers present with full thickness skin loss with exposed bone tendon or muscle. Slough or eschar may be present on some parts of the wound bed and often include undermining and tunneling. The depth of stage IV pressure ulcers varies by anatomical location. The bridge of the nose, ear occiput, and malleolus do not have subcutaneous tissue and these ulcers can be shallow. Stage IV ulcers can extend into muscles and/or supporting structures (e.g., fascia tendon or joint capsule), making osteomyelitis possible. Exposed bone/tendon is visible or directly palpable (Figure 11.6).

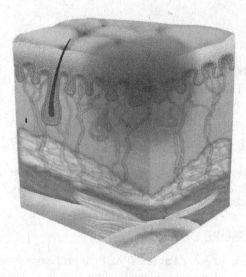

FIGURE 11.2 Stage I pressure injury—Caucasian. (Used with permission of the National Pressure Ulcer Advisory Panel.)

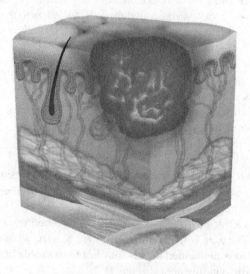

FIGURE 11.3 Stage II pressure injury. (Used with permission of the National Pressure Ulcer Advisory Panel, 2013.)

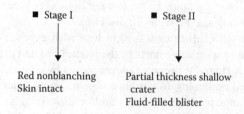

FIGURE 11.4 Differences between Stages I and II.

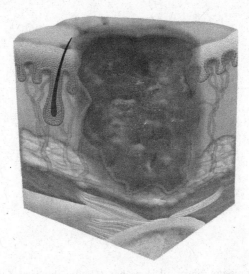

FIGURE 11.5   Stage III pressure injury. (Used with permission of the National Pressure Ulcer Advisory Panel.)

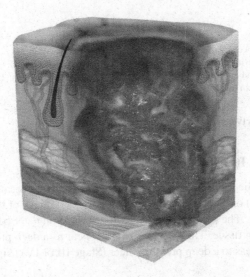

FIGURE 11.6   Stage IV pressure injury. (Used with permission of the National Pressure Ulcer Advisory Panel, 2013.)

11.7.1   Unstageable Pressure Ulcer

Unstageable pressure ulcers are identified when there is full thickness tissue loss and the bone of the ulcer is covered by slough (yellow, tan, gray, green, or brown) and/or eschar (tan, brown, or black) in the wound bed.

Until the slough and/or eshar is debrided to expose the base of the wound, the true depth, and therefore stage, cannot be determined.

Stable eschar on heels serves as the body's natural (biological) cover, and should not be removed (Figure 11.7).

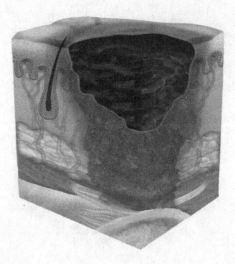

FIGURE 11.7 Unstageable pressure injury—dark eschar. (Used with permission of the National Pressure Ulcer Advisory Panel, 2013.)

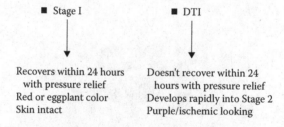

FIGURE 11.8 Difference between Stage I and deep tissue injury (DTI).

11.7.2 SUSPECTED DEEP TISSUE INJURY

Deep tissue injury should be suspected whenever there is a localized area of discolored intact skin (purple or maroon in color) or blood-filled blister(s) due to the damage of the underlying soft tissue from pressure and/or shear. The area may be painful, firm or spongy, or boggy warm or cool compared with the surrounding tissue. These lesions often appear as a deep purple bruise and some of these lesions rapidly progress to a deep pressure ulcer (Stage III or IV) (Figure 11.8).

11.8 ASSESSMENT OF PRESSURE ULCERS

The appearance of a wound gives an indication of the stage of healing such as necrotic, infected, sloughy, granulating, and epithelizing. Some wounds may fit into more than one category as mixed wounds.

The assessment and management of pressure ulcers require a comprehensive and multidisciplinary approach in order to understand patients with ulcers. Focusing on the wound itself is not enough. Understanding the physiological and pathological processes of aging skin helps to understand the development of pressure ulcers in the elderly.

Factors to consider include the patient's underlying pathologies such as obstructive lung disease or peripheral vascular disease; the severity of the patient's primary illness; comorbidities such as dementia or diabetes mellitus; functional status such as activities of daily living and ambulatory status; nutritional status (swallowing difficulties or dentures); and the degree of available social and emotional support.

11.8.1 PUSH Tool

The pressure ulcer scale for healing (PUSH) is an objective tool used to assess wound healing. The PUSH tool is designed to monitor the three parameters that are most indicative of healing:

- (Length × width): Scored 0–10 based on the measurement
- Exudate amount: Scored 0 (none) to 3 (heavy)
- Tissue type: Scored 0 (closed) to 4 (necrotic tissue)

The three subscores are added to obtain the total score, which is then placed on a pressure ulcer-healing graph. A comparison of total scores measured over time provides an indication of the improvement or deterioration in healing; a decreasing score indicates healing, and an increase will signify that the wound is deteriorating. The PUSH tool was developed by the NPAUP as a quick and reliable tool to monitor the change in pressure ulcer status over time. The wound should be evaluated for length, width, depth, presence of sinus tract, necrotic tissue, exudate, and the presence of granulation. The possibility of infection should be considered even if systemic signs of fever and elevated white count are absent.[9]

Pressure ulcer assessment requires meticulous and consistent clinical evaluation. One commonly used mnemonic "MEASURE" provides a framework for assessing ulcers.

11.8.2 MEASURE[10]

Parameter	Parameter Content
M—Measure	Length, width, depth, and area
E—Exudate	Quantity and quality
A—Appearance	Wound bed, tissue type, and amount
S—Suffering	Pain type and level
U—Undermining	Presence or absence
R—Reevaluate	Monitoring all parameters regularly
E—Edge	Condition of wound and surrounding skin

11.8.2.1 Tunneling

Tunneling, as the name implies, is a narrow passageway created by the separation or destruction of fascial planes. Tunneling is measured by inserting a probe into the passageway until resistance is felt. The tunnel depth is the distance from the probe tip to the point at which the probe is level with the wound edge.

11.8.2.2 Undermining

Undermining occurs when the tissue under the wound edges becomes eroded, resulting in a large wound with a small opening. Undermining is measured by inserting a probe under the wound edge directed almost parallel to the wound surfaces and moved in a clockwise direction until resistance is felt, which identifies indicating the deepest point of the wound.

11.8.2.2.1 Braden Scale

The Braden scale is the most commonly used tool for assessing pressure ulcers.

The scale has six subscales:

1. Sensory perception
2. Moisture
3. Activity
4. Mobility

5. Nutrition
6. Friction/shear

The scale is based on the two primary etiologic factors of pressure ulcer development—intensity and duration of pressure and tissue tolerance for pressure.

Sensory perception, mobility, and activity address clinical situations that predispose a patient to intense and prolonged pressure, while moisture, nutrition, and friction/shear address clinical situations that alter tissue tolerance for pressure.[11]

Sensory perception, moisture, activity, mobility, and nutrition have scores from one to four and friction/shear scores from one to three.

Initial patient evaluation with pressure ulcers should include

- General mental and physical health, including life expectancy
- Recent medical and functional status
- Nutritional status, patient diet
- Presence or absence of spasticity or contractures
- History of hospitalization operation or ulcerations
- Bowel and bladder habits and continence status
- Medication and allergies to medication
- Tobacco and recreational drug use
- Functional status for mobility and activities of daily living (ADLs)
- Social and financial support
- Place of residence and use of durable medical equipment (DMEs), and supportive surfaces
- Advance directive, power of attorney, specific cultural, religion, or ethnic issues

11.9 MANAGEMENT OF PRESSURE ULCERS

Evaluating the dressing: Once the wound is clean, it is essential to preserve local humidity to prevent dressing-induced desiccation. A variety of dressings is available; the choice of optimal dressing depends on the state of wound, that is, stage, the amount of secretion, and odor. When evaluating a dressing, various aspects need to be considered: patient comfort, ease of application, effectiveness, and cost.

Patient comfort is of primary importance for any wound management product; it should not be painful upon removal. Dressings that fail to produce sufficient absorbency and allow the leakage of exudate can cause considerable inconvenience, as well as promoting feelings of insecurity in the patient.

Dressings should be easy to apply and should stay in place. The effectiveness of the dressing is very important; if a product does not promote healing, then it does not matter if it is comfortable or easy to apply.

11.9.1 DEBRIDEMENT AND CLEANING

- Debridement is the cornerstone for treating contaminated ulcers. Debridement is done by removing necrotic tissues, slough, and other nonviable components of ulcer to promote healing and to facilitate staging. There are several methods of debridement.
- Surgical (sharp)
- Enzymatic
- Chemical
- Autolytic (permitting the body to perform self-debridement on occlusive dressing)
- Biological (maggots)
- Mechanical (dry on wet; drip or friction)

These methods are used in combination or sequentially. A common practice for extensive Stage III and IV pressure ulcers is to use an initial sharp debridement in combination with a mechanical procedure followed by autolytic methods.

11.10   EVALUATION AND MANAGEMENT OF MEDICAL CONDITIONS

By exploring and treating reversible medical conditions that have the potential to damage skin leading to pressure ulcers, for example, intensive diuretic treatment for congestive heart failure can reduce leg swelling and the associated risk of pressure ulcers. The occlusion of blood vessels in peripheral vascular disease can be treated with angioplasty and further treatment options. The inability to change positions (immobility) without assistance may cause several complications that lead to the development of pressure ulcers. Early mobilization after surgical procedures and acute medical conditions, such as pneumonia and urinary tract infections, is important to prevent pressure ulcers. It is important to remember that a pressure ulcer may appear within hours, but take years to heal.

Pressure-relieving devices, such as mattresses and overlays, cushions, and ankle and/or heel protectors, should be encouraged in the early stages of immobility.

Repositioning is a key factor in the prevention and treatment of pressure ulcers. Recumbent patients should be repositioned every 2 hours, and seated patients, every 15–30 minutes. Physical and occupational therapists should exercise early with a range of motion, stretching, and mobilization programs.

11.10.1   MOISTURE REDUCTION TECHNIQUES IN OLDER ADULTS

Regularly allowing the individual to use the bathroom, changing diapers, and frequently applying cream to the skin can best manage moisture from urinary incontinence. Older males should be evaluated and treated for benign prostate hypertrophy.

11.10.1.1   Nutrition in the Elderly

Several studies have indicated the importance of a balanced nutritional intake, including adequate protein intake for the prevention and treatment of pressure ulcers.

Reduction in the ability to feed oneself and recent weight loss are risk factors for pressure ulcers; the early detection of nutritional deficiencies can prevent dehydration and malnutrition.

11.10.1.2   Nutritional Support

- Nutritional support is critical in preventing and managing pressure ulcer.
- Patients at high risk and those with established ulceration should be assessed and monitored by a dietitian.
- Supplementary feeding, either assisted or enteral (via a nasogastric tube or a percutaneous endoscopic gastrostomy [PEG] tube), may be necessary.
- Supplementation with vitamins and trace elements should be a consideration.
- Adequate hydration is essential

11.10.2   MARKERS FOR IDENTIFYING PROTEIN–CALORIE MALNUTRITION IN PATIENTS WITH PRESSURE ULCERS

The unintentional weight loss of 5% or more in the previous 30 days or of 10% or more in the previous 180 days.

Weight less than 80% of ideal body weight

Serum albumin level less than 3.5 g per dL (35 g per L)[a]

Prealbumin level less than 15 mg per dL (150 mg per L)[a]

Transferrin level less than 200 mg per dL (2 g per L)

Total lymphocyte count less than 1500 per mm³ (1.50 × 109 per L)

Source: Adapted with permission from Hess, CT; *Wound Care.* 4th ed. Springhouse, PA; Springhouse; 2002.

ᵃ Dehydration can falsely elevate serum albumin and prealbumin. Albumin and prealbumin are negative acute phase reactant and may decrease with inflammation. Physiologic stress, cortisol excess, and hypermetabolic states also reduce serum albumin.

11.10.3   LOCAL WOUND CARE FOR PRESSURE ULCERS

The goal of local wound care for pressure ulcers in the elderly is to create a warm, moist wound bed with healthy surrounding tissue to promote wound closure. Protecting the skin surrounding a wound needs constant evaluation. Erythema and heat may be indicative of infection. Erythema alone may result from an allergy to the dressing (contact dermatitis). Periwound protection with moisture barriers or skin sealants is essential to protect from excessive moisture from bowel or bladder incontinence.

Debride necrotic tissue if appropriate. Control infection, minimize pressure, and shear forces. Educate patients and caregivers on wound etiology and risk factor modification, nutritional status, and intervention strategies.

Adjunctive therapies: Adjunctive interventions are appropriate if a pressure ulcer does not show evidence of healing with appropriate standard care. Some of the common ones are

- Electrical stimulation
- Hyperbaric oxygen
- Skin substitutes
- Ultrasound
- Growth factors

11.10.3.1   Electrical Stimulation for Wound Healing

Electrical stimulation may offer a unique treatment option to heal complicated and recalcitrant category, Stage II, III, and IV wounds, improve flap and graft survival, and even improve surgery results. When a wound occurs in the skin, an electrical leak is produced that short-circuits the skin battery at that point, allowing the current to flow out of the moist wound.[12,13]

Electrical stimulation is believed to restart or accelerate the wound-healing process by imitating the natural electrical current that occurs in the skin when it is injured.[14,15]

Transcutaneous electrical nerve stimulation (TENS) consists of a generic application of low frequency pulsed electrical currents transmitted by electrodes through the skin surface.

The theory that a moist wound environment is required for the bioelectric system to function is of clinical significance.

Electrical stimulation affects each phase of wound healing differently, beginning with the inflammatory phase that imitates the wound repair process. In this phase, increasing blood flow can help in the removal of debris by way of phagocytosis. In addition, electrical stimulation enhances tissue oxygenation.

Electrical stimulation also promotes the proliferation phase by stimulating the fibroblasts and epithelial cells needed for tissue repair. Membrane transport improves, which supports the body's natural current and produces collagen, which helps in the stimulation of wound contraction.

Electrical stimulation can increase adenosine triphosphate (ATP) concentration in tissues. Increased DNA synthesis promotes the healing of soft tissue or ulcers, reduces edema, and inhibits the growth of various pathogens.

11.11   PRESSURE-RELIEVING STRATEGIES

Pressure-relieving strategies are the cardinal approach for the prevention and treatment of pressure ulcers.[16] They involve three basic strategies:

- Positioning techniques
- Protective devices
- Support surfaces, and repositioning bed-bound patients

Bed-bound patients should be properly positioned and frequently repositioned every 2 hours in lateral decubitus positions. The patient's head should be maintained at an angle of 30° to minimize pressure in the trochanteric region. The heels are particularly vulnerable; a pillow can be placed under the calf to float the heels off the bed, or suspension boots can be used. Current guidelines state that heels should be off the bed.[17]

The risk of pressure ulcers while sitting is more than from that while reclining in bed, as sitting puts the patient's weight on the relatively small surface areas of the buttocks, thigh, and sole of the feet. It is important for chair-bound patients to change position regularly if they are in a sitting position for long hours. Patients who are able to move should shift their weight every 15 minutes. Patients who are immobile should be positioned in a chair for postural alignment, distribution of weight, balance, and stability, and repositioned every hour. Slouching can cause shearing and friction, placing undue pressure on the sacrum and coccyx. If a patient uses a footstool, it is important that the knees are not above the hips as this can shift the weight from the back of the thighs to the ischial tuberosities.

11.11.1 PROTECTIVE DEVICES

Padding and pillows should be utilized for pressure reduction: heel protectors, foam, and pillows can be used in supine positions, and soft seat cushions can be used when sitting in a chair. Donut-shaped devices should not be used for treating pressure ulcers as these can reduce blood flow to an even wider area of tissue.

11.11.1.1 Support Surfaces

In a comprehensive literature review, researchers found evidence that specially designed support surfaces effectively prevent pressure ulcers.[18] An ideal support surface manages microclimate, tissue loads, and other curative functions. Seat cushions, overlays, mattresses, and integrated bed systems may be used to prevent pressure ulcers. Selecting the type of device or surface is determined by the risk and degree of assistance necessary for repositioning or mobility.

11.12   TREATMENT OF PRESSURE ULCERS ACCORDING TO STAGES

The treatment of pressure ulcers depends on its stage, presence, or absence of infection, and the patient's physical and psychosocial condition.

11.12.1 STAGE I

Stage I usually heals with early interventions and proper care, including

- Pressure redistribution
- Prevention of shear and friction
- Moisture maintenance
- Periodic assessment of skin
- Pain management
- Prevention and treatment of infection
- Keep area clean
- Massage is contraindicated

11.12.2   STAGE II

Promoting wound healing and preventing further skin damage is the main goal of this stage's treatment plan.

* Similar steps are taken as mentioned in Stage I, with a focus on infection prevention by using moist dressing such as transparent film to maintain a clean wound bed.
* Nutritional status should be reevaluated and supplements can be started.
* Surgical treatment is not indicated and debridement is rarely required.

11.12.3   STAGE III

The wound bed should be clean and moist to prevent infections and promote granulation. Monitor closely for local or systemic infection and continue the measures described in Stage I plus debridement, if indicated. Autolytic or enzymatic debridement is recommended for light to moderate exudates. Surgical debridement is necessary if there is necrotic tissue and infection.[19] If the ulcer is covered with necrotic tissue, wound gel can be used. For wound beds without necrotic tissues, foam dressings and cavity fillers are recommended. An alginate dressing is appropriate to use if excessive exudate is present. Stage III ulcers usually heal spontaneously with appropriate cleaning; when treated conservatively, they have a recurrence rate of 32%–77%. Surgical management can reduce the rate of recurrence in some patients.[20]

11.12.4   STAGE IV

The goal of this stage is to promote an environment for new tissue growth, which involves the removal of necrotic tissue and drainage reduction. The wound is assessed for bone involvement and signs of infection and the need for antibiotics. Surgical management is often indicated to prevent complications for large-sized wounds and debridement is often necessary to remove necrotic tissue.

11.12.5   UNSTAGEABLE

Unstageable ulcers should be debrided, except for eschar on the heels, which is not debrided unless infected. The ulcer's stage is reassessed when the base is visible and the wound should be monitored for signs of infection and need for antibiotics. As with all other stages, pain management and patient comfort should be continually addressed.

11.12.6   SUSPECTED DEEP TISSUE INJURY

Suspected deep tissue injuries usually heal with proper care and management, but some deteriorate further. The goal of treatment is to quantify the extent of wound, increase blood circulation, and prevent further breakdown of the skin. All measures mentioned in Stage I apply to all stages, including this one.

11.13   COMPLICATIONS

* Sepsis and septic shock (Figure 11.9)
* Chronic wounds

For many older adults, pressure ulcers may become chronic and remain so for prolonged periods, even for the remainder of the patient's lifetime. A large number of stage III and IV pressure ulcers become chronic wounds and lead to death from ulcer complications such as sepsis or osteomyelitis.

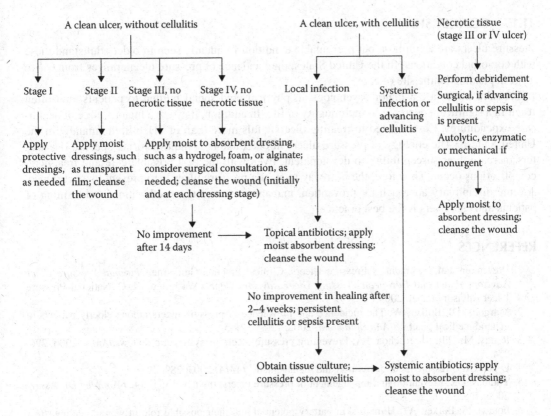

FIGURE 11.9 Algorithm of pressure ulcer treatment. (Hess, CT, *Clinical Guide to Skin and Wound Care*, Wolters Kluwer Health/Lippincott Williams & Wilkins, 2008.)

Wound infection impairs wound healing. Wound infection can show localized signs of infection such as warmth, erythema, local tenderness, purulent discharge, and foul odor; delayed healing can also be a sign of wound infection. MRSA (methicillin-resistant *Staphylococcus aureus*) and VRE (vancomycin-resistant *Enterococcus*) infections can complicate wound healing, and can pose a potential risk to other hospitalized patients. Sinus tracts communicate with deep viscera, including the bowel or bladder. Occasional heterotopic ossification, systemic amyloidosis due to chronic inflammatory state, and malignant transformation of squamous cell carcinoma can occur in chronic pressure ulcers and should always be considered in nonhealing wounds.

11.14 MANAGEMENT OF COMORBIDITIES

Comorbidities increase the susceptibility to pressure ulcers and interfere with the healing process. Better management of comorbid conditions is part of the multidisciplinary approach to pressure ulcer care. Common conditions include diabetes, bowel and bladder incontinence, peripheral vascular disease, hypertension, hypoxia, malignancies, dehydration, poor nutritional status, end stage renal disease (ESRD), depression, and cognitive impairment. Diabetes can cause microvascular disease and loss of protective sensation of the lower extremities. Acute illnesses or exacerbation of comorbid conditions can cause reduced mobility and mental status changes may increase the risk of pressure ulcers. Patients using medications such as chemotherapeutic agents, systemic corticosteroids, and nonsteroidal anti-inflammatory drugs can experience impaired.

11.15 CONCLUSION

Pressure ulcers are a common but preventable condition frequently seen in older adults and those with comorbid conditions. In the United States, the incidence of pressure ulcers ranges from 0% to 40%, depending on the site of care.[21]

Pressure ulcers are a major psychological, physical, and social burden to patients, and often result in a significant decrease to their quality of life. In addition, they are a major source of healthcare expenditures. Costs related to treating ulcers totals more than of $11 billion annually in the United States.[22] The etiology of pressure ulcers in older adults is multifactorial; specific risk factors increase their susceptibility to development. Even with the best possible care and treatment, complications occur. Therefore, the best way to treat a pressure ulcer is to prevent its occurrence. An interdisciplinary approach for prevention, management, treatment, education, and training of patients and caregivers is the best practice.

REFERENCES

1. Prevention and Treatment of Pressure Ulcers. Clinical Practice Guideline. *National Pressure Ulcer Advisory Panel and European Pressure Ulcer Advisory Panel.* Washington D.C. National Pressure Ulcer Advisory Panel; 2009.
2. Margolis, DJ; Bulker, W; The incidence and prevalence of pressure ulcers among elderly patients in general medical practice. *Ann Epidemiol.* 2002; 12(5): 321–5.
3. Reddy, M; Gill, SS; Rochon, PA; Preventing pressure ulcers: A systematic review. *JAMA.* 2006; 296: 974.
4. Lyder, CH; Pressure ulcer prevention and management. *JAMA.* 2003; 289: 223.
5. Thomas, DR; Prevention and management of pressure ulcers, the new f-tag 314. *J Am Med Dir Assoc.* 2006; 7: 523.
6. Foulds, IS; Barker, AT; Human skin battery potential and their possible role in wound healing. *Br J Dermatol.* 1983; 109: 515–22.
7. Reger, SI; Hyodo, A; Reyes, ET; Browne, EZ; Treatment of pressure ulcers by electrical stimulation. *Rehabil Res Dev Program Rep.* 1992; 29: 467–8.
8. Joseph, E; Grey, Keith G; Pressure ulcers. *Harding BMJ.* 2006; 25; 332(7539): 472–5.
9. Livesley, NJ; Chow, AW; Infected pressure ulcers in elderly individuals. *Clin Infect Dis.* 2002; 35: 1390–6.
10. Keast, DH; Bowering, CK; Evans, AW; Mackean, GL; Burrows, C; D'Souza, L; MEASURE: A proposed assessment framework for developing best practice recommendations for wound assessment. 2004; 12(3 Suppl): S1–17.
11. Ayello, EA; Braden, B; How and why to do pressure ulcer risk assessments. *Adv Skin Wound Care.* 2002; 15(3): 125–32.
12. Barker, A; Jaffe, L; Vanable, J; The glabrous epidermis of cavies contains a powerful battery. *Am J Physiol.* 1982; 242(3): R358–66.
13. Vanable, JW Jr.; Integumentary potentials and wound healing. In *Electric Fields in Vertebrate Repair* (eds. Borgens, RB; Robinson, KR; Vanable, JW Jr.; McGinnis, ME), pp. 171–224. Alan R. Liss, Inc.; New York; 1989.
14. Chen, CC; Johnson, MI; McDonough, S; Cramp, F; The effect of transcutaneous electrical nerve stimulation on local and distal cutaneous blood flow following a prolonged heat stimulus in healthy subjects. *Clin Physiol Funct Imaging.* 2007; 27(3): 154–61.
15. Barker, AT; Measurement of direct current in biological fluids. *Med Bio Eng Comput.* 1981; 19: 507–8.
16. Remsburg, RE; Bennett, RG; Pressure-relieving strategies for preventing and treating pressure sores. *Clin Geriatr Med.* 1997; 13(3): 513–41.
17. Emory University School of Medicine Wound, Ostomy and Continence Nursing Education Center. *Skin and Wound Module.* 6th ed. Atlanta, GA; Emory University WOCNEC; 2006.
18. Agostini, JV; Baker, DI; Bogardus, ST; Prevention of pressure ulcers in older patients. In *AHRQ: Making Health Care Safer: A Critical Analysis of Patient Safety Practices.* Public Health Service, US Department of Health and Human Services, Rockville, MD; 2001.
19. Hess, CT; *Clinical Guide to Skin and Wound Care.* Philadelphia, PA; Wolters Kluwer Health/Lippincott Williams & Wilkins; 2008.

20. Conway, H; Griffith, B; Plastic surgery for closure of decubitus ulcers in patients with paraplegia based on experience with 1000 cases. *Am J Surgery.* 1956; 91(6): 946–75.
21. The National Pressure Ulcer Advisory Panel. Pressure ulcer prevalence, cost and risk assessment; consensus development conference statement. *Decubitus.* 1989; 2(2): 24–8.
22. Agency for Healthcare Research and Quality. Preventing pressure ulcers in hospital; A toolkit for improving quality of care. Available at http://www.ahrq.gov/sites/default/files/publications/files/putoolkit.pdf

12 Pain and Its Management in Older Adults

Annie Philip, Diya Goorah, and Rajbala Thakur

CONTENTS

12.1   INTRODUCTION

The objective of this chapter is to provide an overview of pain management in older adults across multiple clinical care settings. Older adults are the fastest-growing section of the world's population. According to the U.S. Census Bureau, there were 40 million people 65 years and older in 2010, comprising 13% of the total U.S. population. Within this segment of the population, 5.5 million were 85 years and older. In 2030, the older population is projected to be twice as large as in 2000, growing from 35 to 72 million, representing 20% of the total U.S. population.[1] The increase in the aging demography will present with complex health problems, making pain management even more challenging than it already is. Although these challenges have unique dimensions in different care settings, namely in acute care settings, nursing homes, and outpatient settings, there are some common factors pertaining to physiology, pain assessment, pharmacokinetics and pharmacodynamics, and available analgesic options in older adults that are uniformly applicable across the care settings. Pain as defined by international association for the study of pain is an "unpleasant sensory and emotional experience associated with actual or potential tissue damage, or described in terms of such damage." Pain, often categorized as acute and chronic, has no consensus in the literature as to the duration beyond which pain is termed as chronic; in clinical practice, chronic pain in older adults is pain lasting for longer than the expected duration of healing from an injury or disease. Examples are ongoing pain secondary to chronic conditions such as arthritis, diabetic neuropathy, or episodic pain flare-ups in a chronic disease state and long-standing angina in persons who are older than 65 years of age. Although pain management should be a priority on humanitarian and ethical grounds, there are a number of deleterious consequences of suboptimal pain management in the context of a biopsychosocial model. Acute pain, not appropriately addressed, has consequences that can be significant for both the patient and healthcare system. Severe pain results in increased stress response, delayed ambulation, and decreased respiratory efforts. These may increase the risk of pneumonia, deep vein thrombosis, pulmonary embolism, myocardial ischemia, poor wound healing, and depressed immune response. Poor pain control places patients at risk for developing long-standing depression, anxiety, and chronic pain syndrome.[2] If pain is not managed well in rehabilitation setting it interferes with physical therapy and ambulation, resulting in slow recovery and increasing length of hospital stay.[3] In addition, poor pain control in postoperative period or trauma-related pain increases the risk of delirium in older frail adults.[4,5] Delirium serves as a particularly poor prognostic sign. Considering the 22%–76% mortality rate in hospitalized patients with delirium, as well as the 35%–40% 1-year mortality, the consequences of poorly managed postoperative pain are quite substantial.[4–6]

12.2   EPIDEMIOLOGY OF PAIN IN OLDER ADULTS

Uncontrolled pain is an obvious quality of life issue across all ages, but epidemiological literature suggests that pain is most prevalent in older adult population. Incidence and prevalence of pain increases with age plateauing in the seventh decade with a modest decline in extremes of age.[7] In a review done by Gibson and colleagues,[7] the prevalence of pain is 30%–65% in those aged 55–65 years declining to 22%–55% in those >85 years of age. However, incidence of specific pain states, such as joint pain, foot, or leg pain, increases exponentially with age up to 90 years.[7–12]

In a study of 1000 community dwelling seniors (median age 75.3 ± 6.7 years), 74% reported pain in the last 30 days, 52% had daily pain, and 26% reported agonizing pain.[13] In another study by Sengstaken and colleagues,[14] 66% of geriatric nursing home residents had chronic pain and the treating physician could not detect the source of pain in about 50% of these patients.

The older adult will have complexities of pain within the inpatient setting. As the population is aging, the number of surgical procedures performed in older adults is expected to increase as is trauma and cancer-related pain. In 2007, approximately 35% of surgical procedures were performed in older adults and 42% of hospitalized patients received at least one procedure compared to 10% in patients younger than 65 years of age.[15]

12.3 PAIN ASSESSMENT

Pain assessment in older adults is challenging. While self-reporting remains the gold standard for cognitively intact older adults, it could be difficult in patients who have mild to moderate cognitive impairment and almost impossible in patients with severe impairment. Hence, assessment requires a comprehensive understanding of social, psychological, and biophysical factors that contribute to the experience of pain. Regardless of the clinical setting, or pain acuity, the goal of a thorough pain assessment in older adults is to identify a cause, conduct a thorough history of comorbid medical and psychosocial factors, perform a physical examination, and initiate a diagnostic workup. This is the only way to help the clinician make an individualized care plan for the patient, which often requires a multidisciplinary approach. Evaluation of the patient's level of function is important as the pain affects the degree of independence, overall quality of life, as well as activities of daily life (ADLs) (eating, bathing, and dressing) and instrumental ADLs (IADL) (light housework, shopping, managing money, and preparing meals). There are a number of reliable and valid instruments available to help the clinician for assessment of pain in older adults but the choice depends on the patient, clinical setting, and available time for evaluation. In patients with cognitive or physical limitations, it is helpful to query family members and/or other caregivers for additional input. Reviewed in the following paragraph are a few of the instruments for pain assessment in older adults.

For cognitively intact older adults

1. The numeric rating scale (NRS, Figure 12.1) has a series of numbers between 0 and 10, with 0 as no pain and 10 as the worst pain ever, representing the entire possible range of pain intensity. NRS, administered verbally or in written format, is both simple and easily understood and effortlessly administered and scored.
2. Another scale that can be used is the visual analog scale (VAS). The VAS (Figure 12.2) has proven reliability in clinical and research settings, and offers advantages of simplicity and ease of administration.[8,9] A line drawn vertically by the patient is measured using a scale and recorded in centimeters or millimeters.
3. The faces pain scale (Figure 12.3) is a self-reported measure of pain intensity developed initially for children from the age of 4 to 16 years but can be used in older adults who are cognitively intact but have mild dementia. The scale uses a series of facial expressions to represent the varying degrees of pain.
4. Verbal rating scale: The verbal rating scale (Figure 12.4) consists of a series of phrases from no pain or least intense pain to very severe pain or most intense pain. The strength of the verbal rating scale is the simplicity and ease of administration.

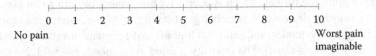

FIGURE 12.1 Numeric rating scale (NRS). (Reprinted from *Essentials of Pain Medicine*, 2nd edn., Jensen MP, Karoly P, Self-report scales and procedures for assessing pain in adults, Copyright 1992, with permission from Elsevier.)

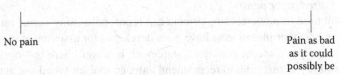

FIGURE 12.2 Visual analog scale (VAS). (Reprinted from *Essentials of Pain Medicine*, 2nd edn., Jensen MP, Karoly P, Self-report scales and procedures for assessing pain in adults, Copyright 1992, with permission from Elsevier.)

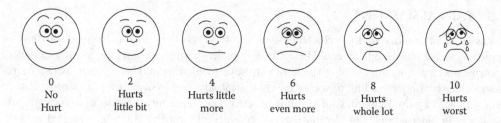

0	2	4	6	8	10
No Hurt	Hurts little bit	Hurts little more	Hurts even more	Hurts whole lot	Hurts worst

FIGURE 12.3   Wong-Baker FACES™ pain rating scale. (Reprinted from *Essentials of Pain Medicine*, 2nd edn., Jensen MP, Karoly P, Self-report scales and procedures for assessing pain in adults, Copyright 1992, with permission from Elsevier.)

Five Point VRS	
None	0
Mild	1
Moderate	2
Severe	3
Very severe	4

FIGURE 12.4   Verbal rating scale. (Reprinted from *Essentials of Pain Medicine*, 2nd edn., Jensen MP, Karoly P, Self-report scales and procedures for assessing pain in adults, Copyright 1992, with permission from Elsevier.)

The McGill pain questionnaire has evidence for validity, reliability, as well as discriminative abilities that are not age related. The short form is easier than the original scale for use in geriatric population and is multidimensional, which is useful for assessment of pain as an experience. This scale includes 11 sensory dimensions (throbbing, shooting, stabbing, sharp, cramping, gnawing, hot-burning, aching, heavy, tender, and splitting) four affective dimensions (tiring-exhausting, sickening, fearful, and punishing-cruel). The intensity is rated as 0—none, 1—mild, 2—moderate, and 3—severe.[10] Derived from the sum of the intensity rank values chosen from the sensory and affective component are the three pain scores. In clinical practice, we commonly use a verbal numerical scale of 0–10 where "0" is no pain and "10" is the worst pain imaginable.

For cognitively impaired older adults

Older adults with mild to moderate impairment can report pain using verbal numerical scale as detailed above. Pain behavior instruments have been developed for assessment in older adults with advanced dementia. As per a recent consensus statement, however, there is "insufficient evidence of reliability and validity at this time to recommend any one tool for broad use across populations and settings" in people with dementia. For these individuals, the caregiver's observation is best. In addition, behavioral cues can be used[16] as listed below:

Facial expressions. Frown, sad, frightened face, grimace, wrinkle forehead, and tightened eyes

Verbalizations and vocalizations. Sighing, moaning, groaning, grunting, calling out, and asking for help, noisy breathing, and verbal abuse

Body movements. Rigid, tense body posture, guarding, fidgeting, pacing, rocking, gait, and mobility changes

Changes in interpersonal interactions. Aggressive, combative, resisting care, withdrawn, socially inappropriate, and disruptive

Changes in activity patterns or routine. Refusing food, appetite change, sleep, rest pattern changes, and sudden cessation of common routines

Mental status changes. Crying, tears, increased confusion, and irritability or distress

In summary, pain assessment measures from the most important to least important are self-reporting, anticipated pain depending on the clinical context as in acute fracture or a particular procedure, observed behaviors, proxy ratings by caregivers, and physiological parameters being the least.

12.4 PHARMACOKINETIC/PHARMACODYNAMIC CHANGES

A detailed description of age-related physiological changes, pharmacokinetics, and pharmacodynamics effect is given in Chapters 1 and 5. Outlined here are some changes in the context of pain and pharmacotherapy. Pain threshold studies have shown that somatosensory thresholds for non-noxious stimuli increase with age, whereas pressure pain thresholds decrease and heat pain thresholds show no age-related changes.[17]

12.4.1 CHANGES IN VOLUME OF DISTRIBUTION

Older adult patients have increased fat mass of 20%–40%, decreased muscle mass, and decreased body water of 10%–15%, all of which play an important role in drug distribution. Many patients are on diuretics, which results in decreased blood volume. Lipophilic medications like fentanyl may have an increased duration of effect. Water-soluble drugs such as morphine, oxycodone, and hydromorphone are not efficiently distributed and this then results in higher plasma concentrations.

A decrease in serum albumin increases the amount of free drug availability, magnified in patients with chronic disease and malnutrition. This causes increased incidence of adverse effects when using high protein-binding analgesics such as nonsteroidal anti-inflammatory medications.

12.4.2 HEPATIC CHANGES

Altered by age are hepatic phase 1 reactions involving oxidation and hydrolysis. Likewise, there is a decline in cytochrome P-450. Furthermore, liver mass decreases by 1% per year after the age of 50. Blood flow to the liver decreases by 33% in individuals over the age of 65. However, there are no significant changes in liver function tests. In addition, here may be a slight decrease in serum albumin levels, leading to an increase in free fraction of protein-bound drugs. Hepatic impairment affects the metabolism of drugs undergoing glucuronidation like morphine and oxymorphone. Although oxymorphone metabolism is independent of P-450, it is being considered as a safer opioid for this patient population.[18]

12.4.3 RENAL CHANGES

Reduction in renal clearance is the largest pharmacodynamic change in older adults. Kidney size decreases by 20%–30% by age 70. The renal tubules decrease in length, number, and thickness. Also decreased is renal blood flow by 10% per decade after age 20 and glomerular filtration rate decreases 10 mL/minute per decade. The decline in glomerular filtration rate begins after age 40 by approximately 1% per year or 1 mL/minute per year decline in creatinine clearance. Renal impairment affects the clearance of opioids like morphine and hyrdromorphone and results in accumulation of metabolites. It also affects the clearance of adjuvant medications used in pain control such as gabapetnin and pregabalin.

12.4.3.1 CNS Changes

Older adults have increased sensitivity to centrally acting drugs such as benzodiazepines and opioids and decreased sensitivity to receptor-specific drugs such as beta-blockers. These changes are probably due to age-related decline in central nervous system (CNS) function.

12.5 ACUTE PAIN MANAGEMENT IN OLDER ADULTS

Effective analgesia can not only improve patient comfort but may also reduce the risk of deleterious consequences as mentioned above. Pain assessment tools should be used and documented consistently across all clinical care settings that are appropriate to patient's cognitive abilities. This will be necessary to overcome barriers that hinder communication regarding unrelieved pain. There are concerns for postoperative cognitive decline associated with the use of general anesthetics, benzodiazepines, and opioid analgesic medications in older adults. Physiological frailty makes the use of regional as well as neuraxial modalities challenging. Providers should recognize that older adult patients might respond differently than their younger counterparts to pain and analgesic medications, due to comorbidities and are more likely to be on multiple medications. Hence, providers need to be extra vigilant about dose titration, to avoid side effects of the drugs such as excessive somnolence, balance problems, and constipation. They should look into optimal utilization of nonpharmacological modalities such as heating pads, ice packs, and/or topical medications whenever possible. In this vulnerable population, a multimodal analgesic strategy should be used to optimize analgesia and minimize side effects. An example of "balanced analgesia" could include combining opioids with nonsteroidal anti-inflammatory drugs (NSAIDs) and neuromodulators such as gabapentin and pregabalin. At the same time, it could mean using regional techniques, such as peripheral nerve blocks and neuraxial analgesia concurrently with systemic pharmacologic options.[19] Unfortunately, a paucity of well-designed studies to delineate an optimal combination of effective therapies has not been conducted. In lieu of focused studies, clinicians must use the available data, extrapolate available information, and individualize therapy based on patient-specific factors. A pain service consult should be requested for patients with inadequately controlled moderate to severe pain related to trauma, surgery, cancer, or acute on chronic pain flare-ups related to various disease states. Intravenous or neuraxial route may be required to control pain initially. Once the patient starts to tolerate oral medications, the analgesic regimen can be changed from intravenous to oral opioid, including oxycodone, hydrocodone, hydromorphone, morphine, tramadol, tapentodol, or combination medications like hydrocodone–acetaminophen or oxycodone–acetaminophen. Uses of oral acetaminophen and/or NSAIDs are recommended for additive effect.

12.5.1 Opioids

Opioids: The mainstay for management of moderate to severe acute pain as a part of multimodal analgesic regimen includes NSAIDs, acetaminophen, and/or local anesthetic blocks. In the immediate postoperative period, intravenous administration is the most common method of delivery and patient-controlled analgesia (PCA). Either intravenous or neuraxial may offer significant advantages. Other routes of delivery include oral, rectal, or via ostomy. Not typically used are transdermal preparations in postoperative settings unless a patient has been on these medications preoperatively. Some novel delivery systems include transbuccal lollipops, sublingual tablets, nasal sprays, and transdermal patient-controlled analgesia.

12.5.1.1 Patient-Controlled Analgesia

This modality permits self-administered delivery of small predetermined doses of analgesic medication at a fixed time interval. This delivery method helps to dilute the effect of variability in an individual's sensitivity to medications and their pain threshold. In addition, it provides patients with a sense of control. The inherent safety lies in the premise that patient will have to be relatively awake to administer the analgesic dose, hence reducing the risk of opioid-induced toxicity in the context of excessive somnolence and respiratory depression.[20] Cognitively intact older adults are perfectly capable of using PCA.[21] Age is not an impediment to effective use of patient-controlled analgesia by surgical patients. In older adults, who are opioid naïve basal infusions should not be used. Basal infusions can be useful for patients with consistently high-dose opioid requirements as in palliative care settings.[22]

As a rule, the basal infusion should not exceed 20%–30% of the total available hourly dose. The most common opioid used is morphine followed by hydromorphone and fentanyl. The usual dose for morphine is a loading dose of 0.1–0.3 mg/kg in divided doses. One-tenth of the total loading dose can be used as a bolus every 10–15 minutes on an as-needed basis. For example, if a patient needed 10 mg of morphine to be comfortable, the prn bolus should be set at 1 mg every 10–15 minutes. Dosing for hydromorphone or fentanyl can be extrapolated using equianalgesic charts. Intravenous PCA is a safe and effective modality for use in cognitively intact older adults albeit they are able to understand and participate in their care, hence appropriate selection is very important.[23]

In addition, other research done in older adults with cognitive impairment in this domain, found that "patient-controlled analgesia can be used successfully in cognitively impaired older adults. Numerous challenges remain however, and additional research can improve the management of pain in this particularly vulnerable population."[24]

The incidence of acute postoperative confusion is as high as 7%–50% and appears to be related mainly to the surgical procedure itself. Close monitoring and evaluation of the patient throughout the perioperative period is required to ensure the appropriate and successful use of PCA in older patients.[22] Other concerns include respiratory depression with an overall incidence of 0.1%–1%. Caution should be exercised in patients with chronic obstructive pulmonary disorder (COPD) or underlying respiratory conditions. Somnolence can result from the use of background infusions and/or concurrent use of other CNS depressant drugs. Opioid antagonists such as naloxone should always be readily available. Nausea, pruritus, constipation, and ileus are other important concerns.

In patients with renal or hepatic impairment, there is a risk of accumulation of the parent compound or an active metabolite. Doses should thus be titrated carefully as this may lead to drug accumulation, increasing the risk of opioid-associated side effects. Fentanyl or hydromorphone are recommended instead of morphine for patients with renal insufficiency or hemodynamic instability.

12.5.2 Acetaminophen

Acetaminophen is used pre- and postoperatively in the management of pain related to major pelvic, abdominal, and orthopedic surgical or trauma-related pain as part of multimodal analgesia.[25] Intravenous acetaminophen (OFIRMEV®) reduces the amount of opioids needed and gives quick and sustained pain relief. Acetaminophen can be safely used as an alternative in patients where NSAIDs are contraindicated or with NSAIDs for an additive analgesic effect. Adult IV and oral dosing are up to 1 g every 6 hours.

12.5.3 Nonsteroidal Anti-Inflammatory Drugs

Ketorolac is the most commonly used intravenous NSAID in the United States and is Food and Drug Administration (FDA) approved for use in acute pain settings. Ibuprofen and indomethacin are not available in intravenous formulation, however, not commonly used. Diclofenac is commonly used globally, but is not available in the United States. Ketorolac 7.5 mg every 6 hours can be tried first, increasing to 15 mg every 6 hours if the lower dose was ineffective. It can be used exclusively or as a part of multimodal analgesic regimen with opioids, acetaminophen, and invasive interventional techniques and has a significant opioid sparing effect. Caution should be exercised in patients with renal impairment, bleeding risk, and cardiovascular issues.

12.5.4 GABAPENTINOIDS

Gabapentin and pregabalin can be considered in patients when conventional analgesic medications are not adequate in managing acute pain. Studies are limited but these medications have demonstrated efficacy in reducing pain and analgesic requirements in some acute pain conditions.[26] These medications are useful in surgeries associated with a higher risk of persistent neuropathic pain, that is, major orthopedic procedures, thoracotomies, mastectomies, and lower abdominal surgeries. Preemptive use of these neuromodulating medications may be very beneficial. Similarly, in acute pain states like herpetic neuralgia pain or pain associated with rib trauma or burns, these medications are useful adjuncts. The usual dose for older adults should be 100–200 mg given the night prior to surgery or 1–2 hours preoperatively and then continued at 100 mg three times daily in the postoperative period. Dose can be further titrated as tolerated with a maximum dose of 900 mg t.i.d. Reduced dosages are recommended in patients with renal impairment.

12.6 INTERVENTIONAL MODALITIES IN ACUTE PAIN MANAGEMENT IN OLDER ADULTS

In addition to the surgery-related pain, there are a number of indications for use of interventional pain management techniques in older adults in acute care settings. Neuraxial analgesia (see Table 12.1) is a useful modality for pain related to trauma such as extremity fractures, pelvic, and/or rib fractures, as well as intractable cancer pain. Single shot techniques are more useful in ambulatory settings, whereas indwelling catheters are commonly used in hospitalized patients with few exceptions.[27]

12.6.1 PERIPHERAL NERVE BLOCKS IN ACUTE PAIN MANAGEMENT

A number of peripheral nerve blocks can be performed in the management of acute postoperative pain, acute trauma pain, or cancer-related pain in older adults. The goal is to optimize pain relief and minimize the need for systemic analgesics, which in turn would minimize the occurrence of systemic side effects for vulnerable populations. The exact type of nerve block would depend on the area of pain or desired surgery as listed in Table 12.2. These blocks can be single shot blocks or a perineural catheter can be left in place to help with pain relief and physical therapy in the postoperative period. Local anesthetic medications are commonly used for acute situations. For cancer pain management, neurolytic agents like alcohol or phenol can be used. In most institutions, ultrasound-guided blocks have become the norm, although these blocks can be performed using anatomical landmarks or electrical nerve stimulation. The type of medication used depends on desired onset and duration of action. Bupivacaine or ropivacaine is used commonly as these agents have a longer duration of effect, with analgesia lasting for about 12–18 hours after a single dose. The total dose of local anesthetic injected must be taken into account to prevent systemic toxicity. The American Society of Anesthesiologists recommends patient monitoring with pulse oximetry, electrocardiography, and blood pressure measurements, while performing these procedures.

12.7 MANAGEMENT OF PAIN IN ACUTE REHABILITATION IN OLDER ADULTS

Adequate management of pain is essential in acute rehabilitation in older adults so that they can adequately participate in physical and occupational therapy to attain the highest level of functioning in spite of their underlying impairment. On admission to the rehabilitation unit, in addition to a comprehensive history and physical examination including cognitive status, pain assessment

TABLE 12.1
Neuroaxial Analgesia

Indication	Epidural catheter:
	Trauma pain related to rib fractures and lower extremities/pelvis fracture
	Any surgery involving thorax, abdomen, pelvis, or bilateral lower extremity
	Intrathecal or epidural catheter:
	Intractable cancer pain involving thoracic, abdomen, pelvis, or lower extremities
	Single shot techniques:
	Short-acting agents such as fentanyl is used for outpatient procedures like lithotripsy, longer-acting agents such as morphine are used or in-patient surgeries like hip arthroplasty or knee surgery
Procedure	A 19-gauge catheter is placed within epidural space or subarchnoid space
	Mixture of opioids and/or local anesthetics delivered via a programmable pump to deliver medications to their site of action in an effort to increase effectiveness and minimize systemic side effects
	Combination therapies are often used; for example, 0.1% bupivacaine with hydromorphone 12 mcg/mL or bupivicaine–fentanyl mixture
	If there are issues related to cognitive side effects from use of opioids or side effects related to sympatholytic effect like hypotension or impaired ambulation due to motor weakness from local anesthetics, then appropriate single agents can be used
	Epinephrine and clonidine can be added to augment local anesthetic effect
	NSAIDs/acetaminophen can be used as supplemental analgesics
Advantages	Frail patients may be better served with epidural analgesia compared to intravenous PCA[27]
	Sympatholytic effect decreases intraoperative blood loss in hip surgery, pelvic, urologic, and other lower extremity surgeries and improves graft patency in vascular surgeries
	Decreases postoperative morbidity/mortality—lower risk of postoperative pneumonia, deep vein thrombosis (DVT), pulmonary emboli, and respiratory depression
	Enables statistically significant superior pain relief compared with intravenous and oral pain regimens
	In cognitively intact adults patient-controlled delivery (patient-controlled epidural analgesia [PCEA]) can be used, whereas only continuous infusion settings can be used in patients with cognitive impairment
	Indwelling catheters are usually reserved for cancer pain management in inpatient settings and implantable pumps are normally used for outpatient management
Disadvantages	Side effects of hypotension, urinary retention, pruritus, respiratory depression, headache, and nausea/vomiting are common and need to be addressed. Less common risks include epidural hematoma or abscess
	Older adults are generally on anticoagulation/antiplatelet agents. Providers should be well aware of the limitations imposed by these, and work in close collaboration with the primary service, nursing services, and pharmacy regarding these issues
	Specialized care is needed for this therapy

using instruments mentioned earlier in this chapter, the severity of the pain, and its temporal relationship with the patients' activities are assessed. This is essential to ensure an effective analgesic intervention.

Guidelines for pain medication use during acute rehabilitation in older adults:

- Obtain and document accurate history of over-the-counter as well as prescription medications, including side effects, used prior to hospitalization.
- Review and document the diagnoses and use of pain and psychotropic medications.
- Discontinue medications that are not needed.
- Discuss with patients and make sure they comprehend the concept of taking medications as needed for moderate to severe pain.
- Simplify medication schedules if possible.
- Educate the patient and family about the indications for medications and their side effects.

TABLE 12.2

Procedures and Indications for Acute Pain

Body Region	Procedure	Pain/Surgery Indication	Comments
Face and neck	Nerve block of trigeminal nerve and its branches Superficial cervical plexus block	Neuralgias in the distribution of trigeminal nerve could be related to postherpetic neuralgia (PHN), idiopathic neuralgia, or dental work Pain related to carotid surgery Cancer pain due to tumor in the area	Local anesthetic like 0.5% bupivacaine can be used for surgical and postsurgical pain In terms of cancer pain, a neurolytic block with 10% phenol can be used after a positive diagnostic block with local anesthetic
Upper extremity	Brachial plexus block can be performed at multiple target points across the plexus	Interscalene for shoulder, distal clavicle, and proximal humerus Supraclavicular/infraclavicular for Mid-distal humerus, elbow, and hand Axillary Distal forearm and hand	Risk of phrenic nerve paralysis, hence be cautious in older patients with COPD Risk of pneumothorax/vascular puncture (minimal with ultrasound guided blocks) Safe except for risk of vascular puncture exists Concentration of local anesthetic can be altered depending on the intent of the block and need for patient participation in physical therapy For cancer pain management, either a perineural catheter can be used or graded neurolysis can be performed through a catheter or directly through a needle
Trunk	Paravertebral nerve blocks	Mastectomy Thoracotomy Intercostal neuralgia due to malignant or nonmalignant causes	Single shot or catheter In cancer-related pain, neurolysis can be safely performed using alcohol or phenol
	Trans abdominal plane (TAP) block	Lower/mid-abdominal surgical pain Acute on chronic abdominal wall pain	Single shot or a catheter can be used under ultrasound guidance. Minimal risk associated with this block
Lower extremity	Lumbar plexus	For hip surgical pain	Risk of vascular puncture or nerve injury[28]
	Femoral nerve block	Anterior thigh or knee, for example, knee arthroscopy, anterior collateral ligament (ACL) reconstruction, femoral shaft fracture repairs, and total knee replacements	
	Sciatic nerve block	Blocked at gluteal level for surgeries on posterior thigh and leg below knee At popliteal fossa for surgeries on leg below knee At ankle for surgeries on distal 1/3 foot	
	Ankle block	Foot and toes	

(Continued)

TABLE 12.2 *(Continued)*

Procedures and Indications for Acute Pain

Body Region	Procedure	Pain/Surgery Indication	Comments
Miscellaneous	Infiltration	Pain related to ambulatory hernia surgery, around ports for laparoscopic surgery and other minor surgeries	Lidocaine, bupivacaine, or a liposomal preparation of bupivacaine (Exaprel) can be injected around the incision. Duration of analgesia around 4–6 hours longer with liposomal preparation
	Intra-articular	Useful in pain related to ambulatory surgeries like knee arthroscopy or shoulder surgeries	Local anesthetics and opioids in combination or as single agents. Morphine in dosages of 1–5 mg has been studied, but the evidence of efficacy is inconclusive

- Determine whether the patient's pain is neuropathic or nociceptive, as this will determine the use of neuromodulators along with acetaminophen, opioids, or NSAIDS for optimal pain control.
- Determine whether the patient's pain is continuous or only associated with movement or activity.
- If the patient's pain is constant but exacerbated with activity, use a scheduled medication for the constant pain and an as-needed medication for the breakthrough or activity-related pain. In context of opioids, use 10% of the total daily opioid dose as short-acting medication that should be taken 20–30 minutes before activity to help with the pain exacerbation.
- If it is determined that the pain occurs with certain activity, then educate the patient about asking providers for pain medications 20–30 minutes before the anticipated activity. Nurses should be proactive in offering the medication before a scheduled activity for inpatients with cognitive impairment.
- If IV medications are used to treat exacerbation of pain, they should be given 2–5 minutes before the expected activity, which can either be delivered by the nurse or PCA.
- In case of a peripheral nerve catheter or intrathecal catheter infusion being used for pain control during the stay in acute rehabilitation, consideration for using local anesthetic concentration of 0.0625% or 0.1% to minimize the risk of motor blockade so patient can safely participate in physical therapy is essential.
- Examine the patient to rule out other causes of pain like spasticity (which should be treated with antispasticity agents like baclofen), pressure ulcers, depression, anxiety, or infections that need to be addressed adequately for optimal pain control.
- Examine patient and determine whether the patient can take medication orally and also whether they are able to swallow tablets or capsules.
- If patient can only take crushed medications in applesauce, then remember that sustained-release medications cannot be crushed. Medications like morphine, oxycodone, and hydromorphone are available in instant-release formulations, which can be crushed and a liquid form is also available, so consider use of these medications. Methadone if used can be crushed and is also available in liquid form. Fentanyl is transdermal and can be used for patients unable to take by mouth (PO). Buccal preparations of fentanyl can be used for episodic or breakthrough pain.

- When opioid medications are being titrated, calculate the 24-hour dose and titrate up depending on the patient's usage every 2–3 days except for titration of methadone, which should be done only every 5–7 days.

When converting from one opioid to another, consider reducing the dose by 30.

12.8   CHRONIC PAIN MANAGEMENT IN OLDER ADULTS

A stepwise, thoughtful, proactive, and integrative approach has the best chance of being successful. A multidisciplinary approach using pharmacotherapy, physical rehabilitation, interventional modalities, alternative medicine modalities, and psychosocial interventions is recommended for optimal pain management. In terms of pharmacotherapy, The World Health Organization analgesic ladder can be applied as one useful analgesic strategy with well-proven efficacy and ease of application. Patients with mild pain can be started on acetaminophen alone or in combination with a mild opioid analgesic such as tramadol or tapentodol. NSAIDs can be used provided there are no contraindications to their use. Patients with moderate pain can be started on short-acting opioid medications and, if tolerated, can be converted to a timed-release preparation if clinically warranted. There are certain pain syndromes that have a disproportionately higher incidence in the older adult population. It is helpful to think in the context of whether a pain syndrome is primarily neuropathic or nociceptive, common examples of such pain syndromes in older adults are listed in Table 12.3. This helps the clinician in initiating appropriate pharmacological management. One would use neuromodulators like gabapentinoids and/or antidepressant medications as first line in neuropathic pain versus primarily analgesic medications or interventions in nociceptive pain syndromes.

TABLE 12.3

Common Pain Syndromes in Older Adults

Neuropathic Pain

Herpes zoster

Postherpetic neuralgia

Radicular pain

Trigeminal neuralgia

Peripheral neuropathies caused by diabetes, HIV, or artherosclerotic disease

Spinal cord injury

Poststroke pain

Neuromuscular disease—amyotropic lateral sclerosis, multiple sclerosis, and Parkinson's disease

Spinal stenosis

Temporal arteritis

Nociceptive Pain

Tendonitis

Myofascial pain

Low back pain—facet arthritis, spondylosis, or sacroiliac joint dysfunction

Osteoarthritis

Osteoporosis and bone fractures

Autoimmune inflammatory arthropathy—rheumatoid arthritis, systemic lupus sclerosis, scleroderma

Gout

Ischemic heart disease

Peripheral vascular disease

Mixed Neuropathic and Nociceptive

Cancer pain

Postlaminectomy pain syndromes

Postoperative pain

12.9 PHARMACOTHERAPY

The American Geriatrics Society's (AGS) updated clinical guideline titled "The Management of Persistent Pain in Older Persons" reiterated that pharmacotherapy continues to be the mainstay of treatment to control pain in older adults;[16] however, there are significant concerns around the use of analgesic medications in this population. Consulting (AGS) Beers criteria for potentially inappropriate medication use as outlined in Table 12.4 is often helpful.

In the following section, the common pharmacological modalities used for pain management in older adults are outlined.

12.9.1 Acetaminophen

Acetaminophen should be considered as a first-line agent for persistent musculoskeletal pain (high-quality evidence, strong recommendation).[43] The recommended dose is 325–500 mg every 4 hours or 500–1000 mg every 6 hours. The maximum daily dose is 3 g daily. Providers should reduce the maximum dose by 50%–75% in patients with hepatic insufficiency or history of alcohol abuse. Note that liver failure is an absolute contraindication for the use of acetaminophen. The exact mechanism of action of the drug is unclear. The proposed mechanism is inhibition of prostaglandins through COX-3 inhibition and/or central 5 hydroxyl tryptophan receptor-dependent antinociceptive action. It interacts with anticoagulants like warfarin, alcohol, and hepatic enzyme inducers like phenytoin and carbamazepine. Advantages for using acetaminophen are that it can have an additive effect when used with NSAIDS and an opioid sparing effect as well. In addition, it does not have any sedative effect. The disadvantages, however, are the hepatotoxicity with acute overdose or excessive chronic use and hypersensitivity/anaphylactic reactions, although that is rare.

12.9.1.1 Nonselective NSAIDs and COX 2 Selective Inhibitors

NSAIDs should be used with caution in select individuals with mild to moderate nociceptive pain (high-quality evidence, strong recommendation).[44] Common NSAID drug dosages include the following:

Salsate—500–750 mg every 12 hours
Celebrex—100 mg once a day
Naproxen—220 mg twice a day
Ibuprofen—200 mg three times per day
Diclofenac—50 mg twice a day or 75 mg extended release daily
Nabumetone—1 g daily

Recommendations are that the initial dose should be 50% of the recommended dose, slowly titrated up while monitoring for side effects. Older persons should use a proton pump inhibitor when taking nonselective NSAIDs. Absolute contraindications to NSAIDs include current active peptic ulcer disease, chronic kidney disease, and heart failure. These medications are relatively contraindicated in patients with coronary artery disease or patients with history of Transient ischemic attack (TIA)s or stroke. The mechanism of action of this drug class is reversible nonspecific COX 1 and COX 2 inhibition and reduction in CNS and peripheral prostaglandin synthesis. NSAIDs interact with angiontensin converting enzyme (ACE) inhibitors, diuretics, methotrexate, anticoagulants, lithium, hypoglycemic agents, and probenecid. Use of NSAIDs is advantageous as it has an opioid sparing effect reducing opioid consumption by 25%–45% in addition to its beneficial anti-inflammatory effects. Adverse effects include gastrointestinal bleeding, renal, hepatic and cardiac adverse effects, peripheral edema, and idiosyncratic cognitive side effects.

TABLE 12.4

Beers Criteria 2012

Organ System/ Therapeutic Category/ Drug(s)	Rationale	Recommendation	Quality of Evidence	Strength of Recommendation	References
Tertiary tricyclic antidepressant (TCA)'s: amitriptyline, imipramine	Highly anticholinergic, sedating, and cause orthostatic hypotension	Avoid	High	Strong	Coupland 2011,[29] Nelson 2011,[30] Sharf 2008[31]
Meperidine	Not an effective oral analgesic in dosages commonly used: may cause neurotoxicity; safer alternatives available	Avoid	High	Strong	Kaiko 1982,[32] Meperidine Package insert
Non-Cox selective NSAIDs, full oral • Aspirin > 325 mg/ day • Diclofenac • Diflunisal • Etodolac • Fenoprofen • Ibuprofen • Ketoprofen • Meclofenamate • Mefenamic acid • Meloxicam • Nabumetone • Naproxen • Oxaprozin • Piroxicam • Sulindac • Tolmetin	Increases risk of gastro intestinal (GI) bleeding/peptic ulcer disease in high-risk groups, including those >75 years old or taking oral or parenteral corticosteroids, anticoagulants, or antiplatelet agents. Use of proton pump inhibitor or misoprostol reduces risk but does not eliminate risk. Upper GI ulcers, gross bleeding, or perforation caused by NSAIDs occur in approximately 1% of patients treated for 3–6 months, and in about 2%–4% of patients treated for 1 year. These trends continue with longer duration of use	Avoid chronic use unless other alternatives are not effective and patient can take gastro-protective agent (proton pump or inhibitor or misoprostol)	All others: moderate	Strong	AGS Pain Guideline 2009,[33] Langman 1994,[34] Lanas 2006,[35] Llorente Melero 2002,[36] Pilotto 2003,[37] Piper 1991[38]

(Continued)

TABLE 12.4 (Continued)
Beers Criteria 2012

Organ System/ Therapeutic Category/ Drug(s)	Rationale	Recommendation	Quality of Evidence	Strength of Recommendation	References
Indomethacin ketorolac, includes parenteral	Increases risk of GI bleeding/ peptic ulcer disease in high-risk groups (see above non-Cox selective NSAIDs). Of all the NSAIDs indomethacin has most adverse effects	Avoid	Indomethacin: moderate ketorolac: high	Strong	Onder 2004[39]
Pentazocine	Opioid analgesic that causes CNS adverse effects, including confusion and hallucinations, more commonly than other narcotic drugs; is also a mixed agonist and antagonist; safer alternatives available	Avoid	Low	Strong	AGS Pain Guideline 2009, Pentazocine Package Insert[40]
Skeletal muscle relaxant • Carisoprodol • Chlorzoxazone • Cyclobenzaprine • Metaxalone • Methocarbamol • Orphenadrine	Most muscle relaxants poorly tolerated by older adults, because of anticholinergic adverse effects, sedation, increased risk of fractures; effectiveness at dosages tolerated by older adults is questionable	Avoid	Moderate	Strong	Billups 2011,[41] Rudolph 2008[42]

12.9.1.2 Opioids

This class of medications is considered in patients with moderate to severe pain with pain-related functional impairment resulting in diminished quality of life (low quality of evidence, strong recommendation). There are a number of opioids available for use in clinical practice with immediate-release and time-release preparations, combination products with acetaminophen, a variety of novel route deliveries including nasal, sublingual, transbuccal, and transdermal preparations. In general, opioid naïve patients should be started on an immediate-release preparation first. Once the tolerability is established and pain control remains an issue, transition to a time-release or long-acting agent can be instituted.

12.9.1.3 Tramadol/Tapentodol

These are atypical opioid medications, considered to be more potent analgesics than NSAIDs with fewer cardiac, renal, and gastrointestinal side effects and with reduced risk of abuse, physical dependence, and tolerance compared to pure opioids. Caution needs to be exercised in patients with renal impairment and these are contraindicated in patients with history of seizures. Dizziness, lethargy, nausea, vomiting, and constipation are common side effects. Tramadol is available as Ultracet (tramadol 37.5 mg/acetaminophen 325 mg), tramadol 50 mg immediate-release tablets, and tramadol extended release. Tramadol dose is 50–100 mg every 6 hours. Maximum daily dose in patients older than 65 years of age is 300 mg/day. Tapentodol is available as immediate as well as extended-release preparation with a *dose* of 50–100 mg every 4–6 hours. Maximum dose is 400–600 mg/day and is indicated for use in patients in whom NSAIDS are contraindicated and tramadol has not been effective.

12.9.2 Pure Opioid Agonists

Pure opioid agonists are used in patients with moderate to severe pain that is not relieved with acetaminophen, NSAIDs, atypical opioids alone, or in combination with adjuvants. They should be started in select patients after a careful assessment is done and therapeutic goals are clearly established. In situations where patients are opioid naïve, starting with immediate-release opioids at the lowest dose and titrating to the desired effect as tolerated is recommended. These formulations are available as single agents as well as combination products. Recommended starting dose is as follows:

Hydrocodone/acetaminophen, 2.5–5 mg every 4–6 hours; hydrocodone sustained release (SR) formulation 10 mg every 12 hours

Oxycodone/acetaminophen, 2.5–5 mg every 4–6 hours; oxycodone immediate release 2.5–5 mg every 4–6 hours and oxycodone SR 10 mg every 12 hours

Morphine immediate release 2.5–10 mg every 4 hours and morphine sustained release 15 mg every 8–24 hours

Oxymorphone immediate release 5 mg every 6 hours and oxymorphone extended release 5 mg every 12 hours

Hydromorphone—1–2 mg every 3–4 hours

Fentanyl patch is a transdermal preparation and should not be used in opioid naïve patients. The starting dose for fentanyl is 12–25 mcg/hour every 72 hours.

Methadone is not recommended for use in opioid naïve patients and should be only used by practitioners who are knowledgeable with its pharmacokinetics. The recommended starting dose is 2.5 mg every 8 hours.

Pure opioid agonists produce analgesia by binding to primarily mu receptors and to kappa receptors. There is no ceiling effect and no major organ toxic effect. Dose limiting adverse effects include nausea, vomiting, constipation, urinary retention, respiratory depression, dizziness, sedation, and cognitive side effects. There is also the potential for opioid abuse and addiction.

12.9.2.1 Topical Medications

Topical medications have significant role as analgesics in older adults because of their favorable side effect profile. These medications should only be applied on intact skin and are inherently safer as systemic absorption is limited.

Topical local anesthetics include lidocaine patch 5%, lidocaine cream and ointment 5%, and mixture of lidocaine 2.5% and prilocaine 2.5%. The lidocaine patch 5% is FDA approved for use in postherpetic neuralgia,[45] and diabetic peripheral neuropathic pain. Maximum dose is 3–4 patches for 12–18 hours and then on and off for 6–12 hours. Lidocaine blocks abnormal activity in the upregulated neuronal sodium channels. It inhibits the expression of nitric oxide resulting in suppression of cytokines release from T cells in addition to acting as a protective barrier against cutaneous stimuli. Adverse effects are minimal and include local burning, dermatitis, pruritus, and rash.

12.9.2.2 Topical NSAIDs

There are many topical NSAIDs such as pennsaid 1.5% topical solution maximum dose—40 drops, four times per day, diclofenac gel 1% maximum dose 16–32 g per day, and diclofenac patch 1.3% maximum dose—1 patch twice a day. Topical NSAIDS have 40% less systemic absorption hence the side effects may be less compared to oral and intravenous route. These work by inhibiting the enzyme COX resulting in inhibition of prostaglandins, thromboxane, and prostacyclin synthesis. Usual adverse effects are local site reaction.

12.9.2.3 Topical Capsaicin

Topical capsaicin is a cream/lotion 0.025% and 0.075% that is available over the counter and can be used three to four times per day. A high-dose capsaicin patch 8% (Qutenza) is FDA approved for use in postherpetic neuralgia,[45] and pain related to diabetic and HIV neuropathy. It is applied in a supervised setting with a maximum dose of four patches after local anesthetic application. In clinical practice, it is used for other chronic neuropathic pain conditions as well. The expected duration of relief is 3–4 months after a single application. Capsaicin acts on vanilloid receptors, a TRPV1 receptor present on afferent nociceptors, leading to depletion of substance P from the presynaptic terminals, which depresses the function of type C nociceptive fibers. Side effects include burning at application site, blisters, and rash.

12.9.2.4 Adjuvant Medications

Adjuvant medications should be considered to enhance the analgesic effects of other medications for nociceptive dominant pain. These medications could be used as first-line agents for neuropathic pain conditions.

Antidepressants. This class of medications is considered for treatment of neuropathic pain as well as myofascial pain. Older adults rarely tolerate doses greater than 75–100 mg per day. Tertiary tricyclic antidepressant (amitriptyline, imipramine, and doxepin) should be avoided in older adults owing to anticholinergic and cognitive side effects. On the other hand, secondary tricyclic antidepressants (nortriptyline and desipramine) can be considered in older adults owing to their less anticholinergic and cognitive side effects. Selective serotonin and norepinephrine reuptake inhibitors can also be used. For example, duloxetine has also been approved for musculoskeletal back pain[46] and painful osteoarthritis of knee[47] in addition to diabetic neuropathic pain and fibromyalgia. The usual starting dose is 20 mg. Venlafaxine at 37.5 mg daily can also be used for the same indications. Analgesic effect is mediated by the blockade of reuptake of serotonin and norepinephrine that results in augmenting the descending inhibition of pain. Adverse effects include cognitive side effects, urinary retention, increased risk of falls, and worsening of anxiety. Venlafaxine is associated with dose-related increase in blood pressure.

Anticonvulsants. This class of medications is used in treatment of neuropathic pain conditions, fibromyalgia, and migraines. These should be started at a low dose and titrated slowly as tolerated in older adults due to a significant risk of cognitive side effects. Gabapentin is used for the treatment of diabetic neuropathic pain, postherpetic neuralgia, and in the treatment of spinal stenosis and postlaminectomy pain syndrome with a dose range from 1800 to 3600 mg per day, in three divided doses. The recommended starting dose for gabapentin is 100 mg at night, increasing in 100 mg increments every 3 days as tolerated. Pregabalin is FDA approved for treatment of pain related to diabetic neuropathy, spinal cord injury, postherpetic neuralgia, and fibromyalgia. Dosing is 150–600 mg per day in two or three divided doses. The recommended starting dose in older population is 50 mg at night and titrating by 50 mg increments every 3–4 days as tolerated. These medications are thought to work on alpha2 delta subunit of voltage gated calcium channels. Weight gain, edema, ataxia, and dizziness are common side effects associated with the use of gabapentinoids.

Topamax. Topamax is FDA approved for migraine prophylaxis. The recommended starting dose is 50 mg once a day, again with slow titration. Dosing should be 100–200 mg per day in two divided doses. Topamax inhibits neuronal hyperactivity along the pain pathways by alteration of voltage-gated calcium channels, sodium channels, and modulation of Gaba amino butyric acid (GABA) and glutamate. Adverse effects include weight loss, paresthesia, and anorexia.

Muscle relaxants. This class of medications should be used in select individuals with extreme caution. Common medications used in this class are baclofen, tizanidine, and cyclobenzaprine (flexeril). Baclofen is a Gaba-b agonist with a starting dose of 5 mg three times per day. Older adults may be unable to tolerate more than 30–40 mg per day. Tizanidine should be started at a dose of 2 mg three times per day. Tizanidine is a centrally acting alpha2 adrenergic agonist and is used in the treatment of spasticity in spinal cord injury and multiple sclerosis. Older adults may be unable to tolerate more than 16 mg per day. Flexeril should be used very cautiously and started at low doses of 5 mg three times per day, with a maximum daily dose of 30 mg per day. The mechanism of action is not well understood but its effect could be due to inhibition of interneuronal activity in the descending reticular formation. General adverse effects associated with this class of medications are somnolence, cognitive effects, and orthostasis. Patients need close monitoring of liver functions when on tizanidine. Flexeril should not be used in patients with close angle glaucoma.

12.10 PHYSICAL REHABILITATION

Physical therapy will help the patient live more independently by helping them with compensatory techniques for disabilities from their primary disorder, preventing secondary injuries, and treating functional deficits. Strength and endurance training, stretching, isometric strengthening, and aerobic exercises should be incorporated. Myofascial release for treatment of myofascial pain is equally important. Use of modalities such as transcutaneous electrical nerve stimulation (TENS) unit could be beneficial.

12.11 INTERVENTIONAL MODALITIES

These modalities can be helpful for specific pain indications as listed in Table 12.5. These include injections of local anesthetics with or without steroids in addition to chemical or thermal neurolysis. These interventions serve a diagnostic as well as a therapeutic purpose. Overall advantage in clinical practice is possible pain relief while minimizing intolerable medication-related side effects.

TABLE 12.5

Procedures and Indications for Chronic Pain

Type of Block	Indications
Trigger point injections	Myofascial pain
Epidural steroid injection	Degenerative disc disease (DDD), spinal stenosis, postlaminectomy pain syndrome
Facet joint/nerve injections including radiofrequency ablation	Facetogenic pain of all spine levels
Intercostal nerve injections	Postthoracotomy pain syndrome, postmastectomy pain syndrome, postherpetic neuralgia, malignancy
Greater and lesser occipital nerve injections	Occipital neuralgia in the context of whiplash injury or other process
Botox injections	Migraine headaches
Sacroiliac joint injection	Sacroiliac joint dysfunction
Stellate ganglion block	Sympathetically mediated head and upper extremity pain like complex regional pain syndrome, intractable facial neuralgic pain, ischemic pain in patients who are not surgical candidates
Lumbar sympathetic block	Sympathetically mediated lower extremity pain in complex regional pain syndrome (CRPS), ischemic limb pain
Celiac plexus block	Abdominal pain due to chronic pancreatitis, pancreatic cancer or cancer related to upper abdominal viscera
TAP block	Chronic abdominal wall pain like postherniorrhaphy pain
Superior hypogastric plexus block	Chronic pelvic pain due to interstitial cystitis, endometriosis or pelvic viscera malignancies
Ganglion impar block and Pudendal nerve block	Rectal, vaginal, and pelvic floor pain, including pain related to rectal cancer
Intra-articular joint injections	Joint pain related to osteoarthritis, both steroid as well as viscosupplementation can be used
Spinal cord stimulator	Postlaminectomy pain, complex regional pain syndrome, intractable angina, peripheral ischemic pain
Intrathecal pump	Spasticity treatment and intractable chronic pain

12.12 COMPLEMENTARY AND ALTERNATIVE MEDICINE MODALITIES

Acupuncture. Acupuncture is helpful in many chronic pain conditions. Qi and meridians are important concepts in acupuncture. Meridians represent various organ systems and qi is the flow of energy across meridians. One of the accepted mechanisms is that analgesic effect of acupuncture is mediated by A-deltaafferent stimulation resulting in the initiation of a cascade of endorphin and monoamine release. This in turn facilitates the descending inhibition of nociception.

Yoga. Yoga increases strength, flexibility, and feelings of well-being and vitality. This significantly reduces pain intensity and use of pain medications. The asanas (poses) and pranayama (mindful breathing techniques) help harmonize the physiological system and initiate a relaxation response in the neuroendocrine system. As the neural discharge is modulated, the state of hyperarousal of the nervous system is attenuated. Yoga helps with affective component of chronic pain, and improves quality of life.[48]

12.13 PSYCHOSOCIAL INTERVENTIONS

Pain-coping techniques such as relaxation, psychotherapy, meditation, imagery and behavioral modification therapy, a strong social support, and better control of anxiety and depression are important in pain management.

12.14 SUMMARY

Pain is an inevitable part of aging and its management in this population is challenging due to barriers to proper pain assessment, under-reporting of pain, multiple medical comorbidities, cognitive decline, limited social support, and physiological changes. Pharmacological interventions remain the mainstay of pain management in older adults. When choosing medications in this population, consider medications with the least side effects, lowest cost, and least daily frequency for optimizing compliance. Recommendations are to start low and go slow while titrating the medications. Use of multimodal therapy is recommended rather than depending solely on pharmacological agents to avoid polypharmacy. The potential merits of each of these agents need to be carefully balanced against each patient's ability to tolerate their side effects. This is a particularly salient consideration given that patients are older or otherwise frail. Invasive modalities may play an important role in the overall management especially in patients with intractable pain. Finally, the role of patient and family education and psychological support cannot be overemphasized, given that the currently available treatments will not be effective for all patients.

The geriatric population poses a unique challenge where the goal is reducing persistent pain and maximizing function while avoiding treatment-related harm (Figures 12.5 and 12.6).

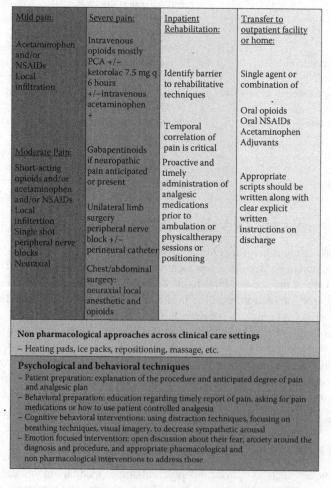

Mild pain:	Severe pain:	Inpatient Rehabilitation:	Transfer to outpatient facility or home:
Acetaminophen and/or NSAIDs Local infiltration	Intravenous opioids mostly PCA +/− ketorolac 7.5 mg q 6 hours +/−intravenous acetaminophen +	Identify barrier to rehabilitative techniques	Single agent or combination of Oral opioids Oral NSAIDs Acetaminophen Adjuvants
Moderate Pain: Short-acting opioids and/or acetaminophen and/or NSAIDs Local infiltertion Single shot peripheral nerve blocks Neuraxial	Gabapentinoids if neuropathic pain anticipated or present Unilateral limb surgery peripheral nerve block +/− perineural catheter Chest/abdominal surgery: neuraxial local anesthetic and opioids	Temporal correlation of pain is critical Proactive and timely administration of analgesic medications prior to ambulation or physicaltherapy sessions or positioning	Appropriate scripts should be written along with clear explicit written instructions on discharge

Non pharmacological approaches across clinical care settings
– Heating pads, ice packs, repositioning, massage, etc.

Psychological and behavioral techniques
– Patient preparation: explanation of the procedure and anticipated degree of pain and analgesic plan
– Behavioral preparation: education regarding timely report of pain, asking for pain medications or how to use patient controlled analgesia
– Cognitive behavioral interventions: using distraction techniques, focusing on breathing techniques, visual imagery, to decrease sympathetic arousal
– Emotion focused intervention: open discussion about their fear, anxiety around the diagnosis and procedure, and appropriate pharmacological and non pharmacological interventions to address those

FIGURE 12.5 Summary of multimodal management of acute pain in older adults.

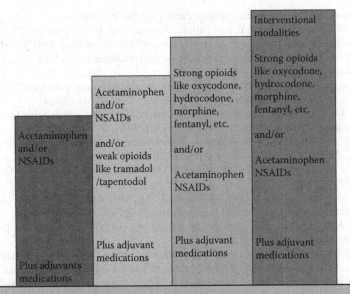

FIGURE 12.6 Modified WHO analgesic ladder in chronic pain management in older adults.

REFERENCES

1. Aging Stats. *Federal Interagency Forum on Aging Related Statistics.* www.aging stats.gov. Retrieved online April 22, 2009, 2006.
2. Management ASoATFoAP. Practice guidelines for acute pain management in the perioperative setting: An updated report by the American Society of Anesthesiologists Task Force on Acute Pain Management. *Anesthesiology.* 2004;100:1573–1581.
3. Pasero C, McCaffery M. Orthopaedic postoperative pain management. *Journal of PeriAnesthesia Nursing.* 2007;22(3):160–174.
4. Vaurio LE, Sands LP, Wang Y, Mullen EA, Leung JM. Postoperative delirium: The importance of pain and pain management. *Anesthesia and Analgesia.* 2006;102(4):1267–1273.
5. Morrison RS, Magaziner J, Gilbert M et al. Relationship between pain and opioid analgesics on the development of delirium following hip fracture. *The Journals of Gerontology Series A: Biological Sciences and Medical Sciences.* 2003;58(1):M76–M81.
6. Inouye SK. Delirium in older persons. *New England Journal of Medicine.* 2006;354(11):1157–1165.
7. Helme RD, Gibson SJ. The epidemiology of pain in elderly people. *Clinics in Geriatric Medicine.* 2001;17(3):417–431.
8. Jensen MP, Karoly P. Self-report scales and procedures for assessing pain in adults. In: Turk DC, Melzack R, editors *Handbook of Pain Assessment,* 2nd edn. New York: Guilford Press; 1992.
9. Richardson J. *Practical Management of Pain.* 3rd edn. St. Louis, Missouri: Mosby Inc.; 2000.

10. Melzack R. The short-form McGill pain questionnaire. *Pain.* 1987;30(2):191–197.
11. Herr KA, Mobily PR, Wallace RB, Chung Y. Leg pain in the rural Iowa 65+ population: Prevalence, related factors, and association with functional status. *The Clinical Journal of Pain.* 1991;7(2):114–121.
12. Borenstein DG. Epidemiology, etiology, diagnostic evaluation, and treatment of low back pain. *Current Opinion in Rheumatology.* 2001;13(2):128–134.
13. Sawyer P, Bodner EV, Ritchie CS, Allman RM. Pain and pain medication use in community-dwelling older adults. *The American Journal of Geriatric Pharmacotherapy.* 2006;4(4):316–324.
14. Sengstaken EA, King SA. The problems of pain and its detection among geriatric nursing home residents. *Journal of the American Geriatrics Society.* 1993;41(5):541–544.
15. Hall MJ, DeFrances CJ, Williams SN, Golosinskiy A, Schwartzman A. National hospital discharge survey: 2007 summary. *National Health Statistics Reports.* 2010;29(29):1–20.
16. Persons APoPPiO. The management of persistent pain in older persons. *Journal of the American Geriatrics Society.* 2002;50(6 Suppl):S205.
17. Lautenbacher S, Kunz M, Strate P, Nielsen J, Arendt-Nielsen L. Age effects on pain thresholds, temporal summation and spatial summation of heat and pressure pain. *Pain.* 2005;115(3):410–418.
18. Pergolizzi JV Jr, Raffa RB, Gould E. Considerations on the use of oxymorphone in geriatric patients. *Expert Opinion on Drug Safety.* 2009;8(5):603–613.
19. Elia N, Lysakowski C, Tramèr MR. Does multimodal analgesia with acetaminophen, nonsteroidal antiinflammatory drugs, or selective cyclooxygenase-2 inhibitors and patient-controlled analgesia morphine offer advantages over morphine alone? Meta-analyses of randomized trials. *The Journal of the American Society of Anesthesiologists.* 2005;103(6):1296–1304.
20. Grass JA. Patient-controlled analgesia. *Anesthesia and Analgesia.* 2005;101(5S):S44–S61.
21. Gagliese L, Jackson M, Ritvo P, Wowk A, Katz J. Age is not an impediment to effective use of patient-controlled analgesia by surgical patients. *The Journal of the American Society of Anesthesiologists.* 2000;93(3):601–610.
22. Lavand'Homme P, De Kock M. Practical guidelines on the postoperative use of patient-controlled analgesia in the elderly. *Drugs and Aging.* 1998;13(1):9–16.
23. Ready LB. PCA is effective for older patients—But are there limits? *The Journal of the American Society of Anesthesiologists.* 2000;93(3):597–598.
24. Licht E, Siegler EL, Reid MC. Can the cognitively impaired safely use patient controlled analgesia? *Journal of Opioid Management.* 2009;5(5):307.
25. Song K, Melroy MJ, Whipple OC. Optimizing multimodal analgesia with intravenous acetaminophen and opioids in postoperative bariatric patients. *Pharmacotherapy: The Journal of Human Pharmacology and Drug Therapy.* 2014;34(S1):14S–21S.
26. Dauri M, Faria S, Gatti A, Celidonio L, Carpenedo R, Sabato AF. Gabapentin and pregabalin for the acute post-operative pain management. A systematic-narrative review of the recent clinical evidences. *Current Drug Targets.* 2009;10(8):716–733.
27. Mann C, Pouzeratte Y, Boccara G et al. Comparison of intravenous or epidural patient-controlled analgesia in the elderly after major abdominal surgery. *The Journal of the American Society of Anesthesiologists.* 2000;92(2):433–441.
28. Raimer C, Priem K, Wiese AA et al. Continuous psoas and sciatic block after knee arthroplasty: Good effects compared to epidural analgesia or i.v. opioid analgesia: A prospective study of 63 patients. *Acta Orthopaedica.* 2007;78(2):193–200.
29. Coupland C, Dhiman P, Morriss R, Arthur A, Barton G, Hippisley-Cox J. Antidepressant use and risk of adverse outcomes in older people: Population based cohort study. *BMJ.* 2011;343:d4551.
30. Nelson JC, Devanand DP. A systematic review and meta-analysis of placebo-controlled antidepressant studies in people with depression and dementia. *Journal of the American Geriatrics Society.* 2011;59(4):577–585.
31. Scharf M, Rogowski R, Hull S et al. Efficacy and safety of doxepin 1 mg, 3 mg, and 6 mg in elderly patients with primary insomnia: A randomized, double-blind, placebo-controlled crossover study. *The Journal of Clinical Psychiatry.* 2008;69(10):1478–1564.
32. Kaiko RF, Foley KM, Grabinski PY et al. Central nervous system excitatory effects of meperidine in cancer patients. *Annals of Neurology.* 1983;13(2):180–185.
33. Adults A. The management of persistent pain in older adults. *Journal of the American Geriatrics Society.* 2002;50(6 Suppl):S205–S224.
34. Langman M, Weil J, Wainwright P et al. Risks of bleeding peptic ulcer associated with individual non-steroidal anti-inflammatory drugs. *The Lancet.* 1994;343(8905):1075–1078.

35. Lanas A, García-Rodríguez L-A, Arroyo M-T et al. Risk of upper gastrointestinal ulcer bleeding associated with selective cyclo-oxygenase-2 inhibitors, traditional non-aspirin non-steroidal anti-inflammatory drugs, aspirin and combinations. *Gut.* 2006;55(12):1731–1738.

36. Llorente MM, Tenías BJ, Zaragoza MA. Comparative incidence of upper gastrointestinal bleeding associated with individual non-steroidal anti-inflammatory drugs. *Revista Espanola de Enfermedades Digestivas: Organo Oficial de la Sociedad Espanola de Patologia Digestiva.* 2002;94(1):7–18.

37. Pilotto A, Franceschi M, Leandro G et al. The risk of upper gastrointestinal bleeding in elderly users of aspirin and other non-steroidal antiinflammatory drugs: The role of gastroprotective drugs. *Aging Clinical and Experimental Research.* 2003;15(6):494–499.

38. Piper JM, Ray WA, Daugherty JR, Griffin MR. Corticosteroid use and peptic ulcer disease: Role of nonsteroidal anti-inflammatory drugs. *Annals of Internal Medicine.* 1991;114(9):735–740.

39. Onder G, Pellicciotti F, Gambassi G, Bernabei R. NSAID-related psychiatric adverse events. *Drugs.* 2004;64(23):2619–2627.

40. Hanlon JT, Backonja M, Weiner D, Argoff C. Evolving pharmacological management of persistent pain in older persons. *Pain Medicine.* 2009;10(6):959–961.

41. Billups SJ, Delate T, Hoover B. Injury in an elderly population before and after initiating a skeletal muscle relaxant. *Annals of Pharmacotherapy.* 2011;45(4):485–491.

42. Rudolph JL, Salow MJ, Angelini MC, McGlinchey RE. The anticholinergic risk scale and anticholinergic adverse effects in older persons. *Archives of Internal Medicine.* 2008;168(5):508–513.

43. Bowsher D, Rigge M, Sopp L. Prevalence of chronic pain in the British population: A telephone survey of 1037 households. *Pain Clinic.* 1991;4(4):223–230.

44. Kaye AD, Baluch A, Scott JT. Pain management in the elderly population: A review. *The Ochsner Journal.* 2010;10(3):179–187.

45. Jones VM, Moore KA, Peterson DM. Capsaicin 8% topical patch (Qutenza)—A review of the evidence. *Journal of Pain and Palliative Care Pharmacotherapy.* 2011;25(1):32–41.

46. Skljarevski V, Desaiah D, Liu-Seifert H et al. Efficacy and safety of duloxetine in patients with chronic low back pain. *Spine.* 2010;35(13):E578–E585.

47. Chappell AS, Ossanna MJ, Liu-Seifert H et al. Duloxetine, a centrally acting analgesic, in the treatment of patients with osteoarthritis knee pain: A 13-week, randomized, placebo-controlled trial. *Pain.* 2009;146(3):253–260.

48. Vallath N. Perspectives on Yoga inputs in the management of chronic pain. *Indian Journal of Palliative Care.* 2010;16(1):1.

13 Polypharmacy and Rational Prescribing

Finding the "Golden Mean" for the "Silver Tsunami"

Mikhail Zhukalin, Christopher J. Williams,
Michael Reed, and Dale C. Strasser

CONTENTS

13.1 BACKGROUND

Older adults as well as other vulnerable patients are particularly susceptible to the deleterious effects of polypharmacy and related inappropriate prescribing practices common in contemporary medicine. Rehabilitation physicians are uniquely positioned within the healthcare system to favorably influence prescribing practices as they manage patients during a transition between acute care and the community, and develop interventions to reduce pain and promote function. Understanding polypharmacy and engaging in rational prescribing is a skill important to every physiatrist and is likely to improve patients' outcomes. This chapter provides an overview of prescribing practices for the older adult, emphasizes selected classes of medications commonly encountered in physiatric practice, and outlines strategies for rational medication management. The title of this chapter emphasizes the clinical appropriateness of specific medications and the interactions of multiple medications (e.g., "finding the golden mean") in the face of rapidly aging population ("the silver tsunami"). While the focus of this chapter is on the benefits of rational prescribing with the older adults, rehabilitation professionals commonly manage other vulnerable groups where the same principles apply such as those with spinal cord injuries, brain injuries, and complex medical conditions.

13.2   INTRODUCTION

Since ancient times, people have been searching for a *panacea*, a remedy that would cure all diseases and prolong life indefinitely. This mystical factor, named after the Greek goddess of universal remedy, was sought by various cultures throughout centuries, to no avail. If such a substance was ever found, it would effectively end the need for discussions of therapeutic agents, treatment algorithms, and side-effect profiles. In the absence of this universal cure-all, every medication needs to be considered with great care, weighing its benefits and potential deleterious effects in the context of individual patients, disease processes, desired goals, current medications, and various intrinsic or extrinsic factors such as the patient's beliefs, attitudes, and socioeconomic circumstance.

Pharmacotherapy has undergone unprecedented growth and development over the last century, becoming a cornerstone of medical education and practice. With ever-growing knowledge of pathophysiology, molecular mechanisms, and genetic variations, more and more avenues become available to target these complex processes. Partly as a result of these advances, along with improved sanitation, nutrition, lower rates of infant mortality, and the development of effective vaccines, the average longevity of humans has increased substantially. According to the CDC's National Center for Health Statistics, life expectancy at birth for the U.S. population reached a record high of 78.8 years in 2012 [1]. At the same time, the United States is experiencing significant increase in the proportion of the older people. According to the U.S. Census Bureau projections, by 2030, more than 20% of U.S. residents will be 65 and over, compared with 13% in 2010 and 9.8% in 1970 (Figure 13.1) [2].

Concurrent with this *Silver Tsunami*, medications prescribed to the older adults have shown a steep increase globally. Recently, Guthrie et al. reported on 15-year trends in prescription practices in Scotland. Database analysis of 310,000 patients between 1995 and 2010 revealed that the proportion of adults dispensed ≥5 drugs doubled to 20.8%, and the proportion dispensed ≥10 tripled to 5.8% with a corresponding increase in the potentially serious drug–drug interactions that doubled to 13% in 2010 [3] (Figures 13.2 and 13.3).

According to the CDC's National Center for Health Statistics 2010 Data Brief [4], over the last decade, the percentage of Americans who took at least one prescription drug in the past month increased by 10%. The use of multiple prescription drugs increased by 20% and the use of five or more drugs increased by 70%. Among older Americans (aged 60 and over), more than 76% used two or more prescription drugs, and 37% used five or more prescription drugs (Figure 13.4).

Multiple factors contribute to the expansion of prescribing practices. For example, expert panels have established evidence-based treatment recommendations, which can involve multiple medications for a host of common conditions such as stroke, hypertension, congestive heart failure, and coronary artery disease. The old adage of a "pill for every ill" transforms into "a number of pills for every ill." In delineating the complex societal forces that influence medication use, Busfield [5] describes the complex interactions of the public, physicians, governmental and regulatory agencies, and the pharmaceutical industry on medication use. Even though these entities have diverse incentives, and an array of goals and external pressures, their collective influence results in even greater medication use.

As people age, they are more likely to suffer from different ailments and chronic diseases, and their physicians prescribe more medications to treat these conditions. This process is prone to exponential growth, and the question becomes "how much is too much?" With an increasing

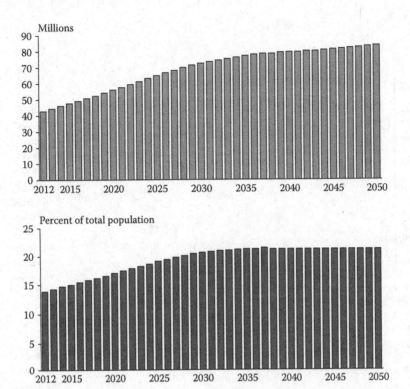

FIGURE 13.1 Population aged 65 and over for the United States: 2012–2015. (From US Census Bureau, 2012 population estimates and 2012 national projections.)

number of medications, there is a corresponding increase in the likelihood of adverse drug effects, drug–drug interactions, and inappropriate use, which in turn correlates with increased morbidity (falls, delirium, loss of function), as well as mortality [6–9]. Considering that the older population is particularly vulnerable to the adverse effects of over-prescribing [10], and that patients over the age of 65 are the largest per capita consumers of prescription medications in the United States, this is a trend that will only increase with aging population [11–18]. These concerns have brought the topic of polypharmacy to the forefront of medical, ethical, and social debate.

Polypharmacy has been defined quite variably. A 2008 review paper by Bushardt et al. found more than 24 distinct definitions of polypharmacy [19]. In general, commonly used definitions include the use of a large number of medications (usually ≥5), the use of potentially inappropriate medications with increased risk of adverse drug effects, the underuse of medications contrary to instructions, and medication duplication [20]. The term "polypharmacy" frequently carries a negative connotation. Still, "rational polypharmacy," where two or more medications with different mechanisms of action, frequently at lower dosages, may be used together in order to achieve a synergistic effect and minimize adverse effects [12]. Given the arguably vague nature of the definition of polypharmacy, some authors have advocated for an alternative definition or lexicon to better define over-prescribing. Terms such as "hyperpharmacotherapy" [19] or "extraordinary prescribing" [21] have been proposed. For the purposes of this chapter, we will use the term "polypharmacy" due to its global recognition and common use in the literature.

In addition to virtually every medication having a set of possible side effects, there is also the possibility of drug–drug interaction, which increases exponentially with the number of medications prescribed. While the chance of two medications having an interaction is approximately 13%, this possibility increases to 38% with four medications, and the risk of having a drug–drug interaction

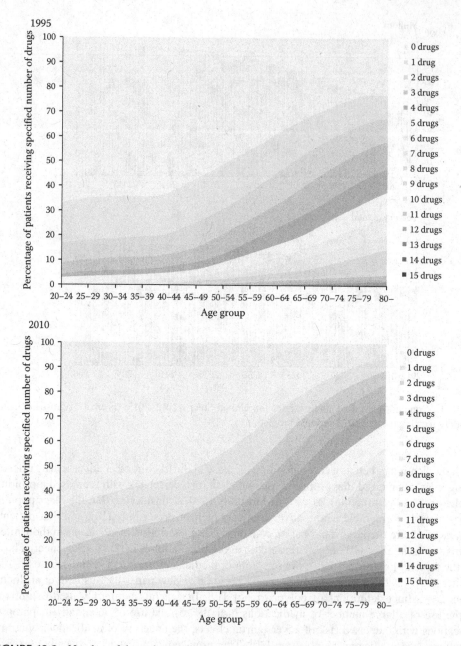

FIGURE 13.2 Number of drug classes dispensed in the 84-day period in 1995 and 2010 by age of patient. (Adapted from Guthrie B et al. *BMC Med* 2015;13:74.)

while taking seven medications simultaneously is estimated to be 82% [15,22]. Therefore, if you see a patient in a hospital ward or in an outpatient clinic taking 9–10 medications (a common occurrence in modern medical practice), you can assume with a high degree of certainty that there is at least one potentially deleterious drug–drug interaction, even if not immediately apparent or easily identifiable.

The trend of increasing prescribing in the aging populations is especially alarming given the growing proportion of older adults within the United States, and the predisposition of the older to

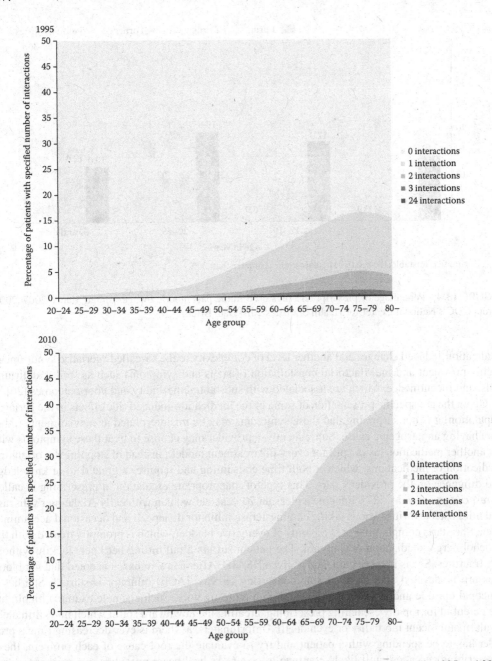

FIGURE 13.3 Number of potentially serious drug–drug interactions in the 84-day period in 1995 and 2010 by age of patient. (Adapted from Guthrie B et al. *BMC Med* 2015;13:74.)

the deleterious effects of polypharmacy and inappropriate prescribing. Of these deleterious effects, some are fairly obvious and straightforward, such as increased risk of gastrointestinal (GI) bleeding with nonsteroidal anti-inflammatory drugs (NSAIDs) or anticoagulants, respiratory depression or somnolence with opioids, and hypotension with antihypertensive medications. Other deleterious effects may be more subtle and difficult to detect since the presentation is nonspecific with symptoms such as confusion, lethargy, light-headedness, depression, constipation, etc. [23–25]. The

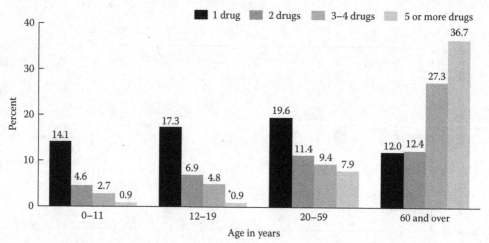

FIGURE 13.4 Percentage of prescription drugs used in the past month, by age: United States, 2007–2008. (From CDC's National Center for Health Statistics 2010 Data Brief.)

medication-induced changes add another level of complexity to the so-called "geriatric syndromes," highly prevalent and multifactorial constellation of signs and symptoms such as frailty, delirium, falls, and incontinence, which are associated with substantial morbidity and poor outcomes [26].

Given the nonspecific presentation of some of the medication-induced side effects in the geriatric population, it is not surprising that these symptoms may be misinterpreted as new ailments rather than having an iatrogenic cause. Subsequently, a provider may choose to treat these symptoms with yet another medication (as in "pill for every ill" treatment model), instead of stopping the offending medication or medications, which is both time consuming and requires a great deal of knowledge and diligence on the provider's part. This type of inappropriate escalation in prescribing is called *"prescribing cascade"* [27]. Imagine a pleasant 70-year-old woman with early Alzheimer's disease and mild osteoarthritis, who is taking cholinesterase inhibitor donepezil and occasional acetaminophen. She starts complaining of symptoms of overactive bladder, which is promptly treated with the anticholinergic medication oxybutynin. The patient suffers a fall hitting her knee, luckily without any fractures. She is in more pain, and is given NSAID. After a few weeks, it is noted that her blood pressure is elevated, and an adenosine-converting enzyme (ACE) inhibitor is started. She has a syncopal episode and is taken to a hospital with a hip fracture. Such a simple example highlights the potential for rapidly escalating prescribing, creating the downward spiral which may ultimately result in significant morbidity or even death. Unfortunately, as there is ever-decreasing time a provider has to be spending with a patient and try to evaluate the root cause of each problem, these "prescribing cascades" will likely continue to occur. As healthcare providers, we must recognize the importance of raising awareness of the problem of polypharmacy and potentially inappropriate prescribing and incorporate this topic into every level of medical education, starting in medical school and continuing throughout the professional career.

13.3 POLYPHARMACY AND REHABILITATION

Rehabilitation physicians frequently manage complex patients with several comorbid conditions and on multiple medications. Physiatrists are uniquely positioned to be on the lookout for polypharmacy and inappropriate prescribing given the multiple problems it poses, including functional decline. This pharmacologic vigilance can span the entire range of the physiatric practice, from acute hospitalization to outpatient clinics. In an acute inpatient rehabilitation setting, physiatrists, alone or in teams with primary care providers and various specialists, can be the ones to undertake "medication list debridement" while monitoring patients in a controlled environment for any unwanted changes. In an outpatient setting, taking the time to review current medications and optimize prescriptions when needed can be an important step in ensuring appropriate care, minimizing morbidity, and maximizing functional gains. Rational prescribing practices can improve the lives of our patients and make the job of a physician more satisfying and fulfilling.

Rehabilitation physicians use pharmacotherapy to treat a wide range of conditions. As a group, we prescribe medications to improve pain, mood, sleep, attention, cognition, spasticity, and bowel or bladder dysfunction, to name a few. Many medications used to treat these conditions may themselves cause problems and should be prescribed with a great deal of caution and substantial knowledge of pharmacology and pathophysiology.

13.4   AGING AND DRUG METABOLISM

When caring for older patients, the changes in physiology and drug metabolism are important to keep in mind and consider in the context of each prescription, as well as comprehensive medication list assessments. These changes include pharmacokinetics (absorption, distribution, metabolism, and excretion); pharmacodynamics (physiologic effects of the mediation), as well as age-related changes in body composition and physiology. Table 13.1 summarizes these changes in older patients.

Even though older patients with multiple comorbidities are frequently the ones being prescribed multiple medications, this group is often underrepresented in the clinical drug trials. There are several reasons for this underrepresentation. Some of these reasons include complex protocols, research focus on aggressive therapies with substantial toxicity, restrictive entry criteria often excluding concurrent conditions and medication, limited expectations of benefits of patients and their families, and lack of financial, logistic, and social support [28]. Van Spall et al. published a study looking at exclusion criteria for RCTs done between 1994 and 2006 in general medical journals with a high

---

TABLE 13.1

Age-Related Physiologic Changes and Potential Pharmacokinetic Consequences

	Age-Related Alterations	Implication(s)
Body composition	↑ Body fat	↑ Vd and longer t1/2 for lipophilic medications
	↓ Total body water	↓ Vd, increased plasma concentration of hydrophilic medications
Protein binding	↓ Serum albumin	↑ Free fraction of in plasma of highly protein-bound acidic medications
Gastrointestinal function	↓ GI motility	Potential increased vulnerability to opiate-related bowel dysmotility
	↓ pH	Rarely clinically significant
Liver function	↓ Hepatic blood flow	↓ First-pass effect, resulting in higher medication bioavailability
Kidney function	↓ Renal blood flow	↓ Renal elimination of medications, resulting in
	↓ Glomerular filtration rate (GFR)	prolonged effects of metabolites
Tissue sensitivity	Changes in receptor number, second-messenger function, and cellular response	Potential ↑ or ↓ in sensitivity to an agent

Source: Geller AI et al. *PM&R* 2012;4(3):198–216.

impact factor [29]. They found that patients were excluded due to age in 72.1% of all trials (38.5% specifically in older adults). Individuals receiving commonly prescribed medications were excluded in 54.1% of trials. Of all exclusion criteria, only 47.2% were graded as strongly justified in the context of the specific RCTs.

13.5 MEDICATIONS COMMONLY ADMINISTERED IN THE OLDER ADULT POPULATION

There is an abundance of medication that is commonly prescribed in the older population. Many of the medications that are used have a significant list of side effects, which are often treated with the addition of other medications. This may lead to a prescribing cascade and increasing polypharmacy [30,31]. In the following section, we will provide a general overview of the medications associated with the highest risk of adverse events. For ease of reference, the common "offenders" are placed in table format at the conclusion of this section.

13.6 PAIN MEDICATIONS

The variety of commonly used pain medications ranges from topical analgesics to intravenous opioids. Here, we discuss the most commonly used oral medications. We focus initially on medications used to treat nociceptive pain (i.e., pain originating from bones, organs, or other tissues), then review medications for neuropathic pain.

Acetaminophen, which is available as an over-the-counter medication, is a first-line medication for pain relief for many acute and chronic conditions such as osteoarthritis [31,32]. Due to the potentially hazardous effects on the liver, the U.S. Food and Drug Administration (FDA) now restricts the amount that can be combined with other medications to 325 mg since, the maximal recommended daily dose is not to exceed 3 g a day [32–34]. Greater restrictions are usually placed on patients taking the blood thinning medication, warfarin, to 2 g per day or those with alcohol consumption greater than two drinks per day [35].

NSAIDs are not only widely prescribed but are also easily accessible over the counter. These medications are a very broad class (i.e., COX-1 vs. COX-2 inhibitors) and are commonly used in the treatment of acute and chronic pain. The most common complications are gastrointestinal bleeding, kidney injury, cardiovascular disease, and hematologic problems [35] and the FDA recommends against the chronic use of NSAIDs in the older adult due to these risks [36–38,93,94].

The use of opioids for the management of chronic pain in the older adult has surged over the last couple of decades [39]. Although the American Geriatric Society (AGS) cautiously recommends opioid therapy in the older adult population with persistent moderate to severe pain, there is little evidence in the literature showing efficacy of opioids in the management of chronic pain [40,41]. The rate of overdose from opioids has risen drastically over the last decade, primarily due to the increase in prescribing practices of opioids for the treatment of chronic pain [39,42]. In the older adult population, the use of opioids caries up to an eightfold increase in the risk of respiratory depression, falls, and fractures [43]. Mild side effects in this class of medications also include nausea, vomiting, somnolence, constipation, altered liver metabolism, and hypogonadism [43]. Opioids are commonly prescribed in combination with acetaminophen. Many over-the-counter medications also contain acetaminophen, which can lead to unintended excessive use of this medications.

Tramadol has become a more commonly prescribed pain medication due to its action as a weak mu-opioid receptor agonist with serotonergic and noradrenergic properties. The increased risk of serotonin syndrome and lowering of the seizure threshold are the major side effects, with nausea being a common clinical side effect associated with tramadol. Because tramadol is only a weak opioid receptor agonist, there is a lower risk of tolerance, dependence, and respiratory depression [44].

The treatment of neuropathic pain (i.e., pain involving the central or peripheral nervous system) in the older adult involves only a few first-line agents. Gabapentin and Pregabalin work in the central nervous system on voltage-dependent calcium channels and are commonly used to treat pain associated with diabetic neuropathy, postherpetic neuralgia, fibromyalgia, and poststroke and spinal cord injury dysesthesia. Common side effects include edema, somnolence, dizziness, and abnormal thinking [45,46]. Both of these medications are excreted by the kidneys and require adjustments in dosing in patients with chronic renal insufficiency.

Serotonin and norepinephrine reuptake inhibitors (SNRIs) (e.g., duloxetine, venlafaxine, and mirtazapine) are a newer class of medications that are more commonly used for the treatment of depression [47]. More recent studies have shown some efficacy in the treatment of chronic pain with neuropathic properties with these agents [48,95]. The side effects of these medications are discussed with the antidepressant medications later in this section. Opioids can be effective agents for neuropathic pain and are discussed elsewhere.

13.6.1 Neurostimulants

Neurostimulants are commonly used in the older adult population to aid in memory, attention, arousal, and processing speed [49] through a variety of mechanisms. For example, they can exert their affects by inhibiting dopamine and norepinephrine reuptake (i.e., methylphenidate), reducing cholinesterase (i.e., donepezil), and by blocking the N-methyl-D-aspartate (NMDA) receptor (i.e., memantine) to name just a few [50]. Understandably, the side effects of these medications vary widely and include confusion, insomnia, headaches, and gastrointestinal symptoms.

13.6.2 Antidepressants

Depression is commonly encountered in the older adult population and can commonly be confused with Alzheimer disease or memory impairment. There are several different types of antidepressants used, with the most common class being the selective serotonin reuptake inhibitors (SSRIs). SSRIs are considered first-line for the treatment of depression and have replaced many of the older classes of medications used to treat depression (i.e., tricyclic antidepressants [TCAs] and monoamine oxidase inhibitors [MAOIs]) due to a better side effect profile. However, these medications are not without risk, and some of the common adverse effects include hyponatremia, increased risk of bleeding, insomnia, sexual dysfunction, and vasoconstriction [47,51,52].

Other medications commonly used to treat depression include SNRIs, for example, duloxetine, venlafaxine, as well as bupropion. SNRIs also carry the risk of serotonin syndrome and the effects of increased norepinephrine effects (i.e., hypertension, dry mouth, restlessness, headache, etc.) [97]. Bupropion has a relatively mild side-effect profile, but has been shown to lower the seizure threshold and cause sexual dysfunction [47]. TCAs and MAOIs are rarely prescribed as the primary treatment of depression due their anticholinergic effects [47].

13.6.3 Sleep Medications

Insomnia and sleep disturbances are reported in up to 40% of the older adult population [53]. Patients with sleep difficulties commonly meet criteria for the diagnosis of depression and other medical conditions such as sleep apnea, congestive heart failure, and restless leg syndrome, which should be ruled out as underlying causes [54]. Clinically, providers usually take a hierarchical approach to the management of sleep disorders. Sleep hygiene is the first-line treatment prior to the addition of medications [55,56]. Melatonin should be considered first due to its mild side effect profile, which may include morning drowsiness, headaches, and vivid dreams. Other medications include sedating antidepressants (e.g., trazodone and mirtazapine), nonbenzodiazepines binding gamma-aminobutyric acid (GABA) receptors (e.g., zolpidem), and benzodiazepines, which also bind GABA receptors (e.g., alprazolam and temazepam) [57]. Trazodone has been shown to cause QT prolongation, orthostatic hypotension, serotonin syndrome, and neuroleptic malignant syndrome. The nonbenzodiazepines have less anxiolytic and anticonvulsant activity, but are associated with cognitive side effects (e.g., hallucinations and amnesia), gastrointestinal symptoms, and the development of drug tolerance and dependence [57]. Benzodiazepines ("benzos") have been found to be particularly harmful in the older adult population due to the increased risk of falls, fracture, tolerance, dependence, and cognitive effects [57–59]. For this reason, the AGS strongly recommends the avoidance of these medications in the older adult. Diphenhydramine and amitriptyline are two medications that are often inappropriately used for sleep and should be avoided in the older adult due to their anticholinergic properties [60,61].

13.6.4 SEXUAL DYSFUNCTION AND BPH MEDICATIONS

There are three FDA approved medications for erectile dysfunction in men (e.g., sildenafil/Viagra, tadalafil/Cialis, and vardenafil/Levitra). All of these medications work by increasing blood flow to the penis and thereby have an increased risk of hypotension. Caution should be used in those who are taking antihypertensive medications, alpha blockers for benign prostatic hyperplasia (BPH) (e.g., tamsulosin), or nitroglycerines [62]. Administration of alpha blockers at bedtime, instead of morning, may limit daytime orthostasis.

13.6.5 ANTIHYPERTENSIVE MEDICATIONS

Hypertension is extremely common in the general population, with a prevalence of 60%–80% in the older adult [63]. Diuretics have the most serious side-effect profile due to the increased risks of hypotension, dizziness, electrolyte disturbances, and falls. Commonly prescribed diuretics include furosemide and hydrochlorothiazide [64]. All antihypertensives have the potential to cause hypotension and orthostasis. Modified guidelines from the JNC-8 suggest that hypertension in those ≥60 years of age, should only be treated if measurements exceed >150 mm Hg for systolic or >90 mm Hg for diastolic pressure [65].

13.6.6 HYPOGLYCEMIC MEDICATIONS

Oral hypoglycemic medications, such as metformin and glipizide, are commonly used to treat diabetes mellitus. Side effects commonly include hypoglycemia, gastrointestinal disturbances, and dizziness. This group of medications is also associated with increased visits to the emergency department [66]. It should also be mentioned that metformin can cause lactic acidosis and should be used with caution in those with renal insufficiency [67].

13.6.7 ANTICOAGULANT AND ANTIPLATELET AGENTS

Anticoagulant and antiplatelet medications are associated with an increased risk of bleeding [68]. These medications are used to treat those with stroke, myocardial infarction, and clotting disorders [69]. Caution should be used when prescribing the medications for the older adult, especially for those with an increased fall risk [70,71]. Anticoagulants are associated with increased visits to the emergency department in the older adult [66].

13.6.8 ANTICHOLINERGIC PROPERTIES

Anticholinergic medications are neither used to treat one specific condition nor do they belong to one class of medications; however, the associated side effects make them an extremely high-risk group of medications in the older adult population. These medications increase morbidity and mortality for the older adult [60]. Medications with the most anticholinergic properties include TCAs, typical antipsychotics, antihistamines (e.g., diphenhydramine, promethazine, and hydroxyzine), paroxetine, methocarbamol, meclizine, scopolamine, agents to treat urinary incontinence (e.g., oxybutynin and tolterodine), and atropine to name a few [60,72]. The degree of anticholinergic properties is clinically measured as the anticholinergic burden (ACB) of a medication. The most common adverse effects of medications with a high ACB (i.e., 1 or 2) include dry mouth, blurred vision, decreased sweating, delirium, sedation, urinary retention, and constipation. In the older adult population, these medications should be avoided and alternatives used whenever possible [60,73,61].

13.6.9 APPETITE STIMULANTS

Unintended weight loss in the older adult contributes to increased morbidity and mortality, due to an increased risk of falls, infections, and depression [74–76]. The underlying etiology for weight loss can be extensive, with depression, cancer, and gastrointestinal disorders as the most common culprits [77–80,96,98]. Polypharmacy in itself, is a relatively common cause of unintended weight loss due to the side effects of many of the medications that are commonly prescribed for this population (e.g., the SSRI fluoxetine) [81]. A thorough physical and mental examination should be done to try and identify any underlying treatable pathology affecting the appetite or metabolic rate [82,83]. The diagnostic workup will likely also include a battery of laboratory tests and imaging studies. Management of unintentional weight loss should be approached initially as conservative as possible. Initial treatment strategies may include identifying environmental factors that may be negatively affecting food consumption, which often can be present in long-term care facilities. Some common environmental factors include staff turnover, dedicated meal times, and feeding protocols [84]. Ensuring that diets are as unrestricted as possible with the help of dieticians and speech therapists is also a key component to increasing caloric intake. Medications are also commonly used to promote weight gain in the older adult; however, many of these agents have not been studied, and the U.S. FDA has not approved the usage of these drugs for the management of weight loss [85]. The most common agents utilized include mirtazapine (i.e., an SNRI antidepressant), dronabinol (i.e., a cannabinoid derivative), and megestrol. Common side effects encountered with these medications include confusion, edema, and constipation [81,84,86]. Megestrol is also associated with an increased risk of thromboembolism and should be used with caution [84,87,88].

13.7 POLYPHARMACY IN CLINICAL SETTINGS

Managing multiple medications is a challenging task in clinical settings particularly with the increased specialization, fragmentation, and time pressures of contemporary healthcare. The notion of "start low and go slow" is a familiar dogma in medicine, especially for geriatric and other vulnerable populations. Reasonable strategies for the management of multiple medications include physician engagement, accurate medication lists, patient-centered process, explicit and implicit criteria for guidance, technology and computer-assisted tools to identify problem areas and offer solutions, and perhaps most importantly, with an attitude of medication debridement [92] (Table 13.2).

TABLE 13.2
Strategies for Managing Polypharmacy in the Older Adult

Physician engagement

Accurate medication lists

Medication assessments—effectiveness and potential side effects

Patient and care-giver engagement in prescribing

Explicit and implicit criteria for guidance

Computer-assisted tools for problem identification and to guide interventions an attitude of *Medication Debridement*

TABLE 13.3

Side Effects and Common Offenders

Side Effect	Common Medication Offenders
Bleeding	NSAIDs (e.g., indomethacin and ketorolac), anticoagulants (e.g., warfarin), and antiplatelets (e.g., aspirin and plavix)
Cardiovascular disease	NSAIDs
Cerebrovascular disease	NSAIDs
Cognitive effects	TCAs, benzodiazepines, antipsychotics, opioids, gabapentin, pregabalin, tramadol, donepezil, anticholinergics, and appetite stimulants (megastrol, dronabinol, and mirtazapine)
Drowsiness	Benzodiazepines, opioids, gabapentin, pregabalin, TCAs, SNRIs (mirtazapine and trazodone), melatonin, zolpidem, antipsychotics, and antihistamines
Peripheral edema	Antihypertensives (e.g., amlodipine), gabapentin, and pregabalin
Gastrointestinal symptoms (e.g., nausea, vomiting, and constipation)	Opioids, tramadol, zolpidem, donepezil, methylphenidate, SNRIs, TCAs, SSRIs, melatonin, and appetite stimulants
Headache	Bupropion, NSAIDs, melatonin, zolpidem, and methylphenidate
Hepatotoxicity	Acetaminophen and gabapentin
Hypertension	Methylphenidate and SNRIs
Hyponatremia	SSRIs and SNRIs
Hypotension	Diuretics (e.g., furosemide and hydrochlorothiazide), tramadol, TCAs (e.g., amitriptyline), opioids, sildenafil, vardenafil, and tadalafil
Insomnia	SSRIs (e.g., paroxetine), SNRIs, and methylphenidate
Lowered seizure threshold	Bupropion and methylphenidate
Peripheral edema	Gabapentin and pregabalin
QT prolongation	Opioids (e.g., methadone), typical antipsychotics, and SNRI (e.g., trazodone)
Renal dysfunction	NSAIDs
Tolerance and dependence	Opioids, benzodiazepines, zolpidem, and tramadol

Note: SSRI, selective serotonin reuptake inhibitor; TCA, tricyclic antidepressant; NSAIDs, nonsteroidal anti-inflammatory drugs; and SNRIs, serotonin and norepinephrine-uptake inhibitor.

While trying to optimize medications, we find it useful to remain cognizant of the common side effects and some of the drugs implicated in producing these side effects. Table 13.3 provides a template for organizing clinical thought process when evaluating potential side effects in correlation with pharmacologic therapy.

13.8   CASE STUDY: A RATIONAL PRESCRIBING INITIATIVE WITH A COMPUTER-ASSISTED DECISION TOOL

We (the authors) developed and implemented a 3-year quality improvement (QI) project to promote rational prescribing in the older adult in an acute inpatient rehabilitation unit in an academic medical center. In weekly interdisciplinary polypharmacy rounds over the course of 1 year, we reviewed medications for all inpatients 65 years of age and older for potentially inappropriate medications. A novel tool to identify potentially inappropriate medications based on the 2012 Beers Criteria [89], the ACB index [90], and population data on emergency hospitalizations [66] were used to guide the discussion. In the preliminary data analysis, potentially inappropriate medications decreased from 3.89 to 1.72 ($p < 0.01$); the ACB score was reduced from 1.70 to 1.25 ($p = 0.03$), and the mean total number of medications decreased from 12.76 to 12.01 ($p = 0.20$) between year 1 ($n = 127$) and year 3 ($n = 138$). The results of this project suggest that interdisciplinary pharmacy rounds coupled with a tool to identify potential offending medications may be an effective means to encourage appropriate prescribing practices [91].

13.9 SILVER TSUNAMIS, GOLDEN MEANS, AND RATIONAL PRESCRIBING

We are in the midst of a *Silver Tsunami* as the number of the older adults increase concurrent with a greater proportion of the population in this age group. Hence, a shrinking number of working age adults is available to assist this larger vulnerable population. There is an opportunity for rehabilitation professionals to expand our traditional interventions of exercise, orthotics, and assistive devices to include medication prescribing.

Rational prescribing connotes a proactive approach to evaluation, intervention, and monitoring of medications. Medications should be selected based on their potential benefits while minimizing undesirable side effects including the all too common drug–drug interactions. After initiation of a medication, beneficial and detrimental effects need to be monitored and adjustments made accordingly. This iterative process is a cornerstone of rational prescribing.

Ample evidence exists on the deleterious effects of polypharmacy. More medications result in greater incidence of medication-induced complications such as falls, fractures, confusion, and decreased safety awareness along with the common side effects of sedation, anxiety, orthostasis, constipation, and disorientation. The unaware professional can easily fall into the prescribing cascade resulting in more meds intended to dampen the side effects of earlier meds. We seek a *Golden Mean* of medications for our *Silver Tsunami* demographic.

13.10 CONCLUSION

Rational medication prescribing in frail, older adult individuals plays a pivotal role in the maintenance and promotion of function in this vulnerable population. Physiatrists and other rehabilitation providers have a unique opportunity to promote rational prescribing and lessen the burden of polypharmacy. The rehabilitation focus on function, interdisciplinary teamwork, and patient-centered care provides an excellent foundation to impact the older adult and other vulnerable groups through the application of straightforward principles outlined in this chapter.

REFERENCES

1. Xu J, Kochanek KD, Murphy SL, Arias E. Mortality in the United States, 2012. NCHS Data Brief, Number 168, October 2014.
2. US Census Bureau, 2012 population estimates and 2012 National projections. http://www.census.gov/population/projections/data/national/2012.html.
3. Guthrie B, Makubate B, Hernandez-Santiago V et al. The rising tide of polypharmacy and drug–drug interactions: Population database analysis 1995–2010. *BMC Med* 2015;13:74.
4. Gu Q, Dillon CF, Burt VL. Prescription drug use continues to increase: U.S. Prescription Drug Data for 2007–2008. NCHS Data Brief, Number 42, September 2010.
5. Busfield J. "A pill for every ill": Explaining the expansion in medicine use. *Soc Sci Med* 2010;70:934–941.
6. Jyrkkä J, Vartiainen L, Hartikainen S, Sulkava R, Enlund H. Increasing use of medicines in elderly persons: A five-year follow-up of the Kuopio 75 Study. *Eur J Clin Pharmacol* 2006;62:151–158.
7. Kojima T, Akishita M, Nakamura T et al. Association of polypharmacy with fall risk among geriatric outpatients. *Geriatr Gerontol Int* 2011;11:438–444.
8. Kragh A, Elmstahl S, Atroshi I. Older adults' medication use 6 months before and after hip fracture: A population-based cohort study. *J Am Geriatr Soc* 2011;59:863–868.
9. Herr M, Robine JM, Pinot J, Arvieu JJ, Ankri J. Polypharmacy and frailty: Prevalence, relationship, and impact on mortality in a French sample of 2350 old people. *Pharmacoepidemiol Drug Saf* 2015;24(6):637–646.
10. Scott I, Jayathissa S. Quality of drug prescribing in older patients: Is there a problem and can we improve it? *Intern Med J* 2010;40:7–18.
11. Hayes BD, Klein-Schwartz W, Barrueto F Jr. Polypharmacy and the geriatric patient. *Clin Geriatr Med* 2007;23:371–390, vii.

12. Gallagher RM. Pain science and rational polypharmacy: An historical perspective. *Am J Phys Med Rehabil* 2005;84(Suppl):S1–3.

13. Eskildsen M, Price T. Nursing home care in the USA. *Geriatr Gerontol Int* 2009;9:1–6.

14. Greenwald DA. Aging, the gastrointestinal tract, and risk of acid-related disease. *Am J Med* 2004;117(Suppl 5A):8S–13S.

15. Page RL II, Linnebur SA, Bryant LL, Ruscin JM. Inappropriate prescribing in the hospitalized elderly patient: Defining the problem, evaluation tools, and possible solutions. *Clin Interv Aging* 2010;5:75–87.

16. Qato DM, Alexander GC, Conti RM, Johnson M, Schumm P, Lindau ST. Use of prescription and over-the-counter medications and dietary supplements among older adults in the United States. *JAMA* 2008;300:2867–2878.

17. Spinewine A, Schmader KE, Barber N et al. Appropriate prescribing in elderly people: How well can it be measured and optimised? *Lancet* 2007;370:173–184.

18. Stegemann S, Ecker F, Maio M et al. Geriatric drug therapy: Neglecting the inevitable majority. *Ageing Res Rev* 2010;9:384–398.

19. Bushardt RL, Massey EB, Simpson TW, Ariail JC, Simpsom KN. Polypharmacy: Misleading but manageable. *Clin Interv Aging* 2008;3(2):383–389.

20. Maggiore RJ, Gross CP, Hurria A. Polypharmacy in older adults with cancer. *Oncologist* 2010;15:507–522.

21. Gillette C, Prunty L, Wolcott J et al. A new lexicon for polypharmacy: Implications for research, practice, and education. *Res Soc Adm Pharm* 2015;11(3):468–471.

22. Goldberg RM, Mabee J, Chan L, Wong S. Drug–drug and drug–disease interactions in the ED: Analysis of a high-risk population. *Am J Emerg Med* 1996;14:447–450.

23. Bootman JL, Harrison DL, Cox E. The health care cost of drug-related morbidity and mortality in nursing facilities. *Arch Intern Med* 1997;157:2089–2096.

24. Gallagher P, Barry P, O'Mahony D. Inappropriate prescribing in the elderly. *J Clin Pharm Ther* 2007;32:113–121.

25. Hanlon JT, Schmader KE, Koronkowski MJ et al. Adverse drug events in high risk older outpatients. *J Am Geriatr Soc* 1997;45:945–948.

26. Inouye SK, Studenski S, Tinetti ME et al. Geriatric syndromes: Clinical, research and policy implications of a core geriatric concept. *J Am Geriatr Soc.* 2007;55(5):780–791.

27. Rochon PA, Gurwitz JH. Optimising drug treatment for elderly people: The prescribing cascade. *BMJ* 1997;315:1096–1099.

28. Bayer A, Fish M. The doctor's duty to the elderly patient in clinical trials. *Drug Aging* 2003;20(15):1087–1097.

29. Van Spall HG, Toren A, Kiss A, Fowler RA. Eligibility criteria of randomized controlled trials published in high-impact general medical journals: A systematic sampling review. *JAMA* 2007;297:1233–1240.

30. Kaufman DW, Kelly JP, Rosenberg L, Anderson TE, Mitchell AA. Recent patterns of medication use in the ambulatory adult population of the United States: The Slone survey. *JAMA* 2002;287:337–344.

31. American Geriatics Society Panel. Pharmacological management of persistent pain in older persons. *J Am Geriatr Soc* 2009;57:1331–1346.

32. Lee WM. Acetaminophen-related acute liver failure in the United States. *Hepatol Res* 2008;38:S3–S8.

33. Larson AM, Polson J, Fontana RJ et al. Acetaminophen-induced acute liver failure: Results of a United States multicenter, prospective study. *Hepatology* 2005;42:1364–1372.

34. Burgess S. FDA limits acetaminophen in prescription combination products; requires liver toxicity warnings. *FDA News Release*. Silver Spring, Maryland: US Food and Drug Administration, Center for Drug Evaluation and Research; 2011.

35. Zhang Q, Bal-dit-Sollier C, Drouet L et al. Interaction between acetaminophen and warfarin in adults receiving long-term oral anticoagulants: A randomized controlled trial. *Eur J Clin Pharmacol* 2011;67:309–314.

36. FDA Drug Safety Communication: FDA strengthens warning that non-aspirin nonsteroidal anti-inflammatory drugs (NSAIDs) can cause heart attacks or strokes; 2015.

37. Schilling A, Corey R, Leonard M, Eghtesad B. Acetaminophen: Old drug, new warnings. *Cleve Clin J Med* 2010;77:19–27.

38. Vandraas KF, Spigset O, Mahic M, Slordal L. Non-steroidal antiinflammatory drugs: Use and co-treatment with potentially interacting medications in the elderly. *Eur J Clin Pharmacol* 2010;66:823–829.

39. Okie S. A flood of opioids, a rising tide of deaths. *N Engl J Med* 2010;363:1981–1985.

40. Manchikanti L, Vallejo R, Manchikanti KN, Benyamin RM, Datta S, Christo PJ. Effectiveness of long-term opioid therapy for chronic non-cancer pain. *Pain Physician* 2011;14:E133–156.

41. Chou R, Ballantyne JC, Fanciullo GJ, Fine PG, Miaskowski C. Research gaps on use of opioids for chronic noncancer pain: Findings from a review of the evidence for an American Pain Society and American Academy of Pain Medicine clinical practice guideline. *J Pain* 2009;10:147–159.

42. Fishbain DA, Cole B, Lewis J, Rosomoff HL, Rosomoff RS. What percentage of chronic nonmalignant pain patients exposed to chronic opioid analgesic therapy develop abuse/addiction and/or aberrant drug-related behaviors? A structured evidence-based review. *Pain Med* 2008;9:444–459.

43. Barber JB, Gibson SJ. Treatment of chronic non-malignant pain in the elderly: Safety considerations. *Drug Saf* 2009;32:457–474.

44. Leppert W. Tramadol as an analgesic for mild to moderate cancer pain. *Pharmacol Rep* 2009;61:978–992.

45. Moore RA, Wiffen PJ, Derry S, McQuay HJ. Gabapentin for chronic neuropathic pain and fibromyalgia in adults. *Cochrane Database Syst Rev* 2011;(3):CD007938.

46. Moore RA, Straube S, Wiffen PJ, Derry S, McQuay HJ. Pregabalin for acute and chronic pain in adults. *Cochrane Database Syst Rev* 2009;(3):CD007076.

47. Price A, Rayner L, Okon-Rocha E et al. Antidepressants for the treatment of depression in neurological disorders: A systematic review and meta-analysis of randomised controlled trials. *J Neurol Neurosurg Psychiatry* 2011;82:914–923.

48. Reisner L. Pharmacological management of persistent pain in older persons. *J Pain* 2011;12(Suppl 1):S21–29.

49. Casey DA, Antimisiaris D, O'Brien J. Drugs for Alzheimer's disease: Are they effective? *Pharm Ther* 2010;35(4):208–211.

50. Emptage RE, Semia TP. Depression in the medically ill elderly: A focus on methylphenidate. *Ann Pharmacother* 1996;30(2):151–157.

51. Diem SJ, Blackwell TL, Stone KL et al. Use of antidepressant medications and risk of fracture in older women. *Calcif Tissue Int* 2011;88:476–484.

52. Jacob S, Spinler SA. Hyponatremia associated with selective serotonin-reuptake inhibitors in older adults. *Ann Pharmacother* 2006;40:1618–1622.

53. Sukying C, Bhokakul V, Udomsubpayakul U. An epidemiological study on insomnia in an elderly Thai population. *J Med Assoc Thai* 2003;86:316–324.

54. Avidan AY. Sleep changes and disorders in the elderly patient. *Curr Neurol Neurosci Rep* 2002;2:178–185.

55. Friedman L, Bliwise DL, Yesavage JA, Salom SR. A preliminary study comparing sleep restriction and relaxation treatments for insomnia in older adults. *J Gerontol* 1991;46:P1–P8.

56. Klink ME, Quan SF, Kaltenborn WT, Lebowitz MD. Risk factors associated with complaints of insomnia in a general adult population. Influence of previous complaints of insomnia. *Arch Intern Med* 1992;152:1634–1637.

57. Glass J, Lanctot KL, Herrmann N, Sproule BA, Busto UE. Sedative hypnotics in older people with insomnia: Meta-analysis of risks and benefits. *BMJ* 2005;331:1169.

58. Zint K, Haefeli WE, Glynn RJ, Mogun H, Avorn J, Sturmer T. Impact of drug interactions, dosage, and duration of therapy on the risk of hip fracture associated with benzodiazepine use in older adults. *Pharmacoepidemiol Drug Saf* 2010;19:1248–1255.

59. van der Hooft CS, Schoofs MW, Ziere G et al. Inappropriate benzodiazepine use in older adults and the risk of fracture. *Br J Clin Pharmacol* 2008;66:276–282.

60. Fox C, Richardson K, Maidment ID et al. Anticholinergic medication use and cognitive impairment in the older population: The Medical Research Council Cognitive Function and Ageing Study. *J Am Geriatr Soc* 2011;59(8):147–183.

61. Boustani MA, Campbell NL, Munger S, Maidment I, Fox GC. Impact of anticholinergics on the aging brain: a review and practical application. *Aging Health* 2008;4(3):311–320.

62. Yuan J, Zhang R, Yang Z et al. Comparative effectiveness and safety of oral phosphodiesterase type 5 inhibitors for erectile dysfunction: A systematic review and network meta-analysis. *Eur Urol* 2013;63(5):902–912. doi: 10.1016/j.eururo.2013.01.012. Epub January 31, 2013.

63. Greenberg A. Diuretic complications. *Am J Med Sci* 2000;319(1):10–24.

64. Aronow WS, Fleg JL, Pepine CJ et al. ACCF/AHA 2011 expert consensus document on hypertension in the elderly: A report of the American College of Cardiology Foundation Task Force on Clinical Expert Consensus Documents. *Circulation* 2011;123(21):2434–506. doi: 10.1161/CIR.0b013e31821daaf6. Epub April 25, 2011.

65. James PA, Oparil S, Carter BL et al. Evidence-based guideline for the management of high blood pressure in adults report from the panel members appointed to the eighth joint national committee (JNC 8). *JAMA* 2014;311(5):507–520. doi:10.1001/jama.2013.284427.

66. Budnitz DS, Lovegrove MC, Shehab N, Richards CL. Emergency hospitalizations for adverse drug events in older Americans. *N Engl J Med* 2011;365:2002–2012.
67. Luna B, Feinglos MN. Oral agents in the management of type 2 diabetes mellitus. *Am Fam Physician* 2001;63(9):1747–1756.
68. Lopes RD, Alexander KP, Manoukian SV et al. Advanced age, antithrombotic strategy, and bleeding in non-ST-segment elevation acute coronary syndromes. *J Am Coll Cardiol* 2009;53:1021–1030.
69. Fitzmaurice DA, Blann AD, Lip GYH. Bleeding risks of antithrombotic therapy. *BMJ* 2002;325:828–831.
70. Gage BF, Fihn SD, White RH. Warfarin therapy for an octogenarian who has atrial fibrillation. *Ann Intern Med* 2001;134(6):465.
71. Garwood CL, Corbett TL. Use of anticoagulation in elderly patients with atrial fibrillation who are at risk for falls. *Ann Pharmacother* 2008;42(4):523–532. doi: 10.1345/aph.1K498. Epub March 11, 2008.
72. Tranulis C, Skalli L, Lalonde P, Nicole L, Stip E. Benefits and risks of antipsychotic polypharmacy: An evidence-based review of the literature. *Drug Saf* 2008;31:7–20.
73. Campbell N, Boustani M, Limbil T et al. The cognitive impact of anticholinergics: A clinical review. *Clin Interv Aging* 2009;4(1):225–233.
74. Murden RA, Ainslie NK. Recent weight loss is related to short-term mortality in nursing homes. *J Gen Intern Med* 1994; 9:648–650.
75. Calle EE, Thun MJ, Petrelli JM, Rodriguez C, Heath CW Jr. Body-mass index and mortality in a prospective cohort of U.S. adults. *N Engl J Med* 1999;341:1097–1105.
76. Ryan C, Bryant E, Eleazer P, Rhodes A, Guest K. Unintentional weight loss in long-term care: Predictor of mortality in the elderly. *South Med J* 1995; 88:721–724.
77. Reife CM. Involuntary weight loss. *Med Clin North Am* 1995;79:299–313.
78. Fabiny AR, Kiel DP. Assessing and treating weight loss in nursing home patients. *Clin Geriatr Med* 1997;13:737–751.
79. Morley JE. Anorexia of aging: Physiologic and pathologic. *Am J Clin Nutr* 1997;66:760–773.
80. Rabinovitz M, Pitlik SD, Leifer M, Garty M, Rosenfeld JB. Unintentional weight loss. A retrospective analysis of 154 cases. *Arch Intern Med* 1986;146:186–187.
81. Fawcett J, Barkin RL. Review of the results from clinical studies on the efficacy, safety and tolerability of mirtazapine for the treatment of patients with major depression. *J Affect Disord* 1998; 51:267–285.
82. Morley JE, Silver AJ. Nutritional issues in nursing home care. *Ann Intern Med* 1995;123:850–859.
83. Markson EW. Functional, social, and psychological disability as causes of loss of weight and independence in older community-living people. *Clin Geriatr Med* 1997;13:639–652.
84. Huffman GB. Evaluating and treating unintentional weight loss in the elderly. *Am Fam Physician* 2002;15;65(4):640–651.
85. Carr-Lopez SM, Phillips SK. The role of medications in geriatric failure to thrive. *Drug Aging* 1996;9:221–225.
86. Volicer L, Stelly M, Morris J, McLaughlin J, Volicer BJ. Effects of dronabinol on anorexia and disturbed behavior in patients with Alzheimer's disease. *Int J Geriatr Psychiatry* 1997;12:913–919.
87. Chen HC, Leung SW, Wang CJ, Sun LM, Fang FM, Hsu JH. Effect of megestrol acetate and propulsid on nutritional improvement in patients with head and neck cancers undergoing radiotherapy. *Radiother Oncol* 1997;43:75–79.
88. Rowland KM Jr, Loprinzi CL, Shaw EG et al. Randomized double-blind placebo-controlled trial of cisplatin and etoposide plus megestrol acetate/placebo in extensive-stage small-cell lung cancer: A North Central Cancer Treatment Group Study. *J Clin Oncol* 1996;(14):1135–1141.
89. Resnick B, Pacala JT. 2012 Beers Criteria. *J Am Geriatr Soc.* 2012;60(4):612–613.
90. Anticholinergic Burden Index, developed by the Aging Brain Program at Indiana University Center for Aging Research. http://www.agingbraincare.org/uploads/products/ACB_scale_-_legal_size.pdf.
91. Williams CJ, Zhukalin, M, Reed M et al. *Rational Prescribing in an Acute Inpatient Rehabilitation Facility: A Three Year Quality Improvement Project*, June 2015, Atlanta, Georgia, Unpublished.
92. Geller AI, Nopkhun W, Dows-Martinez MN et al. Polypharmacy and the role of physical medicine and rehabilitation. *PM&R* 2012;4(3):198–216.
93. Hegeman J, van den Bemt BJ, Duysens J, van Limbeek J. NSAIDs and the risk of accidental falls in the elderly: A systematic review. *Drug Saf* 2009;32:489–498.

94. Weinblatt ME. Nonsteroidal anti-inflammatory drug toxicity: Increased risk in the elderly. *Scand J Rheumatol Suppl* 1991;91:9–17.
95. Bril V, England J, Franklin GM et al. Evidence-based guideline: Treatment of painful diabetic neuropathy: Report of the American Academy of Neurology, the American Association of Neuromuscular and Electrodiagnostic Medicine, and the American Academy of Physical Medicine and Rehabilitation. *PM R* 2011;3:345–352, 352. e1–21.
96. Morley JE, Kraenzle D. Causes of weight loss in a community nursing home. *J Am Geriatr Soc* 1994;42:583–585.
97. Brymer C, Winograd CH. Fluoxetine in elderly patients: Is there cause for concern? *J Am Geriatr Soc* 1992;40:902–905.
98. Wallace JI, Schwartz RS. Involuntary weight loss in elderly outpatients: Recognition, etiologies, and treatment. *Clin Geriatr Med* 1997;13:717–735.

14 Sleep Disorders in Older Adults

Armando Miciano and David Berbrayer

CONTENTS

14.1 GENERAL PRINCIPLES IN OLDER ADULTS

Nearly half of the older adults report difficulty initiating and maintaining sleep. With age, several changes occur that can place one at risk for sleep disturbance including increased prevalence of medical conditions, increased medication use, age-related changes in various circadian rhythms, and environmental and lifestyle changes. Although sleep complaints are common among all age groups, older adults have increased prevalence of many primary sleep disorders including sleep-disordered breathing (SDB), restless legs syndrome (RLS)/periodic limb movement in sleep (PLMS), rapid eye movement (REM), sleep-behavior disorder (RBD), circadian rhythm sleep disorder (CRSD), and insomnia.

Poor sleep results in increased risk of significant morbidity and mortality. The decrements seen in the sleep of the older adult are often due to a decrease in the ability to get needed sleep. However, the decreased ability is less a function of age and more a function of other factors that accompany aging, such as medical and psychiatric illness, increased medication use, advances in the endogenous circadian clock, and a higher prevalence of specific sleep disorders.

It has long been the belief that the amount of sleep needed per night decreases with age. Yet, in a national survey of older adults, the total sleep time reported was, on average, 7 hours a night—the same or more than that reported by younger adults [1]. Nevertheless, older adults do complain about their sleep. In a large epidemiological study of sleep, Foley et al. [2] found that over 50% of older adults had complaints of insomnia, but that chronic sleep disturbances were associated primarily with indications of poor health. At follow-up 3 years later, of the 2000 survivors with chronic insomnia at baseline, about 50% had no symptoms, and improved sleep was associated with improved health [3]. Other studies using rigorous exclusion criteria for comorbidities have found that disturbed sleep is rare in healthy older adults [4]. These studies have confirmed that, while the need for sleep may not change with age, the ability to get the needed sleep does decrease with age. Multiple causes could be responsible for reduced capability to achieve sufficient sleep with age, including medical or psychiatric illnesses, life changes (e.g., retirement, bereavement, and decreased social interactions), environmental changes (e.g., placement in a nursing home), and polypharmacy.

14.2 DSM-5 DEFINITION

The *Diagnostic and Statistical Manual of Mental Disorders*, fifth edition (DSM-5) classification of sleep–wake disorders is intended for use by general mental health and medical clinicians. Sleep–wake disorders encompass 10 disorders or disorder groups: insomnia disorder, hypersomnolence disorder, narcolepsy, breathing-related sleep disorders, circadian rhythm sleep–wake disorders, nonrapid eye movement (NREM) sleep arousal disorders, nightmare disorder, RBD, RLS, and substance/medication-induced sleep disorder. Individuals with these disorders typically present with sleep–wake complaints of dissatisfaction regarding the quality, timing, and amount of sleep. Resulting daytime distress and impairment are core features shared by all these sleep–wake disorders.

The DSM-5's major criteria for diagnosis of *insomnia* include the following:

- Dissatisfaction with sleep quantity or quality, with one or more of the following symptoms: difficulty initiating sleep, difficulty maintaining sleep, and early morning awakening
- The sleep disturbance causes significant distress or impairment in social, occupational, educational, academic, behavioral, or other important areas of functioning
- The sleep difficulty occurs at least 3 nights per week, is present for at least 3 months, and despite adequate opportunity for sleep
- The insomnia does not co-occur with another sleep disorder
- The insomnia is not explained by coexisting mental disorders or medical conditions

DSM-5 pays more attention to coexisting medical conditions when it comes to sleep disorders, to better emphasize when an individual has a sleep disorder warranting independent clinical attention, in addition to any medical and mental disorders that are also present. The American Psychiatric Association (APA) recognizes that coexisting medical conditions, mental disorders, and sleep disorders are interactive and bidirectional in the DSM-5—it is not as important to make assumptions about what causes the sleep disorder. Hence, the diagnosis of *primary insomnia* has been renamed *insomnia disorder*, in order to avoid the differentiation of primary and secondary insomnia. DSM-5 also distinguishes narcolepsy—which is now known to be associated with hypocretin deficiency—from other forms of hypersomnolence. These changes, the APA believes, are warranted by neurobiological and genetic evidence validating this reorganization.

14.3 SLEEP ARCHITECTURE, SLEEP SCIENCE, AND PHYSIOLOGY

A large meta-analysis of 65 overnight studies representing 3577 subjects across the entire age spectrum reported that, with age, the percentage time of REM sleep decreased, while the percentages of light sleep (stage 1 and stage 2 sleep) increased [5]. Furthermore, slow-wave sleep (SWS) had a gradual and linear decrease of 2% per decade in young and middle-aged adults. When only reviewing studies of elderly participants, SWS remained constant after the age of 60 years with no significant continued change with age [5]. Finally, men aged 16–83 years had an average decrease in the total sleep time of 27 minutes per decade from midlife into late age [6]. While these age-related changes are well documented, their consequences are not fully understood or extensively researched. However, in the current theoretical framework, such changes in sleep architecture are considered nonpathological and might reflect age-related neural degeneration [7].

Circadian rhythms, such as core body temperature, hormone secretion, and the sleep–wake cycle, oscillate approximately every 24 hours. In humans, the sleep–wake cycle is regulated by an endogenous pacemaker and exogenous stimuli. The hypothalamic suprachiasmatic nucleus is believed to be this endogenous clock of the brain and is also considered the mediator of circadian rhythms, which are naturally entrained by exogenous stimuli; as people age, their circadian rhythms become weaker, desynchronized, and lose amplitude. It is hypothesized that the deterioration of the suprachiasmatic nucleus and its subsequent weakened functioning contribute to the disruption of circadian rhythms in older adults. The external cues that are necessary to entrain the circadian rhythm of sleep–wake cycles may be weak or missing in older adults. The elderly, especially those who are institutionalized, spend very little time exposed to bright light. Healthy older adults have a daily average of 60 minutes exposure to bright light; those who suffer from Alzheimer and live at home have only 30 minutes, and those who are in nursing homes have 0 minute of bright light exposure zeitgebers (time cues) [8]. The most significant zeitgeber is light.

Older adults often display an advanced circadian tendency, having an earlier bedtime and an earlier wake-up time. Sleep architecture changes include spending an increased proportion of time in stages N1 and N2 sleep (i.e., the lighter stages of sleep) and a decreased proportion of time in stage N3 sleep (i.e., a deeper stage of sleep) and in REM sleep. These architecture changes reflect a decrease in deep, restorative sleep and an increase in light, transitory sleep. In addition, older adults tend to spend slightly less time asleep than their younger counterparts.

14.3.1 SLEEP AND NORMAL AGING

Changes in the phasing of the circadian rhythm can develop in older adults, which can cause changes in the timing of the sleep period. Phase advance is common in older patients, causing them to wake up earlier in the morning and get tired earlier in the evening. Individuals with advanced sleep rhythms will typically fall asleep between 7:00 and 9:00 p.m., correlating with the cyclical drop in body temperature, and wake up about 8 hours later between 3:00 and 5:00 a.m. Due to societal pressure, many older adults with an advanced sleep–wake cycle resist their fatigue and attempt to stay up late, believing that they will wake up later in the morning. Yet these individuals will still wake up early in the morning as a result of their phase advancement. This behavior results in less total time in bed, less sleep time, and daytime sleepiness.

14.4 SLEEP DISORDERS AND INSOMNIA IN THE ELDERLY

The most common primary sleep disorders in the elderly population are as follows: SDB, RLS/periodic limb movements in sleep (PLMS), RBD, CRSD, and insomnia. Figure 14.1 reviews a general approach to sleep disorders [9].

14.4.1 SLEEP-DISORDERED BREATHING

SDB describes a range of respiratory events that occur periodically during sleep, from simple snoring at the milder end of the spectrum to complete cessation of airflow (apnea) at the more severe end. The number of instances of apnea and hypopnea (partial reduction in airflow) per hour of sleep is called the apnea–hypopnea index (AHI). SDB diagnosis is made when a patient has an AHI of >5–10.

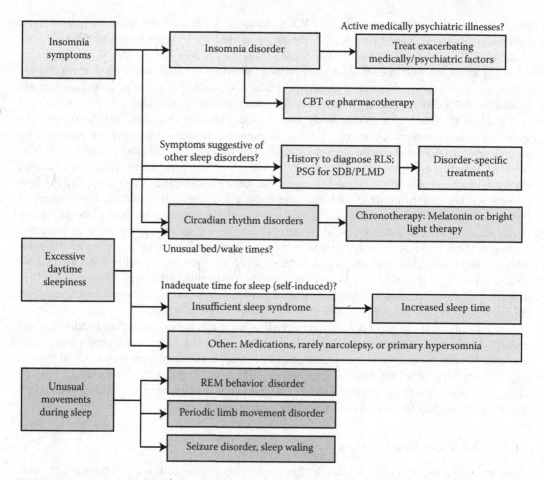

FIGURE 14.1 Diagnostic algorithm for sleep disorders in older persons CBT, cognitive-behavioral therapy; RLS, restless leg syndrome; PSG, polysomnography; SDB, sleep-disordered breathing; PLMD, periodic limb movement disorder; and REM, rapid eye movement. (Adapted from Gooneratne NS, Vitiello MV. *Clin Geriatr Med.* 2014;30(3):591–627.)

SDB is more prevalent in the older population and even more common in elderly nursing home patients, especially among those who suffer from dementia. In a large study of randomly selected community-dwelling elderly people, aged 65–95 years, Ancoli-Israel et al. [10] reported prevalence rates of 62% for an AHI of ≥10, 44% for an AHI of ≥20, and 24% for an AHI of ≥40. In a longitudinal study that followed older adults for 18 years, Ancoli-Israel et al. [11] found that the AHI remained stable and only changed with associated changes in body mass index (BMI). The Sleep Heart Health Study [12] reported that for the ages of 60–69 years, 32% had an AHI of 5–14 and 19% had an AHI of ≥15. For the ages of 70–79 years, 33% had an AHI of 5–14 and 21% had an AHI of ≥15. For the ages of 80–98 years, 36% had an AHI of 5–14 and 20% had an AHI of ≥15. These SDB prevalence results in the elderly are in contrast to the prevalence of SDB among middle-aged adults, which is estimated at 4% for men and 2% for women defined by an AHI of ≥5 with the presence of excessive daytime sleepiness (EDS) [13].

Risk factors for SDB in the aging population include age, gender, and obesity. Other conditions that increase the risk of developing SDB include the use of sedating medications, alcohol consumption, family history, race, smoking, and upper-airway configuration. The main symptoms of SDB in the elderly population are snoring and EDS.

Gooneratne et al. [14] studied elderly subjects with both insomnia and SDB and found that they had more functional impairment, specifically significantly lower daytime functioning and longer psychomotor reaction times, than those with just insomnia alone. Most studies have suggested that older adults with SDB are excessively sleepy and that SDB likely contributes to decreased quality of life (QoL), decreased cognitive function, greater risk of nocturia, hypertension, and cardiovascular disease [15]. The Sleep Heart Health Study found that the risk of developing cardiovascular disease, including coronary artery disease, congestive heart failure (CHF), and stroke, is positively related with the severity of SDB [16]. A recent study in acute ischemic stroke patients reported that SDB was common, particularly in older male patients with diabetes and a nighttime stroke onset [17]. In the older adult, severe SDB (AHI ≥ 30) is consistently reported to cause impairments in attention, concentration, executive tasks, immediate and delayed recall, planning and sequential thinking, and manual dexterity. Older adults with milder SDB (AHI 10–20) may suffer cognitive dysfunction only in the presence of excessive sleepiness [18].

When assessing SDB in the elderly, practitioners should use a stepwise approach. First, a complete sleep history should be obtained focusing on the symptoms of SDB. Special attention should be given to snoring severity, unintentional napping, and EDS. Assessment of sleep disturbances is more effective when the bed partner or caregiver is present since he or she is more likely to be aware of the subject's behavior during sleep. Assessments should consider the presence of other sleep disorders (i.e., RLS) and also sleep-related habits that may confound adequate sleep (i.e., noise or light). The patient's detailed medical history should be reviewed, paying attention to SDB-associated medical conditions, medications, the use of alcohol, and evidence of cognitive impairment. If assessment is suggestive of SDB, an overnight recording should be obtained for confirmation of the disorder.

The most common and proven treatment for SDB is continuous positive airway pressure (CPAP). CPAP compliance could be an issue in all age groups; yet, clinicians should not assume that older adults will be less compliant simply due to their age. Ayalon et al. [19] reported that patients with mild Alzheimer disease (AD) and SDB used CPAP for an average of 5 hours a night, and poor CPAP compliance was associated with the presence of depression—not with age, severity of dementia, or severity of SDB.

In a review of the literature, Weaver and Chasens [20] concluded that in the elderly, CPAP reduces or eliminates apnea and hypopnea; improves sleep architecture; improves daytime sleepiness; improves self-reported symptoms (snoring and gasping); improves motor speed, nonverbal learning, and memory; improves vascular resistance, platelet coagulability, and other factors affecting cardiac function; and has a positive effect on nocturia, reducing the number of voids per night. In general, if the SDB is associated with clinical symptoms, it should be treated regardless of the age of the patient [21].

14.4.2 Restless Legs Syndrome and Periodic Limb Movement in Sleep

RLS is a condition characterized by leg dysesthesia that occurs when the patient is in a relaxed awake or restful state and, thus, is more common during the evening or at night. Patients typically describe RLS as an uncomfortable sensation in their legs that is accompanied by the urge to move. Movement provides temporary relief of this uncomfortable sensation. Other terms that are used to describe this sensation include creepy-crawly, electric current, crazy legs, worms moving, ants crawling, or pain. Similar to PLMS, the etiology of RLS is unknown but is associated with iron deficiency states (including pregnancy), uremia, peripheral neuropathy, and radiculopathy. Diagnosis of RLS is done on the basis of history alone. There exist four essential features of RLS, according to the International Restless Legs Syndrome Study Group [22]: (1) experience the urge to move legs (and/or other parts of body) accompanied or caused by an uncomfortable and/or unpleasant sensation in the body part affected; (2) urge to move or the uncomfortable/unpleasant feeling start and/or worsen during periods of rest, relaxation, or inactivity; (3) urge to move or uncomfortable/unpleasant feeling partially or totally relieved by movement; and (4) urge to move or the uncomfortable sensation worsen in the evening or at night (as compared to the daytime). Asking the question "When you relax in the evening, do you ever have unpleasant, restless feelings in your legs that can be relieved by walking or movement?' could be sufficient for diagnosis.

PLMS, often related to RLS, is characterized by clusters of repetitive leg jerks or kicks during sleep. These leg movements characteristically occur every 20–40 seconds (s) and recur throughout the night. Each jerk or kick may result in an arousal or a brief awakening which causes sleep fragmentation and might lead to complaints of EDS. Since the patients are not aware of these kicks, the complaints might be wrongly interpreted as insomnia. For assessment, a bed partner might be helpful since they are most likely aware of their partner's excessive movements during the night. Diagnosis of PLMS should be based only on an overnight polysomnogram showing a calculated periodic limb movement index (the number of limb movements per hour of sleep) of ≥5. The etiology of PLMS is unknown. In the absence of RLS, there may be little clinical significance to PLMS.

PLMS and RLS are both common in the older adult. The prevalence of both RLS and PLMS increases significantly with age [23]. About 90% of the patients with RLS also have PLMS, but only about 20% of the PLMS patients suffer from RLS.

Pharmacological therapy should be limited to patients who suffer from clinically relevant symptoms. Chronic RLS is usually treated with either a dopamine agonist (pramipexole, ropinirole, and rotigotine) or an $\alpha2\delta$ calcium-channel ligand (gabapentin, gabapentin enacarbil, and pregabalin). Augmentation is the main complication of long-term dopaminergic treatment and frequently requires a reduction in current dopaminergic dose or a switch to nondopaminergic medications [24]. The off-label use of other dopamine agonists (e.g., carbidopa–levodopa) has also been shown to be effective [25].

14.4.3 RAPID EYE MOVEMENT SLEEP BEHAVIOR DISORDER

RBD is a condition in which the skeletal muscle atonia normally found in REM sleep is absent. RBD patients are often described as "acting out their dreams." This disorder is characterized by the display of elaborate movements during REM sleep: kicking, punching, running, and/or yelling. The patient's uncontrolled movements are sometimes aggressive and/or violent, and might result in injuries either to the patient himself and/or the patient's bed partner. The etiology of chronic RBD is currently unknown; yet, it appears to be strongly related to a number of underlying neurological or neurodegenerative disorders (approximately 40% of the RBD cases). Some data suggest that RBD may be the first manifestation and/or indication of a neurodegenerative disease [26]. In one study, 50% of those diagnosed with RBD developed Parkinson's disease (PD) or multiple system atrophy within 3–4 years [27]. RBD is more common in the elderly, with a significantly higher prevalence in older men.

The diagnosis of RBD requires a thorough sleep history which should be conducted in the presence of the patient's bed partner. Recently, a new screening questionnaire was developed and validated [28]. An overnight polysomnography (PSG) recording that includes video recording is helpful in confirming the disorder. Close attention should be paid to the presence of intermittent elevations in muscle tone or limb movements on the electromyogram channel during REM sleep as this is highly suggestive of RBD.

The treatment of RBD should include a safe sleep environment, obtained by the removal of potentially dangerous objects from the bedroom. Both patient and bed partner should be educated in all aspects of the disorder, especially the potential for inadvertent self-harm at night. Removal of a medication that promotes RBD activity, such as selective serotonin-reuptake inhibitor (SSRI) antidepressants, may be beneficial. When associated with a neurodegenerative condition such as PD, multiple sclerosis, or Alzheimer dementia, treatment of the primary disorder, when possible, is appropriate. When drug treatment is thought to be warranted, clonazepam may be used and is effective. The initial dose is generally 0.5 mg at bedtime, with some patients requiring up to 1 mg. Levodopa–carbidopa has been used in patients with RBD and early PD. Dopaminergic agents such as pramipexole have been found to be effective in this disorder and are now emerging as first-line therapy. Regardless of which treatment is used, long-term therapy is usually required because symptoms, once established, tend to persist [29,30].

14.4.4 CIRCADIAN RHYTHM SLEEP DISORDER

CRSDs may be primarily intrinsic (e.g., advanced sleep phase and delayed sleep phase) or situational (e.g., time zone change/jet lag syndrome or shift-work disorder). Correlations have been made between changes in circadian rhythms and advancing age. The circadian rhythm itself also shows evidence of age-related fragmentation, with sleep becoming more desynchronized and likely to impinge on daytime activities. Research suggests that an age-related reduction in sleep promotion of the circadian pacemaker, along with decreased homeostatic pressure for sleep in older adults, may be involved in this desynchronization [31,32].

Commonly, older people experience an advanced sleep phase, which leads to a pattern of an early bedtime and early morning awakening. The alteration in circadian rhythm can be marked in people who are bed-bound. When the internal clock is completely desynchronized, the sleep–wake cycles become irregular, with sleep occurring during the day and wakefulness at night or alternating periods of sleep and wakefulness throughout the 24-hour period.

Wrist actigraphy and/or sleep logs can be used for making a diagnosis and for monitoring treatment response. PSG is indicated when the diagnosis is unclear or another sleep disorder is suspected.

Depending on the specific CRSD, treatments may include appropriately timed bright-light exposure, appropriately timed melatonin use, prescribed sleep scheduling, and other measures. An intervention employing bright-light therapy (BLT) and melatonin treatment has also been tested in elderly patients with dementia and shown to improve some cognitive and noncognitive symptoms of dementia and also sleep efficiency. According to systematic review and meta-analysis, the short-term use of melatonin is not effective in treating most primary sleep disorders but may be effective in treating delayed sleep phase syndrome and circadian rhythm disorders [33,34].

14.4.5 INSOMNIA

According to the International Classification of Sleep Disorders, Third Edition, insomnia is defined as a subjective complaint of difficulty initiating sleep, difficulty maintaining sleep, or early morning awakenings that occur at a minimum of 3 nights per week, for 3 months, and are associated with significant daytime consequences. Examples of these daytime consequences include difficulty concentrating, mood disturbances, fatigue, and worry about sleep. On average, older adults experience insomnia symptoms for several years before receiving a formal diagnosis.

Insomnia (difficulty falling or staying asleep) is often comorbid with medical and psychiatric illness [2]. Studies examining the prevalence of sleep disturbances in patients with chronic medical diseases have reported that the majority of patients with arthritis, chronic pain, and diabetes reported difficulty falling and/or staying asleep. Other health-related diseases that are associated with insomnia include CHF, cancer, nocturia, shortness of breath due to chronic obstructive pulmonary disease (COPD), neurological deficits related to cerebrovascular accidents, and PD. In addition, older adults with multiple medical conditions are more likely to have sleep complaints [1].

Research has recognized that depression and insomnia are closely related to each other; in fact, untreated insomnia may result in depression, and the presence of a depressed mood may even predict insomnia [29]. Ohayon and Roth [31] conducted a large cross-sectional survey and found that 65% of those with major depression, 61% of those with panic disorder, and 44% of those with generalized anxiety disorder also suffered from insomnia. In a recent study by Perlis et al. [35], elderly subjects with persistent insomnia, particularly women, were at greater risk for the development of depression.

TABLE 14.1

Insomnia Severity Index

Please rate the current (i.e., last 2 weeks) severity of your insomnia problems:

1. Have you had difficulty falling asleep?
2. Have you had difficulty staying asleep?
3. Have you had problems waking up too early?
4. How satisfied/dissatisfied are you with your sleep pattern?
5. How noticeable to others do you think your sleep problem is in terms of impairing the quality of your life?
6. How worried/distressed are you about your current sleep problem?
7. To what extent do you consider your sleep problem to interfere with your daily functioning (e.g., daytime fatigue, mood, ability to function at work/daily chores, concentration, and memory)?

Source: Morin CM et al. *Sleep.* 2011;34(5):601–608.

Note: Five-point Likert scale (0, no problem; 4, very severe problem) possible answers for all items. Total score categories: 0–7, no clinically significant insomnia; 8–14, subthreshold insomnia and; 15–21, moderate insomnia; and 22–28, severe insomnia.

14.4.5.1 Agents That Can Cause Insomnia

While the prevalence of insomnia in the general population has been estimated at 10%–20%, studies in older adults have found higher frequencies. In a study of more than 9000 adults over the age of 65 years, 42% of participants had difficulty both falling asleep and staying asleep with a higher prevalence found in those older adults with poor health and who were taking medications for a variety of medical problems [36]. Participants who were depressed were 2.5 times more likely to report insomnia, and those with respiratory symptoms were 40% more likely to do so. The finding that there are a considerable proportion of sleep complaints among older people may be associated with chronic disease and other health problems [36–40].

Insomnia in the older adult is associated with significant morbidity and mortality. Compared to controls, those with difficulty sleeping report decreased QoL and increased symptoms of depression and anxiety [41–45]. Napping during the day and sleeping less than 7 hours a night have been associated with increased risk of falls [46]. Cognitive decline, difficulty ambulating, difficulty with balance, and difficulty seeing are also associated with poor sleep, even after controlling for medication use [47–50]. The relative risk for increased mortality in the older adult has been associated with taking more than 30 minutes to fall asleep and with a sleep efficiency (time asleep as a percentage of time in bed) of less than 80% [51].

Polypharmacy is increasingly common among older adults. In many cases, there is no consideration of the effect of medications on the patients' sleep. Many of the medications that are prescribed for chronic medical and psychiatric conditions can also contribute to, or even cause, insomnia, such as central nervous system stimulants (e.g., modafinil and methylphenidate), antihypertensives (e.g., β-blockers and α-blockers), respiratory medications (e.g., theophylline and albuterol), chemotherapy, decongestants (e.g., pseudoephedrine), hormones (e.g., corticosteroids and thyroid hormones), or psychotropics (e.g., SSRIs, atypical antidepressants and MAO inhibitors). When possible, stimulating medications and diuretics should be taken earlier in the day, and sedating medications should be administered prior to bedtime. Morin et al. in 2011 [52] described an Insomnia Severity Index to evaluate and treat insomnia (Table 14.1).

14.4.5.2 Assessment and Management of Sleep Disorders in Older Persons

The best method for detecting sleep–wake problems in ambulatory older people is simply to inquire about sleep on a regular basis. The clinician may do this initially during the patient visit. An alternative is to allow a staff member to administer a brief sleep questionnaire before or during routine vital signs assessments, perhaps prior to the first visit in all new patients and then at least semi-annually in returning patients. The answers to these questions will then be immediately available to the clinician to review and/or expand upon if necessary. If a bed partner is with the patient, he or she should assist with the answers [53].

The following 12 questions can serve as the initial assessment regarding sleep [53]:

1. What time do you normally go to bed at night? What time do you normally wake up in the morning?
2. Do you often have trouble falling asleep at night?
3. About how many times do you wake up at night?
4. If you do wake up during the night, do you usually have trouble falling back asleep?
5. Does your bed partner say (or are you aware) that you frequently snore, gasp for air, or stop breathing?
6. Does your bed partner say (or are you aware) you kick or thrash about while asleep?
7. Are you aware that you ever walk, eat, punch, kick, or scream during sleep?
8. Are you sleepy or tired during much of the day?
9. Do you usually take one or more naps during the day?
10. Do you usually doze off without planning during the day?
11. How much sleep do you need to feel alert and function well?
12. Are you currently taking any type of medication or other preparation to help you sleep?

If symptoms of a sleep complaint are suggested in this initial screening, further questions may be appropriate to ask when taking a sleep history [54]:

1. Do you have the urge to move your legs or do you experience uncomfortable sensations in your legs during rest or at night?
2. Do you have to get up often to urinate during the night?
3. If you nap during the day, how often and for how long?
4. How much physical activity or exercise do you get daily?
5. Are you exposed to natural outdoor light most days?
6. What medications do you take, and at what time of day and night?
7. Do you suffer any uncomfortable side effects from your medications?
8. How much caffeine (e.g., coffee, tea, and cola) and alcohol do you consume each day/night?
9. Do you often feel sad or anxious?
10. Have you suffered any personal losses recently?

The patient's responses should indicate how to proceed with any further history, focused physical examination, or laboratory investigations. Specific questions, examinations, laboratory tests, procedures, and possible referrals are discussed in more detail in the sections concerning the particular sleep disorders. A flow diagram (Figure 14.2) may be helpful in identifying and treating sleep complaints in older ambulatory individuals [55].

14.4.5.3 Measures to Improve Sleep Hygiene

Sleep restriction therapy entails limiting time in bed to consolidate actual time sleeping. The patient is counseled to reduce the amount of time in bed to correlate closely with actual time sleeping. The recommended sleep times are based on sleep logs kept for 2 weeks before sleep restriction therapy is begun. Thus, an individual who reports spending 8.5 hours in bed, but sleeping only 5.5 of those hours, would be counseled to limit his/her time in bed to 5.5–6 hours. Time allowed in bed is gradually increased by 15–20 minutes increments (approximately once every 5 days if improvement is sustained) as sleep efficiency increases, until the individual's optimal sleep time is obtained.

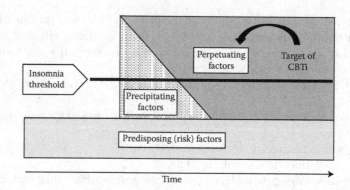

FIGURE 14.2 The 3 P conceptual model of insomnia. Predisposing factors: physical and mental health, family history of insomnia, poverty, and so forth. Precipitating factors: depressive episode, hospitalization, loss of a loved one, moving, and so forth. Perpetuating factors: spending too much time in bed, not following a regular sleep schedule, and so forth. CBTi, cognitive behavior treatment of insomnia. (Adapted from Rodriguez JC, Dzierzewski JM, Alessi CA. *Med Clin North America.* 2015;99(2):431–439.)

In sleep compression, a variant of sleep restriction, patients are counseled to decrease their time in bed gradually to match total sleep time rather than making an immediate substantial change, as is the case in sleep restriction therapy. A number of studies support the efficacy of sleep restriction–sleep compression therapy as a treatment for older patients with chronic insomnia. These approaches can also be combined with other modalities.

People suffering from chronic insomnia may adopt coping strategies that exacerbate the problem. Watching television or reading in bed, worrying about falling asleep, or using the bedroom for vigorous discussions or arguments are examples of behaviors that can impair sleep by producing associations between the bed and bedroom and those activities; the bedroom should be associated only with sleeping and sex. Stimulus control therapy attempts to eliminate these behaviors in the bedroom and thereby strengthen the association between sleep and the bed/bedroom.

The following are helpful instructions for utilizing stimulus control and practicing good sleep hygiene:

1. Develop a sleep ritual such as maintaining a 30-minute relaxation period before bedtime or taking a hot bath 90 minutes before bedtime.
2. Make sure the bedroom is restful and comfortable.
3. Go to bed only if you feel sleepy.
4. Avoid heavy exercise within 2 hours of bedtime.
5. Avoid sleep-fragmenting substances, such as caffeine, nicotine, and alcohol.
6. Avoid activities in the bedroom that keep you awake. Use the bedroom only for sleep and sex; do not watch television from bed or work in bed.
7. Sleep only in your bedroom.
8. If you cannot fall asleep leave the bedroom and return only when sleepy.
9. Maintain stable bed times and rising times. Arise at the same time each morning, regardless of the amount of sleep obtained that night.
10. Avoid daytime napping. If you do nap during the day, limit it to 30 minutes and do not nap, if possible, after 2 pm.

The goal of relaxation therapy is to guide individuals to a calm, steady state when they wish to go to sleep. The methods used include progressive muscle relaxation (tensing and then relaxing each muscle group), guided imagery, diaphragmatic breathing, meditation, and biofeedback.

Cognitive behavior therapy combines multiple behavioral approaches, usually incorporating sleep restriction, stimulus control, and cognitive therapy, with or without relaxation therapy. Sleep hygiene and sleep education are frequently included. Protocols for older adults may vary somewhat from those used for younger patients. All approaches, however, aim to correct the common misperceptions regarding normal aging and sleep by providing information about how much sleep is necessary to maintain health, and the physical and psychological consequences of sleep loss. Motivational strategies to increase compliance are also emphasized.

Some studies report that walking, Tai Chi, acupressure, and weight training improve sleep for some individuals [51,56–58]. However, how these approaches affect sleep is not well understood and is likely to be complex [59]. Also, difficulties inherent in these studies preclude their recommendation as evidence based. Nevertheless, there are many good reasons to encourage regular physical activity in older individuals, given its positive effect on functional and cognitive status.

14.4.5.4 Common Prescription Sleep Medications in Elderly People

Ten drugs have been approved by the FDA for the treatment of insomnia, including benzodiazepines, nonbenzodiazepines, and a melatonin receptor agonist. The selection of any given drug should depend on matching the characteristics of the particular drug with the patient's complaint. All should be started at the lowest available dose.

The benzodiazepines are psychoactive drugs with varying hypnotic, sedative, anxiolytic, anticonvulsant, muscle relaxant, and amnestic properties. Nonbenzodiazepines, also called benzodiazepine receptor agonists, are comparatively new drugs whose actions are similar to those of the benzodiazepines, although they are structurally unrelated. The one approved melatonin receptor agonist has a different mechanism of action. Melatonin receptors, acted upon by endogenous melatonin, are thought to be involved in the maintenance of the circadian rhythm underlying the normal sleep–wake cycle.

The NIH State-of-Science Conference on Insomnia concluded that the benzodiazepine receptor agonists are efficacious in the short-term management of insomnia and that the frequency and severity of any adverse effects are lower than those found in the older benzodiazepines [60]. Older people may be at greater risk for adverse effects because of pharmacokinetic considerations, such as reduced clearance of certain sedative hypnotics. There is also some evidence of pharmacodynamic differences such as increased sensitivity to peak drug effects. Impairment was shown to be dependent on dose and time since dosing.

Other classes of medications have also been used to treat insomnia in the elderly. The 2005 NIH State-of-the-Science Conference on Insomnia concluded that there is no systematic evidence for the effectiveness of many medications, including the antihistamines, antidepressants, antipsychotics, or anticonvulsants used off-label for the treatment of insomnia and warned that the risks of use outweighed the benefits. Trazodone, a frequently prescribed antidepressant for insomnia in older persons, is very sedating, can cause orthostasis, and has no published evidence of sustained efficacy.

Combining both behavioral and pharmacologic therapy may provide for better outcomes than use of either modality alone. Past studies in adults have shown that combination therapy has been efficacious, with medications providing short-term onset relief and behavioral therapy providing longer-term sustained benefit. Only one randomized, controlled clinical trial has evaluated combination therapy in older adults [61]. In this study, combination therapy was not only more efficacious than placebo, but it was also more efficacious than either pharmacologic or behavioral therapy alone. The study concluded that, while combination therapy was effective for the short-term management of insomnia in late life, sleep improvements were better sustained over time with behavioral treatment. While results from the few controlled studies that have been performed on combination therapy are encouraging, there is still enough of a paucity of data to caution against overgeneralization.

14.5 SLEEP APNEA

Sleep apnea, a SDB, is a condition in which people stop breathing while asleep [62]. Apneas (complete cessation of respiration) and hypopneas (partial decrease in respiration) both result in hypoxemia and changes in autonomic nervous system activity, resulting in increases in systemic and pulmonary arterial pressure and changes in cerebral blood flow [63,64]. The episodes are generally terminated by an arousal (brief awakening) which results in fragmented sleep. These arousals are believed to be an important contributor to the symptoms of EDS and the neurocognitive impairment seen in sleep apnea.

Two types of sleep apnea are recognized: obstructive sleep apnea (OSA) and central sleep apnea (CSA). In OSA, the primary pathophysiologic event is obstruction of the upper airway, manifested by greatly diminished or absent airflow in the presence of an effort to breathe. CSA is characterized by recurrent episodes of apnea during sleep resulting from temporary loss of ventilatory effort, due to central nervous system or cardiac dysfunction [65,66]. This latter type of apnea is commonly found in patients with CHF, particularly in those with Cheyne–Stokes respiration. In this discussion, we will primarily focus on the much more common OSA, defined as sleep apnea associated with EDS.

OSA has been described in all age groups. In the adult population, OSA (defined as 10 or more apneas and hypopneas per hour of sleep) occurs in about 15% of men and 5% of women [67]. In older adults, OSA occurs in up to 70% of men and 56% of women [29]. The syndrome is much more common in postmenopausal than premenopausal females, but the prevalence increases in both genders with aging.

EDS and a history of snoring are by far the most common presenting symptoms in most patients with OSA. Other symptoms of OSA include observed apnea, choking or gasping on awakening, morning headache, and nocturia. While most younger OSA patients are obese, the elderly with OSA may not necessarily be obese.

Risk factors for OSA include age, obesity, and anatomic abnormalities affecting the upper airway. In the older population, OSA is also more common among Asians compared to Caucasians. OSA has been associated with heart failure, atrial fibrillation, and stroke, conditions that are more common in the older population. In women, OSA is often associated with a history of hypothyroidism.

Studies show that older adults with OSA are excessively sleepy and that OSA likely contributes to decreased QoL, increased neurocognitive impairment, and greater risk of nocturia and cardiovascular disease. Cardiovascular comorbidities particularly associated with OSA include arterial hypertension, heart failure, and stroke. Often, the hypertension is difficult to control.

Diabetes mellitus is also more common in this population, and there may be an association between apnea and insulin resistance. Depression has also been found as a common comorbidity in women with OSA. Although mortality is increased in untreated apnea patients under the age of 50 years, the impact of OSA on mortality in the older population is unclear.

OSA is managed via a four-step approach: (a) confirming the diagnosis; (b) determining optimal treatment; (c) general management measures; and (d) ongoing, chronic follow-up.

Because OSA is so common in older people, all older patients should be questioned to determine if OSA symptoms are present. The history should be obtained from the patient and a bed partner or caregiver, if possible, and should include questions covering the cardinal symptoms of OSA, specifically EDS, snoring, and observed apnea. Questions about nocturia and cognitive impairment, as well as any comorbidities, should be included as well. Physicians should consider OSA syndrome in individuals who are overweight or have a history of heart disease, hypothyroidism, or stroke.

The Epworth Sleepiness Scale (ESS), although not validated for use in older persons, is useful for documenting daytime drowsiness. Nocturia is a surprisingly common finding in OSA patients. This symptom in males is commonly misinterpreted as being caused by prostatic hypertrophy. OSA should be suspected in all patients with hypertension, especially with hypertension that is resistant to treatment.

The physical should focus on the upper airway, including the nasal and pharyngeal airways, to rule out anatomic obstruction. The skeletal structure of the face must be assessed to exclude the possibility of jaw abnormalities (retrognathia or micrognathia), which may cause OSA in the absence of obesity. Dental structures should be examined if a mandibular advancement device is being considered. Obesity often involves the trunk and neck, and documentation of neck collar size (>17 inches in men and >16 inches in women) may be helpful, especially in males.

Patients suspected of having OSA based on historical features and physical examination will almost always require objective documentation by PSG to confirm the presence and severity of the apnea. The Center for Medicare Services (CMS) and most insurance carriers require PSG for reimbursement of CPAP therapy. Comprehensive PSG includes the measurement of variables to document sleep breathing disorders (oxygen saturation in arterial blood, rib cage and abdominal movement, nasal and oral airflow, and snoring sounds), data regarding sleep and stage of sleep (via electroencephalography, electrooculography, and electromyography), and electrocardiogram and leg electromyogram to document the presence of periodic leg movements. The PSG is usually followed by the data obtained during CPAP titration. Although PSG is usually performed in a laboratory setting, home testing may be covered by CMS in selected patients.

The AHI is the most widely used metric for characterizing the severity of the abnormalities of sleep respiration and is based on the average number of apneas plus hypopneas per hour of sleep in a single-night study. A value of >5 is considered diagnostic for OSA. CMS covers reimbursement for treatment when AHI is >15, or if AHI exceeds 5 and comorbidities (such as sleepiness and/or cardiovascular disease) are present.

When OSA in the older adult is associated with clinical symptoms, particularly hypertension, cognitive dysfunction, nocturia, high levels of SDB, or cardiac disease, then it should be treated, regardless of the age of the patient. Most patients with OSA will probably require referral to or management by sleep specialists, including those with hypoventilation syndromes (e.g., individuals suspected of having obesity hypoventilation, impaired ventilation secondary to neuromuscular diseases, or CSA), those with significant respiratory disease (e.g., COPD, severe asthma, or restrictive diseases), and those with significant cardiac disease such as CHF. Such patients may require complex treatment.

Currently there is no pharmacologic treatment for OSA. CPAP is the best approach and first line of treatment for most patients. CPAP works by stenting open the airway, increasing functional residual capacity of the lungs, possibly increasing pharyngeal dilator activity, and reducing afterload on the heart. Several studies have confirmed that older adults tolerate nightly CPAP use.

The choice of interface type of headgear (nasal or oronasal mask) for securing the mask to the head and necessity for a chinstrap are determined objectively. Response to CPAP is usually assessed as part of comprehensive PSG either during the latter part of the diagnostic study night (split-night study) or during an additional all night study. The CPAP titration is performed in a split-night study after the patient has been asleep for at least 2 hours, and the OSA diagnosis has been confirmed. This involves fitting the patient with an appropriate mask, educating him or her about what is to transpire, and then applying increased levels of pressure until OSA control is attained. Proper fit and education will help compliance and reduce claustrophobia.

A split-night study may not be appropriate if there is insufficient time during the night to make a diagnosis and also determine optimal pressures. In addition, some patients may require a more complex device than a standard fixed-pressure CPAP machine. Only after a review of all diagnostic and therapeutic sleep studies, can the optimal treatment approach be determined. Patients without teeth can sometimes present a challenge for CPAP treatment because of bone resorption in the upper and lower jaws. This situation presents difficulties for optimal mask fitting and makes oral appliances unfeasible.

Alcohol or other agents (e.g., opiates, many anesthetic agents, and the sedative hypnotics) can depress upper-airway tone and may worsen OSA syndrome. Older patients about to undergo surgery should be screened for OSA, at least by history, since they might receive opiates during the perioperative period.

A great deal of evidence supports the strong positive correlation between weight and OSA risk. Weight reduction plays an important role in the management of the obese OSA patient. One study of older OSA patients monitored for 18 years found a reduction in the severity of the apnea with which the weight loss was associated.

Patients with CHF are at risk of developing Cheyne–Stokes respiration, a form of CSA. Cheyne–Stokes respiration can result in severe sleep onset and sleep maintenance insomnia, as well as daytime sleepiness. Older patients with CHF and sleep apnea (particularly CSA) have a 2.7-fold greater risk of reduced survival than patients with CHF or apnea alone.

CHF treatment may improve breathing abnormalities in CSA, but results from a recent randomized clinical trial indicate that CPAP may increase mortality in the first 2 years of treatment. Therefore, CPAP is not currently recommended as a first-line treatment in CHF. Small short-term clinical trials have suggested the effectiveness of oxygen and adaptive servoventilation, a ventilatory support mode specifically designed for CHF breathing abnormalities. No long-term outcome studies are available.

Older people are more likely than younger people to have general surgery and to require general anesthesia. All older patients, especially those with the risk factors for OSA, must be questioned about the possibility of OSA. If they are at high risk, an objective assessment should be made. If OSA is confirmed during the preoperative assessment, nasal CPAP should be initiated prior to hospital admission, and the equipment should be brought to the hospital at admission. The postsurgical period harbors significant risk for such patients because anesthetic agents and opiates can worsen OSA in unprotected individuals.

Oral devices, which move the lower jaw up and forward, can be effective, especially in mild-to-moderate cases. Guidelines for their use are identical to those in younger people. In older individuals, however, special attention must be paid to the examination of the jaws and teeth since at least eight healthy teeth in each of the upper and lower jaws are required to anchor the appliances. At this time, patients without adequate dentition cannot be treated with such appliances.

OSA is a chronic illness and as such requires long-term management. The main symptoms relate to neurocognitive function and daytime sleepiness. The Epworth Sleep Scale (ESS), while not specifically validated in the older population, is the most commonly utilized assessment instrument for daytime sleepiness. With CPAP treatment, an improvement in the ESS score of 2 or more points is expected, as well as an overall improvement in subjective sleepiness assessment. When CPAP is no longer effective or sleepiness returns, the patient should be reevaluated.

Cognitively impaired patients may have difficulty mastering the steps involved in putting on their masks and cleaning their CPAP machines and headgear, although one study of patients with mild to moderate AD living at home showed that these patients were compliant with CPAP treatment. Help either from a family member or from a caregiver is generally necessary. Compliance can be monitored by some of the newer CPAP systems, but the clinical utility of monitoring has not been rigorously determined.

14.6 SLEEP PROBLEMS IN SPECIAL POPULATION

14.6.1 SLEEP PATTERNS IN DEMENTIA

AD is the most frequent cause of dementia in the elderly population. It has been estimated that in 2013, AD affected 4.7 million individuals aged 65 years or older in the United States, a number that is projected to increase to approximately 14 million by 2050 [68]. The classic hallmarks are progressive deterioration of memory, language, and intellect. Sleep and circadian rhythm disorders are very frequent in AD, and it has been reported that up to 45% of the patients may have sleep problems [69–71]. The most frequent disturbances are excessive awakenings (23%), early morning awakening

(11%), EDS (10%), and napping for more than 1 hour during the day (14%) [72]. Such disturbances can appear early in the course of the disease, although they tend to be correlated with the severity of the cognitive decline [70]. Sleep-related breathing disorders (SRBDs) are also very frequent in AD patients and in this group are clearly more prevalent than in the general population [73,74].

Issues that highlight the relevance of the treatment of sleep disorders in patients with AD include the following:

1. Sleep disturbances are associated with increased memory and cognitive impairment [75].
2. Sleep and nighttime behavioral disturbances such as wandering, day/night confusion, getting up repeatedly during the night, and nightmares or hallucinations cause significant caregiver burden and are a primary cause of patient institutionalization [72,76].
3. There is increasing evidence of the role of sleep disturbances in the pathophysiology of AD, and a bidirectional relationship has been proposed [77–79].
4. Normal aging is accompanied by sleep architecture changes, such as increased sleep latency, difficulty in sleep maintenance, decrease in SWS, early morning awakenings, and increased daytime somnolence [80].
5. The sleep disturbances present in patients with AD are similar, but more severe than would be expected by the patient's age [81]. Sometimes, sleep disturbances in AD are so prominent that should be classified as a primary comorbid sleep disorder, such as chronic insomnia. The change that seems most specific to AD is a quantitative decrease in the REM stage [82,83]. In particular, electroencephalogram (EEG) slowing during REM sleep has been proposed as a biological marker of AD [83].
6. The architectural changes present in AD patients are probably related to cognition impairment [84,85]. The cognitive impairment could be different depending on the sleep stage that is altered. For example, Rauchs et al. [86,87] found that the mean intensity of fast spindles was positively correlated, in AD patients, with immediate recall performance, while the amount of SWS was positively correlated with the ability to retrieve recent autobiographical memories.

Abnormalities in sleep–wake patterns and circadian-related disorders are also common in AD patients. [88] In extreme cases, a complete day/night sleep pattern reversal can be observed [89]. Some authors have proposed that the sundowning phenomenon could also be due to a disorder of the circadian rhythm [90–92]. This phenomenon corresponds to an exacerbation of behavioral symptoms of dementia in the late afternoon [93]. The abnormalities in the circadian timing system in AD patients are also manifested in other circadian systems such as body temperature and hormone concentrations [91,94–96]. Stranahan [97] found that disturbances in the circadian timing system also affect the activity of the hippocampus, worsening learning capacities.

SRBDs are also more frequent in patients with AD than in the general population and are present in 40%–70% of these patients [73,74]. In a longitudinal cohort study of sleep disorders using PSG, it was found that the probability of moderate-to-severe SDB was significantly higher in healthy participants with the APOE E4 allele, independent of age, sex, BMI, or race [98]. It has been suggested that SRBD could cause AD [99]. Recently, it has been reported that the presence of SRBD was associated with cognitive decline at an earlier age [100]. Once the dementia is established, the severity of the sleep disturbances seems to be correlated with the severity of the dementia [101]. Apneas alter sleep architecture and lead to a decreased amount of REM sleep and SWS, which causes more frequent awakenings than in patients without apneas [102]. However, Yaffe et al. [103] found that the oxygen desaturation index and the percentage of time in apnea or hypopnea were associated with cognitive decline, but not with sleep fragmentation or sleep duration. These disturbances and the daytime sleepiness could be responsible for additional cognitive symptoms in patients that would be reversible [104–108].

A bidirectional relationship between sleep disturbances and AD has been proposed (Figure 14.3) [109,110]. The physiopathological mechanism is not completely understood, but an association

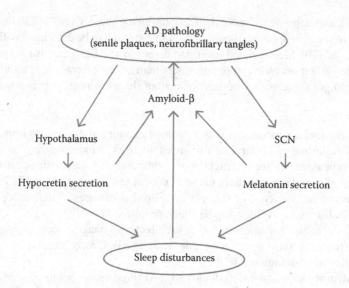

FIGURE 14.3 Bidirectional relationship between sleep and AD pathology. (Adapted from Urrestarazu E, Iriarte J. *Nature and Science of Sleep.* 2016;8:21–33.)

between sleep disturbances and amyloid-β accumulation has been demonstrated in mice [77,78] and humans [111,112]. On the other hand, AD also influences sleep, especially the sleep–wake cycle [113]. Patients with AD suffer some disturbances in the secretion of neurotransmitters related to sleep–wake systems, mainly hypocretins (orexins) and melatonin secretion 130. Hypocretin-1 and Hypocretin-2 are produced by a small cluster of neurons in the posterior hypothalamus [114,115]. The hypocretin system acts as a stabilizing factor in the sleep–wake flip-flop, keeping it in the waking state [116,117]. The disturbances in the secretion of neurotransmitters not only influence the quality of sleep, but they also play a role in the pathogenesis of the AD itself through changes in amyloid-β, originating a complex circle. In fact, it has been reported in mice that physiologic circadian fluctuations of CSF amyloid-β levels are related to the hypocretin system. Melatonin plays a key role not only in sleep disturbances but also in the pathogenesis of AD. Melatonin is a tryptophan metabolite that is synthesized in the pineal gland and has several physiological functions including the regulation of circadian rhythms, clearance of free radicals, improvement of immunity, and inhibition of the oxidation of biomolecules [117]. CSF melatonin levels are already decreased in the preclinical stages of AD [62,63] and continue decreasing further as AD progresses.

The aim of the treatment is to improve the QoL of patients and caregivers. Because of the impact of sleep disorders on cognition, it seems logical to think that the treatment would also improve some cognitive domains. During daytime, AD patients should be encouraged to exercise regularly for at least 30 minutes and walk outdoors. Intake of stimulants such as caffeine or tea should be limited, and naps longer than half an hour or after 1 p.m. should be avoided. Time in bed should be reduced. The schedule for going to sleep and getting up must be regular, and the bedroom should be reserved only for sleeping. Nighttime noise and light exposure and sleep disruptions should be reduced. BLT is a chronotherapeutic intervention used to treat circadian disturbances in AD patients. The most commonly used drugs are melatonin, z-hypnotics such as zolpidem, sedating antidepressants, and antipsychotics. Usually, benzodiazepines are avoided because they may worsen cognitive function. Cholinesterase inhibitors, the first-line treatment for AD, can also improve sleep quality. However, there are few studies assessing the efficacy of these drugs.

Hypnotics are classified into benzodiazepines and nonbenzodiazepines. The side effects of benzodiazepines include daytime sedation, anterograde amnesia, daytime sleepiness, confusion, and risk of falls. Given these risks, they are not recommended for AD patients. They also have a deleterious effect on cognition [118–124].

Sedating antidepressants are used when there is concomitant depression. However, tricyclic antidepressants have anticholinergic activity and may exacerbate the cholinergic disturbances inherent in AD, and should be avoided. They also have other side effects such as somnolence, sedation, and dizziness, which are of great concern in the demented population. Serotonin-reuptake inhibitors with a sedating profile, especially mirtazapine, are also used to treat insomnia. Trazodone is a triazolopyridine antidepressant that offers a dual action on serotonergic receptors by blocking the 2A receptor and inhibiting serotonin reuptake. It improves sleep in patients with depression, but there is insufficient evidence for its use in patients with insomnia without depression. Antipsychotics are frequently administered to control behavioral and neuropsychiatric manifestations of AD. Sometimes, when the first-line treatments have failed, they are also used to treat insomnia. However, they are associated with sedation, increased risk of falls, and might also have serious cardiac side effects. Furthermore, they can aggravate sleep–wake cycle disturbances. Antihistaminic drugs do not seem appropriate to be used in AD patients. They have a wide range of side effects including sedation, cognitive impairment, increased daytime somnolence, and anticholinergic responses.

Acetylcholinesterase inhibitors are a common treatment for AD. Acetylcholine not only plays a key role in memory functions, but it also is related to vigilance states. Levels increase during wakefulness, decrease in non-REM sleep, and rise again in REM sleep. Polysomnographic studies in patients taking acetylcholinesterase inhibitors have shown an increase in the percentage of REM sleep, reduced REM latency, and a decrease in REM sleep slow band power. Galantamine has the best profile regarding sleep and may be the first choice of cholinesterase inhibitor in mild-to-moderate dementia patients in terms of improving sleep quality.

14.6.2 SLEEP DISTURBANCE IN LONG-TERM CARE FACILITY RESIDENTS

Sleep and nighttime behavioral disturbances such as wandering, getting out of bed repeatedly, and day/night confusion are widespread among residents with dementia in adult family homes (AFHs). Residents of AFHs have higher rates of functional and health problems that can contribute to sleep disturbances than do community-dwelling persons with dementia, and paid caregivers have demanding on-the-job responsibilities and schedules not typically faced by family caregivers.

The National Health Provider Inventory (NHPI) estimated that there are more than 34,000 licensed board and care homes, serving the needs of over 600,000 persons, two-thirds of whom are elderly, and one-third of whom have moderate-to-severe cognitive impairment. AFHs are at one end of the board and care facility continuum, being private residences that provide room and board, 24-hour supervision, and assistance with personal care tasks for 2–6 residents not related to the owner or operator. Larger facilities include *adult residential care* (ARC) facilities, which provide board and care for 7 or more adults who need 24-hour assistance and oversight, and *assisted living* (AL) facilities, which provide independent living units with access to personalized care and support services on an as-needed basis. AFHs, which also go by names such as rest homes, adult foster homes, boarding homes, and personal care homes, fill a well-defined niche between AL and nursing homes, and have become a widely accepted alternative to nursing homes for the care of older adults with dementia. Many elderly persons who need residential care choose AFHs over other options because of their small size and homelike environment [53,54,125–134].

Wandering, particularly at night, has been identified as one of the most challenging resident behaviors for AFHs to manage. One study showed that 29% of the residents were waking others up at night in the previous week [135]. In 2003, our research team completed a survey of 101 AFHs in 3 counties in Washington (King et al.) asking about the occurrence of specific sleep or nighttime behavioral disturbances in their residents with dementia [136]. Sixty-eight percent of the surveyed AFHs reported having one or more residents with some form of sleep or nighttime behavioral disturbance, including getting up during the night (83%; excluding 1–2 brief bathroom trips); nocturnal incontinence episodes (72%); waking too early in the morning (71%); talking, yelling, or calling out at night (62%); and wandering or pacing (60%). Eighty-five percent of the surveyed AFHs expressed interest in participating in a study that would teach care providers behavioral strategies for improving sleep problems in their residents.

Administrative and organizational factors unique to AFHs have impacted recruitment and implementation of the ongoing SEP intervention study. Whereas skilled nursing or AL facilities typically assign staff to one of three day, evening, or nighttime shifts, AFHs use a wide variety of facility staffing arrangements. For example, some direct care staff work standard 8-hour shifts under the supervision of an owner-operator who is only occasionally in the home; in other cases, direct care staff work round-the-clock shifts for several days then rotate off for several days and are replaced by other 24-hour rotating staff; in still other situations, the owner-operator may reside in the home with the residents, either as part of an extended-family care system or as the sole care provider 24 hours/day, 7 days/week year-round. In our ongoing AFH study, 24% (6/25) of the participating caregivers work in day shift, 20% (5/25) work in night shift, 28% (7/25) live on an ongoing basis in the AFH residence, and the remainder work a combination or float across shifts. There exists a challenge in providing care to treat insomnia in long-term care facilities. Although common in older adults, sleep complaints are even more prevalent in elders living in nursing homes, and the sleep disturbances experienced by institutionalized older adults are more severe. Factors contributing to sleep impairment in nursing home residents include age-related changes in sleep architecture and circadian rhythms, sleep disorders, dementia, depression, other medical illness, polypharmacy, and institutional and environmental factors. It is important that nursing home residents suffering from sleep problems be evaluated and treated.

14.6.3 Sleep Problems in Elderly with Musculoskeletal Disorders and Chronic Pain

Pain and sleep influence one another. Pain may be exacerbated by sleep disorders [137], while sleep is impaired by pain [138]. The concept of pain-on and pain-off neurons may explain the anatomical interactions of pain and sleep phenomena. These neurons, which are situated in the nucleus raphe magnus, respectively, facilitate and inhibit nociceptive impulses to thalamocortical pathways and are influenced by the wake–sleep cycle: inhibitory pain-off nerve cells are completely activated during deep sleep, whereas excitatory pain-on nerve cells are activated during wakefulness [139]. In this context, serotonin plays a role in promoting both analgesia and deep sleep [140]. Neuroendocrine and autonomic mechanisms may influence and be influenced by pain and sleep. Concerning chronic widespread pain syndromes, sleep disorders and nociceptive afferents are important to elevate the sympathetic tonus, which may lead to vascular remodeling, muscular atrophy, and fatigue [141]. Pain and sleep disturbances may generate or perpetuate cognitive, affective, and motivational dysfunctions, which, in turn, promote hypervigilance and frequent awakenings. This is explained by the sharing of common afferent circuits such as the parabrachial amygdala and parabrachial hypothalamic pathways [142].

Less than 6 hours of sleep may contribute to pain manifestations in the following day [143]. Similarly, sleep deprivation, especially of deep sleep, results in wakening unrefreshed with widespread pain and fatigue in healthy sedentary individuals. In this context, alpha wave (8–10 Hz) activity inappropriately intrudes during delta wave (0.5–3.5 Hz) activity [144–146].

The restoration of adequate sleep is essential to avoid exacerbation of painful symptoms [147]. In the case of REM sleep deprivation, a reduced pain threshold persists for a variable period of time, even after normal sleep has been restored.

Prominent fatigue is very commonly reported by patients and is related to sleep disorders, musculoskeletal pain, anxiety, and fibromyalgia, which occurs in 55% of the patients. The approval of pregabalin, a derivative of γ-aminobutyric acid (GABA) that has analgesic, anticonvulsant, anxiolytic, and sleep-modulating activities, has been a real advance for the management of nonrestorative sleep in fibromyalgia. Up to 80% of the patients with ankylosing spondylitis tend to wake up during the night in need of walking in order to get some relief of low back pain. Morning stiffness differs from osteoarthritis because in rheumatoid arthritis it lasts more than 1 hour and in osteoarthritis less than 30 minutes. Additionally, association between clinical manifestations of the disease and fatigue, EDS, and sleep alterations has been reported.

Sleep studies are only available for carpal tunnel syndrome. Patients may complain of nocturnal and early morning awakenings with hand pain and numbness. Nonrestorative sleep, daytime sleepiness, and polysomnographic findings such as arousals and periodic limb movement indexes tend to improve after surgical treatment of the affected wrist. Many investigators have tried to explain why tendonitis, tenosynovitis, bursitis, and periarthritis tend to worsen at night, as described for shoulder-related disorders, but the reasons are still unclear and deserve more study. Clinical symptoms of osteoarthritis tend to be exacerbated at night and on complaints of abdominal cramps and flatulence persist during the night, awakening the patient. Sleep fragmentation leads to poor sleep, which, in turn, promotes deterioration of intestinal symptoms awakening.

Sleep disorders have been described in more than 75% of the subjects suffering from various forms of rheumatic diseases, and fatigue is observed in up to 98% of the cases. Modifications of pain mediators, such as serotonin and substance P, and of neuroimmune mechanisms, such as inflammatory cytokines (interleukin-1 and tumor necrosis factor-α [TNF-α]) and cell-mediated immunity have also been described. Moreover, there is involvement of neuroendocrine mechanisms, such as the hypothalamic–pituitary–adrenal axis and the thyroid, alongside the autonomic nervous system.

14.6.4 SLEEP PROBLEMS IN ELDERLY WITH NEUROLOGICAL DISORDERS

Sleep disturbances are very common in patients with PD and are associated with a variety of negative outcomes. The evaluation of sleep disturbances in these patients is complex as sleep may be affected by a host of primary sleep disorders, other primary medical or psychiatric conditions, reactions to medications, aging, or the neuropathophysiology of PD itself, for example, amyloid [148].

Disturbances of sleep are highly prevalent in PD, affecting up to 88% of the community-dwelling patients [149]. Furthermore, in studies that examine the impact of PD on QoL, sleep difficulties are independent and important predictors of poor QoL [150]. In fact, most reports suggest that sleep disturbance, depression, and lack of independence are the primary determinants of poor QoL [151]. In addition, sleep disturbances contribute to EDS and poor daytime functioning as well as patients' reduced enthusiasm for daily events. Adverse effects have also been observed in the sleep habits and the QoL of their spousal caregivers [106–108].

The interactions between PD and sleep are complicated. First, many of the degenerative changes that are occurring in the brain may directly affect sleep–wake mechanisms and lead to sleep disruption. In particular, brain neurotransmitters that mediate sleep functions (norepinephrine, serotonin, dopamine, and GABA) are variably damaged in PD. Furthermore, neurotransmitters involved in REM sleep (acetylcholine, serotonin, and norepinephrine) are also variably disrupted in PD. Motor difficulties, such as inability to move in bed, dystonic movements, and pain from leg cramps may all interfere with sleep maintenance. While dopaminergic replacement therapy may improve sleep in patients experiencing nighttime motor dysfunction, it can also disrupt normal sleep architecture and may be stimulating to some patients. As previously discussed, many other primary sleep disorders, such as sleep apnea and restless legs, occur commonly in individuals with PD. Superimposed on these complex interactions are age-related sleep and circadian changes. Approximately 40% of the elderly population experience sleep difficulties, and these problems tend to be more common in those elderly population with physical and psychological problems.

Sleep problems are very prevalent in PD, affecting about three quarters of these individuals. The disturbance most often involves difficulty staying asleep through the night, but it may affect virtually any aspect of sleep. Other co-occurring sleep disorders, such as sleep apnea, REM behavior disorder, and RLS, are also very common. These sleep problems are associated with poor QoL for both the patient and the caregiver [109,152–163].

The treatment of sleep disturbances in PD is largely unstudied, but recommendations based on clinical experience in PD and research studies in other geriatric populations can be made. The first step is proper diagnosis. The next step is to treat the specific sleep disorder or the co-occurring disorder that is interfering with sleep as many conditions, such as RBD and RLS, have specific treatments. Special attention should be paid to depression, which frequently travels with PD and nearly always interferes with sleep. The control of the motor aspects of PD must also be paramount as nighttime movements will interfere with sleep.

14.7 SUMMARY

A careful sleep history needs to be taken in all geriatric patients. The patient's responses should indicate how to proceed with any further history, focused physical examination, or laboratory investigations. Specific questions, examinations, laboratory tests, procedures, and possible referrals need to be considered depending on the pathology. Improvement in recognition and treatment of insomnia in the older adult will improve daytime functioning and help reduce medical and psychiatric comorbidities, especially depression and anxiety. The treatment of OSA in the older adult results in improvements in nocturia and cognition and helps facilitate care in skilled nursing facilities or long-term care. The treatment of RLS affects outcomes such as blood pressure, depression, sleep measures, and health-related QoL in older individuals.

Research is needed to define the timing, duration, and optimal light wavelength of BLT for older adults with advanced sleep-phase disorder. Multicenter, placebo-controlled, randomized studies are necessary to determine the efficacy, safety, and tolerability of long-term therapy with bright light in older adults. Placebo-controlled, randomized clinical trials of the efficacy and safety of melatonin receptor agonists are required in the treatment of irregular sleep-wake disorder (ISWD) in patients with dementia. Basic research to understand the pathophysiology of CRSDs, including the role of genetics, is also a priority. Multicenter trials are needed of the safety and efficacy of pharmacologic therapies in older adults with parasomnias, such as RBD. Trials should be conducted for clonazepam, melatonin, and dopamine agonists. Research is necessary to elucidate the relationship between RBD and PD.

If possible, the history from the bed partner as well as the patient should be obtained. Questions should address EDS, cataplexy, symptom response to napping (if any), presence of dreaming during naps, hypnagogic hallucinations, sleep paralysis, and automatic behaviors. Onset, frequency, and duration of the sleepiness as well as any episodes of remission should be established. Questions about the patient's medical, neurologic and psychiatric illnesses as well as use or recent discontinuation of recreational drugs, prescription drugs, and/or alcohol should be included. Questions about other comorbid sleep disorders such as OSA or RLS are also relevant. A number of subjective sleep questionnaires are available to assess sleep habits, sleep–wake schedules, and sleepiness (e.g., the most commonly used ESS and Karolinska Sleep Scales [KSS]; sleep diaries are also useful assessment tools).

The basic pathophysiologic mechanism(s) of excessive sleepiness due to idiopathic hypersomnia, narcolepsy, and AD needs to be further investigated. There is a need for standardization and validation of multiple sleep latency test (MSLT) studies in older adults. The efficacy of treatment modalities, especially pharmacotherapy (e.g., modafinil, lithium, and sodium oxybate), in older adults for hypersomnia of central origin requires further study. There is a need for better understanding the comorbidities that may be associated with hypersomnias of central origin in older adults (e.g., cognitive deficits and obesity). There is a need for better understanding of how increasing age and comorbidities may modify the symptoms and response to treatment in older adults.

Future research should clarify the consequences of sleep disturbance among nursing home residents, particularly in terms of effects on QoL. The effectiveness of pharmacologic interventions to improve sleep among nursing home residents should be tested, with careful attention to the balance of potential risks and benefits in this vulnerable population. More effective behavioral and other nonpharmacologic interventions must be identified that will help to improve disturbed sleep patterns among nursing home residents. The relationship among insomnia, sedative hypnotic medications, and adverse events, including falls, among nursing home residents must be clarified.

REFERENCES

1. Foley D, Ancoli-Israel S, Britz P et al. Sleep disturbances and chronic disease in older adults: Results of the 2003 National sleep Foundation Sleep in America Survey. *J Psychosom Res.* 2004;56:497–502.
2. Foley DJ, Monjan AA, Brown SL et al. Sleep complaints among elderly persons: An epidemiologic study of three communities. *Sleep.* 1995;18:425–432.
3. Foley DJ, Monjan A, Simonsick EM et al. Incidence and remission of insomnia among elderly adults: An epidemiologic study of 6,800 persons over three years. *Sleep.* 1999;22:S366–S372.
4. Vitiello MV, Moe KE, Prinz PN. Sleep complaints cosegregate with illness in older adults: Clinical research informed by and informing epidemiological studies of sleep. *J Psychosom Res.* 2002;53:555–559.
5. Ohayon MM, Carskadon MA, Guilleminault C et al. Meta-analysis of quantitative sleep parameters from childhood to old age in healthy individuals: Developing normative sleep values across the human lifespan. *Sleep.* 2004;27:1255–1273.
6. Van Cauter EV, Leproult R, Plat L. Age-related changes in slow wave sleep and REM sleep and relationship with growth hormone and cortisol levels in healthy men. *JAMA.* 2000;284:861–868.
7. Prinz PN, Vitiello MV, Raskind MA et al. Geriatrics: Sleep disorders and aging. *N Engl J Med.* 1990;323:520–526.
8. Shochat T, Martin J, Marler M et al. Illumination levels in nursing home patients: Effects on sleep and activity rhythms. *J Sleep Res.* 2000;9:373–380.
9. Gooneratne NS, Vitiello MV. Sleep in older adults: Normative changes, sleep disorders, and treatment options. *Clin Geriatr Med.* 2014;30(3):591–627.
10. Ancoli-Israel S, Kripke DF, Klauber MR et al. Sleep disordered breathing in community-dwelling elderly. *Sleep.* 1991;14:486–495.
11. Ancoli-Israel S, Gehrman P, Kripke DF et al. Long-term follow-up of sleep disordered breathing in older adults. *Sleep Med.* 2001;2:511–516.
12. Young T, Shahar E, Nieto FJ et al. Predictors of sleep-disordered breathing in community-dwelling adults: The Sleep Heart Health Study. *Arch Intern Med.* 2002;162:893–900.
13. Young T, Palta M, Dempsey J et al. The occurrence of sleep disordered breathing among middle-aged adults. *N Engl J Med.* 1993;328:1230–1235.
14. Gooneratne N, Gehrman PR, Nkwuo JE et al. Consequences of comorbid insomnia symptoms and sleep-related breathing disorder in elderly subjects. *Arch Intern Med.* 2006;166:1732–1738.
15. Launois SH, Pepin JL, Levy P. Sleep apnea in the elderly: A specific entity? *Sleep Med Rev.* 2007;11:87–97.
16. Shahar E, Whitney CW, Redline S et al. Sleep-disordered breathing and cardiovascular disease: Cross sectional results of the Sleep Heart Health Study. *Am J Respir Crit Care Med.* 2001;163:19–25.
17. Bassetti CL, Milanova M, Gugger M. Sleep-disordered breathing and acute ischemic stroke: Diagnosis, risk factors, treatment, evolution, and long-term clinical outcome. *Stroke.* 2006;37:967–972.
18. Aloia MS, Ilniczky N, Di Dio P et al. Neuropsychological changes and treatment compliance in older adults with sleep apnea. *J Psychosom Res.* 2003;54:71–76.
19. Ayalon L, Ancoli-Israel S, Stepnowsky C et al. Adherence to continuous positive airway pressure treatment in patients with Alzheimer's disease and obstructive sleep apnea. *Am J Geriatr Psychiatry.* 2006;14:176–180.
20. Weaver TE, Chasens ER. Continuous positive airway pressure treatment for sleep apnea in older adults. *Sleep Med Rev.* 2007;11:99–111.
21. Ancoli-Israel S. Sleep apnea in older adults – Is it real and should age be the determining factor in the treatment decision matrix? *Sleep Med Rev.* 2007;11:83–85.
22. Allen RP, Picchietti DL, Hening WA et al. Restless Legs Syndrome Diagnosis and Epidemiology workshop at the National Institutes of Health, International Restless Legs Syndrome Study Group Restless legs syndrome: Diagnostic criteria, special considerations, and epidemiology. A report from the restless legs syndrome diagnosis and epidemiology workshop at the National Institutes of Health. *Sleep Med.* 2003;4:101–119.
23. Ancoli-Israel S, Kripke DF, Klauber MR et al. Periodic limb movements in sleep in community-dwelling elderly. *Sleep.* 1991;14:496–500.
24. de Biase S, Valente M, Gigli GL. Intractable restless legs syndrome: Role of prolonged-release oxycodone-naloxone. *Neuropsychiatr Dis Treat.* 201623;12:417–25.

25. Hening W, Allen RP, Picchietti DL et al. Restless legs syndrome task force of the standards of Practice Committee of the American Academy of Sleep Medicine: An update on the dopaminergic treatment of restless legs syndrome and periodic limb movement disorder. *Sleep.* 2004;27:560–583.

26. Boeve BF, Silber MH, Ferman TJ et al. Association of REM sleep behavior disorder and neurodegenerative disease may reflect an underlying synucleinopathy. *Mov Disorders.* 2001;16:622–630.

27. Olson EJ, Boeve BF, Silber MH. Rapid eye movement sleep behaviour disorder: Demographic, clinical and laboratory findings in 93 cases. *Brain.* 2000;123:331–339.

28. Stiasny-Kolster K, Mayer G, Schäfer S et al. The REM sleep behavior disorder screening questionnaire – A new diagnostic instrument. *Mov Disorders.* 2007;22:2386–2393.

29. Cole MG, Dendukuri N. Risk factors for depression among elderly community subjects: A systematic review and meta-analysis. *Am J Psychiatry.* 2003;160:1147–1156.

30. Wolkove N, Elkholy O, Baltzan M et al. Sleep and aging: 2. Management of sleep disorders in older people. *CMAJ.* 2007 May 8;176(10):1449–54.

31. Ohayon MM, Roth T. What are the contributing factors for insomnia in the general population? *J Psychosomatic Res.* 2001;51:745–755.

32. Dijk D.J., Duffy J.F., and Czeisler C.A. Contribution of circadian physiology and sleep homeostasis to age-related changes in human sleep. *Chronobiol Int.* 2000;17:285–311

33. Riemersma-van der Lek RF, Swaab DF, Twisk J et al. Effect of bright light and melatonin on cognitive and noncognitive function in elderly residents of group care facilities: A randomized controlled trial. *JAMA.* 2008. 299:2642–55.

34. Buscemi N, Vandermeer B, Hooton N et al. Efficacy and safety of exogenous melatonin for primary sleep disorders: A meta-analysis. *J Gen Intern Med.* 2005;20:1151–8.

35. Perlis ML, Smith LJ, Lyness JM et al. Insomnia as a risk factor for onset of depression in the elderly. *Behav Sleep Med.* 2006;4:104–113.

36. Morin CM, Colecchi C, Stone J et al. Behavioral and pharmacological therapies for late life insomnia. *JAMA.* 1999;281:991–999.

37. Edinger JD, Sampson WS. A primary care "friendly" cognitive behavioral insomnia therapy. *Sleep.* 2003;26:177–182.

38. National Institutes of Health State of the Science Conference Statement on Manifestations and Management of Chronic Insomnia in Adults, June 13–15, 2005. *Sleep.* 2005;28:1049–1057.

39. McCurry SM, Reynolds CF, Ancoli-Israel S et al. Treatment of sleep disturbances in Alzheimer's disease. *Sleep Med Rev.* 2000;4:603–628.

40. Ancoli-Israel S, Klauber MR, Butters N et al. Dementia in institutionalized elderly: Relation to sleep apnea. *J Am Geriatr Soc.* 1991;39:258–263.

41. Stewart R, Besset A, Bebbington P et al. Insomnia comorbidity and impact and hypnotic use by age group in a national survey population aged 16 to 74 years. *Sleep.* 2008;29:1391–1397.

42. Ancoli-Israel S. Insomnia in the elderly: A review for the primary care practitioner. *Sleep.* 2000;23(suppl. 1):S23–S30.

43. Ancoli-Israel S, Roth T. Characteristics of insomnia in the United States: Results of the 1991 National Sleep Foundation Survey. I. *Sleep.* 1999;22(Suppl. 2):S347–S353.

44. Stone KL, Ewing SK, Lui LY et al. Self-reported sleep and nap habits and risk of falls and fractures in older women: The study of osteoporotic fractures. *J Am Geriatr Soc.* 2006;54:1177–1183.

45. Avidan AY, Fries BE, James ML et al. Insomnia and hypnotic use, recorded in the minimum data set, as predictors of falls and hip fractures in Michigan nursing homes. *J Am Geriatr Soc.* 2005;53:955–962.

46. Brassington GS, King AC, Bliwise DL. Sleep problems as a risk factor for falls in a sample of community-dwelling adults aged 64–99 years. *J Am Geriatr Soc.* 2000;48:1234–1240.

47. Cricco M, Simonsick EM, Foley DJ. The impact of insomnia on cognitive functioning in older adults. *J Am Geriatr Soc.* 2001;49:1185–1189.

48. Stone KL, Ancoli-Israel S, Blackwell T et al. Actigraphy-measured sleep characteristics and risk of falls in older women. *Arch Intern Med.* 2008;168(16):1768–1775.

49. Crenshaw MC, Edinger JD. Slow-wave sleep and waking cognitive performance among older adults with and without insomnia complaints. *Physiol Behav.* 1999;66:485–492.

50. Dew MA, Hoch CC, Buysse DJ et al. Healthy older adults' sleep predicts all-cause mortality at 4 to 19 years of follow-up. *Psychosom Med.* 2003;65:63–73.

51. Chen ML, Lin LC, Wu SC et al. The effectiveness of acupressure in improving the quality of sleep in institutionalized residents. *J Gerontol A: Biol Sci Med Sci.* 1998;54:M389–M394.

52. Morin CM, Belleville G, Belanger L et al. The insomnia severity index: Psychometric indicators to detect insomnia cases and evaluate treatment response. *Sleep.* 2011;34(5):601–608.

53. Bloom HG, Ahmed I, Alessi CA et al. Evidence-based recommendations for the assessment of sleep disorders in older persons. *J Am Geriatr Soc.* 2009;57(5):761–789.

54. Pat-Horenczyk R, Klauber MR, Shochat T et al. Hourly profiles of sleep and wakefulness in severely versus mild-moderately demented nursing home patients. *Aging Clin Exp Res.* 1998;10:308–315.

55. Rodriguez JC, Dzierzewski JM, Alessi CA. Sleep problems in the elderly. *Med Clin North America.* 2015;99(2):431–439.

56. King AC, Oman RF, Brassington GS et al. Moderate-intensity exercise and self-rated quality of sleep in older adults. A randomized controlled trial. *JAMA.* 1997;277:32–37.

57. Li F, Fisher KJ, Harmer P et al. Tai Chi and self-rated quality of sleep and daytime sleepiness in older adults: A randomized controlled trial. *J Am Ger Soc.* 2004;52:892–900.

58. Tsay S, Rong J, Lin P. Acupoints massage in improving the quality of sleep and quality of life in patients with end-stage renal disease. *J Adv Nurs.* 2003;42:134–142.

59. McCurry SM, Logsdon RG, Terri L et al. Evidence-based psychological treatments for insomnia in older adults. *Psychol Aging.* 2007;22(1):18–27.

60. National Institutes of Health State of the Science Conference Statement on Manifestations and Management of Chronic Insomnia in Adults. *Sleep.* 2005;28:1049–1057.

61. Morin CM, Hauri PJ, Espie CA et al. Nonpharmacologic treatment of chronic insomnia. An American Academy of Sleep Medicine review. *Sleep.* 1999;22:1134–1156.

62. Phillips B, Kryger MH. Management of obstructive sleep apnea hypopnea syndrome: Overview. In: Kryger M, Roth T, Dement WC, editors. *Principles and Practice of Sleep Medicine.* 4th. Philadelphia, PA: Elsevier; 2005. pp. 1109–1121.

63. Banno K, Kryger MH. Sleep apnea: Clinical investigations in humans. *Sleep Med.* 2007;8:400–426.

64. Somers V, Javaheri S. Cardiovascular effects of sleep-related breathing disorders. In: Kryger M, Roth T, Dement WC, editors. *Principles and Practice of Sleep Medicine.* 4th. Philadelphia, PA: Elsevier; 2005. pp. 1180–1191.

65. White DP. Central sleep apnea. In: Kryger M, Roth T, Dement WC, editors. *Principles and Practice of Sleep Medicine.* 4th. Philadelphia, PA: Elsevier; 2005. pp. 969–982.

66. American Academy of Sleep Medicine. *Diagnostic and Coding Manual.* 2nd. Westchester, IL: American Academy of Sleep Medicine; 2005. International Classification of Sleep Disorders.

67. Young T, Palta M, Dempsey J et al. The occurrence of sleep-disordered breathing among middle-aged adults. *N Engl J Med.* 1993;328:1230–1235.

68. Hebert LE, Weuve J, Scherr PA et al. Alzheimer disease in the United States (2010–2050) estimated using the 2010 census. *Neurology.* 2013;80(19):1778–1783.

69. Pistacchi M, Gioulis M, Contin F et al. Sleep disturbance and cognitive disorder: Epidemiological analysis in a cohort of 263 patients. *Neurol Sci.* 2014;35(12):1955–1962.

70. Moran M, Lynch CA, Walsh C et al. Sleep disturbance in mild to moderate Alzheimer's disease. *Sleep Med.* 2005;6(4):347–352.

71. Cipriani G, Lucetti C, Danti S et al. Sleep disturbances and dementia. *Psychogeriatrics.* 2015;15(1):65–74.

72. Vitiello MV, Borson S. Sleep disturbances in patients with Alzheimer's disease: Epidemiology, pathophysiology and treatment. *CNS Drugs.* 2001;15(10):777–796.

73. Hoch CC, Reynolds CF, 3rd, Kupfer DJ et al. Sleep-disordered breathing in normal and pathologic aging. *J Clin Psychiatry.* 1986;47(10):499–503.

74. Ancoli-Israel S, Klauber MR, Butters N et al. Dementia in institutionalized elderly: Relation to sleep apnea. *J Am Geriatr Soc.* 1991;39(3):258–263.

75. Shin HY, Han HJ, Shin DJ et al. Sleep problems associated with behavioral and psychological symptoms as well as cognitive functions in Alzheimer's disease. *J Clin Neurol.* 2014;10(3):203–209.

76. Gaugler JE, Edwards AB, Femia EE et al. Predictors of institutionalization of cognitively impaired elders: Family help and the timing of placement. *J Gerontol B Psychol Sci Soc Sci.* 2000;55(4):P247–P255.

77. Ju YE, Lucey BP, Holtzman DM. Sleep and Alzheimer disease pathology – A bidirectional relationship. *Nat Rev Neurol.* 2014;10(2):115–119.

78. Guarnieri B, Sorbi S. Sleep and cognitive decline: A strong bidirectional relationship. It is time for specific recommendations on routine assessment and the management of sleep disorders in patients with mild cognitive impairment and dementia. *Eur Neurol.* 2015;74(1–2):43–48.

79. Villa C, Ferini-Strambi L, Combi R. The synergistic relationship between Alzheimer's disease and sleep disorders: An update. *J Alzheimers Dis.* 2015;46(3):571–580.

80. Cooke JR, Ancoli-Israel S. Normal and abnormal sleep in the elderly. *Handb Clin Neurol.* 2011;98:653–665.

81. Peter-Derex L, Yammine P, Bastuji H et al. Sleep and Alzheimer's disease. *Sleep Med Rev.* 2015;19:29–38.

82. Prinz PN, Peskind ER, Vitaliano PP et al. Changes in the sleep and waking EEGs of nondemented and demented elderly subjects. *J Am Geriatr Soc.* 1982;30(2):86–93.
83. Petit D, Gagnon JF, Fantini ML et al. Sleep and quantitative EEG in neurodegenerative disorders. *J Psychosom Res.* 2004;56(5):487–496.
84. Born J, Rasch B, Gais S. Sleep to remember. *Neuroscientist.* 2006;12(5):410–424.
85. Diekelmann S, Born J. The memory function of sleep. *Nat Rev Neurosci.* 2010;11(2):114–126.
86. Rauchs G, Schabus M, Parapatics S et al. Is there a link between sleep changes and memory in Alzheimer's disease? *Neuroreport.* 2008;19(11):1159–1162.
87. Rauchs G, Piolino P, Bertran F et al. Retrieval of recent autobiographical memories is associated with slow-wave sleep in early AD. *Front Behav Neurosci.* 2013;7:114.
88. Song Y, Dowling GA, Wallhagen MI et al. Sleep in older adults with Alzheimer's disease. *J Neurosci Nurs.* 2010;42(4):190–198. quiz 199–200.
89. Bliwise DL. Sleep disorders in Alzheimer's disease and other dementias. *Clin Cornerstone.* 2004;6(Suppl. 1A):S16–S28.
90. Khachiyants N, Trinkle D, Son SJ et al. Sundown syndrome in persons with dementia: An update. *Psychiatry Investig.* 2011;8(4):275–287.
91. Coogan AN, Schutova B, Husung S et al. The circadian system in Alzheimer's disease: Disturbances, mechanisms, and opportunities. *Biol Psychiatry.* 2013;74(5):333–339.
92. Gnanasekaran G. "Sundowning" as a biological phenomenon: Current understandings and future directions: An update. *Aging Clin Exp Res.* 2015;28(3):383–392.
93. Ferrazzoli D, Sica F, Sancesario G. Sundowning syndrome: A possible marker of frailty in Alzheimer's disease? *CNS Neurol Disord Drug Targets.* 2013;12(4):525–528.
94. Giubilei F, Patacchioli FR, Antonini G et al. Altered circadian cortisol secretion in Alzheimer's disease: Clinical and neuroradiological aspects. *J Neurosci Res.* 2001;66(2):262–265.
95. Harper DG, Stopa EG, McKee AC et al. Differential circadian rhythm disturbances in men with Alzheimer disease and frontotemporal degeneration. *Arch Gen Psychiatry.* 2001;58(4):353–360.
96. Videnovic A, Lazar AS, Barker RA et al. "The clocks that time us" – Circadian rhythms in neurodegenerative disorders. *Nat Rev Neurol.* 2014;10(12):683–693.
97. Stranahan AM. Chronobiological approaches to Alzheimer's disease. *Curr Alzheimer Res.* 2012;9(1):93–98.
98. Kadotani H, Kadotani T, Young T et al. Association between apolipoprotein E epsilon4 and sleep-disordered breathing in adults. *JAMA.* 2001;285(22):2888–2890.
99. Pan W, Kastin AJ. Can sleep apnea cause Alzheimer's disease? *Neurosci Biobehav Rev.* 2014;47:656–669.
100. Osorio RS, Gumb T, Pirraglia E et al. Sleep-disordered breathing advances cognitive decline in the elderly. *Neurology.* 2015;84(19):1964–1971.
101. Reynolds CF, 3rd, Kupfer DJ, Taska LS et al. Sleep apnea in Alzheimer's dementia: Correlation with mental deterioration. *J Clin Psychiatry.* 1985;46(7):257–261.
102. Cooke JR, Liu L, Natarajan L et al. The effect of sleep-disordered breathing on stages of sleep in patients with Alzheimer's disease. *Behav Sleep Med.* 2006;4(4):219–227.
103. Yaffe K, Laffan AM, Harrison SL et al. Sleep-disordered breathing, hypoxia, and risk of mild cognitive impairment and dementia in older women. *JAMA.* 2011;306(6):613–619.
104. Kielb SA, Ancoli-Israel S, Rebok GW et al. Cognition in obstructive sleep apnea-hypopnea syndrome (OSAS): Current clinical knowledge and the impact of treatment. *Neuromolecular Med.* 2012;14(3):180–193.
105. Lal C, Strange C, Bachman D. Neurocognitive impairment in obstructive sleep apnea. *Chest.* 2012;141(6):1601–1610.
106. Pal PK, Thennarasu K, Fleming J et al. Nocturnal sleep disturbances and daytime dysfunction in patients with Parkinson's disease and in their caregivers. *Parkinsonism Relat Disord.* 2004;10(3):157–168.
107. Smith MC, Ellgring H, Oertel WH. Sleep disturbances in Parkinson's disease patients and spouses. *J AM Geriatr Soc.* 1997;45:194–199.
108. Lowe AD. Sleep in Parkinson's disease. *J Psychosom Res.* 1998;44(6):613–617.
109. Ripley B, Overeem S, Fujiki N et al. CSF hypocretin/orexin levels in narcolepsy and other neurological conditions. *Neurology.* 2001;57(12):2253–2258.
110. Urrestarazu E, Iriarte J. Clinical management of sleep disturbances in Alzheimer's disease: Current and emerging strategies. *Nat Sci Sleep.* 2016;8:21–33.
111. Spira AP, Gamaldo AA, An Y et al. Self-reported sleep and beta-amyloid deposition in community-dwelling older adults. *JAMA Neurol.* 2013;70(12):1537–1543.

112. Lim AS, Yu L, Kowgier M et al. Modification of the relationship of the apolipoprotein E epsilon4 allele to the risk of Alzheimer disease and neurofibrillary tangle density by sleep. *JAMA Neurol.* 2013;70(12):1544–1551.

113. Musiek ES, Xiong DD, Holtzman DM. Sleep, circadian rhythms, and the pathogenesis of Alzheimer disease. *Exp Mol Med.* 2015;47:e148.

114. Wennstrom M, Londos E, Minthon L et al. Altered CSF orexin and alpha-synuclein levels in dementia patients. *J Alzheimers Dis.* 2012;29(1):125–132.

115. Slats D, Claassen JA, Lammers GJ et al. Association between hypocretin-1 and amyloid-beta42 cerebrospinal fluid levels in Alzheimer's disease and healthy controls. *Curr Alzheimer Res.* 2012;9(10):1119–1125.

116. Dauvilliers YA, Lehmann S, Jaussent I et al. Hypocretin and brain beta-amyloid peptide interactions in cognitive disorders and narcolepsy. *Front Aging Neurosci.* 2014;6:119.

117. Claustrat B, Leston J. Melatonin: Physiological effects in humans. *Neurochirurgie.* 2015;61(2–3):77–84.

118. Benedict C, Byberg L, Cedernaes J et al. Self-reported sleep disturbance is associated with Alzheimer's disease risk in men. *Alzheimers Dement.* 2015;11(9):1090–1097.

119. Ju YE, McLeland JS, Toedebusch CD et al. Sleep quality and preclinical Alzheimer disease. *JAMA Neurol.* 2013;70(5):587–593.

120. Lim AS, Kowgier M, Yu L et al. Sleep fragmentation and the risk of incident Alzheimer's disease and cognitive decline in older persons. *Sleep.* 2013;36(7):1027–1032.

121. Tranah GJ, Blackwell T, Stone KL et al. Circadian activity rhythms and risk of incident dementia and mild cognitive impairment in older women. *Ann Neurol.* 2011;70(5):722–732.

122. Tsapanou A, Gu Y, O'Shea D et al. Daytime somnolence as an early sign of cognitive decline in a community-based study of older people. *Int J Geriatr Psychiatry.* 2015 Jun 15; Epub.

123. Spira AP, Chen-Edinboro LP, Wu MN et al. Impact of sleep on the risk of cognitive decline and dementia. *Curr Opin Psychiatry.* 2014;27(6):478–483.

124. Hahn EA, Wang HX, Andel R et al. A change in sleep pattern may predict Alzheimer disease. *Am J Geriatr Psychiatry.* 2014;22(11):1262–1271.

125. Schnelle JF, Cruise PA, Alessi CA et al. Sleep hygiene in physically dependent nursing home residents. *Sleep.* 1998;21:515–523.

126. Ancoli-Israel S, Jones DW, McGuinn P et al. Sleep disorders. In: Morris J, Lipshitz J, Murphy K, Belleville-Taylor P, editors. *Quality Care for the Nursing Home.* St Louis, MO: Mosby Lifeline; 1997. pp. 64–73.

127. Alessi CA, Schnelle JF. Approach to sleep disorders in the nursing home setting. *Sleep Med Rev.* 2000;4:45–56.

128. Ancoli-Israel S, Gehrman PR, Martin JL et al. Increased light exposure consolidates sleep and strengthens circadian rhythms in severe Alzheimer's disease patients. *Behav Sleep Med.* 2003;1:22–36.

129. Martin J, Stepnowsky C, Ancoli-Israel S. Sleep apnea in the elderly. In: McNicholas WT, Phillipson EA, editors. *Breathing Disorders during Sleep.* London: W.B. Saunders Company Ltd.; 2002. pp. 278–287.

130. Crenshaw MC, Edinger JD. Slow-wave sleep and waking cognitive performance among older adults with and without insomnia complaints. *Physiol Behav.* 1999;66:485–492.

131. Brassington GS, King AC, Bliwise DL. Sleep problems as a risk factor for falls in a sample of community-dwelling adults aged 64–99 years. *J Am Geriatr Soc.* 2000;48:1234–1240.

132. Stone KL, Ancoli-Israel S, Blackwell T et al. Poor sleep is associated with increased risk of falls in older women. *Arch Intern Med.* 2008;168:1768–1775.

133. Dew MA, Hoch CC, Buysse DJ et al. Healthy older adults' sleep predicts all-cause mortality at 4 to 19 years of follow-up. *Psychosom Med.* 2003;65:63–73.

134. Foley DJ, Monjan AA, Brown SL et al. Sleep complaints among elderly persons: An epidemiologic study of three communities. *Sleep.* 1995;18:425–432.

135. Tornatore JB, Hedrick SC, Sullivan JH et al. Community residential care: Comparison of cognitively impaired and noncognitively impaired residents. *Am J Alz Dis Other Dem.* 2003;18(4):240–246.

136. McCurry SM, Logsdon RG, Avery DH et al. Development of behavioral interventions to improve sleep in persons with dementia residing in adult family homes. *Gerontologist.* 2005;45(Special Issue II):129.

137. Chiu YH, Silman AJ, Macfarlane GJ et al. Poor sleep and depression are independently associated with a reduced pain threshold. Results of a population based study. *Pain.* 2005;115:316–321.

138. Ohayon MM. Relationship between chronic painful physical condition and insomnia. *J Psychiatr Res.* 2005;39:151–159.

139. Foo H, Mason P. Brainstem modulation of pain during sleep and waking. *Sleep Med Rev.* 2003;7:145–154.

140. Leung CG, Mason P. Physiological properties of raphe magnus neurons during sleep and waking. *J Neurophysiol.* 1999;81:584–595.

141. Gangwisch JE, Heymsfield SB, Boden-Albala B et al. Short sleep duration as a risk factor for hypertension: Analyses of the first National Health and Nutrition Examination Survey. *Hypertension.* 2006;47:833–839.

142. Wiech K, Ploner M, Tracey I. Neurocognitive aspects of pain perception. *Trends Cogn Sci.* 2008;12:306–313.

143. Lautenbacher S, Kundermann B, Krieg JC. Sleep deprivation and pain perception. *Sleep Med Rev.* 2006;10:357–369.

144. Older SA, Battafarano DF, Danning CL et al. The effects of delta wave sleep interruption on pain thresholds and fibromyalgia-like symptoms in healthy subjects; correlations with insulin-like growth factor I. *J Rheumatol.* 1998;25:1180–1186.

145. Lentz MJ, Landis CA, Rothermel J et al. Effects of selective slow wave sleep disruption on musculoskeletal pain and fatigue in middle aged women. *J Rheumatol.* 1999;26:1586–1592.

146. Onen SH, Alloui A, Gross A et al. The effects of total sleep deprivation, selective sleep interruption and sleep recovery on pain tolerance thresholds in healthy subjects. *J Sleep Res.* 2001;10:35–42.

147. Tang NK. Cognitive-behavioral therapy for sleep abnormalities of chronic pain patients. *Curr Rheumatol Rep.* 2009;11:451–460.

148. Huang Y, Potter R, Sigurdson W et al. Beta-amyloid dynamics in human plasma. *Arch Neurol.* 2012;69(12):1591–1597.

149. Factor SA, McAlarney T, Sanchez-Ramos JR et al. Sleep disorders and sleep effect in Parkinson's disease. *Mov Disord.* 1990;5:280–285.

150. Scaravelli T, Gasparoli E, Rinaldi F et al. Health related quality of life and sleep disorders in Parkinson's disease. *Neurol Sci.* 2003;24(3):209–210.

151. Karlsen KH, Tanberg E, Arsland D et al. Health related quality of life in Parkinson's disease: A prospective longitudinal study. *J Neurol Neurosurg Psychiatry.* 2000;69:584–589.

152. Slats D, Claassen JA, Verbeek MM et al. Reciprocal interactions between sleep, circadian rhythms and Alzheimer's disease: Focus on the role of hypocretin and melatonin. *Ageing Res Rev.* 2013;12(1):188–200.

153. de Lecea L, Kilduff TS, Peyron C et al. The hypocretins: Hypothalamus-specific peptides with neuro-excitatory activity. *Proc Natl Acad Sci USA.* 1998;95(1):322–327.

154. Peyron C, Tighe DK, van den Pol AN et al. Neurons containing hypocretin (orexin) project to multiple neuronal systems. *J Neurosci.* 1998;18(23):9996–10015.

155. Mieda M, Tsujino N, Sakurai T. Differential roles of orexin receptors in the regulation of sleep/wakefulness. *Front Endocrinol (Lausanne)* 2013;4:57.

156. Tsujino N, Sakurai T. Role of orexin in modulating arousal, feeding, and motivation. *Front Behav Neurosci.* 2013;7:28.

157. Kang JE, Lim MM, Bateman RJ et al. Amyloid-beta dynamics are regulated by orexin and the sleep-wake cycle. *Science.* 2009;326(5955):1005–1007.

158. Fronczek R, van Geest S, Frolich M et al. Hypocretin (orexin) loss in Alzheimer's disease. *Neurobiol Aging.* 2012;33(8):1642–1650.

159. Dauvilliers Y, Baumann CR, Carlander B et al. CSF hypocretin-1 levels in narcolepsy, kleine-levin syndrome, and other hypersomnias and neurological conditions. *J Neurol Neurosurg Psychiatry.* 2003;74(12):1667–1673.

160. Deuschle M, Schilling C, Leweke FM et al. Hypocretin in cerebrospinal fluid is positively correlated with tau and pTau. *Neurosci Lett.* 2014;561:41–45.

161. Schmidt FM, Kratzsch J, Gertz HJ et al. Cerebrospinal fluid melanin-concentrating hormone (MCH) and hypocretin-1 (HCRT-1, orexin-A) in Alzheimer's disease. *PLoS One.* 2013;8(5):e63136.

162. Mishima K, Tozawa T, Satoh K et al. Melatonin secretion rhythm disorders in patients with senile dementia of Alzheimer's type with disturbed sleep-waking. *Biol Psychiatry.* 1999;45(4):417–421.

163. Wu YH, Swaab DF. The human pineal gland and melatonin in aging and Alzheimer's disease. *J Pineal Res.* 2005;38(3):145–152.

Section III

---

*Systemic Disorders in
Geriatric Rehabilitation*

15 Dysphagia in Older Adults and Its Management

Sandhya Seshadri

CONTENTS

15.1 INTRODUCTION

Oropharyngeal dysphagia is a swallowing disorder that results in difficulties with the passage of food, liquids, and secretions from the mouth to the esophagus. Symptoms of dysphagia include drooling, difficulty chewing, manipulating the bolus, and propelling it to the posterior aspect of the oral cavity, coughing before, during, or after swallowing, and moving the bolus through the pharynx. The term oropharyngeal dysphagia is sometimes used interchangeably with deglutition disorder and dysphagia. In this chapter, we will use the term dysphagia to mean oropharyngeal dysphagia. As the word suggests, oropharyngeal refers primarily to the oral (mouth) region and the pharynx, and is different from esophageal dysphagia. Speech-language pathologists (SLPs) diagnose and treat persons with oropharyngeal dysphagia, while gastroenterologists usually diagnose and treat persons with esophageal dysphagia.

Dysphagia may result in an unsafe swallow—which can result in aspiration (passage of secretions, food, and liquids into the larynx and lower respiratory tract), choking due to an inability to clear the food through the pharynx—or an inefficient swallow that can lead to malnutrition and dehydration. Several diseases such as stroke that are common among older adults can result in dysphagia. Every year approximately half a million people are diagnosed with dysphagia due to neurological disorders (1,12). An estimated 43%–54% of stroke patients with dysphagia experience aspiration and 37%–50% develop pneumonia (12,35,41). The medical outcomes of dysphagia for older adults include aspiration, aspiration pneumonia (lower respiratory tract infection secondary to aspiration), malnutrition, dehydration, and, in some cases, death (7,18). While an unsafe swallow can lead to aspiration, an inefficient swallow can lead to malnutrition and dehydration and pose serious threats to older adults. It is reported that more than half of frail older adults are at significant risk for malnutrition, and as many as 75% of adults with dysphagia are at risk for malnutrition and dehydration (35). In one study, the prevalence of malnutrition/risk for malnutrition among independently living older adults with dysphagia was 2.72 times higher than among those without dysphagia (39). In addition to poor medical outcomes, dysphagia affects the social and psychological well-being and quality of life of older adults. Eating and drinking are often social events and older adults with dysphagia can experience anxiety and depression, leading them to withdraw from social interactions. In a study on the social and psychological impact of dysphagia among 360 older adults with subjective dysphagia symptoms in clinics and nursing homes across four countries in Europe, 41% reported mealtime-related anxiety and 36% reported decreased participation in activities that entailed eating with others (13).

15.2   EPIDEMIOLOGY

The risk of diseases such as stroke and cancer increases with age. Accordingly, 10%–30% of adults over the age of 65 are estimated to have dysphagia (6). Among community-dwelling older adults, the prevalence of dysphagia ranges from 13.8% to 33% (10,15,39). The prevalence of dysphagia may be higher than reported in the literature, as data are usually gathered from self-reported questionnaires and many older adults have the mistaken belief that dysphagia is an inherent part of aging and do not report their symptoms (22). On the other hand, the incidence of dysphagia among older adults continues to increase and is commensurate with the increase in the population of older adults. In an epidemiologic study on aging and dysphagia, the dysphagia referral rates at a university hospital doubled between 2000 and 2007 from a total of 428 in 2000 to 858 in 2007 (20). In fact, referrals for older adults between 60 and greater than 90-years old, were approximately 70% of total referrals for dysphagia (20).

15.3   NORMAL SWALLOWING, DYSPHAGIA, AND PRESBYPHAGIA

Effective dysphagia management and treatment warrant an understanding of the differences between normal swallowing, dysphagia, and presbyphagia.

15.3.1   NORMAL SWALLOWING

SLPs who diagnose dysphagia distinguish between the four stages of normal swallowing, namely, the oral preparatory, oral, pharyngeal, and esophageal stages. These four stages are separated to better assess and understand the swallowing mechanism, even though they are interdependent and are part of one integrated process. The oral preparatory stage involves the preparation of the bolus (food) for the swallow, beginning with the placement of food in the mouth followed by lip closure; oral musculature tension; and mandibular, anterior velar, and lingual movements. In a synchronized manner, each part of the oral cavity (lips, teeth, tongue, jaw, and velum) contributes to the preparation of the bolus. The oral stage commences when the bolus is prepared and propelled to the posterior aspect of the oral cavity before the swallow is triggered. The pharyngeal stage begins when the swallow is triggered and involves velopharyngeal closure, base of tongue excursion, upward and anterior hyolaryngeal movement with inversion of the epiglottis, and adduction of the vocal cords. The esophageal stage commences with the relaxation of the upper-esophageal sphincter and the passage of the bolus into the esophagus. Some symptoms of dysphagia may warrant an assessment of the esophageal stage to ensure that the cause of pharyngeal symptoms do not lie in the esophagus. For example, patients may complain of feeling food "stuck in the throat" (a globus sensation) or may point to the sternum as the source of discomfort. Sometimes these symptoms are suggestive of gastroesophageal reflux and esophageal dysphagia. If a patient's symptoms are predominantly related to the esophageal stage of the swallow, a referral may be made to a gastroenterologist or to an otolaryngologist, depending on the nature of the deficits and the presenting symptoms.

15.3.2 DYSPHAGIA

Given the complexity of the swallowing mechanism patients may experience difficulties and demonstrate deficits in any or all of the stages of the swallow leading to the diagnosis of dysphagia. Thus, a diagnostic report may include stage and severity of dysphagia with a description of the characteristics of the deficits. Symptoms of dysphagia and the deficits identified may include drooling, difficulty chewing food; prolonged mastication of food; a wet vocal quality after the swallow; multiple swallows for a single bite of food; frequent throat clearing while eating; coughing before, during, or after the swallow; and food residue in the mouth after a swallow. The presence of these and other difficulties with swallowing has a direct bearing on the health of older adults if left undiagnosed and untreated as they can lead to respiratory illnesses, malnutrition, and dehydration. In frail older adults, these symptoms can cause further weakness and a worsening health trajectory. Thus, a comprehensive dysphagia evaluation often includes patient-reported symptoms obtained during a patient interview and a description of both objective symptoms and inferred deficits based on the evaluation. Signs and symptoms of aspiration, such as coughing before, during, or after a swallow, may be indicative of deficits at different stages of the swallow: for example, an inability to manage the bolus in the oral preparatory or oral stages, resulting in premature spillage; an unprotected airway due to an inadequate epiglottic inversion during the pharyngeal stage; or aspiration of residue in the pyriform sinuses or vallecular spaces. Similarly, poor dentition and the symptoms of decreased ability to chew foods, prolonged mastication, and difficulty with manipulating the bolus in the oral cavity may suggest that the older adult may be at risk for decreased oral intake and poor nutrition. In older adults, several factors can contribute to these signs and symptoms and it is important to differentiate between deficits and normal age-related changes.

15.3.3 PRESBYPHAGIA

Presbyphagia refers to normal age-related changes that occur in the swallowing mechanism and may place an older adult at risk for dysphagia. Age-related changes include the loss of dentition and increased lingual atrophy with decreased lingual strength (6,15), delays in pharyngeal transit time (29,31), and delays in the closing of the laryngeal vestibule during the swallow, resulting in the bolus being adjacent to an open airway (23,37). Normal aging can also result in decreased taste, smell, lingual pressure, and enlarged cervical osteophytes that impinge on the pharyngeal wall. Age-related changes to the swallowing mechanism may place the older adult at a higher risk for dysphagia especially in the presence of other factors such as decreased cognition, multiple-morbidities, poly-pharmacy, and frailty.

15.4   DYSPHAGIA AND AGING

It is known that more than 50% of adults over the age of 65 years suffer from three or more chronic conditions, which often leads to complex clinical management and greater resource utilization (2). Multiple comorbidities may entail the ingestion of multiple medications. While aging does not lead to decreased salivary flow, diseases and ingestion of certain medications can result in decreased saliva production (33). More than 2000 drugs are known to cause xerostomia (dry mouth and reduced salivary flow), and this, in turn, can place an older adult at risk for dysphagia (6,31) making it difficult to manipulate food in the oral cavity and form a cohesive bolus. In addition, some drugs can affect the mental alertness necessary to participate in the act of eating and swallowing (6,31,42). Xerostomia may indirectly affect the respiratory health of an older adult. The oropharynx is known to contain florae that remain stable in healthy individuals. The saliva produced by the parotid glands not only protects and lubricates the oral cavity but also contains antimicrobials that prevent disease that could result from the presence of oral pathogens (5). Patients with head and neck cancer who have had surgery and radiation can also demonstrate signs of xerostomia. Thus, diseases, treatments, and medications can lead to decreased saliva and decreased antimicrobial protection, causing colonization of pathogens. Dental diseases such as plaque and gingivitis are the result of the colonization of normal oral pathogens (5). Older adults with poor dentition and poor oral hygiene are at risk for pneumonia if they aspirate their oral secretions. While it was previously believed that aspiration pneumonia was the consequence of food and liquids entering the lungs, it is now known that aspiration pneumonia could also occur when pathogen-laden secretions enter the lungs.

Many medical conditions that are common among older adults can impact swallowing and cause dysphagia. In one study, 20%–92% of patients with chronic obstructive pulmonary disease (COPD) self-reported swallowing abnormalities (28). In another study, older adults with well-controlled medical problems, particularly hypertension, had longer pharyngeal transit times (the time taken for the bolus to pass through the pharynx) during a swallow compared to those without medical problems (18). A longer pharyngeal transit time can leave the airway unprotected and lead to aspiration. Other factors prevalent among older adults, such as sarcopenia (muscle weakness), frailty, failure to thrive, and poor oral health are also associated with dysphagia and can affect respiratory function and adequacy of nutrition and hydration (15,31,43). Thus, presbyphagia, multiple comorbidities, poor oral hygiene, frailty, decreased muscle strength, decreased cognition and alertness, and poly-pharmacy can place older adults at risk for dysphagia and make the assessment and management of the symptoms of dysphagia challenging.

15.5   TYPES OF DYSPHAGIA ASSESSMENT METHODS AND TOOLS

As dysphagia impacts several aspects of an older adult's health, the assessment of the swallowing function needs to be comprehensive. A safe swallow entails both a robust oral and pharyngeal anatomy and physiology and an alert participation in the act of eating with adequate cognition. Thus, most dysphagia assessments will include a review of the patient's social, psychological, and medical history; a comprehensive examination of the oral-peripheral mechanism; a cognitive-linguistic assessment; and trials of different textures of food and liquids. In addition, for older adults, the assessment may include a review of normal eating patterns, preferred foods, the type and extent of social support that is available to them, and their current living situation (e.g., whether they live independently in the community, at a skilled nursing facility, or at an assisted living facility). A comprehensive assessment is important to ensure that recommendations for management can be implemented with the least amount of difficulty. Table 15.1 provides a list of assessment types, methods, and tools that are used either in isolation or in combination when completing a dysphagia evaluation.

TABLE 15.1

Dysphagia Assessment Types, Methods, and Tools

Types of Assessment	Assessment Methods and Tools
Bedside swallow evaluation	Review of medical, social, and psychological history
	Oral-peripheral examination
	Cognitive-linguistic assessment
	PO trials
Instrumental assessments	Modified barium swallow study (MBSS)
	Fiberoptic endoscopic evaluation of swallowing (FEES)
Scales and tests	Mann assessment of swallowing ability (MASA)
	Modified barium swallow impairment profile (MBSImp)
	Volume-viscosity swallow test (V-VST)
	Penetration–aspiration scale

15.5.1 TYPES OF ASSESSMENT

When there are concerns about the safety or efficiency of an older adult's swallow, a referral for a dysphagia evaluation is usually made to the SLP. Depending on the facility where the referral is made, there may be variations in the type of assessment that an SLP completes. The preliminary step prior to any assessment, regardless of the type of assessment used, is a review of the patient's social, psychological, and medical history. It is important to review the medical history to better understand the underlying etiology of dysphagia, as this will impact the clinical decisions for management of the symptoms. For example, knowing whether a patient suffered a stroke, had a head injury, or a neurodegenerative disease can help a clinician anticipate the type of swallowing and cognitive deficits that may be present and determine the manner in which to best elicit patient report of symptoms and prior treatments, if any, of dysphagia. Similarly, it is important to know the patient's premorbid nutritional intake, dysphagia history, history of unexpected weight loss, presence of symptoms of gastroesophageal reflux, and practices of ingesting over-the-counter medications such as antacids. It is equally important to know the social and psychological history, as the extent and type of social support available, living conditions, financial burdens experienced by the patient, presence of depression or other psychological disorders, and ingestion of antipsychotic medication can influence clinical decision making during the stages of evaluation and treatment. Finally, it is very important to know the cognitive status of the patient and level of functional independence. Particularly for older adults, a diagnosis of dementia can influence clinical decision-making for management of dysphagia symptoms.

15.6 BEDSIDE SWALLOW EVALUATION

In many hospitals and nursing homes, the assessment process begins with a bedside swallow evaluation or screening conducted by an SLP. After a review of pertinent medical, social, and psychological history, informal observations of the patient are usually completed. These observations may include information on the patient's level of alertness, the extent to which he/she can independently sit upright, give appropriate responses to questions, his/her level of cooperation, indications of breathing difficulties, and general appearance (e.g., signs of a frail, weak, or fatigued appearance). These observations are usually made within the first few minutes of entering a patient's room and engaging the patient in general conversation. Thus, the patient's cognition, memory, comprehension, language, and intelligibility are informally assessed while engaging the patient in conversation. These observations are important because, for example, the presence of receptive language deficits (difficulty with comprehension) may influence the extent to which the patient may be able to follow therapy or dysphagia management instructions. Similarly, the presence of unintelligible speech (dysarthria) may suggest lingual weakness and would warrant an assessment of lingual mobility and strength. Sometimes, if there is concern about a patient's cognitive status, a detailed cognitive-linguistic evaluation may be completed. In addition, assessments of visual deficits, indications of visual neglect, and vocal quality are also made. For example, a breathy vocal quality may indicate incomplete vocal cord closure and place the patient at risk for aspiration during the swallow.

Following these observations, the bedside evaluation is completed, which includes an oral-peripheral examination and trials of foods and liquids of varying consistencies. The oral-peripheral examination includes an examination of the anatomy and an assessment of the function of oral structures. Observations are made of abnormalities (such as lesions, sores, and facial droop), signs of asymmetry, dentition, oral hygiene, adequacy of moisture in the oral cavity, and halitosis. The function of oral structures is completed through the assessment of the movement patterns and the strength of the lips, tongue, mandible, and palate. Thus, lingual movement is assessed through an observation of the lateralization and protrusion of the tongue tip. In addition, the assessment includes mandible and lip movement during phonation, symmetry and strength of velopharyngeal closure, diadochokinetic rates, buccal strength, vocal quality, respiratory drive, and strength of a volitional and a reflexive cough. Hyolaryngeal excursion may be perceived during a dry swallow of saliva by lightly placing a finger at the thyroid notch. Once the oral exam is completed, and it is determined that the patient is alert enough to participate in oral trials of foods and/or liquids, the patient may be offered trials of foods and liquids of different consistencies. The types and textures of foods and liquids offered to the patient may depend on the information gathered prior to the oral trials. The trials may begin with consistencies that the patient may be able to chew and swallow easily such as thickened liquids or pudding. During the oral trials, an assessment is made of the patient's ability to open the mouth, maintain lip closure to prevent anterior loss of the bolus, chew and control the bolus, the time taken to chew and initiate the swallow, whether swallowing and respiration appear coordinated, whether there exists any residue in the oral cavity after the swallow, and whether there are any changes in vocal quality after the swallow or signs or symptoms of aspiration (8). Based on the bedside evaluation, recommendations may be made for the type of texture modification of foods and liquids that would result in a safe and efficient swallow along with referrals for further instrumental assessments and/or consultations from other services such as nutrition, or gastroenterology. Documentation of the bedside swallow evaluation varies from one facility to another and is usually based on the protocols followed by the facility where the patient is seen. Some facilities may use scales such as the Mann assessment of swallowing ability (MASA), (26) to allow consistency in bedside assessments by different SLPs. In addition, the bedside swallow evaluation may include cervical auscultation to assess the sounds of swallowing with a stethoscope, and/or use pulse oximetry to measure arterial oxygenation with a drop in SpO_2 indicating aspiration (8).

15.6.1 Instrumental Assessments

There are two objective instrumental assessments that are commonly used as diagnostic tools: the modified barium swallow study (MBSS) (sometimes referred to as videofluoroscopy or a pharyngogram) and the fiberoptic endoscopic evaluation of swallowing (FEES). These tools offer clinicians an opportunity to objectively assess the anatomical structures of swallowing, their physiology, and the nature of deficits. Both instruments offer relevant and objective information on the pharyngeal stage of swallowing.

15.6.2 Modified Barium Swallow Study

Dr. Jeri Logemann introduced the technique of evaluating the swallow function using videofluoroscopy (24) commonly known as the MBSS. A team of professionals, usually an SLP and a radiologist (there may be variations in the composition of the team from one facility to another) collaborate to assess the swallow function of a patient under fluoroscopy. The MBSS allows the team to objectively view the anatomy and physiology of the swallow and review the possible causes for deficits identified during a bedside or informal assessment. During the instrumental assessment, the team may trial therapeutic and postural techniques that elicit the safest and most efficient swallow. Often MBBS is used to rule out aspiration and it is very useful to view any episodes of silent aspiration.

During an MBBS, the patient may stand or sit between an upright table and the fluoroscope. The fluoroscope is positioned such that it can be moved up and down to view the swallow in real time (8). The patient's swallowing may be viewed in the lateral and/or anterior–posterior aspect. The patient is offered barium of different consistencies while the team views images of the swallow in real time. If there is a suspicion of risk of aspiration prior to the assessment, or if there is evidence of laryngeal penetration or aspiration during the assessment, the texture of the food or liquid may be modified. The modified texture is then viewed to determine whether it results in any differences or improvement in the swallow function. The order of presentation of different textures of foods and liquids is usually based on the information gathered prior to the study. In addition, the patient may be asked to swallow foods and liquids using therapeutic postures that may improve the swallow efficiency or safety. Postural adjustments are part of the compensatory strategies used to manage the symptoms of dysphagia. With older adults, it is important to not only spend additional time explaining the procedure but also to ascertain whether the patient demonstrates adequate comprehension. Dementia, poor receptive language skills, mild cognitive impairment, poor attention, poor respiratory status, and difficulty staying alert may preclude the use of MBSS with an older adult.

Older adults may experience difficulties with swallowing large solid foods or may complain of a globus sensation. This can result from multiple issues, such as poor mastication skills, impulsive behaviors associated with eating (such as, taking large bites or eating too quickly), weakened pharyngeal musculature, xerostomia, or presence of other physical anomalies such as a cervical osteophyte (bony growth of the cervical vertebrae). It is not uncommon for older adults to present with cervical osteophytes that may impinge on the pharyngeal wall, giving rise to a globus sensation or narrowing of the pharyngeal passage, making it difficult to swallow solid foods. With the use of an MBSS, these anomalies can be viewed and recommendations can be made for the resolution or minimization of the symptoms. In addition, sometimes a Zenker's diverticulum (pharyngeal pouch) or a cricopharyngeal bar may also be identified during an MBSS.

While there are benefits to using the MBSS to assess a patient's swallow, it must be used only if it will affect the way that dysphagia symptoms are managed. The MBSS evaluation report may vary across facilities, but often includes the steps of the procedure adopted, the observations made during the oral, pharyngeal, and sometimes, esophageal stages of the swallow. Specific observations may include the length of time of the swallow; the extent of airway protection; observations of laryngeal penetration and aspiration; whether the laryngeal penetration occurred before, after, or during the swallow; coordination of swallowing and respiration; evidence of pharyngeal or oral residue; structural abnormalities; extent of hyolaryngeal excursion and epiglottic inversion, and upper-esophageal sphincter opening. Each of these observations contributes to the clinical decisions on the most effective means by which the patient's symptoms of dysphagia may be managed.

15.6.3 Fiberoptic Endoscopic Evaluation of Swallowing

FEES enables a direct view of the structures and function of the swallowing mechanism (19). Introduced by Dr. Langmore, FEES offers the SLP an opportunity to view many of the oral and pharyngeal structures from the superior aspect, assess the patient's swallowing of different consistencies of real foods and liquids (as opposed to the barium used during a swallow evaluation with an MBSS), and the patient's response to different techniques and postures to manage the symptoms of dysphagia (8). The procedure involves the passage of an endoscope with a light source and camera through the left or right nares following the contours of the nares to the soft palate, at the level of the nasopharynx. To minimize discomfort, the endoscope is usually lubricated with a lubricating gel. Numbing sprays and medications that are used to minimize discomfort during other endoscopic examinations cannot be used during FEES, as they may interfere with and alter sensation, and impact swallowing. The endoscope is 3–4 mm in diameter and is positioned above the vocal folds such that the SLP can view the images of the velum, the oropharynx, the hypopharynx, the larynx, and the superior aspect of the trachea on a computer monitor attached to the endoscope (8). The position of the endoscope may be periodically shifted to obtain a better view of some structures of swallowing and speech. In addition, the pharyngeal stage of the swallow, including aspiration of foods/liquids and residue of foods and liquids in the pyriform sinuses and vallecular spaces can be viewed. In a normal swallow, the view is obscured during a half-second period known as "white out." A shorter or absent white out period may indicate inadequate airway closure. The swallowing function can be assessed along with sensory testing of the structures and aspiration before and after the swallow. Aspiration during the swallow can be inferred from the location of the residue.

Both instruments (MBSS and FEES) provide useful information on the swallowing function of a patient with dysphagia. Some of the advantages of FEES are that it is portable, it may be easier to position patients for the study, real foods and liquids can be used during trials, and it is less costly compared to the MBSS. However, some patients cannot withstand the discomfort of an endoscope, and caution needs to be exercised when passing the endoscope through the nares, due to the risk of laryngospasms. Thus, a clinician may choose one instrument over another based on several factors, including patient tolerance, patient's cognitive status, cost, and effectiveness in aiding clinical decision making for management of symptoms.

15.6.4 STANDARDIZED SCALES

To facilitate systematic and reliable means of assessing and measuring the swallowing mechanism, one or more standardized scales may be used. The use of standardized scales or instruments is variable and based on the practices adopted by different facilities. In this section, two tests of swallowing that can facilitate the bedside swallow evaluation and two tests that can facilitate a swallow examination using the MBSS are described. The purposes of these scales/tests are to improve inter-rater reliability and provide a common language among clinicians. The two bedside swallow assessment scales described are the MASA (26) and the volume-viscosity swallow test (V-VST) (36) for clinical screening of dysphagia and aspiration, and the two tests that can be used during an MBSS are the modified barium swallow impairment profile (MBSImp) (27), and the penetration–aspiration scale (38).

15.6.5 MANN ASSESSMENT OF SWALLOWING ABILITY

The MASA was developed to provide a standardized assessment of the nature and severity of dysphagia in patients with neurogenic disorders (26). It comprises 24 items and allows an assessment of oral-motor aspects of swallowing; language comprehension; assessment of the oral and pharyngeal stages of swallowing including bolus preparation and pharyngeal clearance; and a risk rating for aspiration. Based on the assessment, recommendations for the safest diet can be made. A version of the test that measures the nature and severity of dysphagia among patients with head and neck cancer is also available.

15.6.6 VOLUME-VISCOSITY SWALLOW TEST

This screening tool was designed to address the clinical signs of impairment in the efficiency and safety of swallow of liquids. As a bedside screening method, it allows for an assessment of different volumes and viscosities of boluses. The patient is offered the bolus via a syringe and efficacy is assessed based on the clinical signs of efficacy of labial seal, presence of oral or pharyngeal residue, and piecemeal deglutition (multiple swallows). The safety of swallow is assessed based on the presence of vocal quality changes, coughs, or a decrease in SpO_2. The trials commence with nectar-thick liquids that are offered in increasing volumes of 5-, 10-, and 200-mL boluses. Safe swallow of all volumes leads to the assessment of regular liquids that are offered in the same progression of increasing volumes. The screening ends with an assessment of pudding-like thick liquids.

15.6.7 MODIFIED BARIUM SWALLOW IMPAIRMENT PROFILE

The MBSImp (27) was developed to minimize variability in the reporting of dysphagia evaluations using the MBSS. The lack of standardization along with variability in training of SLPs in conducting a MBSS created ambiguity in understanding of impairments and functional outcomes. The MBSImp aims to standardize training, protocol, assessment, language used, and analysis and reporting methods. It entails an assessment of 17 physiological components in three domains—oral impairment, pharyngeal impairment, and esophageal impairment—through a scoring scale with three to five scores for each of the 17 components that describe the level of impairment.

15.6.8 PENETRATION–ASPIRATION SCALE

The penetration–aspiration scale (38) is a standardized scale that uses an eight-point, equal appearing interval scale to measure laryngeal penetration and aspiration observed during an MBSS. A score of 1 would indicate a normal swallow with no material swallowed entering the airway and a score of 8 would indicate silent aspiration of swallowed material below the level of the vocal folds with no response from the patient.

15.7 MANAGEMENT AND TREATMENT OF DYSPHAGIA

The ultimate goal of any dysphagia assessment tool or method is to determine the best path for managing symptoms and rehabilitation. Over the years, the risks associated with aspiration and aspiration pneumonia have driven facilities to require that dysphagia assessments primarily focus on a patient's safety for oral intake. Previously, the determination of aspiration often led to patients being npo (nil per os, a medical recommendation to withhold all oral foods and liquids). Feeding tubes (percutaneous endoscopic gastric [PEG] tubes or gastric [G] tubes) were then placed in patients, as alternative forms of nutrition to minimize the risk of oral aspiration. Often older adults with dementia, who lived in institutional settings and were diagnosed with dysphagia, had feeding tubes placed as a means to promote nutrition and prevent aspiration. However, there is evidence now that feeding tubes do not eliminate the risk of aspiration as patients can aspirate oral, nasal, and pharyngeal secretions that can result in pneumonia. In addition, oral care may be neglected when a patient has a feeding tube. Poor oral hygiene can lead to pneumonia as a result of aspiration of pathogen-laden oral secretions. In a study on the risk factors for aspiration pneumonia, researchers found that the strongest predictor of aspiration pneumonia was dependence on others for feeding and oral care (19).

The goals of dysphagia management are not only to minimize aspiration and risks for choking but also to promote nutrition and hydration through oral means as much as possible. To achieve these goals, patients may be provided with compensatory strategies such as a recommendation to eat and drink texture-modified foods and liquids, use certain postures during swallowing, use facilitation techniques, and/or dysphagia therapy focusing on exercise-based interventions. Dysphagia management and therapy usually begin at the site where the diagnosis was made. Dysphagia following an acute event that led to hospitalization often leads to the determination of the safest diet in the hospital and may include therapy, depending on the facility. Sometimes, older adults may be diagnosed with dysphagia as outpatients and may seek outpatient therapy for the management of symptoms and rehabilitation.

Many older adults do not seek care for their symptoms of dysphagia, either because they believe that swallowing difficulties are part of aging or because they believe that therapy is expensive and time consuming (9,22). Improvements in swallowing can be achieved through techniques that facilitate the management of symptoms, enable safe and efficient swallowing, and improve swallowing function through dysphagia therapy. Modification of the texture of foods and liquids and utilization of specific postures, swallowing techniques, adaptive utensils, and methods that impact the rate of intake are ways by which swallowing difficulties can be managed and compensated for. Facilitation techniques such as surface electrical stimulation, thermal stimulation, and biofeedback tools such as surface electromyography (sEMG), Iowa Oral Performance Instrument (IOPI), and the SwallowSTRONG device are methods used during therapy to facilitate improvements in swallow. Dysphagia therapy often includes exercise-based interventions such as effortful pitch glide, jaw-opening exercises, head lift exercises, lingual effort exercises, and Shaker exercises. Stretching and therapies to facilitate and improve jaw opening or laryngeal range of motion may also be included in therapy.

15.7.1 COMPENSATORY STRATEGIES

To compensate for impairments identified during the swallow assessments, several compensatory strategies are used. Some of these strategies include recommendations for alternating foods and liquids during a meal, swallowing multiple times for each bite, or eating only texture-modified diets.

15.7.2 TEXTURE-MODIFIED DIETS

In hospitals, the first compensatory strategy adopted is texture modification of the patient's diet. Since severe oropharyngeal dysphagia can lead to tube feeding, texture-modified diets are used to compensate for weak pharyngeal muscles and/or oropharyngeal anomalies, to promote oral intake, nutrition, and hydration, and to minimize prandial aspiration, whenever possible. While the initial motivation for promoting texture-modified diets was to minimize the risk for aspiration or choking, it is important to note that texture-modified diets and other strategies are used not only to minimize the risk for aspiration, but also to facilitate an efficient swallow. Just as dysphagia assessments should not be viewed as "pass/fail" examinations that determine whether a patient can continue an oral intake or not, dysphagia management strategies should also be viewed as ways to not only minimize aspiration risk, but also to improve the efficiency of the swallow and minimize the risk of malnutrition and dehydration.

The term for modifying the texture of foods and liquids varies across healthcare facilities and across countries (9). Some of the terms used include *modified texture food* (17), or *dysphagia diet*, or *diet-consistency modification*. In this chapter, all diets that include the texture modification of foods and liquids to manage the symptoms of dysphagia will be referred to as *texture-modified diets*, with the term texture-modified foods referring to solid foods and thickened liquids referring to the modification of liquids. The American Dietetic Association published the National Dysphagia Diet in 2002: the levels of diets as defined by in this publication are commonly used in many facilities in the United States. Table 15.2 provides a list of types of texture-modified foods and thickened liquids.

TABLE 15.2

Texture-Modified Diets

Texture-modified foods	Level 1 pureed
	Level 2 mechanically altered
	Level 3 advanced
	Level 4 regular
Thickened liquids	Spoon thick (>1750 cP)
	Honey thick (351–1750 cP)
	Nectar thick (51–350 cP)
	Thin (1–50 cP)

The levels listed in the National Dysphagia Diet include pureed (level 1), mechanically altered (level 2), advanced (level 3), and regular (level 4). In addition, liquids modified through the addition of thickening agents are classified based on measurement units of viscosity called centipoise (cP). Thus, the ranges for liquids were identified as thin (1–50 cP), nectar-like (51–350 cP), honey-like (351–1750 cP), and spoon thick (>1750 cP) (14).

Patients have expressed a dislike for thickened liquids (11) and the practice of thickening liquids can have serious implications for older adults who may be at risk for dehydration due to decreased fluid intake. In one study, 75% of patients who were recommended thickened liquids reduced their intake of liquids due to dislike for the taste (25). Pureed foods (level 1) are often prepared by adding water to foods and may have fewer calories (16). The recommendation of a diet of pureed foods for older adults may need to be supplemented with nutritional supplements and such patients may need to be closely monitored to ensure adequate nutritional intake.

15.7.3   ORAL CARE AND FREE WATER PROTOCOL

Some facilities have adopted the "Frazier Free Water Protocol" (32) as a way to improve hydration among patients who have been recommended thickened liquids as part of dysphagia management. Based on frequent rejection of thickened liquids by patients, a protocol allowing water between meals to some patients was developed by the SLP staff at Frazier Rehabilitation Hospital in 1984. After the implementation of the protocol, the staff of the hospital found that the incidence of pneumonia among patients on the protocol, over a period of 18 months, was very low. The protocol has been refined over the years and includes a screening for water by an SLP, and an instrumental swallow examination to assess the severity of dysphagia. Detailed guidelines list the manner and times when patients with dysphagia who aspirate on thin liquids are to be given water. For patients who have been recommended oral diets, water is offered when requested between meals and 30 minutes after a meal (32). The guidelines also call for aggressive oral care for patients who are dependent on others for their oral care.

While some facilities have adopted the free water protocol, others have resisted it because there are no randomized control trials that have provided unequivocal evidence in support of it. Nonetheless, oral care is recognized as an important part of dysphagia management, particularly for older adults with poor dentition and dental hygiene for whom aggressive oral care is critical. SLPs may sometimes discuss the free water protocol with patients who receive outpatient therapy and older adults receiving dysphagia therapy are usually guided on the importance of oral care.

15.7.4   RATE OF INTAKE AND ADAPTIVE UTENSILS

As a compensatory strategy, SLPs may also recommend techniques to modify the rate of intake of food and liquids. In addition to requiring patients to be seated upright or supported to sit as upright as possible during meals or when eating or drinking, SLPs may recommend the use of strategies to slow the rate of intake. Patients at risk for aspiration may be recommended to use teaspoons instead of large spoons to reduce the volume of intake of foods, to take small sips, and to use small cups without straws to minimize aspiration. Older adults with Parkinson's disease or with a tremor may experience difficulties holding a spoon or a cup. Many adaptive utensils to facilitate stability during eating are commercially available and maybe recommended.

15.7.5   POSTURES AND MANEUVERS

In addition to the recommendation that patients with dysphagia sit upright (with or without support) during all acts of eating and drinking to maximize the benefits of gravity, some postures and maneuvers to facilitate a safe or improved swallow may be recommended. Changing the position of the head during a swallow can change the dimensions of the pharynx and the direction of the bolus as it passes through the pharynx. The chin tuck is a commonly used postural adjustment. The patient is taught to lower their chin to approximate the chest with the head in a midline position (to mimic the act of looking down) while swallowing. For some patients, this position may protect the airway during a swallow or may narrow the pharynx and improve pharyngeal clearance of the bolus. While this is a popular postural adjustment, it is not meant for all patients, and recommendations are usually based on the type of deficits that have compromised swallowing safety. Another postural adjustment is head rotation or head turn, where the patient is required to turn the head to the weaker side. For patients who present with unilateral weakness, turning the head to the weaker side changes the direction of the bolus to the stronger side and minimizes the risk of aspiration or choking from residue on the weaker side. Sometimes a head tilt posture may also be used to direct the bolus to the stronger side.

Maneuvers are often recommended to protect the airway and include the supraglottic swallow maneuver, the Mendelsohn maneuver, and the effortful swallow. To perform the supraglottic swallow maneuver, patients are required to take a deep breath, hold it, swallow while holding the breath and exhale, and cough or clear the throat after the swallow. For patients who demonstrate a reduced laryngeal elevation during the swallow, the Mendelsohn maneuver may be recommended. In this maneuver, the patient is asked to hold the swallow at its height thereby prolonging the time of hyolaryngeal elevation. The effortful swallow is useful for patients who may demonstrate pharyngeal weakness: the maneuver literally entails having the patient swallow hard. For older adults with dysphagia, it is important to ensure adequate comprehension of these compensatory strategies and ability to follow them. While postural adjustments and swallow maneuvers have positive effects in promoting safe swallows, they can increase social isolation among older adults, as using these adjustments and maneuvers when eating and drinking in public, is often embarrassing for patients.

15.7.6 FACILITATION TECHNIQUES

SLPs may use techniques such as surface electrical stimulation (sEMG) and thermal stimulation to facilitate improvements in swallowing function. sEMG is a biofeedback technique that measures myoelectric impulses. The signal is fed into a device and displayed as a waveform on a monitor for the patient, which helps to improve awareness of muscular contractions during swallowing (8). It is often used to improve coordination and facilitate recruitment of muscles where there is weakness.

Sometimes, thermal stimulation techniques may be used to facilitate improvements in the swallow function. During therapy sessions, the anterior faucial pillars are stroked by a chilled laryngeal mirror or swab, providing cold, tactile, and pressure stimulation. The underlying principle for using thermal stimulation is to stimulate the sensory nerves to facilitate the initiation of a swallow as swallowing is a sensory motor activity. Sometimes chemical stimuli (dipping the laryngeal mirror in citric acid instead of ice) have also been used. Evidence for the success of these methods has been mixed, with some studies reporting success and others reporting no treatment effects (40).

15.8 DYSPHAGIA REHABILITATION

Several exercise-based interventions exist for the improvement of swallowing. These interventions are used as part of dysphagia rehabilitation across facilities such as acute-care hospitals, rehabilitation centers and outpatient clinics, or provided in the home to community-dwelling older adults. Despite wide variations in durations, types of therapeutic interventions, and study designs, dysphagia therapies have positive outcomes (40). According to the National Outcomes Measurement System (NOMS), approximately 60% of adults who needed alternative means of nutrition such as feeding tubes, improved with dysphagia therapy to the extent that they were able to recommence oral intake and no longer needed feeding tubes (3). SLPs may use interventions in isolation or in combination to maximize the potential for recovery. Cognition and physical ability to consistently practice the exercises can influence clinical decision making with regard to the use of exercise-based interventions with older adults. Some of these exercises include the lingual resistance exercises, the effortful pitch glide, Shaker exercise (head lift), Masako maneuver, and jaw-opening exercise.

Lingual resistance exercises have been noted to be beneficial in improving swallowing in older adults. Aging can affect isometric pressure and strength of lingual muscles. In one study, healthy older adults participated in an 8-week lingual resistance exercise program (34). The program consisted of compressing the IOPI, a bulb filled with air, and placing it between the tongue and the hard palate. Using biofeedback, study participants increased the pressure applied to the IOPI bulb. All study participants' demonstrated significant increases in isometric and swallowing pressures. In a subsequent study with patients with dysphagia, significant increases in isometric tongue strength were observed and scores on the penetration–aspiration scale were significantly reduced for 3 mL liquids after 4 weeks and for 10 mL liquids after 8 weeks, indicating a reduction in signs of aspiration and penetration (34). There is evidence that forceful lingual pressure also increases pharyngeal pressure (21), and this has positive implications for patients with weak pharyngeal squeeze during a swallow. Several devices exist for facilitating lingual and oropharyngeal strengthening including the tongue depressor, IOPI, KayPentax Digital Swallowing Workstation, and the SwallowSTRONG Management System. The standard strengthening protocol requires 10 lingual presses against the sensor, three times a day, 3 days a week, for 8 weeks and hence requires a time commitment from patients.

Another exercise that targets the pharynx is the pharyngeal squeeze maneuver where patients sustain the vowel "e" with the greatest intensity possible. In a recent study, researchers assessed the effects of effortful pitch glide by combining the pharyngeal squeeze maneuver with the pitch glide, where the patient is required to glide up in pitch reaching a falsetto, targeting both laryngeal and pharyngeal muscles (30). Results indicate that this exercise targets muscles that enable laryngeal elevation and muscles in the pharynx that are relevant to swallowing.

Aging is known to result in delays in the opening of the upper-esophageal sphincter during swallowing. To improve upper-esophageal sphincter opening during the swallow, the Shaker exercise (head lift) is used. The patient is required to lie flat on his/her back on a bed, without a pillow, lift the head to look at the toes while keeping the shoulders on the bed, and sustain the posture for a specific number of seconds. In a systematic review on the effects of the head lift exercise, numerous studies reported on increased upper-esophageal sphincter opening after an exercise-based intervention using the Shaker exercise of the head lift (4). The Massako maneuver is another exercise that is used during therapy. In this exercise, patients are required to protrude the tongue and bite gently on the anterior portion while swallowing their saliva. For the jaw-opening exercise, the patient is instructed to open the jaw to the widest possible extent and hold that position for a determined number of seconds. This is another exercise-based intervention that is used to facilitate hyolaryngeal elevation and upper-esophageal sphincter opening.

All exercise-based interventions require effort and commitment to effectively improve swallowing function. In developing a treatment plan, an assessment of the older adult's physical and cognitive abilities to complete the rigors of the interventions must be completed along with an assessment of his/her level of motivation, financial concerns, social support, and physical barriers to attending therapy sessions regularly.

15.9 CONCLUSION

The assessment and management of dysphagia in older adults warrants an understanding of aging and the risks that older adults face when diagnosed with dysphagia. While traditional methods of assessment and management do not distinguish between younger and older adults, there is a growing body of literature in the area of dysphagia in older adults including interventions that are beneficial. Older adults often present with multiple comorbidities, polypharmacy, and age-related changes to the swallowing mechanism, which place them at a higher risk for dysphagia. A diagnosis of dysphagia, can lead to a worsening health trajectory for older adults if unattended, not monitored or not followed with appropriate interventions. There is a need not only to include aspects of aging into comprehensive evaluations of swallowing in older adults, but also to assess the risks for malnutrition, dehydration, and social isolation when developing dysphagia management and rehabilitation plans that include texture-modified diets.

REFERENCES

1. Agency for Health Care Policy and Research. *Diagnosis and Treatment of Swallowing Disorders (Dysphagia) in Acute-Care Stroke Patients.* Agency for Health Care Policy and Research, 1999. Retrieved from http://archive.ahrq.gov/clinic/tp/dysphtp.htm.
2. American Geriatrics Society Expert Panel on the Care of Older Adults with Multimorbidity. Guiding principles for the care of older adults with multimorbidity: An approach for clinicians. *Journal of the American Geriatrics Society* 60, no. 10, 2012: E1–E25.
3. American Speech-Language and Hearing Association (ASHA). *Treatment Efficacy Summary: Swallowing Disorders (Dysphagia) in Adults.* Retrieved from http://www.asha.org/uploadedFiles/public/TESDysphagiainAdults.pdf, 2014.
4. Antunes, E. B. and N. Lunet. Effects of the head lift exercise on the swallow function: A systematic review. *Gerodontology* 29, no. 4, 2012: 247–57.
5. Ashford, J. and M. Skelly. Oral care and the elderly. *Perspectives on Swallowing and Swallowing Disorders* 17, no. 1, 2008: 19–26.
6. Barczi, S. R., P. A. Sullivan, and J. Robbins. How should dysphagia care of older adults differ? Establishing optimal practice patterns. *Seminars in Speech and Language* 21, no. 4, 2000: 347–61.
7. Cichero, J. A. and K. W. Altman. Definition, prevalence and burden of oropharyngeal dysphagia: A serious problem among older adults worldwide and the impact on prognosis and hospital resources. *Nestle Nutrition Institute Workshop Series* 72, 2012: 1–11.
8. Cichero, J. A. and B. E. Murdoch (eds). *Dysphagia: Foundation, Theory and Practice.* Chichester; New York: Wiley, 2006.
9. Cichero, J. A., C. M. Steele, J. Duivestein, P. Clavé, J. Chen, J. Kayashita, R. Dantas et al. The need for international terminology and definitions for texture-modified foods and thickened liquids used in dysphagia management: Foundations of a global initiative [In English]. *Current Physical Medicine and Rehabilitation Reports* 1, no. 4, 2013: 280–91.
10. Clave, P., L. Rofes, S. Carrion, O. Ortega, M. Cabre, M. Serra-Prat, and V. Arreola. Pathophysiology, relevance and natural history of oropharyngeal dysphagia among older people. *Nestle Nutrition Institute Workshop Series* 72, 2012: 57–66.
11. Davis, L. A. Quality of life issues related to dysphagia. *Topics in Geriatric Rehabilitation* 23, no. 4, 2007: 352–65.
12. Doggett, D. L., K. A. Tappe, M. D. Mitchell, R. Chapell, V. Coates, and C. M. Turkelson. Prevention of pneumonia in elderly stroke patients by systematic diagnosis and treatment of dysphagia: An evidence-based comprehensive analysis of the literature. *Dysphagia* 16, no. 4, 2001: 279–95.
13. Ekberg, O., S. Hamdy, V. Woisard, A. Wuttge-Hannig, and P. Ortega. Social and psychological burden of dysphagia: Its impact on diagnosis and treatment. *Dysphagia* 17, no. 2, 2002: 139–46.
14. Garcia, J. M., E. Chambers, Z. Matta, and M. Clark. Viscosity measurements of nectar- and honey-thick liquids: Product, liquid, and time comparisons. *Dysphagia* 20, no. 4, 2005: 325–35.
15. Humbert, I. A. and J. Robbins. Dysphagia in the elderly. *Physical Medicine and Rehabilitation Clinics of North America* 19, no. 4, 2008: 853–66, ix–x.
16. Keller, H., L. Chambers, H. Niezgoda, and L. Duizer. Issues associated with the use of modified texture foods. *The Journal of Nutrition, Health and Aging* 16, no. 3, 2012: 195–200.
17. Keller, H. H., L. W. Chambers, D. A. Fergusson, H. Niezgoda, M. Parent, D. Caissie, and N. Lemire. A mix of bulk and ready-to-use modified-texture food: Impact on older adults requiring dysphagic food. *Canadian Journal on Aging* 31, no. 3, 2012: 335–48.
18. Kendall, K. A., R. J. Leonard, and S. McKenzie. Common medical conditions in the elderly: Impact on pharyngeal bolus transit. *Dysphagia* 19, no. 2, 2004: 71–7.
19. Langmore, S. E., K. Schatz, and N. Olson. Fiberoptic endoscopic examination of swallowing safety: A new procedure. *Dysphagia* 2, 1988: 216–19.
20. Leder, S. B. and D. M. Suiter. An epidemiologic study on aging and dysphagia in the acute care hospitalized population: 2000–2007. *Gerontology* 55, no. 6, 2009: 714–8.

21. Lenius, K., J. Stierwalt, L. L. LaPointe, M. Bourgeois, G. Carnaby, and M. Crary. Effects of lingual effort on swallow pressures following radiation treatment. *Journal of Speech, Language and Hearing Research* 58, no. 3, 2015: 687–97.

22. Leow, L., M. Huckabee, T. Anderson, and L. Beckert. The impact of dysphagia on quality of life in ageing and Parkinson's disease as measured by the swallowing quality of life (Swal-Qol) questionnaire. *Dysphagia* 25, no. 3, 2010: 216–20.

23. Leslie, P., M. J. Drinnan, G. A. Ford, and J. A. Wilson. Swallow respiratory patterns and aging: Presbyphagia or dysphagia? *The Journals of Gerontology Series A* 60, no. 3, 2005: 391–5.

24. Logemann, J. A. *Evaluation and Treatment of Swallowing Disorders*. San Diego, California: College-Hill Press, 1983.

25. Macqueen, C., S. Taubert, D. Cotter, S. Stevens, and G. Frost. Which commercial thickening agent do patients prefer? *Dysphagia* 18, 2003: 46–52.

26. Mann, G. *MASA: The Mann Assessment of Swallowing Ability*. San Diego, California: Singular Publishing Group, 2002.

27. Martin-Harris, B., M. Brodsky, Y. Michel, D. Castell, M. Schliecher, J. Sandidge, and R. Maxwell. MBS measurement tool for swallow impairment—MbSimp: Establishing a standard. *Dysphagia* 23, no. 4, 2008: 392–405.

28. McKinstry, A., M. Tranter, and J. Sweeney. Outcomes of dysphagia intervention in a pulmonary rehabilitation program. *Dysphagia* 25, no. 2, 2010: 104–11.

29. Mendell, D. A. and J. A. Logemann. Temporal sequence of swallow events during the oropharyngeal swallow. *Journal of Speech, Language, and Hearing Research* 50, no. 5, 2007: 1256–71.

30. Miloro, K. V., W. G. Pearson, Jr., and S. E. Langmore. Effortful pitch glide: A potential new exercise evaluated by dynamic MRI. *Journal of Speech, Language, and Hearing Research* 57, no. 4, 2014: 1243–50.

31. Ney, D. M., J. M. Weiss, A. J. Kind, and J. Robbins. Senescent swallowing: Impact, strategies, and interventions. *Nutrition in Clinical Practice* 24, no. 3, 2009: 395–413.

32. Panther, K. The Frazier free water protocol. *Perspectives on Swallowing and Swallowing Disorders* 14, 2005: 4–9.

33. Pelletier, C. A. Chemosenses, aging, and oropharyngeal dysphagia: A review. *Topics in Geriatric Rehabilitation* 23, no. 3, 2007: 249–68.

34. Robbins, J., R. E. Gangnon, S. M. Theis, S. A. Kays, A. L. Hewitt, and J. A. Hind. The effects of lingual exercise on swallowing in older adults. *Journal of the American Geriatrics Society* 53, no. 9, 2005: 1483–9.

35. Rofes, L., V. Arreola, J. Almirall, M. Cabre, L. Campins, P. Garcia-Peris, R. Speyer, and P. Clave. Diagnosis and management of oropharyngeal dysphagia and its nutritional and respiratory complications in the elderly. *Gastroenterology Research and Practice* 2011 (2011). doi: 10.1155/2011/818979.

36. Rofes, L., V. Arreola, and P. Clave. The volume-viscosity swallow test for clinical screening of dysphagia and aspiration. *Nestle Nutrition Institute Workshop Series* 72, 2012: 33–42.

37. Rofes, L., V. Arreola, M. Romea, E. Palomera, J. Almirall, M. Cabre, M. Serra-Prat, and P. Clave. Pathophysiology of oropharyngeal dysphagia in the frail elderly. *Neurogastroenterology and Motility* 22, no. 8, 2010: 851–8, e230.

38. Rosenbek, J. C., J. A. Robbins, E. B. Roecker, J. L. Coyle, and J. L. Wood. A penetration–aspiration scale. *Dysphagia* 11, no. 2, 1996: 93–8.

39. Serra-Prat, M., G. Hinojosa, D. Lopez, M. Juan, E. Fabre, D. S. Voss, M. Calvo et al. Prevalence of oropharyngeal dysphagia and impaired safety and efficacy of swallow in independently living older persons. *Journal of the American Geriatrics Society* 59, no. 1, 2011: 186–7.

40. Speyer, R., L. Baijens, M. Heijnen, and I. Zwijnenberg. Effects of therapy in oropharyngeal dysphagia by speech and language therapists: A systematic review. *Dysphagia* 25, no. 1, 2010: 40–65.

41. van der Maarel-Wierink, C. D., J. N. Vanobbergen, E. M. Bronkhorst, J. M. Schols, and C. de Baat. Meta-analysis of dysphagia and aspiration pneumonia in frail elders. *Journal of Dental Research* 90, no. 12, 2011: 1398–404.

42. Youmans, S. R. and J. A. Stierwalt. Normal swallowing acoustics across age, gender, bolus viscosity, and bolus volume. *Dysphagia* 26, no. 4, 2011: 374–84.

43. Zeanandin, G., O. Molato, F. Le Duff, O. Guerin, X. Hebuterne, and S. M. Schneider. Impact of restrictive diets on the risk of undernutrition in a free-living elderly population. *Clinical Nutrition* 31, no. 1, 2012: 69–73.

16 Vision Impairment and Its Management in Older Adults

Rajeev S. Ramchandran, Holly B. Hindman,
and Silvia Sörensen

CONTENTS

16.1 INTRODUCTION

The population over 60 years is forecast to cross one billion by 2020 and two billion by 2050 worldwide.[1] The rapidly growing number of older Americans in the next two decades has been coined the "gray tsunami" with the overall population expected to reach 72.1 million by 2030. The prevalence of preventable vision loss proportionately affects more of the older adult US population. In fact, 54% of ophthalmology office visits are for people 65 years and older. Moreover, ophthalmology visits account for the highest percentage of specialty office visits for adults over 65 years.[2] Vision loss is a leading disability for individuals over age 60 with over 15 million and over 94 million being affected in developed and developing countries, respectively. The four most common causes of vision loss in both the developing and developed worlds in those over 60 are from refractive errors that often can be corrected by glasses, cataract, treated with cataract surgery, macular generation, and glaucoma.[1]

From US-based population studies[3] in the year 2000, there were an estimated one million blind (20/200 or worse in the best-corrected eye) and 2.4 million with low vision (<20/40 in the better seeing best-corrected eye) in people over 40 years of age in the United States. The percentage of blind persons among Americans over 60 years of age is double that of those younger than 60. Moreover, age-specific blindness increases exponentially from 0.36% of the population age 65%–69% to 7% of the population over 80 years of age. Similarly, the percentage of those with low vision exponentially increases from 1.1% for those 65–69 years of age to 16.7% for those over 80. By 2020, the number of persons blind and with low vision is expected to increase to 1.6 and 3.9 million[4] in these age groups, respectively.

The above criteria for vision impairment is based on Snellen visual acuity measure, which may not be as sensitive as other instruments, such as contrast sensitivity, in identifying elderly individuals with vision loss. Self-reported vision loss in the over 65 years US populations is more than 12% compared to 5.5% for those 18–44 years.[4] Cataract, refractive error, and dry eye syndrome are the leading causes of vision loss in the elderly and vision restoring treatment is readily available. However, the other common causes of blindness in the elderly are permanent if not detected and treated early. These include age-related macular degeneration (AMD), the leading cause of blindness in Americans over age 65; diabetic retinopathy (DR), the leading cause of blindness in the working age population which includes those between 20 and 74 years; and glaucoma, the leading cause of blindness among African Americans and Hispanics. Other common pathology leading to vision loss in older adults include retinal vein occlusion and optic neuropathy and hemianopia due to stroke. These chronic eye diseases are more prevalent among older adults and result in more vision loss with increasing age. By 2030, 50% of seniors will have at least one visually significant ocular disease that could account for about 50% of the health care budget for older adults.[5] Direct medical expenses for older adults with vision impairment cost the United States $8.3 billion a year.[6] It is estimated that the amount spent toward caring for a blind person is about $5.4 billion annually.[7] Of course, the personal cost of going blind to an individual and their loved ones is immeasurable.

16.2 VISUAL SYSTEM

The visual system is part of the central nervous system and enables organisms to see by interpreting information from visible light received by the eye and interpreted by the brain to build a representation of the world. The visual system forms representations and perceptions of visual information and distance and guides movements. To achieve normal vision, the eyes and associated structures must be normal in structure and function. The light rays must be focused well. The neurological pathways from the retina via the optic nerve to the visual cortex must be intact. The brain must be capable of interpreting the information received.

Any abnormality of structure, development, or function will result in vision loss. The risk of abnormalities due to aging or disease increases exponentially after age 65. Since many diseases affecting the structure and function of the eye have a quiescent phase before they effect vision, seeing an eye care specialist for regular dilated eye examinations at least once every 5 years after age 40 and yearly if diabetic is advised. Examination of older adults may be limited by ability to position their head in a traditional slit lamp due to cervical arthritis or being in a wheel chair or bed bound. Bedside style eye examinations using a hand-held slit lamp and indirect ophthalmoscope is used in these cases. This may limit completeness of examination, but usually allows for adequate diagnosis and management plan that considers the patient's level of cognition, physical health, and requirements for vision.

After age 40, the need for reading glasses due to presbyopia increases and almost everyone after age 50 require reading glasses. Thus as a person ages, he/she are more likely to interact with eye care professionals. An optician is a licensed professional for the making and fitting of glasses. An optometrist is an eye care professional who has a strong foundation of optics and is very good at assessing refractive error and performing a general eye examination, and fits and prescribes contact lenses and glasses. An ophthalmologist is a physician who has completed medical school and undergone rigorous medical and surgical training to provide comprehensive eye care. An ophthalmologist may be a generalist who performs cataract surgery and other general eye procedures along with

care for medical diseases of the eye. An ophthalmologist may also specialize in the various components of the eye and visual system, such as the cornea or retina, or specific disease of the eye such
as uveitis or glaucoma. If vision loss is not treatable, a person may be referred to a vision therapist
who specializes in vision rehabilitation or low vision therapy. These individuals use various special
lenses, prisms, and magnifying devices to maximize a person's existing vision potential.

16.3   AGING AND THE EYE

As the eye ages, it undergoes natural changes, which can adversely affect vision by altering ocular
structures and interfering with the pathway traveled by light to the retina. The same changes that
affect the skin affect the epithelium of the eyes as well. The fibrous Tenon's capsule thins as does
the epithelium of the conjunctiva. Years of sun exposure may discolor the conjunctiva and sclera
and lead to proliferation of fibrous and elastic tissue leading to pterygium and pinguecula. Similar
exposure to the skin of the eye lids and periocular region lead to actinic changes, decreased elasticity, and even skin cancers. As the skin and connective tissue of the eye lids age, they become
more lax which may result in turning in, entropion, or turning out, ectropion, of the eye lid margin leading to abnormality in tear film maintenance, which can affect the cornea. These eye lid
changes may necessitate surgical correction. Aging changes can also lead to corneal changes due
to changes in the endothelial layer leading to decreased ability to actively pump fluid from the
stroma and keep it clear. Loss of tear consistency and quantity due to diminished functioning of
tear glands may also lead to corneal pathology and lack of clarity. Arcus senilis or lipid deposits
in the corneal periphery can also occur, but this change is cosmetic with little or no effect on
vision.

The pupillary response also becomes less brisk with smaller pupillary size due to decreased
reactivity of the dilator muscles letting less light into the eye. As the eye ages, the lens thickens and
becomes heavier. This is due to nuclear sclerosis, which is the most common form of cataract in
those over 65 years. Nuclear sclerosis occurs when the continual production of lens fibers compacts
around the nucleus causing a hard lens. With aging, the lens proteins transform and precipitate
causing the lens to become yellow or brown in color. This normal aging process can be hastened by
ultraviolet exposure and leads to a myopic shift due to change in its refractive index. These changes
cause light to be scattered through the lens causing less light to reach the retina and can dim the
vision.

Diminished accommodation of the lens, known as presbyopia, is first noticed between 40 and
50 years and increases with age. Presbyopia causes difficulty focusing on near images and requires
the use of magnifying or plus lenses or reading glasses. As the lens hardens with aging, it becomes
less flexible and its curvature changes.[8] These changes coupled with weakened ability of the ciliary
body to manipulate the lens lead to presbyopia.[9] Although reading glasses and contact lenses have
been the mainstay of treatment for presbyopia. Accommodative intraocular lens implants and
unique refractive surgical procedure to alter the shape and way light bends through the cornea have
and are being developed.

With increased age, collagen in the body breaks down and the eye is not immune to these
changes. Not only do epithelial changes result, but also the vitreous fluid that fill the cavity between
the lens and retina also breaks down or undergoes syneresis as the eye ages. Generally, by about
65–70 years of age, the vitreous has separated from the retina over the macular and optic nerve as a
posterior vitreous detachment. This can result in floaters in one vision that can be fairly obtrusive.
The separating vitreous may also pull hard enough on the retina at areas of strong vitreoretinal
adhesions to cause a retinal tear that can lead to a retinal detachment if not treated timely with laser.
A retinal detachment requires receiving intraocular tamponade and keeping one's head in a certain
position for up to a week to ensure retinal reattachment. Often a retinal detachment requires intraocular surgery, which can lead to and hasten cataract formation in the eye that has not undergone
cataract surgery.

Changes to the vasculature and retinal structure also occur with aging especially in those genetically or environmentally predisposed to developing such changes. Atherosclerosis affects the small arteries and veins of the retina and optic nerve and can lead to vascular occlusions causing ischemia and loss of vision from the death of astrocytes and photoreceptors. Age-related deposits, called drusen, can occur under the macular or central region of the retina due to genetic predisposition and other unknown factors. These deposits may be associated with AMD, which can eventually rob one of their central vision.

16.4   VISUAL FUNCTION AND AGING

Vision is a complex entity that is often subjective in its measurement and definition. A common way to measure vision is by measuring visual acuity on a standardized vision chart. Visual acuity measures the ability to distinguish details and measures the clarity of vision. While one's visual acuity may be very good even at older ages, contrast sensitivity or the ability to see low contrast patterns, such as faces, is an example of a measure of vision that is very sensitive to aging and can decrease overtime after age 60 years, often due to the presence of a cataract. Measuring the visual field is another way to assess ocular function, and the area of vision may be reduced peripherally, paracentrally, or centrally due to retinopathy, macular degeneration, or glaucoma, loss of optic nerve tissue associated often with relative increased intraocular pressure and aging in the eye. Aging may also impact the oculomotor ability for fixation and tracing. These involve the ability to focus on a fixed point and are important for reading. Recovery of visual function after being subject to bright light or glare is more of a problem in the older population often due to cataract. Stereo acuity or fine detail depth perception and color vision may also be impacted due to changes associated with aging affecting the eye and visual system.

There are many issues related to vision loss that go beyond just the functional impairment of being able to perform activities of daily living (ADLs) and navigate safely in one's environment. Vision loss can lead to social isolation. It is linked to increased risk of falls and hospitalizations. There is greater risk for physical and mental health problems, such as depression and anxiety. Low literacy, including health literacy and employment also are seen in populations with low vision. Vision loss poses a tremendous economic burden in the United States with four million people with poor vision costing society $130 billion annually. An effective way to think about eye disease leading to vision loss is in terms of their impact on loss of function. A functional classification of eye disease groups eye diseases or pathology as causing (1) diffuse image blur; (2) central or paracentral field defects; and (3) peripheral field defects.

16.5   CAUSES OF DIFFUSE IMAGE BLUR

In diffuse image blur, the vision is blurred or distorted over the entire field with varying degrees of density and contrast sensitivity. Symptoms include complaints of blurring, haze, glare, poor contrast, and vision that are limited by direct and amount of ambient light, especially in the case of glare.[10] The most common cause of diffuse image blur in the older adult population is refractive error. This can be due to needing glasses or due to cataract. Visual impairment in one-third of nursing home residents can be reversed by treatment of uncorrected refractive error. A study by Owsley et al. has shown that dispensing spectacles to nursing home residents leads to improved vision-targeted health-related quality of life, less-reported difficulty in the visual ADLs, and decreased depressive symptoms.[11]

16.5.1   CATARACT AND REFRACTIVE ERROR

A cataract forms when the crystalline lens in the eye becomes cloudy to the various insults, such as trauma, intraocular inflammation, increased oxygenation of the vitreous after vitrectomy surgery, or aging-related changes. In the United States and the developing world, cataract is still the leading cause of poor vision found in 50% of the blind population.[10] Risk factor for cataract includes ultraviolet B exposure, diabetes, smoking, excessive drinking, certain medications, such as steroids, history of intraocular surgery or ocular trauma, and having a family history of cataract. Therefore, people who are prone to prolonged sun exposure are asked to wear a hat or sunglasses. Healthy living such as avoiding smoking and limiting one's alcohol intake along with care of systemic medical conditions, such as good glycemic control in diabetes are advocated to limit or delay cataract formation.

Eventually, if one lives long enough, everyone will develop a cataract that may or may not be visually significant. If one has blurring of vision, difficulty with glare, or requiring more light to read, they may have a cataract and should be evaluated by their eye doctor. At the doctor's visit, your vision, need for glasses, eye pressure, density of cataract, retina, and optic nerve will be measured and examined. A cataract may make the eye more myopic or near-sighted and prescribing new glasses is all that may be needed. Alternatively, the ophthalmologist may determine whether the cataract is visually significant and requires surgical correction. If this is the case, measurements of the eye are taken to record the length of the eye, curvature of the cornea, and calculate the appropriate lens power of the implantable lens used as a replacement to the cloudy crystalline lens that is removed during cataract surgery. Other ocular pathology that may influence vision can also be identified with the preoperative evaluation. These include common diseases such as glaucoma and macular degeneration and less-common pathology such as Fuchs' corneal dystrophy and pseudo-exfoliation syndrome, both of which are more common in older eyes. The latter two can lead to complications such as corneal edema and loss of zonular support and subsequent lens prolapse as well as small pupils, making cataract surgery challenging.

A cataract can be classified by the location of the opacity in the lens, including the nucleus, cortex, and subcapsular regions. Nuclear clouding is the most common type of cataract in older adults with an average age of 79 years.[12] Over 22 million Americans have been diagnosed with cataract and by age 80, more than 50% of all Americans have cataracts.[4] As the population ages, the number of Americans diagnosed with cataract will increase by 50%.[13] As a progressive disease, there is a continual steady decline of vision overtime with studies showing a cumulative progression rates of about 20%–50% for the various types of cataracts.[14–17]

Cataract surgery has rapidly advanced over the last two decades to become an outpatient procedure performed in ambulatory care centers. It is the most common surgery done in America. Cataracts are easily treated by cataract surgery performed in operating rooms under sterile conditions. The most common form of cataract surgery in the United States is phacoemulsification, which uses ultrasound energy to remove the lens in sections after which a foldable intraocular lens is placed in the capsular bag once containing the crystalline lens. The developing world primarily uses small incisional extracapsular surgery, in which the lens is removed as a single entity leaving the capsular bag intact to allow for an intraocular lens to be placed at the same time. This procedure can be best performed when cataracts are more mature than those typically seen in the United States. Months to years after the intraocular lens is placed and less common in elder patients, a film of epithelial cells can grow across the lens implant, called a posterior capsular opacity. Today, there are lenses that can give patients intermediate and far vision that are termed accommodating intraocular lenses. These lenses, which are usually not covered by medical insurance, are another option to the standard single focus lenses that are usually used to correct the eyes for distance vision. If a standard lens is implanted for distance vision, then reading glasses are likely needed to see object up close as standard lenses do not accommodate. Most cataract surgeries are done using topical or local anesthesia and this helps the many older adults having surgery avoid the systemic effects of general anesthesia. However, if arthritis and spinal alignment affecting head positioning are encountered, general anesthesia may be needed to allow the patient to assume the proper supine position for the surgeon to perform surgery.

As the world population ages, the number of cataract surgeries performed will rapidly rise. By 2020, over 25 million cataract surgeries will be performed worldwide.[10] Complications from cataract are rare (from <1% for infections up to a few percentage points for retinal detachments in high myopic people as recorded in population studies), but include intraocular infection or endo-phthalmitis, retinal tear or detachment, lens prolapse, intraocular or suprachoroidal hemorrhage, cystoid macular edema of the retina, and increased intraocular pressure. As more surgeries are performed in all regions of the world, implementation and dissemination of standard practices to control infection and other complications are needed. Improved visual function from cataract surgery is achieved as a result of better optically corrected vision, correction of refractive error, reduced glare, increased depth perception, improved color vision, and increased contrast sensitiv-ity. Physical function also improves with cataract surgery, allowing one to perform ADLs better. One sizable study showed that the greatest improvements in visual function allowed individuals to achieve better daytime and nighttime driving and self-care activities.[18] Mental and emotional health also improves with cataract surgery. Self-esteem and increased socialization as well as less fear of blindness have resulted from cataract surgery. Cataract surgery is also very cost effective. A typical cataract surgery in the United States costs between $2 and $3000 and provides nearly $100,000 net present value return on investment during a lifetime.[19] This makes cataract surgery a very valuable procedure in a capitated population health model.

16.5.2 Dry Eye Syndrome

Dry eye syndrome is a disease of the ocular surface and tear film that is prevalent in older adults. Women are commonly affected more than men, and 5%–30% of the older adult population experi-ence symptomatic dry eye.[20] The syndrome, also called keratoconjunctivitis sicca, is a multifacto-rial disease of the tear film and ocular surface resulting in eye discomfort and compromised visual quality. Dysfunction of any component of the lacrimal gland, ocular surface, eyelids, and nervous system can cause dry eyes. Patients with dry eye experience blurred vision, foreign body sensation, pain, injection, epiphora, and, in severe cases, loss of vision.

Disruption of the balance between proper tear production and tear drainage, can lead to dry-ness. Systemic and topical medication use is much higher in older adults and can cause deficient tear production. The CDC reported that greater than 76% of Americans 60 years or older used two or more prescription drugs and 37% used five or more between 2007 and 2008.[21,22] Prescription drugs used more commonly by older adults including topical drops for glaucoma, antidepressants, diuretics, dopaminergic drugs for Parkinson's disease, antimetabolites, frequently used in treating rheumatoid arthritis, as well as over-the-counter topical eye drops with preservatives, deconges-tants, antihistamines, and vitamins are linked with causing or exacerbating dry eye.[23–25] Along with polypharmacy, the higher prevalence of autoimmune diseases (Sjogren's syndrome and rheumatoid arthritis) and decreased corneal sensitivity contribute to decreased tear film, which in severe cases can have vision-threatening consequences. Lacrimal gland dysfunction from low levels of the androgens, including dehydroepiandrosterone sulfate (DHEAS), in some older men and more commonly in postmenopausal women leads to dry eye. Deficiency of estrogen, which stimulates meibomian glands, occurs in postmenopausal women and can contribute to dry eye.[26–30]

Increased evaporation of tear film due to age-related changes in eyelid positioning (laxity, floppy eyelid syndrome, retraction, and lagophthalmos), meibomian gland dysfunction, rosacea, abnormal corneal sensation, and decreased blink reflex are more common in older adults.[24,31,32] Malpositioned eye lids may be surgically corrected to avoid chronic blepharitis, chronic conjunctivitis, and super-ficial punctate keratopathy as without such correction, 50%–70% have been observed to develop dry eye syndrome.[31] Conjunctivochalasis contributes to poor tear outflow and is characterized by redundant bulbar conjunctiva interposed between the globe and the eyelid.[32] The prevalence of conjunctivochalasis increases dramatically with age from less than 71.5% in patients 50 years or younger to greater than 98% in patients above 61 years of age.[33] Changes in corneal sensitivity, also more common in older adults, include hypersensitivity with increased ocular surface discomfort, and decreased sensitivity, which increased the risk of exposure keratopathy and associated complications. Neurodegenerative diseases, such as Parkinson's disease, can cause decreased blink rate and reflex, which also leads to greater risk for exposure keratopathy. Aging also increases oxidative stress through increased inflammation and decreased ability of the body's antioxidants to counteract free radicals. This alters the regenerative capacity of cells such as corneal epithelium, especially in dry eye conditions.[34] Poorly healing epithelium can rapidly evolve into severe corneal conditions, such as erosions, keratitis, or ulcers, which cause vision loss in the older adults.

In the aging eye, risk factors such as polypharmacy, androgen deficiency, decreased blink rates, and oxidative stress can predispose the patient to developing dry eye that is frequently more severe, has higher economic costs, and leads to poorer quality of life. As dry eye disease is a significant burden to the aging population, early screening, prompt attention, and targeted cost-effective treatment can make a difference in a patient's mental health, self-confidence,[35] and functional status. For smokers, smoking cessation is advocated as the smoke that not only physically affects the ocular surface, but also the oxidative elements of the smoke are damaging to the glands responsible for tear film production. Treatments at dry eye syndrome are aimed at treating the aqueous and oil-based deficiencies of tear film as well as correcting eyelid malposition to support better tear film composition and maintenance. If there is an aqueous deficiency, then artificial tears, preferably without preservatives such as benzalkonium chloride (BAK) that can destabilize the tear film, humidifiers, and punctal plugs to block the tear drainage duct are recommended. If an oil layer dysfunction is present, then warm compresses and lid hygiene, oral antibiotics or anti-inflammatory medications, such as nonsteroidals and cyclosporine, may be prescribed. Nutritional supplementation with omega-3 fatty acids at higher concentrations may be beneficial, but discussion with the ophthalmologist and primary care team should occur before dietary changes are made.

While high-contrast visual acuity may not be greatly affected and the degree of visual acuity loss in dry eye patients is commonly mild-to-moderate, individuals with dry eye can suffer from discomfort and/or functional vision changes that can be debilitating. In one study, subjects with severe dry eye reported a quality-of-life rating similar to that reported in other studies for moderate-to-severe angina or dialysis.[36] Dry eye is also linked to chronic pain syndromes[37] and associated with poorer general health,[38] and can lead to greater problems in daily activities by factors 2-3 ×, over those of normal.[39] Dry eye disease also has significant economic burden to older adults. In patients over 50 years of age, the health care system spends $3.84 billion to support cost of ocular lubricants, cyclosporine, punctal plugs, nutritional supplements, and professional healthcare visits for those with dry eye.[40]

16.6 CAUSES OF CENTRAL OR PARACENTRAL FIELD DEFECTS

Diseases of the eye, common in older adults, may cause central or paracentral field defects while leaving a relatively normal peripheral field. Symptoms of central vision loss include variable difficulty reading, recognizing faces, seeing detail, and affect normal ability. Retinal diseases, such as AMD, are common cause of central scotomas. Some of these diseases, such as DR can lead to complete field and vision loss.

16.6.1 AGE-RELATED MACULAR DEGENERATION

AMD is a leading cause of permanent vision loss for Americans age 50 and older.[1] Approximately, 15 million Americans have some level of AMD.[2] The Beaver Dam Eye Study showed that 46% of those aged 75 years or more developed some stage of AMD over 10 years of follow-up.[41] Approximately, two million Americans aged 40 or over have advanced or vision threatening macular degeneration and this number will rise to three million by 2020 as the populations continues to age.[42] AMD is a progressive eye condition that impacts central vision causing difficulty conducting daily tasks such as driving, reading, and recognizing faces. It is more common in people of

Northern European ancestry, those with family history of AMD, those with increased Ultraviolet B exposure, and those with cardiovascular disease. AMD is responsible for almost 46% of the cases of legal blindness in those over 40 years of age in the United States.

The most common form of AMD is "dry" AMD, found in 85% of those with AMD, but is responsible for 10% of the vision loss from this disease.[42] Dry AMD occurs when the cells of the macula, the central region of the retina responsible for sharp vision suffer damage from physiologic changes that can lead to eventual loss with loss of underlying retinal pigment epithelium (RPE) cells (geographic and nongeographic atrophy). Dry AMD is associated with the presence of small yellow deposits called drusen, which form under the retina and are a sign of abnormal functioning and health of the RPE. RPE serves to support and phagocytize components of photoreceptors and retinal pigments and support the process of sight. RPE pigmentary changes are also seen more commonly in later forms of dry AMD. "Wet" or neovascular AMD evolves from underlying early or more commonly intermediate dry AMD and often causes more rapid vision loss. It is found in 15% of those diagnosed with AMD, but is responsible for causing 90% of the vision loss from AMD.[42] In this form of the disease, tiny new blood vessels grow under and into the retina. These abnormal blood vessels allow exudates and transudate fluid to enter into the retina and surrounding structures upsetting the anatomy of the retina and causing vision loss.

Early AMD has almost no effect on vision and is defined as having small or few medium drusen in the macula with little or no pigment changes of the RPE. These eyes have very low risk of progressing to advanced AMD. Intermediate AMD is defined as the presence of either many medium-sized drusen or one or more large drusen in the macula region of the retina with or without RPE changes. Eyes with intermediate AMD have been found to have between 9% and 45% chance of developing advanced AMD over 5 years.[43] According to the Age-related Eye Disease Study, AREDS and AREDS-2 (addition of lutein and zeaxanthin with the exclusion of beta-carotene) vitamin supplementation helped to lower the risk of developing advanced AMD in eyes with intermediate AMD by 25% over 5 years.[44,45] Thus, this vitamin supplementation along with weekly self-testing of each eye with an Amsler grid is recommended. These vitamin supplements were not found to limit disease progression significantly relative to natural history in eyes with early AMD. Eating healthy for the eyes, including large portions of fruits, tree nuts, and vegetables, such as green leafy vegetables, is advised for all individuals to ensure eye health. Beta-carotene supplementation is not advised for smokers due to the association of increased lung cancer rates in such individuals taking beta-carotene supplements. Avoiding or stopping smoking is also beneficial to reduce the risk of developing and having AMD progress.

Advanced AMD is defined as either having an area of geographic atrophy in the retina resulting from loss of RPE and photoreceptors (advanced dry AMD) or the development of choroidal neovascular membranes (wet AMD), which are abnormal and fragile networks of blood vessels that develop from the choroidal layer under the retina. Exudative fluid leaks from these vessels and disrupt retinal anatomy crucial for good vision, which is seen as distortion by those affected. Both forms of advanced AMD can cause severe vision loss with loss of central vision. Currently, there are no approved or well-studied effective treatments for advanced dry AMD, although clinical trials are ongoing. Intravitreal anti-vascular endothelial growth factor (VEGF) agents, such as off-label bevacizumab (Genentech, Inc., South San Francisco, California), ranabizumab (Genentech, South San Francisco, California), and aflibercept (Regeneron Pharmaceuticals, Inc., Tarrytown, New York) have been shown to arrest the progression of vision loss and even improve vision in individuals with neovascular ("wet") AMD. These treatments need to be administered repeatedly, starting monthly, and are done so in the United States as an in-office procedure.[46] Other treatments that have been tried with less effect include photodynamic therapy and intravitreal steroids.

People with early and intermediate AMD, and even some with advanced AMD, often do not experience any symptoms or changes in their vision. Individuals ages 60 and over need to have a comprehensive dilated eye examination with subsequent eye examinations every year or every 2 years depending on whether AMD or other eye diseases were identified. Identifying AMD early allows people to modify their behavior, such as quitting smoking and increasing cardiovascular fitness, and dietary habits to limit their risk of developing advanced AMD. These examinations also identify individuals with intermediate AMD, who would benefit from taking AREDS or AREDS-2 vitamins to limit disease progression and potential vision loss.

16.6.2 DIABETIC RETINOPATHY

Diabetes mellitus (DM) is a worldwide pandemic that currently affects nearly 180 million people. An estimated 370 million are expected to be afflicted by this disease by 2030. Type I or juvenile diabetes accounts for 5% of the disease burden. The other 95% of diabetics have type II or adult onset diabetes, which accounts for the increasing prevalence of this disease due to the rise in obesity and sedentary life styles. DM primarily affects those older than 30 years of age. Moreover, DM is often silent early in the disease course. The United States Center for Disease Control and Prevention reports that an estimated 24 million Americans or 8% of the total US population have DM. One-third of these individuals is unaware that they have the disease. The prevalence of DM in the United States is expected to rise to 12% by the year 2025. If uncontrolled, the high level of blood sugar in people with DM, due to the inability to produce insulin (type I) or ineffectiveness of insulin (type II), leads to end organ damage, including retinal vascular damage known as retinopathy. This makes regular monitoring of blood sugar a universal must for people with this disease. Multiple clinical trials have shown that the level of blood sugar control is directly related to the severity of retinopathy and other end organ damage.[47–51] Other eye diseases that are more frequent in people with DM include glaucoma and cataracts.

The most feared complication from DM is vision loss, which is due to DR. In the United States, DR is the most common cause of blindness in the working age population (age 20–74) and currently affects over five million Americans. Nearly, 5% of these individuals have advanced DR that could lead to severe vision loss. As the population ages, by 2020, six million US residents will have DR and 1.34 million of these residents will have vision-threatening disease. DR rates in people 65 years of age or older are expected to quadruple by 2050, from 2.5 to 9.9 million.[52] Epidemiologic studies have indicated that the rates of DR are present in 30%–40% of all populations of Americans 30 years of age and older. Nearly 90% of diabetics requiring insulin have some level of retinopathy after 10 years. Of those with DR for 15 years, including many over age 60, 10% are severely visually handicapped and 2% are legally blind.[53,54] Annually, 7200 persons become permanently blind from DR in the United States.[55] The National Federation of the Blind estimates that the average lifetime cost to society for each person who becomes blind is nearly $1 million.[56] Of course, the personal cost of going blind to an individual and their loved ones is immeasurable.

DR is a microvascular disease that has distinct stages. DR first develops as mild nonproliferative diabetic retinopathy (NPDR) with microaneurysms, and can progress to moderate and severe NPDR with time, poor glycemic control, and high blood pressure. Poor glycemic control leads to damage to vascular endothelial cells and loss of associated anatomic structures that support the integrity of capillaries. This results in poor microvascular circulation resulting in ischemia of retinal tissue. The ischemic retina releases VEGF, which increases tissue and vascular permeability allowing for retinal edema and hemorrhages. These changes lead to diabetic macular edema (DME), the major cause of vision loss in DR. VEGF also stimulates neovascularization. In this way, DR progresses to severe NPDR and then proliferative diabetic retinopathy (PDR). PDR can lead to vision loss by causing vitreous hemorrhage and tractional retinal detachments. Mild and moderate (NPDR) usually do not cause vision problems unless there is concurrent macular edema, which can occur at any stage. Severe NPDR may quickly progress to PDR over a few years in patients with poor glycemic control, which increases the risk of vision loss.

DR is often silent until it becomes severe and affects vision, at which time treatment by a retinal specialist is crucial to prevent severe visual handicap and/or permanent blindness. Treatments for DR include laser therapy and more recently intravitreal steroid or anti-VEGF injections (similar to

AMD), and/or surgery. Laser therapy has been a standard of care for over two decades for DME and PDR. It is often associated with local scotomas in areas of treated retina, but it has been shown to robustly limit vision loss in a majority of individuals.[57,58] Intravitreal steroids have been used for DME with improvement of vision in many patients. However, steroid-response glaucoma and cataract in phakic individuals may limit the use of steroids. For patients who can routinely keep follow-up appointments, intravitreal anti-VEGF agents are now the choice treatment for vision-threatening DR as studies have shown improved vision without risk of scotomas, cataract, or development of glaucoma in the short term.[59,60] Routine follow-up may be difficult for older adults due to transportation issues and other health issues that may be life threatening and require hospitalization.

Fortunately, tight regulation of blood sugar by regulating one's diet, regular exercise, and adhering to appropriate medical therapy, along with regular dilated eye examinations by a trained eye care specialist can prevent vision loss even after many years of having DM. While diabetic patients must see their primary care provider at least yearly and often more frequently to obtain care and prescriptions necessary for survival, primary care providers are not trained or equipped to perform the required dilated retinal examination. Screening for DR with dilated retinal examinations is a specialized skill performed by eye care specialists and allows for appropriate treatment of vision-threatening DR with laser, intraocular medical therapy, and/or surgery to prevent permanent blindness. With the advent of increasingly affordable digital imaging technology, retinal imaging had become more accepted as an alternative to live screening in underserved populations. In addition, images of the retina serve as a tangible and real demonstration of the damage of elevated blood sugar levels on the body's blood vessels as the eye is the only place in the body where one can noninvasively observe small blood vessels, such as capillaries, which are damaged in DM. These images are used by eye care providers to counsel diabetic patients on their risk of vision loss and thus can motivate patients to better control their blood sugar and systemic disease.[61]

Due to the importance of regular eye examinations in this population, the American Academy of Ophthalmology recommends yearly dilated eye examinations for all persons diagnosed with DM. Annual dilated eye examinations are also an important Healthcare Effectiveness Data and Information Set (HEDIS) criteria developed by the National Committee for Quality Assurance (NCQA) used by federal agencies and health insurance companies to measure the quality of care provided to the diabetic population. Furthermore, regular eye examinations are advocated for all adults, especially after the age of 30 to detect and timely treat vision-threatening conditions such as macular degeneration, glaucoma, cataract, and need for glasses.

16.7   CAUSES OF ALTITUDINAL AND PERIPHERAL FIELD DEFECTS

Numerous diseases or pathologies affecting the retina and optic nerve that may occur more commonly with age can cause field loss in the peripheral retina. Some of these, such as retinal vascular occlusions (RVO), optic neuropathies, and retinal detachment, may involve the entire visual field in their severest forms.

16.7.1   RETINAL VASCULAR OCCLUSIONS

RVO are the second most common cause of blindness affecting the retinal blood vessels after DR. The major risk factor for an RVO is age. Most RVOs occur after age 50. Diabetes, hypertension, other risk factors of cardiovascular disease, and glaucoma, which are all more common in older adults, are the underlying factors for developing an RVO. An RVO can involve a branch or the entire retinal arterial or venous circulation and is named accordingly as branch retinal artery occlusion (BRAO), central retinal artery occlusion (CRAO), branch retinal vein occlusion (BRVO), and central retinal vein occlusion (CRVO).[62] Artery occlusions are embolic in nature, with plaques traveling from larger clots in the heart chambers or carotid artery. Venous occlusions are thrombotic in nature and develop locally from alterations in vascular flow due to the wall of the retinal arteries, thickened due to atherosclerosis, pushing on the more malleable retinal veins as arteries, and veins travel in the same intimal sheath at crossing points.[63]

Vision loss is relative to the regions of ischemic retina supplied by the affected vessel. When the central retinal vessel is affected, loss of vision in the entire visual field occurs. Arterial occlusions result in permanent vision loss with no treatment proving effective. Anecdotal reports of removing intraocular fluid or giving intraocular pressure lowering medicines to lower the pressure in the eye so as to move the embolus and relive the blockage, and of vascular specialists using intra-arterial tissue plasminogen activator delivered into the ophthalmic artery have been reported but not well studied.[64] A vein occlusion has a better visual prognosis and the main reason for decreased vision is macular edema although neovascularization and vitreous hemorrhage can also occur, as seen in DR. These sequelae of vein occlusion are the target of treatments, which are the same as those used to treat DR. Intravitreal steroids, intravitreal anti-VEGF, and focal laser (for BRVO) have varying success in improving vision from the sequelae of vein occlusions.[65–70] Serial intravitreal anti-VEGF injections are the treatment of choice for most patients who can make monthly appointments and receive these treatments, as they have shown the best visual outcome with the less side effects of glaucoma, cataract, or visual field defect. Vision loss may be permanent after an RVO, especially if it is arterial and thus prevention of an occurrence in the other eye is stressed. There is up to a 1% risk per year of developing an RVO in the fellow eye.[71–73] Development of an RVO is a marker for poorer overall systemic health, increased mortality, and increased use of medical resources. Thus, utilization of care and expenditures are higher for those experiencing an RVO.[74]

16.7.2 Optic Neuropathy and Cerebral Lesions

Ischemic insults on the optic nerve result in optic neuropathy and lesions affecting the parietal or occipital lobes can result in peripheral or hemispheric vision loss. If the all nerve fibers in the optic nerve are compromised, complete vision loss results. Older adults are at higher risk due to the increased risk of atherosclerotic disease and other systemic diseases, including cancer. Cerebral vascular accidents, compression and tissue destruction from cerebral neoplasms or aneurysms, and traumatic brain injury, which increase with age, can led to visual field loss. The specific region of field loss is relative to the region of the visual pathway affected with manifestation on the opposite field of the side of the brain affected. There are currently no medical or surgical interventions to correct this field loss. In addition to visual field loss, oculomotor coordination and alignment of the eyes and blink response may be affected if the cranial nerves controlling these movements have been affected. Double vision and exposure keratopathy may result. Occupational and visual rehabilitation via retraining have been helpful as is time. If visual recovery occurs, it usually does so within the first 6 months.

Ischemic optic neuropathy is classified as nonarteritic or arteritic in nature and usually occurs in people above age 50 with increasing prevalence. The nonarteritic variety or NAION is painless and more common and is thought to be due to vascular insufficiency or infarction and usually leave the patient with an attitudinal visual field defect affecting the lower or upper vertical hemisphere. However, 25% of patients had a central visual field defect.[75] Risk factors include hypertension and diabetes among other vascular factors and males and females are equally affected. Vision usually worsens over 2 weeks and stabilizes at 2 months, but visual recovery has been seen up to 6 months. Visual recovery may be better than 20/50 in many eyes, but nearly a quarter of those eyes studied were still legally blind (20/200 or worse). Oral prednisone, 80 mg a day tapered over a few months may hasten and result in improved anatomic and visual recovery.[76] Intravitreal anti-VEGF agents have also been used to treat vision loss in NAION with varying degrees of effectiveness.[77]

Arteritic ION or AION is rarer than NAION and is usually seen in those over 70 years of age. Females may be disproportionately affected. AION occurs due to inflammation of the arterial wall and can be seen in giant-cell arteritis or temporal arteritis. An altitudinal filed defect usually occurs and visual acuity loss is severe. The significant painless vision loss is often permanent with

15%–30% of affected eyes regaining any vision even with prednisone therapy. The vision loss may be associated with jaw claudication, scalp tenderness, arthritis, arthralgia, myalgia, weight loss, and increased fatigue. An elevated C-reactive protein and erythrocyte sedimentation rate can nearly confirm the diagnosis if corroborated with history. A temporal artery biopsy is done to confirm the diagnosis. Treatment is aimed at quelling the inflammation to prevent an AION in the fellow eye as visual recovery is poor. Oral or intravenous prednisone is used and tapered very slowly over a course of 6 months to a year at times. Chronic steroid use has more detrimental side effects in older adults, who already may have trouble sleeping, gastro-esophageal reflux, and bone density loss due to osteoporosis. Timely diagnosis and treatment with prednisone is key to avoid involvement of the fellow eye.[78]

16.7.3 Retinal Holes, Retinal Tear, and Rhegmatogenous Retinal Detachment

Posterior vitreous separation or detachment (PVD) is a natural occurrence that usually occurs between age 45 and 65 in the general population.[79] If symptomatic, typical signs are flashes and floaters. People with a symptomatic PVD should have a dilated eye examination within a day of symptoms as it can signal that a retinal tear has developed, especially if vitreous or retinal hemorrhage is seen.[80] These tears can develop into a retinal detachment that will cause a visual field defect. This defect starts peripherally and corresponds to the area of detached retina. If the macula is involved, central vision will be affected. Thus, it is important to seek timely care from a retinal specialist if one notices visual field defect before the detachment increases in size. The risks of a retinal detachment include having had cataract surgery in the eye, which is more likely in older adults, as well as being myopic and having had a retinal detachment in the fellow eye.

Separation of the vitreous from the retina can also cause a retinal hole or separation at the fovea, known as a macular hole. A full thickness macular hole causes a central field defect with reduced visual acuity to 20/100 or worse, which is considered legally blind. Population studies indicate that over half of patients with macular hole are between 65 and 74 years of age.[81] Retinal detachments and macular holes are repaired surgically with intraocular gas tamponade that require the patient to keep their head in a certain position up to a week. This may be difficult for older adults, especially those with arthritis or stiffness in their necks and backs. Thus, sometimes silicone oil tamponade is used, which does not require as extensive positioning, but necessitates another surgical procedure to remove the oil in order for the vision to be fully rehabilitated.

16.7.4 Glaucoma

Glaucoma is an optic neuropathy thought to be related to the relative value of the intraocular pressure, which is felt to be too high for the health of optic nerve tissue in those with the disease. Intraocular pressure can increase when the passage of aqueous fluid out of the eye is blocked. Globally, glaucoma, both open-angle and angle closure, is the second leading cause of blindness. The term angle refers to the space between the iris and cornea at which the entrance to the trabecular meshwork that drains the aqueous fluid is found. Approximately, 8.4 million people are blind due to glaucoma worldwide, and 2% of the US population over 40 years of age has open-angle glaucoma (OAG).[82,83] Afro-Caribbean and African Americans are most at risk for developing OAG.[84] Most people with angle closure glaucoma (ACG) are of Asian descent with 20.2 million people being affected globally and 15.5 million of these living in Asia.[85] Cases of OAG will increase from 2.2 to 3.3 million by 2020 and this is larger because of the aging population[86–87] as aging is both a risk factor for OAG and ACG.[88–95]

As OAG and to some degree ACG, except for acute attacks of angle closure, lead to painless vision loss, having a complete eye examination to assess the risks for developing glaucoma, including anatomy of the eye, family history, and age is needed. In general, people need to see an eye doctor at least once every 5 years to have their eyes examined once they turn 40 and once every

2 years after age 65. If there are risk factors for glaucoma or glaucoma is suspected then more frequent follow-ups are needed. Vision loss starts in the peripheral visual field and can be very advanced when the patient starts to notice vision loss in their central field. Thus, following a patient with glaucoma requires periodic visual field tests and eye examinations. Treatments for glaucoma involve procedures that lower intraocular pressure as increased relative intraocular pressure for an individual's optic nerve is thought to cause the disease to progress. Topical drops, administered daily to lower the production and increase the outflow of aqueous humor and laser surgery and operating room-based intraocular surgery to improve drainage of aqueous fluid are the mainstays of treatment. Older adults may have a hard time following up with frequent treatment visits to their eye care specialists and placing drops in their eyes. Moreover, the topical medications may have side effects, such as disruption of the ocular surface leading to dry eye syndrome and periocular skin discoloration. Total irreversible blindness is possible if the optic nerve fibers all succumb to the disease. Thus, educating vulnerable communities such as seniors about glaucoma and the need for timely eye care along with provision of better access to eye care is needed.

16.8   EFFECTS OF VISION LOSS IN OLDER ADULTS

Vision is critical for many ADLs and to maintain independence. Driving is a large part of one's independence in the United States and good vision is crucial to safe driving. In New York State, one needs to have a visual acuity of 20/40 or better in each eye for a commercial driver's license, 20/40 or better in one eye for an unrestricted noncommercial driver's license, 20/70 or better in one eye for a restricted driver's license limiting one to daylight driving only, and a continuous horizontal field of 140°. These are legal definitions of being qualified to drive, but visual processing issues and visual alertness for changing environments along with the ability to scan one's environment for potential hazards are all affected by vision impairment, which may make driving hazardous for the impaired driver and those around them. The visually impaired have greater difficulty with mobility, especially if their peripheral vision is affected. Their increased reading difficulty interferes with their ability to access information and may cause errors in self-administration of medications. Not being able to read, drive, and even see the television or computer can limit one's ability to self-care.[96-98] Individuals with vision impairment are likely to be admitted into a nursing home 3 years earlier than the average age individuals.[99]

Even with mild vision loss, the risk of falling is also increased by twofold. Falls are the leading cause of injury-related death and disability in those aged 65 and older and in the United States one in three older adults fall each year. Older adults are hospitalized for falls five times more than for other causes and women are three times more likely than men to be hospitalized for a fall-related injury. Thus, a fall check list should be initiated in care settings of vision impaired older adults. Due to the increased risk of falls, mild vision impairment also increases the risk of hip fracture by fourfold.[100-102] In the United States, 8.5% of hip fractures occur in elderly patients with mild-to-moderate vision loss (visual acuity between 20/30 and 20/80), whereas only 3% of hip fractures occur in older patients with a visual acuity of 20/25 or better.[103] Hip fractures can lead to decreased independence, functional status, and quality of life. Hip fractures also lead to increased mortality. The increased risk of falling and fracturing one's hip is not only due to decreased visual acuity, but also due to glare, altered depth perception, loss of peripheral visual field, and decreased night vision that occur with age-related changes and pathology in the eye.

Vision impairment impacts quality of life and increases social isolation.[104-111] With mild vision loss, the risk of depression is increased threefold.[104,112-115] In addition, older adults with depression may present with vision loss or other somatic symptoms. Vision loss may worsen dementia symptoms (analogous to "sun downing"). Vision loss may also be the presenting sign of Alzheimer's dementia (visual variant). Treatment of vision loss may slow progression of dementia, especially if both are recognized early. Thus, involving eye care specialists in the care of older adults with or at risk for depression and dementia is beneficial.

16.9   VISION REHABILITATION

Even when efforts are made to have older adults seek timely eye care, there may be little that can be done to reverse vision impairment due to ocular pathology. These individuals left with low vision, or visual impairment not corrected by standard glasses, or medical/surgical treatment, may be helped with reading aids and assistive technology. Older adults are disproportionately affected. In the United States, 70% of adults with severe vision impairment, vision less than 20/160 in the better seeing eye, are over 80 years of age.[116] The population over age 65 will reach 80 million by 2050 in the United States and 3.5% of this population will require vision rehabilitation.[117]

Comprehensive vision rehabilitation services include low vision evaluations and social work services to assess the needs of individuals with vision loss. The low vision specialist is often an optometrist and occupational therapist who can provide optical and nonoptical equipment to help with vision rehabilitation therapy. This therapy may use adaptive technology to assist orientation and mobility, occupational needs, and career training. The specific training is determined by functional loss and individual goals. Optical lenses, telescopes, and electronic devices are used to maximize the use of remaining vision. Magnification is helpful to read large print and see things at a distance. These devices may be higher power microscopes or hand-held magnifiers, computer-based video magnifiers using specialized software, or hand-held or spectacle-based telescopes or higher power plus lenses. Adaptive technology, including screen readers, computer technology, talking devices, and talking smart phones, cell phones, watches, and tablets are all being employed to assist those with vision impairment better navigate and interact with their environment.

In New York State, low vision specialists work with driving rehabilitation specialists to help people use telescoping devices to qualify for a special driver's license, which allows for greater mobility and quality of life. Intraocular telescopes are also being surgically implanted in one eye by ophthalmologists for some individuals with end-stage AMD and severe bilateral vision loss. These implanted devices require low vision specialists to help train recipients to effectively using their new field of vision in the implanted eye. Other tools for vision rehabilitation include prisms for image relocation, improved contrast and glare control using video magnifiers, task illumination, filers, and software to alter the color and size of print on an electronic device. Simple visual skills such as eccentric viewing training and scanning for hemianopia are helpful for those with visual field loss. Home visits by therapists are also helpful as is the support provided by social workers and mental health providers to help individuals emotionally adjust to their vision loss. Art therapy has shown to be beneficial for some individuals facing emotional difficulty from their vision loss. Staying linked to a community and activities that are meaningful to the individual who has lost vision are also beneficial.

16.10   EYE CARE IN SPECIFIC OLDER ADULT COMMUNITIES

While many older adults may remain living on their own for much of their life, independent and assisted living facilities (ALFs), referred to together as senior living facilities (SLFs) will be a more popular choice of residence. In the 38,000 ALFs nationwide, there are currently about one million persons living there with an average age of 86.9 years. This population will double by 2030.[118,119] Older patients with visual impairment are more likely to have severe problems with daily activities, mobility, pain, and discomfort, anxiety, depression, and self-care and thus may need to reside in SLFs or nursing homes.[120] Eichenbaum and colleagues documented increased prevalence of cataract, AMD, glaucoma in Americans 65 years and older residing in nursing homes compared with non-nursing home residents of similar age.[121] Elliot and colleagues published a study on vision impairment in ALFs, which demonstrated vision impairment in at least 70% of an Alabama ALF population. Review of residents' medical records showed that nearly 90% of screened residents had a documented eye problem.[122] This study relied on residents having seen an eye care provider as eye disease data were gathered by abstraction of medical records. Thus, the actual prevalence of eye disease, although high in this population, may even be underreported, as eye disease is often asymptomatic until advanced stages. Moreover, the authors could not accurately assess the cause of vision impairment documented by their vision screening as they did not evaluate best corrected vision, perform a concurrent dilated eye examination or use real-time diagnostic imaging. Thus, it is unclear from the work of Elliot and colleagues how many of those with vision impairment in the ALF were receiving care from an ophthalmologist and how many had previously undiagnosed eye disease.

A 2009 review by the US Preventive Health Task Force[123] demonstrated ample high-quality evidence of ability to effectively treat the common eye diseases in older adults especially if diagnosed early. However, this report concluded that good evidence is lacking for the role of visual acuity and other nonimage-based diagnostic screening techniques, such as Amsler grid testing of one's central vision, in improving vision or preventing vision loss. A reported 44% of older adults living in nursing homes have documented eye examinations in their medical records despite 90% of these individuals having health insurance.[124] The annual eye examination rate may even be less among residents in SLFs. Residents in these facilities are responsible for managing their own health care to a large extent, as SLFs are not federally regulated, as in the case of nursing homes, to ensure that their residents follow a certain regimen of wellness or preventive health, including eye care.

The primary barriers for patients to access timely eye care include; lack of awareness of needing eye examinations, inequitable distribution of eye care providers, and the additional costs in terms of travel, and extra medical fees associated with seeing another care provider. The barriers to see an eye care specialist may be greater for those in SLFs whose residents may not have ready access to transportation. In addition, this population may not be aware of the need for timely eye examinations. These barriers may be overcome by providing diagnostic capability at the residential site. A small UK-based prospective study in nursing home residents demonstrated the effectiveness of using a hand-held retinal (fundus) camera to detect eye pathology in this population with notable issues of patient mobility and media opacity affecting image quality.[125,126]

16.11 SUMMARY

Older adults are a growing segment of the US population. Even a simple check of visual acuity and refraction for the need of glasses is an important first step in the care of any older adult complaining of decreased vision. Older adults are susceptible to many eye diseases, especially those that are age related. An estimated 95% of blindness from AMD, DR, and glaucoma in older adults is preventable with early interventions and treatment. However, these eye diseases are often asymptomatic until they become advanced and result in permanent vision loss.[127] Early detection through regular surveillance for eye disease is thought to be necessary to ensure vision health in older adults. The American Academy of Ophthalmology recommends dilated eye examinations by an ophthalmologist at least every 2 years for the 65 years and over population and every year for those with diabetes.[128] Only 60% percent of the Medicare diabetic population routinely obtains yearly eye examinations.[129] Thus, increasing access to eye care by addressing knowledge and service gaps is needed. Vision loss increases the risk of isolation, depression, makes one less independent, and more susceptible to falls. To decrease this burden, timely diagnosis and treatment for detected vision-related problems is recommended. When vision loss is permanent, low vision services and vision rehabilitation may be appropriate to keep older adults functioning with good quality of life and lessen potential morbidity and mortality.

REFERENCES

1. UNFPA. 2012. *Ageing in the Twenty-First Century: A Celebration and a Challenge.* Available at: http://unfpa.org/ageingreport/ (accessed June 10, 2014).
2. National Ambulatory Medial Care Survey. Available at: http://www.cdc.gov/nchs/ahcd.htm (accessed June 10, 2014).

3. The Eye Diseases Prevalence Research Group. 2004. Causes and prevalence of visual impairment among adults in the United States. *Archives of Ophthalmology* 122:477–485.
4. Prevent Blindness America. 2008. *Vision Problems in the U.S. Prevalence of Adult Vision Impairment and Age-Related Eye Disease in America, update to the 4th ed.* Chicago, Illinois: Prevent Blindness America 23. Available at: www.preventblindness.net/site/DocServer/VPUS_208_update. pdf?docID=1561 (accessed June 10, 2014).
5. Eichenbaum, J. W. 2012. Geriatric vision loss due to cataract, macular degeneration, and glaucoma. *The Mount Sinai Journal of Medicine* 79:276–294.
6. Rein, D. B., P. Zhang, K. E. Wirth et al. 2006. The economic burden of major adult visual disorders in the United States. *Archives of Ophthalmology* 124:1754–1760.
7. Frick, K. D., E. W. Gower, J. H. Kempen et al. 2007. Economic impact of visual impairment and blindness in the United States. *Archives of Ophthalmology* 125:544–550.
8. Truscott, R. J. 2009. Presbyopia: Emerging from a blur towards an understanding of the molecular basis for this most common eye condition. *Experimental Eye Research* 88(2):241–247. doi: 10.1016/j.exer.2008.07.003.
9. Strenk, S. A., L. M. Strenk, and J. F. Koretz. 2005. The mechanism of presbyopia. *Progress in Retinal and Eye Research* 24(3):379–393. doi: 10.1016/j.preteyeres.2004.11.001.
10. Available at: http://www.cdc.gov/visionhealth/basic_information/eye_disorders.htm (accessed January 15, 2016).
11. Owsley, C., G. McGwin, K. Scilley et al. 2007. The visual status of older persons residing in nursing homes. *Archives of Ophthalmology* 125:925–930.
12. Lewis A., N. Congdon, B. Munoz et al. 2004. Cataract surgery and subtype in a defined, older population: The SEECAT Project. *The British Journal of Ophthalmology* 88:1512–1517.
13. Congdon N., J. R. Vingerling, B. E. Klein et al. 2004. Prevalence of cataract and pseudophakia/aphakia among adults in the United States. *Archives of Ophthalmology* 122:487–494.
14. Leske, M. C., S. Y. Wu, B. Nemesure et al. 2004. Nine-year incidence of lens opacities in the Barbados Eye Studies. *Ophthalmology* 111:483–490.
15. McCarty, C. A., B. N. Mukesh, P. N. Dimitrov et al. 2003. Incidence and progression of cataract in the Melbourne Visual Impairment Project. *American Journal of Ophthalmology* 136:10–17.
16. Leske, M. C., L. T. Chylack Jr, Q. He et al. 1997. Incidence and progression of cortical and posterior subcapsular opacities: The Longitudinal Study of Cataract. The LSC Group. *Ophthalmology* 104:1987–1993.
17. Leske, M. C., L. T. Chylack Jr, S. Y. Wu et al. 1996. Incidence and progression of nuclear opacities in the Longitudinal Study of Cataract. *Ophthalmology* 103:705–712.
18. Bassett, K., K. Noertjojo, P. Nirmalan et al. 2005. RESIO revisited: Visual function assessment and cataract surgery in British Columbia. *Canadian Journal of Ophthalmology* 40:27–33.
19. Cutler, D. M. and M. McClellan. 2001. Is technological change in medicine worth it? *Health Affairs* (Millwood) 20:11–29.
20. Smith, J. A., J. Albenz, C. Begley et al. 2007. The epidemiology of dry eye disease: Report of the epidemiology subcommittee of the international Dry Eye Work Shop. *Ocular Surface* 5(2):93–107.
21. Gu, Q., C. F. Dillon, and V. L. Burt. 2010. Prescription drug use continues to increase: US prescription drug data for 2007–2008. *NCHS Data Brief* 42:1–8.
22. National Center for Health Statistics. Health, United States. Available at: http://www.cdc.gov/nchs/ (accessed June 5, 2013).
23. Somogyi, A., D. Hewson, M. Muirhead et al. 1990. Amiloride disposition in geriatric patients: Importance of renal function. *British Journal of Clinical Pharmacology* 29:1–8.
24. Moss, S. E., R. Klein, and B. Klein. 2008. Long-term incidence of dry eye in an older population. *Optometry and Vision Science* 85(8):668–674.
25. Leung, E. W., F. A. Medeiros, and R. N. Weinreb. 2008. Prevalence of ocular surface disease in glaucoma patients. *Journal of Glaucoma* 17(5):350–355.
26. Sullivan, D. A., R. V. Jensen, T. Suzuki et al. 2009. Do sex steroids exert sex-specific and/or opposite effects on gene expression in lacrimal and meibomian glands? *Molecular Vision* 15:1553–1572.
27. Suzuki, T., F. Schirra, S. M. Richards et al. 2006. Estrogen's and progesterone's impact on gene expression in the mouse lacrimal gland. *Investigative Ophthalmology and Visual Science* 47:158–168.
28. Valtysdottir, S. T., L. Wide, and R. Hallgren. 2003. Mental wellbeing and quality of sexual life in women with primary Sjogren's syndrome are related to circulating dehydroepiandrosterone sulphate. *Annals of the Rheumatic Diseases* 62(9):875–879.
29. Azcarate, P. M., V. D. Venincasa, A. Galor et al. 2014. Androgen deficiency and dry eye syndrome in the aging male. *Investigative Ophthalmology and Visual Science* 55:5046–5053.

30. Labrie, F., A. Bélanger, L. Cusan et al. 1997. Marked decline in serum concentrations of adrenal C19 sex steroid precursors and conjugated androgen metabolites during aging. *Journal of Clinical Endocrinology and Metabolism* 82(8):2396–2402.

31. Damasceno, R. W., M. H. Osaki, P. E. Dantas et al. 2011. Involutional entropion and ectropion of the lower eyelid: Prevalence and associated risk factors in the elderly population. *Ophthalmic Plastic and Reconstructive Surgery* 27(5):317–320.

32. Meller D. and S. C. G. Tseng. 1998. Conjunctivochalasis: Literature review and possible pathophysiology. *Survey of Ophthalmology* 43(3):225–232.

33. Mimura, T., S. Yamagami, T. Usui et al. 2009. Changes of conjunctivochalasis with age in a hospital-based study. *The American Journal of Ophthalmology* 147(1):171.e1–177.e1.

34. Dogru, M., T. Wakamatsu, T. Kojima et al. 2009. The role of oxidative stress and inflammation in dry eye disease. *Cornea* 28(1):S70–S74.

35. Tong, L., S. Waduthantri, T. Y. Wong et al. 2010. Impact of symptomatic dry eye on vision-related daily activities: The Singapore Malay Eye Study. *Eye* 24(9):1486–1491.

36. Buchholz, P., C. S. Steeds, L. S. Stern et al. 2006. Utility assessment to measure the impact of dry eye disease. *Ocular Surface* 4(3):155–161.

37. Schaumberg, D. A. 2012. Epidemiology of dry eye disease and the patient's perspective. *Johns Hopkins Advanced Studies in Ophthalmology* 9(1):4.

38. Mertzanis, P., L. Abetz, K. Rajagopalan et al. 2005. The relative burden of dry eye inpatients' lives: Comparisons to a U.S. normative sample. *Investigative Ophthalmology and Visual Science* 46(1):46–50.

39. Miljanović, B., R. Dana, D. A. Sullivan et al. 2007. Impact of dry eye syndrome on vision-related quality of life. *American Journal of Ophthalmology* 143(3):409–415.

40. Yu, J., C. V. Asche, and C. J. Fairchild. 2011. The economic burden of dry eye disease in the United States: A decision tree analysis. *Cornea* 30(4):379–387.

41. Klein, R., B. E. Klein, and K. L. Linton. 1992. Prevalence of age-related maculopathy: The Beaver Dam Eye Study. *Ophthalmology* 99:933–943.

42. Friedman, D. S., B. J. O'Colmain, B. Munoz et al. 2004. Prevalence of age-related macular degeneration in the United States. *Archives of Ophthalmology* 122:564–572.

43. Chew, E. Y., T. E. Clemons, E. Agron et al., Age-Related Eye Disease Study Research Group. 2014. Ten-year follow-up of age-related macular degeneration in the age-related eye disease study: AREDS report number 36. *JAMA Ophthalmology* 132:272–277.

44. Age-Related Eye Disease Study Research Group. 2001. A randomized, placebo-controlled, clinical trial of high-dose supplementation with vitamins C and E, beta carotene, and zinc for age-related macular degeneration and vision loss: AREDS report number 8. *Archives of Ophthalmology* 119:1417–1436.

45. Age-Related Eye Disease Study 2 Research Group. 2013. Lutein + zeaxanthin and omega-3 fatty acids for age-related macular degeneration: The Age-Related Eye Disease Study 2 (AREDS2) randomized clinical trial. *JAMA* 309:2005–2015.

46. Vedula, S. and M. Krzystolik. 2008. Anti-vascular endothelial growth factor for neovascular age-related macular degeneration. *Cochrane Database of Systematic Reviews* 8:CD005139.

47. King, H., R. E. Aubert, and W. H. Herman. 1998. Global burden of diabetes, 1995–2025: Prevalence, numerical estimates, and projects. *Diabetes Care* 21(9):1414–1431.

48. Klein, R., B. E. Klein, S. E. Moss et al. 1984. The Wisconsin Epidemiologic Study of Diabetic Retinopathy: II. Prevalence and risk of diabetic retinopathy when age at diagnosis is less than 30 years. *Archives of Ophthalmology* 102:520–526.

49. Klein, R., B. E. Klein, S. E. Moss et al. 1984. The Wisconsin Epidemiologic Study of Diabetic Retinopathy: III. Prevalence and risk of diabetic retinopathy when age at diagnosis is 30 or more years. *Archives of Ophthalmology* 102:527–532.

50. The Diabetes Control and Complications Trial Research Group. 1995. The relationship of glycemic exposure (HbA1c) to the risk of development and progression of retinopathy in the Diabetes Control and Complications Trial. *Diabetes* 44:968–483.

51. UK Prospective Diabetes Study (UKPDS) Group. 1998. Intensive blood-glucose control with sulphonyl-ureas or insulin compared with conventional treatment and risk of complications in patients with type 2 diabetes (UKPDS 33). *Lancet* 352:837–853.

52. Saaddine, J. B., A. A. Honeycutt, K. M. Narayan et al. 2008. Projection of diabetic retinopathy and other major eye diseases among people with diabetes mellitus: United States, 2005–2050. *Archives of Ophthalmology* 126(12):1740–1747.

53. Zhang, X., B. J. B. Saaddine, C. Chou et al. 2010. Prevalence of diabetic retinopathy in the United States, 2005–2008. *JAMA* 304(6):649–656.
54. Centers for Disease Control and Prevention, National Diabetes Fact Sheet. Available at: www.cdc.gov/diabetes/pubs/pdf/ndfs_2011.pdf (accessed August 21, 2011).
55. Klein, B. E. 2007. Overview of epidemiologic studies of diabetic retinopathy. *Ophthalmic Epidemiology* 14:179–183.
56. Available at: http://www.nfb.org/nfb/blindness_statistics.asp (accessed July 31, 2011).
57. Early Treatment Diabetic Retinopathy Study Research Group. 1987. Treatment techniques and clinical guidelines for photocoagulation of diabetic macular edema: Early Treatment Diabetic Retinopathy Study Report Number 2. *Ophthalmology* 94(7):761–774.
58. The Early Treatment Diabetic Retinopathy Study Research Group. 1987. Techniques for scatter and local photocoagulation treatment of diabetic retinopathy: Early Treatment Diabetic Retinopathy Study Report No. 3. *International Ophthalmology Clinics* 27(4):254–264.
59. Diabetic Retinopathy Clinical Research Network. 2015. Panretinal photocoagulation vs intravitreous ranibizumab for proliferative diabetic retinopathy: A randomized trial. *JAMA* 314(20):2137–2146. doi: 10.1001/jama.2015.15217.
60. Diabetic Retinopathy Clinical Research Network, Wells J. A., A. R. Glassman, A. R. Ayala et al. 2015. Aflibercept, bevacizumab, or ranibizumab for diabetic macular edema. *New England Journal of Medicine* 372(13):1193–1203. doi: 10.1056/NEJMoa1414264.
61. Salti, H., J. Cavallerano, N. Salti et al. 2011. Nonmydriatic retinal image review at time of endocrinology visit results in short-term HbA1c reduction in poorly controlled patients with diabetic retinopathy. *Telemedicine and e-Health* 17(6):415–419.
62. Buehl, W., S. Sacu, and U. Schmidt-Erfurth. 2010. Retinal vein occlusions. *Developments in Ophthalmology* 56:54–72.
63. Weinberg, D., D. G. Dodwell, and S. A. Fern. 1990. Anatomy of arteriovenous crossings in branch retinal vein occlusion. *American Journal of Ophthalmology* 109:298–302.
64. Ghazi, N. G., Noureddine, B., Haddad, R. S., Jurdi, F. A., and Bashshur, Z. F. 2003. Intravitreal tissue plasminogen activator in the management of central retinal vein occlusion. *Retina* 23(6):780–784.
65. Branch Vein Occlusion Study Group. 1984. Argon laser photocoagulation for macular edema in branch vein occlusion. *American Journal of Ophthalmology* 98:271–282.
66. Ip, M. S., I. U. Scott, P. C. VanVeldhuisen et al., Score Student Research Group. 2009. A randomized trial comparing the efficacy and safety of intravitreal triamcinolone with observation to treat vision loss associated with macular edema secondary to central retinal vein occlusion: SCORE Study Report 5. *Archives of Ophthalmology* 127:1101–1114.
67. Heier, J. S., P. A. Campochiaro, L. Yau et al. 2012. Ranibizumab for macular edema due to retinal vein occlusions: Long-term follow-up in the HORIZON trial. *Ophthalmology* 119:802–809.
68. Haller, J. A., F. Bandello, R. Belfort Jr et al., Ozurdex GENEVA Study Group. 2010. Randomized, sham-controlled trial of dexamethasone intravitreal implant in patients with macular edema due to retinal vein occlusion. *Ophthalmology* 117:1134–1146.
69. Haller, J. A., F. Bandello, R. Belfort Jr et al., Ozurdex GENEVA Study Group. 2011. Dexamethasone intravitreal implant in patients with macular edema related to branch or central retinal vein occlusion twelve-month study results. *Ophthalmology* 118:2453–2460.
70. Campochiaro, P. A., J. S. Heier, L. Feiner et al., BRAVO Investigators. 2010. Ranibizumab for macular edema due to branch retinal vein occlusions: Six-month primary end point results of a phase III study. *Ophthalmology* 117:1102–1112.
71. Rogers, S., R. L. McIntosh, M. Cheung et al., International Eye Disease Consortium. 2010. The prevalence of retinal vein occlusion: Pooled data from population studies from the United States, Europe, Asia, and Australia. *Ophthalmology* 117:313–319.
72. Jaulim, A., B. Ahmed, T. Khanam et al. 2013. Branch retinal vein occlusion: Epidemiology, pathogenesis, risk factors, clinical features, diagnosis, and complications: An update of the literature. *Retina* 33:901–910.
73. Central Vein Occlusion Study Group. 1997. Natural history and clinical management of central retinal vein occlusion. *Archives of Ophthalmology* 115:486–491.
74. Suner, I. J., J. Margolis, K. Ruiz et al. 2014. Direct medical costs and resource use for treating central and branch retinal vein occlusions in commercially insured working-age and Medicare populations. *Retina* 34:2250–2258.
75. Rizzo, J. F. and S. Lessell. 1991. Optic neuritis and ischemic optic neuropathy. Overlapping clinical profiles. *Archives of Ophthalmology* 109(12):1668–1672.

76. Hayreh, S. S. and M. B. Zimmerman. 2008. Nonarteritic anterior ischemic optic neuropathy: Natural history of visual outcome. *Ophthalmology* 115(2):298–305 e292.

77. Atkins, E. J., B. B. Bruce, N. J. Newman et al. 2010. Treatment of nonarteritic anterior ischemic optic neuropathy. *Survey of Ophthalmology* 55(1):47–63.

78. Hayreh, S. S., P. A. Podhajsky, and P. Zimmerman. 1998. Ocular manifestations of giant cell arteritis. *American Journal of Ophthalmology* 125:509–520.

79. Snead, M. P., D. R. Snead, S. James et al. 2008. Clinicopathological changes at the vitreoretinal junction: Posterior vitreous detachment. *Eye (London)* 22:1257–1262.

80. Sarrafizadeh, R., T. S. Hassan, A. J. Ruby et al. 2001. Incidence of retinal detachment and visual outcome in eyes presenting with posterior vitreous separation and dense fundus-obscuring vitreous hemorrhage. *Ophthalmology* 108:2273–2278.

81. Eye Disease Case–Control Study Group. 1994. Risk factors for idiopathic macular holes. *American Journal of Ophthalmology* 118:754–761.

82. Quigley, H. A. and A. T. Broman. 2006. The number of people with glaucoma worldwide in 2010 and 2020. *British Journal of Ophthalmology* 90:262–267.

83. Friedman, D. S., R. C. Wolfs, B. J. O'Colmain et al., Eye Disease Prevalence Research Group. 2004. Prevalence of open-angle glaucoma among adults in the United States. *Archives of Ophthalmology* 122:532–538.

84. Sommer, A., J. M. Tielsch, J. Katz et al. 1991. Racial differences in the cause-specific prevalence of blindness in east Baltimore. *New England Journal of Medicine* 325:1412–1417.

85. Subak-Sharpe, I., S. Low, W. Nolan et al. 2010. Parmocological and environmental factors in primary angle-closure glaucoma. *British Medical Bulletin* 93:125–143.

86. Klein, B. E. and R. Klein. 2013. Project prevalence of age-related eye diseases. *Investigative Ophthalmology and Visual Science* 54:ORSF5–ORSF13. doi:10.1167/iovs.13-12789.

87. Vajaranant, T. S., S. Wu, M. Torres et al. 2012. The changing face of primary open-angle glaucoma in the United States: Demographic and geographic changes from 2011 to 2050. *American Journal of Ophthalmology* 154:303–314.

88. Tielsch, J. M., A. Sommer, J. Katz et al. 1991. Racial variations in the prevalence of primary open-angle glaucoma: The Baltimore Eye Survey. *JAMA* 266:369–374.

89. Leske, M. C., A. M. Connell, A. P. Schachat et al. 1994. The Barbados Eye Study: Prevalence of open-angle glaucoma. *Archives of Ophthalmology* 112:821–829.

90. Quigley, H. A., S. K. West, J. Rodriguez et al. 2001. The prevalence of glaucoma in a population-based study of Hispanic subjects: Proyecto VER. *Archives of Ophthalmology* 119:1819–1826.

91. Mitchell, P., W. Smith, K. Attebo et al. 1996. Prevalence of open-angle glaucoma in Australia: The Blue Mountains Eye Study. *Ophthalmology* 103:1661–1669.

92. Wensor, M. D., C. A. McCarty, Y. L. Stanislavsky et al. 1998. The prevalence of glaucoma in the Melbourne Visual Impairment Project. *Ophthalmology* 105:733–739.

93. Seah, S. K., P. J. Foster, P. T. Chew et al. 1997. Incidence of acute primary angle-closure glaucoma in Singapore. An island-wide survey. *Archives of Ophthalmology* 115:1436–1440.

94. Foster, P. J., J. Baasanhu, P. H. Alsbirk et al. 1996. Glaucoma in Mongolia: A population-based survey in Hovsgol province, northern Mongolia. *Archives of Ophthalmology* 114:1235–1241.

95. Bengtsson, B. 1981. The prevalence of glaucoma. *British Journal of Ophthalmology* 65:46–49.

96. Drummond, S. R., R. S. Drummond, and G. N. Dutton. 2004. Visual acuity and the ability of the visually impaired to read medication instructions. *British Journal of Ophthalmology* 88:1541–1542.

97. Feinberg, J. L., P. A. Rogers, and D. Sokol-McKay. 2009. Age-related eye disease and medication safety. *Annals of Long-Term Care* 17:17–22. Available at: www.annalsoflongtermcare.com/content/age-related-eye-disease-and-medication-safety?page=0,0 (accessed January 24, 2016).

98. American Society of Consultant Pharmacists Foundation and American Foundation for the Blind. 2008. *Guidelines for Prescription Labeling and Consumer Medication Information for People with Vision Loss.* Available at: http://ascpfoundation.org/downloads/Rx-CMI%20Guidelines%20vision%20loss-FINAL2.pdf (accessed January 24, 2016).

99. Wang, J. J., P. Mitchell, W. Smith et al. 2001. Incidence of nursing home placement in a defined community. *The Medical Journal of Australia* 174:271–275.

100. Ivers, R. Q., R. G. Cumming, P. Mitchell et al. 1998. Visual impairment and falls in older adults: The Blue Mountains Eye Study. *Journal of the American Geriatrics Society* 46(1):58–64.

101. Klein, B. E., R. Klein, K. E. Lee et al. 1998. Performance-based and self-assessed measures of visual function as related to history of falls, hip fractures, and measured gait time: The Beaver Dam Eye Study. *Ophthalmology* 105(1):160–164.

102. McCarty, C. A., C. L. Fu, and H. R. Taylor. 2002. Predictors of falls in the Melbourne visual impairment project. *Australian and New Zealand Journal of Public Health* 26(2):116–119.
103. Felson, D. T., J. J. Anderson, M. T. Hannan et al. 1989. Impaired vision and hip fracture. The Framingham study. *Journal of the American Geriatrics Society* 37(6):495–500.
104. West, S. K., B. Munoz, G. S. Rubin et al. 1997. Function and visual impairment in a population-based study of older adults. The SEE project. Salisbury Eye Evaluation. *Investigative Ophthalmology and Visual Science* 38:72–82.
105. Hassell, J. B., E. L. Lamoureux, and J. E. Keeffe. 2006. Impact of age related macular degeneration on quality of life. *British Journal of Ophthalmology* 90:593–596.
106. Weih, L. M., J. B. Hassell, and J. Keeffe. 2002. Assessment of the impact of vision impairment. *Investigative Ophthalmology and Visual Science* 43:927–935.
107. Lamoureux, E. L., J. B. Hassell, and J. E. Keeffe. 2004. The determinants of participation in activities of daily living in people with impaired vision. *American Journal of Ophthalmology* 137:265–270.
108. Lamoureux, E. L., J. B. Hassell, and J. E. Keeffe. 2004. The impact of diabetic retinopathy on participation in daily living. *Archives of Ophthalmology* 122:84–88.
109. Burmedi, D., S. Becker, V. Heyl et al. 2002. Emotional and social consequences of age-related low vision: A narrative review. *Visual Impairment Research* 4:47–71.
110. Lee, P. P., K. Spritzer, and R. D. Hays. 1997. The impact of blurred vision on functioning and well-being. *Ophthalmology* 104:390–396.
111. Lamoureux, E. L., J. F. Pallant, K. Pesudovs et al. 2007. The effectiveness of low-vision rehabilitation on participation in daily living and quality of life. *Investigative Ophthalmology and Visual Science* 48:1476–1482.
112. Silverstone, B., M. Lang, B. P. Rosenthal et al. (eds). 2000. *The Lighthouse Handbook on Vision Impairment and Vision Rehabilitation*. New York: Oxford University Press.
113. Rovner, B. W. and R. J. Casten. 2002. Activity loss and depression in age-related macular degeneration. *American Journal of Geriatric Psychiatry* 10:305–310.
114. Rovner, B. W., R. J. Casten, and W. S. Tasman. 2002. Effect of depression on vision function in age-related macular degeneration. *Archives of Ophthalmology* 120:1041–1044.
115. Mogk, L. G., A. Riddering, D. Dahl et al. 2000. Depression and function in adults with visual impairments. In: Stuen, C., Arditi, A., Horowitz, A. et al. (eds), *Vision Rehabilitation: Assessment, Intervention, and Outcomes*. Exton, Pennsylvania: Swets & Zeitlinger, pp. 663–665.
116. Congdon, N., B. O'Colmain, C. C. Klaver et al. 2004. Causes and prevalence of visual impairment among adults in the United States. *Archives of Ophthalmology* 122:477–485.
117. Agency for Healthcare Research and Quality. 2004. Vision Rehabilitation for Elderly Individuals with Low Vision or Blindness. Available at: www.cms.hhs.gov/InfoExchange/Downloads/RTCvisionrehab.pdf (accessed January 24, 2016).
118. United States Department of Health and Human Services. 2007. *Residential Care and Assisted Living Compendium*. Available at: aspe.hhs.gov/daltcp/reports/2007/07alcom.htm (accessed October 30, 2013).
119. National Center for Assisted Living. 2001. *Facts and Trends: The Assisted Living Sourcebook*. Washington, DC: National Center for Assisted Living.
120. van Nispen, R. M. A., M. R. de Boer, J. G. J. Hoeijmakers et al. 2009. Co-morbidity and visual acuity are risk factors for health-related quality of life decline: Five-month follow-up EQ-5D data of visually impaired older patients. *Health and Quality of Life Outcomes* 7:18–27.
121. Eichenbaum J. W., W. B. Burton, G. M. Eichenbaum et al. 1999. The prevalence of eye disease in nursing home and non-nursing home geriatric populations. *Archives of Gerontology and Geriatrics* 28(3):191–204.
122. Elliot, A. F., G. McGwin, and C. Owsley. 2013. Vision impairment among older adults in assisted living facilities. *Journal of Aging and Health* 25(2):364–378.
123. Chou, R., T. Dana, and C. Bougatsos. 2009. Screening older adults for impaired visual acuity: A review of the evidence for the U.S. Preventive Services Task Force. *Annals of Internal Medicine* 151:44–58.
124. Owsley, C., G. McGwin, K. Scilley et al. 2007. The visual status of older persons residing in nursing homes. *Archives of Ophthalmology* 125:925–930.
125. Hartnett, M. E., I. J. Key, N. M. Loyacano et al. 2005. Perceived barriers to diabetic eye care: Qualitative study of patients and physicians. *Archives of Ophthalmology* 123:387–391.
126. Frazier, M. and R. N. Kleinstein. 2009. Access and barrier to vision, eye, and health care. In: *Optometric Care within the Public Health Community*. Cadyville, New York: Old Post Publishing. webpages.charter.net/oldpostpublishing/oldpostpublishing/Section 4, Access and Barriers to Eye and Health Care/Sect 4, Access and Barriers by Frazier and Kleinstein.pdf. Accessed January 11, 2016.

127. Varma, R., N. Bressler, Q. V. Doan et al. 2013. Awareness of diabetic retinopathy and eye exams in the US based on NHANES 2005–2008. Paper Presented at the 73rd Scientific Sessions of the American Diabetes Association, Chicago, Illinois, June 21–25.
128. American Academy of Ophthalmology Retina Panel. 2009. *Preferred Practice Pattern Guidelines. Diabetic Retinopathy.* San Francisco, California: American Academy of Ophthalmology. (4th printing 2012). Available at: www.aao.org/ppp (accessed January 18, 2016).
129. National Center for Quality Assurance. 2009. HEDIS performance measures. Available at: www.ncqa.org/tabid/855/Default.aspx (accessed October 30, 2013).

17 Arthritis and Common Musculoskeletal Conditions

Jennifer H. Paul, Katarzyna Iwan, and Claudia Ramirez

CONTENTS

17.1 OSTEOARTHRITIS

17.1.1 EPIDEMIOLOGY, BACKGROUND, AND RISK FACTORS

Osteoarthritis (OA), the "wear and tear arthritis," is a common disease, which most often affects knees, hips, and hands and can be associated with significant morbidity. OA is estimated to affect more than 27 million people in the United States and for those over the age of 65 more than half are living with OA. In the case of knee arthritis, prior to age 55, men and women are equally affected, however, after 65 years of age, women tend to be more affected. OA usually occurs due to repetitive use of the joints causing microtrauma and commonly affects weight-bearing joints. The pathophysiology includes inflammation due to increased proteoglycan synthesis and release of cytokines and metalloproteinases. Disease progression occurs as a result of imbalance between pro- and anti-inflammatory cytokines. This cytokine imbalance leads to an increase in proteolytic enzymes, which leads to the destruction of cartilage. Loss of cartilage leads to joint space narrowing, bone cyst formation, subchondral sclerosis, and osteophytes. Clinically, the patient can experience pain, tenderness, stiffness, loss of flexibility, swelling, and a grating sensation.[1]

There are several risk factors/causes of OA including aging, female sex, bone deformities, obesity, occupation, sports activities, sedentary lifestyle, muscle weakness, genetic factors, previous trauma, calcium crystals, infection, inflammatory joint conditions (rheumatoid arthritis), neuromuscular/neuropathic disorders, metabolic disorders (osteoporosis), endocrine disorders (acromegaly), hemoglobinopathies (sickle cell disease), and bone disorders (Paget disease, avascular necrosis).[2,3]

Symptoms of OA include pain, loss of function, crepitus, swelling/effusion, muscle wasting, and joint deformity (genu varum). Hand OA can lead to Bouchard's nodes and Heberden's nodes and patients with knee arthritis develop quadriceps weakness and decreased knee range of motion. As a result of these symptoms, patients are at risk for obesity, falls, chronic pain syndromes, fatigue and depression, as well as other diseases related to a sedentary lifestyle.[4]

17.1.2 DIAGNOSIS

17.1.2.1 History

Patients should be asked how long their symptoms have been present, progression overtime, history of trauma, whether pain worsened with activity and improved with rest, as well as associated symptoms such as stiffness and swelling.

17.1.2.2 Physical Examination

The physical examination should include looking for any deformity/malalignment of the joint and any muscle atrophy. The joint should be assessed for any lesions and palpated for warmth, effusion, and crepitus. One should look for any locations of tenderness including the medial and lateral joint lines and the patellar facets of the knees. For the hip examination, one should assess for lateral tenderness over the greater trochanter, as well as tenderness in the lumbar spine/buttock and anterior muscular tenderness. The examination should look at range of motion limitations and should test for ligamentous laxity and other causes of pain, including synovial swelling in the hands suggestive of possible inflammatory arthritis. An acutely swollen, erythematous, warm, and tender joint can suggest possible infection. Gait and activities of daily living (ADLs) should also be assessed including the need for an assistive device.

17.1.3 LABORATORY STUDIES

Possible testing may include erythrocyte sedimentation rate (ESR) and C-reactive protein (CRP). Synovial fluid may be analyzed for other causes of joint pain and the assessment may include assessing for organisms, elevated white blood cell count, as well as assessing for crystals.

17.1.4 IMAGING

Plain radiographs can be very helpful when diagnosing arthritis. Typically, imaging for OA includes plain radiographs that are helpful for all stages of knee OA except for very early stage OA.

There are currently several ways to diagnose and classify knee OA. The Kellgren–Lawrence grading scale is commonly used and is broken up into four grades:

1. *Grade 1.* Doubtful narrowing of joint space and possible osteophytic lipping.
2. *Grade 2.* Definite osteophytes and definite narrowing of joint space.
3. *Grade 3.* Moderate multiple osteophytes, definite narrowing of joint space, some sclerosis, and possible deformity of bone contour.
4. *Grade 4.* Large osteophytes, marked narrowing of joint space, severe sclerosis, and definite deformity of bone contour.[4]

Magnetic resonance imaging (MRI) can be helpful for assessment of soft tissue injuries and avascular necrosis (AVN).[5]

Computerized tomography (CT) gives more bony detail and can provide more information about intra-articular bodies. Bone scans can be helpful to differentiate other causes of joint pain.

17.1.5 TREATMENT

Treatment goals include controlling pain and swelling, minimizing disability, improving quality of life, preventing the progression of disease, and educating the patient about the disease. Treatment goals should be individualized based on a patient's goals, their level of function/activity, the joints involved, and severity of the disease, occupational/vocational needs, and coexisting medical problems. Treatment options include activity modifications, physical therapy, modalities, oral and injected medications, as well as biological agents.

17.1.5.1 Activity

Activity modification is essential. It is important to provide education about activities that can increase arthritis pain such as excessive use of stairs. For hand OA, it is helpful to instruct in joint protection techniques. It is also helpful to emphasize that rest is important for up to 24 hours following an acute flare, but after 24 hours, increase in activity is generally recommended. Physical therapy including both land and aqua therapy is essential for patients. Supervised formal physical therapy programs seem to be more likely to succeed. The focus is on strengthening, improving range of motion especially, gait training, and evaluating need for assistive device. Ability to perform ADLs should also be evaluated. There is high-quality evidence that exercise and weight reduction reduces pain and improves physical function in patients with OA of the knee and hip. Studies show that even a small amount of weight loss can help significantly with a patient's pain and risk for progression of the disease. It is strongly recommended that patients with symptomatic knee or hip OA who are overweight be counseled regarding weight loss. Patients should participate in cardiovascular (aerobic) and resistance exercise. Aquatic therapy may be preferred to land therapy by some patients. Generally, encourage low impact conditioning exercises such as walking, swimming, biking, elliptical, and tai chi programs. Weight loss is best achieved through both diet and exercise. Dieticians can play an important role in helping these patients lose weight.[6]

17.1.5.2 Modalities and Devices

Modalities such as transcutaneous electrical nerve stimulation (TENS) unit, thermotherapy, and ultrasound can be helpful for some patients with OA. Paraffin baths may be used by hand therapists to help manage hand OA. Other patients may benefit from assistive devices such as canes and walkers. Appropriate footwear is very important. Good cushioned stable shoes are recommended. Braces such as medial compartment unloader braces can help with knee pain especially when there is a feeling of instability or unequal compartment joint space narrowing. Medial OA is one of the most common subtypes of knee OA. One type of treatment for medial knee OA involves reducing medial loading to ease the physical stress applied to that compartment of the joint by placing a lateral wedge in the shoe. However, recent studies report no significant improvement in knee arthritic pain using lateral wedges.[6] Some studies reveal that patellar taping can enhance pain relief for knee OA. For hand OA, it can be helpful to provide splints for patients with trapeziometacarpal joint OA.[7-9]

17.1.5.3 Supplements and Medications

Supplements such as glucosamine chondroitin are commonly used by patients trying to treat arthritic pain. Studies have been somewhat inconclusive at this time regarding their benefits.[9] Topical medications are often suggested due to decreased risks of drug interaction and serious side effects. Topical medications often used include lidocaine ointment/Lidoderm patches, Voltaren gel, and capsaicin. Tylenol is typically the first medication used to try to treat arthritis pain, given it is generally well tolerated. The maximum dose recommended is 3 g per day divided into at least three doses. If Tylenol is not effective, nonsteroidal anti-inflammatory drugs (NSAIDs) such as Mobic and Celebrex are attempted. Tramadol can also be helpful. Narcotics are usually used for acute flares and for patients with end-stage arthritis failing other treatments.[6]

17.1.5.4 Complementary and Alternative Medicine

Some patients find acupuncture, chiropractic maneuvers, and massage beneficial for arthritis pain, however, studies are conflicting about long-term benefits.[10]

17.1.5.5 Psychology

Patients may benefits from psychosocial interventions. Pain psychologists can be helpful in managing chronic pain.

17.1.5.6 Corticosteroid Injections

Intra-articular steroid injections have been commonly used in the treatment of painful knee and hip OA, two of the most commonly affected joints. For knee OA, there is evidence of short-term benefit of intra-articular steroid injection to provide pain relief for up to 3–4 weeks, however, for some relief lasts longer (8+ weeks). Studies have shown there may be a number of predictors of response to intra-articular steroid injections, including knee joint effusion, aspiration of fluid prior to the injection, absence of synovitis, using ultrasound guidance technology, Kellgren–Lawrence severity, and severity of knee pain.[11]

17.1.5.7 Viscosupplementation

Intra-articular hyaluronic acid (HA) is a US Food and Drug Administration-approved treatment (since 1997) for knee OA; however, its efficacy remains controversial. Viscosupplementation is also used for other joints. In arthritic joints, synovial fluid has a diminished HA concentration and lower viscosity and decreased elasticity. These injections are believed to restore the elasticity and improve pain and function in patients with arthritis. Viscosupplementation can be an alternative to treatment such as medications and corticosteroid injections when they are contraindicated, not tolerated, or ineffective. Typically, one injection per week for 3–5 weeks is a common approach.

Pain relief following the injections is expected to last 6 months. Injections can be repeated at that time.[1,12]

17.1.5.8   Platelet-Rich Plasma

Platelets contain growth factors and cytokines that are important in inflammation reduction, necrotic cell removal, soft tissue healing, and bone mineralization. Steps in administering include obtaining blood through a usual venous draw, putting the blood through a centrifuge to obtain plasma with a high concentration of platelets, and then injecting the platelet-rich plasma (PRP) into the arthritic joint. Transforming growth factor-beta, present in PRP, has been associated with chondrogenesis in cartilage repair. PRP increases chondrocyte proliferation and may have clinical effects on degenerative cartilage. PRP increased HA concentration, stabilizing angiogenesis in 10 patients with osteoarthritic knees.[1,13]

17.1.5.9   Surgical Intervention

Total knee arthroplasty and total hip arthroplasty are considered after conservative treatments have failed. Surgery can be contraindicated in the setting of medical comorbidities including obesity or due to a patient's unwillingness/inability to complete the postoperative rehabilitation process.

17.1.6   Upcoming Research

The newest advances in arthritis treatments include the following: biologic treatments including PRP as discussed previously, stem cell therapy, vitamin C/D, and new developments in acupuncture techniques.

17.2   RHEUMATOID ARTHRITIS

17.2.1   Epidemiology, Background, and Risk Factors

Rheumatoid arthritis is a chronic, systemic inflammatory polyarthritis of autoimmune origin. If inflammation persists without treatment, it can lead to proliferation of tissues, and erosion of cartilage and bone, which leads to synovial damage and joint fusion. Imaging evidence of rheumatoid arthritis is seen as early as 2 years of disease activity.[14–17] The importance of recognizing and treating rheumatoid arthritis early is important to prevent loss of mobility and function. The elderly are at an increased risk of debility due to late recognition of rheumatoid arthritis as this population is prone to OA, osteoporosis, fractures, degenerative joint disease, cardiovascular disease, and multiple other comorbidities. The etiology of rheumatoid arthritis is unknown and new research continues to emerge. According to the Centers for Disease Control and Prevention (CDC), an estimated 22% of Americans suffer from arthritis and specifically 0.4%–1.3% from rheumatoid arthritis.[16,17] Incidence is high in Hispanic and Latino groups with Puerto Ricans showing the highest age-adjusted prevalence of arthritis.[16,17] In addition, prevalence of rheumatoid arthritis is highest in females, people aged 65 years and older, and people who are obese. Patients with rheumatoid arthritis have higher mortality rate and lifespan is shortened by 3–18 years.[17]

17.2.2   Diagnosis

The diagnosis of rheumatoid arthritis begins with a medical history, thorough physical examination, and laboratory workup. The American College of Rheumatology (ACR)/European League against Rheumatism (EULAR) criteria were modified in 2010 to include both acute and chronic disease. This criteria includes number and size of involved joints, serological abnormality, elevated CRP/ESR, and symptoms lasting at least 6 weeks.[14,15,17] In addition to these criteria, patients are classified as having rheumatoid arthritis if they present with imaging evidence of erosive disease and have a compatible history or have longstanding disease and previously fulfilled the above-mentioned criteria.[14,17]

History focuses on the location of involved joints. Peripheral joints are more commonly affected and include the metacarpophalangeal (MCP), metatarsophalangeal (MTP), proximal interphalangeal (PIP), and wrists. Morning joint stiffness lasts more than 30 minutes and improves with activity. Symptoms that have been present for less than 6 weeks may be due to an acute viral polyarthritis. Rheumatoid arthritis is associated with systemic symptoms such as fever, fatigue, depression, anorexia, malaise, weight loss, and anemia. Rheumatoid arthritis is a progressive, debilitating disease if left untreated, especially in the elderly population, therefore, it is important to assess functional capacity.[14,15,17]

Physical examination should focus on assessing for inflammation of the joint lining or synovitis. Joints have a limited range of motion and are soft, warm, boggy, and tender to palpation. A comprehensive examination involves 28 joints, focusing on the small joints of the hands and feet.[14,15,17] Extra-articular manifestations of rheumatoid arthritis are assessed. Moreover, symptoms of other systemic diseases on the differential are ruled out.[17]

17.2.3 Extra-Articular Manifestations

Approximately 40% of patients with rheumatoid arthritis have involvement of extra-articular systems.[16] These changes are hypothesized to be caused by the same cytokines that are responsible for synovial pathology. Positive rheumatoid factor or anti-cyclic citrullinated peptide (CCP) and smoking history are associated with extra-articular manifestations.[16] Such patients have increased severity of disease with increased morbidity and premature mortality.

Osteopenia is due to synovitis, immobility, and use of glucocorticoid steroids, which cause thinning of cortical bone. Decreased bone mineral density is found in rheumatoid arthritis patients as compared to controls regardless of glucocorticoid use.[18,19] Research has shown that glucocorticoids have an additive effect and patients are more prone to stress fractures, compression fractures, and loss of height as compared to controls.[18,19] A study of 287 rheumatoid arthritis patients showed that 22% had bone mineral density greater than 2.5 standard deviations below average at the hip, lumbar spine or of both sites indicating increased risk of osteopenia.[17-19] Men with rheumatoid arthritis also appear to have a lower bone mass. Providers should have a low threshold to start bisphosphonates.

Synovitis is associated with diminished joint mobility and therefore can cause muscle weakness, especially in the quadriceps. Moreover, chronic glucocorticoid steroids use can cause a proximal myopathy. 20%–35% of rheumatoid arthritis patients have nodules, which are commonly found on pressure points, such as the olecranon.[16,17] Eye manifestations include episcleritis and scleritis but these are less common.[16,17]

Lung involvement is common and has many presentations. Rheumatoid arthritis can cause lung disease of different histological and clinical presentations. Pleural disease is common in rheumatoid arthritis and usually presents as pleural thickening or small pleural effusions. Autopsy results identified pleural disease in 38%–73% of patients with rheumatoid arthritis, but only 5%–21% of those affected reported symptoms.[20,21] Pleural involvement is most common in chronic disease and in men.[22] It coexists with rheumatoid nodules and interstitial lung disease in up to 30% of patients.[22] Rheumatoid pleuritis and pleural effusions usually do not require specific treatment and resolve spontaneously or with treatment of joint disease.[22] Other manifestations include upper and lower airway obstruction, rheumatoid nodules, drug-induced toxicity due to methotrexate, and infection related to immunosuppression.[20,21] Moreover, there is a slightly increased risk of lung cancer than the general population.[20] Research has not shown an increased prevalence of pulmonary infections but there is an association with higher morbidity and mortality.[23] Patients should be vaccinated against streptococcal pneumonia and influenza on a yearly basis.

Rheumatoid arthritis is a risk factor for coronary artery disease and coronary events. Less than 10% of patients have a clinical episode of pericarditis but up to 30% have echo evidence of pericardial effusions.[16,24] There is a twofold increase in the occurrence of venous thromboembolism.[25] The prevalence of atherosclerotic disease is also greater than in the general population.[16,24] This was illustrated in a study that compared nonsmoking rheumatoid arthritis patients with controls, which showed an association between rheumatoid arthritis and peripheral artery abnormalities (19% vs. 5%).[16,25]

17.2.4 DIFFERENTIAL DIAGNOSIS

Differentiating rheumatoid arthritis from other connective tissue diseases is difficult. Degenerative joint disease does not have constitutional symptoms and is usually relieved by rest. OA affects the distal interphalangeal (DIP) and carpometacarpal joints. The classic presentation is stiffness that is worse with activity. Moreover, typical radiologic findings include osteophytes, joint space narrowing, subchondral cysts, and sclerosis. Gouty arthritis is intermittent and monoarticular, however, it can become a chronic polyarticular process. Gout is distinguished from pseudogout by the presence of urate crystals, whereas the later has calcium pyrophosphate crystals. Infectious polyarthritis can usually be differentiated by presence of fever, duration of symptoms, and presence of organism within the joint fluid or blood. It is important to rule out HIV, gonorrhea, human parvovirus B19, HBV, HCV, rubella, alphavirus, and Lyme. Hepatitis can have a positive Rheumatoid factor (RF) but always negative anti-CCP. Lyme disease usually affects large joints and is associated with migratory arthralgias.

Reactive arthritis is an HBL-27 positive, asymmetric, mono/oligoarthritis that is most commonly found in the knee joint. It is characterized by sacroiliitis and enthesopathy, which is inflammation of the site where tendon inserts into bone. Systemic rheumatological diseases such as systemic lupus erythematosus (SLE), Sjogren's syndrome, or dermatomyositis may be difficult to distinguish but are identified by other features such as rashes, myositis, nephritis, and specific antibodies. Unlike rheumatoid arthritis, CRP is always within normal limits. Generalized pain and muscle aches are the dominant features of polymyalgia rheumatica, hypermobility syndrome, and fibromyalgia. There is a lack of synovitis, antibodies, or acute phase reactant.

17.2.5 LABORATORY STUDIES

Diagnostic criteria for rheumatoid arthritis include presence of serological and acute phase reactants on laboratory workup. Rheumatoid factor is present in 70%–80% of patients but it has poor specificity.[14,15] It is found in higher titers in older individuals and in patients with other inflammatory diseases, such as SLE. Antibodies against citrullinated peptides have a much higher specificity, ranging from 95% to 98%, and a similar sensitivity to rheumatoid factor.[14,15] Acute phase reactants, such as ESR and CRP, represent the degree of inflammation and are elevated in active disease. Their presence can rule out differential diagnoses such as OA and fibromyalgia. Further laboratory analysis includes antinuclear antibody (ANA), anti-dsDNA, anti-Sm, complete blood count (CBC), and serum uric acid. Arthrocentesis and synovial fluid analysis involves cell count and differential, crystals, gram stain, and culture.

Seronegative rheumatoid arthritis is negative for rheumatoid factor or anti-CCP. It has a different disease progression and response to medications. Rheumatoid arthritis that has been present for less than 6 weeks or inactive disease will not have positive laboratory results.[14,15]

17.2.6 IMAGING

Rheumatoid arthritis can be identified and diagnosed on X-rays. Imaging shows cartilage loss, joint space narrowing, erosions, edema, joint effusion, tenosynovitis, ulnar deviation, swan neck, and boutonniere deformities.[14,17] X-rays are utilized as a baseline for monitoring disease progression.[17]

Ultrasound and MR imaging of joints is more sensitive and can help diagnose seronegative or inactive disease. A chest X-ray and CT scan of the chest can help to identify extra-articular manifestations such as pleural effusion, pneumothorax, pericardial fluid, subpleural nodules, and loculated fluid.

17.2.7 TREATMENT

Early recognition, prompt diagnosis and treatment prevent irreversible disease progression and joint injury. Within 2 years of disease, 80% of patients show space narrowing and 66% show erosions.[14,15,17] Medications are chosen according to past response, severity of disease, and stage of therapy.

Nonpharmaceutical treatments include exercise, physical and occupational therapy, nutrition and reduction of cardiovascular disease, and osteoporosis. Occupational and physical therapy play a pivotal role in maintenance or range of motion and strength, in addition to fabrication of splints and other adaptive equipment to maintain function.

Acute flares are treated with analgesic and anti-inflammatory medications such as steroids. Intra-articular glucocorticoid injections may be effective in treating single joints and avoid the need for prolonged systemic therapy.[26] Widespread flares may be treated by increasing the dose of oral steroids with the intention of reduction once the flare is under control. Pulse intravenous steroids are limited to severe flares associated with vasculitis.[26] In patients who receive glucocorticoids, we taper the medication as rapidly as tolerated once disease control is achieved and can be maintained, with the ideal goal of discontinuing systemic glucocorticoid therapy.[26]

As soon as rheumatoid arthritis is diagnosed, disease-modifying antirheumatic drugs (DMARDs) or disease modifying antirheumatic drugs should be initiated. DMARDs are divided into nonbiologic (hydroxychloroquine, methotrexate, sulfasalazine, and leflunomide) and biologic (etanercept, infliximab, adalimumab, rituximab, anakira, and tocilizumab) which target cytokines, their receptors, and other cell surface molecules.[17,27,28] Before starting a patient on DMARD therapy, laboratory testing should include a liver function panel, tuberculosis skin testing, and a visit to the ophthalmologist.[17,27,28] An escalation in dose or a modification in drugs is warranted if the patient is flaring frequently or severely. In patients resistant to initial DMARD therapy, an additional DMARD is added to the ongoing regimen or the patient is switched to a different DMARD, while also treating the active inflammation with anti-inflammatory drug therapy.[27,28]

The Be-St trial showed that at 3 and 12 months functional improvement was significantly better in those who received initial combination therapy.[29] Monotherapy was associated with more radiographic progression.[29] The FIN-RACo trial revealed that a significantly greater proportion of patients in the initial combination group had achieved minimal disease activity (63% vs. 43%) and remission by ACR criteria (37% vs. 19%).[30] In addition, radiographic progression was significantly less in the group receiving initial combination therapy compared with the group on monotherapy for at least 2 years.[30] New research focuses on target DMARDs such as tofacitinib inhibiting signaling through Janus kinase.[27,28]

17.3 ROTATOR CUFF TENDINOPATHY

17.3.1 EPIDEMIOLOGY, BACKGROUND, AND RISK FACTORS

The shoulder is the most mobile joint in the body and therefore more prone to injury.[31] It is stabilized by muscles that originate in the scapula and wrap around inserting into the humerus creating a cuff. Common causes of rotator cuff muscle or tendon injury include normal wear and tear, falls, poor posture, lifting/pulling, and repetitive stress. In the Health ABC study, 18.9% of elderly men and women reported shoulder pain.[31] The incidence of rotator cuff tendinopathy (RCT) rises in individuals who are greater than 40 years old and increases with age.[32] Other risk factors include female gender, previous injury, smoking, physical labor, and participating in competitive sports.[32] The elderly population is significantly affected as they are more likely to have chronic changes in the shoulder joint. Aging tendons develop micro-tears, calcifications, and fibrovascular changes.

The rotator cuff comprise four muscles that include the supraspinatus, infraspinatus, subscapularis, and teres minor. These muscles are responsible for abduction, internal/external rotation, glenohumeral joint stability, and humeral head translation.[33] The supraspinatus is most commonly injured.[33] RCT can be classified according to traumatic or nontraumatic. The former is due to increased force, overload, or direct laceration. The latter comprises chronic changes from previous injury and poor vascularization due to age, comorbidities, and tobacco use. Small tears have an inflammatory component that causes further degenerative changes making healing more difficult. Chronic RCT can lead to full thickness tears and labral injuries.

17.3.2   Diagnosis

It is important to rule out other causes of shoulder pain as RCT can lead to many of these conditions and management differs significantly. Other possible etiologies include cervical radiculopathy, acromioclavicular OA, subacromial bursitis, bicipital tendinopathy, rotator cuff tear, glenoid labrum tear, and adhesive capsulitis. RCT is most commonly associated with anterior glenohumeral dislocation.[33,34] History, clinical presentation, and imaging can help to rule out other conditions. A common complication of RCT is adhesive capsulitis. This is also referred to as "frozen shoulder" and is due to inflamed and stiff connective tissues surrounding the shoulder joint. Motion is restricted and chronic pain can last for years.

17.3.3   Assessment

The Western Ontario Rotator Cuff index is a disease-specific quality of life measurement tool for patients with rotator cuff disease.[32] It encompasses several aspects of RCT including physical symptoms, sports/recreational activities, vocational activities, lifestyle, and emotional burden.[32] In addition, it is vital to complete a thorough history and physical examination focusing on points outlined below.

17.3.3.1   History
1. When the injury occurred?
2. Mechanism, acute/chronic, location, radiation, quality of pain, what aggravates or relieves pain?
3. Prior shoulder injuries?
4. What therapies have been tried to date?
5. Assess ability to dress, reach behind back, brush hair, and donning a jacket?
6. Pain while sleeping on affected shoulder?

17.3.3.2   Physical Examination
1. Inspection for deformity, atrophy or bruising, palpation for edema, crepitus, or effusion.[33]
2. Active and passive range of motion.
3. Strength (e.g., empty can test).
4. Impingement (e.g., Hawkins test and Neer/painful arc test).
5. Labrum testing (e.g., O'brien test and apprehension test).
6. Examine opposite shoulder and cervical spine.

17.3.4   Laboratory Studies

Possible testing may include a general laboratory workup to assess for diabetes mellitus, rheumatologic disease, and small vessel disease.

17.3.5 Imaging

Plain radiographs do not usually reveal RCT but are usually performed as a first step in the assessment of shoulder injury. Three views are obtained and include the anterior–posterior, axillary, and supraspinatus outlet view. Radiographs can be useful when a patient fails conservative treatment, to determine anatomy for joint injection, and in recurrent cases.

The gold standard for initial evaluation of tendinopathy is musculoskeletal ultrasound. It is a quick, noninvasive, dynamic, and inexpensive method of imaging with a high sensitivity.[35,36] It allows the clinician to assess tendons while they are mobile and compare them to the opposite shoulder.[35,36] Changes noted on ultrasound include hypo-echogenicity and tendon thickening.

MRI is used when conservative treatments have failed, when there is high clinical suspicion for a tear or when the diagnosis is unclear.[36] Tears and degeneration are represented by a high intensity signal in the tendon.[36]

17.3.6 Treatment

Many treatment options for RCT exist but few are supported by strong evidence. The goal of treatment is to control pain, prevent progression, and improve quality of life.

17.3.6.1 Acute Management

The initial treatment consists of

1. Icing the shoulder to decrease inflammation and edema, in addition to analgesic properties.
2. Rest is recommended to reduce activities that can aggravate symptoms; that is, overhead reaching.
3. NSAIDs for a period of 7–10 days. The use of NSAIDs for an extended period of time remains controversial as some clinicians believe blocking of the inflammatory response inhibits healing.[37]

Gels, patches, and topical NSAIDs have been shown to provide some symptomatic relief but it has not been shown to be more effective than placebo. This modality may be beneficial if there is underlying OA in the glenohumeral joint. Alternate therapies include electrical stimulation, therapeutic ultrasound, and laser therapy. None of the aforementioned modalities have been supported by evidence.[38]

17.3.6.2 Physical Therapy

A number of physical therapy techniques have been used to treat RCT but no clinical trials exist to support use in rehabilitation. Initial physical therapy focuses on range of motion exercises to maintain mobility and prevent adhesive capsulitis, a common complication of RCT. The therapist then works on strengthening and stretching exercises to restore proper muscle activation and strength balance among the rotator cuff muscles. This is done using open kinetic chain exercises, therabands, muscle recruitment patterns, postural, and scapulohumeral kinesis techniques.

Preliminary studies have shown the benefit of eccentric exercise but further study is needed.[39] Eccentric exercise focuses is the application of a load to create a muscle contraction during the lengthening of a muscle.[39] Several studies suggest that eccentric exercise stimulates healing and provides effective rehabilitation of tendinopathy.[39]

17.3.6.3 Subacute Management

Partial tears or irreparable tears in elderly individuals are treated with conservative treatments. If no improvement is reached within 3 months or if patient cannot participate in physical therapy secondary to pain, other treatment options are considered. This includes local anesthetics, glucocorticoids,

PRP, or HA injections. The first injection attempted is a single, subacromial injection of lidocaine and steroid.[40–42]

There is no good evidence to suggest that glucocorticoid injections provide significant benefit but this is usually the next modality attempted.[40–43] There are a few studies that show a small benefit, although, no difference has been reported when comparing to NSAIDs.[41–43] A randomized controlled trial in Turkey found that, at 1-year follow-up, a PRP injection was found to be no more effective in improving quality of life, pain, disability, and shoulder range of motion than placebo in patients with chronic RCT who were treated with an exercise program.[43] On the contrary, a study comparing subacromial sodium hyaluronate (HA) injections with rehabilitation showed an overall reduction in pain at weeks 2, 4, and 12 in the HA group, therefore, it may be a safe and effective treatment for patients suffering from RCT.[44] Of note, this study was done in a middle-aged population without confounding rotator cuff pathology such as OA and glenohumeral instability. Physical therapy may play a pivotal role in the elderly population in whom these pathologies are common.

Another option is topical nitrate therapy. It is thought to cause local vasodilation, therefore, increasing blood flow to the damaged tendon.[45] It is important to note that nitrates are contraindicated in patients with hypotension, anemia, allergy to nitrate therapy, ischemic heart disease, phosphodiesterase inhibitor therapy (e.g., Viagra), pregnancy, and angle-closure glaucoma.[45] A common side effect of this treatment is headache.[45]

17.3.6.4 Chronic Treatment

An orthopedic referral is warranted when a patient fails conservative treatment for 6–9 months or when a tendon tear is suspected. Three common surgical interventions include debridement, acromioplasty to relieve impingement, and rotator cuff repair. These treatments are considered in active, highly functioning individuals.[46] Medications, injections, and rehabilitation are preferred in the elderly in order to maintain strength, range of motion, and function.

17.3.7 Upcoming Research

Randomized control trial involving extracorporeal shock-wave therapy appear to provide minimal relief when treating calcific tendinopathy, which is more common in the elderly population.[47]

17.4 HIP FRACTURES

17.4.1 Epidemiology, Background, and Risk Factors

Hip fractures in the elderly can be life altering.[48] Overall, 30 day mortality is 9%, development of medical complications increases the rate further, pneumonia alone increases mortality to 43% and heart failure increases it to 65%[49] and mortality at 1 year is 15%–20%.[50,51] The cost of treatment of hip fractures is in the billions[52] and expected to increase given rate of aging of the US population. Annually, in the United States, there are approximately 341,000 people who sustain a hip fracture with approximately 258,000 hospital admissions for fractures in people 65 years of age and older.[48,50,51] The rate of fracture doubles every 5–6 years after the age of 60 years, almost half of fractures take place in adults over the age of 80 years and most fractures in the geriatric population are associated with falls.[48,50]

There are three different types of hip fractures: (a) intracapsular which involve the head and neck of the femur; (b) intertrochanteric, which involve the area between the neck of the femur and the lesser trochanter; and (c) subtrochanteric, which include the area between the lesser trochanter and 5 cm distal to lesser trochanter.[53] Given the vascular supply, with intracapsular fractures, there is a risk of avascular necrosis, which will play a role in deciding the appropriate surgical intervention.

Risk factors include falls, race (white), gender (females), increased age, osteoporosis, heart failure, smoking, alcohol abuse, neurological impairment, institutional living, maternal history of hip fracture, previous hip fracture, tall stature, impaired vision, low body weight, and use of medications that decrease bone mass (steroids, antihypertensives, and antiepileptics). Risk factors for a second fall include age, impaired cognition, decreased bone mass, impaired senses, and impaired mobility.[48,50,52] Hip fractures in the geriatric population are most commonly seen after a fall. Patient may complain of hip pain and difficulty ambulating but may also have vague buttocks, knee, thigh, or groin pain with normal ambulation.

17.4.2 DIAGNOSIS

17.4.2.1 History

Eliciting further details about associated trauma or event will be important, including prodromal symptoms, which may indicate need for further neurological, cardiac, pulmonary, infectious, or oncologic workup as well as preinjury functional status (ambulation and ADLs), which will assist with treatment and disposition algorithm.[54] The former in addition to standard inquiry of past, medical, surgical, and social history, as well as current medications.

17.4.2.2 Physical Examination

1. *Vitals.* Tachycardia and hypotension can indicate blood loss, up to 1.5 L blood loss can be seen with hip fractures.[50]
2. *Inspection.* In the setting of a fall important to conduct a primary survey to evaluate for other injuries, evaluate for skin lesions, ecchymosis, hematoma, edema, deformity, asymmetry, suppleness of thigh, limb positioning, and leg length discrepancy. In the setting of a fracture, the hip is commonly abducted, externally rotated, and shortened, in the case of a subtrochanteric fracture, the proximal fragment can be seen in flexion and externally rotated due to muscle attachments.[54] Patient may also have inability to weight bear.
3. *Palpation.* Tenderness to palpation along hip, pain with internal and external rotation.
4. *Neurovascular examination.* Sensation, strength, reflexes, and pulses may be normal; however, examination may be limited by pain.

17.4.3 LABORATORY STUDIES

No one lab is available to diagnose hip fractures. A complete blood cell count and basic metabolic panel may help to evaluate blood loss and volume status. Standard preoperative labs and additional labs will be determined by need for further workup given circumstances surrounding fracture.

17.4.4 IMAGING

17.4.4.1 Plain Radiograph

Initial x-ray imaging includes anterior posterior (AP) and oblique of pelvis, AP and lateral of hip, and AP and cross-table lateral of involved femur.[50,54]

17.4.4.2 Computed Tomography

CT scans can be obtained by orthopedic surgeons as follow-up to plain radiographs to evaluate fracture post reduction and to assess for intra-articular fragments. It can also help to evaluate unstable patients who cannot tolerate MRI.

17.4.4.3 Magnetic Resonance Imaging

MRI and technetium bone scans can be helpful in identifying nondisplaced or occult fractures in cases where there is a strong clinical suspicion but initial plain radiographs are negative.

17.4.5 Treatment

Hip fractures are an orthopedic emergency! Acutely, it is important to address the basic aging and body composition (ABC) of trauma care, obtain imaging, and consult an orthopedic surgeon. Recommendations on conservative versus surgical management and choice of surgical procedure will depend on patient's age, medical and functional history, prognosis for rehabilitation, type of fracture, severity of fracture, and surgeon's preference.[52] Acute medical treatment will involve management of comorbidities, minimization of risk factors associated with delirium and pain control to facilitate participation in therapy, and minimize complications associated with decreased mobility.

17.4.5.1 Nonsurgical Treatment

This may be considered appropriate option if fracture is stable and can be followed with serials radiographs, patients is bed bound at baseline, and in patients who are poor surgical candidates.

17.4.5.2 Surgical Treatment

Will need to obtain appropriate preoperative evaluations and optimize patient for surgery in a timely fashion, ideally reaching the operating room within 48 hours, as delaying surgery increases both 1 month and 1 year mortality rate and a delay greater than 36 hours reduces likelihood of returning to independent living.[49,50] Management options include closed reduction, traction, arthroplasty, or open reduction internal fixation (ORIF).[55] Postoperative surgery-related complications include bleeding, wound infection, AVN, nonunion, malunion, and chronic pain.[50]

17.4.5.3 Rehabilitation

When a hip fracture as well as its surgical treatment impacts mobility and ADLs, a short stay in inpatient rehabilitation provides the concentrated therapies that may facilitate a return to the community. Patients begin working with physical therapy on postoperative day 1 to work on bed mobility, transfers, ambulation and use of gait aids in setting of weight-bearing restrictions which is determined by the surgeon based on the type of fracture and surgical treatment.[53] Depending on comorbid conditions patient may also benefit from evaluation by occupational therapy to evaluate need for assistance with ADLs.

17.4.6 Prevention/Patient Education[48,52]

Prevention and treatment of medical conditions associated with hip fractures is critical as 50% of patients will have a second fracture within 3–5 years. Providers should evaluate calcium and vitamin D levels, screen for osteoporosis using dual-energy x-ray absorptiometry (DEXA) scan, prescribe calcium (1000–1500 mg/day) and vitamin D supplementation (400–800 IU/day) and bisphosphonates, encourage smoking cessation and yearly eye examinations, discuss alcohol use, and review medications to minimize issues with polypharmacy as well as other conditions, which increase fall risk.

Providers should encourage geriatric patients to participate in exercise programs that focus on balance and stability, such as Tai Chi, to reduce risk of falls, weight-bearing exercises to help increase bone density, and muscle strengthening to assist with transfers and ambulation.[48,55] Patients would also benefit from continued physical therapy to improve gait stabilization, flexibility, and use of assistive devices. Environmental modifications reduce risk of falls such as addition of grab bars in the bathroom, placement of skid mats, fortifying rails for stairs, having adequate lighting, and ensuring clear paths where patient ambulates (no loose carpets, rugs, and toys).[51]

17.4.7 Upcoming Research

Research has been initiated on the use of hip protectors (specially designed underwear with padding) for fracture prophylaxis with mixed results and on the efficacy of prophylactic fixation in patients at risk for contralateral hip fracture.[56,57]

17.5   SPINAL STENOSIS

17.5.1   EPIDEMIOLOGY, BACKGROUND, AND RISK FACTORS

Lumbar spinal stenosis (LSS) is a condition that involves central canal, lateral recess, and/or neural foramen narrowing, which when symptomatic can lead to radiculopathy or neurogenic claudication. It is a common condition in the geriatric population with an estimated 8%–11% incidence rate in the United States.[58] The etiology of LSS can be divided into congenital and acquired; the latter involving degenerative changes of facet joints and discs, spondylolisthesis, iatrogenic causes, post-traumatic, malignancy, and metabolic bone disorders.[59] The most common etiology is degenerative LSS, given this, will focus discussion on that topic.

There are a series of events that result in spinal stenosis, which are addressed by the Kirkaldy-Willis degenerative spine cascade theory that looks at the interaction between the facet joints and the intervertebral disc in establishing a three-joint complex. This complex undergoes three phases in a parallel fashion: dysfunctional phase, instability phase, and stabilization phase. The phases include development of annular fissures and tears secondary to repetitive microtrauma, which predisposes the disc to herniation and loss of height followed by development of facet joint synovitis, hypomobility, cartilage degeneration, and capsular laxity causing loss of mechanical integrity at the three-joint complex. The final phase involves further disc space narrowing, fibrosis, osteophyte formation, and endplate destruction.[60–63]

17.5.2   DIAGNOSIS

17.5.2.1   History

Onset is usually insidious, back and leg pain is worse with standing, walking, or other activities that require lumbar extension and improve with sitting and lumbar flexion.[63–66] This presentation of symptoms is known as neurogenic claudication and should be distinguished from vascular claudication by the lack of vascular and skin changes as well as variability with position as listed above. Pain may be described as a burning, sharp, shooting, tight, or sore sensation. Symptoms can vary depending on involvement of single or multiple nerve roots.

1. *Red flags.* Provider should also assess for red flags, which merit urgent workup and potentially urgent treatment. These include fevers, chills, night sweats, and pain worse at night, unintentional weight loss, bowel or bladder issues, saddle anaesthesia, motor weakness and point tenderness which may indicate presence of infection, malignancy, cauda equina, or fracture.

The above components of the history are all in addition to standard inquiry of past medical, surgical, and social history, as well as current medications.

17.5.2.2   Physical Examination

1. *Vitals.* Usually within normal limits, abnormalities may indicate alternative diagnosis.
2. *Inspection/palpation.* Loss of lumbar lordosis, patient may prefer forward flexed posture; there is generally no appreciable erythema or ecchymosis as the pathology is deeper.
3. *Range of motion.* Pain may be reproduced or exacerbated with lumbar extension and improved with flexion.
4. *Neurological examination.* Sensation, strength, reflexes may be normal or mildly impaired. Care should be taken to distinguish give way weakness due to pain versus frank weakness. Patient may have impaired heel, toe, or tandem gait.
5. *Provocative maneuvers.* Straight leg raise and flexion abduction external rotation (FABER) testing are typically negative.

17.5.3　Laboratory Studies

No one diagnostic study or biomarker available to diagnose spinal stenosis.

17.5.4　Imaging

17.5.4.1　Plain Radiographs

Initial x-ray imaging should include AP and lateral view of lumbar spine to evaluate for spondylo-listhesis, disc space narrowing, end plate sclerosis, and facet joint arthropathy.[59,63–66]

17.5.4.2　Computed Tomography

CT scans may be ordered when MRI is contraindicated (pacemakers and aneurysm clips) or in postoperative patients. It can be paired with a lumbar myelogram.

17.5.4.3　Magnetic Resonance Imaging

MRI is very effective at evaluating canal, lateral recess, and foraminal narrowing as well as visualizing disc, nerve root, facet joint pathology, and ligamentum flavum hypertrophy. A lumbar spinal canal diameter of less than 10 mm is considered stenotic.

17.5.5　Treatment

Conservative treatment is the initial strategy, once red flags have been excluded, and involves patient education, use of oral medications, physical therapy, and epidural injections.[64,65]

17.5.5.1　Patient Education

Provide patient information of pathology involved in LSS; discuss avoidance of positions that exacerbate symptoms—predominantly those that involve lumbar extension.

17.5.5.2　Medications

Pain and symptoms control is important to ensure mobilization and participation in therapy. Range of oral medications includes NSAIDs such as meloxicam, short course of oral steroids for acute exacerbations, neuromodulators such as gabapentin, and antidepressants such as nortriptyline. Given the comorbidities of many geriatric patients and the potential side-effect profile of those oral medications, which include gastrointestinal (GI) intolerance, increased risk of bleeding, worsening hypertension (HTN), congestive heart failure (CHF), drowsiness, and sedation, the ability to utilize these may be limited.

17.5.5.3　Rehabilitation

When lumbar stenosis as well as its surgical treatment impacts mobility and ADLs, a short stay in inpatient rehabilitation provides the concentrated therapies that may facilitate a return to the community. A prescription should be provided for physical therapy to focus on pain tolerance, endurance, core strengthening, neutral- to flexion-based lumbar stabilization, posture, range of motion, flexibility, gait stabilization, and use of assistive devices.

17.5.5.4　Injections

Efficacy of epidural steroid injections is equivocal, however, given assumption that inflamed and compressed nerves may benefit from local anesthetic and anti-inflammatory treatment it continues to be a therapeutic option.

17.5.5.5　Surgical Treatment

Surgical treatment is deemed appropriate for patients who develop cauda equina, those who have progressive neurological impairment and recalcitrant pain not responsive to conservative therapies.[64,65,67] Options include laminectomy with and without spinal fusion. Laminectomy has been found to be helpful in patients with greater leg than back pain.

17.5.6 UPCOMING RESEARCH

Limited research data are available on biomarkers for spinal stenosis, use of lumbar corsets, benefit of epidural steroid injections, or benefit of supplemental fusion after decompression.

17.6 GREATER TROCHANTERIC PAIN SYNDROME

17.6.1 EPIDEMIOLOGY, BACKGROUND, AND RISK FACTORS

Accurate diagnosis and treatment of hip pain is essential for improving health and quality of life for the older population.[68] Greater trochanteric pain syndrome (often referred to as greater trochanteric bursitis) was first described in the 1930s. It is a common condition and is most often seen in elderly and middle-aged adults. Peritrochanteric bursitis has been typically thought to be the cause of the lateral hip pain and tears of the gluteus medius and minimus tendons may contribute. Gluteus medius tears are found in up to 22% of elderly patients. The iliotibial band (ITB) and tensor fascia lata are also thought to be a source of greater trochanteric pain syndrome.[69,70]

Greater trochanteric bursitis is one of the most common pain syndromes in older adults and affects 10%–25% of the general population.[69,71]

There are several factors implemented as causes of greater trochanteric pain syndrome including aging, female sex (F:M = 4:1), leg length discrepancy, lower back pain, knee/hip/lumbar spine OA, ITB tightness, strain of hip external rotators, obesity, and activity level (seen both in those who are sedentary and in runners).[71,72]

17.6.2 DIAGNOSIS

17.6.2.1 History

There is an extensive differential diagnosis for lateral hip pain and that may include lumbar spine pathology, fibromyalgia, bursitis, gluteus medius and minimus tears, hip OA, stress fractures of the proximal femur, trauma, avascular necrosis, and femoral nerve irritation.[70]

History should include areas of pain including the lower back and groin region. Patients with greater trochanteric pain syndrome typically present with chronic lateral hip pain. The area is often tender to palpation. Pain is exacerbated by lying on the affected side or with weight-bearing activities such as walking. Flexion, abduction, and external rotation of the hip often provokes the lateral hip pain.[68]

17.6.2.2 Physical Examination

Physical examination should include looking for any deformity or skin changes at the hip. One should assess the extremity for any muscle atrophy. Tenderness is typically present over the greater trochanter in greater trochanteric pain syndrome. One should do a full neurologic examination including strength testing (including hip abductors), sensory testing, and deep tendon reflexes. The lumbar spine should be assessed. Hip and knee range of motion abnormalities should be noted. Single leg stance as well as gait should be evaluated (looking for Trendelenburg gait).

17.6.3 LABORATORY STUDIES

Laboratory testing is not typically done for the diagnosis of greater trochanteric pain syndrome. However, systemic symptoms may lead one to test for markers of infection or inflammation such as CBC, CRP, and ESR.

17.6.4 IMAGING

17.6.4.1 Plain Radiographs

X-ray imaging is typically obtained first to assess for other causes of hip pain including OA and fracture. Calcification of the abductor tendons may be seen at the site of insertion to the greater trochanter.[71]

17.6.4.2 Ultrasound

Ultrasound can assess for gluteus medius/minimus tendon thickening, tendinopathy, and partial/full thickness tears. Calcific tendinopathy of the gluteal tendons can be aspirated and injected under ultrasound guidance.[71]

17.6.4.3 Magnetic Resonance Imaging

MRI of the hip in patients with greater trochanteric pain syndrome typically reveals a combination of peritrochanteric edema/bursal fluid and gluteus minimus/medius pathology. However, these findings are not specific for greater trochanteric pain syndrome and are also found in individuals without hip pain.[70] MRI can recognize partial/full thickness tears, tendon calcification, and fatty muscle atrophy. Edema suggests gluteal tendinopathy. One can see thickening or increased intra-substance signal intensity on T2-weighted scans when there is tendinopathy. One may also see fatty atrophy, bony irregularity, and tendon calcification over the greater trochanter. A partial tear is evidenced by focal tendon interruptions. Whereas a complete tear is seen with tendon discontinuity and possibly an avulsed bony fragment.[71]

17.6.5 TREATMENT

Greater trochanteric bursitis is often managed conservatively. Common management includes activity modification, weight loss, ice, physical therapy, ultrasound, nonsteroidal anti-inflammatory medications, and corticosteroid injections. With these measures, usually greater than 90% of patients report improvement in their pain. However, greater trochanteric pain syndrome often recurs and further management may only provide partial temporary improvement in pain. Occasionally, patients with ongoing pain will choose to proceed with surgical intervention.[69]

17.6.5.1 Rehabilitation

Treatment for greater trochanteric pain syndrome in an institution should start with basic range of motion exercises and avoidance of pressure on the affected side. Rehabilitation should progress to include education on a home exercise program for continued success in the community. Further home or outpatient physical therapy may be needed upon discharge.

17.6.5.2 Activity

Activity modification and relative rest is recommended. For the outpatient setting, a formal physical therapy program should then be considered. The physical therapy program for greater trochanteric pain syndrome works on piriformis and ITB stretching, gluteal strengthening, straight leg raises, and assisted squats.[69]

17.6.5.3 Modalities and Devices

Ice/heat as well as ultrasound is commonly used for this condition.[71] Low-energy shock-wave therapy has also been studied and has proven to show some benefit, however, improvements are often temporary and studies have significant limitations in the literature.[69]

17.6.5.4 Supplements and Medications

Anti-inflammatory medications may be very beneficial in patients diagnosed with greater trochanteric pain syndrome.[71]

17.6.5.5 Complementary and Alternative Medicine

Some patients find acupuncture, chiropractic treatment, and massage beneficial for their pain.

17.6.5.6 Psychology

One may choose to refer their patients with refractory pain to pain psychology.

17.6.5.7 Cortisone Injections

Usually, one corticosteroid injection provides a significant improvement in pain and function.[69] Injections typically provide short-term relief (3 months); however, it appears that they do not affect long-term resolution of pain at 1 year.[73]

17.6.5.8 Surgical Intervention

Surgery is indicated for severe refractory cases. Surgical management may involve lengthening/release of the ITB and fascia lata (proximal Z-plasty, proximal longitudinal release, and distal Z-plasty). For others, treatment may involve a bursectomy or trochanteric reduction osteotomy. Repairing tears of gluteus medius and gluteus minimus have been shown to improve pain.[69]

17.6.6 UPCOMING RESEARCH

The newest advances in treatments include the following: biologic treatments including PRP, the use of ultrasound guided injection techniques, and new arthroscopic approaches. Further research is needed in these areas.[71,74]

REFERENCES

1. Cerza F et al. Comparison between hyaluronic acid and platelet-rich plasma, intra-articular infiltration in the treatment of gonarthrosis. *Am J Sports Med* 2012; 40(12): 2822–7.
2. Yucesoy B et al. Occupational and genetic risk factors for osteoarthritis: A review. *Work* 2015; 50(2): 261–273. doi: 10.3233/WOR-131739.
3. Felson DT et al. Weight loss reduces the risk for symptomatic knee osteoarthritis in women. The Framingham Study. *Ann Intern Med* 1992; 116(7): 535–9.
4. Ersoz M et al. Relationship between knee range of motion and Kellgren–Lawrence radiographic scores in knee osteoarthritis. *Am J Phys Med Rehabil* 2003; 82(2): 110–5.
5. Kornaat PR et al. Osteoarthritis of the knee: Association between clinical features and MR imaging findings. *Radiology* 2006; 239(3): 811–17.
6. Hochberg MC et al. American College of Rheumatology 2012 recommendations for the use of nonpharmacologic and pharmacologic therapies in osteoarthritis of the hand, hip, and knee. *Arthritis Care Res (Hoboken)* 2012; 64(4): 465–74.
7. Jamtvedt G et al. Physical therapy interventions for patients with osteoarthritis of the knee: An overview of systematic reviews. *Phys Ther* 2008; 88(1): 123–36. Epub November 6, 2007.
8. Parkes MJ et al. Lateral wedge insoles as a conservative treatment for pain in patients with medial knee osteoarthritis: A meta-analysis. *JAMA* 2013; 310(7): 722–30. doi:10.1001/jama.2013.243229.
9. Hathcock JN, Shao A. Risk assessment for glucosamine and chondroitin sulfate. *Regul Toxicol Pharmacol* 2007; 47(1): 78–83.
10. Selfe TK, Taylor AG. Acupuncture and osteoarthritis of the knee: A review of randomized, controlled trials. *Fam Community Health* 2008; 31(3): 247–54.
11. Maricar N et al. Predictors of response to intra-articular steroid injections in knee osteoarthritis—A systemic review. *Rheumatology (Oxford)* 2013; 52(6): 1022–32. Epub 2012 December 22, 2012.
12. Lo G et al. Intra-articular hyaluronic acid in treatment of knee osteoarthritis: A meta-analysis. *JAMA* 2003; 290(23): 3115–21.
13. Sampson S et al. Injection of platelet-rich plasma in patients with primary and secondary knee osteoarthritis: A pilot study. *Am J Phys Med Rehabil* 2010; 89(12): 961–9.
14. Aletaha D et al. Rheumatoid arthritis classification criteria: An American College of Rheumatology/European League against Rheumatism collaborative initiative. *Arthritis Rheum* 2012; 62: 2569.

15. Anderson J et al. Rheumatoid arthritis disease activity measures: American College of Rheumatology recommendations for use in clinical practice. *Arthritis Care Res* 2012; 64(5): 640–7.

16. Turesson C et al. Extra-articular disease manifestation in rheumatoid arthritis: Incidence trends and risk factors over 46 years. *Ann Rheum Dis* 2003; 62(8): 722.

17. http://www.cdc.gov/arthritis/basics/rheumatoid.htm.

18. Haugeberg G et al. Clinical decision rules in rheumatoid arthritis: Do they identify patients at high risk of osteoporosis? Testing clinical criteria in a population based cohort of patients with rheumatoid arthritis recruited from the Oslo Rheumatoid Arthritis Register. *Ann Rheum Dis* 2002; 61(12): 1085–9. doi: 10.1136/ard.61.12.1085.

19. Ørstavik RE et al. Vertebral deformities in rheumatoid arthritis: A comparison with population-based controls. *Arch Intern Med* 2004; 164(4): 420–5. doi: 10.1001/archinte.164.4.420.

20. Tsuchiya Y et al. Lung diseases directly associated with rheumatoid arthritis and their relationship to outcome. *Eur Respir J* 2011; 37(6): 1411–7. doi: 10.1183/09031936.00019210.

21. Nannini C et al. Incidence and mortality of obstructive lung disease in rheumatoid arthritis: A population-based study. *Arthritis Care Res* 2013; 65(8): 1243–50. doi: 10.1002/acr.21986.

22. Balbir-Gurman A et al. Rheumatoid pleural effusion. *Semin Arthritis Rheum* 2006; 35(6): 368–78. doi: 10.1016/j.semarthrit.2006.03.002.

23. Blumentals WA et al. Rheumatoid arthritis and the incidence of influenza and influenza-related complications: A retrospective cohort study. *BMC Musculoskelet Disord* 2012; 13: 158. doi: 10.1186/1471-2474-13-158.

24. Turesson C et al. Severe extra-articular disease manifestations are associated with an increased risk of first ever cardiovascular events in patients with rheumatoid arthritis. *Ann Rheum Dis* 2007; 66(1): 70–5. doi: 10.1136/ard.2006.052506.

25. del Rincon I et al. Lower limb arterial incompressibility and obstruction in rheumatoid arthritis. *Ann Rheum Dis* 2005; 64(3): 425–32. doi: 10.1136/ard.2003.018671.

26. Gorter SL et al. Current evidence for the management of rheumatoid arthritis with glucocorticoids: A systematic literature review informing EULAR recommendations for the management of rheumatoid arthritis. *Ann Rheum Dis* 2010; 69(6): 1010–4. doi: 10.1136/ard.2009.127332.

27. Singh JA et al. 2012 update of the 2008 American College of Rheumatology recommendations for the use of disease-modifying antirheumatic drugs and biologic agents in the treatment of rheumatoid arthritis. *Arthritis Care Res* 2012; 64(5): 625–39. doi: 10.1002/acr.21641.

28. Nam JL et al. Current evidence for the management of rheumatoid arthritis with biological disease-modifying anti-rheumatic drugs: A systematic literature review informing the EULAR recommendations for the management of RA. *Ann Rheum Dis* 2010; 69(6): 976–86. doi: 10.1136/ard.2009.126573.

29. Goekoop-Ruiterman YP et al. Clinical and radiographic outcomes of four different treatment strategies in patients with early rheumatoid arthritis (the BeSt study): A randomized, controlled trial. *Arthritis Rheum* 2005; 52(11): 3381–90.

30. Rantalaiho V et al. The good initial response to therapy with a combination of traditional disease-modifying antirheumatic drugs is sustained over time: The eleven year results of the Finnish rheumatoid arthritis combination therapy trial. *Arthritis Rheum* 2009; 60(5): 1222–31. doi: 10.1002/art.24447.

31. Vogt MT et al. Neck and shoulder pain in 70- to 79-year-old men and women: Findings from the Health, Aging and Body Composition Study. *Spine J* 2003; 3: 435–41.

32. Chakravarty K, Webley M. Shoulder joint movement and its relationship to disability in the elderly. *J Rheumatol* 1993; 20(8): 1359–61.

33. http://www.orthobullets.com/sports/3032/glenohumeral-joint-anatomy-stabilizer-and-biomechanics.

34. Robinson CM, Shur N, Sharpe T, Ray A, Murray IR. Injuries associated with traumatic anterior gleno-humeral dislocations. *J Bone Joint Surg Am* 2012; 94: 18–26.

35. Smith TO, Back T, Toms AP, Hing CB. Diagnostic accuracy of ultrasound for rotator cuff tears in adults: A systematic review and meta-analysis. *Clin Radiol* 2011; 66: 1036–48.

36. Teefey SA et al. Detection and quantification of rotator cuff tears: Comparison of ultrasonographic, magnetic resonance imaging, and arthroscopic findings in seventy-one consecutive cases. *J Bone Joint Surg Am* 2004; 86-A: 708.

37. Andreas BM, Murrell GA. Tendinopathy: What works, what does not, and what is on the horizon. *Clin Orthop Relat Res* 2008; 466(7): 1539–54.

38. de Witte PB, Henseler JF, Nagels J, Vliet Vlieland TP, Nelissen RG. The Western Ontario rotator cuff index in rotator cuff disease patients: A comprehensive reliability and responsiveness validation study. *Am J Sports Med* 2012; 40: 1611–19.

39. Murtaugh B et al. Eccentric training for the treatment of tendinopathies. *Curr Sports Med Rep* 2013; 12: 175–82.
40. Alvarez CM et al. A prospective, double-blind, randomized clinical trial comparing subacromial injection of betamethasone and xylocaine to xylocaine alone in chronic rotator cuff tendinosis. *Am J Sports Med* 2005; 33(2): 255–62.
41. Buchbinder R et al. Corticosteroid injections for shoulder pain. *Cochrane Database Syst Rev* 2003; (1): CD004016. doi: 10.1002/14651858.CD004016.
42. Koester MC, Dunn WR, Kuhn JE, Spindler KP. The efficacy of subacromial corticosteroid injection in the treatment of rotator cuff disease: A systematic review. *J Am Acad Orthop Surg* 2007; 15(1): 3–11.
43. Kesikburun S et al. Platelet-rich plasma injections in the treatment of chronic rotator cuff tendinopathy: A randomized, controlled trial with 1 year follow up. *Am J Sports Med* 2013; 41: 2609–16.
44. Mellora G, Bianchi P, Porcellini G. Ultrasound-guided subacromial injections of sodium hyaluronate for the management of rotator cuff tendinopathy: A prospective comparative study with rehabilitation. *Musculoskelet Surg* 2013; 97: 49–56.
45. Paoloni JA et al. Topical glyceryl trinitrate application in the treatment of chronic supraspinatus tendinopathy: A randomized, double-blinded, placebo-controlled trial. *Am J Sports Med* 2005; 33: 806–13.
46. Gerber C, Wirth SH, Farshad M. Treatment options for massive rotator cuff tears. *J Shoulder Elbow Surg* 2011; 20(2 Suppl): S20–S29. doi: 10.1016/j.jse.2010.11.028.
47. Huisstede BM et al. Evidence for effectiveness of extracorporeal shock-wave therapy (ESWT) to treat calcific and non-calcific rotator cuff tendinosis—A systematic review. *Man Ther* 2011; 16: 419.
48. Hip fractures among older adults. Centers for Disease Control and Prevention. Updated September 20, 2016. Retrieved from http://www.cdc.gov/homeandrecreationalsafety/falls/adulthipfx.html.
49. Pollack P. Don't let hip fractures kill. American Association of Orthopaedic Surgeons Now. n.d. Retrieved from http://www.aaos.org/news/aaosnow/jan13/clinical9.asp.
50. Davenport M, Mills T. Hip Fracture in Emergency medicine. Medscape. n.d. Retrieved from http://emedicine.medscape.com/article/825363-overview.
51. Slear T. Hip Fracture survival and recovery. AARP. n.d. Retrieved from http://www.aarp.org/health/conditions-treatments/info-10-2011/hip-fractures-survival.html.
52. Brunner L, Eshilian-Oates L, Kuo, T. Hip fractures in adults. Am Fam Physician 2003; 67(3): 537–42. Retrieved from http://www.aafp.org/afp/2003/0201/p537.html.
53. Hip fractures. Ortho Info. American Academy of Orthopedic Surgeons. n.d. Retrieved from http://orthoinfo.aaos.org/topic.cfm?topic=A00392.
54. Koval KF, Zuckerman JD. *Handbook of Fractures*, 3rd edn. Philadelphia, Pennsylvania: Lippincott Williams and Wilkins; 2006: 303–45.
55. Sinaki M. Osteoporosis. In: Braddom RL, ed. *Physical Medicine and Rehabilitation*. 4th edn. Philadelphia, PA: Elsevier Saunders; 2011: 919.
56. Faucett SC, Genuario JW, Tosteson AN, Koval KJ. Is prophylactic fixation a cost-effective method to prevent a future contralateral fragility hip fracture? *J Orthop Trauma* 2010; 24(2): 65–74.
57. http://www.cochrane.org/CD001255/MUSKINJ_hip-protectors-for-preventing-hip-fractures-in-older-people.
58. Shamie AN. Lumbar spinal stenosis: The growing epidemic. AAOS Now. 2011. Available at: http://www.aaos.org/news/aaosnow/may11/clinical10.asp (accessed December 15, 2013).
59. Freeman TL, Freeman ED. Musculoskeletal medicine. In: Cuccurulo SJ, ed. *Physical Medicine and Rehabilitation Board Review*. 2nd edn. New York: Demos Medical Publishing, 2010: 306–11.
60. Patel RK. Lumbar degenerative disk disease. Medscape. 2012. Available at: http://emedicine.medscape.com/article/309767-overview (accessed July 7, 2013).
61. Laplante B, DePalma MJ. Spine osteoarthritis. *PM&R* 2011; 4(5 Suppl): S28–S36.
62. Middleton K, Fish DE. Lumbar spondylosis: Clinical presentation and treatment approaches. *Curr Rev Musculoskelet Med* 2009; 2: 94–104.
63. Everett CR, Ramirez CR, Perkowski M. Lumbar disc disorders. PM&R Knowledge NOW 2013. Available at: http://now.aapmr.org/msk/disorders-spine/Pages/Lumbar-disc-disorders.aspx (accessed December 13, 2013).
64. Katz JN, Harris MB. Lumbar spinal stenosis. *N Engl J Med* 2008; 358: 818–25.
65. Chen AL, Spivak JM. Degenerative lumbar spinal stenosis. *Phys Sportsmed* 2003; 31: 1–13.
66. Barr KP, Harast MA. Low back pain. In: Braddom RL, ed. *Physical Medicine and Rehabilitation*. 4th edn. Philadelphia, PA: Elsevier Saunders; 2011; pp. 902–3.
67. Angela MF, Jennie MS, Terry N, Jill LC, Wes C, Paul NS. Greater trochanteric pain syndrome: Defining the clinical syndrome. *Br J Sports Med* 2013; 47(10): 649–53. doi: 10.1136/bjsports-2012-091565.

68. Fearon A et al. Greater trochanteric pain syndrome: Defining the clinical syndrome. *Br J Sports Med* 2013; 47(10): 649–53.
69. Lustenberger D et al. Efficacy of treatment of trochanteric bursitis: A systemic review. *Clin J Sports Med* 2011; 21(5): 447–53.
70. Blankenbaker D et al. Correlation of MRI findings with clinical findings of trochanteric pain syndrome. *Skeletal Radiol* 2008; 37(10): 903–9.
71. Del Buono A et al. Management of the greater trochanteric pain syndrome: A systemic review. *Br Med Bull* 2012; 102: 115–31.
72. Segal N et al. Greater trochanteric pain syndrome: Epidemiology and associated factors. *Arch Phys Med Rehabil* 2007; 88: 988–92.
73. Brinks A et al. Corticosteroid injections for greater trochanteric pain syndrome: A randomized controlled trial in primary care. *Ann Fam Med* 2011; 9(3): 226–34.
74. McEvoy J et al. Ultrasound-guided corticosteroid injections for treatment of greater trochanteric pain syndrome: Greater trochanteric bursa versus subgluteus medius bursa. *AJR Am J Roentgenol* 2013; 201(2): W313–7.

18 Osteoporosis and Exercise in the Older Adult

Roger P. Rossi, Talya K. Fleming, Krishna J. Urs, and Sara J. Cuccurullo

CONTENTS

18.1 INTRODUCTION

Osteoporosis is the most common bone and skeletal disease, and a major cause of fracture with often consequent permanent disability and increased mortality. It is most common in older, postmenopausal women, but it is not uncommon in men and can occur at any age (1). In osteoporosis, there is a progressive loss of bone mass and structural changes in bone architecture that lead to bone fragility (2).

While osteoporosis can be easily identified at its early stages and there are effective pharmacological and nonpharmacological interventions to prevent its progression, it is often identified only after a fracture. The majority of older individuals at risk for developing osteoporosis are not routinely screened for the disease (3).

There are a number of medications that have been developed to delay onset, treat, or prevent progression of osteoporosis. It is however increasingly evident that physical activity, lifestyle modification, and especially exercise are essential in the treatment and prevention of osteoporosis.

In this chapter, we will review the basic disease concepts and discuss the principles and application of exercise and other interventions in the management and prevention of osteoporosis.

18.2 EPIDEMIOLOGY

The National Osteoporosis Foundation (NOF) estimates that up to 54 million U.S. adults aged 50 years and older are affected by osteoporosis or low bone mass, with approximately 10 million adults living with osteoporosis and over 43 million demonstrating low bone mass (3). With the aging of the U.S. population, it is also estimated that by 2020 the number of older adults with low bone mass or osteoporosis will increase to 64.4 million, and to over 71.2 million by 2030 (4).

Osteoporosis becomes more prevalent with age and while it is recognized in all racial groups, it is more common in Caucasians and Asians (5). It is estimated that as many as 50% of Caucasian postmenopausal women and 25% of older men are at risk for an osteoporosis-related fracture (6). Women are at a significantly higher risk for primary osteoporosis, with the risk of developing osteoporosis and fractures increasing dramatically after menopause. There is a high risk of osteoporosis-related fractures, especially femoral and vertebral fracture, in older women (7). Although osteoporosis has a female-to-male ratio of 4:1, men can also develop osteoporosis, but in the majority of cases the disease in men is secondary to other medical, nutritional, or metabolic disorders (8).

An estimated 2 million fractures occur each year in the United States among individuals with osteoporosis, resulting in more than 432,000 hospital admissions, 2.5 million medical office visits, and an estimated 180,000 nursing home admissions (3). Vertebral fractures are common osteoporotic fractures with 66% of vertebral fractures occurring after bending, lifting, or even sneezing (9).

The resultant effect of these fractures are significant, and include but are not limited to back pain, shortened stature, cervical lordosis, thoracic kyphosis (dowager's hump) with secondary restrictive lung disease, severe postural changes, restriction of intra-abdominal space, with consequent disability, loss of independence, and increased mortality (10).

Hip fractures are most common in women in their eighth decade of life. There are approximately 300,000 hip fractures yearly, 90% of which occur after a fall with an associated mortality of 20% during the first year. Up to 50% of patients with hip fracture require long-term assistance with activities of daily living and 20% require long-term placement (9).

Wrist fractures (Colles fractures) have a bimodal age distribution, with young adults and older individuals being most affected. They often result from a low-impact fall, and 85% of women who suffer distal radius fractures have shown to have low bone mineral density (BMD) and 51% have osteoporosis (11).

Other osteoporosis-associated fractures in decreasing order include forearm, proximal humerus, other femoral sites, ribs, pelvis, tibia, fibula, metatarsal bone, and calcaneus with varying consequences on overall morbidity and mortality (12).

18.3   ETIOLOGY AND PATHOPHYSIOLOGY

Different bones and skeletal sites have varying ratios of two predominant bone structures, cortical (compact) to trabecular (cancellous or spongy) bone. Cortical bones have a dense outer shell and comprise osteons or haversian systems that account for the more compact structure of the bone. Spongy bones are mostly made of trabeculae and are found mainly at the end of long bones and at the inner parts of flat bones. The cancellous to cortical bone ratio is about 75:25 in the vertebra, 50:50 in the intertrochanteric region of the hip (13), and 95:5 in the shaft or diaphysis of the radius (14).

In osteoporosis, there is a reduction of skeletal mass caused by an imbalance between bone resorption and bone formation. In adults, approximately 25% of trabecular bone and 3% of cortical bone are resorbed and remodeled every year. Skeletal osteoclasts are responsible for bone resorption removing older or damaged bone structures, while osteoblasts secrete and mineralize osteoid and are activated for new bone formation. Normal bone remodeling requires a tight coupling of bone resorption to bone formation to guarantee no alteration in bone mass or quality after each remodeling cycle (15). The rate and efficiency of bone remodeling varies with age and is different in men and women, and is affected by a number of regulating factors.

In osteoporosis, the balance between osteoclastic and osteoblastic activity is lost, with increased remodeling and relative decrease of osteoblastic function that results in net bone loss over time (2). This imbalance leads to trabecular perforation and reduced connectivity of the trabecular bone structure. There is also thinning and increased porosity of the cortices with the conversion of the normal plate-like trabeculae into thinner rod-like structures (14). These changes eventually cause increased bone fragility and higher fracture risk (14). As bone loss initiates at the bone surfaces, changes in bone mass occur earlier and to a greater extent in trabecular bone than in skeleton regions that are primarily cortical (14).

Age, gender, and endocrine factors are especially important in maintaining bone health. After the third decade of life, and more severely with advancing age, bone resorption exceeds bone formation with consequent osteopenia and osteoporosis. This loss of bone mass is much more marked in women, who lose significantly more trabecular bone than cortical bone (9). By 90 years of age, women lose 25% of their peak cortical bone mass compared to 18% in men and 55% of their trabecular bone (in central sites) compared to 46% in men (16).

Bone development is influenced by many physiologic factors including physical activity, body size, and sex hormones. Specifically, testosterone reduces bone resorption and a higher lifetime exposure to testosterone reduces the risk of osteoporosis. This gender advantage may first become important during puberty with a prolonged surge of testosterone production in males and longer bone maturation period, so that at skeletal maturity, men have 5%–10% greater bone mass than women (16). Estrogens also affect bone homeostasis, and estrogen receptors are expressed in both osteoblasts and osteoclasts (17) and higher levels of estrogen promote bone integrity. The effect of estrogens on bone remodeling also occurs through modulation of cytokines activity, and especially IL-1, IL-6, and tumor necrosis factor (TNF)–alpha (18). Estrogens also influence bone mineralization and estrogen deficiency renders bones more sensitive to parathyroid hormone (PTH), resulting in increased calcium resorption from bone. This in turn decreases PTH secretion, 1,25-dihydroxyvitamin D production, and calcium absorption and ultimately causes demineralization, especially of trabecular bone (19).

Lower estrogen production after menopause leads to enhanced bone resorption and decreased bone formation with bone loss that becomes significant in the first years after menopause (17). The change in estrogen levels also leads to rapid remodeling in menopause with an increased risk for fracture as the newly produced bone is less mineralized and structurally less solid (20).

Changes in calcium metabolism also affect bone integrity and bone homeostasis. Abnormal vitamin D and PTH activity are often identifiable contributing factors of bone fragility (21). Decreased bone mineralization (osteopenia) is seen not only in metabolic and endocrine disorders affecting calcium, PTH, and vitamin D, but can also be affected by nutrition and activity status.

Finally, concomitant muscle wasting or sarcopenia, usually age related, coexists with osteoporosis contributing to general vulnerability and frailty and may be an independent risk factor and indirectly lead to inactivity and bone fragility (18).

18.3.1 OSTEOPOROSIS-RELATED FRACTURES

Fractures occur when bone undergoes direct trauma or excess mechanical stress. Osteoporotic fractures refer to fractures that occur in bones rendered fragile by osteoporosis. Often in osteoporosis, fractures can result from low-energy trauma such as falls from a sitting or standing position. Nearly all hip fractures are related to falls, usually low-energy falls (22).

Fractures can be divided into two main categories: 27% are vertebral fractures of the spine, while the other 73% are nonvertebral fractures. Total incident fractures by skeletal site are vertebral (27%), wrist (19%), hip (14%), pelvic (7%), and other (33%) (23). Nonvertebral fractures, which typically occur in cortical bone (e.g., fractures of the hip, legs, upper arms, and forearms), were estimated to account for 73% of the total number of fractures and 94% of healthcare costs (24). Total costs by fracture type were vertebral (6%), hip (72%), wrist (3%), pelvic (5%), and other (14%) (23).

Several studies have assessed the effect on BMD and bone mineral content after exercise in postmenopausal women. Women who exercised had on average 0.85% less bone loss than those who did not exercise. Those who engaged in combinations of exercise types had on average 3.2% less bone loss than those who did not exercise. Postmenopausal women who exercised had on average 1.03% less bone loss than those who did not exercise. Individuals who exercised by strength training had on average 1.03% less bone loss than those who did not. Improvements can also be seen in older men. A 12-month high-impact unilateral exercise intervention was feasible and effective for improving femoral neck BMD, bone mineral content and geometry in older men (25).

Despite attempts at primary prevention, fractures resulting from osteoporosis are common. In the United States, the number of osteoporosis-related fractures was estimated to exceed 2 million in 2005 and total costs estimated at $17 billion (23). The burden of fragility fractures is expected to grow with the aging population. By 2025, the annual incidence and cost of fragility fractures in the United States is projected to increase by 50% (23). Men account for 29% of fractures and 25% of costs (23). Women aged 65 years and older accounted for 74% of all fractures and bore the overwhelming share (89%) of related total costs (24).

18.4 CLINICAL CONSIDERATIONS IN OSTEOPOROSIS

18.4.1 CLASSIFICATION OF OSTEOPOROSIS

Osteoporosis can be classified according to pathology and bone morphology, clinical subtypes, or etiology. The most common classification is based on body distribution, with distinction between generalized and localized bone involvement, and etiology, with a distinction between primary and secondary osteoporosis due to medication or other disorders affecting bone homeostasis (1).

18.4.1.1 Primary Osteoporosis

Primary osteoporosis is the most common type of osteoporosis, and is classified as Type I and Type II, although there is considerable overlap between the two types, and there is limited clinical value in differentiating between the two types. Osteogenesis imperfecta and idiopathic juvenile osteoporosis are also considered primary forms of osteoporosis.

> *Type 1 (Postmenopausal Osteoporosis):* This occurs in postmenopausal women, typically 15–20 years after menopause (age 55–65 years), and is characterized by increased trabecular bone more than cortical bone loss. It is associated more frequently with vertebral body, hip, and distal forearm fractures.
>
> *Type 2 (Senile Osteoporosis):* It occurs in women and men older than 70 years, and more commonly in females than males with a 2:1 ratio. It is frequently associated with fractures of the hip, spine, pelvis, and long bones. Unlike Type I, trabecular and cortical bones are equally affected.

18.4.1.2 Osteogenesis Imperfecta

Osteogenesis imperfecta is a rare form of congenital osteoporosis due to deficiency of Type I collagen formation and consequent bone fragility with brittle bones that are prone to fracture. The majority of cases of osteogenesis imperfecta are by mutations in the *COL1A1* and *COL1A2* genes (26).

18.4.1.3 Idiopathic Juvenile Osteoporosis

Idiopathic juvenile osteoporosis is a rare form of osteoporosis that occurs in children between the ages of 8 and 10 years at times of rapid growth and typically prior to puberty. There is no known cause for this type of osteoporosis, in which there is too little bone formation or excessive bone loss and can lead to kyphosis or other malformations and to bone fractures. Most children experience complete recovery and maintain normal bone function in adulthood (27).

18.4.1.4 Secondary Osteoporosis

Secondary osteoporosis can occur at any age, with men and women being equally affected. It is a complication of a number of other medical diseases or drugs affecting bone metabolism. Among these, the most common are endocrine disorders, especially hyperparathyroidism, hyperthyroidism, and nutritional or metabolic disorders affecting vitamin D metabolism. Osteoporosis is also a frequent complication of cancer, especially leukemias. Among drug-induced osteoporosis, chronic use of corticosteroids, thyroid replacement, anticonvulsants (especially barbiturates and valproic acid) or antineoplastic chemotherapeutics such as aromatase inhibitors are among the most common.

Table 18.1 summarizes the diverse causes of secondary osteoporosis and the most common drugs associated with it.

Other forms of secondary osteoporosis include those secondary to prolonged immobilization (28) and the localized reduction of bone mass associated with reflex sympathetic dystrophy (RSD), with radiographic changes that may occur in the first 3–4 weeks occurring as patchy demineralization of the affected area (28).

TABLE 18.1

Common Causes of Secondary Osteoporosis in Adults

Endocrine or Metabolic Causes	Nutritional/ Gastrointestinal Conditions	Drugs	Disorders of Collagen Metabolism	Other
Acromegaly	Alcoholism	Antiepileptics[a]	Ehlers–Danlos	AIDS/HIV
Diabetes mellitus	Anorexia nervosa	Aromatase inhibitors	syndrome	Ankylosing spondylitis
Type I	Calcium deficiency	Chemotherapy/	Homocystinuria	Chronic obstructive
Type II	Chronic liver	immunosuppressants	due to	pulmonary disease
Growth hormone	disease	Depo-Provera	cystathionine	Gaucher disease
deficiency	Malabsorption	Glucocorticoids	deficiency	Hemophilia
Hypercortisolism	syndromes/	Gonadotropin-releasing	Marfan syndrome	Hypercalciuria
Hyperparathyroidism	malnutrition	hormone agonists	Osteogenesis	Immobilization
Hyperthyroidism	(including celiac	Heparin	imperfecta	Major depression
Hypogonadism	disease, Crohn's	Lithium		Myeloma and some
Hypophosphatasia	disease, and	Proton pump inhibitors		cancers
Porphyria	gastric resection	Selective serotonin		Organ transplantation
Pregnancy	or bypass)	reuptake inhibitors		Renal insufficiency/
	Total parenteral	Thiazolidinediones		Failure
	nutrition	Thyroid hormone (in		Renal tubular acidosis
	Vitamin D	supraphysiologic doses)		Rheumatoid arthritis
	deficiency	Warfarin		Systemic mastocytosis
				Thalassemia

Source: Watts, N. et al. 2010. *Endocr Pract* 16(3): 1–37. http://aace.com/files/osteo-guidelines-2010.pdf, with permission from the American Association of Clinical Endocrinologists.

Note: AIDS, acquired immunodeficiency syndrome; HIV, human immunodeficiency virus.

[a] Phenobarbital, phenytoin, primidone, valproate, and carbamazepine have been associated with low bone mass.

18.5 RISK ASSESSMENT OF OSTEOPOROSIS

There are a number of risk factors for osteoporosis, which can be identified as nonmodifiable, for example, gender or age, and modifiable, such as poor nutrition, alcohol intake, and smoking. Recognizing the modifiable risk factors is important in the prevention and management of osteoporosis.

18.5.1 NONMODIFIABLE RISK FACTORS

The most important nonmodifiable risk factors are age and female gender. Women have a smaller bone mass and lose bone more rapidly than men, with greater bone loss occurring after menopause, approaching up to 5% loss per year (9). While age has a variety of effects on bone health, the age-related loss of estrogen on women and testosterone in men is the most important factor, with a more severe effect induced by estrogen loss (29).

Race is also a notable risk factor, with Caucasians and Asians being at higher risk of developing osteoporosis than other racial groups (30). A positive genetic profile increases an individual's risk of developing osteoporosis with individuals with a family history of osteoporosis, and especially those with a history of fracture, being at a higher risk. While not strictly considered a genetic disease, at least 30 gene mutations have been associated with the development of osteoporosis (21).

Individuals with previous fractures also have an increased risk of any type fracture by 86% compared to those without prior fracture (31).

Other nonmodifiable risk factors include short stature, diminished peak bone mass (PBM) at skeletal maturity, estrogen loss due to menopause or hysterectomy, and primary or secondary hypogonadism in men (28).

18.5.2 MODIFIABLE RISK FACTORS

The majority of osteoporotic fractures are due to falls. A higher risk of falling exists in individuals with muscle weakness due to neurological disorders, cognitive impairment, gait disturbance, balance, visual deficits, dehydration, sedating medications and other medication side effects, or in those with prior history of falling (32).

High alcohol intake, defined as greater than two drinks a day, has also been associated with a 40% increased risk for an osteoporotic fracture (33).

Smokers are at an increased fracture risk, as smoking is directly toxic to bone formation, with evidence of lower BMD and greater annual rate of bone loss (34).

Poor nutrition is also a known risk factor for osteoporosis. Malnutrition in general, and especially a diet with insufficient intake of calcium, vitamins, especially vitamins D, A, K, E, and C, and low in protein is associated with osteoporosis. Interestingly however, high dietary consumption of animal proteins is associated with increased risk of fractures (35). Other relevant nutritional deficiencies include low dietary phosphorus, magnesium, zinc, iron, fluoride, and copper. Diet-related high blood acidity may also negatively affect bone metabolism (36). A high consumption of soft drinks has been associated with osteoporosis in older women (37). An excessive caffeine intake has also been linked to higher risk of osteoporosis (38).

Low body mass index, less than 20 (kg/m^2) regardless of weight loss, sex, and age, is associated with a greater bone loss and fracture risk (39). Interestingly, osteoporosis is less common in overweight people (40).

Sedentary lifestyle is a significant contributing factor for increased prevalence of osteoporosis (41).

A number of other medical diseases are associated with osteoporosis, and modifiable risk factors exist for those disorders that indirectly benefit bone health and may prevent osteoporosis.

Table 18.1 lists common diseases associated with osteoporosis.

18.6 DIAGNOSIS OF OSTEOPOROSIS

In many patients, a diagnosis of osteoporosis is established only at the time of a bone fracture. In many cases however, osteoporotic fractures, especially vertebral fractures, may be asymptomatic or not clinically obvious, and the physical examination may reveal a skeletal deformity or pain present only on mobilization. Femoral fractures or distal forearm fractures are usually painful and functionally disabling. Not infrequently, fractures occur spontaneously or after minimal trauma.

Evidence of bone structure abnormalities suggestive of osteoporosis can be determined through a variety of diagnostic tests that can assess the severity of bone disease and predict the relative risk of fracture by measuring BMD. In all patients with suspected osteoporosis laboratory studies to establish baseline values and to look for potential secondary causes of osteoporosis are warranted.

Quantitative BMD can be determined with dual-energy x-ray absorptiometry (DXA) and quantitative computed tomography (QCT) scanning. In the United States, QCT of the hip and DXA of the spine or hip are the accepted diagnostic methods in the evaluation of osteoporosis.

18.6.1 RADIOGRAPHY

Often the preliminary diagnostic study is a plain radiograph that can identify bone fractures and offer an initial assessment of bone health. Frequently, the reason for a radiographic study is back pain and lateral spine series may detect occult vertebral fractures.

Radiographic studies are not sensitive to detect osteoporosis and cannot be used to assess BMD. Only after at least 30% of BMD is lost, will the typical radiographic changes of osteoporosis, or lucency, become apparent. The late radiographic appearance correlates to the late cortical bone involvement, as in earlier disease stages the bone loss is mostly present in trabecular bone (42).

18.6.2 LABORATORY STUDIES

A number of laboratory studies should be performed in individuals with osteoporosis to assess bone and calcium metabolism and exclude common secondary causes.

Serum calcium, phosphate, magnesium, 25(OH) vitamin D, and alkaline phosphatase should be measured in all patients and can detect common causes of secondary bone loss, while they may be normal in primary osteoporosis. However, contributing calcium and bone metabolism disorders are also commonly associated with osteoporosis and can be detected in a surprisingly high number of healthy women (43).

Thyroid-stimulating hormone (TSH) level, complete blood count (CBC), and liver function tests can be helpful in detecting common causes of osteoporosis. More specific tests include 24-hour urine calcium level and PTH, testosterone and gonadotropin levels, urinary free cortisol level, serum protein electrophoresis (SPEP), antigliadin, and antiendomysial antibodies.

Markers of bone turnover may also be used to assess rate of bone turnover (for instance, in postmenopausal osteoporosis) or to monitor treatment response.

18.6.3 DUAL-ENERGY X-RAY ABSORPTIOMETRY

This test is considered the most cost-effective and reliable instrument to measure BMD, and is a low-cost and low-risk study. DXA tests BMD in the lumbar spine, hip and proximal femur, and can predict the risk of osteoporotic fractures. When used for repeated measurements over time, it can also help monitor disease progression or response to treatment. Osteoporosis does not manifest uniformly throughout the skeleton, but different bone structures usually have different degrees of BMD. While measurement of BMD can predict the overall fracture risk, measurement at a particular anatomical location can more accurately predict the fracture risk at that site.

The World Health Organization's (WHO) definitions of osteoporosis are based on BMD measurements in postmenopausal women and men older than 50 years, with derived T-scores and Z-scores that are used to define osteopenia and osteoporosis. A T-score is the number of standard deviations (SD) from the mean PBM of young adults with the same race and gender. The Z-score is instead the number of SD of the patient's bone density from the BMD of adults of the same age, gender, and ethnicity (44). A normal bone density is defined by a T-score between −1 SD and +1 SD from normal BDM. In osteopenia, the T-score is between −1 and −2.5, while in osteoporosis, the T-score is less than 2.5 SD (45).

Bone densitometry is recommended for all women aged 65 years and older and men aged 70 years and older regardless of clinical risk factors, postmenopausal women and women in menopausal transition with risk factors for fracture, men aged 50–69 years with risk factors for fracture, adults with diseases predisposing or associated with osteoporosis, and adults taking steroids or other medications that can cause bone loss (46).

For each SD reduction in BMD, the relative fracture risk is increased 1.5–3 times. Of note, about half of osteoporotic fractures occur in women with a T-score greater than −2.5, and the other half occur in those with a T-score lower than −2.5, the WHO's cutoff for DXA-based diagnosis of osteoporosis.

18.6.4 QUANTITATIVE COMPUTED TOMOGRAPHY

QCT can also be utilized to measure spinal BMD and can be performed with common CT scanners. It is less commonly used than DXA despite similar costs and accuracy (47). Although QCT has a higher radiation exposure than DXA, it is especially accurate in evaluating vertebral bones, as the scan can detect trabecular bone loss.

The scan may also help identify fractures and areas of callus formation that indicate healing fractures. One of the advantages of QCT is that it measures both cortical and trabecular BMD and the results are expressed as direct measurements of precise volumetric mineral density calculated in mg/cm^3, without the need for calculating T- or Z-scores.

18.6.5   OTHER DIAGNOSTIC TESTS

Other diagnostic tests are used in the diagnostic process of osteoporosis. Among these is magnetic resonance imaging (MRI), which not only can precisely identify fractures, but is also helpful in detecting indirect signs of osteoporosis, such as occult stress fractures of the proximal femur. Quantitative ultrasonography (QUS) of the calcaneus, tibia, and patella is another inexpensive diagnostic modality to assess bone health. It is not as precise as DXA or other modalities, and cannot be used to monitor disease progression. Single-photon emission computed tomography (SPECT) is accurate and specific for bone lesions, and represents a tomographic (CT-like) bone imaging technique that offers better image contrast and more accurate lesion localization than planar bone scanning. It increases the sensitivity and specificity of bone scanning for detection of lumbar spine lesions by 20%–50% over planar techniques.

18.6.6   FRACTURE RISK ASSESSMENT TOOL

The Fracture Risk Assessment Tool (FRAX) was developed by the World Health Organization (WHO) task force in 2008 as a prediction tool for assessing an individual's risk of fracture in order to provide general clinical guidance for treatment decisions. The goal is to incorporate non-BMD clinical risk factors into an overall assessment of an individual's fracture risk, with or without knowledge of BMD.

The FRAX score is considered the most accurate tool to estimate the risk and probability of fracture in the next 10 years in untreated men and women aged 40–90 years (48). It is recommended that all postmenopausal women and men aged 50 years and older should be evaluated for osteoporosis risk in order to determine the need for BMD testing and/or vertebral imaging (3).

The U.S. Preventive Services Task Force (USPSTF) recommends testing women 65 years or older without previous known fractures and women 60–64 years of age with a risk factor. The USPSTF has not made recommendations for screening in men (9). Based on FRAX estimates, it has been estimated that the 10-year fracture risk for a 65-year-old white woman without specific additional risk factors is 9.3% (49).

The FRAX score is a composite measure that is calculated from a number of variables, including age, gender, body mass index (computed from height and weight), and independent risk variables that comprise a prior fragility fracture, parental history of hip fracture, current smoking, previous or current long-term use of oral glucocorticoids (defined as use of >5 mg/day of prednisone for >3 months), rheumatoid arthritis, secondary osteoporosis, and daily alcohol consumption of three glasses or more. If available, femoral neck (hip) BMD can additionally be entered, preferably as a T-score.

18.7   PREVENTION AND TREATMENT OF OSTEOPOROSIS

Prevention of osteoporotic fractures and the consequent disability, morbidity, mortality, and expenses associated with these fractures is a significant global health objective (50). It is essential to identify individuals at risk for osteoporosis and initiate preventive intervention at the earliest possible time. Intervening on modifiable risk factors such as smoking or excessive alcohol consumption, associated medical problems such as hyperthyroidism or hyperparathyroidism, or use of drugs, can effectively reduce the risk of osteoporotic fractures.

TABLE 18.2

Recommended Daily Allowances of Calcium and Vitamin D

Age	Calcium (mg/day)	Vitamin D (IU/day)
1–3 years	700	600
4–8 years	1000	600
9–13 years	1300	600
14–18 years	1300	600
19–30 years	1000	600
31–50 years	1000	600
51–70 years, male	1000	600
51–70 years, female	1200	600
Over 70 years	1200	800

Source: Institute of Medicine of the National Academies. Report Brief. Dietary Reference Intakes for Calcium and Vitamin D. Revised March 2011.

General lifestyle interventions, including adequate dietary intake of calcium and vitamin D, and increasing physical activity, especially weight-bearing exercise aimed at increasing muscle strength, should be recommended to all individuals at risk for osteoporosis (51). The role of exercise in preventing osteoporosis and delaying its progression is increasingly recognized as a key factor in the overall approach to osteoporosis treatment, and will be addressed later in this chapter.

18.7.1 NUTRITION

Nutrition can be an important factor in reducing the risk of osteoporosis. Maintaining appropriate intake of dietary calcium, vitamin D, and other nutrients can help maintain overall bone health. The National Academy of Sciences has developed dosing recommendations for calcium and vitamin D by age group.

Table 18.2 summarizes the recommended daily doses of calcium and vitamin D for different age groups (52).

Incorporating a well-balanced diet including dairy, fruits, vegetables, and fish is important to getting the recommended daily allowance of vitamins and minerals. Some foods are also fortified with extra vitamins and minerals. If nutritional deficiencies are apparent, a multivitamin may be needed as a dietary supplement.

18.8 PHARMACOLOGICAL TREATMENT

A number of pharmacological agents have been developed to treat osteoporosis. While there is no drug or intervention that can effectively reverse or cure osteoporosis, proper intervention may slow or stop its progression. Although most drugs are well tolerated, there are a number of side effects and potential long-term risks that dictate the need for proper selection and individualized treatment.

There is a general consensus on identifying patients in need for pharmacological treatment. The NOF has defined guidelines recommending treatment for postmenopausal women and men aged 50 years or older with

- History of hip or vertebral fractures (either clinical or radiographic evidence of fracture)
- T-score of −2.5 or less at the femoral neck or spine after appropriate evaluation to exclude secondary causes

- Low bone mass (T-score between −1.0 and −2.5 at the femoral neck or spine) and a 10-year probability of a hip fracture of 3% or greater or a 10-year probability of a major osteoporosis-related fracture of 20% or greater based on the U.S.-adapted WHO algorithm (3)

Among the several families of agents available, the most common and widely used drugs are the bisphosphonates. Other drugs include raloxifene, an estrogen-receptor modulator; teriparatide, a recombinant PTH; denosumab, an inhibitor of osteoclasts' maturation; and calcitonin.

Treatment guidelines recommend using bisphosphonates as first line of treatment, limiting the use of the other drugs to individuals who are not responding or cannot tolerate bisphosphonate (50).

All patients who are started on treatment for osteoporosis should also receive adequate intake of calcium and vitamin D supplementation.

18.8.1 BISPHOSPHONATES

Bisphosphonates are the most commonly used agents for the treatment of osteoporosis. These drugs work by inhibiting osteoclast-mediated bone resorption through a direct action on osteoclasts, and can be administered orally or intravenously to subjects unable to tolerate oral formulations.

The relative efficacy of the drugs in this class is not known, but in clinical studies and long-term observation series, these drugs have shown to be effective in significantly reducing risk of fracture, with evidence of higher risk reduction for vertebral than for hip fractures (53).

Although these drugs are usually well tolerated, they can cause esophagitis and other side effects. There are specific instructions to be followed when the drugs are taken orally that include taking the drug in the sitting position, with at least 8 ounces of water and at least 40 minutes prior to eating. Long-term complications of bisphosphonates include osteonecrosis of the jaw and atypical femoral fractures.

Table 18.3 summarizes the different bisphosphonates available in the United States (54).

18.8.2 SELECTIVE ESTROGEN-RECEPTOR MODULATORS

Selective estrogen-receptor modulators (SERMS) are drugs that exert estrogenic protective activity on bones, and on breast and uterus. While the use of these drugs has been associated with higher incidence of deep vein thrombosis and stroke, they are considered safer than estrogen replacement. They also appear to be protective in breast cancer. They bind to bone estrogen receptors and affect bone structure by decreasing bone resorption. Raloxifene (Evista) was the first SERM agent approved for the treatment and prevention of osteoporosis in postmenopausal women.

Recently, the FDA approved a product with bazedoxifene (a novel SERM) and conjugated estrogens for prevention of osteoporosis and treatment of vasomotor symptoms in postmenopausal women (55). Hormone replacement therapy (HRT) is no longer considered an acceptable treatment for osteoporosis due to the high incidence of severe complications, including stroke, myocardial infarction, deep vein thrombosis, and breast cancer (56).

18.8.3 PARATHYROID HORMONE

The recombinant human PTH (1–34). Teriparatide (Forteo) is the only available anabolic agent for the treatment of osteoporosis. Its effect is exerted by activating osteoblasts and increasing serum calcium. It is indicated for the treatment of women with postmenopausal osteoporosis and in men with idiopathic or hypogonadal osteoporosis that did not tolerate or did not respond to other treatments. It may be especially indicated in more severe osteoporosis, and for those at high risk of fracture. It may also be helpful in accelerating bone repair after a fracture (57). Before initiating treatment with teriparatide, levels of serum calcium, PTH, and 25(OH) D need to be monitored.

TABLE 18.3

Bisphosphonates Available for Use in the United States

Generic Name	Brand Name	Strength	Form	Dose
Alendronate	Binosto	70 mg	Effervescent tabs for oral solution	70 mg once weekly
Alendronate	Fosamax	5, 10, 35, 40, 70 mg	Tablet	Treatment: 10 mg once daily or 70 mg once weekly
		70 mg/75 mL	Oral solution	Prevention: 5 mg once daily or 35 mg once weekly
Alendronate/ cholecalciferol (Vitamin D3)	Fosamax Plus D	70 mg/2800 IU 70 mg/5600 IU	Tablet	Treatment: 70 mg/2800 IU or 70 mg/5600 IU once weekly
Risedronate	Actonel	5, 30, 35, 75, 150 mg	Tablet	Prevention and treatment: 5 mg once daily or 35 mg once weekly or one 75 mg tab taken on 2 consecutive days per month or 150 mg once a month
Risedronate	Atelvia	35 mg	Delayed-release tablet	Treatment: 35 mg once weekly
Ibandronate	Boniva	150 mg	Tablet	Prevention and treatment: 150 mg once monthly
		3 mg/3 mL	Injection	Treatment: 3 mg IV once every 3 months
Zoledronic acid	Reclast	5 mg/100 mL	Injection	Treatment: 5 mg IV infusion once year
				Prevention: 5 mg IV infusion once every 2 years

Source: Monthly Prescribing Reference. 2015. Haymarket Media, Inc. Available at http://www.empr.com/clinical-charts/osteoporosis-treatments/article/123840.

Teriparatide cannot be given for more than 2 years, and is contraindicated in patients with preexisting hypercalcemia, severe kidney disease, and history of primary or secondary bone tumor.

18.8.4 CALCITONIN

The use of the hormone calcitonin (Fortical, Miacalcin) is also reserved for the treatment of osteoporotic patients who cannot tolerate or do not respond to other agents. Its efficacy is due to direct inhibition of osteoclastic activity and modulation of calcium reabsorption. It is available as a nasal spray and subcutaneous injection and its efficacy in nonvertebral fractures has not been established. There is also evidence that patients treated with calcitonin have a higher incidence of malignancies (58).

18.8.5 DENOSUMAB

Denosumab (Prolia, Xgeva) is a humanized monoclonal antibody that targets the receptor activator of the nuclear factor-kappa B ligand (RANKL) that has a key role in osteoclast differentiation and activation. As RANKL is overactive in autoimmune and inflammatory disorders, RANKL antibodies may be especially effective in patients with osteoporosis associated with immune and inflammatory disorders (59). Its use is indicated to increase bone mass in postmenopausal women and men with history of osteoporotic fracture and high risk of fracture that are intolerant to other

TABLE 18.4

Known Effect in Preventing Fractures by Anatomical Site

Medication	Fracture Risk Reduction		
	Vertebral	Nonvertebral	Hip
Alendronate (Fosamax)	Yes	Yes	Yes
Risedronate (Actonel)	Yes	Yes	Yes
Zoledronic acid (Reclast)	Yes	Yes	Yes
Denosumab (Prolia)	Yes	Yes	Yes
Teriparatide (Forteo)	Yes	Yes	a
Calcitonin (Miacalcin)	Yes	a	a
Raloxifene (Evista)	Yes	a	a
Ibandronate (Boniva)	Yes	a	a

Source: Watts, N. et al. 2010. *Endocr Pract* 16(3): 1–37. http://aace.com/files/osteo-guide-lines-2010.pdf, with permission from the American Association of Clinical Endocrinologists.

a Insufficient evidence.

available osteoporosis therapies, or in whom osteoporosis therapies have failed (60). It is also used to increase bone mass in men receiving androgen deprivation therapy for prostate cancer who are at risk of fracture, and in women with breast cancer treated with aromatase inhibitors and at risk for fractures (32).

Table 18.4 describes known effect of different drugs in preventing fractures in specific anatomical sites.

18.9 ROLE OF EXERCISE IN OSTEOPOROSIS

Exercise is particularly important in the prevention and management of osteoporosis, and results in specific adaptations to muscle and bone physiology. Because overall physical activity and exercise typically decrease with aging, the exercise prescription is of special significance in the osteoporotic individual. Many effects of debility result from a lack of exercise, and goal-directed exercise can be used to improve bone and muscle health, balance, coordination, task-specific function, and mood (61).

18.9.1 Exercise Effects on the Biology of Bone and Muscle

The biological mechanisms behind bone and muscle health are very complex. Bone strength depends on a number of interrelated factors, including the amount of bone tissue (size and mass), the structure of bone (spatial distribution, shape, and microarchitecture) and the intrinsic properties of the bone material (porosity, matrix mineralization, collagen traits, and microdamage) (62).

Bone remodeling consists of a balance of building new bone and resorption of old bone. The cycle of bone homeostasis causes an overall increase or decrease in bone mass. Bone strain is a measure of bone deformation and is a key determinant in the adaptive response of bone to loading. Strain magnitude and the rate of change in bone strain are positively related to increases in bone mass. Bone strains that exceed the minimum effective strain for modeling will result in a net increase in bone mass, whereas strains falling below the minimum effective strain for remodeling will result in a decrease in bone mass. Bone strains falling between these threshold values generally will result in no net change in bone mass (63).

Exercise is recognized as a contributor to overall bone strength. Evidence-based analyses of trials in children and adolescents indicate that physical fitness programs that feature regular weight-bearing exercise can result in 1%–8% improvements in bone strength at the loaded skeletal sites (64). The benefits of exercise can also be appreciated later in life. In premenopausal women with high exercise compliance, improvements ranging from 0.5% to 2.5% have been reported (64). There continues to be a need for further well-designed, long-term randomized controlled trials with adequate sample sizes to quantify the effects of exercise on whole bone strength and its structural determinants throughout life (64).

Sarcopenia is defined as the age-related loss of muscle mass associated with the normal aging process. Loss of muscle mass decreases strength, can adversely affect balance and coordination, and decreases overall participation in functional activities of daily living. It also impacts function and disability by increasing risk of falls and fall-related consequences like traumatic fractures. Decline in muscle mass is more common in inactive individuals, but can also be seen in those who participate in exercise. Some common causes of sarcopenia are lack of exercise, suboptimal hormonal levels (e.g., estrogen, testosterone, growth hormone, and insulin-like growth factor-1), and insufficient dietary or nutritional protein. Tarantino et al. (65) suggest that the prevalence of sarcopenia increased dramatically with age from 4% of men and 3% of women aged 70–75 years to 16% of men and 13% of women aged 85 years or older.

Although different biological structures, osteoporosis and sarcopenia are interrelated: muscle produces mechanical stress causing a load on bone. Decreased stress on bone makes bones more vulnerable to loss of bone mass. Microarchitectural deficits in the trabecular bone can eventually lead to osteoporosis.

18.9.2 BONE HEALTH AND EXERCISE THROUGHOUT THE LIFESPAN

Bone loss with age is an expected natural process. Bone mass peaks at ages 25–30 years and declines gradually thereafter in both men and women. The amount of bone in older people is determined by the PBM, together with the rate of bone loss with age. PBM is determined by many factors, including diet (particularly calcium nutrition), exercise, gender, and genetic makeup (66). Regardless of age, adequate calcium intake, and exercise can limit bone loss and increase bone and muscle strength.

Early childhood—The body builds the most bone during these years. Children need food rich in calcium and vitamin D. A healthy diet and exercise helps bones grow. The U.S. Department of Health and Human Services recommends that children and adolescents participate in at least 1 hour of physical activity per day (7 hours/week), including daily moderate- or vigorous-intensity aerobic physical activity. Bone- and muscle-strengthening activity should be performed at least 3 days per week (67). Although weight-bearing exercise appears to enhance bone mineral accrual in children, this has yet to be defined (68).

Puberty—Puberty is a crucial time in the development of the bony skeleton and PBM. Half of total body calcium stores in women and up to two-thirds of calcium stores in men are made during puberty (69). Weight-bearing exercise during the teen years is critical to achieving maximum bone strength. Young women who exercise excessively can lose enough weight to cause hormonal changes that stop menstrual periods, leading to amenorrhea. This loss of estrogen can cause bone loss at a time when young women should be enhancing their PBM. In developed countries, at least 90% of PBM is accrued by 19–20 years of age. The relative risk of fracture increases as much as 2.6-fold for each 1 SD decrease in bone mass. An increase of 10% in PBM in the population is estimated to decrease risk of fracture in the elderly by 50% (70).

Early adulthood (ages 20–30 years)—Bones reach PBM and are strongest in early adulthood. Although the skeletal system no longer forms new bone as easily as before, bones will reach their peak strength during these crucial years. During this phase, it is important to continue good nutrition and exercise habits. Adequate calcium intake and exercise support achieving peak bone

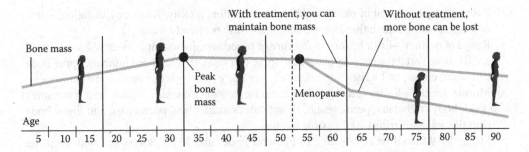

FIGURE 18.1 Bone mass through the lifespan: Exercise helps prevent osteoporosis. (Reproduced with permission from Krames Staywell. http://www.nlm.nih.gov/medlineplus/magazine/issues/winter11/images/timeline.jpg.)

density. It is recommended that adults perform at least 30 minutes of weight-bearing activity, 4 or more days per week. In addition, muscle-strengthening activities are recommended at least 2 days weekly (69).

Early to middle adulthood (age 30 years to menopause)—During early to middle adulthood, bone mass declines slightly as the body makes enough new bone to maintain bone mass. After the skeletal system reaches PBM, there is a trend to gradually lose bone. Prior to age 40, bony remodeling occurs, and the bone removed is almost completely replaced. Gradually, less bone is replaced after age 40, resulting in a net loss of bone mass. Continuing a healthy diet and maintaining an exercise program are fundamental to limiting bone loss. In addition, exercise is essential to preserve muscle mass, which strengthens surrounding bone and helps prevent falls (69).

After menopause—Menstruation stops during menopause. The body makes less estrogen, which starts the phase of primary bone loss. As levels of estrogen fall considerably, women experience a sharp decline in bone mass. In the 10 years after menopause, women can lose 40% of the inner trabecular bone and 10% of the outer cortical bone (69). This loss in bone mass reduces bone strength and increases fracture risk. This hormonal loss for women in middle age also helps to explain why osteoporosis is much more common in women than in men.

Older adults—Later in life, the rate of bone loss increases. After the age of 70 years, men are more likely to experience low bone mass and fractures. During this stage, attention must be placed on fall risk and prevention. Falls are the leading cause of injury in older adults in the United States (69). The weakened and fragile bones of osteoporosis can easily break after a fall. Subsequent consequences often lead to the many reasons why seniors may be hospitalized and become disabled. This cascade often results in loss of independence, and can necessitate a change in living arrangements, such as placement in a nursing home or assisted living facility.

Figure 18.1 illustrates changes in bone mass with age.

18.9.3 Exercise Prescription for Osteoporosis

An organized approach is central to the management of osteoporosis. The overall goals are (1) diagnosis and treatment (pharmacological and nonpharmacological), (2) optimizing function, (3) risk factor assessment and modification, (4) other assessments (quality of life and societal implications), and (5) secondary prevention.

18.10 COMPONENTS OF HISTORY AND PHYSICAL EXAMINATION

The importance of a thorough history and physical examination cannot be underestimated. The following is a systematic way to approach gathering information necessary to create a safe and effective exercise program for the osteoporotic individual:

- Pain—The assessment of pain should include location, quality, frequency, duration, intensity, aggravating/alleviating factors, and interventions already tried.
- Range of motion—Prior history of fracture or procedure, for example, open reduction internal fixation, vertebroplasty, kyphoplasty, spine (cervical, thoracic, and lumbar), upper body (shoulder, elbow, and wrists/fingers), and lower body (hips/pelvis, knees, and ankles/toes).
- Muscle length—Spine (cervical flexors and extensors, lumbar flexors, and extensors), upper body (trapezius, periscapular, rhomboids, serratus, and pectoralis), and lower body (hip flexors, hamstrings, and gastrocnemius).
- Strength—Manual muscle testing of bilateral upper and lower extremities with focus on muscles that provide core strength (abdominals, gluteus medius, and gluteus maximus). Caution must be used with resistance for individuals with severe osteoporosis and in the postoperative patient for risk of fracture.
- Posture—Note resting posture, ability to correct/maintain malposition, prior recognized loss of height, spine (kyphosis and scoliosis), upper body (scapular position), and lower body (pelvic tilt).
- Balance—Choose an appropriate assessment tool based on the patient's functional level and ability (e.g., weight shifting, single-leg stance, tandem stance, and Romberg).
- Function—Bed mobility, transfers, household ambulation, community ambulation, uneven surfaces, and stairs.
- Gait—Abnormalities/patterns, footwear, need for assistive device, and appropriate for current assistive device.
- Knowledge of condition/symptoms—Body mechanics, joint protection, home exercise program and exercise advancement, appropriate footwear, positioning, posture awareness, symptom management, and environmental modifications (lighting, rugs, stairs, and ramps).

The above outline is modified from Brigham and Women's Hospital, Inc. Department of Rehabilitation Services. Standard of Care: Osteoporosis (71).

18.10.1 Types of Exercise for Prescription

Physical activity is defined as any movement beyond resting levels. This includes activities of daily living. In comparison, exercise is defined as structured activity with a particular goal (e.g., physical, psychological, and social benefits) (72). The field of physical therapy is a subdivision of the field of rehabilitation medicine that utilizes targeted goal-directed interventions and specifically designed exercises and equipment to improve an individual's physical abilities.

There are different categories of exercises that can be used to achieve a certain goal. Most exercise prescriptions for osteoporosis will include a combination of aerobic, strength/resistance training, and functional activities designed to improve posture and balance.

Open kinetic chain exercises are exercises where the hand or foot is not fixed to a surface but is allowed to move throughout the exercise. These exercises can include single-joint exercises, which create isolation movements, and in comparison more shearing forces. Some examples include upper body—biceps curls (primarily targeting biceps), and lower body—leg extension (primarily targeting quadriceps).

An alternative to open kinetic chain is closed kinetic chain exercises. Closed kinetic chain exercise are exercises where the hand (or more proximally arm) or foot (or more proximally leg) are fixed and do not move because it remains in contact to a surface (e.g., ground, footplate, and machine handle). These exercises usually incorporate multijoint and compound movements. Some examples include upper body—pushups (cocontraction of pectorals, latissimus, deltoids, biceps, triceps, core abdominals, low back, and forearm/hand muscles) and lower body—lunge (cocontraction of gluteal muscles, hip flexors, quadriceps, hamstrings, and ankle/foot muscles). Some benefits of closed kinetic chain exercise are that they create compressive forces, which more closely mimic activities of daily living.

A weight-bearing activity is when the body is required to move against gravity while staying upright. High-impact weight-bearing activities involve sharp, ballistic movements that cause increased loads along the length of the bones. In contrast, low-impact weight-bearing activities have one foot remaining on the ground during the activity. This creates less loading along the length of the bone. Nonimpact exercises do not create specific forces along bones, and are best to improve posture, balance, and task-specific functional activities.

Strength resistance training are exercises that cause the muscle to contract against an external resistance. The end result may be an increase in strength, tone, muscle mass, and/or endurance. Resistance exercises can include resistance machines with preprogrammed weight, free weights, elastic bands, or use of one's own body weight.

18.10.2 Important Considerations for Exercise with Osteoporosis

While exercise is extremely important, the goal is to increase function by careful implementation of a deliberate plan of treatment. Incorrect posture, sequence, or technique may result in injury and loss of overall function. The following recommendations can be followed from early adulthood to senior living. Most individuals benefit from a formal initial evaluation by a healthcare professional who will give specific recommendations while taking into consideration other comorbid conditions (e.g., coronary artery disease, diabetes mellitus, osteoarthritis, history of falls, and previous fractures).

- Exercise should be regular to get the best benefit.
- Wear sensible and comfortable clothing and footwear.
- Include a preexercise warm up and postexercise cool down period.
- Begin with a low-intensity exercise program and gradually increase. Maintain activity intensity that does not cause or exacerbate pain.
- Always implement your exercise routine with good posture: chin parallel to the floor, back of the neck is long, shoulders rounded back to open the chest, ribs lifted up from the hips, abdominals tight, neutral pelvic tilt, knees soft, and weight distributed evenly. Proper position and form should be maintained throughout the exercise. This will reduce the risk of joint, tendon, ligament, and muscle injury as well as overuse injury. Choose exercises that will decrease your risk of falls.
- Keep the environment free of obstacles that will increase risk of falls. Ensure a comfortable temperature. Take into consideration outdoor weather conditions, for example, uneven surfaces, rain, ice, and snow.
- To reduce the risk of exercise-related fracture in individuals diagnosed with osteoporosis, avoid activities that (1) cause twisting, bending, or compression movements (e.g., golf, rowing, tennis, sit-ups, toe touches, and some yoga poses), (2) use high-impact, rapid, and jerky movements, or (3) cause forced spinal flexion motions (e.g., sit-ups, forward bend to touch your toes).

The majority of studies of exercise and osteoporosis revealed only minor reported side effects of muscle soreness and generalized pain. Clinical decision algorithms exist for osteoporotic individuals at high fragility fracture risk, those with previous fracture, and those consuming systemic corticosteroids for a total period of 3 months or more during the prior year, at a prednisone-equivalent dose of greater than or equal to 7.5 mg daily (73).

Available examples of specific exercises can be found on the following websites:

National Osteoporosis Foundation—http://nof.org/
National Osteoporosis Society—https://www.nos.org.uk/

Table 18.5 summarizes exercise prescription in different age groups.

TABLE 18.5

Exercise Prescription in Different Age Groups

	Children/Adolescents	Adults—Low Risk for Fracture	Adults—High Risk for Fracture
Goals for bone health	Increase bone mass with movements that include high strain and high forces in directions, which stimulate bone mass, encourage developmentally appropriate and enjoyable activity, which create healthy habits	Preservation of bone health with movements that include high forces in directions the bone is accustomed to, maintain healthy activity habits	Prevent disease progression, reduce pain, maintain healthy activity habits, and reduce risk of falls
Intensity	Moderate to vigorous	Moderate to high	Low to moderate
Duration	60 minutes/day	30 minutes/day	30–60 minutes/day
Frequency	7 days/week	3–5 days/week	3–5 days/week
Type—Aerobic	Aerobic and weight-bearing exercises	Aerobic and weight-bearing 3–5 days/week	Aerobic and weight-bearing 3–5 days/week
Type—Impact	High impact	High to low impact depending on activity level and risk	Low to no impact
Type—Strength/ resistance		Resistance exercise 2–3 days/week at moderate to high intensity • Moderate intensity (60%–80% repetition maximum) for 8–12 repetitions • High intensity (80%–90% repetition maximum) for 5–6 repetitions (91)	Resistance exercise 2–3 days/week at moderate intensity • Moderate intensity (60%–80% repetition maximum) for 8–12 repetitions (91)
Type—posture/balance	Encourage sports with psychomotor challenges, agility, and plyometric exercises	Dynamic exercises that engage core, upper and lower body—coordination, flexibility	As often as needed, at least 1 day/week: focus on task specific functional activities that promote stability
Examples	Unstructured activities: playground games, skipping, jogging, and running Structured activities: soccer, basketball, racquetball, tennis, and age-appropriate resistance training	Walking, jogging, stair climbing, dancing, aerobics, tennis, basketball, and running	Walking, stretching, yoga, tai chi, water aerobics, upright cycling, and line dancing

18.11 SPECIFIC CONSIDERATIONS FOR INDIVIDUALS WITH VERTEBRAL COMPRESSION FRACTURE

Vertebral compression fractures are characterized by loss of height of the vertebral body of the spine and acute pain. The pain of an acute fracture can typically last at least 4–6 weeks with intense pain at the site of fracture. Chronic pain may also occur in patients with multiple compression fractures, vertebral body height loss, and low bone density.

Short-term goals are to reduce pain, and improve overall posture and mobility. Vertebral compression fractures leading to a loss of height and spinal deformation can compromise ventilatory capacity and result in a forward shift in the center of gravity. If fractures are numerous and severe, they can lead to significant height loss and curvature, causing shortness of breath, protruding stomach, digestion problems, and stress incontinence. The resultant postural deformity and restrictions lead to a reduced intra-abdominal space (72). Patients may benefit from trunk and postural mobility exercises to enhance movement, and correct posture, as well as instruction in deep breathing.

Individuals with known osteoporosis should avoid forceful and repetitive trunk twisting and flexion activities (73). Long-term objectives are to improve core and trunk strengthening, improve endurance, and reduce pain. Secondary prevention is also of importance. This phase includes the identification and modification of risk factors to prevent the risk of future falls and morbidity.

18.12 NONINTERVENTIONAL APPROACH TO TREATMENT FOR INDIVIDUALS WITH VERTEBRAL COMPRESSION FRACTURE: SPECIAL THERAPEUTIC TECHNIQUES

18.12.1 AQUATIC EXERCISE

The role of exercise for individuals with osteoporosis is to increase the function of underlying neuromuscular structures and to reduce fracture risk. Aqua therapy in a warm pool can improve flexibility and muscle strength. Although a nonweight-bearing form of exercise, the advantage of aquatic exercise is that land-based compressive overloads on the spine are low in aquatic environments due to the physical properties of the buoyancy of the water (74). In a study of aquatic exercise intervention, the intervention group without fractures showed better results than the control group without fractures in flexibility tests, spine extension strength, hip flexor strength, left and right handgrip strength, and decrease in the number of falls and pain perception ($p < 0.05$) (74). The intervention group without fractures also obtained better results for right handgrip strength and decreased pain perception in comparison to the control group with fractures (74).

18.12.2 KINESIOTAPING

The method of kinesiotaping is a therapeutic technique that uses adhesive tape applied in an anatomic manner to provide benefits such as modification of muscle tone, correct posture, develop proper movement patterns, and improve flow of lymphatic fluids. Greater thoracic kyphosis is associated with increased biomechanical loading of the spine, which is potentially problematic in individuals with osteoporotic vertebral fractures. Greig et al. demonstrated that the application of therapeutic postural tape induces an immediate reduction in thoracic kyphosis in individuals with osteoporotic vertebral fracture. They found however, that the reduction in thoracic kyphosis was not associated with any changes in trunk muscle activity or balance during a quiet standing task (75). Further studies are needed to evaluate the underlying relationship between position and spinal muscle activation in osteoporotic vertebral fractures.

18.12.3 NEUROMUSCULAR ELECTRICAL STIMULATION

Neuromuscular electrical stimulation has been used in spinal cord injury research to increase BMD or prevent bone loss in paralyzed human limbs. The application of functional electrical stimulation cycling exercise (FESCE) involves active loading toward the extremities (76). Intervention with FESCEs in the early stages of spinal cord injury can partly attenuate BMD loss in the distal femur, but not in the femoral neck. Additional studies are needed to evaluate the benefits of functional electrical stimulation exercise protocols to improve BMD in populations at risk for osteoporosis.

18.12.4   Low-Intensity Pulse Ultrasound

Low-intensity pulsed ultrasound (LIPUS) has been used to improve fracture healing, and has been approved for several years by the United States Food and Drug Administration. Some preclinical and clinical evidence indicates that fracture healing can be improved by this technique, which appears to be generally safe. There are several suggested mechanisms of action of LIPUS. Clinical studies generally support its usefulness in accelerating fracture healing (77). Initial research from weekly radiography, histomorphometry, microcomputed tomography, and mechanical testing showed the treatment groups with better healing responses than their control groups. Comparing the normal and the osteoporotic treatment groups, a significantly higher ($p = 0.015$) callus width (week 4), higher ratio of increment in bone volume to tissue volume ratio value (7.4% more), faster response of endochondral ossification, and a higher stiffness measurement were observed in the osteoporotic treatment group (78). There is ongoing research to better determine the optimal protocol for LIPUS use.

18.12.5   Whole Body Vibration

Vibration is an oscillatory motion about an equilibrium point (79). Whole-body vibration exercise is a forced oscillation that transfers energy from a vibration surface to a human body or body part. The energy is transmitted across a vibrating platform on which static poses are held or dynamic exercises can be performed, depending on the type and force of the machine. The vibrations generated by motors underneath the platform are transmitted to the person on the machine (80). It is hypothesized that whole-body vibration therapy may offer advantages to individuals who cannot continue or do not want to continue or initiate pharmacological treatment to increase bone density or who cannot tolerate higher levels of exercise. Whole-body vibration therapy for the prevention and treatment of osteoporosis is still investigational with little known about benefits and harms (81).

18.13   NONINTERVENTIONAL APPROACH TO TREATMENT FOR INDIVIDUALS WITH VERTEBRAL COMPRESSION FRACTURE: SPINAL ORTHOSES

When conservative pain medication, activity modification, and basic therapeutic interventions are not sufficient for pain relief, a spinal orthosis may be used to provide support while boney healing occurs.

The primary goal of bracing osteoporosis-related vertebral fractures is to prevent pain from movement by stabilization of the spine. Spinal orthotic use may reduce back fatigue and provide an opportunity for early mobilization with reduction of the period of bed rest after an acute vertebral compression fractures. Bracing is typically necessary during the initial 6–8 weeks postfracture, until the acute pain resolves (82). Despite being widespread, there remains no consensus regarding type and length of orthotic use (83).

Table 18.6 summarizes spinal orthosis.

18.14   INTERVENTIONAL APPROACH TO TREATMENT FOR INDIVIDUALS WITH VERTEBRAL COMPRESSION FRACTURE: VERTEBROPLASTY AND KYPHOPLASTY

There are times when noninterventional approaches to management of vertebral compression fractures are not sufficient to achieve adequate pain relief and mobility. Vertebral augmentation procedures are increasingly common as more individuals are diagnosed with vertebral compression fracture and efficacy and safety of the techniques improves. Surgery for treating osteoporotic vertebral fractures usually consists of a percutaneous minimally invasive procedure known as vertebroplasty

TABLE 18.6
Spinal Orthoses

Name	Characteristics	Photo

Jewett spinal orthosis	• Three-point pressure system = anterior sternum pad and suprapubic pad, plus posterior dorsolumbar pad, which stabilizes hyperextension
	• *Caution for excess hyperextension forces on low spine may exacerbate lumbar spondylosis or posterior element fractures
	• Limits flexion, less control of side bending or rotation
	• Clinical indications:
	  • Anterior wedge compression fracture
	  • Multilevel compression fracture
		Jewett hyperextension orthosis
		(a) Anterior view. (b) Lateral view.
		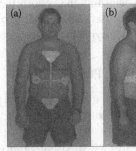
		(Cuccurullo, S. 2015 [92])

CASH (cruciform anterior spinal hyperextension) orthosis	• Anteriorly, a cross-shaped vertical and horizontal metal uprights with sternal, pubic, posterior, and anterolateral pads and a strap around the posterior thoracolumbar region
	• Limits flexion, less control of side bending or rotation
	• Clinical indications:
	  • Anterior wedge compression fracture
	  • Multilevel compression fracture
		CASH (cruciform anterior spinal hyperextension orthosis) TLSO
		(a) Anterior view. (b) Lateral view.
		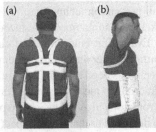
		(Cuccurullo, S. 2015 [92])

Knight–Taylor brace	• Two paraspinal bars that extend superiorly and are attached to an interscapular band, which serves as an attachment site for the axillary straps. The anterior abdominal support is secured to the two lateral uprights with corset lacing • Limits flexion, extension, and lateral bending • Clinical indications: • Stable thoracic or lumbar fracture	Knight–Taylor brace (a) Posterior view. (b) Lateral view. 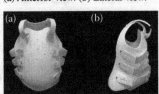 (Cuccurullo, S. 2015 [92])

TLSO (thoraco-lumbo-sacral orthosis)	• Made with molded polyethylene plastic or plaster of Paris, one piece with a single opening or in two pieces with lateral openings (clam shell)
	• Designed to distribute pressure over a wider area
	• Clinical indications:
	  • Burst-type fractures
	  • Multilevel compression fracture
	  • Complex multiplanar fractures
		Clam shell TLSO
		(a) Anterior view. (b) Lateral view.

or kyphoplasty. The purposes of surgical treatment are the rapid relief of pain, the restoration of the vertebral body height and the prevention of the kyphosis deformity (83). To guide placement, both procedures utilize fluoroscopy, which provides real-time radiograph images of the procedure.

With vertebroplasty, a bone needle is passed through either unilateral or bilateral pedicles directly into the vertebral body. A small amount of cement, most commonly, polymethylmethacrylate, is introduced into the area. Once injected, the cement hardens quickly and acts to stabilize the vertebral fragments in their current position (83). The restoration of vertebral body height is more likely to be achieved by vertebroplasty in acute fractures (83). One of the most common complications of vertebroplasty is the leakage of the cement (83).

Although similar, kyphoplasty is different in that a balloon catheter is passed through the cannula. Once in position, the balloon catheter is inflated to increase the collapsed space, create a defined cavity, and restore height to the collapsed vertebra. After removing the balloon, the space created is filled with cement, of which the most commonly used is polymethylmethacrylate (83). Pain relief (as measured by the visual analog scale) and functional outcome improve significantly up to 2 years, even if kyphoplasty is performed 1 month after the diagnoses, when conservative treatment failed (83). Restoration of the vertebral body height is achieved in 47% of cases, higher than in vertebroplasty procedures. At postoperative time, restoration is up to 15.4%, remaining stable up to 3 years follow-up. The control of the vertebral body height reduces the risk of secondary spine deformity in kyphosis (83). Patients operated by kyphoplasty can return to daily activities faster than conservatively treated patients, with a difference of 60 days (83). Cement leakage is less frequent after kyphoplasty procedure (83).

18.15 FALL PREVENTION

In the United States, it is estimated that about one in three adults over age 65 years will experience a fall each year, with those surviving, up to 30% suffering moderate to severe injuries that commonly reduce mobility and independence (84). Multifactorial causes of falls in the elderly include deficits with motor function, vision, proprioception, vestibular, medical comorbidities, polypharmacy, and environmental factors. Approximately 10%–15% of falls result in fractures (Ensrud). Fractures of the hip, wrist, pelvis, proximal humerus, ankle, and elbow are frequently due to falls (24). Reducing the risk of falls includes an assessment of risk factors, safety evaluation, and educating individuals on fall prevention techniques.

Skeletal trauma may be reduced either by preventing falls or by minimizing their consequences (85). Evaluating environmental causes in the home and the community is a way to incorporate meaningful intervention in reducing falls and associated consequences.

There has been ongoing attention given to environmental factors that can help reduce the risk of hip fractures. One of the more common interventions has been the use of hip protectors. External hip protectors, also known as hip protector pads or hip pads, are plastic shields (firm), or foam pads (soft) designed to distribute impact force from the bony greater trochanter over the surrounding soft tissue. The three main designs are (1) underwear with sewn in hip protectors, (2) underwear that hold removable shields, and (3) belts worn on the outside of clothing. Older studies indicate that among ambulatory older adults who are at an increased risk for hip fracture, the risk of fracture can be reduced by 60% by the use of anatomically designed external hip protectors (86). A recent Cochrane Review comparison of older people living in nursing care facilities suggests that providing a hip protector probably decreases the chance of a hip fracture slightly, may increase the small chance of a pelvic fracture slightly, and probably has little or no effect on other fractures or falls. In comparison, for older people living at home in the community, providing a hip protector probably has little or no effect on hip fractures (87). As has been the concern for several years, one of the limitations is the inconsistency in compliance with use.

Another area of research has investigated the potential shock absorber characteristics of different flooring textiles. Wooden carpeted floors were associated with the lowest number of fractures per 100 falls when compared to wooden uncarpeted floors, concrete carpeted floors, and concrete uncarpeted floors. The risk of fracture resulting from a fall was significantly lower compared to all other floor types (odds ratio 1.78, 95% CI 1.33–2.35) (88). Further research is needed to determine how other environmental factors may affect the fracture rate after a fall. Some considerations include patient BMD measurement, fall risk related to carpeted versus uncarpeted flooring, location of fall (e.g., bathroom versus hallway), availability of object to interrupt descent (e.g., grab bar or small space), and the likelihood of assistance to prevent falls (e.g., more likely to have assistance with bathroom tasks).

18.16 PSYCHOSOCIAL AND EMOTIONAL IMPACT OF OSTEOPOROSIS

In the elderly, a hip fracture may make an individual four times more likely to die within 3 months. Often times, the injury can cause an increase in comorbid complications resulting in worsened overall health. One in five people with a hip fracture ends up in a nursing home within a year. Many others become isolated, depressed, or frightened to leave home because they fear they will fall (89). Patients with one vertebral fracture are at increased risk of peripheral fracture and further vertebral fracture.

As vertebral height is lost, patients experience discomfort from the rib cage pressing downward on the pelvis. Patients develop a thoracic kyphosis, a lumbar lordosis, and a protuberant abdomen with prominent horizontal skinfold creases. The reduced thoracic space may result in decreased exercise tolerance and reduced abdominal space may give rise to early satiety and weight loss. Sleep disorders may also occur. Patients lose self-esteem. Self-care may become increasingly difficult. Distorted body image and poor health perception may eventually lead to the inability to care for oneself (90).

In the acute phase, adequate management of pain associated with fracture is paramount to reduce symptoms and mobilize the patient. Long-term goals are to maintain or increase skeletal mass and improve mobility and function (90). If not treated adequately, depression may occur as a result of loss of function and chronic pain. Without proper return of function, anxiety regarding fear of falling may be overwhelming and result in a lack of desire for mobility.

18.17 CONCLUSION

The identification and treatment of osteoporosis requires a comprehensive and holistic approach incorporating multiple interventions, including education, pharmacology, nutritional and environmental awareness, modification of potential factors that enhance risk of fragility fractures, as well as interventional techniques and supportive spinal orthotics. The benefits of exercises in chronic disease prevention, delay of progression, and treatment have gained significant awareness in the medical and lay literature.

There remains, however, an uncertainty as to the minimum amount of exercise and physical activity required to successfully achieve optimal effects. Research is ongoing as to how much, how often, and what intensity and type of exercise should be prescribed for the older adults.

REFERENCES

1. Holroyd, C., E. Dennison and C. Cooper. 2015. Epidemiology and classification of osteoporosis. *Rheumatology*, 6th ed. M.C. Hochberg, A.J. Silman, J.S. Smolen et al. 197: 1633–40. Mosby, an imprint of Elsevier, Ltd., Philadelphia, PA.
2. Bono, C.M. and T.A. Einhorn. 2003. Overview of osteoporosis: Pathophysiology and determinants of bone strength. *Eur Spine J* 12(Suppl 2): S90–6.
3. National Osteoporosis Foundation. Clinician's Guide to Prevention and Treatment of Osteoporosis: 2014 Issue, Version 1. Available at http://nof.org/files/nof/public/content/file/2791/upload/919.pdf. (Accessed February 23, 2015).

4. National Osteoporosis Foundation. 2014. NOF Releases Updated Data Detailing the Prevalence of Osteoporosis and Low Bone Mass in the U.S. Available at http://nof.org/news/2948. (Accessed June 2, 2014).
5. NIH Osteoporosis and Related Bone Diseases National Resource Center. 2014. Handout on Health. Available at http://www.niams.nih.gov/Health_Info/Bone/Osteoporosis/osteoporosis_hoh.asp#2 (Accessed June 10, 2015).
6. Sweet, M., J.M. Sweet, M.P. Jermiah et al. 2009. Diagnosis and treatment of osteoporosis. *Am Fam Phys* 79(3): 193–200.
7. Robbins, J., A.K. Aragaki, C. Kooperberg et al. 2007. Factors associated with 5-year risk of hip fracture in postmenopausal women. *JAMA* 298(20): 2389–98.
8. Cawthon, P.M. 2011. Gender differences in osteoporosis and fractures. *Clin Orthop Relat Res* 469(7): 1900–5.
9. Greenspan, S.L. 2016. Osteoporosis. *Andreoli and Carpenter's Cecil Essentials of Medicine*, 9th ed. I.J. Benjamin, R.C. Griggs, E.J. Wing et al. 75: 757–63. Elsevier Saunders Inc., Philadelphia, PA.
10. Watts, N., J. Bilezikian, P. Camacho et al. 2010. American Association of Clinical Endocrinologists medical guidelines for clinical practice for the diagnosis and treatment of postmenopausal osteoporosis. *Endocr Pract* 16(3): 1–37. http://aace.com/files/osteo-guidelines-2010.pdf.
11. Blakeney, W.G. 2010. Stabilization and treatment of Colles' fractures in elderly patients. *Clin Interv Aging* 5: 337–44.
12. Elia, G.D., G. Roselli, L. Cavalli et al. 2010. Severe osteoporosis: diagnosis of non-hip non-vertebral (NHNV) fractures. *Clin Cases Miner Bone Metab* 7(2): 85–90.
13. Clohisy, J., P. Beaule, C. dellavalle et al. 2014. *The Adult Hip: Hip Preservation Surgery*. 2nd edition. Lippincott Williams & Williams, Philadelphia, PA, 521.
14. Brandi, M.L. 2009. Microarchitecture, the key to bone quality. *Brain* 48(4): 3–8.
15. Umland, E.M. 2008. An update on osteoporosis epidemiology and bone physiology. *Univ Tenn Adv Stud Pharm* 5(7): 210–4.
16. Streeten, E.A., S. Jaimungal, and M.C. Hochberg. 2015. Pathophysiology of osteoporosis. *Rheumatology*, 6th ed. M.C. Hochberg, A.J. Silman, J.S. Smolen et al. 199: 1650–5. Mosby, an imprint of Elsevier, Ltd., Philadelphia, PA.
17. Willson, T., S.D. Nelson, J. Newbold et al. 2015. The clinical epidemiology of male osteoporosis: A review of the recent literature. *J Clin Epidemiol* 7: 65–76.
18. Tarantino, U., J. Baldi, M. Celi et al. 2013. Osteoporosis and sarcopenia: the connections. *Aging Clin Exp Res* 25(1): S93–5.
19. Feng, X. and J.M. Mcdonald. 2011. Disorders of bone remodeling. *Annu Rev Pathol* 6: 121–45.
20. Seeman, E. and P.D. Delmas. 2006. Bone quality—The material and structural basis of bone strength and fragility. *N Engl J Med* 354(21): 2250–61.
21. Raisz, L.G. 2005. Pathogenesis of osteoporosis: Concepts, conflicts, and prospects. *J Clin Invest* 115(12): 3318–25.
22. Bukata, S.V., B.F. Digiovanni, S.M. Friedman et al. 2011. A guide to improving the care of patients with fragility fractures. *Geriatric Orthop Surg Rehabil* 2(1): 5–37.
23. Burge, R., B. Dawson-Highes, D.H. Solomon et al. 2007. Incidence and economic burden of osteoporosis-related fractures in the United States, 2005–2025. *J Bone Miner Res* 22(3): 465–75.
24. Ensrud, K. 2013. Epidemiology of fracture risk with advancing age. *J Gerontol A: Biol Sci Med Sci* 68(10): 1236–42. First published online July 5, 2013.
25. Allison, S., J. Folland, W.J. Rennie et al. 2013. High impact exercise increased femoral neck bone mineral density in older men: A randomized unilateral intervention. *Bone* 53(2): 321–8.
26. Pope, T.L. 2015. Osteogenesis imperfecta. In: *Musculoskeletal Imaging: Osteogenesis Imperfecta*, 2nd ed. J. Teh and R. Smith, 83: 894–4. E14. Saunders: an imprint of Elsevier Inc., Philadelphia, PA.
27. Lorenc, R.S. 2007. Idiopathic juvenile osteoporosis-a model of skeletal disorder leading to fragility fractures in otherwise healthy children. *Bone* 40(6): 15–7.
28. Hoffer, B., S.J. Cuccurullo, K.J. Urs et al. 2015. Osteoporosis. *Physical Medicine and Rehabilitation Board Review*, 3rd ed. S.J. Cuccurullo, pp. 902–13. Demos Medical Publishing LLC, New York.
29. Waugh, E.J., M.A. Lam, G.A. Hawker et al. 2009. Risk factors for low bone mass in healthy 40–60 year old women: A systematic review of the literature. *Osteop Inten* 20(1): 1–21.
30. Melton, L.J. 3rd 2003. Epidemiology worldwide. *Endocrinol Metab Clin North Am* 32(1): 1–13.
31. Ojo, F., S.A. Snih, L.A. Ray et al. 2007. History of fractures as predictor of subsequent hip and nonhip fractures among older Mexican American. *J Natl Med Assoc* 99(4): 412–8.

32. Cosman, F., S.J. De Beur, M.S. Leboff et al. 2014. Clinician's guide to prevention and treatment of osteoporosis: Position paper, osteoporosis international with other metabolic bone diseases. J.A. Kanis and R. Lindsay, *Osteoporosis Int* 25(10): 2359–81. Springer.

33. Kanis, J.A., H. Johansson, O. Johnell et al. 2005. Alcohol intake as a risk factor for fracture. *Osteoporosis Int* J.A. Kanis and R. Lindsay, 16(7): 737–42. Springer.

34. Deal, C.L. and A.G. Abelson. 2015. Management of osteoporosis. *Rheumatology*, 6th ed. M.C. Hochberg, A.J. Silman, J.S. Smolen et al. 201: 1663–73. Mosby, an imprint of Elsevier, Ltd., Philadelphia, PA.

35. Feskanich, D., W.C. Willett, M. J. Stampfer et al. 1996. Protein consumption and bone fractures in women. *Am J Epidemiol* 143(5): 472–9.

36. Ilich, J.Z. 2000. Nutrition in bone health revisited: A story beyond calcium. *J Am Coll Nutr* 19(6): 715–37.

37. Tucker, K.L., K. Morita, N. Qiao et al. 2006. Colas, but not other carbonated beverages, are associated with low bone mineral density in older women: The Framingham Osteoporosis Study. *Am J Clin Nutr* 84(4): 936–42.

38. Ferri, F.F. 2016. Osteoporosis. *Ferri's Clinical Advisor*. F. F. Ferri 907–9. Elsevier, Inc.

39. Chowdhury, B. and B. Kundu. 2014. Body mass index as predictor of bone mineral density in postmenopausal women in India. *Int J Public Health Sci* 3(4): 276–80.

40. Shapses, S.A. and C.S. Riedt. 2006. Bone, body weight, and weight reduction: What are the concerns? *J Nutr* 136(6): 1453–6.

41. Mcgraw, R.L. and J.E. Riggs. 1994. Osteoporosis, sedentary lifestyle, and increasing hip fractures: Pathogenic relationship or differential survival bias. *Calcif Tissue Int* 55(2): 87–9.

42. Resnick, D. and Kransdorf, M. 2005. Osteoporosis. *Bone and Joint Imaging*, 3rd ed. Renick, D. and Kransdorf, M. eds. Elsevier Saunders, Philadelphia, PA: 551.

43. Tannenbaum, C., J. Clark, K. Schwartzman et al. 2002. Yield of laboratory testing to identify secondary contributors to osteoporosis in otherwise healthy women. *J Clin Endocrinol Metab* 87(10): 4431–7.

44. WHO Scientific Group. 2003. Prevention and Management of Osteoporosis. Http://whqlibdoc.who.int/trs/who_trs_921.pdf.

45. Kanis, J.A. 1994. Assessment of fracture risk and its application to screening for postmenopausal osteoporosis: Synopsis of a WHO report. WHO Study Group. *Osteoporos Int* 4(6): 368–81.

46. Schousboe, J.T., J.A. Shepherd, J.P. Bilezikian et al. 2013. Executive summary of the 2013 international society for clinical densitometry position development conference on bone densitometry. *J Clin Densitom* 16(4): 455–66.

47. Nayak, S., M.S. Roberts, S.L. Greenspan. 2011. Cost-effectiveness of different screening strategies for osteoporosis in postmenopausal women. *Ann Intern Med* 155(11): 751–61.

48. Lewiecki, E.M., J.E. Compston, P.D. Miller et al. 2011. FRAX clinical task force of the 2010 joint international society for clinical densitometry and international osteoporosis foundation position development conference. *J Clin Densitom* 14(3): 223–5.

49. Bansal, S., J.L. Pecina, S.P. Merry et al. 2015. US Preventative Services Task Force FRAX threshold has a low sensitivity to detect osteoporosis in woman ages 50–64 years. *Osteoporos Int* 26(4): 1429–33.

50. Qaseem, A., V. Snow, P. Shekelle et al. 2008. Pharmocologic treatment of low bone density or osteoporosis to prevent fractures: A clinical practice guideline from the American College of Physicians. *Ann Intern Med* 149(6): 404–15.

51. Sandhu, S.K. and G. Hampson. 2011. The pathogenesis, diagnosis, investigation, and management of osteoporosis. *J Clin Pathol* 64(12): 1042–50.

52. Institute of Medicine of the National Academies. Report Brief. Dietary Reference Intakes for Calcium and Vitamin D. Revised March 2011.

53. Eriksen, E.F., A. Díez-Pérez, and S. Boonen. 2014. Update on long-term treatment with bisphosphonates for postmenopausal osteoporosis: a systematic review. *Bone* 58: 126–35. Doi:10.1016/j.bone.2013.09.023.

54. Monthly Prescribing Reference. 2015. Haymarket Media, Inc. Available at http://www.empr.com/clinical-charts/osteoporosis-treatments/article/123840.

55. Komm, B.S. and A.A. Chines. 2012. Bazedoxifene: The evolving role of third-generation selective estrogen-receptor modulators in the management of Postmenopausal osteoporosis. *Ther Adv Musculoskelet Dis* 4(1): 21–34.

56. Rossouw, J.E., G.L. Anderson, R.L. Prentice et al. 2002. Risks and benefits of estrogen plus progestin in healthy postmenopausal women: Principal results From the Women's Health Initiative randomized control trial. *JAMA* 288(3): 321–33.

57. Peichl, P., L.A. Holzer, R. Maier et al. 2011. Parathyroid hormone 1-84 accelerates fracture-healing in pubic bones of elderly osteoporotic women. *J Bone Joint Surg Am* 93(17): 1583–7.

58. Postmark Drug Safety Information for Patients and Providers-Questions and Answers: Changes to the Indicated Population for Miacalcin (calcitonin-salmon). U.S. Food and Drug Administration. Available at http://www.fda.gov/Drugs/drugsafety/postmarketdrugsafetyinformationforpatientsand-providers/ucm388641.htm.

59. Anastasilakis, A.D., K.A. Toulis, S.A. Polyzos et al. 2012. Long-term treatment of osteoporosis: Safety and efficacy appraisal of denosumab. *Ther Clin Risk Manag* 8: 295–306.

60. Mcclung, M.R., E.M. Lewiecki, S.B. Cohen et al. 2006. Denosumab in postmenopausal women with low bone mineral density. *N Engl J Med* 354(8): 821–31.

61. Vina, J., F. Sanchis-Gomar, V. Martinez-Bello et al. 2012. Exercise acts as a drug; the pharmacological benefits of exercise. *Br J Pharmacol* 167(1): 1–12.

62. Griffith, J.F. and H.K. Genant. 2008. Bone mass and architecture determination: State of the art. *Best Pract Res Clin Endocrinol Metab* 22(5): 737–64.

63. Kasturi, G. and R. Adler. 2011. Osteoporosis: Nonpharmacologic management. *PM&R* 3(6): 562–72.

64. Nikander, R., H. Sievänen, A. Heinonen et al. 2010. Targeted exercise against osteoporosis: A systematic review and meta-analysis for optimising bone strength throughout life. *BMC Med* 8: 47.

65. Tarantino, U., J. Baldi, M. Celi et al. 2013. Osteoporosis and sarcopenia: The connections. *Aging Clin Exp Res* 25(1): 93–5.

66. O'Flaherty, E. 2000. Modeling normal aging bone loss, with consideration of bone loss in osteoporosis. *Toxicol Sci* 55(1): 171–88.

67. Lavizzo-Mourey, R. 2012. Physical Activity Guidelines for Americans Midcourse Report Subcommittee of the President's Council on Fitness, Sports and Nutrition. *Physical Activity Guidelines for Americans Midcourse Report: Strategies to Increase Physical Activity among Youth.* Washington, DC: U.S. Department of Health and Human Services.

68. Hind, K. and M. Burrows. 2007. Weight-bearing exercise and bone mineral accrual in children and adolescents: A review of controlled trials. *Bone* 40(1): 14–27.

69. Campbell, B. 2012. Healthy Bones at Every Age. American Academy of Orthopedic Surgeons. Available at http://orthoinfo.aaos.org/pdfs/A00127.pdf (Accessed August 10, 2015).

70. Lappe, J., P. Watson, V. Gilsanz et al. 2015. The longitudinal effects of physical activity and dietary calcium on bone mass accrual across stages of pubertal development. *J Bone Miner Res* 30: 156–64.

71. Bodily, D. 2007. Brigham and Women's Hospital, Inc. Department of Rehabilitation Services. Standard of Care: Osteoporosis. Available at http://www.brighamandwomens.org/Patients_Visitors/pcs/rehabilita-tionservices/Physical%20Therapy%20Standards%20of%20Care%20and%20Protocols/General%20-%20Osteoporosis.pdf (Accessed August 10, 2015).

72. National Osteoporosis Society. 2014. Exercise and osteoporosis. How exercise can help with bone health, fragile bones and fractures. Available at http://www.nos.org.uk/~/document.doc?Id=770 (Accessed July 11, 2015).

73. Chilibeck, P.D., H. Vatanparast, S.M. Cornish et al. 2011. Evidence-based risk assessment and recommendations for physical activity: Arthritis, osteoporosis and low back pain. *Appl Physiol Nutr Metab* 36(S1): S49–S79.

74. Fronza, F., L. Moreira-Pfrimer, R. Nolasco dos Santos et al. 2013. Effects of high-intensity aquatic exercises on bone mineral density in postmenopausal women with and without vertebral fractures. *Am J Sports Sci* 1(1): 1–6.

75. Greig, A.M., K.L. Bennell, A.M. Briggs et al. 2008. Postural taping decreases thoracic kyphosis but does not influence trunk muscle electromyographic activity or balance in women with osteoporosis. *Man Ther* 13(3): 249–57.

76. Lai, C.H., W. Chang, W. Chan et al. 2010. Effects of functional electrical stimulation cycling exercise on bone mineral density loss in the early stages of spinal cord injury. *J Rehabil Med Suppl* 42(2): 150–4.

77. Kasturi, G. and R. Adler. 2011. Mechanical means to improve bone strength: Ultrasound and vibration. *Curr Rheumatol Rep* 13(3): 251–6.

78. Cheung, W., W.C. Chin, L. Quin et al. 2012. Low intensity pulsed ultrasound enhances fracture healing in both ovariectomy-induced osteoporotic and age-matched normal bones. *J Orthop Res* 30(1): 129–36.

79. Rauch, F., H. Sievänen, S. Boonen et al. 2010. Reporting whole-body vibration intervention studies: Recommendations of the International Society of Musculoskeletal and Neuronal Interactions. *J Musculoskelet Neuronal Interact* 10(3): 193–8.

80. Rittweger, J. 2010. Vibration as an exercise modality: How it may work, and what its potential might be. *Eur J Appl Physiol* 108(5): 877–904.

81. Wysocki, A., M. Butler, T. Shamliyan et al. 2011. *Whole-Body Vibration Therapy for Osteoporosis.* Technical Brief No. 10. (Prepared by the University of Minnesota Evidence-based Practice Center under Contract No. HHSA 290 2007 10064 1.) AHRQ Publication No. 11(12)-EHC083-EF. Rockville, MD: Agency for Healthcare Research and Quality. Available at http://www.effectivehealthcare.gov/reports/final.cfm.

82. Longo, U., M. Loppini, L. Denaro et al. 2012. Osteoporotic vertebral fractures: Current concepts of conservative care. *Br Med Bull* 102(1): 171–89.

83. Moroni, A. 2014. An overview on the approaches to osteoporotic vertebral fractures management. *J Osteoporos Phys Act* 2: 114.

84. Marks, R. 2014. Falls among the elderly: Multi-factorial community-based falls-prevention programs. *J Aging Sci* 2: e109.

85. WHO Scientific Group on the Prevention and Management of Osteoporosis (2000: Geneva, Switzerland) 2003. Prevention and Management of Osteoporosis: Report of a WHO Scientific Group (PDF). 2007-05-31.

86. Kannus, P., J. Parkkari, S. Niemi et al. 2000. Prevention of hip fracture in elderly people with use of a hip protector. *N Engl J Med* 343(21): 1506–13.

87. Santesso, N., A. Carrasco-Labra, R. Brignardello-Peterson et al. 2014. Hip protectors for preventing hip fractures in older people. *Cochrane Database Syst Rev* (3). Art. No.: CD001255.

88. Simpson, A., S. Lamb, P.J. Roberts et al. 2004. Does the type of flooring affect the risk of hip fracture? *Age Ageing* 33(3): 242–6.

89. United States Department of Health and Human Services. 2012. *The Surgeon General's Report on Bone Health and Osteoporosis: What It Means to You.* U.S. Department of Health and Human Services, Office of the Surgeon General, Bethesda, MD.

90. Silverman, S. 1992. The clinical consequences of vertebral compression fracture. *Bone* 13(2): S27–31.

91. Thompson, W.R., N.F. Gordon, and L.S. Pescatello. eds. 2010. Exercise prescription for other clinical populations: Guidelines for exercise testing and prescription. In *American College of Sports Medicine*, 8th ed. Lippincott Williams and Wilkins, Philadelphia, PA.

92. Uustal H, Baergo E, Joki J. 2015. Prosthetics and Orthotics. In *Physical Medicine and Rehabilitation Board Review*, 3rd edition. ed. S. Cuccurullo, pp. 546–7. Demos Medical Publishing LLC, New York.

19 Diabetes in Older Adults and Its Management

Susanne U. Miedlich and Steven D. Wittlin

CONTENTS

19.1 INTRODUCTION

Diabetes prevalence increases with age (1). In patients over age 65 years, the prevalence in the United States has been reported to exceed 25% (1). Nevertheless, because most clinical trials exclude patients over the age of 70 years, many recommendations for management of diabetes are based on expert opinion or are based on subgroup analysis of larger studies (2). This is especially true for type 1 diabetes, for which controlled clinical trials are virtually nonexistent in the "older" population. Moreover, as also pertains to all topics discussed in this volume, "older" or "elderly" refers to a very heterogeneous group of people (2). Some studies in "older adults" include individuals over the age of 55 years. Thus, treatment plans for older people with diabetes need to be individualized, for they may relate to triathletes or the chronically disabled. This last, important point must be kept in mind when devising treatment regimens as well as therapeutic targets.

19.2 CLASSIFICATION

Older patients with diabetes may have type 1, type 2, or secondary diabetes (3). An extreme example of the latter is postpancreatectomy. A common cause of secondary diabetes is "glucocorticoid-induced."

Type 1A diabetes is an autoimmune disorder associated with pancreatic beta-cell destruction. Insulin production is extremely low. Generally, for research purposes, a stimulated C-peptide <1.0 ng/mL is usually required for inclusion in clinical trials (4). Recent studies suggest that there is often some small, residual insulin production (5). Type 1B diabetes is not often seen in the West and does not seem to be autoimmune (4). The importance of diagnosing type 1 diabetes is that ALL patients with type 1 diabetes, currently, must be treated with insulin replacement. Thus, as will be discussed below, any older patient with type 1 diabetes MUST be given an "insulin regimen." Because type 1 diabetes may develop at any age, the term "juvenile diabetes" is no longer used.

Type 2 diabetes refers to the remainder of patients with diabetes. There is a strong familial predisposition, so that if one of two identical twins develops type 2 diabetes, the second has a >90% chance of developing the disease. These patients develop diabetes because their beta cells cannot produce sufficient insulin to meet their requirements for glycemic/metabolic regulation (3). People with type 2 diabetes are usually resistant to insulin and, as a group, are obese. These people constitute more than 90% of older patients with diabetes in whom diabetes prevalence increases with age. Unless specifically indicated, most of the remainder of this chapter deals with type 2 diabetes. An interesting form of diabetes, which has been described in the past 23 years, is Latent Autoimmune Diabetes in Adults (LADA). These patients were originally described among a population of people with type 2 diabetes. Such patients were leaner, had glutamic acid decarboxylase or islet cell antibodies, higher HbA1C, and >90% required insulin within 6 years versus 16% of type 2 patients who were antibody-negative (6). Disagreement exists as to whether these LADA patients have type 1, type 2, or their own peculiar form of diabetes. Moreover, the natural history of diagnosed type 2 diabetes is progressive beta cell dysfunction, often requiring insulin treatment (6,7).

19.3 PATHOPHYSIOLOGY OF DIABETES IN THE ELDERLY

Insulin secretion, as measured by several parameters, decreases in the "elderly" (8). Insulin sensitivity also diminishes, but this diminution is mainly accounted for by correction for total body fat or visceral fat (8). The total body clearance of insulin diminishes in the "elderly," and hepatic extraction accounts for a greater percentage. Moreover, after correction for activity level, insulin sensitivity is not appreciably different between younger and older people (9). As an illustration, in the Diabetes Prevention Program (DPP), the effect of lifestyle intervention to prevent progression from prediabetes to diabetes was greatest among those over 60 years of age (10). Summary: In older patients with type 2 diabetes, one sees both impaired insulin secretion and impaired insulin sensitivity. However, the effect of age on the latter seems mainly attributable to decreased activity level and seems reversible with lifestyle intervention.

19.4 SPECIFIC DIABETES ISSUES TO BE CONSIDERED IN THE ELDERLY

Diabetes is associated with greater risk of amputation, cardiovascular disease (CVD), visual impairment, chronic kidney disease, and cognitive dysfunction. The comorbidities and chronic complications from diabetes lead to special problems in the older adult, as has been clearly outlined in two recent consensus reports, and the 2016 ADA guidelines (2,11–14). These include cognitive dysfunction, neuropathy, falls and fractures, visual problems, hearing problems, gait disturbances, balance difficulties, issues of polypharmacy, urinary incontinence, and consequences of hypoglycemia. Whether diabetes increases the risk of depression or not is controversial and will not be addressed here (15,16). All of these comorbidities must be taken into account when devising a treatment plan.

19.4.1 Hypertension

Patients with diabetes have an increased prevalence of hypertension (HTN) (11), which must be addressed on an individualized basis. In the past, preference has been given to inhibitors of the renin–angiotensin system because of "renoprotective effects" (17,18). Combined use of angiotensin-converting enzyme inhibitor (ACEI) and angiotensin receptor blockade (ARB) has not been shown to be beneficial and is associated with more adverse events (19). More recently, emphasis has been placed on reaching a target blood pressure. The controversy arises as to the appropriate target. The Action to Control Cardiovascular Risk in Diabetes—Blood Pressure–Lowering Arm (ACCORD-BP (20)) and a recent Swedish meta-analysis (21) suggest that the target should be less than 140 mm Hg systolic, whereas the recently completed Systolic Blood Pressure Intervention Trial (SPRINT) (22) demonstrated that targeting 120/80 was superior to 140/80. Note: The SPRINT trial specifically excluded people with diabetes. Also, in ACCORD-BP, lower blood pressure did reduce the risk of stroke (20). Summary: In keeping with one of the themes of this chapter, treatment goals should be individualized. A blood pressure target of <140 systolic appears to be prudent. Beyond that, in the older patient with diabetes, one must weigh the risks and benefits of more aggressive blood pressure lowering.

19.4.2 Cardiovascular Disease and Dyslipidemia

Although the relative risk of cardiovascular disease (CVD) is attenuated with age, the prevalence of CVD increases with age, and the hazard ratio for CVD in patients over 60 years of age with diabetes is still nearly double the nondiabetic population (23). There are no statin trials exclusively in elderly people with diabetes, none in type 1 diabetes, and precious few with diabetes-only population (24). Nevertheless, subgroup analysis of multiple studies suggests that most older patients with diabetes should receive moderate- to high-dose statin therapy, despite the increased risk of diabetes in statin users: Benefits markedly outweigh the risk (11,25). Aspirin therapy has been recommended for all patients with diabetes over 50 years of age (11). Again, treatment regimens should be individualized. Results from the recently published Bypass Angioplasty Revascularization Investigation (BARI) 2D trial confirm the benefit and feasibility of multiple risk factor control in type 2 diabetes patients (26). Mean age of patients in this study was 62 years (26).

19.4.3 Falls and Fractures

Older patients with diabetes show an increased propensity to fall, reviewed in Reference 27, as well as an increased risk of osteoporosis (28). Certainly, orthostasis from antihypertensive medications, autonomic dysfunction, peripheral neuropathy, other gait disturbances, medication interactions, and visual impairment all contribute to propensity to fall in older patients with diabetes. In addition to usual fall precautions, careful foot examinations, Semmes–Weinstein monofilament testing should be performed, as well as simple and bedside cardiac autonomic function testing—especially for orthostasis (29). Patients should have at least annual dilated eye exams in this age group. As much as 20% of older people with diabetes have visual impairment.

19.4.4 NUTRITION AND EXERCISE

Diet and exercise are the cornerstones of treatment of type 2 diabetes. In the older patient, as in all patients with diabetes, nutritional recommendations need to be individualized. In frail, elderly patients, assuring adequate nutrition is paramount. On the other hand, in a patient in their 60s who is otherwise well, and is overweight, reduced caloric intake by 300–500 kcal would be part of the meal plan. Either group classes or "one-on-one" sessions with a nutritionist/dietician are beneficial in the latter case, while evaluation of adequacy of diet by the nutritionist is advisable in the case of the nonobese individual. As stated in the pathophysiology section, much of the insulin resistance in the older patient is due to lack of exercise. Therefore, a reasonable exercise program, that the patient can adhere to, and is safe, is advisable. This has been shown to have a beneficial effect on body composition. A reasonable prescription is about 30 minutes of exercise 4–6 days a week if attainable (30,31).

19.5 MANAGEMENT OF TYPE 2 DIABETES IN THE ELDERLY

19.5.1 GOALS OF THERAPY

As mentioned previously, elderly patients with type 2 diabetes are at an increased risk for a multitude of pathologies. Increased frailty and musculoskeletal as well as sensory impairment will increase a patient's risk for falls, injuries, and fractures. These are associated with significant morbidity, mortality, and substantial healthcare costs. Thus, in the elderly patient, careful consideration should be given to potential benefits and risks of any specific diabetes therapy with respect to both health outcomes and costs.

One must consider what benefits can be expected from diabetes therapy. Overall, significantly fewer microvascular complications and diabetes-related deaths were demonstrated after about 10 years in newly diagnosed patients with type 2 diabetes when treated to a target fasting glucose level <108 mg/dL (intensive therapy; achieved HbA1C of 7%) as compared to <270 mg/dL (conventional therapy; achieved HbA1C of 7.9%), as shown in the landmark UK Prospective Diabetes Study (UKPDS) trial (32,33). In addition, the intensive metformin arm of this study also had fewer macrovascular complications ($p = 0.02$) (32); a trend toward fewer myocardial infarctions was noted in the intensive sulfonylurea/insulin arm ($p = 0.053$) (33). The latter effect did become significant, but only after another 10 years when glycemic targets were not controlled for anymore (34). Thus, a patient with a life expectancy of less than 10–20 years may not experience these benefits of relatively tight diabetes control. Furthermore, even though the number of photocoagulations and cataract extractions was significantly reduced in the intensive therapy group, overall visual acuity, deterioration of visual acuity, or incidence of blindness were not different in the two treatment groups of the UKPDS study (33). Later studies, namely Action in Diabetes and VAscular Disease: Preterax aNd Diamicron Modified Release Controlled Evaluation (ADVANCE), ACCORD, and Veterans Affairs Diabetes Trial (VADT) (35–37) in patients with a prior history of type 2 diabetes (8–11.5 years), as compared to newly diagnosed patients in the UKPDS trial (32,33), did not find significant differences in either macrovascular and most microvascular complications except for a reduction in diabetic nephropathy (35,37) in patients of intensive versus conventional therapy arms (HbA1C 6.4%–6.9% versus 7.3%–8.4% in intensive and conventional therapy arms, respectively). It should be added though that the mean study duration of ADVANCE and VADT trials was only about 5 years (35,37). In fact, the ACCORD study had to be stopped prematurely due to increased mortality of patients in the intensive therapy arm (36).

Next, what are potential hazards of diabetes therapy? As expected, diabetes medications as well as tighter glycemic targets increase the risk of hypoglycemia (incidence of any hypoglycemia was as high as 30% with intensive insulin therapy as compared to 0.9% in the conventional therapy arm per UKPDS study (33)). Per ADVANCE and VADT studies, the occurrence of hypoglycemia was at least twice as high (>40%) in the intensive as compared to the conventional therapy arms (35,37). Interestingly, with the implementation of tighter glycemic targets following the publication of the UKPDS study, the overall incidence of hypoglycemia rose threefold between 1998 and 2005 (38). Furthermore, insulin was the second most common medication associated with adverse events reported to the Food and Drug Administration (FDA) (38). Insulin was also the second most common medication associated with emergency department visits of patients >65 years, 95.4% due to hypoglycemia; 25.1% of these patients required hospitalization (39). Data from a German registry showed that even in patients exclusively treated with oral diabetes medications, hypoglycemia occurred significantly more often in those aged >70 years compared to their younger peers <60 years (incidence 12.8% and 9%, respectively, $p < 0.01$, (40)). The authors also identified the presence of stroke, congestive heart failure (CHF), depression, and sulfonylurea use as predictors of hypoglycemia (40). In addition, reduced baseline cognitive function, but also longer diabetes duration, presence of albuminuria, and African American ethnicity were identified as risk factors for severe hypoglycemia (41,42). Interestingly, although severe hypoglycemia was noted more often in the intensive as compared to the conventional therapy arm of the ACCORD trial (42), the actual achieved HbA1c was not different in patients with or without severe hypoglycemia suggesting that patients who experienced severe hypoglycemia were also hyperglycemic. Nonetheless, aiming for less stringent glycemic goals in elderly patients, especially in those with impaired cognition may be a more sensible approach to therapy. Of note, baseline cognitive impairment was neither a predictor nor a sequela of severe hypoglycemia in young adult type 1 diabetes patients of the Diabetes Control and Complications Trial (DCCT)/Epidemiology of Diabetes Interventions and Complications (EDIC) trial (43,44). Quite the contrary, higher levels of HbA1c were associated with a decline in psychomotor efficiency and motor speed (44) in young adult type 1 diabetes patients.

A factor that might be contributory to increased risk and morbidity of hypoglycemia in the elderly is decreased hypoglycemia awareness. Autonomic but not neuroglycopenic symptoms are reduced in the elderly (45), but no difference in either autonomic or neuroglycopenic symptoms was noted between nondiabetic and diabetic elderly patients (46). Differences in counter-regulatory hormones have been described in elderly type 2 diabetics compared to normal individuals, but the noted differences in glucagon, epinephrine, and cortisol responses to hypoglycemia were not consistent throughout the studies (reviewed in Reference 46).

To summarize: When considering therapeutic options for the elderly patient with type 2 diabetes, one should first determine life expectancy, comorbidities, and goal of therapy. Symptom control and strict avoidance of hypoglycemia and/or volume depletion (or in other words maintenance of quality of life and avoidance of hospitalization) should be major goals in frail and/or cognitively impaired patients with comorbid conditions such as CVD, heart failure, depression, and a life expectancy of less than 10 years. For this population, an HbA1C of about 8% (approximating an average glucose of 183 mg/dL, which is around the threshold for renal glucose excretion and, thus, should not result in major fluid loss) appears to be a safe target to maintain quality of life and avoid hospitalization. In biologically "younger" patients with a life expectancy of more than 10–20 years and fewer comorbidities, somewhat tighter goals between 7% and 7.5% should be targeted instead. No significant benefit but an increased risk of adverse outcomes may be expected when targeting an HbA1C below 7%. Thus, avoidance of hypoglycemia should always be a major consideration of therapy. Ideally, medications with a low risk of hypoglycemia, as discussed below, should be first-line therapies in older patients due to concerns of relative hypoglycemia unawareness in this population and, potentially, associated adverse health outcomes. Diet and exercise are the cornerstones of treatment of type 2 diabetes.

19.5.2 Noninsulin Medications for Type 2 Diabetes

19.5.2.1 Metformin (Biguanides)

While the first descriptions of hypoglycemic effects of biguanides in animals date back to the 1920s (reviewed in Reference 47), its hypoglycemic effects in humans were only described in the late 1950s and early 1960s (47,48). Phenformin, a biguanide used extensively in Europe in the 1960s, was withdrawn from the market in 1977 due to its increased risk of lactic acidosis (49). Lactic acidosis with metformin is a concern but overall a very rare complication (see below). Biguanides, or metformin in particular, reduce hepatic gluconeogenesis; they also increase peripheral muscle glucose uptake and, thus, mediate impressive reductions in fasting glucose, glycosylated hemoglobin (>2% reductions), and less dramatic yet significant reductions in insulin but not glucagon levels (50). In the large-scale UKPDS study, diabetic patients on metformin had significantly fewer diabetes-related endpoints after 10 years (relative risk reduction 32% (32)). Furthermore, the benefit of intensive diabetes control was significantly greater in the metformin than in the sulfonylurea/insulin arm (32). Surprisingly, microvascular endpoints such as progression of albuminuria or retinopathy were not, or only marginally, different between the metformin and conventional therapy arm of the UKPDS trial (32). Here, the benefit of intensive therapy was much greater in patients treated with sulfonylurea/insulin (33). This difference carried through to the follow-up study published in 2008 (10-year therapy to goal, 10-year follow-up without initial therapy goal, final HbA1C slightly but significantly lower only in previously assigned intensive sulfonylurea/insulin arm (34)). At the end of the latter study, significantly less microvascular complications were again seen in the previously intensive therapy sulfonylurea/insulin arm but not in the metformin arm (34). On the other hand, macrovascular endpoints were now significantly reduced in both previously intensive therapy arms (metformin and sulfonylurea/insulin (34)). Another study that compared glycemic outcomes of type 2 diabetic patients treated with metformin or pioglitazone similarly noted no change in urinary albumin in patients treated with metformin despite a reduction in HbA1C of about 1.5% (51). On the other hand, patients in the pioglitazone group showed both a significant reduction in HbA and a reduction in albuminuria (51).

In regards to adverse effects, gastrointestinal (GI) side effects with metformin are fairly common (4%–8%) but rarely lead to major complications (52). The overall risk of lactic acidosis on therapy with metformin is low. A recent meta-analysis and critical review of metformin studies concludes that (a) metformin therapy by itself may slightly elevate lactate levels though not enough to cause lactic acidosis and (b) the overall risk of lactic acidosis is not significantly increased (reviewed in Reference 53). Also, the overall incidence of lactic acidosis in metformin-treated patients with normal kidney function or mild, moderate, and severe renal impairment was not significantly different and mostly related to other comorbidities (54), leading to an adjustment of treatment recommendations per the United Kingdom's National Institute of Clinical Excellence (NICE) and American Diabetes Association (ADA) such that metformin is not recommended if the glomerular filtration rate (GFR) is <45 mL/min or if the patient is at risk for sudden deterioration of kidney function (55,56).

The risk of hypoglycemia/year, a major adverse event especially in the older population, as alluded to earlier, is low for patients treated with metformin (4.2% in metformin group versus 0.9% in conventional group, 12.1%–17.5% in sulfonylurea group, 34% in insulin group; data from the UKPDS study (32)). Vitamin B12 deficiency may unusually occur with metformin use (57).

Summary: Except for GI side effects, metformin represents an excellent option for diabetes therapy in the elderly population; it appears overall safe, even in the presence of mild-to-moderate renal impairment and leads to a significant cardiovascular risk reduction within 10 years. The risk for hypoglycemia with metformin therapy is very low. However, it should be used with caution in patients at risk for hypoxia or hypoperfusion, especially in the presence of moderate-to-severe renal impairment (potential risk of lactic acidosis).

Dosing: metformin: 500–2500 mg per day (1000 mg/day with lower GFR).

19.5.2.2 Sulfonylureas and Meglitinides

About 60 years ago sulfonylureas were first described for their hypoglycemic actions in diabetic patients (58,59). They act by binding to and inhibiting the sulfonylurea receptor (SUR), a component of the ATP-dependent potassium channel on pancreatic beta cells leading to depolarization, calcium influx, and subsequent insulin secretion (reviewed in Reference 60). Per UKPDS and UKPDS follow-up study, newly diagnosed type 2 diabetes patients treated with either sulfonylurea or insulin to an HbA1C of about 7% (compared to 7.9%) benefited both in terms of microvascular and macrovascular complications, though the latter effect became only apparent during the follow-up study when the glycemic control was not tightly controlled anymore (HbA1C 8.5% in previously conventional versus 7.9% in intensive therapy arm, $p < 0.001$ (33,34)). An area of debate has been whether sulfonylurea drugs negatively interfere with cardiac ischemic preconditioning (short repetitive myocardial ischemias reduce myocardial necrosis following a subsequent lasting coronary artery occlusion; thus, it is thought to be a cardioprotective mechanism, reviewed in Reference 61). Studies show that pretreatment with sulfonylureas, and in particular glibenclamide, prevented above myocardial preconditioning in mice and ischemic ECG and echocardiographic changes in humans (reviewed in Reference 61). A meta-analysis of observational studies points to an increased risk of cardiovascular events in patients treated with sulfonylureas (62). However, randomized controlled trials do not recapitulate this effect. Patients treated with glibenclamide in the UKPDS study did not have more cardiac events than patients in the conventional group (33). In fact, patients in the intensive therapy arm, treated with either sulfonylurea or insulin, had significantly fewer myocardial infarctions than patients in the conventional arm at the end of the UKPDS follow-up study (34). However, a later study of diabetic patients on metformin therapy to which either glimepiride or the DPP4-inhibitor linagliptin was added showed a different trend (63). That is, patients in the metformin plus glimepiride arm did have significantly more cardiovascular events compared to patients in the metformin plus linagliptin arm (63). A difference in BMI could explain the above noted differences: The patients who benefited from sulfonylurea therapy in the UKPDS study (though only after more than 10 years) were nonobese (33), whereas patients in the latter study (63) were mildly obese on average. In line with this hypothesis, a high BMI (≥30) was identified as a risk factor for cardiovascular events in the observational studies pointing to adverse outcomes in patients treated with sulfonylureas (62).

A major disadvantage of sulfonylureas over alternative medications in elderly patients is the relatively high risk of hypoglycemia. In the UKPDS study, the rate of hypoglycemia/year was 12.1%–17.5% in patients treated with sulfonylureas, but only 4.2% in patients treated with metformin (32). The previously mentioned noninferiority study of glimepiride versus linagliptin demonstrated hypoglycemias in 36% of patients treated with glimepiride but in only 7% of patients treated with linagliptin (HbA1C not different in both groups (63)). Last but not least, it should be mentioned here that sulfonylureas are eliminated through the kidneys and thus accumulate in the presence of renal insufficiency. Consequently, the rate of hypoglycemia is expected to be even higher under those circumstances. In a recently published, large database analysis of patients on sulfonylureas in Germany and Austria, the rate of severe hypoglycemia almost doubled when GFR dropped <30 mL/min (64). In this context, both glyburide and glimepiride yield active liver metabolites with long half-lives (9–10 hours), whereas glipizide does not produce an active liver metabolite and has a shorter half-life (per prescribing information). Thus, glipizide should be preferred in patients with mild renal impairment.

Interestingly, derivatives of the nonsulfonylurea moiety of glibenclamide, so-called meglitinides (repaglinide and nateglinide), were found to inhibit the SUR similarly to sulfonylureas and have been used successfully in diabetes patients for over 30 years now with similar effects on glycemic control (HbA1C reductions of about 1%, reviewed in References 65 and 66). Contrary to sulfonylureas, they inhibit SUR only in the presence of glucose and have a short half-life (reviewed in Reference 65). Accordingly, the risk of hypoglycemia is very low and meglitinides have been used safely in patients with mild-to-moderate renal impairment (reviewed in Reference 65).

Summary: Sulfonylureas have been used in patients with type 2 diabetes for over 50 years. They are quite effective and have been associated with significantly reduced microvascular complications, though again with a latency of about 10 years. Whether they affect macrovascular complications, either positively or negatively, remains an area of debate; beneficial effects may be limited to nonobese patients. Sulfonylureas clearly increase the risk for hypoglycemia, especially in the presence of renal impairment. Purely from a safety standpoint, when selecting an oral insulin-secretagogue, meglitinides should be considered in preference to sulfonylureas more often in elderly patients. They are safer to use in patients with mild-to-moderate renal impairment and cause less hypoglycemias. The major advantages of sulfonylureas, and the source of their popularity, are their cost (inexpensive), and their excellent short-term efficacy in reducing blood sugar.

Dosing: glipizide: 2.5–40 mg/day, glyburide: 2.5–20 mg/day, glimepiride: 2–8 mg/day, repaglinide: 0.5–4 mg/meal, nateglinide: 60–120 mg/meal.

19.5.2.3 Thiazolidinediones

The first evidence of hypoglycemic actions of thiazolidinediones (TZDs) stems from experiments in obese diabetic mice and rats and dates back to 1983 (67). The first trials, in patients with diabetes, were conducted in the early 1990s (68,69). In diabetic patients, the TZDs lowered glucose levels (HbA1C reductions between 0.5% and 1%), yet they did not stimulate but reduce insulin secretion thus improving insulin sensitivity. They also reduced hepatic glucose production (68,69). In short, they appeared extremely promising for their use in obese patients with insulin resistance, a population on the rise since the late 1970s. By now we know that TZDs act by binding to peroxisome proliferator-activated receptors (PPAR), the nuclear receptors that heterodimerize with retinoid x receptor (RXR) and bind to DNA together with additional coregulators and, thus, control transcription of multiple genes involved in fatty acid and glucose metabolism and also inflammation and differentiation (reviewed in Reference 70).

TZD therapy is associated with fluid retention and was completely abolished in knockout mice where PPAR was selectively deleted in the collecting ducts of the kidneys (71). Another off-target action is TZD-induced bone loss. Patients on TZDs, mostly females, experienced more fractures and had small but significant reductions in bone density compared to placebo- or metformin-treated patients (reviewed in Reference 72). This is a particularly important hazard in the elderly, who are more prone to falls and fractures. PPAR-mediated regulation of (a) mesenchymal stem cell differentiation into adipocytes rather than osteoblasts and (b) enhanced osteoclast differentiation are thought to mediate this effect (reviewed in Reference 72). As the above-noted effects of fluid retention and bone loss are noted as early as 1–2 years after start of therapy with TZDs (72), they represent major concerns, especially in older patients with a history of heart failure and/or frail patients at risk for fractures.

What are the benefits of TZDs? After only 3 years, patients in the PROactive study (41) treated with pioglitazone compared to placebo (difference in HbA1C 0.5% between groups) had slightly, but significantly ($p = 0.027$) fewer combined secondary outcomes (nonfatal myocardial infarctions, strokes, and all-cause deaths) pointing to an early cardiovascular benefit of TZD therapy. Of note, a significant difference in cardiovascular events with metformin or sulfonylurea/insulin was observed only after 10–20 years of therapy (32,33)). Interestingly, another randomized, prospective study of rosiglitazone with a slightly different design (Rosiglitazone Evaluated for Cardiovascular outcomes in ORal agent combination therapy for type 2 Diabetes [RECORD], open label, non-inferiority, rosiglitazone plus metformin, or sulfonylurea versus metformin plus sulfonylurea) did not show any difference in cardiovascular events after 5 years (73). Of note, both TZD studies noted "a trend" toward fewer strokes in patients treated with pio- or rosiglitazone (73,74). Another double-blind randomized controlled trial, comparative to RECORD in the choice of agents, the A Diabetes Outcome Progression Trial (ADOPT) study (75), showed improved and more sustained glycemic control in addition to improved insulin sensitivity and subsequently less insulin use in newly diagnosed diabetic patients treated with rosiglitazone compared to glyburide or metformin. The fact that in the ADOPT study significantly less insulin use was noted in the TZD compared to the metformin arm but even more so compared to the glyburide arm (also observed in the RECORD study (73)) may suggest preservation of beta cell function with TZDs that is superior to metformin and even more sulfonylureas (75). No difference in cardiovascular events was noted between all treatment arms after 4 years in the ADOPT trial (75). In the recently published Insulin Resistance Intervention after Stroke (IRIS) trial (which only included patients with insulin resistance, NOT diabetes, and prior stroke or TIA) pioglitazone significantly reduced the risk of stroke or myocardial infarction (76).

In all of the above studies (73–75), the use of TZDs was associated with an overall low risk of hypoglycemia, and a significantly lower risk compared to patients on glyburide (73,75). A relatively increased risk of congestive heart failure (CHF) and edema was noted in patients treated with TZDs compared to metformin and sulfonylurea (73,75). However, it should be mentioned that the absolute risk of CHF with TZD therapy remains rather low (<4%) compared to the overall risk of hypoglycemia (incidence in all groups between 10% and 39%, (73,75)). An increased risk of fractures was only observed in women treated with TZDs (about 9%–11% (73,75)).

A retrospective observational study (77) noted an increased risk of bladder cancer in the TZD compared to a sulfonylurea cohort after 5 years of therapy. Of note, no significantly increased risk of bladder cancer was noted after 5 years in the TZD arms of the two prospective studies (73,74). However, longer prospective studies are needed to determine whether TZD use clearly alters the risk of cancer or cardiovascular events.

Summary: TZDs appear to be a reasonable alternative to metformin therapy, especially in insulin-resistant patients. The current data also suggest an early cardiovascular benefit, at least with pioglitazone, as well as a relative preservation of beta cell function. TZDs should be avoided in patients at risk for heart failure and in women at risk for fractures. In elderly women with frequent falls or propensity to fall, the latter point should be seriously considered.

Dosing: pioglitazone: 15–45 mg/day; rosiglitazone: 2–8 mg/day.

19.5.2.4 GLP-1 Analogues

The secretion of glucagon-like peptides (GLPs) from the gut was first described in 1968 and was attributed to L-cells, endocrine cells, similar to the ones found in pancreatic islets, with a predominant localization in the distal ileum (reviewed in Reference 78). Upon secretion, stimulated by nutrient ingestion, GLPs activate their respective GLP1- or GLP-2 receptors, class B G protein-coupled receptors (GPCR), which then activate G proteins with subsequent signaling through cAMP and protein kinase A (reviewed in Reference 78). Activation of GLP1-receptors stimulates pancreatic insulin secretion and synthesis, reduces glucagon secretion, and also reduces appetite and delays gastric emptying, exocrine pancreatic, and gastric acid secretion (reviewed in Reference 78). Appetite-reducing actions promote weight loss and are presumably mediated via direct activation of hypothalamic GLP-1 receptors rather than activation of peripheral vagal neurons (79,80). All of these actions mediate powerful glucose-lowering actions while promoting weight loss, drawing considerable attention to the development of GLP-1 receptor agonists (GLP-1RA) for therapy of both diabetes and/or obesity. Endogenous GLP-1 is rapidly cleaved (within 2 minutes) by dipeptidyl peptidase 4 (DPP4) to inactive metabolites, thus greatly limiting its usefulness as a drug (reviewed in Reference 78). Research efforts have thus focused on developing agonists that are resistant to DPP4 cleavage. The first available GLP-1RA was resistant to DPP4 cleavage due to a mutation of the cleavage site, exendin 4, was isolated from the venom of a lizard (Heloderma suspectum or gila monster). The synthesized amide version of exendin 4, exenatide, was approved for diabetes therapy in 2005 (reviewed in Reference 78). Since then, four more long-acting GLP-1RA have been approved for diabetes therapy (liraglutide, albiglutide, dulaglutide, and lixisenatide; (81)). In addition, a higher-dose preparation of liraglutide has now also been approved for therapy of obesity without diabetes (12/2014, per prescribing information). So far, the prospective studies with GLP-1RA show HbA1C reductions of up to 1.5% as well as an average weight loss of 3 kg (reviewed in Reference 81). Associated lower blood pressures, improved lipid profiles (reviewed in Reference 82), and also improved left ventricular function (83,84) suggest that GLP-1RA may confer an early benefit regarding cardiovascular outcomes. A meta-analysis of available placebo-controlled trials of GLP-1RA suggested a 25%–30% cardiovascular risk reduction in patients treated with a GLP1-RA (85). More important, a large prospective trial just confirmed significantly fewer cardiovascular events in high-risk diabetic patients when treated with liraglutide over placebo after about 4 years (86).

The most common side effects with GLP-1RA relate to their inhibition of gastric emptying and are reported in up to 29% of patients treated with liraglutide (87), though they usually improve over time. Thus, nausea/vomiting was only noted in about 5% of liraglutide-treated patients after 2 years of active therapy (88). The publication of case reports of pancreatitis with GLP-1RA, first seen in a patient on exenatide (89), caused a major concern and led to a black box warning for both GLP-1RA and DPP4-inhibitors (discussed below). Of note, a meta-analysis of available randomized controlled trials as well as observational studies did not confirm a significantly increased risk of pancreatitis for either exenatide or liraglutide, though none of the studies were powered (nor will they ever be) to detect significant differences for these overall very rare outcomes (reviewed in Reference 90). Similarly, an increased incidence of C-cell hyperplasia and medullary thyroid tumors in rat studies with GLP-1RA has not been substantiated in monkey (91) and human studies so far (reviewed in Reference 90).

As with metformin and TZDs, the risk of hypoglycemia with GLP-1RAs is relatively low (3%–12%, reviewed in Reference 81). In addition, placebo-controlled studies show preserved beta-cell function with GLP-1RA (92,93). Furthermore, in the Liraglutide versus Glimepiride Monotherapy for Type 2 Diabetes (LEAD-3) study (87), more than twice as many patients dropped out due to ineffective therapy in the glimepiride compared to the liraglutide arm, pointing to the preservation of beta-cell function with GLP-1RAs (87).

Last but not least, most GLP-1RAs can be used safely in patients with mild-to-moderate renal impairment (reviewed in Reference 94). However, the commonly noted GI side effects of GLP-1RAs can be enhanced in patients with moderate or severe renal impairment and they can subsequently lead to volume depletion as well as acute renal failure. Thus, caution is recommended when used in this population.

Summary: GLP-1RAs provide an excellent option for diabetes therapy especially in the ever-growing obese population with a rather low risk of hypoglycemia, associated weight loss, a potential for beta-cell preservation, as well as relative safety in patients with mild-to-moderate renal impairment. Caution should be exercised in patients who experience GI side effects as they could result in significant volume depletion and thus increase morbidity, and potentially mortality, especially in the older population. Consideration of GI side effects is especially important in older individuals with poor diets or poor appetites. Available clinical studies point to a reduced risk of cardiovascular events with GLP-1RAs, which is promising. Note that all GLP-1RAs at the time of this writing are administered by pen injection.

Dosing:

Shorter-acting GLP-1RA: exenatide: 5–10 mcg BID, liraglutide: 0.6–1.8 mg/day, lixisenatide: 10–20 mcg/day.

Longer-acting GLP-1RA: extended-release exenatide: 2 mg weekly, dulaglutide: 0.75–1.5 mg weekly, albiglutide: 30–50 mg weekly.

19.5.2.5 DPP-4 Inhibitors

In mice, hypoglycemic effects of the dipeptidyl peptidase 4 inhibitor (DPP-4) sitagliptin were first described in 2005 (95). Treatment of diabetic patients with a single dose of sitagliptin confirmed postprandial glucose reductions as well as a greater than 80% inhibition of DPP-4 (96). Glucose reductions were associated with a twofold elevation in GLP-1, a significant increase in C-peptide and insulin but a reduction in glucagon levels (96) as expected for GLP-1R activation. However, in comparison to the DPP-4-resistant GLP-1RAs discussed above, the glycemic effects of the new DPP-4 inhibitors are not quite as potent. Overall, therapy with DPP-4 inhibitors reduces the HbA1C by about 0.5% (reviewed in Reference 97). That said, they have an excellent side-effect profile. In the cited study, GI adverse effects or hypoglycemia were not different in the DPP-4 inhibitor compared to the placebo arm (98). In comparison, hypoglycemia was 5–10 times less common with DPP-4 inhibitors when compared to either sulfonyurea or insulin therapy (63,99,100). In another study, diarrhea and nausea were significantly less common in patients treated with sitagliptin (a DPP-4 inhibitor) compared to metformin (101), which makes this class an attractive first-line treatment option for patients who do not tolerate metformin.

A long-term study (up to 4 years) does not suggest a hazardous effect on cardiovascular outcomes, including CHF in patients treated with sitagliptin compared to placebo (98). The authors do mention a trend toward a slightly higher occurrence of pancreatitis in the sitagliptin arm, though the difference was not statistically significant ($n = 23$ in sitagliptin arm, $n = 12$ in placebo arm, $p = 0.07$ (98)). Another study with alogliptin reports no change in cardiovascular outcomes during follow-up of up to 2.5 years with a similar risk of hypoglycemia compared to the placebo group; no pancreatitis cases were reported (102). Further studies are underway (reviewed in Reference 103).

Most DPP-4 inhibitors can be used safely in patients with moderate-to-severe CKD, albeit at reduced doses (note: linagliptin does not require this dose reduction), with similar effects on glycemic control and no increase in adverse events (reviewed in Reference 94).

Summary: DPP-4 inhibitors are quite safe though somewhat less effective compared to metformin, sulfonylurea, and GLP-1RA. A large body of data support their benefits on glycemic control with few hazards thus far.

Dosing: sitagliptin: 100 mg daily, linagliptin: 5 mg daily, alogliptin: 6.25–25 mg daily.

19.5.2.6 SGLT-2 Inhibitors

Derivatives of phlorizin, a natural plant glucoside and nonselective inhibitor of sodium-glucose-cotransporters (SGLT), were first used in diabetic rats and found to alleviate fasting but predominantly postprandial hyperglycemia without affecting insulin secretion (104). SGLT-1 and -2 are predominantly expressed in small intestine and kidney, respectively (reviewed in Reference 105). Both SGLT-1 and -2 function similarly by facilitating glucose transport driven by a sodium gradient (reviewed in Reference 105). However, SGLT1 also mediates galactose absorption and has about a ten-fold higher affinity for glucose compared to SGLT2 (reviewed in Reference 105). In the kidney, both SGLT-1 and -2 are expressed within the brush border membrane of the proximal tubules. Whereas the low-affinity transporter (SGLT-2) is expressed more proximally and directs 80%–90% of all glucose reabsorption, the high-affinity transporter (SGLT-1) is expressed more distally and mediates 10%–20% of renal glucose reabsorption (reviewed in Reference 105). In the small intestine, only SGLT-1 is expressed where it mediates both absorption of glucose and galactose into the blood (reviewed in Reference 105). Thus, inhibiting these transporters results in decreased glucose absorption from the gut and also enhanced glucose excretion through the kidneys. As inhibition of SGLT-1 causes glucose and galactose malabsorption as well as diarrhea, research has focused on the development of selective SGLT-2 inhibitors. Currently, three are FDA-approved (canagliflozin, dapagliflozin, empagliflozin; reviewed in Reference 106). In clinical studies, they have been shown to reduce HbA1C by 0.7%–1.9%, with greater effects seen in patients with higher baseline HbA1C (reviewed in Reference 106). In clinical studies, SGLT-2 inhibitors are generally well tolerated with less than 5% of the patients discontinuing the medication due to adverse effects (107–109). The most common side effect of these drugs, seen predominantly in women, is an increased risk of genital infections (4%–22% compared to 0.4%–5% in placebo arms (107–112)). Because increased renal glucose excretion is associated with fluid loss, volume depletion is a concern. However, so far the above studies have not substantiated an increased risk of symptomatic volume depletion, although overall most studies noted small, transient increases in BUN, Hct, or creatinine compared to placebo, consistent with a diuretic effect of SGLT-2 inhibitors (107–112). Precisely, this diuretic effect makes SGLT-2 inhibitors an attractive add-on medication for patients with coexisting heart failure, hypertension, or for patients on TZDs (known to cause fluid retention, see above discussion). In fact, when dapagliflozin was added to pioglitazone, an additional HbA1C reduction was achieved with little weight gain compared to patients treated with pioglitazone alone who gained an average of 3 kg (112). Furthermore, the first study examining cardiovascular endpoints (follow-up to 4 years) in a patient population at high cardiovascular risk reported significantly fewer composite cardiovascular events as well as fewer hospitalizations for CHF (111). In addition, SGLT-2 inhibitors carry little intrinsic risk of hypoglycemia with overall events being similar to placebo (108–110).

Recent case reports have raised concerns for an increased risk of ketoacidosis with SGLT-2 inhibitors (113,114). However, the above large study that reported decreased cardiovascular events with empagliflozin did not find a significantly increased incidence of ketoacidosis though "a trend" was noted (one case in placebo versus four cases in empagliflozin arm (111)). Furthermore, another analysis of combined data from prospective studies with canagliflozin, conducted by Janssen Research and Development, LLC (maker of canagliflozin, over 17,500 patients), showed an extremely small incidence of ketoacidosis cases overall, which, however, occurred more in the canagliflozin arm (0.07%–0.11% in the canagliflozin arm versus 0.03% in the comparator arm (115)). Compared to patients without ketoacidosis, patients with ketoacidosis had a longer duration of diabetes, lower BMI, higher HbA1C, lower GFR, were older, and predominantly male (115). Elevated glucagon secretion (in response to the SGLT-2 inhibitor), relative insulin deficiency, together with increased renal glucose excretion, are thought to trigger increased lipolysis and ketogenesis (reviewed in Reference 116). In addition, reduced ketonuria as a direct sequela of renal SGLT-2 inhibition may play a role (reviewed in Reference 116).

Summary: SGLT-2 inhibitors comprise the latest approved class of diabetes medications with potent effects on HbA1C reduction. They carry little risk of hypoglycemia, which makes them very attractive for treating older patients. They may offer additional long-term benefits for cardiovascular outcomes, in particular in patients with comorbid conditions such as CHF or hypertension. Caution is recommended in women at risk for genital infections as well as in frail, older, insulin-dependent patients in whom volume depletion may be an issue. They may confer an increased risk of ketoacidosis. All of the available SGLT-2 inhibitors are given once daily.

Dosing: canagliflozin: 100–300 mg/day, empagliflozin: 10–25 mg/day, dapagliflozin: 5–10 mg/day.

19.5.2.7 Alpha-Glucosidase Inhibitors

Acarbose and miglitol are reversible inhibitors of intestinal alpha-glucosidases and, thus, delay glucose absorption (reviewed in Reference 117). They were first shown to decrease postprandial hyperglycemia in the late 1970s (118,119). Based on their mechanism of action, it was found that they also caused sucrose malabsorption with subsequent fermentation of nonabsorbed carbohydrates by colonic bacteria, causing flatulence (118,119). Flatulence and/or diarrhea have been reported in 10%–50% of patients on acarbose (reviewed in Reference 120). Overall reductions in HbA1C are about 0.8% (reviewed in Reference 120). Additional benefits are a slight weight loss (0.5–1 kg) and no inherent risk for hypoglycemia (120,121). Also, in the Study TO Prevent Non-Insulin Dependent Diabetes Mellitus (STOP-NIDDM) diabetes prevention trial, significantly fewer cardiovascular events as well as fewer cases of diabetes were noted in patients with impaired glucose tolerance treated with acarbose for 3 years (122). The latter effect was comparable to results achieved in the metformin arm of the DPP trial (about 25% relative risk reduction of diabetes incidence with metformin (30)).

Summary: alpha-glucosidase inhibitors are comparable to DPP-4 inhibitors in regards to glycemic control. They do cause frequent, though usually mild and time-limited, GI side effects but may in fact confer an early cardiovascular benefit, at least in patients with prediabetes. However, more studies are needed to confirm the above-noted promising trends. They are relatively safe agents, with minimal systemic absorption. The likelihood of several weeks of GI upset may be of concern in older individuals who are having poor food intake or are malnourished.

Dosing: acarbose or miglitol: 25–100 mg/meal.

19.5.2.8 Bile Acid Sequestrants

Bile acid sequestrants are nonabsorbable resins that bind and sequester bile acids in the intestine, thus diverting them from the enterohepatic cycle. As a consequence, low-density lipoprotein (LDL) delivery to the liver is increased to compensate for the reduction of the bile acid pool (reviewed in Reference 123). These events translate into a 10%–15% reduction of LDL levels and led to the approval of bile acid sequestrants for the therapy of hypercholesterolemias (reviewed in

Reference 123). The first evidence of a glucose-lowering effect of bile aid sequestrants, in particular cholestyramine, dates back to 1994 (124). Colesevelam was later approved for diabetes therapy. The exact mechanisms of the hypoglycemic actions of bile acid sequestrants are not entirely understood but may involve the bile acid receptor FXR (nuclear farnesoid X receptor) and FGF19 pathway (fibroblast growth factor 19), stimulation of incretin secretion through TGR5 (also known as GPBAR1 or G protein-coupled bile acid receptor 1), and possibly modulation of gut microbiota composition (reviewed in Reference 123).

In several randomized controlled trials of diabetic patients treated with colesevelam, a 0.5% HbA1C reduction was observed on average (reviewed in References 125 and 126). As expected, colesevelam also mediated a decrease in LDL of about 13% in these patients (reviewed in Reference 125). Existing studies in diabetic patients were not powered to detect differences in cardiovascular outcomes (reviewed in References 125 and 126). Of note, in patients with primary hypercholesterolemia (but not diabetes), cholestyramine has been shown to significantly reduce cardiovascular events after 7 years (127). Because bile acid sequestrants act in the intestine without being absorbed they are safe to use in patients with renal of hepatic failure. For the same reason, reported adverse effects are of gastrointestinal nature (constipation and flatulence) though overall uncommon (reviewed in References 125 and 126). Colesevelam rarely causes hypoglycemia and it is weight neutral (reviewed in References 125 and 126).

Summary: bile acid sequestrants are comparable to DPP-4 inhibitors in their potency to lower HbA1C; they also lower LDL, are overall well tolerated, and are safe to use in patients with hepatic or renal impairment. Hypoglycemia is extremely rare. Thus, they might be an excellent choice for the elderly diabetic patient. Caution is advised in patients with a history of constipation—not an uncommon problem in older patients. No cardiovascular outcome data are available for bile acid sequestrants in diabetic patients.

Dosing: colesevelam: 3750 mg/day (may be given in divided doses).

19.5.2.9 Dopamine Agonists

The first reports of dopamine agonists affecting glucose metabolism date back to the late 1970s (for instance (128,129)). Interestingly, in patients with a long duration of diabetes or dependent on insulin, the glucose-lowering effects of bromocriptine (a dopamine agonist) were not seen (128,130). Animal studies and data from patients treated with typical as well as atypical antipsychotics (both are antagonists of dopamine type 2 receptors) suggest that antagonizing hypothalamic dopamine receptors mediates increased peripheral sympathetic activity, insulin resistance, increased glucose production, as well as fat oxidation (reviewed in Reference 131). Activation of hypothalamic dopamine receptors by bromocriptine, on the other hand, has the opposite effects and thus lowers glucose levels (reviewed in Reference 131).

In a study of obese patients with type 2 diabetes, both a significant glucose-lowering effect and a 1 kg weight loss and improvement in insulin resistance were observed during an 18-week study (132). Follow-up studies in mostly obese diabetics did not report a weight change but reproduced significant HbA1C reductions of about 0.8%, with the degree mostly dependent on the starting of HbA1C and bromocriptine dose (133–137). In a recent, small study of morbidly obese, highly insulin-resistant patients, addition of bromocriptine resulted in a 27% reduction in insulin use at comparable glycemic control (138). Furthermore, a 1-year placebo-controlled trial of high-risk diabetic patients (diabetes duration about 8 years, majority with comorbidities like HTN and hyperlipoproteinemia) pointed to an early cardiovascular benefit of bromocriptine. The number of composite CV events was significantly reduced in the bromocriptine compared to the placebo arm (relative hazard ratio 0.48–0.6 with bromocriptine compared to placebo (136,137)).

Another benefit of bromocriptine is a low incidence of hypoglycemia (6.9% in bromocriptine versus 5.3% in placebo arm (136)). Bromocriptine can be used in patients with advanced CKD as it is mostly excreted through the biliary system (reviewed in Reference 131). Also, glucose-lowering effects of bromocriptine were observed in patients with CKD stage 4 (139).

What about hazards? The biggest disadvantage of bromocriptine therapy is its side-effects profile, with nausea being the most common adverse effect noted (up to 32%, although mostly transient (136)). Compared to other diabetes medications, a relatively high percentage of patients (24%) discontinued bromocriptine due to adverse effects, which compares to 10%–16% discontinuations in studies of TZDs and GLP-1RA (74,140).

Overall, bromocriptine appears to be a rather safe medication and comparable to DPP-4 inhibitors in its glycemic effects with one large study pointing to an early cardiovascular benefit. However, most of the studies published to date are relatively small, and compared to other diabetes medications the frequency of reported side effects with use of bromocriptine (in particular nausea) is rather high. More important, when considering bromocriptine in older patients, GI upset, dizziness, depression, and fatigue have been reported with this medication.

Dosing: bromocriptine (Cycloset): 0.8–4.8 mg daily.

19.5.3 Insulin for Type 2 Diabetes

Pros and cons of different insulin therapies are discussed in detail in the section related to type 1 diabetes below.

19.5.4 Selecting an Agent in the Older Patient with Type 2 Diabetes

A major emphasis of the ADA and the European Association for the Study of Diabetes (EASD) has been individualization of therapy. Nowhere is this more important than in selecting an agent to treat the older patient. Skill in using or not using a pen injector may influence the decision to use a GLP-1RA. The sequelae and risk of hypoglycemia will determine the desirability of the inexpensive sulfonylureas, as will renal and liver function. Edema or risk of falls will influence whether or not one chooses a TZD. Bowel abnormalities will exclude many of the aforementioned agents that have GI side-effects. B12 deficiency or GFR <45 mL/minute should dissuade one from using metformin. With these thoughts in mind, some guiding principles may be suggested. All things being equal, metformin is generally considered the initial agent of choice. If one does not reach goal, then a second agent should be added, rather than switching agents. If one still does not reach goal, then either a third oral agent or an injectable should be given (either basal insulin or GLP-1RA). Beyond this, multidose insulin therapy (see type 1 diabetes section) is the desired regimen.

19.6 MANAGEMENT OF TYPE 1 DIABETES IN THE ELDERLY

As indicated in the introduction, people with type 1 diabetes make little or no insulin. The discovery of insulin in 1921 changed a disease with about 100% mortality into a manageable disorder. Today, with imperfect tools, we attempt, with insulin replacement therapy, to mimic, as best as possible, physiologic insulin delivery. One of the biggest difficulties is that whereas physiologically insulin is released rapidly into the portal system and about 50% is removed by the liver before entry into systemic circulation (141,142), subcutaneous insulin absorption is relatively slow (see below), and it is absorbed directly into the systemic circulation, thus reversing the hepatic/systemic insulin ratio. In summary, our attempts at "physiologic insulin replacement" are not really physiologic.

As opposed to older patients with type 2 diabetes, most people with type 1 diabetes have, almost necessarily, had their diabetes for a very long time—often from childhood or adolescence. Hence, the older term "juvenile diabetes." As such, their habits in using insulin are very ingrained, as are their thoughts regarding blood glucose targets. This may result in some resistance, when adjusting glucose targets to avoid hypoglycemia. Also, many patients over the age of 60 years acquired their basic diabetes education before the advent of insulin pumps, insulin analogues, and multidose insulin regimens, and even human insulin. Many or most have chronic microvascular complications from their diabetes. People with type 1 diabetes also have a greater risk of macrovascular disease, although, as indicated previously, there really are no prospective statin intervention trials completed in people with type 1 diabetes.

Benbow et al. studied 55 patients meeting criteria for "elderly brittle diabetes" during a survey in the UK: they were all aged above 60 years and took insulin. Brittle was defined as "glycemic instability leading to life disruption" (143). Mean age was = 74 years, and 71% were female. They noted the following: "mixed glycemic instability" in 44%, recurrent diabetic ketoacidosis in 29%, recurrent hypoglycemia in 27%, and 84% lived independently (143). Bain et al. described the "golden years" cohort in 2003 (144). These were 400 individuals with type 1 diabetes in the UK who were medal-holders for having diabetes for more than 50 years. Characteristics were 54% male, 46% female, mean age = 68.9 years, mean BMI = 25.0 kg/m^2, and mean insulin dose = 0.52 units/kg (144). Despite doing so well, mean HbA1C was 7.6% (nl = 3.8%–5.0%), and, most interestingly, NO ONE had a normal HbA1C (144)! Thus, one would conclude from these two studies (143,144) that in older patients with type 1 diabetes, at least in the UK, patients tend to be lean, patients tend to be insulinopenic, both DKA and hypoglycemia may be problems, problematic or "brittle" patients tend to be adherent, and such patients almost always have elevated HbA1C's. However, since the DCCT, treatment targets and regimens have been more aggressive.

The guiding principles of managing type 1 diabetes are that because such people make no insulin, (1) at least basal insulin must ALWAYS be provided, (2) an attempt at "physiological insulin replacement" is desirable, and (3) type 1 diabetes is not a dietary disorder; it is due to insulin deficiency. As such, the diet should be as close to "normal" as possible, while avoiding an excessive glycemic load at any meal. This begs the question: What does "physiological insulin replacement" look like? In people without diabetes, a basal amount of insulin is secreted throughout the day with a diurnal rhythm (142). It regulates hepatic glucose production as well as fat and protein catabolism. Slightly more insulin is needed toward dawn and less in the middle of the night. At mealtime, a burst of insulin is rapidly released in two phases, presumably a readily releasable pool and newly synthesized insulin, respectively. Each of these components, that is, basal and prandial insulin, accounts for about 50% of insulin secreted. At the present time, aside from using an insulin pump, there is no single insulin species "smart enough" to effectively provide all of the components of physiological insulin secretion. Hence, the development of the basal-bolus concept.

Prior to the late 1970s, there were no fingerstick blood glucose testing devices or measurement of long-term diabetes control, that is, HbA1C. Hence, there was dispute over the relationship between glucose control and diabetes complications. This was resolved with the publication in 1993 of the DCCT trial results (145) showing that an approximately 2% reduction in HbA1C achieved by using multidose insulin or pumps versus what was then "conventional"—twice daily "split and mixed" insulin—achieved remarkable reductions in retinopathy, neuropathy, and nephropathy. Long-term follow-up of these patients (DCCT/EDIC) (146) demonstrated persistence of these benefits as well as a major reduction in cardiovascular outcomes. Optimization of blood glucose control to near-normal glucoses, when feasible, using basal–bolus insulin or pumps thus became the goal. However, the HbA1C reductions achieved were at the expense of a tripling in the occurrence of severe hypoglycemia—defined as resulting in altered level of consciousness (147). This problem has only recently been partially overcome by the use of REAL-time continuous glucose monitoring and sensor-augmented insulin pump therapy with or without threshold-suspend (148). Clearly, increasing severe hypoglycemia is unacceptable in the older patient population. At the time of this writing, US Medicare does not reimburse for REAL-time continuous glucose monitoring. Therefore, older people who have long tried to normalize their blood sugar now must be asked to relax their blood glucose targets. Persuading people with type 1 diabetes to do so can sometimes be challenging.

19.6.1 Intensive Diabetes Management

The components of intensive diabetes management, which are appropriate for type 1, thin, or insulin-requiring type 2, or LADA patients are knowledge of carbohydrate counting, an insulin/carbohydrate ratio, a correction algorithm (insulin sensitivity factor), a target blood glucose, a fast/rapid-acting insulin at mealtime, and a basal insulin or, alternatively, an insulin pump. Patients must be taught "sick-day rules," treatment of hypoglycemia, what to do for exercise and for snacks. Note that this does not specify what the target glucose is. Therefore, one can adjust the target based on factors such as frailty, hypoglycemia awareness or unawareness, presence or absence of CVD, and so on. In a patient who is fit, 62 years old with no significant complications, a near-normal blood sugar might be an appropriate target. In a patient who has had two strokes, chronic kidney disease, and mild dementia, a target glucose of 150–180 mg/dL may be appropriate to minimize risk of hypoglycemia, while avoiding glucosuria. Given the increased prevalence of dementia in older patients with diabetes, one must adjust the complexity of the regimen accordingly. In patients who are "tech-savvy," calculators and "apps" have been developed to assist with this. However, unfortunately, many older patients do not fall into this category. The compromise has been to use a fixed mealtime "baseline" fast/rapid-acting insulin at meals rather than having the patient count carbohydrates. Yet, unless the patient can have a fairly consistent carbohydrate intake, this system will necessarily result in erratic blood sugars. An ideal solution does not exist to date. Hopefully, in the near future, "smart insulins" that release insulin in response to glucose, closed-loop insulin pumps, encapsulated islets, or islet-cell transplantation will help our patients to better manage/cure their type 1 diabetes. Until then, we are left with optimizing the insulins discussed below.

19.6.2 Basal Insulins

The original basal insulins were isophane (NPH), PZI, and ultralente insulins. These were originally animal-derived and lasted at least 24 hours. With the development of human insulins in the 1980s it was found that the duration of action of these preparations was shortened. The variability of absorption exceeded 50%, and human isophane insulin has a distinct peak at 4–8 hours (reviewed in Reference 149). Thus, none of these insulins were ideal for basal insulin replacement. These problems led to the development of basal insulin analogues that have less of a peak and a more predictable absorption.

The first basal analogue developed and marketed was insulin glargine. There is a glycine for asparagine substitution at position 21 on the A-chain and two arginines at the C-terminal end of the B-chain. At a dose of 0.4 units/kg, the duration of action is approximately 21–22 hours. When patient data are aggregated, it appears peakless, although some patients show a distinct peak. The two arginines result in an isoelectric point of about pH 6.7. As such, it is soluble at acid pH; thus the preparation in the vial is acidic: pH = 4.0. Glargine precipitates at physiologic pH, resulting in its prolonged action (150). The glargine is metabolized to M1 and M2 metabolites. The M1 metabolite is the primary circulating species of glargine, with minimal levels of parent glargine or M2 found (151). The M1 metabolite has a much lower affinity for the IGF-1 receptor than does parent glargine. Glargine is administered once daily. It has been shown to reduce hypoglycemia versus isophane insulin (149). A U-300 (3 times the concentration, i.e., 300 units/mL) preparation is currently being marketed. It has comparable efficacy to U-100 glargine, but with slightly less hypoglycemia events (152).

A second basal insulin analogue is insulin detemir, which has a myristic acid at position B29 and a deletion of the threonine at position B30. It has a Cmax of 6–8 hours. These changes allow a longer hexamerization period in the subcutaneous tissues, as well as binding to albumin in the circulation, allowing for less variability in its effect (153). At doses of 0.4 units/kg and the above duration of activity, insulin detemir appears to last for about 24 hours. At lower doses it does not (154) and requires twice-daily dosing. It reportedly has more reproducible absorption than insulin glargine (155) and does not cross the placenta. The latter, of course, is of no importance when dealing with older patients.

Insulin degludec was approved by the FDA in 2015. It contains an added hexadecanoic acid at LysB29 using a linker of glutamic acid. As a result, it is injected as a dihexamer containing phenol and zinc. These hexamers combine to form multihexamers in the depot as phenol is removed. Finally, in the subcutaneous space, as zinc is removed, the multihexamers break up into absorbable dimers and eventually monomers. The result is a very protracted duration of action of insulin degludec, more predictable absorption, with less hypoglycemia (156–158). As opposed to glargine, whose acid pH makes combining it with other preparations difficult, insulin degludec has been formulated with insulin aspart (see below) and liraglutide. It is injected once daily.

19.6.3 Fast and Rapid-Acting Insulins

When regular insulin is injected into the subcutaneous space, it exists as hexamers coordinated by zinc. These hexamers are not absorbed. The hexamers dissociate into dimers and monomers in order to be absorbed. This takes time and allows for variability in absorption (159). Furthermore, insulin is absorbed fastest from the abdomen and slowest from the thigh and buttock. The result is that regular insulin must be injected about 30 minutes before a meal and still may have a "tail" after the postmeal glucose rise has ended. Furthermore, most patients did not wait the requisite 30 minutes before eating. The results were postmeal hyperglycemia and late hypoglycemia (149). The peak of regular insulin is about 2 hours with a duration of 6–10 hours when given as 0.4 units/kg (149).

Therefore, rapid-acting insulin analogues were developed that prevented hexamerization of the insulin, resulting in so-called monomeric insulins. Currently, three such species (insulin lispro, insulin apart, and insulin glulisine) are on the market. For the sake of brevity and because their pharmacodynamics are so similar, their pharmacodynamics will be considered as one. They do have different excipients. In short, the time to peak, and duration of action are about twice as fast as regular insulin when dosed at 0.4 units/kg. They result in significantly less hypoglycemia than does regular insulin (149).

19.6.4 Insulin Pumps

Insulin pumps have been used in patients with type 1 and 2 diabetes and in the elderly patients successfully. Insulin pumps have been reported to reduce hypoglycemias, although such studies specifically in the elderly patients have not been carried out. Before initiating pump therapy, one should be sure that the patient has good cognition, can count carbohydrates, has adequate manual dexterity, can actually read the meter and the pump, and cognitively, can make independent judgments. Older couples may "comanage" the insulin pump (author's personal experience). Given potential difficulties, insulin pump therapy should be used under the supervision of a diabetes professional. Threshold-suspend insulin pumps further reduce hypoglycemias (148), but unfortunately, at the time of this writing, are not insured by Medicare in the United States. Recently, "apps" have become available to assist in the management of diabetes in general and pumps in particular.

19.6.5 Building a Regimen

So, how would one calculate/devise an insulin regimen in an older individual? As stated above, the same techniques as used in a younger individual should be used, but, in the older, less than optimally healthy individual, higher glucose targets should be used, and, when appropriate, simplified regimens. In a patient who is relatively lean, with type 1 diabetes, a dose of 0.5–1.0 units/kg of insulin (TOTAL DAILY DOSE = TDD) is usual. Approximately 50% of this dose would be given as basal insulin and the remainder divided into doses approximately proportional to the carbohydrate loads of the three meals. Ideally, the mealtime bolus is given at an insulin/carbohydrate (I/CHO) ratio. A "guesstimate" of the I/CHO is 500 divided by the TDD. A correction factor or insulin sensitivity factor (ISF) is added to the dose calculated for the I/CHO. A usual ISF is calculated as 1500–1800 divided by the TDD. As an example, in an 80 kg person with type 1 diabetes, the TDD could be 80 kg × 0.6 kg = 48 units; 24 units would be given as basal insulin, and then the ISF = 1800 divided by 48 = ~1 unit/40 mg/dL over target. The I/CHO = 500/48 = ~1 unit/10 g CHO. The two are added to determine the mealtime dose. If the patient cannot count carbohydrates, then one could divide the remaining 24 units of mealtime insulin (48 units total insulin – 24 units basal = 24 units) into three meals, that is, 8 units/meal plus correction (see References 160 and 161). In a very healthy person, with more than 10 years life expectancy, one could use a target glucose of somewhere in the vicinity of 100–150 mg/dL, whereas in a frail patient with a shorter life expectancy, a target of 150–180 mg/dL or even higher may be appropriate. If oral intake is in question, the rapid-acting insulin may be given after completion of the meal. Dose adjustment of the basal insulin is based on fasting finger-stick glucose, whereas prandial insulin dose is adjusted based either on the postmeal glucose, or more usually, the following preprandial or bedtime glucose. Thus, a standard monitoring regimen would be at least before each meal and at bedtime. In patients with type 2 diabetes, if they are lean, a similar regimen is used. If they are obese, then often 1.0 units/kg or more TDD is required. If one is only using basal insulin to treat type 2 diabetes, in addition to oral medications, then one may either start conservatively at 12 units in the morning or at bedtime—based on the fasting blood sugar with upward titration as necessary—or 0.2 units/kg with upward titration as given above. Sometimes, one may use an oral agent that affects mainly postmeal glucose (e.g., alpha-glucosidase inhibitor, meglitinide, DPP-4 inhibitor, or SGLT-2 inhibitor) in combination with a basal insulin.

19.6.6 HYPOGLYCEMIA IN THE OLDER PATIENT WITH DIABETES

Older patients have a higher incidence of hypoglycemia unawareness and severe hypoglycemia (38–42). Use of newer insulin analogues reduces the risk of hypoglycemia as noted above (162). Older men had a greater incidence of cognitive impairment and delayed recognition of hypoglycemia (162). In the Diabetes and Aging Study (163) severe hypoglycemia occurred in 9.3%–13.8% of patients. Risk was highest in patients with a near-normal HbA1C and patients with a high HbA1C. The least risk of severe hypoglycemia occurred in those patients with an HbA1C 7.0%–7.9%. Mean age was 59.5 years (163). It therefore seems prudent in older patients with less than a 10-year life expectancy to target an HbA1C < 8.0%, and in the frail elderly with poor health, an HbA1C < 8.5%, as recommended by ADA and the International Diabetes Federation (IDF; 13,164). In the event of hypoglycemia, 20 g of glucose would be expected to raise blood sugar by 20 mg/dL in 20 minutes (20-20-20 rule). If the patient cannot take oral glucose, then glucagon should be administered.

19.7 MANAGEMENT OF DIABETES IN THE SKILLED NURSING FACILITY

A major tenet of diabetes education and management is patient empowerment. The situation for residents of the Skilled Nursing Facility (SNF) is almost antithetical to this principle. Usually, it is the staff who administer medications and insulin. Thus, insulin regimens tend to be simplified; that is, they are independent of carbohydrate intake, and patients are often unaware of their treatment regimen. Furthermore, insulin and glucose record-keeping tend to be for the benefit of documentation rather than for ease of interpreting trends in diabetes management. Patient's oral intake may be very variable, and swallowing may be suspect. Timing of insulin and meals may be disrupted. Patients may be unaware of, or unable to communicate readily, signs or symptoms of hypoglycemia. Finally, when patients are sent for diabetes specialty visits, the patients rather than nurses come to the visit, although the patients may have little input into their own management and assessment of blood glucose trends. Records are often handwritten, legibility poor, and interpretation difficult.

The patient in the SNF needs to have individualized goals and therapeutic regimens. Avoidance of hypoglycemia is of primacy, while attempting to adequately maintain blood sugars below the glucosuric threshold. Decisions in selecting oral agents need to take into consideration not only hepatic and renal function but also drug–drug interactions. Adequate nutritional intake needs to be ensured. A balance needs to be struck between avoiding high glycemic index foods and providing foods that the patient prefers. In this setting, insulin secretagogues carry a high risk of hypoglycemia and are probably less preferable. As previously emphasized, HbA1C targets will depend on patient functionality, comorbidities, and life expectancy. Often, this means accepting an HbA1C of 8% or sometimes even higher.

In patients receiving insulin, as explained above, the higher the dose, the longer the duration of action, and the more variable the absorption. Therefore, it is the authors' bias that multidose insulin is often preferable to and safer than a single, large injection of basal insulin. Current-day syringe needles and pens are vastly less painful than those of previous generations. If multidose insulin therapy is needed, the same principles that apply to type 1 or insulin-requiring type 2 diabetes obtain, but higher target blood glucoses should be used, for example, 150–180 mg/dL. A prandial fast/rapid-acting insulin dose based on an insulin/carbohydrate ratio is desirable but often not achievable in the SNF setting. In that case, a fixed dose of mealtime insulin, with a correction factor (ISF) must be used. It is imperative, in this case, that oral intake be assured. If oral intake is uncertain, then the insulin should be administered only upon completion of the meal. Obviously, increased or decreased activity will influence basal insulin requirements. Given a fixed dose of basal insulin, snacks may be useful before exercise, for example, physical therapy. Bedtime rapid-acting insulin and "sliding-scale" basal insulin (or for that matter, any "sliding-scale" insulin) should be discouraged. If the patient has type 1 diabetes, basal insulin cannot be withheld! Blood sugar should be checked before each meal and at bedtime, if a multidose insulin regimen is used. On the other hand, fingersticks hurt a lot more than injections, so that if a patient has stable glucose levels on an oral agent fingerstick blood glucoses should be obtained only in so far as they will influence treatment. Again, individualization is key.

Electronic health records may decrease medication errors, alert providers of drug–drug interactions, and provide legible, sequential meal and glucose logs. If the patient has their own glucose meter, downloading that meter every 1–2 days allows for adjustment of the treatment regimen. Use of telemedicine holds the promise of allowing the specialist to interact with the nursing staff, who are delivering the care and implementing the diabetes regimen, in addition to communicating with the patient, thus improving care.

19.8 SUMMARY

Diabetes and its comorbidities provide a unique set of challenges in the management of older patients. A realistic assessment of the patient's physical, cognitive, and psychosocial well-being must precede formulation of any therapeutic plan. The International Diabetes Federation (IDF) categorizes patients usefully into functionally independent, functionally dependent (A. frail, B. dementia), and end-of-life care (164). Functionally independent, however, may include a wide range of patients—from those who are sedentary at home, to those who are healthy and exercise daily. Selection of treatment agents, diet, and exercise regimens, as well as glucose targets, will all depend on this categorization. Individualization and common sense need always be applied and there must be a willingness to adjust treatment regimens and goals as the patient's health, cognitive, and psychosocial situation changes. It is a challenging yet rewarding endeavor.

REFERENCES

1. Cheng YJ, Imperatore G, Geiss LS et al. Secular changes in the age-specific prevalence of diabetes among U.S. adults: 1988–2010. *Diabetes Care* 2013; 36:2690–2696.
2. Kirkman MS, Briscoe VJ, Clark N et al. Diabetes in older adults. *Diabetes Care* 2012; 35:2650–2664.
3. American Diabetes Association Diabetes Care. 2. Classification and diagnosis of diabetes. *Diabetes Care* 2016; 39(Suppl 1):S13–S22.
4. Palmer JP, Fleming GA, Greenbaum CJ et al. C-peptide is the appropriate outcome measure for type 1 diabetes clinical trials to preserve beta-cell function: Report of an ADA workshop, 21–22 October 2001. *Diabetes* 2004; 53:250–264.

5. Keenan HA, Sun JK, Levine J et al. Residual insulin production and pancreatic ss-cell turnover after 50 years of diabetes: Joslin Medalist Study. *Diabetes* 2010; 59:2846–2853.

6. U.K. prospective diabetes study 16. Overview of 6 years' therapy of type II diabetes: A progressive disease. U.K. Prospective Diabetes Study Group. *Diabetes* 1995; 44:1249–1258.

7. Wittlin SD. Treating the spectrum of type 2 diabetes: Emphasis on insulin pump therapy. *Diabetes Educ* 2006; 32:39S–46S.

8. Basu R, Breda E, Oberg AL et al. Mechanisms of the age-associated deterioration in glucose tolerance: Contribution of alterations in insulin secretion, action, and clearance. *Diabetes* 2003; 52:1738–1748.

9. Amati F, Dube JJ, Coen PM et al. Physical inactivity and obesity underlie the insulin resistance of aging. *Diabetes Care* 2009; 32:1547–1549.

10. Diabetes Prevention Program Research Group, Crandall J, Schade D et al. The influence of age on the effects of lifestyle modification and metformin in prevention of diabetes. *J Gerontol A: Biol Sci Med Sci* 2006; 61:1075–1081.

11. American Diabetes Association Diabetes Care. 8. Cardiovascular disease and risk management. *Diabetes Care* 2016; 39(Suppl 1):S60–S71.

12. American Diabetes Association Diabetes Care. 9. Microvascular complications and foot care. *Diabetes Care* 2016; 39(Suppl 1):S72–S80.

13. American Diabetes Association Diabetes Care. 10. Older adults. *Diabetes Care* 2016; 39(Suppl 1):S81–S85.

14. Kirkman MS, Briscoe VJ, Clark N et al. Diabetes in older adults: A consensus report. *J Am Geriatr Soc* 2012; 60:2342–2356.

15. Anderson RJ, Freedland KE, Clouse RE et al. The prevalence of comorbid depression in adults with diabetes: A meta-analysis. *Diabetes Care* 2001; 24:1069–1078.

16. Fisher L, Gonzalez JS, Polonsky WH. The confusing tale of depression and distress in patients with diabetes: A call for greater clarity and precision. *Diabet Med* 2014; 31:764–772.

17. Effects of ramipril on cardiovascular and microvascular outcomes in people with diabetes mellitus: Results of the HOPE study and MICRO-HOPE substudy. Heart Outcomes Prevention Evaluation Study Investigators. *Lancet* 2000; 355:253–259.

18. Ravid M, Brosh D, Levi Z et al. Use of enalapril to attenuate decline in renal function in normotensive, normoalbuminuric patients with type 2 diabetes mellitus. A randomized, controlled trial. *Ann Intern Med* 1998; 128:982–988.

19. ONTARGET Investigators, Yusuf S, Teo KK et al. Telmisartan, ramipril, or both in patients at high risk for vascular events. *N Engl J Med* 2008; 358:1547–1559.

20. Group AS, Cushman WC, Evans GW et al. Effects of intensive blood-pressure control in type 2 diabetes mellitus. *N Engl J Med* 2010; 362:1575–1585.

21. Brunstrom M, Carlberg B. Effect of antihypertensive treatment at different blood pressure levels in patients with diabetes mellitus: Systematic review and meta-analyses. *BMJ* 2016; 352:i717.

22. Group SR, Wright JT Jr, Williamson JD et al. A randomized trial of intensive versus standard blood-pressure control. *N Engl J Med* 2015; 373:2103–2116.

23. Halter JB, Musi N, McFarland Horne F et al. Diabetes and cardiovascular disease in older adults: Current status and future directions. *Diabetes* 2014; 63:2578–2589.

24. Colhoun HM, Betteridge DJ, Durrington PN et al. Primary prevention of cardiovascular disease with atorvastatin in type 2 diabetes in the Collaborative Atorvastatin Diabetes Study (CARDS): Multicentre randomised placebo-controlled trial. *Lancet* 2004; 364:685–696.

25. Betteridge DJ, Carmena R. The diabetogenic action of statins—Mechanisms and clinical implications. *Nat Rev Endocrinol* 2016; 12:99–110.

26. Bittner V, Bertolet M, Barraza Felix R et al. Comprehensive cardiovascular risk factor control improves survival: The BARI 2D Trial. *J Am Coll Cardiol* 2015; 66:765–773.

27. Vinik AI, Vinik EJ, Colberg SR et al. Falls risk in older adults with type 2 diabetes. *Clin Geriatr Med* 2015; 31:89–99, viii.

28. Epstein S, Defeudis G, Manfrini S et al. Diabetes and disordered bone metabolism (diabetic osteodystrophy): Time for recognition. *Osteoporos Int* 2016; 27:1931–1951.

29. Vinik AI. The conductor of the autonomic orchestra. *Front Endocrinol (Lausanne)* 2012; 3:71.

30. Knowler WC, Barrett-Connor E, Fowler SE et al. Reduction in the incidence of type 2 diabetes with lifestyle intervention or metformin. *N Engl J Med* 2002; 346:393–403.

31. Pownall HJ, Bray GA, Wagenknecht LE et al. Changes in body composition over 8 years in a randomized trial of a lifestyle intervention: The look AHEAD study. *Obesity (Silver Spring)* 2015; 23:565–572.

32. Effect of intensive blood-glucose control with metformin on complications in overweight patients with type 2 diabetes (UKPDS 34). UK Prospective Diabetes Study (UKPDS) Group. *Lancet* 1998; 352:854–865.

33. Intensive blood-glucose control with sulphonylureas or insulin compared with conventional treatment and risk of complications in patients with type 2 diabetes (UKPDS 33). UK Prospective Diabetes Study (UKPDS) Group. *Lancet* 1998; 352:837–853.

34. Holman RR, Paul SK, Bethel MA et al. 10-year follow-up of intensive glucose control in type 2 diabetes. *N Engl J Med* 2008; 359:1577–1589.

35. Group AC, Patel A, MacMahon S et al. Intensive blood glucose control and vascular outcomes in patients with type 2 diabetes. *N Engl J Med* 2008; 358:2560–2572.

36. Group AS, Gerstein HC, Miller ME et al. Long-term effects of intensive glucose lowering on cardiovascular outcomes. *N Engl J Med* 2011; 364:818–828.

37. Duckworth W, Abraira C, Moritz T et al. Glucose control and vascular complications in veterans with type 2 diabetes. *N Engl J Med* 2009; 360:129–139.

38. Moore TJ, Cohen MR, Furberg CD. Serious adverse drug events reported to the Food and Drug Administration, 1998–2005. *Arch Intern Med* 2007; 167:1752–1759.

39. Budnitz DS, Shehab N, Kegler SR et al. Medication use leading to emergency department visits for adverse drug events in older adults. *Ann Intern Med* 2007; 147:755–765.

40. Bramlage P, Gitt AK, Binz C et al. Oral antidiabetic treatment in type-2 diabetes in the elderly: Balancing the need for glucose control and the risk of hypoglycemia. *Cardiovasc Diabetol* 2012; 11:122.

41. de Galan BE, Zoungas S, Chalmers J et al. Cognitive function and risks of cardiovascular disease and hypoglycaemia in patients with type 2 diabetes: The action in diabetes and vascular disease: Preterax and Diamicron modified release controlled evaluation (ADVANCE) trial. *Diabetologia* 2009; 52:2328–2336.

42. Punthakee Z, Miller ME, Launer LJ et al. Poor cognitive function and risk of severe hypoglycemia in type 2 diabetes: Post hoc epidemiologic analysis of the ACCORD trial. *Diabetes Care* 2012; 35:787–793.

43. Austin EJ, Deary IJ. Effects of repeated hypoglycemia on cognitive function: A psychometrically validated reanalysis of the diabetes control and complications trial data. *Diabetes Care* 1999; 22:1273–1277.

44. The Diabetes Control and Complications Trial/Epidemiology of Diabetes Interventions and Complications (DCCT/EDIC) Study Research Group, Jacobson AM, Musen G et al. Long-term effect of diabetes and its treatment on cognitive function. *N Engl J Med* 2007; 356:1842–1852.

45. Meneilly GS, Cheung E, Tuokko H. Altered responses to hypoglycemia of healthy elderly people. *J Clin Endocrinol Metab* 1994; 78:1341–1348.

46. Meneilly GS, Cheung E, Tuokko H. Counterregulatory hormone responses to hypoglycemia in the elderly patient with diabetes. *Diabetes* 1994; 43:403–410.

47. Gottlieb B, Auld WH. Metformin in treatment of diabetes mellitus. *Br Med J* 1962; 1:680–682.

48. Sterne J. [Treatment of diabetes mellitus with N,N-dimethylguanylguanidine (LA. 6023, glucophage)]. *Therapie* 1959; 14:625–630.

49. Biguanides and lactic acidosis in diabetics. *Br Med J* 1977; 2:1436.

50. Stumvoll M, Nurjhan N, Perriello G et al. Metabolic effects of metformin in non-insulin-dependent diabetes mellitus. *N Engl J Med* 1995; 333:550–554.

51. Schernthaner G, Matthews DR, Charbonnel B et al. Efficacy and safety of pioglitazone versus metformin in patients with type 2 diabetes mellitus: A double-blind, randomized trial. *J Clin Endocrinol Metab* 2004; 89:6068–6076.

52. DeFronzo RA, Goodman AM. Efficacy of metformin in patients with non-insulin-dependent diabetes mellitus. The Multicenter Metformin Study Group. *N Engl J Med* 1995; 333:541–549.

53. Inzucchi SE, Lipska KJ, Mayo H et al. Metformin in patients with type 2 diabetes and kidney disease: A systematic review. *JAMA* 2014; 312:2668–2675.

54. Richy FF, Sabido-Espin M, Guedes S et al. Incidence of lactic acidosis in patients with type 2 diabetes with and without renal impairment treated with metformin: A retrospective cohort study. *Diabetes Care* 2014; 37:2291–2295.

55. Shaw JS, Wilmot RL, Kilpatrick ES. Establishing pragmatic estimated GFR thresholds to guide metformin prescribing. *Diabet Med* 2007; 24:1160–1163.

56. Lipska KJ, Bailey CJ, Inzucchi SE. Use of metformin in the setting of mild-to-moderate renal insufficiency. *Diabetes Care* 2011; 34:1431–1437.

57. Aroda VR, Edelstein SL, Goldberg RB et al. Long-term metformin use and vitamin B12 deficiency in the diabetes prevention program outcomes study. *J Clin Endocrinol Metab* 2016; 101:1754–1761.

58. Brown FR Jr, Friskey RW, Grindle L et al. Treatment of diabetic patients; observations on the use of carbutamide and tolbutamide. *Calif Med* 1956; 85:285–288.
59. Brown FR Jr, Friskey RW, Kinsell LW et al. Observations with sulfonylureas in diabetes. *Metabolism* 1956; 5:864–867.
60. Bryan J, Aguilar-Bryan L. Sulfonylurea receptors: ABC transporters that regulate ATP-sensitive K(+) channels. *Biochim Biophys Acta* 1999; 1461:285–303.
61. Meier JJ, Gallwitz B, Schmidt WE et al. Is impairment of ischaemic preconditioning by sulfonylurea drugs clinically important? *Heart* 2004; 90:9–12.
62. Forst T, Hanefeld M, Jacob S et al. Association of sulphonylurea treatment with all-cause and cardio-vascular mortality: A systematic review and meta-analysis of observational studies. *Diab Vasc Dis Res* 2013; 10:302–314.
63. Gallwitz B, Rosenstock J, Rauch T et al. 2-year efficacy and safety of linagliptin compared with glimepiride in patients with type 2 diabetes inadequately controlled on metformin: A randomised, double-blind, non-inferiority trial. *Lancet* 2012; 380:475–483.
64. Schloot NC, Haupt A, Schutt M et al. Risk of severe hypoglycemia in sulfonylurea-treated patients from diabetes centers in Germany/Austria: How big is the problem? Which patients are at risk? *Diabetes Metab Res Rev* 2015; 32:316–324.
65. Dornhorst A. Insulinotropic meglitinide analogues. *Lancet* 2001; 358:1709–1716.
66. Chan SP, Colagiuri S. Systematic review and meta-analysis of the efficacy and hypoglycemic safety of gliclazide versus other insulinotropic agents. *Diabetes Res Clin Pract* 2015; 110:75–81.
67. Fujita T, Sugiyama Y, Taketomi S et al. Reduction of insulin resistance in obese and/or diabetic animals by 5-[4-(1-methylcyclohexylmethoxy)benzyl]-thiazolidine-2,4-dione (ADD-3878, U-63,287, ciglitazone), a new antidiabetic agent. *Diabetes* 1983; 32:804–810.
68. Iwamoto Y, Kuzuya T, Matsuda A et al. Effect of new oral antidiabetic agent CS-045 on glucose toler-ance and insulin secretion in patients with NIDDM. *Diabetes Care* 1991; 14:1083–1086.
69. Suter SL, Nolan JJ, Wallace P et al. Metabolic effects of new oral hypoglycemic agent CS-045 in NIDDM subjects. *Diabetes Care* 1992; 15:193–203.
70. Sauer S. Ligands for the nuclear peroxisome proliferator-activated receptor gamma. *Trends Pharmacol Sci* 2015; 36:688–704.
71. Zhang H, Zhang A, Kohan DE et al. Collecting duct-specific deletion of peroxisome proliferator-activated receptor gamma blocks thiazolidinedione-induced fluid retention. *Proc Natl Acad Sci USA* 2005; 102:9406–9411.
72. Billington EO, Grey A, Bolland MJ. The effect of thiazolidinediones on bone mineral density and bone turnover: Systematic review and meta-analysis. *Diabetologia* 2015; 58:2238–2246.
73. Home PD, Pocock SJ, Beck-Nielsen H et al. Rosiglitazone evaluated for cardiovascular outcomes in oral agent combination therapy for type 2 diabetes (RECORD): A multicentre, randomised, open-label trial. *Lancet* 2009; 373:2125–2135.
74. Dormandy JA, Charbonnel B, Eckland DJ et al. Secondary prevention of macrovascular events in patients with type 2 diabetes in the PROactive Study (PROspective pioglitAzone Clinical Trial In mac-roVascular Events): A randomised controlled trial. *Lancet* 2005; 366:1279–1289.
75. Kahn SE, Haffner SM, Heise MA et al. Glycemic durability of rosiglitazone, metformin, or glyburide monotherapy. *N Engl J Med* 2006; 355:2427–2443.
76. Kernan WN, Viscoli CM, Furie KL et al. Pioglitazone after ischemic stroke or transient ischemic attack. *N Engl J Med* 2016; 374:1321–1331.
77. Mamtani R, Haynes K, Bilker WB et al. Association between longer therapy with thiazolidinediones and risk of bladder cancer: A cohort study. *J Natl Cancer Inst* 2012; 104:1411–1421.
78. Holst JJ. The physiology of glucagon-like peptide 1. *Physiol Rev* 2007; 87:1409–1439.
79. Sisley S, Gutierrez-Aguilar R, Scott M et al. Neuronal GLP1R mediates liraglutide's anorectic but not glucose-lowering effect. *J Clin Invest* 2014; 124:2456–2463.
80. Secher A, Jelsing J, Baquero AF et al. The arcuate nucleus mediates GLP-1 receptor agonist liraglutide-dependent weight loss. *J Clin Invest* 2014; 124:4473–4488.
81. Harris KB, McCarty DJ. Efficacy and tolerability of glucagon-like peptide-1 receptor agonists in patients with type 2 diabetes mellitus. *Ther Adv Endocrinol Metab* 2015; 6:3–18.
82. Fisher M. Glucagon-like peptide 1 receptor agonists and cardiovascular risk in type 2 diabetes: A clini-cal perspective. *Diabetes Obes Metab* 2015; 17:335–342.
83. Sokos GG, Nikolaidis LA, Mankad S et al. Glucagon-like peptide-1 infusion improves left ventricu-lar ejection fraction and functional status in patients with chronic heart failure. *J Card Fail* 2006; 12:694–699.

84. Read PA, Hoole SP, White PA et al. A pilot study to assess whether glucagon-like peptide-1 protects the heart from ischemic dysfunction and attenuates stunning after coronary balloon occlusion in humans. *Circ Cardiovasc Interv* 2011; 4:266–272.

85. Monami M, Cremasco F, Lamanna C et al. Glucagon-like peptide-1 receptor agonists and cardiovascular events: A meta-analysis of randomized clinical trials. *Exp Diabetes Res* 2011; 2011:1–10.

86. Marso SP, Daniels GH, Brown-Frandsen K et al. Liraglutide and cardiovascular outcomes in type 2 diabetes. *N Engl J Med* 2016; 375:311–322.

87. Garber A, Henry R, Ratner R et al. Liraglutide versus glimepiride monotherapy for type 2 diabetes (LEAD-3 Mono): A randomised, 52-week, phase III, double-blind, parallel-treatment trial. *Lancet* 2009; 373:473–481.

88. Garber A, Henry RR, Ratner R et al. Liraglutide, a once-daily human glucagon-like peptide 1 analogue, provides sustained improvements in glycaemic control and weight for 2 years as monotherapy compared with glimepiride in patients with type 2 diabetes. *Diabetes Obes Metab* 2011; 13:348–356.

89. Denker PS, Dimarco PE. Exenatide (exendin-4)-induced pancreatitis: A case report. *Diabetes Care* 2006; 29:471.

90. Alves C, Batel-Marques F, Macedo AF. A meta-analysis of serious adverse events reported with exenatide and liraglutide: Acute pancreatitis and cancer. *Diabetes Res Clin Pract* 2012; 98:271–284.

91. Bjerre Knudsen L, Madsen LW, Andersen S et al. Glucagon-like Peptide-1 receptor agonists activate rodent thyroid C-cells causing calcitonin release and C-cell proliferation. *Endocrinology* 2010; 151:1473–1486.

92. Retnakaran R, Kramer CK, Choi H et al. Liraglutide and the preservation of pancreatic beta-cell function in early type 2 diabetes: The LIBRA trial. *Diabetes Care* 2014; 37:3270–3278.

93. Zinman B, Gerich J, Buse JB et al. Efficacy and safety of the human glucagon-like peptide-1 analog liraglutide in combination with metformin and thiazolidinedione in patients with type 2 diabetes (LEAD-4 Met + TZD). *Diabetes Care* 2009; 32:1224–1230.

94. Scheen AJ. Pharmacokinetics and clinical use of incretin-based therapies in patients with chronic kidney disease and type 2 diabetes. *Clin Pharmacokinet* 2015; 54:1–21.

95. Kim D, Wang L, Beconi M et al. (2R)-4-oxo-4-[3-(trifluoromethyl)-5,6-dihydro[1,2,4]triazolo[4,3-a] pyrazin-7(8H)- yl]-1-(2,4,5-trifluorophenyl)butan-2-amine: A potent, orally active dipeptidyl peptidase IV inhibitor for the treatment of type 2 diabetes. *J Med Chem* 2005; 48:141–151.

96. Herman GA, Bergman A, Stevens C et al. Effect of single oral doses of sitagliptin, a dipeptidyl peptidase-4 inhibitor, on incretin and plasma glucose levels after an oral glucose tolerance test in patients with type 2 diabetes. *J Clin Endocrinol Metab* 2006; 91:4612–4619.

97. Tran L, Zielinski A, Roach AH et al. Pharmacologic treatment of type 2 diabetes: Oral medications. *Ann Pharmacother* 2015; 49:540–556.

98. Green JB, Bethel MA, Armstrong PW et al. Effect of sitagliptin on cardiovascular outcomes in type 2 diabetes. *N Engl J Med* 2015; 373:232–242.

99. Aschner P, Chan J, Owens DR et al. Insulin glargine versus sitagliptin in insulin-naive patients with type 2 diabetes mellitus uncontrolled on metformin (EASIE): A multicentre, randomised open-label trial. *Lancet* 2012; 379:2262–2269.

100. Goke B, Gallwitz B, Eriksson JG et al. Saxagliptin vs. glipizide as add-on therapy in patients with type 2 diabetes mellitus inadequately controlled on metformin alone: Long-term (52-week) extension of a 52-week randomised controlled trial. *Int J Clin Pract* 2013; 67:307–316

101. Aschner P, Katzeff HL, Guo H et al. Efficacy and safety of monotherapy of sitagliptin compared with metformin in patients with type 2 diabetes. *Diabetes Obes Metab* 2010; 12:252–261.

102. Zannad F, Cannon CP, Cushman WC et al. Heart failure and mortality outcomes in patients with type 2 diabetes taking alogliptin versus placebo in EXAMINE: A multicentre, randomised, double-blind trial. *Lancet* 2015; 385:2067–2076.

103. Ferrannini E, DeFronzo RA. Impact of glucose-lowering drugs on cardiovascular disease in type 2 diabetes. *Eur Heart J* 2015; 36:2288–2296.

104. Rossetti L, Smith D, Shulman GI et al. Correction of hyperglycemia with phlorizin normalizes tissue sensitivity to insulin in diabetic rats. *J Clin Invest* 1987; 79:1510–1515.

105. Wright EM, Loo DD, Hirayama BA. Biology of human sodium glucose transporters. *Physiol Rev* 2011; 91:733–794.

106. Abdul-Ghani MA, Norton L, DeFronzo RA. Renal sodium-glucose cotransporter inhibition in the management of type 2 diabetes mellitus. *Am J Physiol Renal Physiol* 2015; 309:F889–F900 ajprenal 00267 02015.

107. Forst T, Guthrie R, Goldenberg R et al. Efficacy and safety of canagliflozin over 52 weeks in patients with type 2 diabetes on background metformin and pioglitazone. *Diabetes Obes Metab* 2014; 16:467–477.

108. Bailey CJ, Gross JL, Pieters A et al. Effect of dapagliflozin in patients with type 2 diabetes who have inadequate glycaemic control with metformin: A randomised, double-blind, placebo-controlled trial. *Lancet* 2010; 375:2223–2233.
109. Haring HU, Merker L, Seewaldt-Becker E et al. Empagliflozin as add-on to metformin plus sulfonyl-urea in patients with type 2 diabetes: A 24-week, randomized, double-blind, placebo-controlled trial. *Diabetes Care* 2013; 36:3396–3404.
110. Jabbour SA, Hardy E, Sugg J et al. Dapagliflozin is effective as add-on therapy to sitagliptin with or without metformin: A 24-week, multicenter, randomized, double-blind, placebo-controlled study. *Diabetes Care* 2014; 37:740–750.
111. Zinman B, Wanner C, Lachin JM et al. Empagliflozin, cardiovascular outcomes, and mortality in type 2 diabetes. *N Engl J Med* 2015; 373:2117–2128.
112. Rosenstock J, Marx N, Kahn SE et al. Cardiovascular outcome trials in type 2 diabetes and the sulpho-nylurea controversy: Rationale for the active-comparator CAROLINA trial. *Diab Vasc Dis Res* 2013; 10:289–301.
113. Hine J, Paterson H, Abrol E et al. SGLT inhibition and euglycaemic diabetic ketoacidosis. *Lancet Diabetes Endocrinol* 2015; 3:503–504.
114. Hayami T, Kato Y, Kamiya H et al. Case of ketoacidosis by a sodium-glucose cotransporter 2 inhibitor in a diabetic patient with a low-carbohydrate diet. *J Diabetes Investig* 2015; 6:587–590.
115. Erondu N, Desai M, Ways K et al. Diabetic ketoacidosis and related events in the canagliflozin type 2 diabetes clinical program. *Diabetes Care* 2015; 38:1680–1686.
116. Taylor SI, Blau JE, Rother KI. SGLT2 inhibitors may predispose to ketoacidosis. *J Clin Endocrinol Metab* 2015; 100:2849–2852.
117. van de Laar FA. Alpha-glucosidase inhibitors in the early treatment of type 2 diabetes. *Vasc Health Risk Manag* 2008; 4:1189–1195.
118. Caspary WF. Sucrose malabsorption in man after ingestion of alpha-glucosidehydrolase inhibitor. *Lancet* 1978; 1:1231–1233.
119. Walton RJ, Sherif IT, Noy GA et al. Improved metabolic profiles in insulin-treated diabetic patients given an alpha-glucosidehydrolase inhibitor. *Br Med J* 1979; 1:220–221.
120. DiNicolantonio JJ, Bhutani J, O'Keefe JH. Acarbose: Safe and effective for lowering postprandial hyperglycaemia and improving cardiovascular outcomes. *Open Heart* 2015; 2:e000327.
121. Chiasson JL, Josse RG, Hunt JA et al. The efficacy of acarbose in the treatment of patients with non-insulin-dependent diabetes mellitus. A multicenter controlled clinical trial. *Ann Intern Med* 1994; 121:928–935.
122. Chiasson JL, Josse RG, Gomis R et al. Acarbose for prevention of type 2 diabetes mellitus: The STOP-NIDDM randomised trial. *Lancet* 2002; 359:2072–2077.
123. Sonne DP, Hansen M, Knop FK. Bile acid sequestrants in type 2 diabetes: Potential effects on GLP1 secretion. *Eur J Endocrinol* 2014; 171:R47–R65.
124. Garg A, Grundy SM. Cholestyramine therapy for dyslipidemia in non-insulin-dependent diabetes mel-litus. A short-term, double-blind, crossover trial. *Ann Intern Med* 1994; 121:416–422.
125. Ooi CP, Loke SC. Colesevelam for type 2 diabetes mellitus. *Cochrane Database Syst Rev* 2012; 12:CD009361.
126. Handelsman Y. Role of bile acid sequestrants in the treatment of type 2 diabetes. *Diabetes Care* 2011; 34(Suppl 2):S244–S250.
127. The Lipid Research Clinics Coronary Primary Prevention Trial results. I. Reduction in incidence of coronary heart disease. *JAMA* 1984; 251:351–364.
128. Thomas M, Tri VH, Perrault M. Action of bromocriptine on glucose metabolism in diabetics. *Sem Hop* 1977; 53:1857–1862.
129. Thomas M, Tri VH, Ribeiro F et al. Effects of bromocriptine CB 154 on glycoregulation in diabetics. *Ann Med Interne (Paris)* 1977; 128:685–690.
130. Scobie IN, Kesson CM, Ratcliffe JG et al. The effects of prolonged bromocriptine administration on PRL secretion GH and glycaemic control in stable insulin-dependent diabetes mellitus. *Clin Endocrinol (Oxf)* 1983; 18:179–185.
131. Defronzo RA. Bromocriptine: A sympatholytic, d2-dopamine agonist for the treatment of type 2 diabe-tes. *Diabetes Care* 2011; 34:789–794.
132. Cincotta AH, Meier AH. Bromocriptine (Ergoset) reduces body weight and improves glucose tolerance in obese subjects. *Diabetes Care* 1996; 19:667–670.
133. Pijl H, Ohashi S, Matsuda M et al. Bromocriptine: A novel approach to the treatment of type 2 diabetes. *Diabetes Care* 2000; 23:1154–1161.

134. Aminorroaya A, Janghorbani M, Ramezani M et al. Does bromocriptine improve glycemic control of obese type-2 diabetics? *Horm Res* 2004; 62:55–59.

135. Ghosh A, Sengupta N, Sahana P et al. Efficacy and safety of add on therapy of bromocriptine with metformin in Indian patients with type 2 diabetes mellitus: A randomized open labeled phase IV clinical trial. *Indian J Pharmacol* 2014; 46:24–28.

136. Gaziano JM, Cincotta AH, O'Connor CM et al. Randomized clinical trial of quick-release bromocriptine among patients with type 2 diabetes on overall safety and cardiovascular outcomes. *Diabetes Care* 2010; 33:1503–1508.

137. Gaziano JM, Cincotta AH, Vinik A et al. Effect of bromocriptine-QR (a quick-release formulation of bromocriptine mesylate) on major adverse cardiovascular events in type 2 diabetes subjects. *J Am Heart Assoc* 2012; 1:e002279.

138. Roe ED, Chamarthi B, Raskin P. Impact of bromocriptine-QR therapy on glycemic control and daily insulin requirement in type 2 diabetes mellitus subjects whose dysglycemia is poorly controlled on high-dose insulin: A Pilot Study. *J Diabetes Res* 2015; 2015:834903.

139. Mejia-Rodriguez O, Herrera-Abarca JE, Ceballos-Reyes G et al. Cardiovascular and renal effects of bromocriptine in diabetic patients with stage 4 chronic kidney disease. *Biomed Res Int* 2013; 2013:104059.

140. Buse JB, Rosenstock J, Sesti G et al. Liraglutide once a day versus exenatide twice a day for type 2 diabetes: A 26-week randomised, parallel-group, multinational, open-label trial (LEAD-6). *Lancet* 2009; 374:39–47.

141. Leahy JL. Intensive insulin therapy in Type 1 diabetes. In: Leahy JL, Cefalu WT, eds. *Insulin Therapy.* Boca Raton, FL: CRC Press, Taylor & Francis Group; 2002, 87–112.

142. Ritzel RA, Butler PC. Physiology of glucose homeostasis and insulin secretion. In: Leahy JL, Cefalu WT, eds. *Insulin Therapy.* Boca Raton, FL: CRC Press, Taylor & Francis Group; 2002, 61–72.

143. Benbow SJ, Walsh A, Gill GV. Brittle diabetes in the elderly. *J R Soc Med* 2001; 94:578–580.

144. Bain SC, Gill GV, Dyer PH et al. Characteristics of type 1 diabetes of over 50 years duration (the Golden Years Cohort). *Diabet Med* 2003; 20:808–811.

145. The effect of intensive treatment of diabetes on the development and progression of long-term complications in insulin-dependent diabetes mellitus. The Diabetes Control and Complications Trial Research Group. *N Engl J Med* 1993; 329:977–986.

146. The Diabetes Control and Complications Trial (DCCT)/Epidemiology of Diabetes Interventions and Complications (EDIC) Study Research Group. Intensive diabetes treatment and cardiovascular outcomes in type 1 diabetes: The DCCT/EDIC Study 30-year follow-up. *Diabetes Care* 2016; 39:686–693.

147. Epidemiology of severe hypoglycemia in the diabetes control and complications trial. The DCCT Research Group. *Am J Med* 1991; 90:450–459.

148. Bergenstal RM, Klonoff DC, Garg SK et al. Threshold-based insulin-pump interruption for reduction of hypoglycemia. *N Engl J Med* 2013; 369:224–232.

149. Wittlin SD, Woerle HJ, Gerich JE. Insulin pharmacokinetics. In: Leahy JL, Cefalu WT, eds. *Insulin Therapy.* Boca Raton, FL: CRC Press, Taylor & Francis Group; 2002, 73–86.

150. Bolli GB, Di Marchi RD, Park GD et al. Insulin analogues and their potential in the management of diabetes mellitus. *Diabetologia* 1999; 42:1151–1167.

151. Bolli GB, Hahn AD, Schmidt R et al. Plasma exposure to insulin glargine and its metabolites M1 and M2 after subcutaneous injection of therapeutic and supratherapeutic doses of glargine in subjects with type 1 diabetes. *Diabetes Care* 2012; 35:2626–2630.

152. Matsuhisa M, Koyama M, Cheng X et al. New insulin glargine 300 U/ml versus glargine 100 U/ml in Japanese adults with type 1 diabetes using basal and mealtime insulin: Glucose control and hypoglycaemia in a randomized controlled trial (EDITION JP 1). *Diabetes Obes Metab* 2016; 18:375–383.

153. Tibaldi JM. Evolution of insulin: From human to analog. *Am J Med* 2014; 127:S25–S38.

154. Plank J, Bodenlenz M, Sinner F et al. A double-blind, randomized, dose-response study investigating the pharmacodynamic and pharmacokinetic properties of the long-acting insulin analog detemir. *Diabetes Care* 2005; 28:1107–1112.

155. Heise T, Nosek L, Ronn BB et al. Lower within-subject variability of insulin detemir in comparison to NPH insulin and insulin glargine in people with type 1 diabetes. *Diabetes* 2004; 53:1614–1620.

156. Jonassen I, Havelund S, Hoeg-Jensen T et al. Design of the novel protraction mechanism of insulin degludec: an ultra-long-acting basal insulin. *Pharm Res* 2012; 29:2104–2114.

157. Heise T, Hermanski L, Nosek L et al. Insulin degludec: four times lower pharmacodynamic variability than insulin glargine under steady-state conditions in type 1 diabetes. *Diabetes Obes Metab* 2012; 14:859–864.

158. Heller S, Mathieu C, Kapur R et al. A meta-analysis of rate ratios for nocturnal confirmed hypoglycae-mia with insulin degludec vs. insulin glargine using different definitions for hypoglycaemia. *Diabet Med* 2016; 33:478–487.

159. Brange J, Owens DR, Kang S et al. Monomeric insulins and their experimental and clinical implica-tions. *Diabetes Care* 1990; 13:923–954.

160. Bode B. Insulin regimens. In: Bode B, ed. *Medical Management of Type 1 Diabetes*. 4th ed. Alexandria, VA: American Diabetes Association; 2004, 57–64.

161. Wolpert H. Figuring out your bolus doses. In: Wolpert H, ed. *Smart Pumping for People with Diabetes*. Alexandria, VA: American Diabetes Association; 2002, 40–56.

162. Lee P, Chang A, Blaum C et al. Comparison of safety and efficacy of insulin glargine and neutral prot-amine hagedorn insulin in older adults with type 2 diabetes mellitus: Results from a pooled analysis. *J Am Geriatr Soc* 2012; 60:51–59.

163. Lipska KJ, Warton EM, Huang ES et al. HbA1c and risk of severe hypoglycemia in type 2 diabetes: The diabetes and aging study. *Diabetes Care* 2013; 36:3535–3542.

164. Cho NH, Colagiuri S, Distiller L, Dong B et al. *Managing Older People with Type 2 Diabetes—Global Guideline*. Brussels, Belgium: International Diabetes Federation; 2013, 6–94.

20 Cardiovascular Disease

Matthew Dounel and K. Rao Poduri

CONTENTS

20.1 CARDIAC REHABILITATION AND SECONDARY PREVENTION

20.1.1 INTRODUCTION

Heart disease is the leading cause of death globally with 17.3 million deaths and among U.S. men and women is a cause of substantial morbidity and mortality. Each year about 1 million people survive heart attacks in the United States. Additionally, more than 7 million people have stable angina, more than 1 million patients have had angioplasty, and almost half a million patients have had bypass surgery.

In comparison with the general population, survivors of a heart attack have a higher incidence of sudden death and illness, including another heart attack, angina, heart failure (HF), and stroke. Cardiac rehabilitation improves patient outcomes and quality of life after a heart attack by providing a multidisciplinary approach to reducing cardiovascular risk and preventing secondary cardiac events and serious sequelae. The aim of cardiac rehabilitation is to restore and improve function, minimize disability, reduce cardiac risk factors, and optimize cardiac conditioning. These goals are achieved through a prescribed education and exercise program individualized to patients with cardiac disease with the goal to resume their normal activities of daily living and minimize their risk of progression of cardiac disease.[1-4]

20.2   DEMOGRAPHICS

Coronary heart disease (CHD) is the leading cause of death in adults in the United States, accounting for about one-third of all deaths in subjects over age 35. The 2010 Heart Disease and Stroke Statistics update of the American Heart Association (AHA) reported that the 2006 overall death rate from cardiovascular disease (CVD) was 262.5 per 100,000. The update reported that 17.6 million persons in the United States have CHD, including 8.5 million with myocardial infarction and 10.2 million with angina pectoris. The reported prevalence increases with age for both women and men.

Mortality rates for CVD and CHD in men and women have fallen in most developed countries by 24%–50% since 1975, although the decline has slowed since 1990. The Global Burden of Disease Study 2013 estimated that 17.3-million deaths worldwide in 2013 were related to cardiovascular diseases (CVDs) (CVD in selected countries between 1970 and 2009), a 41% increase since 1990 (Figure 20.1).[5,6]

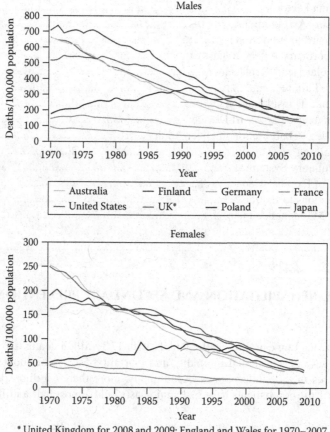

* United Kingdom for 2008 and 2009; England and Wales for 1970–2007.

FIGURE 20.1   Death rates for CHD. Age adjusted to the European Standard Population. (Reproduced from NHLBI Fact Book, 2011. National Heart Lung and Blood Institute. Available at: http://www.nhlbi.nih.gov/about/factbook/toc.ht.)

In the 1960s cardiac rehabilitation programs were first developed once the benefits of ambulation during prolonged hospitalization for coronary events had been recognized. Subsequently after discharge from the hospital, the process of physical reconditioning was continued at home. Concern about the safety of unsupervised exercise after discharge led to the development of highly structured rehabilitation programs that were supervised by physicians and included electrocardiographic (ECG) monitoring. The focus of these programs was almost exclusively on exercise.[7,8]

Currently, cardiac rehabilitation focuses not only on medically supervised exercises but also on other essential elements, including improving patients' function given their cardiac impairments, patient evaluation, lifestyle modification, physical activity, and nutritional counseling, psychosocial counseling or referral, and risk factor management and reduction, including cholesterol level, blood pressure, weight, diabetes, and smoking.[2-4,9]

There is a 20%–30% reduction in all-cause mortality rates with decreased mortality at up to 5 years postparticipation in cardiac rehabilitation. Furthermore, individuals who participated in a cardiac rehabilitation program report reduced symptoms including angina, dyspnea, and fatigue in addition to improving adherence to preventive medications for their respective cardiac conditions.

Participation in a cardiac rehabilitation program is associated with reduced hospitalizations and use of medical resources, improved health-related quality of life, and enhanced ability to perform the activities of daily living. In addition, participants in a cardiac rehabilitation program report an increased ability to return to work or engage in leisure activities and to improved psychosocial symptoms including depression and anxiety.[8,10,11]

Despite the benefits demonstrated, cardiac rehabilitation remains underutilized, particularly among women and minorities. Only 14%–35% of eligible heart attack survivors and 31% of patients after coronary bypass surgery participate in a cardiac rehabilitation program. The utilization rate for cardiac rehabilitation among people over 65 years of age in the United States is approximately 12%.[12,13]

Low patient participation rates in cardiac rehabilitation can be attributed to the lack of a referral or a strong endorsement from the patient's physician, limited follow-up or facilitation of enrollment after referral, and lack of program availability and access, and lack of perceived need for rehabilitation. Additional factors for poor participation in cardiac rehabilitation programs include patient conflicts with work or home responsibilities, hours of operation that conflict with work demands, scarcity of programs in rural areas in low income communities. Other limiting factors include lack of access to public transportation and parking, gender-dominated cardiac rehabilitation programs with little racial diversity among staff, and language barriers between patients and healthcare providers.[14,15]

20.3 RISK FACTOR MODIFICATION: PRIMARY AND SECONDARY PREVENTION

An important component of any cardiac rehabilitation is achievement of a patient's healthier lifestyle through a program with a goal of cardiac risk factor modification. Cardiac risk factors can be divided into two major categories: reversible and irreversible risk factors. Irreversible risk factors include male gender, past history of vascular disease, age, and family history. Reversible risk factors include physical inactivity, obesity, hyperlipidemia, smoking cigarettes, and conditions such as diabetes mellitus type-2 and hypertension. The patient and family should be educated on the presence of their risks, and if appropriate family counseling should be provided.

A comprehensive secondary prevention program in cardiac rehabilitation for patients requires an aggressive reduction of risk factors through nutritional counseling, weight management, and adherence to prescribed drug therapy. Previously published guidelines from the AHA, American College of Cardiology, U.S. Public Health Service, and American Association of Cardiovascular and Pulmonary Rehabilitation about prevention of heart attack and death in CVD patients summarize evidence-based strategies and recommendations for controlling risk factors. Clinical trials during the past two decades have provided conclusive evidence of reduced mortality in patients with cardiovascular disease via the reduction of individual risk factors by pharmacological and nonpharmacological interventions. Early and aggressive identification and treatment of reversible risk factors is essential in individuals with significant reversible risks. Modification of reversible risk factors is part of a cardiac rehabilitation program, and should be part of a, "heart healthy" lifestyle for all individuals.[16–22]

Patients who receive cardiac rehabilitation programs typically have psychosocial dysfunction which includes depression, anger, anxiety disorders, and social isolation. Observational studies have demonstrated associations between psychosocial disorders and the risk of initial or recurrent cardiovascular events. These conditions should be identified and, when appropriate, treatment should be initiated including therapy and medical management. These interventions are an integral part of a cardiac rehabilitation program to improve the psychological well-being and quality of life of cardiac patients.[23–25]

20.4 REHABILITATION MANAGEMENT AND TREATMENT

The American Association of Cardiopulmonary Rehabilitation and the AHA have delineated core components that all cardiac rehabilitation programs should provide for secondary prevention efforts.[20] The goal of these components is to minimize cardiovascular risks, promote healthy behavior, patient adherence, and promote an active lifestyle for patients with CVD.

Cardiac rehabilitation is divided into three stages or phases. The first phase is considered the acute phase, which is during the inpatient period immediately following the cardiac event leading up to discharge and is characterized by early mobilization. The second phase is the rehabilitation phase which is initiated after the healing of the cardiac event is completed and characterized by aerobic conditioning and an intensive education program. The third phase is devoted to the maintenance of aerobic conditioning that has been maintained in phase II through a program of scheduled exercises. Secondary prevention and risk factor modification is provided and reemphasized throughout all three phases of rehabilitation.

20.5 PHASE I (INPATIENT PHASE)

20.5.1 HISTORY AND INTRODUCTION

Six weeks of bed rest were the recommendation for patients with myocardial infarction (MI) in the 1930s. Chair therapy was introduced in the 1940s, and by the early 1950s, 3–5 minutes of daily walking was advocated, beginning at 4weeks. Gradually clinicians began to recognize that early ambulation avoided many of the complications of bed rest, including deconditioning and pulmonary embolism (PE). However, there were concerns about the safety of unsupervised exercise which led to the development of structured, physician-supervised rehabilitation programs, which included clinical supervision, as well as ECG monitoring.

In the 1950s, Hellerstein presented a comprehensive rehabilitation of patients recovering from an acute cardiac event. He advocated a multidisciplinary approach to the rehabilitation program. His approach was adopted by cardiac rehabilitation programs throughout the world. Despite multiple advances, Hellerstein's original ideas have not been improved upon significantly. Multifactorial intervention targeted secondary prevention; incorporating aggressive risk factor modification has become an integral part of present day cardiac rehabilitation.[26]

Cardiac rehabilitation is recommended for patients with an acute coronary syndrome, recent myocardial revascularization, HF, or stable angina pectoris. The following indications are now covered by the Center for Medicare and Medicaid Services and many third party payers in the United States:

- Acute MI within the preceding 12 months
- Coronary artery bypass graft (CABG)

- Stable angina pectoris
- Heart valve repair/replacement
- Percutaneous coronary intervention (PCI) with or without stenting
- Heart or heart–lung transplant
- Chronic HF

Other candidates for cardiac rehabilitation/secondary prevention programs include those with diabetes, peripheral arterial disease, pulmonary artery hypertension, and congenital heart disease.[27–31]

Approximately 10%–20% of eligible patients following MI participate in formal structured cardiac rehabilitation in the United States and the United Kingdom. The primary reason is likely low rates of referral (20%–30%). Women, nonwhites, and patients over age 65 (and particularly older than 75) have particularly low rates. Other predictors of suboptimal participation include poor functional status, higher body mass index, tobacco use, and depression, long distance to facilities, low health literacy, and inflexible work schedules.[25,32,33]

Participation in a cardiac rehabilitation is associated with significant reductions in all-cause mortality and cardiac mortality. Cardiac rehabilitation is also associated with improvements in exercise tolerance, cardiac symptoms, lipid levels, cigarette smoking cessation rates (in conjunction with a smoking cessation program), stress levels, improved medical regimen compliance, and improved psychosocial well-being, as well as being cost effective.[7,34–36]

Phase IA is considered for patients recovering after a cardiac event or after vascularization who are hospitalized prior to discharge home. The main goal of a phase-I program is to provide an early mobilization program and condition a patient to perform most activities of daily living at home after discharge which is considered to be up to 4 METs.

A select population of patients in phase IA will be transitioned to phase IB which is considered for patients recovering after a cardiac event or after revascularization who are admitted to an acute or subacute rehabilitation facility prior to their discharge home. It is more common to see patients with cardiac disease in individuals with advanced age or individuals who have significant comorbidities that make mobilization more difficult. In this phase many of the rehabilitation specialists will care for these patients. The guidelines for exercise are often are the same as for phase 1 patients, however the period of recovery is considered longer. Exercise intensity limited to a safe target heart rate (HR) determined by a low level exercise tolerance test (ETT) or from known limitations from revascularization performed prior to discharge to a rehabilitation setting. The level of exercises can usually be determined to be at 70% maximum HR or a 5-MET level is acceptable. In individuals greater than 40 years of age it generally represents a HR of 130 beats per minute (bpm) or 5 METs, and for individuals less than 40 years of age, 140 bpm or 7 METs. A Borg rating of perceived exertion (RPE) of 7 (modified scale) and 15 (scale) can also be utilized to determine maximum tolerated exercise.[37–40]

20.6 PHASE II (TRAINING PHASE)

In the outpatient setting, cardiac rehabilitation programs provide secondary prevention initiatives in addition to supervised exercise training. The goal of these programs is to speed the recovery from acute cardiovascular events such as MI, myocardial revascularization, or hospitalization for HF, or heart or valve surgery, and to improve quality of life.

The components of a cardiac rehabilitation program include a comprehensive long-term program involving the following core components: (1) medical evaluation and baseline patient assessment; (2) exercise training and physical activity counseling; (3) coronary risk factor modification and secondary prevention which incorporates nutritional counseling and weight management; (4) psychosocial support; and (5) patient education regarding medication compliance.[2,3,41,42] These five core components are usually delivered by a dedicated team including a medical director, physician extenders and nurse clinicians, exercise physiologists and exercise professionals, nutritionists, counselors, and social workers.

A majority of outpatient cardiac rehabilitation programs consist of a program that patients participate in electrocardiogram-monitored, hour-long exercise sessions three times weekly for up to 8–12 weeks, and in some instances longer. The objectives of these sessions are to develop and teach an individualized exercise program for the patient that is considered to be both safe and effective, and to initiate targeted interventions that are aimed at reducing coronary risk factors, as well as identifying and managing psychosocial problems for these patients.[35,43,44]

Outpatient cardiac rehabilitation is typically ordered by health professionals for their patients who are candidates for outpatient cardiac rehabilitation. The first visit can be scheduled as early as the first week after hospitalization for an uncomplicated MI or PCI. Patients with a complicated hospital course or who received coronary artery bypass grafting may have to wait longer before starting depending on the referral of the health professional. Several studies have suggested that early enrollment can improve subsequent attendance and outcomes.[45–48]

20.6.1 Exercise Prescription

The objective of exercise in a cardiac rehabilitation program is to assess the patient's baseline ability and limitations, and to develop an exercise program. The risk of cardiovascular complications from exercise training should be evaluated before starting an exercise program. The AHA has published risk stratification guidelines to stratify prospective patients into four categories of risk according to clinical characteristics that includes contraindications for exercise.

Once exercise prescription has been developed, health professionals should observe the patient's response to that exercise program and encourage transition into a phase III exercise program which is a long-term participation in regular unsupervised exercise.

The components of an exercise prescription include the mode, frequency, duration, and intensity of exercise.

Mode—the mode of exercise should be aerobic exercise such as walking, jogging, cycling, machine stair climbing, and other endurance activities that require the use of large muscle groups. These exercises should be enjoyable to the patient for maximal compliance with the exercise prescription. Low impact activities are recommended because of a lesser risk of physical injury. Selected exercise modalities must take into account physical limitations and musculoskeletal conditions of the participants.

Frequency and duration—the recommended frequency of exercise in an outpatient cardiac rehabilitation program is at least three times a week but preferably to be on most days of the week, which would be necessary to achieve improvement in functional capacity. Outpatient cardiac rehabilitation programs can vary in their duration, however 12 weeks is common for most programs.[35,44,49,50]

Content — there are three phases for each exercise session:

- *Warm up session.* This component usually is for 5–10 minutes. Warm-up exercises can consist of stretching, flexibility movements, and aerobic activity that gradually increase the HR into the target range. There is a gradual increment in oxygen demand that minimizes the risk of exercise-related cardiovascular complications.
- *Training session.* This component consists of at least 20 minutes with an aim of 30–45 minutes of continuous or discontinuous aerobic activity.
- *Cool-down session.* This component consists of 5–10 minutes. The cool-down period involves low-intensity exercise and permits a gradual recovery from the conditioning phase. Transient decrease in venous return, reducing coronary blood flow when HR and myocardial oxygen consumption remain high can be a result of the omission of a cool-down session in an outpatient cardiac rehabilitation program. Adverse consequences can also include hypotension, angina, ischemic ST–T changes, and ventricular arrhythmias.[51]

Intensity—The intensity of exercise can range from 40% to 85% of functional capacity (VO_2max), which corresponds to 55%–90% of maximal HR (estimated as 220 minus the age in years, or more accurately measured at the highest exercise intensity on the maximal exercise test).

There are several methods for determination of the target HR. Selection of the intensity of the exercise program based upon a fixed percentage of maximal HR is the method commonly utilized to guide exercise intensity. A percentage range is calculated from the maximal heart rate (percent HRmax) reached at peak exercise during a symptom-limited ETT. Exercise intensity has been categorized using the percent HRmax as light (<60%), moderate (60–79), and heavy (80%).[49]

Energy expenditure for an exercise session is related to both intensity and duration. In general, lower intensity exercise should be performed for a longer duration. Symptom-limited patients may begin with discontinuous exercise and progress to 20–30 minutes of continuous exercise. The duration is increased before increasing the intensity.

Participants in a supervised outpatient cardiac rehabilitation program rotate among a variety of dynamic exercise modalities including treadmill, bicycle, arm ergometer, rowing machine, etc. The energy expenditure and HR response for a supervised session are related to the intensity of the activity and the amount of muscle mass used to perform the activity.

Many patients in an outpatient cardiac rehabilitation program may be on beta blockers, which reduce the cardiac output (CO) response to exercise predominantly by limiting HR. Although resting HR, submaximal, and maximal exercise HRs are reduced by beta blockers, traditional HR methods may be used to prescribe exercise intensity based on the patient's maximal HR measured during an exercise test performed on medication.

Symptom-limited exercise test refers to a submaximal testing modality often conducted before initiating a cardiac rehabilitation program to establish a baseline fitness level, determine maximal HR, and assess the safety of exercise by observing symptoms and ECG indications of ischemia or cardiac arrhythmia. A symptom-limited exercise test is terminated at the onset of symptoms related to CHD, usually chest pain or shortness of breath. The HR level from the symptom-limited exercise test becomes the maximal HR, and the exercise training HR is a given rate for the given exercise prescription.[52] There is a relationship between exercise HR and VO_2 or MET (metabolic equivalent of training). One MET is defined as 3.5 mL O_2 uptake/kg min^{-1}, which is the resting oxygen uptake in a sitting position.[53]

Borg scale—RPE: Exercise intensity can also be prescribed using the RPE. This is a validated method that most patients can learn and apply with unsupervised exercise. On the RPE scale of 6–20, an RPE of 12–13 (somewhat hard) corresponds to 60% VO_2max and an RPE of 16 (hard to very hard) corresponds to 85% VO_2max. The exercise intensity for healthy adults is usually 60%–70% of functional capacity (using VO_2max, maximal METs, or HR maximum reserve) or a 12–13 level of the RPE scale. Individuals with a low-baseline fitness level, which is often the case with cardiac patients, should begin at a lower percentage of capacity. Patients with stable angina may have an exercise prescription based upon 60%–70% of the HR at which ischemic ST segment changes or anginal symptoms appear.[54-56]

Exercise progression: Another component of an exercise prescription is the progression of exercise. There is no standard format for exercise progression, but should be individualized according to patient motivation, goals, symptoms, tolerance, baseline fitness level, and musculoskeletal limitations.[57]

Once the aerobic exercise targets have been attained, many cardiac rehabilitation programs incorporate resistance training as well. The primary goals of resistance training are to increase muscle strength, endurance, and mass, and enhance a patient's ability to perform household and vocational tasks.

Resistance exercises are referenced to the individual's measured or estimated maximal strength or the "one-repetition maximum," or the maximal weight a patient can lift once. A recommendation for resistance training for cardiac patients includes 30%–40% of the one-repetition maximum for upper body exercises and 40%–50% of one-repetition maximum for lower body exercises; with 12–15 repetitions per set, performed two to three times weekly.[56]

Cardiac rehabilitation programs typically address the traditional modifiable risk factors of smoking, hypertension, diabetes, and lipid abnormalities. The success of these interventions depends largely upon patient compliance; therefore, patient compliance with medications, exercise, diet, and smoking cessation should be assessed regularly by the outpatient rehabilitation team. When staff identifies poor compliance; the etiology should be identified and encouragement and alternatives should be provided.

The aim of nutritional counseling is aimed at achieving weight loss or control and an improved lipid profile and blood pressure level. Lifestyle modification interventions with patient include discussion on dietary habits, food choices, and how to implement an individualized dietary plan. Strategies on sodium restriction and diabetes control should also be included.

The aim of smoking cessation and prevention of relapse include patient education about the risks of continued smoking; referral to smoking cessation group programs; nicotine patch therapy, nicorette gum, or other pharmacotherapy; self-help literature and encouragement by the primary care providers. Effective smoking cessation can be difficult to achieve because of the strong psychological and physiologic dependence that occurs with this patient population.[44,58]

The optimal pharmacologic management of diabetes, hypertension, and dyslipidemia are usually instituted in parallel by the physician. In the absence of a contraindication, all patients are prescribed medications as indicated for their treatment and their risk factors and for secondary prevention. The role of the outpatient cardiac rehabilitation program with regard to these conditions is to continue the educational process, monitor compliance with recommended therapies, and monitor outcomes.

A major component of a cardiac rehabilitation program is the identification and management of the variety of psychosocial and vocational problems that arise as a consequence to a cardiac event or cardiac diagnosis. Depression, anxiety, and denial of medical conditions are common in patients following MI, occurring in up to 20% of patients. Patients with depression can have lower exercise capacity, less energy, more fatigue, and a reduced quality of life and sense of well-being. Furthermore, younger women are at increased risk for depression.[58–61] Individual or group psychotherapy and sometimes pharmacotherapy are beneficial for treatment. Trained health personnel including psychologists, psychiatrists, and social workers should be available within the cardiac rehabilitation program or on a referral basis to best manage these specific issues.

20.7   ALTERNATIVE OUTPATIENT PROGRAMS

Alternative approaches to the delivery of supervised cardiac rehabilitation include home-based programs with monitoring of exercise, community-based setting programs, disease management, and lifestyle health coaching interventions delivered by nonphysician health professionals using the telephone and Internet, and other Internet-based case management systems. The long-term assessment of the effectiveness of these approaches and the optimal mode of their delivery remain unknown. The attractiveness of these models is the potential to provide cardiac rehabilitation to low- and moderate-risk coronary patients.[27,62–65]

20.8   CARDIAC REHABILITATION IN SELECT POPULATIONS

28.8.1   Angina Pectoris

For patients with stable angina syndrome a cardiac rehabilitation program should be encouraged. The goal of cardiac rehabilitation for patients with angina is to utilize the training effectively to improve the efficiency of exercise performance below the anginal threshold. Exercise can result in a lower oxygen requirement for a given workload, thereby improving exercise tolerance, promoting a sense of well-being, and reducing symptoms. The increase in work capacity achieved will often lead to an increase in functional capacity that can significantly decrease the disability caused by recurrent chest pain that patients would experience from angina.

Furthermore, with exercise there is a possible benefit of reduction of atherosclerotic lesions and increased cardiac collateralization that is cardio-protective and symptom reducing. Prior to the initiation of a cardiac rehabilitation exercise program, a full level ETT should be done in order to determine the target and maximum HRs and rule out potential life threatening events. Cardiac rehabilitation programs can be initiated at phase II as this patient population has not suffered an actual infarction.

A cardiac rehabilitation program is also beneficial in secondary prevention incorporating the management of risk factors for coronary heart disease such as lipids, blood pressure, obesity, and diabetes mellitus.[66–69]

20.8.2 CARDIAC ARRHYTHMIAS

The risk of death from cardiac arrhythmia during rehabilitation is low. According to one study, in 25,420 patients with 743,471 hours of exercise training, there was a risk of one myocardial arrest event for every 1.3 million therapy hours and one cardiac event for every 49,565 patient hours of exercise. For patients with life-threatening arrhythmias, the automatic implantable cardiac defibrillator (AICD) has been increasingly used to improve safety. The modification of an exercise program with patients with AICD is mostly to set to avoid the HR at which the AICD should fire. An exercise stress test and cardiac precautions with target HR set below the trigger threshold are recommended modifications to the exercise program. Patients with AICD who participated in a cardiac rehabilitation program have been shown to have a good functional outcome. Furthermore, an important component of patients with AICD who participate in a cardiac rehabilitation program is reassurance and support about the safety of exercise, there is a role of cognitive-behavioral modification program for anxiety about recurrent arrhythmias.[70–72]

20.8.3 MYOCARDIAL INFARCTION

The main goal of a phase I program is to provide early mobilization and condition a patient to perform most activities of daily living at home after discharge which is considered to be up to 4 METs. The basics of an early mobilization program is outlined in the Wenger Protocol and was designed to transition individuals post-MI from bed rest to climbing two flights of stairs with current programs achieving this goal in 3–5 days. The target for early mobilization reflects the current trend to decrease length of stay in addition to the recognition of the early benefits of mobilization.

According to the Wenger Protocol patients are encouraged to be sitting out of bed in a chair as soon as medically stable usually by day 1–2. By day 2 or 3, patients are initiated on an ambulation program for short distances along with advancement of ADL (activities of daily living) training to include bathroom privileges. By approximately day 3, patients progress with their ambulation program with increased distances, stair negotiation is initiated, and a home exercise program is introduced. After a successful completion of a low level ETT for risk stratification on day 4 or 5, the patient completes learning home exercises and is discharged.

An educational program relating to risk factor modification should be introduced since many patients are ready to receive advice on risk factor reduction prior to discharge.

Early mobilization should be initiated with appropriate cardiac monitoring under the supervision of a trained physical therapist and occupational therapist. The post-MI HR rise should be kept to within 20 beats per minute (bpm) of baseline and the systolic blood pressure rise within 20 mm Hg of baseline and any decrease of systolic blood pressure of 10 mm Hg or more should be considered worrisome and exercise halted.[37,38]

20.8.4 POSTCORONARY ARTERY BYPASS SURGERY

Coronary artery bypass (CABG) surgery is recommended for patients with obstructive coronary artery disease whose survival will be improved compared to medical therapy or percutaneous coronary intervention (PCI). Furthermore, patients with angina pectoris that is refractory to medical therapy may receive a recommendation for CABG if PCI cannot be performed. CABG involves the construction of one or more grafts between the arterial and coronary circulations. Graft patency, advancement of disease in the native vessels, and comorbid conditions are major predictors of long-term mortality, particularly in patients aged 65 years or older.[73] The benefits of cardiac rehabilitation in the post bypass patient population include increased ischemic threshold, improved left ventricular function, increased coronary collaterals, decreased serum lipids, decreased serum catecholamines, decreased platelet aggregation and increased fibrinolysis, and improved psychological status.[74]

The major complications associated with CABG are death, MI, wound infection, prolonged requirement for mechanical ventilation, acute kidney injury, and bleeding requiring transfusion or reoperation.[75–78] Atrial fibrillation (AF) is an additional postoperative complication and is usually self-limited if the patient did not have a prior history of AF.[79] A frequent complication of CABG is a low CO, primarily due to left ventricular dysfunction and is often transient and responds to fluid replacement and/or a brief period of inotropic support.[80]

Additional complications include pericarditis after CABG, which is due to pericardial injury and known as a postpericardiotomy syndrome. The most frequent complaint is chest pain, occurring a few days to several weeks after surgery. In most cases, the effusion is small and clinically insignificant; however, the pericardial effusion may be large, resulting in tamponade and hemodynamic instability requiring urgent therapy with pericardiocentesis or reoperation. Postoperative anticoagulation may increase the risk of tamponade in patients who develop an effusion.[81–83] Neurological complications include brachial plexus injury, stroke, intracranial hemorrhage, encephalopathy, delirium, and seizures.[84–87] Patients with postcoronary artery bypass grafting should be closely monitored for complications and have a cardiac rehabilitation program individualized to address their complications in a cardiac rehabilitation program.

Cardiac rehabilitation after CABG can be thought of as being similar to a post-MI rehabilitation program. Phase I rehabilitation begins in the intensive care unit with a goal for mobilization on day 1 if the patient has not had a stable postoperative course or severe HF. The program is often initiated with sitting upright, active leg exercises, and subsequent mobilization out of bed. The patient subsequently progresses to supervised ambulation for distances to 150–200 ft with patients advancing to independent ambulation by day 3. Early mobilization provides several benefits of reducing deleterious effects of immobilization including decreasing risk of DVT (deep vein thrombosis), PE, and cardiac deconditioning.

Subsequent to discharge the patient and medical team develop a program that allows the patient to be self-monitored at home with gradual progression to previous levels of activity. In addition identification and prevention of secondary risk factors are incorporated into the program. Patients who are at high risk and those that require intensive interventions may require an inpatient phase IB rehabilitation program before transitioning into the outpatient setting. Patients in the IB setting can include those with neurological complications. Phase IB programs and outpatient programs for patients at high risk should be tailored to the needs of the patient in coordination with their cardiologist and/or cardiothoracic surgeon.

The phase II post-CABG program is usually conducted at home or in an outpatient setting under the supervision of physicians. Appropriate risk stratification is conducted to place patients in low-, medium-, or high-intensity programs. A low-intensity program is a progressive ambulation program with 2–4-MET energy expenditures and a target HR 65%–75% of maximum HR. Moderate-intensity programs can be progressive ambulation programs from 3 to 6.5-MET energy expenditures and a target HR 70%–80% HR maximum. High-intensity programs can incorporate a walk–jog program from 5 to 8.5-MET energy expenditure levels with a target HR of 75%–85% HRmax. For patients who are receiving a beta blocker HR usually can be set at 20 bpm above resting HR or can be determined through an ETT. An ETT can be safely performed at 3–4 weeks after CABG. The goal of the exercise test is to determine the maximum functional capacity, maximum HR, exercise blood pressure response, exercise induced arrhythmias, and anginal threshold. Patients in phase II program can transition into the phase III program where they are provided with a home exercise program with appropriate monitoring by their supervising physicians.[74,88–91]

For those patients who undergo an open heart surgery with a median sternotomy, precautions are important. The strongest force that challenges the sternum is the pectoralis muscles. These muscles pull in opposing directions holding down the wire sutures. Sternal disruption can occur in 2%–8% of the population with a median sternotomy. Patients are at risk if they have risk factors that hinder bone healing including smoking, obesity, steroids, osteoporosis, and diabetes mellitus. Patients should receive instructions in sternal precautions within the first few days after surgery. These instructions include the proper method of going from supine to sitting position, which includes rolling on one side and propping oneself up on an elbow instead of attempting a partial sit-up. Patients are instructed to utilize their legs rather than pushing down with their arms which can exert an unequal pull on their sternum. Self-hugging or hugging a pillow when coughing or sneezing can help to brace the sternotomy incision. Sternal precautions should be rigorously followed for at least 3 months after surgery and lifting should be limited to <10 lb. Avoidance of simultaneous bilateral shoulder flexion, abduction to >90° is recommended. Also important is to advise patients not to drive or sit in a passenger seat behind an airbag for 4 weeks.

Patients who undergo a sternotomy have to follow the recommended precautions postoperatively.[92–94] These precautions are dependent upon the surgeon and the institution and should be obtained from the surgeon at the institution where the patient had undergone the procedure.

20.8.5 VALVULAR HEART REPLACEMENT

The overall training program for patients undergoing valve replacement is similar to the post-CABG patient. Patients who undergo a median sternotomy should undergo sternal precautions to prevent sternal disruption. An issue that is present with patients after valve replacement is the presence of postoperative anticoagulation for mechanical valves. Patients on anticoagulation therapy are at risk of bruising and hemarthrosis. Therefore, it is recommended that this patient population avoid high-impact exercises to avoid these complications and include a component of education regarding injury avoidance.

In addition, patients who are maybe at risk of patient–prosthetic mismatch (PPM) may have a lower predicted exercise capacity than patients without PPM. Individualized exercise prescriptions based on cardiologist assessment are recommended before a patient initiates a cardiac rehabilitation program.[95,96]

20.8.6 HEART FAILURE

Patients with HF often have limited exercise capacity because of dyspnea and fatigue. Symptoms of exercise-induced dyspnea may be interpreted by patients as worsening of their disease and make them fearful of exercise.[97] Furthermore, depression is prevalent in this population. The HF-ACTION trial in which the Beck Depression Inventory II was administered to 2322 patients at entry, 28% of patients had scores of 14 or higher, which is considered clinically significant for depression. Exercise training modestly improved the depression scores compared to the control group at 3 months with a smaller response at 1 year.[98]

Cardiac rehabilitation can improve functional capacity and quality of life in patients with HF and it should be offered to patients with stable class II to III HF who do not have advanced arrhythmias and or other limitations to exercise. This recommendation applies to patients with HF with reduced ejection fraction (HFrEF) as well as to patients with HF with preserved ejection fraction (HFpEF), although the evidence is not as strong for patients with HFpEF. Currently, there is not enough data to recommend cardiac rehabilitation for patients with class IV HF.[99,100]

In the United States, the Centers for Medicare and Medicaid Services (CMS) and most insurers provide coverage for outpatient cardiac rehabilitation services for patients with stable chronic HF with left ventricular ejection fraction ≤35% and New York Heart Association class II to IV symptoms with treatment with optimal HF therapy for at least 6 weeks. Stable is defined as no recent (≤6 weeks) or planned (≤6 months) major cardiovascular hospitalizations or procedures.[101]

HF-ACTION, the largest trial of exercise training in patients with HFrEF found that exercise training was well tolerated and safe. Aerobic interval training has been the type of training best studied in patients with left ventricular dysfunction and the type of exercise applied in HF-ACTION.

Aerobic activity is defined by movement through space and includes treadmill walking, cycling, upper body ergometry, dancing, swimming, and playing sports. With a variety of training modalities, patients may remain more engaged and find exercise enjoyable. Aerobic exercise blocks can alternate with intervals of rest. Resistive training has been less well studied in HF due to concerns about increasing vascular resistance and diastolic stiffness.[102,103]

20.8.7 Cardiac Transplantation

Although there are advances in the survival of cardiac transplant recipients, published reports have consistently shown abnormal levels of functional capacity post-transplantation. There is usually a rise in exercise capacity that occurs at approximately 2 months post-transplant in which many patients are able to return to their activities with improved quality of life. However, in this patient population, exercise function remains approximately 30%–40% below normal.[104–106]

Cardiac transplant candidates should initiate an exercise program as soon as possible after transplant listing and prior to cardiac transplant. The cardiac rehabilitation program should include both aerobic training as well as resistive exercise.[99,102,107,108]

If the program is instituted pre-transplantation, the patient will be familiar with range of motion exercises and should be able to reinitiate exercises with minimal reeducation shortly after transplantation. In addition, if the pre-transplant patient is in a better conditioned state, the few days of inactivity after transplant will do little to reverse this level of conditioning.

Pre-transplant cardiac rehabilitation programs can be divided into different groups; stable outpatients, patients on home inotropic therapy, and patients with a left ventricular assist device (LVAD).

For stable outpatients, a prescribed exercise program is recommended as an adjuvant to pharmacologic therapy during the entire pre-transplantation waiting period. For patients on home inotropic therapy, a monitored program in a cardiac rehabilitation center is recommended since inotropes can stimulate or worsen arrhythmias. For hospitalized patients who become dependent upon inotropic support therapy a similar type of program can be instituted in the hospital. In a controlled intensive care setting with appropriate medical supervision, a set routine consisting of bicycle, treadmill, upper body ergometry, and free weights can be carried out safely. For hospitalized patients on inotropic support who are being monitored hemodynamically, physical activity will vary depending upon the patients' mobility restrictions. Range of motion and leg movement exercises can be performed at the bedside with appropriate clinical supervision and restrictions. Furthermore, incentive spirometry will help insure that the ventilatory muscles remain active.[2,27,42,99,102,109]

In the immediate post-transplant period, the recommendations can be categorized prior to removal of chest tubes or pacer wires, once out of bed, once ambulation has begun, and prior to discharge. Exercise consists mainly of passive and active range of motion accompanied by incentive spirometry to facilitate pulmonary hygiene, prior to removal of the chest tubes and pacer wires.

Leg raising and hip girdle exercises can become useful as a preparation to transfer weight from sitting to standing when the patient is out of the bed to a chair. A trial of ambulation is initiated when the patient is able to stand which is initiated in the patient's room and progressing to the ward with appropriate telemetry monitoring. Intensity can be assessed by rate of perceived exertion, more commonly using the RPE (Borg) scale.[110]

If no allograft rejection occurs and prior to discharge, the patient may be able to exercise on a stationary bicycle ergometer and/or treadmill. A predischarge cardiopulmonary exercise test should be performed to better define an exercise prescription for an outpatient cardiac rehabilitation program for the phase II training phase.

The post-transplantation exercise prescription should include all the essentials of an exercise prescription including intensity, duration, frequency, and progression. Patients receiving rehabilitation programs should also be given specific exercise modalities, incorporating aerobic exercises and resistance training after at least the first 6 weeks post-transplantation, the time required to permit healing of the sternal incision with precautions determined by the referring surgeon. Although less well studied in transplant recipients, resistance exercise can be performed safely with appropriate sternal precautions and can increase strength and flexibility for tasks of daily living. It is recommended, therefore, that a resistance program be added to the aerobic training regimen.

The intensity can be determined by the Borg (RPE) scale. The RPE scale at the anaerobic threshold is used to prescribe intensity since the HR will not be commensurate to the effort because of cardiac denervation. Early in a cardiac program an outline detailing a progressive increase in exercise activity is important for improvement in function. An RPE of 11–13 often results in early deconditioning. Thus, every effort should be made to increase the intensity to at least RPE 13–15 to approach the ventilatory threshold, which may also improve with exercise.

The duration of the session including warm-up and cool-down is essential with a minimum of 20-minutes at the prescribed intensity. The frequency of exercise should be performed in a supervised setting three times per week for a minimum of 6–8 weeks with some programs constructed for up to a 12-week period. An extension of this duration of the program is often necessary to take into account early episodes of rejection or infection, which may preclude the opportunity to exercise for several days at a time.[111]

After the initial program of cardiac rehabilitation is completed, a repeat cardiopulmonary exercise test should be performed in order to update the exercise prescription. Patients should be encouraged to adopt exercise and activity as a way of life. Adherence to physical activity should be monitored in a similar fashion to adherence to the medical regimen.

20.8.8 LEFT VENTRICULAR ASSIST DEVICE

Continuous flow ventricular support devices which are primarily left ventricular assist devices (LVADs) and less frequently for biventricular support (biventricular assist devices [BiVAD]) are increasingly used for the management of patients with end stage HF stage D both as a bridge to transplantation and as destination therapy.[104–106,112]

LVADs work in parallel with the left ventricle actively contributing to the systemic circulation directly through ejection across the aortic valve and indirectly through LVAD filling. The growing role of ventricular assist devices, particularly those with continuous flow, in the physiology and rehabilitation of those patients needs to be readdressed. In addition, as LVAD implantation is on the rise as a bridge to a decision for cardiac transplantation, particularly in older patients.[113]

HF patients are debilitated, bedbound, malnourished, and are often dependent on intravenous medications to support the circulation at rest prior to surgery. Following LVAD implantation, these patients become ambulatory and could benefit from intensive rehabilitation including physical therapy. Formal cardiac rehab programs post-LVAD have not been well described and most rehabilitation centers are unfamiliar with the operation of LVADs. Close collaboration between the device and rehabilitation centers is needed to develop successful rehabilitation programs. There is minimal data on the impact of aerobic training in this patient population.[114]

Early and late mobilization may improve quality of life in this growing population that may be very limited in their functional capacity. According to the AHA statements on cardiac rehabilitation, further investigations are needed to determine the effect of exercise training in patients receiving mechanical circulatory support as the data is not clear.[2,27,115]

20.8.9 Cardiac Rehabilitation in Older Adults

Older patients, regardless of age derived clinical benefit from cardiac rehabilitation programs. Exercise recommendations, similar to those made for younger individuals, need to take into account the physical ability of the patient, comorbidities, and any potential risk to exercise.[10,32]

Elderly patients following hospitalization for a coronary event such as an acute coronary syndrome or HF are at increased risk of disability, including a repeat cardiovascular event. The efficacy and safety of cardiac rehabilitation have been demonstrated in various patient populations, including the elderly as defined as age greater than 65 years.[116]

There are special considerations due to age related cardiovascular changes in the elderly population. The changes include a decrease in maximal oxygen consumption due to a loss of muscle mass; an impaired efficiency of maximal peripheral oxygen extraction; and a decline in maximal HR, which is compensated for by an increase in stroke volume (SV) in order to maintain CO. In addition, special consideration should be given for comorbidities that may include arthritis and peripheral vascular disease, resulting in impaired mobility.

Elderly patients being considered for an exercise program should be evaluated for potential risks with physical activity and determine whether any contraindications to exercise exist which may require modest modifications for physical activity.[117–123]

In developing an appropriate exercise prescription for this population there needs to be a greater emphasis and more time devoted to warm-up activities, including flexibility and range of motion exercises, which enable musculoskeletal and cardiorespiratory readiness for exercise. Furthermore, older adults are at a greater risk for hypotension because of the delayed baroreceptor responsiveness with aging from cool-down activities. Cool-down activities allow gradual dissipation of the heat load of exercise and subsidence of exercise-induced peripheral vasodilatation, and may lead to hypotension.[124]

There is a decrease in skin blood flow in aging, which lowers the efficiency of sweating and temperature regulation during exercise. A reduction in the intensity of exercise is recommended for elderly patients in hot or humid environments.

Exercise HR returns more gradually to resting values in the elderly patient, hence a longer period of rest between various components of exercise or a low-intensity activity alternated with periods of higher-intensity exercise is recommended.

The following modification to the outpatient exercise prescription is recommended for elderly patients. Aerobic training is initially begun at low intensity, for example at, 2–3 METs, with a gradual increase in both exercise intensity and duration to limit discomfort and injury. Only mild fatigue should be engendered by an exercise training session. Musculoskeletal complications can be minimized by avoidance of running, jumping, and other high-impact aerobic activities.[125]

The ideal exercise regimen for elderly patients has not yet been determined. The exercise program should be dynamic, enjoyable, easily accessible, and without adverse sequelae. Brisk walking constitutes a substantial percentage of the lower maximal oxygen uptake of elderly patients and is therefore an effective and safe physical conditioning stimulus. Strength training, designed to improve muscle function and increase muscle mass, also enhances aerobic capacity and it is an additional component of value in the exercise rehabilitation of the elderly coronary patient.

The American College of Sports Medicine has specific recommendations for physical activity and exercise in older adults which include aerobic training, muscle strengthening, flexibility, and balance training. Aerobic activities can include activities such as moderate-intensity aerobic physical activity (30 minutes 5 days/week) or vigorous-intensity aerobic activity (20 minutes 2 days/week). Muscle strengthening activity can include weight training that allows 10–15 repetitions for each exercise using major muscle groups. Flexibility activities should improve flexibility and are recommended to be at least 2 days/week for 10 minutes/day. The objective of balance exercises is to reduce the risk of injury from falls, and older adults should perform exercises that maintain or improve balance.[124,126,127]

Patients can be taught to control the intensity of their exercise by counting their pulse, using of the RPE, or by the "talk test." Patients are instructed to exercise only to an intensity that permits them to continue talking to an exercising companion.[128]

20.9 EXERCISE TRAINING

Epidemiologic studies have shown an inverse association between physical activity and CHD incidence and mortality. Fitness also appears to be important, as a graded relation has been noted between the degree of fitness and the reduction in coronary risk. The benefits of aerobic exercise are mediated through hemodynamic and metabolic effects.[56,129–134]

Understanding of physiology would assist in proper exercise prescription. Exercise requires coordination with ventilation, CO, and systemic and pulmonary blood flow to meet the metabolic demands of contracting muscles. Physiological homeostasis is needed to preserve cellular oxygenation along with acid–base homeostasis during exercise to adapt rapidly to changes in tissue demands.

Skeletal muscles are organized in motor units, in which each motor unit is innervated by a single motor neuron. The muscle fibers within a given motor unit are classified as type I or type II fibers. Type I fibers or slow twitch fibers are dense in mitochondria, have a high content of oxygen binding protein myoglobin, and a high content of oxidative enzymes for producing adenosine triphosphate (ATP). Type II or fast-twitch fibers are further categorized as types IIA and IIB. Type IIA fibers are similar to type I in their myoglobin content and oxidative enzyme capacity. Type IIB fibers have a low content of myoglobin and high anaerobic, glycolytic capacity and are typically recruited for short-term, heavy work.[135,136]

The main sources for energy to produce the ATP used by skeletal muscle during exercise are glycogen, glucose, and free fatty acids with glycogen being the predominant source of energy.

20.9.1 CIRCULATORY SYSTEM

The ability to deliver oxygen to the muscles is accomplished by an increase in the extraction of oxygen by exercising muscle, HR, and SV, as well as a decrease in the systemic and pulmonary vascular resistance. This accomplishes the goal of the circulatory system to deliver oxygen to the muscles.

The delivery of oxygen to the muscles by the circulatory system (VO_2) is expressed in a rearrangement of the Fick equation:

$$VO_2 = CO \times (CaO_2 - CvO_2)$$

In this equation, CO is defined as the cardiac output (which is the product of HR × SV) and ($CaO_2 - CvO_2$) is defined as the systemic oxygen extraction or the difference in O_2 content between arterial and mixed venous blood. The increased activity of muscle during exercise results in increased oxygen extraction in the peripheral circulation.

The arteriovenous oxygen difference ($CaO_2 - CvO_2$) is calculated by the following equation:

$$(CaO_2 - CvO_2) = 1.34 \times \text{hemoglobin concentration} \times (\text{arterial oxygen saturation} - \text{mixed venous oxygen saturation})$$

The maximal CO, which facilitates transport of oxygen from the alveolus to skeletal muscle, determines the maximal oxygen uptake (VO_2max) and aerobic capacity to a large degree.

The ability to maintain CaO_2 while simultaneously depressing CvO_2 during exercise are circulatory functions that require the respective matching of blood flow to ventilation and tissue metabolism.

CO increases during incremental exercise through changes in both HR and SV. In healthy adults, CO is generally the limiting factor in the VO_2max. The maximal HR decreases as a function of age, as predicted by the following equation:[137,138]

$$\text{Maximal HR} = 220 - \text{age (in years)}$$

20.10   ASSESSMENT OF EXERCISE CAPACITY

Cardiopulmonary exercise testing (CPET) can provide detailed information of an individual's response to exercise. CPET entails an incremental exercise test that is symptom-limited which involves a continuous increase in workload up until the patient has symptoms which can include dyspnea or fatigue which would make the patient exercise at a higher workload. The test entails a collection of the patient's physiologic data which would include oxygen uptake, carbon dioxide output, tidal volume, minute ventilation, ECG tracings, as well as pulse oximetry, and are measured throughout the test and during the first several minutes of recovery.[136–139]

The individual's functional aerobic capacity can be defined as their maximum oxygen uptake. The maximum oxygen uptake (VO_2max, L/minute) is a reflection of the maximal ability at which an individual can take in, transport, and utilize oxygen. VO_2max is considered the "gold standard" laboratory measure of cardiorespiratory fitness and is considered the most important parameter measured during functional exercise testing. Typically, incremental bilateral exercises such as a treadmill are used to provide the VO_2max and provide an overall assessment of exercise capacity.[140–143]

The VO_2max is identified by a plateau of VO_2 when VO_2 is graphed versus work however, this plateau typically occurs in a subset of subjects and patients during a maximal incremental protocol. Therefore, in cases where VO_2max is not achieved, peak VO_2, averaged over 30 of the final 60 seconds of exercise, is the more appropriate term to describe the highest achieved oxygen uptake during exercise.

VO_2max is typically indexed to an individual's body weight (mL/kg min^{-1}) and can be expressed in metabolic equivalents of training (MET), which are multiples of normal baseline oxygen uptake at rest. One MET is normal baseline oxygen uptake at rest and is equal to 3.5 mL/kg min^{-1}.[144–147]

20.11   CONTRAINDICATIONS TO EXERCISE

The AHA has published a summary outlining the absolute and relative contraindications for exercise testing and training. It is divided into absolute and relative contraindications. The absolute contraindications include cardiac and noncardiac disease. The relative contraindications can be superseded if benefits outweigh the risks.

The AHA has published a summary outlining the absolute and relative contraindications for exercise testing and training. It is divided into absolute and relative contraindications. Absolute contraindications can include cardiac and noncardiac disease.

Cardiac disease can include acute MI within 2 days, unstable angina, uncontrolled cardiac arrythmias which can result in symptoms or hemodynamic compromise, symptomatic severe aortic stenosis, uncontrolled symptomatic HF, acute myocarditis, acute pericarditis, acute endocarditis, and acute aortic dissection.

Noncardiac absolute cardiac contraindications can include acute pulmonary embolus, acute pulmonary infarction, or acute noncardiac disease that can affect the performance of exercise or be aggravated by exercise such as renal failure or infection.

Relative contraindications can include cardiac and noncardiac disease. The relative contraindications can be superseded if the benefits outweigh the risks. Cardiac disease can include left main coronary artery stenosis or its equivalent, moderate stenotic valvular heart disease, severe hypertension (systolic $\geq$200 mm Hg and/or diastolic $\geq$110 mm Hg), tachyarrhythmias or bradyarrhythmias including AF with uncontrolled ventricular rate, high degree atrioventricular block, and hypertrophic cardiomyopathy and other cardiac forms of outflow tract obstruction.

Relative noncardiac contraindications can include electrolyte abnormalities, mental or physical impairment leading to the inability to cooperate, or noncardiac conditions that may be a relative contraindication for exercise.[35,148]

20.12   PHASE III OR MAINTENANCE PHASE

The maintenance phase in cardiac rehabilitation is the most important part of cardiac rehabilitation because once the patient stops exercising the benefits that are obtained from phase II are lost in a few weeks. The program should emphasize exercise that is integrated into a patient's lifestyle to facilitate patients' compliance. In addition, there needs to be an emphasis on secondary prevention and provision of necessary interventions for life style modifications.

ECG monitoring is not necessary during the maintenance phase for exercise. For patients advised to perform moderate level exercises, instructions are provided to perform ongoing exercises at the target rate for at least 30 minutes three times a week. For low level exercises, patients are advised to exercise five times a week.

20.13   CONCLUSION

In summary, cardiac rehabilitation can be considered a spectrum that is divided into three phases. Phase I is characterized by inpatient care, phase II as outpatient care, and phase III as a maintenance program. Throughout the process secondary risk factor modification and prevention is emphasized along with improvement of function and exercise training. The outcome in a patient's participation in a cardiac rehabilitation program is associated with significant reduction in all-cause mortality and cardiac mortality.

REFERENCES

1. Rosamond W, Flegal K, Friday G et al. Heart disease and stroke statistics—2007 update: A report from the American Heart Association Statistics Committee and Stroke Statistics Subcommittee. *Circulation* 2007; 115:e69–e171.
2. Balady GJ, Williams MA, Ades PA et al. Core components of cardiac rehabilitation/secondary prevention programs: 2007 update. A scientific statement from the American Heart Association Exercise, Cardiac Rehabilitation, and Prevention Committee, the Council on Clinical Cardiology; the Councils on Cardiovascular Nursing, Epidemiology, and Prevention, and Nutrition, Physical Activity, and Metabolism; and the American Association of Cardiovascular and Pulmonary Rehabilitation. *Circulation* 2007; 115:2675–2682.
3. Leon AS, Franklin BA, Costa F et al. Cardiac rehabilitation and secondary prevention of coronary heart disease: An American Heart Association scientific statement from the Council on Clinical Cardiology (Subcommittee on Exercise, Cardiac Rehabilitation, and Prevention) and the Council on Nutrition, Physical Activity, and Metabolism (Subcommittee on Physical Activity), in collaboration with the American Association of Cardiovascular and Pulmonary Rehabilitation. *Circulation* 2005; 111:369–376.
4. American Heart Association. *Heart Disease and Stroke Statistics—2007 Update*. Dallas, TX: American Heart Association; 2007.
5. Nichols M, Townsend N, Scarborough P, Rayner M. Cardiovascular disease in Europe 2014: Epidemiological update. *Eur Heart J* 2014; 35:2950.
6. GBD 2013 Mortality and Causes of Death Collaborators. Global, regional, and national age-sex specific all-cause and cause-specific mortality for 240 causes of death, 1990–2013: A systematic analysis for the Global Burden of Disease Study 2013. *Lancet* 2015; 385:117.

7. Geol K, Lennon RJ, Tilbury RT et al. Impact of cardiac rehabilitation on mortality following PCI. *Circulation* 2011; 123:2344–2352.

8. Taylor RS, Unal B, Critchley JA, Capewell S. Mortality reductions in patients receiving exercise-based cardiac rehabilitation: How much can be attributed to cardiovascular risk factor improvements? *Eur J Cardiovasc Prev Rehabil* 2006; 13(3):369–374.

9. Rosamond W, Flegal K, Friday G et al. Heart disease and stroke statistics—2007 update: A report from the American Heart Association Statistics Committee and Stroke Statistics Subcommittee. *Circulation* 2007; 115:e69–e171.

10. Suaya JA, Stason WB, Ades PA et al. Cardiac rehabilitation and survival in older coronary patients. *J Am Coll Cardiol* 2009; 54:25–33.

11. Stephens MB. Cardiac rehabilitation. *Am Fam Physician* 2009; 80(9):955–959.

12. Milani RV, Lavie CJ. Impact of cardiac rehabilitation on depression and its associated mortality. *Am J Med* 2007; 120(9):799–806.

13. Williams MA, Ades PA, Hamm LF et al. Clinical evidence for a health benefit from cardiac rehabilitation: An update. *Am Heart J* 2006; 152(5):835–841.

14. Suaya JA, Shepard DS, Normand SL, Ades PA, Prottas J, Stason WB. Use of cardiac rehabilitation by Medicare beneficiaries after myocardial infarction or coronary bypass surgery. *Circulation* 2007; 116:1653–1662.

15. Centers for Disease Control and Prevention (CDC). Receipt of outpatient cardiac rehabilitation among heart attack survivors—United States, 2003. *Morb Mortal Wkly Rep* 2008; 57:89–94.

16. Taylor RS, Brown A, Ebrahim S, Jolliffe J, Noorani H, Rees K, Skidmore B, Stone JA, Thompson DR, Oldridge N. Exercise-based rehabilitation for patients with coronary heart disease: Systematic review and meta-analysis of randomized trials. *Am J Med* 2004; 116:682–697.

17. Balady GJ, Ades PA, Comoss P, Limacher M, Pina IL, Southard D, Williams MA, Bazzarre T. Core components of cardiac rehabilitation/secondary prevention programs: A statement for healthcare professionals from the American Heart Association and American Association of Cardiovascular and Pulmonary Rehabilitation Writing Group. *Circulation* 2000; 102:1069–1073.

18. Smith SC Jr, Blair SN, Bonow RO et al. AHA/ACC Scientific Statement: AHA/ACC guidelines for preventing heart attack and death in patients with atherosclerotic cardiovascular disease: 2001 update. A statement for healthcare professionals from the American Heart Association and the American College of Cardiology. *Circulation* 2001; 104:1577–1579.

19. Wenger NK, Froelicher ES, Smith LK et al. *Clinical Practice Guidelines No. 17: Cardiac Rehabilitation as Secondary Prevention.* Rockville, MD: US Department of Health and Human Services, Public Health Service, Agency for Health Care Policy and Research, National Heart, Lung and Blood Institute; 1995. AHCPR Publication 96-0672.

20. American Association of Cardiovascular and Pulmonary Rehabilitation. *Guidelines for Cardiac Rehabilitation and Secondary Prevention Programs.* 4th ed. Champaign, IL: Human Kinetics; 2004.

21. Ades PA. Cardiac rehabilitation and secondary prevention of coronary heart disease. *N Engl J Med* 2001; 345:892–902.

22. Mukherjee D, Fang J, Chetcuti S, Moscucci M, Kline-Rogers E, Eagle KA. Impact of combination evidence-based medical therapy on mortality in patients with acute coronary syndromes. *Circulation* 2004; 109:745–749.

23. Rozanski A, Blumenthal JA, Kaplan J. Impact of psychological factors on the pathogenesis of cardiovascular disease and implications for therapy. *Circulation* 1999; 99:2192–2217.

24. Berkman LF, Blumenthal J, Burg M et al., Enhancing Recovery in Coronary Heart Disease Patients Investigators (ENRICHD). Effects of treating depression and low perceived social support on clinical events after myocardial infarction: The Enhancing Recovery in Coronary Heart Disease Patients (ENRICHD) Randomized Trial. *JAMA* 2003; 289:3106–3116.

25. Ades PA, Huang D, Weaver SO. Cardiac rehabilitation participation predicts lower rehospitalization costs. *Am Heart J* 1992; 123:916–921.

26. Bethell HJ. Cardiac rehabilitation: From Hellerstein to the millennium. *Int J Clin Pract* 2000; 54(2):92–97.

27. Balady GJ, Ades PA, Bittner VA et al. Referral, enrollment, and delivery of cardiac rehabilitation/secondary prevention programs at clinical centers and beyond: A presidential advisory from the American Heart Association. *Circulation* 2011; 124:2951.

28. Kwan G, Balady GJ. Cardiac rehabilitation 2012: Advancing the field through emerging science. *Circulation* 2012; 125:e369.

29. Mazzini MJ, Stevens GR, Whalen D et al. Effect of an American Heart Association Get With the Guidelines program-based clinical pathway on referral and enrollment into cardiac rehabilitation after acute myocardial infarction. *Am J Cardiol* 2008; 101(8):1084–1087.

30. Arena R, Williams M, Forman DE et al. Increasing referral and participation rates to outpatient cardiac rehabilitation: The valuable role of healthcare professionals in the inpatient and home health settings: A science advisory from the American Heart Association. *Circulation* 2012; 125:1321.

31. www.cms.hhs.gov/mcd/viewdecisionmemo (Accessed on August 21, 2006).

32. Wenger NK. Rehabilitation of the patient with coronary heart disease. In: *Hurst's the Heart*. 11th ed. Fuster V, Alexander RW, O'Rourke RA (Eds.), New York: McGraw-Hill; 2004, pp.1517–1527.

33. Menezes AR, Lavie CJ, Milani RV et al. Cardiac rehabilitation in the United States. *Prog Cardiovasc Dis* 2014; 56:522.

34. Taylor RS, Brown A, Ebrahim S et al. Exercise-based rehabilitation for patients with coronary heart disease: Systematic review and meta-analysis of randomized controlled trials. *Am J Med* 2004; 116:682–692.

35. Fletcher GF, Balady GJ, Amsterdam EA et al. Exercise standards for testing and training: A statement for healthcare professionals from the American Heart Association. *Circulation* 2001; 104:1694–1740.

36. Fidan D, Unal B, Critchley J et al. Economic analysis of treatments reducing coronary heart disease mortality in England and Wales, 2000–2010. *QJM* 2007; 100:277–289.

37. Kavanagh T, Shephard RJ, Doney H, Pandit V. Intensive exercise in coronary rehabilitation. *Med Sci Sports* 1973; 5:34–39.

38. Pashkow FJ. Issues in contemporary cardiac rehabilitation: A historical perspective. *J Am Coll Cardiol* 1993; 21:822–834.

39. Pashkow FJ, Pashkow PS, Schafer MN. *Successful Cardiac Rehabilitation: The Complete Guide for Building Cardiac Rehab Programs*. 1st ed. Loveland, CO: The Heart Watchers Press; 1988, pp. 211–212.

40. Humphrey R, Bartels MN. Exercise Cardiovascular Disease and chronic heart failure: A focused review. *Arch Phy Med Rehabil* 2001; 82(3 Suppl 1):S76–S81.

41. Wenger NK. Current status of cardiac rehabilitation. *J Am Coll Cardiol* 2008; 51:1619.

42. Wenger NK, Froelicher ES, Smith LK et al. Clinical Practice Guideline No. 17. Rockville, MD: U.S. Department of Health and Human Services, Agency for Healthcare Policy and Research, and the National Heart, Lung, and Blood Institute; 1995. AHCPR Publication No. 96-0672.

43. Squires RW, Gau GT, Miller TD et al. Cardiovascular rehabilitation: Status, 1990. *Mayo Clin Proc* 1990; 65:731.

44. Cardiac Rehabilitation Programs. A statement for healthcare professionals from the American Heart Association. *Circulation* 1994; 90:1602.

45. Zullo MD, Jackson LW, Whalen CC, Dolansky MA. Evaluation of the recommended core components of cardiac rehabilitation practice: An opportunity for quality improvement. *J Cardiopulm Rehabil Prev* 2012; 32:32.

46. Russell KL, Holloway TM, Brum M et al. Cardiac rehabilitation wait times: Effect on enrollment. *J Cardiopulm Rehabil Prev* 2011; 31:373.

47. Soga Y, Yokoi H, Ando K et al. Safety of early exercise training after elective coronary stenting in patients with stable coronary artery disease. *Eur J Cardiovasc Prev Rehabil* 2010; 17:230.

48. Pack QR, Mansour M, Barboza JS et al. An early appointment to outpatient cardiac rehabilitation at hospital discharge improves attendance at orientation: A randomized, single-blind, controlled trial. *Circulation* 2013; 127:349.

49. Kenney WL, Humphrey RH, Bryant CX et al. *American College of Sports Medicine Guidelines for Exercise Testing and Prescription*. 5th ed. Baltimore: Williams & Wilkins; 1995.

50. Antman EM, Anbe DT, Armstrong PW et al. ACC/AHA guidelines for the management of patients with ST-elevation myocardial infarction. http://circ.ahajournals.org/content/110/9/e82.full.pdf (Accessed on April 10, 2016).

51. Dimsdale JE, Hartley LH, Guiney T et al. Postexercise peril. Plasma catecholamines and exercise. *JAMA* 1984; 251:630.

52. Fletcher GF, Ades PA, Kligfield P et al. Exercise standards for testing and training: A scientific statement from the American Heart Association. *Circulation* 2013; 128:873.

53. Paskow FJ, Dafoe W (Eds.). *Clinical Cardiac Rehabilitation: A Cardiologist Guide*. 2nd ed. Baltimore, MD: Williams and Wilkins; 1999.

54. Borg G. *Physical Performance and Perceived Exertion*. Lund, Sweden: Gleerup; 1992.

55. Centers for Disease Control and Prevention. Perceived exertion (Borg rating of perceived exertion scale). http://www.cdc.gov/physicalactivity/basics/measuring/exertion.htm (Accessed on April, 10, 2016).

56. Thompson PD, Buchner D, Pina IL et al. Exercise and physical activity in the prevention and treatment of atherosclerotic cardiovascular disease: A statement from the Council on Clinical Cardiology (sub-committee on exercise, rehabilitation, and prevention) and the Council on Nutrition, Physical Activity, and Metabolism (subcommittee on physical activity). *Circulation* 2003; 107:3109.

57. Pescatello LS, Arena R, Riebe D, Thompson PD. *ACSM's Guidelines for Exercise Testing and Prescription.* Philadelphia, PA: Wolters Kluwer/Lippincott Williams & Wilkins; 2014.

58. Wenger NK, Hellerstein HK (Eds.). *Rehabilitation of the Coronary Patient.* 3rd ed., Chapter 16, pp. 291–307. New York: Churchill Livingstone; 1992.

59. Milani RV, Lavie CJ, Cassidy MM. Effects of cardiac rehabilitation and exercise training programs on depression in patients after major coronary events. *Am Heart J* 1996; 132:726.

60. Mallik S, Spertus JA, Reid KJ et al. Depressive symptoms after acute myocardial infarction: Evidence for highest rates in younger women. *Arch Intern Med* 2006; 166:876.

61. Lichtman JH, Froelicher ES, Blumenthal JA et al. Depression as a risk factor for poor prognosis among patients with acute coronary syndrome: Systematic review and recommendations: A scientific statement from the American Heart Association. *Circulation* 2014; 129:1350.

62. Taylor RS, Dalal H, Jolly K et al. Home-based versus centre-based cardiac rehabilitation. *Cochrane Database Syst Rev* 2010; (1): CD007130. doi: 10.1002/14651858.CD007130.pub2.

63. Lear SA, Singer J, Banner-Lukaris D et al. Randomized trial of a virtual cardiac rehabilitation program delivered at a distance via the Internet. *Circ Cardiovasc Qual Outcomes* 2014; 7:952.

64. Turk-Adawi K, Grace SL. Smartphone-based cardiac rehabilitation. *Heart* 2014; 100:1737.

65. Varnfield M, Karunanithi M, Lee CK et al. Smartphone-based home care model improved use of cardiac rehabilitation in postmyocardial infarction patients: Results from a randomised controlled trial. *Heart* 2014; 100:1770.

66. Thompson PD. Exercise prescription and proscription for patients with coronary artery disease. *Circulation* 2005; 112(15):2354.

67. Gielen S, Schuler G, Hambrecht R. Exercise training in coronary artery disease and coronary vasomotion. *Circulation* 2001; 103(1):E1–E6.

68. Niebauer J, Hambrecht R, Marburger C et al. Impact of intensive physical exercise and low fat diet on collateral vessel formation in stable angina pectoris and angiographically confirmed coronary artery disease. *Am J Cardiol* 1995; 76(11):771–775.

69. Lash JM, Nixon JC, Unthank JL. Exercise training effects on collateral and microvascular resistances in rat model of arterial insufficiency. *Am J Physiol* 1995; 268(1 Pt 2):H125–137.

70. Fitchet A, Doherty PJ, Bundy C et al. Comprehensive cardiac rehabilitation programme for implantable cardioverter-defibrillator patients: A randomised controlled trial. *Heart* 2003; 89(2):155–160.

71. Pycha C, Gulledge AD, Hutzler J et al. Psychological response to the implantable defibrillator. *Psychosomatics* 1986; 27:841–845.

72. Frizelle DJ, Lewin RJ, Kaye G et al. Cognitive behavioral rehabilitation programme for patients with an implanted cardioverter defibrillator: A pilot study. *Br J Health Psychol* 2004; 9(pt 3):381–392.

73. Shahian DM, O'Brien SM, Sheng S et al. Predictors of long-term survival after coronary artery bypass grafting surgery: Results from the Society of Thoracic Surgeons Adult Cardiac Surgery Database (the ASCERT study). *Circulation* 2012; 125(12):1491.

74. Juneau M, Geneau S, Marchand C et al. Cardiac rehabilitation after coronary bypass surgery (review). *Cardiovasc Clin* 1991; 21(2):25–42.

75. Estafanous FG, Loop FD, Higgins TL, Tekyi-Mensah S, Lytle BW, Cosgrove DM 3rd, Roberts-Brown M, Starr NJ. Increased risk and decreased morbidity of coronary artery bypass grafting between 1986 and 1994. *Ann Thorac Surg* 1998; 65(2):383.

76. Hammermeister KE, Burchfiel C, Johnson R, Grover FL. Identification of patients at greatest risk for developing major complications at cardiac surgery. *Circulation* 1990; 82(5 Suppl):IV380.

77. Magovern JA, Sakert T, Magovern GJ, Benckart DH, Burkholder JA, Liebler GA, Magovern GJ Sr. A model that predicts morbidity and mortality after coronary artery bypass graft surgery. *J Am Coll Cardiol* 1996; 28(5):1147.

78. Fortescue EB, Kahn K, Bates DW. Development and validation of a clinical prediction rule for major adverse outcomes in coronary bypass grafting. *Am J Cardiol* 2001; 88(11):1251.

79. Crystal E, Connolly SJ, Sleik K, Ginger TJ, Yusuf S. Interventions on prevention of postoperative atrial fibrillation in patients undergoing heart surgery: A meta-analysis. *Circulation* 2002; 106(1):75.

80. Yau TM, Fedak PW, Weisel RD, Teng C, Ivanov J. Predictors of operative risk for coronary bypass operations in patients with left ventricular dysfunction. *J Thorac Cardiovasc Surg* 1999; 118(6):1006.

81. Weitzman LB, Tinker WP, Kronzon I, Cohen ML, Glassman E, Spencer FC. The incidence and natural history of pericardial effusion after cardiac surgery—An echocardiographic study. *Circulation* 1984; 69(3):506.

82. Meurin P, Weber H, Renaud N, Larrazet F, Tabet JY, Demolis P, Ben Driss A. Evolution of the postoperative pericardial effusion after day 15: The problem of the late tamponade. *Chest* 2004; 125(6):2182.

83. Kuvin JT, Harati NA, Pandian NG, Bojar RM, Khabbaz KR. Postoperative cardiac tamponade in the modern surgical era. *Ann Thorac Surg* 2002; 74(4):1148.

84. Hogue CW Jr, Barzilai B, Pieper KS, Coombs LP, DeLong ER, Kouchoukos NT, Dávila-Román VG. Sex differences in neurological outcomes and mortality after cardiac surgery: A society of thoracic surgery national database report. *Circulation* 2001; 103(17):2133.

85. Roach GW, Kanchuger M, Mangano CM, Newman M, Nussmeier N, Wolman R, Aggarwal A, Marschall K, Graham SH, Ley C. Adverse cerebral outcomes after coronary bypass surgery. Multicenter Study of Perioperative Ischemia Research Group and the Ischemia Research and Education Foundation Investigators. *N Engl J Med* 1996; 335(25):1857.

86. Aldea GS, Mokadam NA, Melford R Jr, Stewart D, Maynard C, Reisman M, Goss R. Changing volumes, risk profiles, and outcomes of coronary artery bypass grafting and percutaneous coronary interventions. *Ann Thorac Surg* 2009; 87(6):1828.

87. Racz MJ, Hannan EL, Isom OW et al. A comparison of short- and long-term outcomes after off-pump and on-pump coronary artery bypass graft surgery with sternotomy. *J Am Coll Cardiol* 2004; 43(4):557.

88. Pollock ML, Foster C, Anholm JD et al. Diagnostic capabilities of exercise testing soon after cardiac revascularization surgery. *Cardiology* 1982; 69:358.

89. Dubach P, Froelicher V, Klein J et al. Use of exercise test to predict prognosis after coronary artery bypass grafting. *Am J Cardiol* 1989; 63:530.

90. Wainright RJ, Brennand-Roper DA, Maisey MN et al. Exercise thanllium-201 myocardial scintiography in the follow up of aortocoronary bypass graft surgery. *Br Heart J* 1980; 43:56.

91. Hartley HL. Exercise of the cardiac patient. *Cardiol Clin* 1993; 11:277–284.

92. Robicsek F, Fokin A, Cook J, Bhatia D. Sternal instability after midline sternotomy. *Thorac Cardiovasc Surg* 2000; 48:1–8.

93. Brocki BC, Thorup CB, Andeasen JJ. Precautions related to midline sternotomy in cardiac surgery: A review of mechanical stress factors leading to sternal complications. *Eur J Cardiovasc Nurs* 2010; 9:77–84.

94. Westerdahl E, Moller M. Physiotherapy supervised mobilization and exercise following cardiac surgery: A national questionnaire survey in Sweden. *J Cardiothorac Surg* 2010; 5:67.

95. Bleiziffer S, Eichinger WB, Hettich I et al. Impact on patient–prosthesis mismatch on exercise capacity in patients after bioprosthetic valve aortic valve replacement. *Heart* 2008; 94:637–641.

96. Sakamato H, Watanabe Y. Does patient–prosthesis mismatch affect long term results after valve replacement? *Ann Thorac Cardiovasc Surg* 2010; 16:163–167.

97. Kokkinos PF, Choucair W, Graves P et al. Chronic heart failure and exercise. *Am Heart J* 2000; 140:21.

98. Blumenthal JA, Babyak MA, O'Connor C et al. Effects of exercise training on depressive symptoms in patients with chronic heart failure: The HF-ACTION randomized trial. *JAMA* 2012; 308:465.

99. Piña IL, Apstein CS, Balady GJ et al. Exercise and heart failure: A statement from the American Heart Association Committee on exercise, rehabilitation, and prevention. *Circulation* 2003; 107:1210.

100. Yancy CW, Jessup M, Bozkurt B et al. 2013 ACCF/AHA guideline for the management of heart failure: A report of the American College of Cardiology Foundation/American Heart Association Task Force on Practice Guidelines. *J Am Coll Cardiol* 2013; 62:e147.

101. https://www.cms.gov/medicare-coverage-database/details/nca-decision-memo.aspx?NCAId=270 (Accessed on April 12, 2016).

102. O'Connor CM, Whellan DJ, Lee KL et al. Efficacy and safety of exercise training in patients with chronic heart failure: HF-ACTION randomized controlled trial. *JAMA* 2009; 301:1439.

103. Wisløff U, Støylen A, Loennechen JP et al. Superior cardiovascular effect of aerobic interval training versus moderate continuous training in heart failure patients: A randomized study. *Circulation* 2007; 115:3086.

104. Osada N, Chaitman BR, Donohue TJ et al. Long-term cardiopulmonary exercise performance after heart transplantation. *Am J Cardiol* 1997; 79:451.

105. Degre SG, Niset GL, De Smet JM et al. Cardiorespiratory response to early exercise testing after orthotopic cardiac transplantation. *Am J Cardiol* 1987; 60:926.

106. Daida H, Squires RW, Allison TG et al. Sequential assessment of exercise tolerance in heart transplantation compared with coronary artery bypass surgery after phase II cardiac rehabilitation. *Am J Cardiol* 1996; 77:696.

107. Giannuzzi P, Temporelli PL, Tavazzi L et al. EAMI—Exercise training in anterior myocardial infarction: An ongoing multicenter randomized study. Preliminary results on left ventricular function and remodeling. The EAMI Study Group. *Chest* 1992; 101:315S.
108. Giannuzzi P, Tavazzi L, Temporelli PL et al. Long-term physical training and left ventricular remodeling after anterior myocardial infarction: Results of the exercise in anterior myocardial infarction (EAMI) trial. EAMI Study Group. *J Am Coll Cardiol* 1993; 22:1821.
109. Whellan DJ, O'Connor CM, Pina I. Training trials in heart failure: Time to exercise restraint? *Am Heart J* 2004; 147:190.
110. Borg G. Perceived exertion as an indicator of somatic stress. *Scand J Rehabil Med* 1970; 2:92.
111. Brubaker PH, Berry MJ, Brozena SC et al. Relationship of lactate and ventilatory thresholds in cardiac transplant patients. *Med Sci Sports Exercise* 1993; 25:191.
112. Renlund DG, Taylor DO, Ensley RD et al. Exercise capacity after heart transplantation: Influence of donor and recipient characteristics. *J Heart Lung Transplant* 1996; 15:16.
113. Weiss ES, Nwakanma LU, Patel ND, Yuh DD. Outcomes in patients older than 60 years of age undergoing orthotopic heart transplantation: An analysis of the UNOS database. *J Heart Lung Transplant* 2008; 27:184.
114. Marzolini S, Grace SL, Brooks D et al. Time-to-referral, use, and efficacy of cardiac rehabilitation after heart transplantation. *Transplantation* 2015; 99:594.
115. Corrà U, Pistono M, Mezzani A et al. Cardiovascular prevention and rehabilitation for patients with ventricular assist device from exercise therapy to long-term therapy. Part I: Exercise therapy. *Monaldi Arch Chest Dis* 2011; 76:27.
116. Pasquali SK, Alexander KP, Peterson ED. Cardiac rehabilitation in the elderly. *Am Heart J* 2001; 142:748.
117. Fleg JL. Aerobic exercise in the elderly: A key to successful aging. *Discovery Med* 2012; 13:223.
118. Shephard RJ. The scientific basis of exercise prescribing for the very old. *J Am Geriatr Soc* 1990; 38:62.
119. Fleg JL, Lakatta EG. Role of muscle loss in the age-associated reduction in VO_2 max. *J Appl Physiol* 1988; 65:1147.
120. McGuire DK, Levine BD, Williamson JW et al. A 30-year follow-up of the Dallas Bedrest and Training Study: I. Effect of age on the cardiovascular response to exercise. *Circulation* 2001; 104:1350.
121. Blumenthal JA, Emery CF, Madden DJ et al. Cardiovascular and behavioral effects of aerobic exercise training in healthy older men and women. *J Gerontol* 1989; 44:M147.
122. Shephard RJ. Habitual physical activity levels and perception of exercise in the elderly. *J Cardiopulm Rehabil* 1989; 9:17.
123. Jonsson PV, Lipsitz LA, Kelley M, Koestner J. Hypotensive responses to common daily activities in institutionalized elderly. A potential risk for recurrent falls. *Arch Intern Med* 1990; 150:1518.
124. Pollock M, Wilmore J (Eds.). *Exercise in Health and Disease: Evaluation and Prescription for Prevention and Rehabilitation.* 2nd ed. Philadelphia: WB Saunders; 1990.
125. Pollock ML, Carroll JF, Graves JE et al. Injuries and adherence to walk/jog and resistance training programs in the elderly. *Med Sci Sports Exercise* 1991; 23:1194.
126. Bruce RA, Larson EB, Stratton J. Physical fitness, functional aerobic capacity, aging, and response to physical training or bypass surgery in coronary patients. *J Cardiopulm Rehabil* 1989; 9:24.
127. Nelson ME, Rejeski WJ, Blair SN et al. Physical activity and public health in older adults: Recommendation from the American College of Sports Medicine and the American Heart Association. *Circulation* 2007; 116:1094.
128. Borg GA. Psychophysical bases of perceived exertion. *Med Sci Sports Exercise* 1982; 14:377.
129. Blair SN. Physical activity, fitness, and coronary heart disease. In: *Physical Activity, Fitness, and Health.* Bouchard C, Shephard RJ, Stephens T (Eds.). Chapter 39, pp. 579–589. Champaign: Human Kinetics Publishers; 1994.
130. Paffenbarger RS Jr, Hyde RT, Wing AL et al. The association of changes in physical-activity level and other lifestyle characteristics with mortality among men. *N Engl J Med* 1993; 328:538.
131. Wannamethee SG, Shaper AG, Alberti KG. Physical activity, metabolic factors, and the incidence of coronary heart disease and type 2 diabetes. *Arch Intern Med* 2000; 160:2108.
132. Sandvik L, Erikssen J, Thaulow E et al. Physical fitness as a predictor of mortality among healthy, middle-aged Norwegian men. *N Engl J Med* 1993; 328:533.
133. Gulati M, Pandey DK, Arnsdorf MF et al. Exercise capacity and the risk of death in women: The St James Women Take Heart Project. *Circulation* 2003; 108:1554.
134. Myers J, Prakash M, Froelicher V et al. Exercise capacity and mortality among men referred for exercise testing. *N Engl J Med* 2002; 346:793.

135. Fry AC, Allemeier CA, Staron RS. Correlation between percentage fiber type area and myosin heavy chain content in human skeletal muscle. *Eur J Appl Physiol Occup Physiol* 1994; 68:246.
136. Wasserman K, Hansen JE, Sue DY et al. Physiology of exercise. In: *Principles of Exercise Testing and Interpretation: Including Pathophysiology and Clinical Applications.* 5th ed. Philadelphia, PA: Wolters Kluwer, Lippincott, Williams & Wilkins; 2011.
137. Graham TE, Saltin B. Estimation of the mitochondrial redox state in human skeletal muscle during exercise. *J Appl Physiol* 1989; 66:561.
138. Whipp BJ, Wasserman K. Oxygen uptake kinetics for various intensities of constant-load work. *J Appl Physiol* 1972; 33:351.
139. Poole DC, Gaesser GA. Response of ventilatory and lactate thresholds to continuous and interval training. *J Appl Physiol* 1985; 58:1115.
140. ERS Task Force, Palange P, Ward SA et al. Recommendations on the use of exercise testing in clinical practice. *Eur Respir J* 2007; 29:185.
141. Fishman A, Martinez F, Naunheim K et al. A randomized trial comparing lung-volume-reduction surgery with medical therapy for severe emphysema. *N Engl J Med* 2003; 348:2059.
142. Wensel R, Opitz CF, Anker SD et al. Assessment of survival in patients with primary pulmonary hypertension: Importance of cardiopulmonary exercise testing. *Circulation* 2002; 106:319.
143. Kawut SM, O'Shea MK, Bartels MN et al. Exercise testing determines survival in patients with diffuse parenchymal lung disease evaluated for lung transplantation. *Respir Med* 2005; 99:1431.
144. Bassett DR Jr, Howley ET. Limiting factors for maximum oxygen uptake and determinants of endurance performance. *Med Sci Sports Exercise* 2000; 32:70.
145. Hansen JE, Sue DY, Wasserman K. Predicted values for clinical exercise testing. *Am Rev Respir Dis* 1984; 129:S49.
146. Koch B, Schäper C, Ittermann T et al. Reference values for cardiopulmonary exercise testing in healthy volunteers: The SHIP study. *Eur Respir J* 2009; 33:389.
147. Jones NL, Makrides L, Hitchcock C et al. Normal standards for an incremental progressive cycle ergometer test. *Am Rev Respir Dis* 1985; 131:700.
148. Gibbons RJ, Balady GJ, Bricker JT et al. ACC/AHA 2002 guideline update for exercise testing: Summary article: A report of the American College of Cardiology/American Heart Association Task Force on Practice Guidelines (Committee to Update the 1997 Exercise Testing Guidelines). *Circulation* 2002; 106:1883.

21 Pulmonary Disease in the Geriatric Population

Mary Anne M. Morgan

CONTENTS

21.1 INTRODUCTION

The prevalence of pulmonary disease increases with age and contributes significantly to the morbidity and mortality of the geriatric population. Elderly patients with lung disease are disproportionately physically debilitated,[1] are hospitalized at a disproportionate rate, and comprise a substantial proportion of the growing population of older adults.[2] In fact, chronic obstructive pulmonary disease (COPD) ranks as the third most common cause of death in the United States[3] and worldwide[4] and is among the top five causes of disability in the adult population.[5,6] As our population continues to age, and as people live longer with increasingly complex constellations of diseases, an enhanced understanding of geriatric pulmonary physiology is critical as we seek to maximize health and independence in older patients, both primary goals of rehabilitation medicine.

In this chapter, we will review the effect of aging on the lungs, focusing on the impact of both physiologic and pathologic aging. We will then turn to four chronic pulmonary disorders affecting the geriatric population: COPD, asthma, bronchiectasis, and interstitial lung disease (ILD). Within each section, we will address specific issues facing rehabilitation practitioners caring for older patients with these diseases. As the most common pulmonary disease affecting the elderly, and also the disease for which evidence supporting the benefits of structured rehabilitation is most robust, COPD will serve as our model for examining the impact of incorporating principles of rehabilitation medicine into core management of the disease.

21.2 THE AGING LUNG

Pulmonary function begins to decline as early as the third decade due to a host of physiologic and environmental factors. As life progresses, the lung is subjected to a constant onslaught of environmental toxins, including tobacco smoke, air pollution, dusts, and infection, all of which contribute to the observed reduction in physiologic lung capacity that accompanies aging. Because of these cumulative effects, older individuals face increased odds of developing respiratory limitation, if not overt respiratory impairment. An understanding of the expected physiology of the aging lung will allow us to differentiate changes in respiratory function that are expected and physiologic (i.e., normal aging), versus those that are pathologic and warrant further intervention.

21.2.1 NORMAL AGING

Aging is accompanied by a decrement in physiologic lung reserve. This stems from multiple factors, including altered respiratory mechanics, decline in respiratory muscle strength, modified control of ventilation, narrowing of the window for gas exchange, and waning immunity. These changes heighten the vulnerability of older adults—particularly those with history of heavy smoke exposure or history of underlying lung disease—to progressive respiratory impairment, particularly when confronting conditions of increased metabolic demand, such as infection or cardiac dysfunction. The "normal" loss of pulmonary reserve must be considered when evaluating a patient for participation in a structured rehabilitation program in order to avoid either over-testing or inappropriate pharmacotherapy on the one hand, and overlooking important, potentially treatable conditions on the other. An appreciation of lung physiology will allow us to better define both goals and limitations for rehabilitation in the geriatric population.

21.2.2 RESPIRATORY MECHANICS IN THE ELDERLY

21.2.2.1 Structural Changes in the Lung and Chest Wall with Age

Age-related changes in pulmonary physiology are orchestrated by structural changes in the airways, the lung tissue, and the chest wall.

Airway changes include loss of mean airway diameter, primarily due to weakening of the connective tissue network supporting airway patency. This smaller airway diameter causes increased airways' resistance, leading to decreased expiratory flow rates and, ultimately, airflow limitation. In addition, diminished elastic recoil in the lung matrix[7] with aging results in premature closure of the small airways with exhalation. This premature closure shortens effective expiratory time, and can contribute to the phenomenon of "air trapping," or inadequate emptying of the lungs between breaths, particularly in adults with obstructive lung disease. Air trapping, or "dynamic hyperinflation," occurs primarily when respiratory effort is increased, such as during exertion or acute illness, and correlates strongly with the sensation of breathlessness.

Changes in chest wall compliance further impact the normal respiratory physiology of aging. Over the course of the life span, the chest wall—comprised of the bones, muscles, and cartilage—becomes progressively more stiff as kyphoscoliosis, calcification of intercostal cartilages, and narrowing or decreased mobility of costovertebral joints develop. This progressive chest wall rigidity leads to increased reliance upon diaphragmatic and abdominal muscles to match the increased ventilatory demands of stress or exercise. Although diaphragm muscle mass does not atrophy significantly with aging, studies suggest that diaphragm strength decreases by about 25% with age, even in healthy individuals.[8,9] This may be due to flattening of the normal diaphragmatic curve with aging. This loss of curvature decreases the force generated by the muscle during exhalation, sneezing, and, importantly, coughing.[10] In addition, diaphragmatic defects/hernias and central adiposity predispose older adults to respiratory fatigue and inadequate carbon dioxide elimination in situations requiring increased ventilation, such as exercise or with the increased metabolic demands of illness. This excessive reliance on "abdominal breathing" can be of particular impact in individuals who are unable to assume a full upright posture, either related to spinal curvature or to being bed or wheelchair-bound.

Loss of muscle strength with aging contributes to age-related reductions in pulmonary reserve. In contrast to the diaphragm, the intercostal muscles, particularly those responsible for exhalation and coughing, begin to degenerate after the fifth decade even in otherwise healthy individuals.[11] Other muscles responsible for coordinating the respiratory effort are similarly affected. Muscle fatiguing with repeated exertion likely also contributes to decreased functional reserve with exercise.

21.2.2.2 Changes in Pulmonary Function with Age

The structural changes in the lung tissue, airways, and chest wall give rise to predictable changes in lung function tests. Starting in the third decade, the forced expiratory volume in the first second of exhalation (FEV_1) drops by roughly 25–50 mL per year in nonsmokers, with greater declines in smokers.[12,13] This annual decline accelerates after age 65, due to the combination of factors discussed earlier (decreased airway diameter, decreased elastic recoil in the lung, decreased chest wall compliance, and decreased expiratory muscle force). Although the forced vital capacity (FVC, or the total volume of air exhaled with a forceful breath) also declines, the FEV_1 declines to a greater degree such that the ratio of FEV_1 to FVC (FEV_1/FVC) falls, a spirometric parameter that suggests airflow obstruction.

As noted earlier, increased airways resistance and increased airway collapsibility at low lung volumes contribute to premature airway closure, whereby the distal airways begin to close earlier during the expiratory cycle in the aged lung. This causes an increase in residual volume (RV, or volume of air remaining in the lung after full exhalation) of up to 50% by the age of 70.[14,15] The vital capacity (VC, or volume of breath delivered during regular breathing) decreases concomitantly. This inverse relationship of VC and RV hold total lung capacity (TLC) fairly constant across the lifespan, but the volume of breath that is actually being exchanged is decreased (Figures 21.1 and 21.2).

These changes—decline in FEV_1, decrease in FEV_1 to FVC ratio, decrease in VC, and increase in RV—impose substantial limitations on the aging lung when it confronts increased demands,

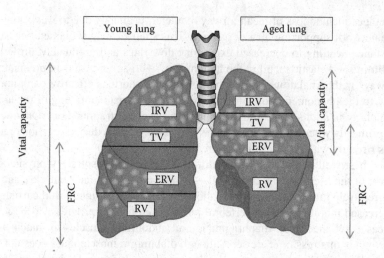

FIGURE 21.1 Schematic of lung volume changes with aging. Note decreases in inspiratory reserve volume (IRV), expiratory reserve volume (ERV), and therefore VC. RV increases, as does functional residual capacity (FRC). TLC and TV remain roughly the same.

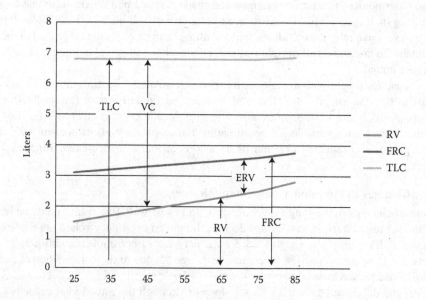

FIGURE 21.2 Change in pulmonary function with age. Aging results in progressive decline in VC and corresponding increase in functional residual capacity, maintaining TLC. TLC: total lung capacity; VC: vital capacity; ERV: expiratory reserve volume; RV: residual volume; FRC: functional residual capacity.

either by virtue of illness or exercise. Adjusting for these changes when designing a geriatric exercise program (e.g., implementing shorter "interval" exercises rather than continuous exercise of longer duration) will allow the older individual to achieve exercise goals without causing harm or excessive fatigue.

21.2.2.3 Changes in Gas Exchange with Age
Structural changes in the lung tissue and chest wall impact gas exchange in the older individual. Changes in capillary distribution and density, increased collagen deposition along alveolar walls,

and loss of alveolar surface area for gas exchange contribute to the higher alveolar–arterial oxygen gradient and reduced gas diffusing capacity (measured as DLCO [diffusing capacity for carbon monoxide]) observed.[16] In addition, enhanced small airway closure, particularly in dependent portions of the lungs, increases ventilation–perfusion mismatching. These processes increase susceptibility to hypoxemia, particularly in conditions of increased metabolic oxygen demand, such as exercise or illness. Numerous studies have documented age-related declines in arterial oxygen content (PaO_2).[15] The effect of this decline in baseline PaO_2 on measured oximetry is magnified when either decreased cardiac output or increased metabolic demand is encountered.

Carbon dioxide exchange (ventilation) also varies across the lifespan, although the carbon dioxide content of the blood ($PaCO_2$) typically does not. In order to maintain stable blood CO_2 levels, the aging lung must adapt to an increasing proportion of the lung not participating in ventilation (i.e., "dead space" fraction) by increasing either the frequency (respiratory rate, RR) or the depth of the breath (tidal volume, TV). Particularly with exercise, when dead space fraction increases further,[17] this can be burdensome for the aging lung.

21.2.2.4   Changes in Control of Ventilation with Age

Multiple studies have investigated the changes in ventilation that occur across the lifespan. In the healthy older adult, a blunted response to both hypoxemia and hypercapnia has been observed.[18] This body of work suggests that there is a significant decrease in the expected rise in minute ventilation (a product of RR and TV) when healthy older individuals confront either hypoxia or hypercapnia.[19] This is due primarily to decreased chemosensitivity to hypercapnia, with decreased central respiratory drive in response to gas exchange perturbations also playing a role.[7] This altered sensitivity to imbalances in gas exchange—the primary driver of dyspnea in the nonelderly population—means that hypoxia or hypercapnia may not be the strongest determinant of air hunger in the older individual. This decreased awareness of hypoxemia or hypercapnia delays the opportunity to intervene when older patients begin to develop respiratory insufficiency, and may make enhanced monitoring during exercise necessary.

21.2.2.5   Changes in Respiratory Physiology in Response to Exercise with Aging

Although the ventilatory response to hypercapnia is blunted as we age, the ventilatory response to exercise is enhanced. This contributes to an increased work of breathing, tachypnea, and breathlessness during exercise. Rapid, shallow breathing during exercise in turn perpetuates narrowing and premature closure of the small airways, resulting in increased RV and hyperinflation. Further, the widened A-a oxygen gradient, reduced diffusing capacity, and increased V–Q mismatching predisposes the elderly exerciser, particularly those with underlying lung disease, to hypoxemia. Interestingly, however, the decline in exercise capacity with age in the healthy elderly individual is thought to be more strongly linked to an altered cardiovascular response to exercise, rather than to changes in pulmonary physiology *per se*.[20] Of course, this may not be true in the older individual with chronic lung disease (Figure 21.3)

21.2.3   Assessment of Pulmonary Function in the Older Adult

Testing to evaluate respiratory impairment includes spirometry, which can be performed using a portable device with appropriate coaching, along with measurements of lung volume, diffusing capacity (both of which require more sophisticated equipment), and gas exchange via the arterial blood gas. Oximetry measurements before and during exercise are easy to obtain and provide useful information.

The mechanics and interpretation of spirometry are beyond the scope of this chapter, but several comments should be made when it comes to interpreting lung function testing in the older individual.

- Change in respiratory mechanics
  1. Decreased functional airway diameter/increased airways resistance
  2. Decreased chest wall compliance
  3. Decreased muscle strength (diaphragm, intercostals, etc.)
- Decrease in gas exchange
  1. Widened A-a gradient, decreased PaO_2, increased V–Q mismatching
  2. Increased minute ventilation to achieve stable $PaCO_2$
- Modified control of ventilation
  1. Blunted response to hypoxia and hypercapnia
  2. Increased ventilatory response to exercise
- Waning immunity = increased vulnerability to infection
  1. Decreased cough reflex
  2. Decreased immune function

FIGURE 21.3   Causes of decreased lung reserve of aging.

	FEV_1	FVC	FEV_1/FVC	Bronchodilator response*	DLCO	TLC	RV/TLC
COPD	Low	Normal or low	Reduced	Typically negative	Typically low	Normal or increased	Normal or increased
Asthma	Low or normal	Normal or low	Reduced or preserved	Typically positive	Typically normal	Normal or increased	Normal or increased
ILD	Low	Low	Preserved	Negative	Low	Low	Normal
Bronchiectasis	Normal or low	Normal or low	Preserved or reduced	Can be positive or negative	Normal or low	Any	Normal or increased

* Of note, a positive bronchodilator response is defined as an improvement in FEV_1 or FVC of at least 12% and 200 cc after administration of an inhaled short-acting bronchodilator.

FIGURE 21.4   Simplified synopsis of expected lung function test findings in four common diseases. Here FEV_1 = forced expiratory volume in 1 second; FVC = forced vital capacity; DLCO = diffusing capacity for carbon monoxide; TLC = total lung capacity. Severity of obstruction and restriction are judged based on the FEV_1 percent predicted. Severity of diffusion impairment in based on the DLCO.

Obtaining valid results requires demonstration of intertesting reproducibility, such that at least three consecutive spirometric maneuvers are advised. This can be both time consuming for the practitioner and physically difficult for the older adult, who may have physical and/or cognitive impairments that interfere with test performance. Maintaining forced exhalation for a minimum of 6 seconds, initiating a breath and exhaling forcefully on command, and breath holding for diffusion measurement can also be challenging. Inexperience either on the part of the tester or the individual interpreting the test can result in misleading diagnoses. It should be emphasized that, although portable equipment is relatively simple, inexpensive, and convenient when compared to testing performed in a fully equipped pulmonary function lab, the results obtained may not always accurately reflect the clinical scenario.

Caveats aside, pulmonary function testing is an excellent tool for establishing the presence of respiratory limitation and for defining its etiology. Recently, pulmonary function test interpretation strategies have been refined, in part due to the recognition of misleading (false-positive and false-negative) interpretations in patients at extremes of age. Currently, the patient's performance on a given test is contrasted with a reference population of individuals matched by age, height, gender, and race, with a "lower limit of normal" cutoff (defined as the bottom fifth percentile of the population), rather than a "fixed" percentile of predicted (e.g., 70%) cutoff. This derived from the recognition that obstructive lung disease was overdiagnosed in the older population given the "normal" and expected decline in the ratio of FEV_1/FVC described earlier.[21,22] It was similarly recognized that the range of "normal" in the older adult was more broad, owing in part to greater variability in test performance (Figure 21.4).[23]

21.3 PULMONARY DISEASES AFFECTING THE OLDER PATIENT IN REHABILITATION

As noted, older patients with chronic lung disease often find themselves trapped in a recurring cycle of hospitalizations, increasing physical disability, and progressive inactivity. This portion of the chapter will review four common chronic lung diseases affecting the older adult, providing a brief overview of their evaluation and management and emphasizing specific factors that may be of use to the rehabilitation practitioner.

21.3.1 CHRONIC OBSTRUCTIVE PULMONARY DISEASE

The burden of COPD has increased steadily worldwide over the last three decades despite welcome trends in reduced tobacco consumption. It has become increasingly a disease of the elderly, with rising prevalence in the sixth decade and beyond.[24,25] As noted earlier, COPD is the third most common cause of death in the United States, and by the year 2020 it is projected to be the fourth leading cause of disability.[26] Indeed, it has been estimated that adults with COPD have a 10-fold higher risk of disability than age-matched members of the general population,[27] and are more disabled than those afflicted by other common chronic diseases like heart disease and diabetes.[28] COPD is a leading cause of hospitalization in the United States, accounting for at least 20% of hospitalizations in patients aged 65 and older.[29] Finally, and importantly, physical inactivity has emerged as a strong independent risk factor for poor outcome in COPD, including mortality.[30] Unlike factors such as past tobacco abuse or comorbid heart disease, physical inactivity in patients with COPD is eminently modifiable, a fact which has appropriately placed rehabilitation efforts at the center of the campaign to better manage this disease.

COPD is an umbrella term encompassing conditions marked by airflow obstruction with varying degrees of reversibility. Here, we will focus on the subsets of emphysema and chronic bronchitis, typically deemed the "irreversible" phenotype(s) of COPD, as asthma will be addressed in the next section. It should be acknowledged that an overlap exists between the obstructive disease phenotypes, and that the dichotomy of "asthma vs. COPD" is likely an oversimplification, particularly in the older population.

21.3.1.1 Clinical Presentation and Evaluation

Symptoms of COPD include coughing, wheezing, chronic sputum production, and exertional dyspnea. Hypoxia and hypercapnia may also be present. The primary risk factor for the development of COPD is exposure to cigarette smoke,[31] but a history of exposure to occupational pollutants or to heavy dusts should also be elicited. Comorbidities of heart and/or vascular disease frequently accompany this disease, given shared risk factors. Anxiety and depression are common in patients with COPD as well.[32]

Pulmonary function tests are the gold standard for diagnosing COPD and for grading severity.[33,34] A combination of airflow obstruction and reduced diffusion capacity, along with the appropriate clinical scenario, clinches the diagnosis. While not essential, lung volume measurement often reveals increased RV as a proportion of total lung capacity (RV/TLC ratio), suggesting air trapping. The latter measurement correlates strongly with exertional dyspnea.

Since lung function, and in particular FEV_1 to FVC ratio, declines physiologically with age, the current American Thoracic Society/European Respiratory Society (ATS/ERS) guidelines employs the bottom fifth percentile of the normal distribution to define obstruction. This minimizes the frequency of "false" diagnoses of COPD in the older population. However, this more stringent criteria may miss some milder cases of COPD, particularly in an otherwise fit older individual. As mentioned earlier, performance on testing may be hampered by age-related cognitive or physical difficulties. A clinical (i.e., nonspirometric) diagnosis is occasionally needed.

21.3.1.2 Management of COPD

The goals of COPD treatment are to curb the rapid decline in lung function characteristic of the disease; to maximize an individual's ability to participate in life by relieving disabling dyspnea, improving exercise tolerance, and improving health-related quality of life; to reduce the frequency and severity of exacerbations; and to reduce hospitalizations and, ultimately, mortality. Pharmacologic and nonpharmacologic interventions must be interwoven to best meet these goals.

Treatment of COPD should follow established clinical practice guidelines.[35] These are not age-specific. In brief, the essential components of COPD management are (1) smoking cessation; (2) pharmacologic therapy, including inhaled bronchodilators for patients with respiratory symptoms and reduced FEV_1, inhaled anticholinergics and/or long-acting beta agonists (LABAs) if $FEV_1 < 60\%$ and symptoms, and combinations of inhaled steroid with long-acting beta agonist (LABA) and anticholinergic therapy for patients with persistent symptoms and/or reduced lung function; (3) Supplemental oxygen in patients with severe resting hypoxemia ($PaO_2 < 55$ mm Hg or $SpO_2 < 88\%$); (4) vaccinations against influenza[36] and pneumococcus; and (5) pulmonary rehabilitation in selected patients. This latter recommendation carries the strongest level of evidence in patients with moderately to severely impaired lung function (designated as having $FEV_1 < 50\%$ predicted), but should, per recent guidelines, be considered in patients with less severe, but symptomatic disease (Figure 21.5).

21.3.1.2.1 Pharmacologic Interventions in COPD

The pharmacologic cornerstone of COPD management is the inhaled bronchodilator, alone or in combination. Evidence does not suggest universal support for one specific inhaler over another, and all have side effects and toxicities. A stepwise approach is preferred in order to assess response and avoid cumulative drug toxicity.

A full review of pharmacologic management of COPD is beyond the scope of this chapter. All long-acting inhaled therapies (LABAs, corticosteroids, and anticholinergics) have been shown to reduce expected annual decline in lung function,[37] and therapeutic combinations of inhalers, particularly in patients with moderate to severe disease, appear to augment airflow, reduce exacerbations

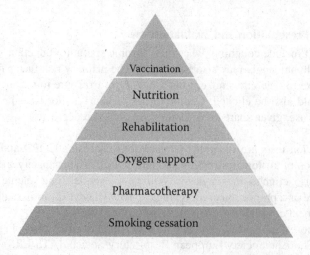

FIGURE 21.5 Foundation of COPD management.

and hospitalizations, improve quality of life,[38] and lower COPD-related mortality.[39] Noninhaled medications, such as theophylline, roflumilast, and intermittent macrolide therapy, also play a role in management of COPD, but are generally adjunctive to the inhaled therapies. For patients with severe or end-stage disease, low dose oral corticosteroid maintenance therapy is sometimes necessary, although evidence supporting its use is lacking.

Medication nonadherence is common in COPD,[40] a multifactorial issue that is amplified in the geriatric population. In addition to universal issues of cost and accessibility, successful usage of inhaled medications is frequently hampered by older patients' difficulty achieving drug delivery; many older patients, even those without underlying lung disease, lack the inspiratory muscle strength to draw the medication into the distal airways,[41,42] rendering it ineffective. Additionally, difficulties with inhaler activation due to arthritis or lack of manual dexterity, as well as the complexity of timing drug delivery with onset of inhalation, can be limiting for older patients. Using a spacer device, a chamber that inserts on to the end of many of the common inhalers, can improve drug delivery[43] and reduce the common inhaled steroid side effect of oropharyngeal thrush. Many inhalers are now available in a nonplunger breath-activated model, making arthritic or dexterity limitations less of an issue. Taking time to instruct the patient on how to use the inhaler, observing their technique, and checking back in to ensure continued proper technique is critical. If the patient is unable to use inhalers, converting to nebulized therapy is an option, but the benefits have not been as rigorously studied.

21.3.1.2.2   Management of COPD Exacerbations

Exacerbations of COPD—heralded as increase in coughing, breathlessness, or sputum volume/character—are a common precipitant for hospitalizations and subsequent rehabilitation. Given the high prevalence of COPD in patients involved in rehabilitation, along with the frequency of repeat exacerbations during recovery, increased vigilance for acute decompensation is needed. Exacerbations are commonly precipitated by infection,[44] although changes in medication, medication nonadherence, and aspiration events can cause decompensations in patients with COPD. Based on data from the ECLIPSE (Evaluation of COPD Longitudinally to Identify Predictive Surrogate Endpoints) study, the single best predictor of COPD exacerbation was a history of exacerbation, regardless of disease severity,[45] suggesting that there is a particular phenotype of "COPD exacerbator."

Management of acute exacerbations of COPD (AECOPD) is comprised primarily of enhanced bronchodilators, often in nebulized form and given at increased frequency, along with provision of systemic steroids, systemic antibiotics for patients with moderate or severe disease,[46] supplemental oxygen if needed, and surveillance for CO_2 retention with use of noninvasive ventilation if indicated. Hospitalization is often needed, and mechanical ventilation may be required.

21.3.1.2.3   Nonpharmacologic Interventions in COPD

Although medications are important in the management of COPD, nonpharmacologic interventions should not be overlooked. The most important nonmedication interventions for management of COPD are reviewed here.

21.3.1.3   Smoking Cessation

Smoking cessation counseling should be the foundation of COPD management, even in the elderly. At any age, smoking cessation slows the decline in lung function wrought by tobacco exposure[47] and reduces chronic coughing, sputum production, and infectious exacerbations. Men who stop smoking at age 65 can potentially add two years of life expectancy, whereas women who quit at 65 can gain 3.7 years,[48] yet physicians are less likely to discuss smoking cessation with older patients.[49] Discussing smoking cessation at any contact with the medical system has been shown to incrementally increase the patient's likelihood of quitting, and the opportunity should not be missed in the older patient undergoing rehabilitation, whether for pulmonary disease or other illness. The major smoking cessation aids currently available—nicotine replacement, bupropion, and varenicline—appear to be effective, safe, and well tolerated in patients aged 65–75 in clinical trials.[50, 51]

21.3.1.4 Supplemental Oxygen

It is well established that the use of supplemental oxygen for patients with resting $PaO_2 < 55$ mm Hg improves not only survival, but also exercise tolerance and cognitive function.[52,53] Other studies have demonstrated quality of life improvements, benefits in sleep, and reduction in secondary polycythemia and nocturnal tachyarrhythmias.[54] In addition, the use of nocturnal oxygen in patients with stable COPD has been shown to be safe with respect to precipitating CO_2 retention.[55] Regular assessments of ambulatory and nocturnal oxygen saturation are recommended during the care of the patient with moderate to severe COPD, particularly during recovery from acute illness.

21.3.1.5 Nutrition, Airway Clearance, and Immunizations

Other important facets of COPD management include nutritional support, assistance with secretion clearance (see Section 21.3.3), and vaccinations. Malnutrition is common as COPD progresses, and contributes to respiratory muscle weakness and diminished immune system reserve. Cachexia itself, defined as BMI < 17 in men and <14 in women, has been found to be an independent predictor of mortality in patients with COPD.[56] Engaging nutritional support services has been shown to be effective in improving exercise performance in malnourished COPD patients.[57] Since respiratory infection is the primary cause of acute exacerbation, vaccinations against typical etiologic agents (such as influenza and pneumococcus) are encouraged (Figure 21.6).

21.3.1.6 Rehabilitation of the Older Patient with COPD

Patients with COPD experience exaggerated age-related declines in lung function and corresponding heightened increases in exertional dyspnea and exercise intolerance. These symptoms are attributable to the changes in pulmonary function described earlier: namely, decreased airway diameter, enhanced by the loss of the tethering support structures due to progression of emphysema, along with increased mucoid secretions in the airways themselves; decreased efficiency of the respiratory muscular apparatus related not only to normal age-related changes but also to excessive flattening of the diaphragm; decreased gas exchange capabilities due to destruction of alveoli and thickening of the alveolar–capillary membranes (scarring); and increased dynamic hyperinflation.

These changes disrupt the balance between respiratory load and the respiratory pump, resulting in exertional dyspnea and respiratory insufficiency. The struggle to breathe with exertion initiates a downward spiral of inactivity leading to cardiovascular deconditioning, accelerated muscle depletion, progression of dyspnea, further inactivity and, ultimately, disability. It should be mentioned that physical inactivity is not unique to advanced COPD; it is already pronounced in patients with mild

---

- Obstructive lung disease frequently but not always associated with history of tobacco exposure
- Symptoms include exertional dyspnea, wheezing, and cough with or without sputum production
- Exam frequently reveals decreased breath sounds or wheezes, evidence of hyperinflation, and hypoxia; pulmonary function tests reveal obstructive pattern, often with impaired diffusing capacity
- Nonpharmacologic management centers around avoidance of cigarette smoke, provision of supplemental oxygen or other respiratory support (BIPAP or CPAP) as needed, enrollment in pulmonary rehabilitation, immunizations, and nutritional support
- Pharmacologic management includes inhaled steroids, anticholinergics, and beta agonists, alone or in combination, along with other adjunctive medications
- Acute exacerbations should be managed with enhanced bronchodilators, steroids ± antibiotics; hospitalization may be necessary

---

FIGURE 21.6 COPD: Key points.

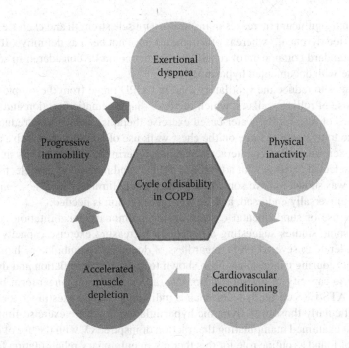

FIGURE 21.7   Spiral of disability in COPD.

or moderate COPD,[58] even preceding the onset of dyspnea.[59] In addition, research into the nature of COPD-related disability reveals that the "nonrespiratory" realm of reduced muscle strength and lower extremity dysfunction are at least as critical as lung function impairment in causing exercise intolerance and disability.[60] Indeed, the quadriceps cross-sectional area has been found to be a predictor of mortality in patients with COPD independent of lung function.[61] Rehabilitation must therefore take into account not only respiratory limitations in patients with COPD, but also coexisting nonrespiratory impairments (Figure 21.7).

21.3.1.7   Pulmonary Rehabilitation for COPD: A Model for Chronic Lung Disease

Pulmonary rehabilitation has arguably the greatest impact of any current therapy on reducing disability and improving exertional capacity in patients with COPD[62] and has gained acceptance as a key facet of COPD management. As emphasized in the 2013 Statement on Pulmonary Rehabilitation published by the ATS/ERS, it is a "comprehensive intervention" of "patient-tailored therapies, which include, but are not limited to, exercise training, education, and behavior change."[63] Multiple studies have documented the many positive effects of pulmonary rehabilitation in COPD, including improvements in exertional dyspnea, exercise tolerance, and quality of life,[64–66] along with reductions in healthcare utilization, including hospitalizations (frequency and/or length) and hospital readmissions for repeat exacerbations.[67] Despite its many other benefits, pulmonary rehabilitation has not been shown to consistently improve lung function or impact mortality. Large randomized trials examining its impact on survival are needed.

In COPD, reduced gas exchange and dynamic hyperinflation are common and powerful determinants of diminished exercise capacity. Techniques to reduce dynamic hyperinflation include breathing retraining and inspiratory muscle training. Training in breathing techniques (such as pursed-lip breathing or so-called "yoga" breathing") was evaluated by a Cochrane meta-analysis and was found to result in improved exercise capacity, without a consistent effect on dyspnea.[68] Inspiratory muscle training, specifically designed to combat the flattened diaphragm's mechanical disadvantage during exercise, has met with mixed results but is advocated by some experts as a helpful component. One meta-analysis examining the effect of inspiratory muscle training on patients with stable COPD found significant increases in inspiratory muscle strength and exercise capacity, with a decrease in reported dyspnea,[69] whereas other studies have not been as definitive. It is not currently advocated as a standard component of rehabilitation, but could be considered in selected patients, particularly those with documented hyperinflation.

Other techniques to reduce the ventilatory load in COPD range from the simple to the complex, and include the use of rolling walkers, which improve diaphragmatic function and facilitate use of accessory muscles of respiration; water-based exercise therapies, which may reduce hyperinflated lung volumes due to hydrostatic force on the chest wall; use of continuous positive airway pressure (CPAP) during exercise, which counteracts dynamic hyperinflation and results in improved exercise capacity in selected patients with advanced COPD[70]; and neuromuscular electrical stimulation (NMES), which was shown to have some benefit in severely limited patients.[71] None of these techniques has been universally endorsed, and further investigation is needed.

The universal use of supplemental oxygen during pulmonary rehabilitation is similarly controversial, with some studies suggesting a benefit in increasing exercise capacity (endurance) in patients with moderate to severe COPD, regardless of documented ambulatory hypoxia. In COPD, increasing the FiO_2 during exercise has been shown to reduce hyperinflation and dyspnea, thereby increasing exercise capacity in the short term. Overall, however, no longer-term benefit has been established. The ATS/ERS currently recommends individual oximetry testing to identify those who may benefit, particularly those with dynamic hyperinflation or severe exercise-limiting dyspnea.[72] Other studies that examined manipulating the fraction of inspired O_2 with the use of helium–oxygen mixtures have not found a routine role for this therapy in pulmonary rehabilitation for patients with COPD.

Methods of assessing and improving exercise capacity in the patient with COPD have been developed and validated. Ambulation has been shown to be as effective a tool for increasing aerobic capacity as use of exercise equipment (such as the stationary bicycle or stepper), and the 6-minute walk distance (6MWD) has become a standard tool for assessing physical activity. Resistance training, of both the lower and upper extremities, has been shown to confer additional benefit and improve general functioning, including the ability to complete the activities of daily living (ADL), and has become a standard component of exercise training in pulmonary rehabilitation.[73] Unsupported arm exercises have been shown to reduce dyspnea during performance of ADLs,[74] and balance training is appropriate in the selected COPD patient with a history of falls. Finally, interval training[75] and muscle partitioning[76] appear to increase the duration and intensity of exercise in patients with severe respiratory limitation. Interval training (walking for three 10-minute blocks rather than one 30-minute block, for example) also appears to increase exercise adherence in patients with COPD, but longer-term benefit has yet to be defined. Muscle partitioning (cycling with one leg at a time, for example) has been shown to improve endurance while reducing the ventilatory load.

The educational component of pulmonary rehabilitation for patients with COPD should not be overlooked. Breathing exercises, avoidance of tobacco and other precipitants of lung decline, medication and oxygen adherence, early recognition of exacerbations, and encouragement of healthy nutrition and physical activity should be emphasized. Multiple studies support additive improvement in endurance and quality of life measures when educational techniques are combined with structured exercise.[77] Many patients also report that the sense of community derived from the group education sessions is helpful.

21.3.1.8 Remaining Questions

Although pulmonary rehabilitation improves exercise performance and quality of life measures in patients with COPD, this is not always accompanied by a sustained improvement in physical activity in daily life. Questions remain regarding optimal duration of therapy; intensity, method, and frequency of follow-up; and how best to prolong the many short-term gains attained during rehabilitation. Determining how to encourage our patients with respiratory disease to continue to

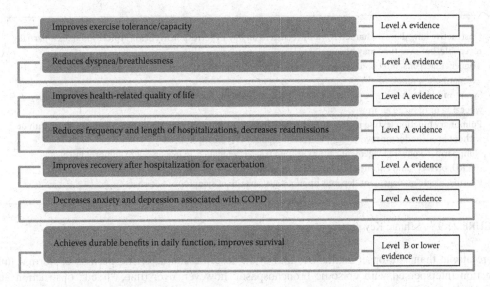

FIGURE 21.8 Benefits of pulmonary rehabilitation in COPD. (Adapted from Pulhan, MA et al. 2011. *Cochrane Database Syst Rev.* (10):CD005305.)

use the tools obtained during structured rehabilitation is an essential area of research if we hope to achieve a lasting benefit as they live with this chronic disease (Figure 21.8).

21.3.2 ASTHMA

Although often viewed as a disease of the young, asthma has a bimodal distribution, with a bump in incidence in patients in their sixth and seventh decades.[78] For the past three decades, the burden of asthma deaths has been greatest in the elderly, yet asthma's substantial morbidity is overshadowed by the multitude of other illnesses afflicting the geriatric population. A bias toward diagnoses of COPD and congestive heart failure after age 65 may obscure the recognition of asthma in this population. Other factors, such as altered perception of bronchospasm, can lead the older adult to underreport symptoms or to describe them differently than the younger asthmatic. Providers may underutilize diagnostic testing, such as pulmonary function tests with bronchodilator reversibility, that would establish a diagnosis. Finally, typical but mild asthma symptoms in older patients may be incorrectly ascribed to more "geriatric" conditions, even in the face of reversible airflow obstruction.[79] Heightened awareness of the prevalence and morbidity of asthma in the geriatric population is needed.

21.3.2.1 Clinical Presentation and Evaluation

Asthma is characterized as chronic airway inflammation leading to recurrent episodes of airway hyperresponsiveness and reversible airflow obstruction. These "twitchy airways" result in the classic symptoms of wheezing, chest tightness, coughing, and dyspnea. Symptoms are classically intermittent, as when a "trigger" is encountered, but can become persistent. When symptomatic, airflow obstruction (decreased ratio of FEV_1 to FVC) is typically seen and is generally at least partially reversible with inhalation of a bronchodilator (the concept behind the so-called bronchodilator reversibility test, performed as part of the pulmonary function assessment). The sporadic nature of the disease can make diagnosis challenging. In an older patient with normal baseline spirometry in whom asthma is being considered, bronchoprovocational testing can be safely used.[80]

Older asthmatic patients include both "early onset" asthmatics whose disease progressed or relapsed, and those whose symptoms arose in late adulthood. Lifelong asthmatics tend to be

- Obstructive lung disease characterized by recurrent airway hyperresponsiveness. Typically is at least partially reversible, but over time may become "fixed"
- Triggers (allergens, infection, changes in temperature/humidity, exposure to smoke or other inhalants, exertion) often reported
- Symptoms include episodic wheezing, chest tightness, cough, and dyspnea; exam often reveals expiratory wheezing or reduced air flow
- Pulmonary function testing may be normal if asymptomatic or show variable degrees of obstruction, with or without bronchodilator reversibility. Diffusion capacity is typically normal
- Nonpharmacologic management centers around trigger avoidance, management of comorbidities (GERD, obesity), and encouraging breathing awareness
- Pharmacologic management depends upon nature/severity of symptoms. See chart

FIGURE 21.9   Asthma: Key points.

more atopic than late-onset asthmatics and often describe characteristic periods of normal lung function interspersed with episodic bronchospasm; however, over time, "fixed" obstruction and chronic hyperinflation can develop, making differentiating between COPD and asthma challenging. Similarly, patients with symptom onset in their later years, and particularly those with a history of cigarette exposure, may be erroneously diagnosed with COPD, particularly if bronchodilator reversibility testing is not done.[79] Eliciting a history of typical symptom triggers, such as exercise, infection, pollens or other aeroallergens, exposure to dusts/fumes, changes in ambient temperature or humidity, and animal contacts, can be helpful in identifying older patients with the asthma phenotype, as can a history of atopy or exposure to airway irritants such as molds or wood burning stoves.[81] Finally, although a history of heavy tobacco exposure can point toward a diagnosis of COPD over asthma, it should be noted that up to 50% of older people with asthma are current or former smokers.[82]

The classic symptoms of wheezing, coughing, and chest tightness are no different in older individuals with asthma, but the older asthmatic is more likely to describe dyspnea at the same degree of airflow limitation, perhaps because of the cumulative effect of increased airways resistance in the aging lung. Interestingly, the older asthmatic may become more adapted to chronic airflow limitation and so may have lesser recognition of acute bronchospasm than younger patients.[83] At the same time, the older asthmatic may also have heightened susceptibility to bronchospasm, as manifested by a larger percentage drop in FEV_1 during an exacerbation. Fortunately, age alone is not a significant predictor of the acute bronchodilator response in asthma[84]; rather, the duration of asthma symptoms appears to be the best indicator of reversibility.

Older asthmatics are more likely than younger asthmatics to endorse symptoms suggestive of chronic bronchitis (chronic productive coughing, chest congestion), and bronchiectasis may develop. The latter condition manifests as a more severe asthma phenotype, and afflicted patients require more hospitalizations and progress to respiratory failure more frequently (Figure 21.9).[85]

21.3.2.2   Management of Asthma in the Older Adult

General principles of asthma management include avoidance of triggers, symptom monitoring, patient education, and pharmacologic therapy. The National Asthma Education and Prevention Program (NAEPP) and the Global Initiative for Asthma (GINA) guidelines suggest that determining asthma severity is essential to guiding therapy, followed by stepwise adjustment of therapy depending on subsequent assessments of asthma control. The goal of asthma therapy in older patients is to address symptoms, preserve, or enhance activity level, decrease exacerbations and hospitalizations, and optimize pulmonary function with minimal adverse effects from medications. As in COPD, older asthmatic patients with poorly controlled symptoms are more likely to report depression and decreased quality of life.[82]

The choice of pharmacologic therapy depends primarily on the severity of disease, but should also take into account difficulties with inhaler use, cost, and the adverse effect of complexity on medication adherence. As in the earlier discussion on COPD, ensuring correct inhaler technique is critical for efficacy of inhaled medications, and substantial effort should be directed toward ensuring that the older asthmatic is able to generate the negative inspiratory force needed to mobilize these medications to the small airways. Again, using a spacer device may optimize drug delivery. Watching patients use their inhaler is essential and frequent reassessments should be done, given changes in cognition, manual dexterity, and lung function with aging. As in COPD, at times nebulized therapy may be necessary if the patient is unable to use inhalers.

21.3.2.2.1 Pharmacologic Interventions in Asthma

A stepwise approach to initiating asthma therapy is recommended, with the general principle that the medications should be titrated—either "up" or "down"—based on the fluctuating nature of symptoms. This so-called "step up" and "step back" therapy requires vigilance on the part of the patient, who should note the frequency with which they are using their short-acting or rescue inhaler, along with the frequency of nocturnal and/or activity-limiting symptoms, and on the part of the provider. The use of questionnaires, such as the Asthma Control Test, is helpful in this regard.

In asthma, the first line agent for persistent disease is the inhaled corticosteroid, whose use is associated with reduced mortality and hospitalizations in older adults with persistent asthma.[86] A rescue agent, or short-acting beta agonist, should also be prescribed. If disease is not controlled, the steroid dose can either be up-titrated or a LABA added ("step up"). It should be noted that a LABA should not be prescribed as monotherapy in asthmatics, and that caution should be used if the patient has recalcitrant tachyarrhythmia. An alternative "step up" is a leukotriene-modifying agent. These medications can be particularly helpful in older, allergic asthmatics.[87] For the severe asthmatic with frequent exacerbations, the long-acting anticholinergic medication tiotropium has recently been added to the GINA algorithm. As in COPD, the oral agent theophylline is an adjunctive therapy, but caution should be exercised due to the narrow therapeutic window and multitude of drug–drug interactions. Anti-IgE (immunoglobulin E) therapy is currently approved in moderate to severe allergic asthmatics inadequately controlled on inhaled glucocorticoids. In the appropriate patient, this therapy reduces exacerbations, improves symptoms, and reduces rescue medication usage; however, a high rate of discontinuation was observed in older asthmatics.[88] Additional monoclonal antibodies, including the anti-IL 5 agents, are under investigation and will likely be useful in the older asthmatic with severe disease.[89]

21.3.2.2.2 Management of Asthma Exacerbations

Systemic steroids and increased frequency of bronchodilator use are the initial steps in managing acute exacerbations of asthma, typically manifested as increased wheezing, coughing, and/or dyspnea. Peak expiratory flow (PEF) is also likely to be reduced. Given the older asthmatic's decreased awareness of bronchospasm, a delay in recognition is more likely. As a result, and in part due to comorbid conditions, the older asthmatic is more likely to require emergency care. Persistent wheezing or dyspnea despite nebulized short-acting bronchodilators, and/or PEF <50% of patient's best, should prompt evaluation; if no response to an initial round of bronchodilators or to an oral steroid, or if the patient appears to be deteriorating rapidly, transfer to an acute care setting should not be delayed (Figure 21.10).

21.3.2.2.3 Other Interventions in Asthma

Although trials evaluating effectiveness of environmental modifications in older adults are lacking, avoiding allergens and/or addressing them with the use of antihistamines and nasal steroids is accepted practice. Anti-reflux measures may be of particular importance in managing the older asthmatic.[90] Immunizations against influenza and pneumococcus are also endorsed. Close symptom monitoring may be more important in the older asthmatic, who is more likely to underrecognize and

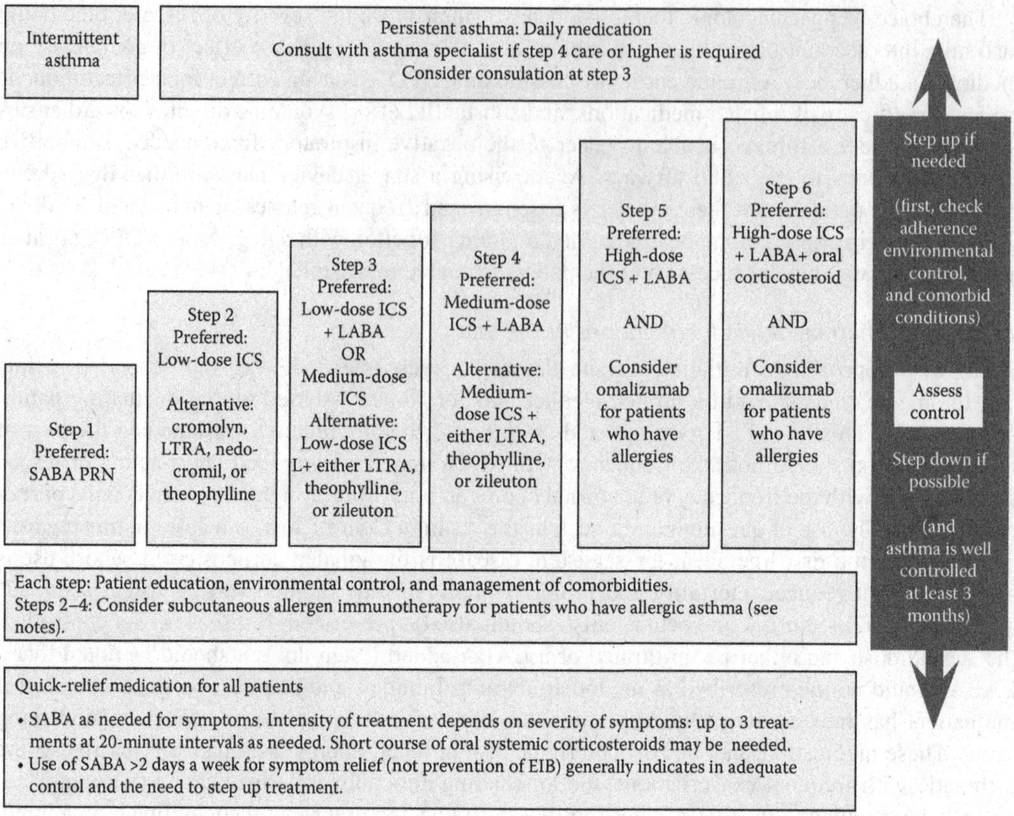

| Intermittent asthma | Persistent asthma: Daily medication
Consult with asthma specialist if step 4 care or higher is required
Consider consulation at step 3 | | | | |

					Step 6 Preferred: High-dose ICS + LABA+ oral corticosteroid AND Consider omalizumab for patients who have allergies
				Step 5 Preferred: High-dose ICS + LABA AND Consider omalizumab for patients who have allergies	
			Step 4 Preferred: Medium-dose ICS + LABA Alternative: Medium- dose ICS + either LTRA, theophylline, or zileuton		
		Step 3 Preferred: Low-dose ICS + LABA OR Medium-dose ICS Alternative: Low-dose ICS L+ either LTRA, theophylline, or zileuton			
	Step 2 Preferred: Low-dose ICS Alternative: cromolyn, LTRA, nedo- cromil, or theophylline				
Step 1 Preferred: SABA PRN					

Step up if needed

(first, check adherence environmental control, and comorbid conditions)

Assess control

Step down if possible

(and asthma is well controlled at least 3 months)

Each step: Patient education, environmental control, and management of comorbidities.
Steps 2–4: Consider subcutaneous allergen immunotherapy for patients who have allergic asthma (see notes).

Quick-relief medication for all patients

• SABA as needed for symptoms. Intensity of treatment depends on severity of symptoms: up to 3 treatments at 20-minute intervals as needed. Short course of oral systemic corticosteroids may be needed.
• Use of SABA >2 days a week for symptom relief (not prevention of EIB) generally indicates in adequate control and the need to step up treatment.

Key: Alphabetical order is used when more than one treatment option is listed within either preferred or alternative therapy.
EIB, exercise-induced bronchospasm; ICS, inhaled corticosteroid; LABA, long-acting inhaled beta$_2$ agonist; LTRA, leukotriene-receptor antagonist; and SABA, inhaled short-acting beta$_2$ agonist.

FIGURE 21.10 Stepwise approach to asthma treatment.[9] (From National Heart, Lung, and Blood Institute, National Institutes of Health.)

underreport subtle changes in function, particularly if memory loss is present.[91] Patient education about the nature of the illness, and in particular the warning signs of an exacerbation, is an essential component to asthma care, and family involvement is helpful. The use of a peak flow meter for monitoring of lung function should be considered in the older asthmatic.

21.3.2.3 Important Points Regarding Rehabilitation in the Older Asthmatic

Older asthmatics are more frequently hospitalized than younger asthmatics and are more likely to curtail physical activity as a result of airflow obstruction, increased work of breathing, and exercise-induced bronchoconstriction. Even when the medication regimen is optimized, many asthmatics have low exercise tolerance, resulting in low levels of physical activity.[92] Poor asthma control is itself associated with functional impairment and reduced ability to participate in the ADL. Lower physical activity levels are in turn associated with increased risk of asthma exacerbations,[93] resulting in increased hospitalizations and deepening of disability. Interrupting this cycle by improving exercise tolerance through a formalized rehabilitation program has the potential to improve outcomes for older asthmatics.

Multiple studies have reported a variety of physiologic benefits of exercise training for asthmatics. Improvements in cardiovascular conditioning, walk distance, and quality of life measurements have all been noted.[94,95] Other studies have suggested that inspiratory muscle training—a technique described in the section on COPD—may lead to improved exercise tolerance by reducing dynamic hyperinflation.[96] Breathing retraining exercises may be similarly beneficial and are easier to teach and for the patient to maintain. Finally, the use of a short-acting bronchodilator prior to exercise is suggested in patients with exercise-induced bronchoconstriction. It is currently recommended that a rehabilitation program for asthmatics encompass both exercise training and breathing exercises, similar to that for COPD, along with asthma-specific education regarding recognizing and avoiding triggers, monitoring symptoms and PEF rate, and action plans for decompensation.

21.3.3 BRONCHIECTASIS

"This affection of the bronchia is always produced by chronic catarrh, or by some other disease attended by long, violent, and often repeated fits of coughing."[97]

Bronchiectasis is an incurable respiratory condition marked by abnormal and irreversible dilatation of the airways. This "outstretching of the bronchi" leads to chronic chest congestion and impaired mucociliary clearance, intractable yet inadequate cough, and recurrent respiratory infections. Distorted airway architecture facilitates the growth of pathogens, including *Pseudomonas aeruginosa, Haemophilus influenzae,* and *Mycobacterium avium,* which in turn perpetuates an inflammatory milieu that further exacerbates airway destruction, resulting in a vicious cycle of infection and inflammation characterized by frequent exacerbations and, typically, progressive disease.

Although present in younger populations (classically in cystic fibrosis and other genetic disorders of mucociliary function), the prevalence of bronchiectasis increases with age. The reasons for this are numerous, and include (1) history of repeated infections; (2) altered host immune defense; (3) impairment of the cough line of defense, resulting in compromised sputum clearance; (4) decreased nutritional state; and (5) comorbid conditions such as recurrent aspiration, gastroesophageal reflux disease, malignancy, autoimmune disease, and interstitial and obstructive lung disease.

Although not as common as COPD or asthma in the elderly, bronchiectasis carries a mortality of approximately 20%.[98] The true prevalence of bronchiectasis is unknown due to underrecognition, but Weycker et al. found that it is dramatically more prevalent in adults over age 75 than in younger adults.[99]

Several factors predispose the elderly patient to the development of respiratory infection, which in turn compounds bronchiectasis. One critical factor is the weakening of the cough as we age. The lung has the greatest epithelial surface area of any organ and therefore shoulders a disproportionate risk of exposure to microbes, either inhaled from ambient air or aspirated from the oropharynx. Coughing is the primary line of defense against this constant assault. As noted earlier, changes in respiratory dynamics, including the loss of diaphragmatic curvature and the increasing rigidity of the chest wall, decrease the effectiveness of coughing as a mechanism of clearing the airway. Mucociliary transport and salivary flow also decline with age, contributing to reduced clearance of pathogens. Finally, multifactorial alterations in immune function—related to underlying illness, use of immunosuppressing medications, chronic malnutrition, and alterations in B and T cell number and function, so-called "immunosenescence"[100,101]—also contribute to the increased incidence and severity of respiratory infection in the older adult (Figure 21.11).

21.3.3.1 Clinical Presentation and Evaluation

Bronchiectasis should be suspected when individuals present with persistent cough productive of mucopurulent sputum, a symptom bronchiectasis shares with chronic bronchitis. In contrast to the latter, however, patients with bronchiectasis have evidence of airway enlargement and distortion on high-resolution computed tomography (HRCT) scan. Other common symptoms include hemoptysis (either mild or severe), chest pain, and dyspnea; generalized constitutional symptoms of fatigue, fevers/chills, night sweats, and unintentional weight loss are often present, particularly in the older bronchiectatic. Auscultory findings include coarse crackles, wheezing, and, occasionally, "pops

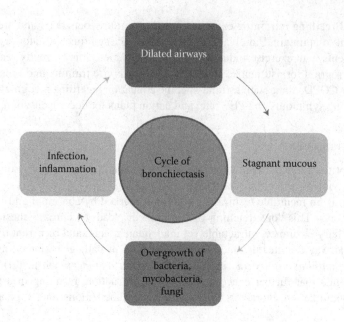

FIGURE 21.11 Cycle of bronchiectasis.

and squeaks." Clubbing can be seen, and pectus excavatum or other chest wall abnormalities are relatively commonplace. Lung function studies demonstrate a variable degree of obstructive and/ or restrictive impairment, with abnormalities of gas exchange (as indicated by reduced diffusing capacity for carbon monoxide/DLCO or PaO_2) increasingly common with more severe disease. Interestingly, sputum volume is said to be the best correlate for quality of life and lung function decline in patients with bronchiectasis.[102]

21.3.3.2 Management of Bronchiectasis in the Older Adult

Bronchiectasis treatment involves (1) assessing for and treating underlying conditions, such as coexisting obstructive lung disease, rheumatoid arthritis or other autoimmune disease, hypogammaglobulinemia, and/or ILD; (2) assisting airway clearance; (3) maintaining a high index of suspicion for acute infectious exacerbations; (4) addressing reductions in pulmonary function as able; (5) providing nutritional, and, if needed, oxygen support; and (6) immunizations.

Airway clearance is the foundation of bronchiectasis management, the rationale being that improved mucociliary clearance may eliminate or at least ameliorate the mucous stagnation associated with bacterial colonization, reducing risk of recurrent infection and minimizing further airway destruction. The goal of chest physiotherapy is to enhance expectoration of sputum from the lungs. A variety of techniques are available, including postural drainage and cupping, active cycle of breathing techniques (so-called "huff coughing"), oscillatory positive expiratory pressure (PEP) devices (such as the "flutter valve"), mechanical tools applied to the chest wall (such as the percussion vest), and cough-assist devices. In the geriatric population, the first approach may be challenging due to decreased mobility, postural disequilibrium, chronic pain, and respiratory fatiguing. Oscillatory devices are relatively inexpensive and simple to use, and can be used as often as necessary. The percussion vest and the cough-assist device are more costly and require the assistance of trained personnel or family, but may be reasonable to use in the rehabilitation setting if resources are available. Importantly, as of this writing, there is no compelling data that any one of these techniques is clearly superior to the others, so an individualized approach based on patient tolerance and preference is recommended. A recent Cochrane meta-analysis on airway clearance in bronchiectasis found a paucity of data on the effect of these techniques on reducing frequency of exacerbations, with some suggestion that they may improve quality of life, including symptoms of breathlessness, coughing, and congestion, and also may improve lung function. Fortunately, no adverse effects were linked to the use of these techniques.[103]

Alternative methods of airway clearance include the use of nebulized substances such as mannitol, hypertonic, or normal saline. Experience with these interventions in non-CF (cystic fibrosis) bronchiectasis is fairly limited, but several studies were recently published that suggest at least partial benefit. In a study evaluating routine inhaled mannitol on exacerbation rates in adults with bronchiectasis, no benefit in reducing exacerbation rate was found; however there was a delay to first exacerbation and a reported improved quality of life in patients on the mannitol protocol.[104] A recent Cochrane review found that nebulized hypertonic saline had no benefit over regular saline,[105] but either substance in the appropriate patient can improve mucous clearance and quality of life, particularly when used as an adjunct to other methods of chest physiotherapy. Finally, a different Cochrane review on mucolytic agents found harm (increased exacerbation frequency) when DNase (deoxyribonuclease) was used by patients with non-CF bronchiectasis.[106]

Patients with bronchiectasis frequently develop progressive airflow obstruction, likely due to a combination of airway distortion and internal airway narrowing due to chronic mucous impaction/plugs. Although not studied in large clinical trials, several small trials have suggested that inhaled corticosteroids may be helpful in improving dyspnea, cough, sputum volume, and airways hyperreactivity, particularly in patients with frequent exacerbations and more purulent sputum.[107,108] Although the addition of a LABA may further improve symptoms of cough and dyspnea, a recent study cautioned that LABA usage in bronchiectasis increased risk of hemoptysis.[109]

Early recognition of infectious exacerbations is paramount in preventing progression of the disease. Patients and caregivers should be vigilant for changes in sputum amount, frequency, or character, along with more subtle infectious signs in the older bronchiectatic such as anorexia, fatigue, and weight loss. Complicating diagnosis of an acute infectious exacerbation is the fact that many patients exhibit airway colonization with bacteria that can also cause disease, most commonly *P. aeruginosa* or *M. avium,* and deciding when to treat with antibiotics in such cases is not easy. When an infection is diagnosed, prompt initiation of antibiotics is crucial, and more prolonged courses are often used, although with less-than-robust supporting data. Although likely less effective than in cystic fibrosis, nebulized antibiotics can be used in the appropriately selected patient with bronchiectasis. Additionally, systemic steroids may be needed if bronchospasm is prominent.

Prevention of exacerbations in patients with bronchiectasis is an area of active interest. Immunizations are critical, as is addressing underlying immunodeficiency (such as immunoglobulin deficiency). Although absolute immunoglobulin deficiency is likely less common in the older bronchiectatic, the previously discussed immunosenescence of aging enables pathogenic bacteria to flourish in the bronchiectatic airways and thereby trigger frequent exacerbations. The use of thrice weekly macrolide therapy for combined immunomodulatory, mucociliary clearance, and antibiotic effect is supported in non-CF bronchiectasis for reducing exacerbations, sputum volume, and, in some patients, decline in lung function.[101–112] Monitoring for cardiac arrhythmias is necessary. The longer-term effects of chronic macrolide use on bronchiectasis have not been assessed. Daily or cycling antibiotics, both oral and inhaled, have been used in an attempt to prevent exacerbations but have not been well-studied. Patients colonized with *Pseudomonas* may derive benefit from inhaled antibiotics, primarily in lessening symptoms and improving clearance of the bacteria, but these results are either mild or only transient, and intolerance is not rare.[113,114] Further studies are needed to investigate the role of these therapies in non-CF bronchiectasis. Other anti-inflammatory therapies, including statins, are currently under investigation as possible tools in bronchiectasis. As always, those who smoke should receive cessation counseling (Figure 21.12).

21.3.3.3 Important Points about Rehabilitation in Bronchiectasis

Although a distinct disease from COPD, bronchiectasis shares similarities of primary pulmonary but secondary muscle involvement, resulting in varying degrees of airflow obstruction, impaired

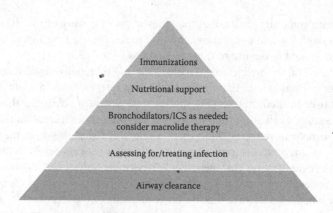

FIGURE 21.12   Management of bronchiectasis.

exercise capacity, tendency toward exacerbation, accelerated muscle wasting, and malnutrition. In one prospective randomized controlled trial examining a structured exercise program with and without inspiratory muscle training for patients with bronchiectasis, improvements in exercise capacity were noted, as were improvements in quality of life measures when exercise was combined with inspiratory muscle training.[115] Other studies have shown that exercise training in patients with non-CF bronchiectasis (including an older cohort) reduces the frequency of exacerbations. The authors postulated several reasons for this benefit, including respiratory muscle conditioning and improved mucous clearance.[116] A smaller study showed similar benefits when combined with chest physiotherapy, including improved exercise tolerance and health-related quality of life.[117]

Rehabilitation in the older patient with bronchiectasis should focus not only on improving exercise capacity, but also on maintaining good pulmonary hygiene with airway clearance techniques described above. An effort should be made to clear the airways as able prior to the onset of exercise, although exertion itself is often a powerful stimulus for mucous clearance. Dynamic hyperinflation should be minimized using breathing techniques, self-pacing, and a short-acting bronchodilator prior to exercise if bronchospastic. On the basis of the above evidence, inspiratory muscle training may have a role. The educational component should center around recognizing early signs of exacerbation, using airway clearance techniques, and maintaining good nutrition (Figures 21.13 and 21.14).

- Bronchiectasis is characterized by abnormal airway dilatation
- Symptoms include persistent, often productive cough, chest congestion, frequent infection, and dyspnea; fatigue, weight loss, and night sweats are also common
- Exam findings include coarse crackles, wheezes, and "pops and squeaks"; lung function testing often reveals obstruction, restriction, and/or impaired gas exchange
- Diagnosis is secured by characteristic airway dilatation on high-resolution CT scan
- Nonpharmacologic management centers around evaluating for underlying conditions, airway clearance techniques, nutritional support, and immunizations
- Pharmacologic management includes
  1. Assessing for/treating infection
  2. Correcting airway inflammation/obstruction with inhaled steroids and/or bronchodilators
  3. Using macrolide therapy and/or chronic inhaled antibiotics to control inflammation

FIGURE 21.13   Bronchiectasis: Key points.

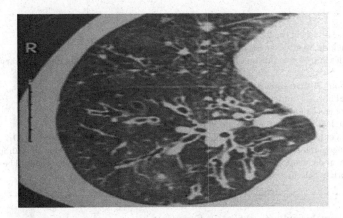

FIGURE 21.14 HRCT image showing bronchiectasis, or dilation of the small airways.

21.3.4 INTERSTITIAL LUNG DISEASE

The diffuse parenchymal lung diseases, or interstitial lung diseases (ILDs), are a heterogenous group of disorders in which the lung interstitium and/or alveolar spaces are variably inflamed or fibrotic. Because it is the most common ILD affecting the elderly patient, the focus in this section will be on Idiopathic Pulmonary Fibrosis (IPF).

21.3.4.1 Clinical Presentation and Evaluation

IPF is associated with advancing age, and diagnosis of IPF in individuals less than 50 years of age is uncommon. Although IPF carries a poor prognosis, even in the face of several new treatment options, prognosis worsens with age.[118] Most patients with IPF present with symptoms of breathlessness and dry cough; physical exam often reveals hypoxemia and coarse basilar crackles. Pulmonary function tests show restriction (i.e., proportionately reduced FEV_1 and FVC, or preserved FEV_1/FVC), along with reduced diffusing capacity (DLCO). The diagnosis can be secured by the presence on HRCT of "classic" findings of subpleural fibrosis, peripheral honeycombing, traction bronchiectasis, and minimal inflammatory change.[119] Alternative causes of this pattern, such as underlying rheumatologic disorders, hypersensitivity processes, or exposures (including to medications), must be ruled out. Video-assisted thoracoscopic biopsy is needed if the diagnosis cannot be established clinically/radiographically.

21.3.4.2 Management of IPF

Patients with IPF experience relentless progression of breathlessness. Until recently, no pharmacotherapeutic options have been available to halt the inexorable decline in lung function, and management has centered around correcting hypoxemia, avoiding infection, treating comorbid conditions such as reflux and right heart dysfunction, addressing symptoms of dyspnea with palliative measures, and encouraging maintenance of physical activity. Lung transplantation has also been an option, with the upper age limit for consideration recently extended to 75 years of age.[120] Recently, two anti-fibrotic medications, nintedanib and pirfenidone, have been shown to slow disease progression in patients with mild to moderate IPF, including an older cohort.[121,122] Both medications carry their own adverse effect profile, particularly given the higher likelihood of drug–drug interactions and/or metabolic derangements in the older adult, but consideration for their use in the appropriate patient should not be withheld due to advanced age.

Patients with IPF may suffer acute deteriorations. Etiologies such as infection, pulmonary embolism, pneumothorax, and decompensated heart failure should be sought and treated appropriately.

- Diffuse disease affecting the lung interstitium
- Symptoms include breathlessness, dry cough
- Coarse crackles and hypoxemia on exam; restriction and impaired diffusion on pulmonary function testing
- High-resolution CT scan shows:
  1. Subpleural fibrosis (honeycombing)
  2. Bronchiectasis (traction)
  3. Relative lack of inflammatory change (ground glass)
- Management centers around correction of hypoxia, evaluation for comorbidities (GERD [gastroesophageal reflux disease], heart failure), treatment of dyspnea, enrollment in pulmonary rehabilitation, and consideration of anti-fibrotic therapies. Lung transplantation should be considered in the appropriate patient.

FIGURE 21.15   Idiopathic pulmonary fibrosis: Key points.

However, the clinical course of IPF is often marked by periods of acute decline whose cause is not identified despite a thorough investigation; these are associated with a poor prognosis. Typical symptoms include subacute progression of dyspnea, cough, and hypoxia; often fever or a viral-type syndrome is described. Respiratory insufficiency can be severe and may require noninvasive or invasive ventilation.[123] After excluding other, treatable causes of these decompensations, a trial of systemic corticosteroids is often given,[124] although evidence in support of this is admittedly lacking. Death after an acute exacerbation of IPF is unfortunately common.

For older patients with IPF, the disease rarely exists in isolation, and comorbid conditions can augment the disease-specific decline in exercise tolerance arising from progressive restriction and hypoxia. Addressing gastroesophageal reflux, decompensated heart failure, and psychological distress may do much to improve the patient's well-being, as can incorporation of a palliative approach for managing troubling symptoms of coughing and breathlessness. Although survival studies in IPF for supplemental oxygen therapy are lacking, it is fair to conclude from studies in COPD that the use of supplemental oxygen for hypoxic patients will at minimum enhance exercise capacity and sleep quality (Figure 21.15).

21.3.4.3   Important Points Regarding Rehabilitation of Patients with IPF

Many patients with IPF experience significant exertional dyspnea and hypoxemia that inhibit their ability to remain active. Causes of dyspnea include exaggeration of the normal physiologic increase in chest wall stiffness and decrease in lung elastance that accompany aging, resulting in an inability to increase TV in response to exercise. Rapid, shallow breathing—the classic breathing pattern of the patient with restrictive lung disease—leads to reduced inspiratory time, which can lead to alveolar hypoventilation and dynamic hypoinflation (in contrast to the dynamic hyperinflation seen in obstructive lung disease). Hypoxemia relating to ventilation–perfusion mismatching and diffusion impairment caused by capillary bed destruction and fibrosis are disease hallmarks. These changes are further exacerbated by ventilatory muscle weakness, coexisting cardiovascular disease, and anxiety.[125] As the disease progresses, individuals become progressively more sedentary and lose noninspiratory muscle strength, such that physical exertion becomes ever more demanding. In one small study of patients with ILD, leg fatigue was the principal cause of exercise cessation in 17%, with more than half of patients stating that it was at least equivalent to dyspnea as a reason for stopping exercise.[126]

Several studies have demonstrated that patients with ILD, including IPF, benefit from a program of guided exercise training. Multiple small, randomized controlled trials have indicated that improvements in walk distance, dyspnea scores, and quality of life occur after exercise training in patients with ILD.[127,128] Even patients with severe functional impairment benefit.[129,130] Importantly, a meta-analysis by the Cochrane group demonstrated that pulmonary rehabilitation is not only safe in ILD, but that improvements in functional exercise capacity, dyspnea, and quality of life were seen quickly. Unfortunately, the evidence was deemed of low to moderate quality due to a paucity of large or randomized trials.[131] It has yet to be seen whether exercise training in patients with ILD will result in durable benefit in either exercise capacity or in dyspnea, and it does appear that the magnitude of the benefit may not be comparable to that seen in COPD. A randomized, multicentered trial examining this benefit is underway.[132]

Because of the rapid, shallow breathing pattern of restrictive lung disease, patients with ILD should be instructed on breathing techniques designed to slow breathing (such as so-called yoga breathing). They will often experience profound exercise-induced hypoxemia, and continuous monitoring with escalating oxygen flow to achieve peripheral oxygen saturations of at least 88% may be required. An emphasis on pacing during exercise may be needed, and interval training or partitioning involved muscles may be beneficial. Cardiovascular effects of chronic hypoxemia should be evaluated and treated. Finally, if bronchiectasis is prevalent, airway clearance techniques may be helpful. The educational component should center around the use of supplemental oxygen, pacing and breath retraining, and symptom management, including discussion of palliative techniques for addressing dyspnea.

21.4　REHABILITATION IN THE OLDER PATIENT WITH PULMONARY DISEASE

Rehabilitation—defined as an evidence-based, multidisciplinary comprehensive intervention to reduce symptoms, optimize function by encouraging adherence to health-enhancing behaviors, and reduce healthcare utilization—is an important management tool for all patients with chronic lung disease, irrespective of age. Although the focus of this chapter was not on pulmonary rehabilitation *per se,* burgeoning interest in this modality in the management of COPD has bolstered our knowledge of the importance of exercise training for patients with chronic lung disease. In COPD, there is robust evidence that pulmonary rehabilitation confers significant improvements in exercise capacity, in symptoms such as dyspnea and fatigue, and in health-related quality of life. It also appears to reduce healthcare use, in both patients with stable disease and in the immediate period following an exacerbation.[133] These improvements likely relate not only to muscle strengthening, as manifested by improvements in objective markers of walking distance and general activity level, but also to favorable effects on other aspects of general functional status, including education on managing a chronic disease and its symptoms, and its role in alleviating isolation and improving depression. The aging of our population, the prevalence of chronic respiratory disease, and the need for a multipronged approach will place rehabilitation at the forefront of our efforts to minimize disability and promote quality of life in the older population.

REFERENCES

1. Pitta F, Troosters T, Spruit MA. 2005. Characteristics of physical activities in daily life in chronic obstructive pulmonary disease. *Am J Respir Crit Care Med* 171:972–977.
2. Burney P, Jithoo A, Kato B et al. 2014. Burden of Obstructive Lung Disease (BOLD) Study. Chronic obstructive pulmonary disease mortality and prevalence: The associations with smoking and poverty—a BOLD analysis. *Thorax* 69:465–473.
3. Kochanek KD, Xu J, Murphy SL, Miniño AM, Kung H. 2011. Deaths: Final data for 2009. *Natl Vital Stat Rep* 60(3):1–116.
4. Lozano R, Naghavi M, Foreman K et al. 2012. Global and regional mortality from 235 causes of death for 20 age groups in 1990 to 2010: A systemic analysis for the Global Burden of Disease Study 2010. *Lancet* 380:2095–2128.
5. Tinetti ME, McAvay GJ, Murphy TE et al. 2012. Contribution of individual diseases to death in older adults with multiple diseases. *J Am Geriatr Soc* 60(8):1228–1456.

6. Eisner M, Iribarren C, Blanc P et al. 2011. Development of disability in chronic obstructive pulmonary disease: Beyond lung function. *Thorax* 66:109–114.

7. Chan ED, Welsh CH. 1998. Geriatric respiratory medicine. *Chest* 114:1704–1733.

8. Tolep K, Higgins N, Muza S et al. 1995. Comparison of diaphragm strength between healthy adult elderly and young men. *Am J Respir Crit Care Med* 152(2):677–682.

9. Enright PL, Kronmal RA, Manolio TA et al. 1994. Respiratory muscle strength in the elderly: Correlates and reference values. *Am J Respir Crit Care Med* 149(2):430–438.

10. Pokey MI, Hamnega C-H, Hughes PD et al. 1998. Influence of acute lung volume change on contractile properties of human diaphragm. *J Appl Physiol* 85(4):1322–1328.

11. Mizuno M. 1991. Human respiratory muscles: Fiber morphology and capillary supply. *Eur Respir J* 4:587–601.

12. Janssens J-P. 2005. Aging of the respiratory system: Impact on pulmonary function tests and adaptation to exertion. *Clin Chest Med* 26:469–484.

13. Vestbo J, Edwards LD, Scanlon PD et al. 2011. Changes in forced expiratory volume in 1 second over time in COPD. *N Engl J Med* 365:1184–1192.

14. Vaz Fragazo C, Gill T. 2012. Respiratory impairment and the aging lung. *J Gerontol A: Biol Sci Med Sci* 67A(3):264–275.

15. Le Blanc P. 1970. Effects of age and body position on "airway closure" in man. *J Appl Physiol* 284:448–451.

16. Guenard H, Marthan R. 1996. Pulmonary gas exchange in elderly subjects. *Eur Respir J* 9:2573–2577.

17. American Thoracic Society, American College of Chest Physicians. 2003. Statement on cardiopulmonary exercise testing. *Am J Respir Crit Care Med* 167:211–277.

18. Peterson DD. 1981. Effects of aging on ventilatory and occlusion pressure responses to hypoxia and hypercapnia. *Am Rev Respir Dis* 124:387–391.

19. Brischetto MJ, Milman RP, Peterson DD et al. 1984. Effect of aging on ventilatory response to exercise and CO2. *J Appl Physiol: Respir Environ Exercise Physiol* 56(5):1143–1150.

20. Mahler DA, Cunningham LN, Curfman GD. 1986. Aging and exercise performance. *Clin Geriatr Med* 2:431–451.

21. Pellegrino R, Viegi G, Brusasco V. 2005. Series "ATS/ERS task force: Standardisation of lung function testing": Interpretation of lung function tests. *Eur Respir J* 26:948–968.

22. Luoto JA, Elmsthal S, Wollmer P, Pihlsgard M. 2015. Incidence of airflow limitation in subjects 65–100 years of age. *Eur Respir J* 46(6). doi: 10.1183/13993003.00635-2015 Published 17 December 2015.

23. Sanojevic S, Wade A, Stoks J et al. 2008. Reference ranges for spirometry across all ages. *Am J Respir Crit Care Med* 177:253–260.

24. Mannion DM, Homa DM, Akinbami LJ et al. 2002. Chronic obstructive pulmonary disease surveillance—United States, 1971–2000. *MMWR Surveill Summ* 51(6):1–16.

25. Kosacz N et al. 2012. Chronic obstructive pulmonary disease among adults—United States. *MMWR Surveill Summ* 61(46):938–943.

26. Murray CJ, Lopez AD. 1997. Alternative projections of mortality and disability by cause 1990–2020: Global Burden of Disease Study. *Lancet* 349(9064):1498–1504.

27. Eisner M, Iribarren C, Blanc P et al. 2011. Development of disability in chronic obstructive pulmonary disease: Beyond lung function. *Thorax* 66:109–114.

28. Eisner MD, Yelin EH, Trupin L et al. 2002. The influence of chronic respiratory conditions on health status and work disability. *Am J Public Health* 92:1506–1513.

29. Mannino DM. 2002. COPD: Epidemiology, prevalence, morbidity and mortality, and disease heterogeneity. *Chest* 121(5 Suppl):121S–126S.

30. Waschki B, Kirsten A, Holz O et al. 2011. Physical activity is the strongest predictor of all-cause mortality in patients with COPD: A prospective cohort study. *Chest* 140:331–342.

31. Pauwels RA, Buist AS, Calverley PM, Jenkins CR, Hurd SS. 2001. Global strategy for the diagnosis, management, and prevention of chronic obstructive pulmonary disease. NHLBI/WHO Global Initiative for Chronic Obstructive Lung Disease (GOLD) Workshop summary. *Am J Respir Crit Care Med* 163(5):1256–1276.

32. Yohannes AM, Baldwin RC, Connolly MJ. 2000. Depression and anxiety in elderly outpatients with chronic obstructive pulmonary disease: Prevalence, and validation of the BASDEC screening questionnaire. *Int J Geriatr Psychiatry* 15(12):1090–1096.

33. WHO (World Health Organization) Global strategy for diagnosis, management, and prevention of COPD 2008. http://www.goldcopd.com/Guidelineitem.asp?l1=2&l2=1&intId=989.

34. Celli BR, MacNee W, Agusti A et al. 2004. Standards for the diagnosis and treatment of patients with COPD: A summary of the ATS/ERS position paper. *Eur Respir J* 23(6):932–946.

35. Qaseem, A, Wilt JJ, Weinberger SE. 2011. Diagnosis and management of stable chronic obstructive pulmonary disease: A clinical practice guideline update from the American College of Physicians, American College of Chest Physicians, American Thoracic Society, and European Respiratory Society. *Ann Intern Med* 55(3):179–192.

36. Nichol KL, Margolis KL, Wuorenma J et al. 1994. The efficacy and cost effectiveness of vaccination against influenza among elderly persons living in the community. *N Engl J Med* 331(12):778–784.

37. Celli BR, Thomas NE, Anderson JA et al. 2008. Effect of pharmacotherapy on rate of decline of lung function in chronic obstructive pulmonary disease: Results from the TORCH study. *Am J Respir Crit Care Med* 178:332–338.

38. Tashkin DP, Celli B, Senn S et al. (UPLIFT Study Investigators). 2008. A 4-year trial of tiotropium in chronic obstructive pulmonary disease. *N Engl J Med* 359(15):1543–1554.

39. Lee TA, Wilke C, Joo M et al. 2009. Outcomes associated with tiotropium use in patients with chronic obstructive pulmonary disease. *Arch Intern Med* 169(15):1403.

40. Ramsey SD. 2000. Suboptimal medical therapy in COPD: Exploring the causes and consequences. *Chest* 117(2 suppl):33S–37S.

41. Jarvis S, Ind PW, Shiner RJ. 2007. Inhaled therapy in elderly COPD patients; time for re-evaluation? *Age Ageing* 36(2):213–218.

42. Jannsens W, VandenBrande P, Hardeman E et al. 2008. Inspiratory flow rates at different levels of resistance in elderly COPD patients. *Eur Respir J* 31(1):78–83.

43. Ho SF, O'Mahoney MS, Steward JA et al. 2004. Inhaler technique in older people in the community. *Age Ageing* 33(2):185–188.

44. Sethi S. 2004. Bacteria in exacerbations of chronic obstructive pulmonary disease. *Proc Am Thorac Soc* 1:109.

45. Hurst JR, Vestbo J, Anzueto A et al. 2010. Evaluation of COPD Longitudinally to Identify Predictive Surrogate Endpoints (ECLIPSE) Investigators. Susceptibility to exacerbation in chronic obstructive pulmonary disease. *N Engl J Med* 363(12):1128.

46. Global Initiative for Chronic Obstructive Lung Disease (GOLD). Global strategy for the diagnosis, management, and prevention of COPD: Updated 2015. http://www.goldcopd.org.

47. Gourlay SG, Benowitz NL. 1996. The benefits of stopping smoking and the role of nicotine replacement therapy in older patients. *Drugs Aging* 9(1):8–23.

48. Taylor DH Jr, Hasselblad V, Henley SJ et al. 2002. Benefits of smoking cessation for longevity. *Am J Public Health* 92(6):990–996.

49. Maguire CP, Ryan J, Kelly A et al. 2000. Do patient age and medical condition influence medical advice to stop smoking? *Age Ageing* 29(3):264–266.

50. Jorenby DE, Hays JT, Rigotti NA et al. 2006. Efficacy of varenicline, an alpha4beta2 nicotinic acetylcholine receptor partial agonist, vs placebo or sustained-release bupropion for smoking cessation: A randomized controlled trial. *JAMA* 296(1):56–63.

51. Gonzales D, Rennard SI, Nides M et al. 2006. Varenicline, an alpha4beta2 nicotinic acetylcholine receptor partial agonist, vs sustained-release bupropion and placebo for smoking cessation: A randomized controlled trial. *JAMA* 296(1):47–55.

52. Nocturnal Oxygen Therapy Trial Group. 1980. Continuous or nocturnal oxygen therapy in hypoxemic chronic obstructive lung disease: A clinical trial. *Ann Intern Med* 93(3):391–398.

53. Report of the Medical Research Council Working Party. 1981. Long term domiciliary oxygen therapy in chronic hypoxic cor pulmonale complicating chronic bronchitis and emphysema. *Lancet* 1(8222):681–686.

54. Chalker RB, Celli BR. 1993. Special considerations in the elderly patient. *Clin Chest Med* 13:437–452.

55. Goldstein RS, Ramcharan V, Bowes G et al. 1984. Effect of supplemental nocturnal oxygen on gas exchange in patients with severe obstructive lung disease. *N Engl J Med* 310:425–429.

56. Chailleux E, Laaban JP, Veale D. 2003. Prognostic value of nutritional depletion in patients with COPD treated by long-term oxygen therapy: Data from the ANTADIR observatory. *Chest* 123(5):1460.

57. Ferreira IM, Brooks D, White J, Goldstein R. 2012. Nutritional supplementation for stable chronic obstructive pulmonary disease. *Cochrane Database Syst Rev* 12:CD000998.

58. Gouzi F, Prefaut C, Abdellauoui A et al. 2011. Evidence of an early physical activity reduction in chronic obstructive pulmonary disease patients. *Arch Phys Med Rehabil* 92:1611–1617.

59. Van Remoortel H, Homikx M, Demeyer H et al. 2013. Daily physical activity in subjects with newly diagnosed COPD. *Thorax* 68:962–963.

60. Eisner M, Iribarren C, Blanc P et al. 2011. Development of disability in chronic obstructive pulmonary disease: Beyond lung function. *Thorax* 66:109–114.
61. Marquis K, Debigare R, Lacasse Y et al. 2002. Midthigh muscle cross-sectional area is a better predictor of mortality than body mass index in patients with chronic obstructive pulmonary disease. *Am J Respir Crit Care Med* 166(6):809–813.
62. Spruit MA, Pitta F, McAuley E et al. 2015. Pulmonary rehabilitation and physical inactivity in patients with chronic obstructive pulmonary disease. *Am J Respir Crit Care Med* 192(8):924–933.
63. Spruit MA, Singh SH, Garvey C et al. 2013. ATS/ERS task force on pulmonary rehabilitation. An official American Thoracic Society/European Respiratory Society statement: Key concepts and advances in pulmonary rehabilitation. *Am J Respir Crit Care Med* 188:e13–e64.
64. Nici L, Donner C, Wouters E et al. 2006. American Thoracic Society/European Respiratory Society statement on pulmonary rehabilitation. *Am J Respir Crit Care Med* 173(12):1390–1413.
65. Guell R, Casan P, Belda J et al. 2000. Long-term effects of outpatient rehabilitation of COPD: A randomized trial. *Chest* 117(4):976–983.
66. Paz-Diaz H, Montes de Oca M, Lopez JM et al. 2007. Pulmonary rehabilitation improves depression, anxiety, dyspnea and health status in patients with COPD. *Am J Phys Med Rehabil* 86(1):30–36.
67. Seymour JM, Moore L, Jolley CJ et al. 2010. Outpatient pulmonary rehabilitation following acute exacerbations of COPD. *Thorax* 65(5):423–428.
68. Holland AE, Hill CJ, Jones AY, McDonald CF. 2012. Breathing exercises for chronic obstructive pulmonary disease. *Cochrane Database Sys Rev* 10:CD008250.
69. Geddes EL, Obrien K, Reid WD et al. 2008. Inspiratory muscle training in adults with chronic obstructive pulmonary disease: An update of a systematic review. *Respir Med* 102:1715–1729.
70. ODonnell DE, Sanii R, Younes M. 1988. Improvement in exercise endurance in patients with chronic airflow limitation using continuous positive airway pressure. *Am Rev Respir Dis* 138:1510–1514.
71. Vivodtzev I, Pepin JL, Vottero G et al. 2006. Improvement in quadriceps strength and dyspnea in daily tasks after 1 month of electrical stimulation in severely deconditioned and malnourished COPD. *Chest* 129(6):1540–1548.
72. Sruit MA, Singh S, Garvey C et al. 2013. An official American Thoracic society/European Respiratory Society statement: Key concepts and advances in pulmonary rehabilitation- an executive summary. *Am J Respir Crit Care Med* 188(8):13–64.
73. Andiranopoulos V, Klijn P, Franssen F, Spruit M. 2014. Exercise training in pulmonary rehabilitation. *Clin Chest Med* 35:313–322.
74. Pan L, Guo YZ, Yan JH et al. 2012. Does upper extremity exercise improve dyspnea in patients with COPD: A meta-analysis. *Respir Med* 106:1517–1525.
75. Beauchamp MK, Nonoyama M, Goldstein RS et al. 2010. Interval versus continuous training in individuals with chronic obstructive pulmonary disease—A systematic review. *Thorax* 65(2):157–164.
76. Dolmage TE, Goldstein RS. 2006. Response to one-legged cycling in patients with COPD. *Chest* 129(2):325–332.
77. Ries AL, Kaplan RM, Limberg TM, Prewitt LM. 1995. Effects of pulmonary rehabilitation on physiologic and psychosocial outcomes in patients with chronic obstructive pulmonary disease. *Ann Intern Med* 122(11):823–832.
78. Akinbami LJ, Moorman JE, Liu X. 2011. *Asthma Prevalence, Health Care Use, and Mortality: United States, 2005–2009.* National Health Statistics Reports; no 32. Hyattsville, MD: National Center for Health Statistics.
79. Bellia V, Battaglia S, Catalano F et al. 2003. Aging and disability affect misdiagnosis of COPD in elderly asthmatics: The SARA study. *Chest* 123(4):1066–1072.
80. Cutitta G, Cibella F, Bellia V et al. 2001. Changes in FVC during methacholine-induced bronchoconstriction in elderly patients with asthma: Bronchial hyperresponsiveness and aging. *Chest* 119(60): 1685–1690.
81. Thorn J, Brisman J, Torén K. 2001. Adult-onset asthma is associated with self-reported mold or environmental tobacco smoke exposures in the home. *Allergy* 56(4):287–292.
82. Enright PL, McClelland RL, Newman AB et al. 1999. Underdiagnosis and undertreatment of asthma in the elderly. Cardiovascular Health Study Research Group. *Chest* 116(3):603–613.
83. Cuttitta G, Cibella F, Bellia V et al. 2001. Changes in FVC during methacholine-induced bronchoconstriction in elderly patients with asthma: Bronchial hyperresponsiveness and aging. *Chest* 119(6):1685–1690.
84. Braman S, Hanania, N. 2007. Asthma in older adults. *Clin Chest Med* 28:685–702.
85. Shichilone N, Pedone C, Battaglia S et al. 2014. Diagnosis and management of asthma in the elderly. *Eur J Intern Med* 25:336–342.

86. Schmier JK, Halpern MT, Jones ML. 2005. Effects of inhaled corticosteroids on mortality and hospitalization in elderly asthma and chronic obstructive pulmonary disease patients: Appraising the evidence. *Drugs Aging* 22(9):717.

87. Korenblat PE, Kemp JP, Scherger JE, Minkwitz MC, Mezzanotte W. 2000. Effect of age on response to zafirlukast in patients with asthma in the Accolate Clinical Experience and Pharmacoepidemiology Trial (ACCEPT). *Ann Allergy Asthma Immunol* 84(2):217.

88. Korn S, Schumann C, Kropf C et al. 2010. Effectiveness of omalizumab in patients 50 years and older with severe persistent allergic asthma. *Ann Allergy Asthma Immunol* 105(4):313–319.

89. Shichilone N, Ventura M, Bonini M et al. 2015. Choosing wisely: Practical considerations on the treatment efficacy and safety of asthma in the elderly. *Clin Mol Allergy* 13(7):1–14.

90. Bardana EJ. 1993. Is asthma really different in the elderly patient? *J Asthma* 30:77–79.

91. Petheram IS, Jones DA, Collins JV. 1982. Assessment and management of acute asthma in the elderly: A comparison with younger asthmatics. *Postgrad Med J* 58:149–151.

92. Ritz T, Rosenfield D, Steptoe A. 2010. Physical activity, lung function, and shortness of breath in the daily life of individuals with asthma. *Chest* 138(4):913–968.

93. Garcia-Aymerich J, Varraso R, Anto JM et al. 2009. Prospective study of physical activity and risk of asthma exacerbations in older women. *Am J Respir Crit Care Med* 179:999–1003.

94. Mendes FA, Goncalves RC, Nunes MP et al. 2010. Effects of aerobic training on psychosocial morbidity and symptoms in patients with asthma. *Chest* 138(2):331–337.

95. Turner S, Eastwood P, Cook A et al. 2011. Improvements in symptoms and quality of life following exercising training in older adults with moderate/severe persistent asthma. *Respiration* 81:302–3010.

96. Turner LA, Mickleborough TD, McConeell AK et al. 2011. Effect of inspiratory muscle training on exercise tolerance in asthmatic individuals. *Med Sci Sports Exercise* 43(11):2031–2038.

97. Laennec RTH (Forbes J, Trans.). 1962. *A Treatise on the Disease of the Chest.* New York: Library of the New York Academy of Medicine, Hafner Publishing.

98. Goeminne PC, Nawrot TS, Ruttens D, Seys S, Dupont LJ. 2014. Mortality in non-cystic fibrosis bronchiectasis: A prospective cohort analysis. *Respir Med* 108:287–296.

99. Weycker D, Edelsberg J, Oster G et al. 2005. Prevalence and economic burden of bronchiectasis. *Clin Pulm Med* 12:205–209.

100. Meyer K. 2005. Aging. *Proc Am Thorac Soc* 2:433–439.

101. Donowitz GR, Cox HL. 2007. Bacterial community acquired pneumonia in older patients. *Clin Geriatr Med* 23:515–534.

102. Martinez-Garcia MA, Perpina-Tordera M, Roman- Sanchez P et al. 2005. Quality-of-life determinants in patients with clinically stable bronchiectasis. *Chest* 128:739–745.

103. Lee AL, Burge AT, Holland AT for the Cochrane Collaboration. 2015. Airway clearance techniques for bronchiectasis. *Cochrane Database Syst Rev* 2015(11). Art. No.: CD008351. doi: 10.1002/14651858. CD008351.pub3.

104. Bilton D, Tino G, Barker AF et al. 2014. B-305 Study Investigators. Inhaled mannitol for non-cystic fibrosis bronchiectasis: A randomised, controlled trial. *Thorax* 69:1073–1079.

105. Hart A, Sugumar K, Milan SJ, Fowler SJ, Crossingham I. 2014. Inhaled hyperosmolar agents for bronchiectasis. *Cochrane Database Syst Rev* 5:CD002996.

106. Wilkinson M, Sugumar K, Milan SJ, Hart A, Crockett A, Crossingham I. 2014. Mucolytics for bronchiectasis. *Cochrane Database Syst Rev* 5:CD001289.

107. Tsang KW, Tan KC, Ho PL et al. 2005. Inhaled fluticasone in bronchiectasis: A 12 month study. *Thorax* 60(3):239–243.

108. Martínez-García MA, Perpiñá-Tordera M, Román-Sánchez P, Soler-Cataluña JJ. 2006. Inhaled steroids improve quality of life in patients with steady-state bronchiectasis. *Respir Med* 100(9):1623–1632.

109. Lee JK, Lee J, Prak SS et al. 2014. Effect of inhalers on the development of hemoptysis in patients with non-cystic fibrosis bronchiectasis. *Int J Tuberc Lung Dis* 18:363–370.

110. Altenburg J, deGraaf C, Stienstra Y et al. 2013. Effect of azithromycin maintenance treatment on infectious exacerbations among patients with non-cystic fibrosis bronchiectasis: The BAT randomized controlled trial. *JAMA* 309(12):1251–1259.

111. Wong C, Jayaram L, Karalus N et al. 2012. Azithromycin for prevention of exacerbations in non-cystic fibrosis bronchiectasis (EMBRACE): A randomised, double-blind, placebo-controlled trial. *Lancet* 380:660–667.

112. Rogers GB, Bruce KD, Martin ML, Burr LD, Serisier DJ. 2014. The effect of long-term macrolide treatment on respiratory microbiota composition in non-cystic fibrosis bronchiectasis: An analysis from the randomized, double-blind, placebo-controlled BLESS trial. *Lancet Respir Med* 2(12):988–996.

113. Scheinberg P, Shore E. 2005. A pilot study of the safety and efficacy of tobramycin solution for inhalation in patients with severe bronchiectasis. *Chest* 127(4):1420–1426.
114. Murray MP, Govan JR, Doherty CJ et al. 2011. A randomized controlled trial of nebulized gentamicin in non-cystic fibrosis bronchiectasis. *Am J Respir Crit Care Med* 183(4):491.
115. Newall C, Stockley RA, Hill SL. 2005. Exercise training and inspiratory muscle training in patients with bronchiectasis. *Thorax* 60(100):889–890.
116. Lee AL, Hill CJ, Cecins N et al. 2014. The short and long term effects of exercise training in non-cystic fibrosis bronchiectasis—A randomized controlled trial. *Respir Res* 15:44.
117. Mandal P, Sidhu MK, Kope L et al. 2012. A pilot study of pulmonary rehabilitation and chest physiotherapy versus chest physiotherapy alone in bronchiectasis. *Respir Med* 106(12):1647–1654.
118. King TE Jr, Tooze JA , Schwarz MI , Brown KR , Cherniack RM. 2001. Predicting survival in idiopathic pulmonary fibrosis: Scoring system and survival model. *Am J Respir Crit Care Med* 164(7):1171–1181.
119. Fell CD, Martinez FJ , Liu LX et al. 2010. Clinical predictors of a diagnosis of idiopathic pulmonary fibrosis. *Am J Respir Crit Care Med* 181(8):832–837.
120. Weill D, Benden C , Corris PA et al. 2015. A consensus document for the selection of lung transplant candidates: 2014—An update from the Pulmonary Transplantation Council of the International Society for Heart and Lung Transplantation. *J Heart Lung Transplant* 34(1):1–15.
121. Richeldi L, du Bois RM, Raghu G et al. 2014. INPULSIS Trial Investigators. Efficacy and safety of nintedanib in idiopathic pulmonary fibrosis. *N Engl J Med* 370(22):2071–2082.
122. King TE Jr, Bradford WZ, Castro-Bernardini S et al. 2014. ASCEND Study Group. A phase 3 trial of pirfenidone in patients with idiopathic pulmonary fibrosis. *N Engl J Med* 370(22):2083–2092.
123. Collard HR, Moore BB, Flaherty KR et al. 2007. Idiopathic Pulmonary Fibrosis Clinical Research Network Investigators. Acute exacerbations of idiopathic pulmonary fibrosis. *Am J Respir Crit Care Med* 176(7):636–643.
124. Raghu G, Collard HR, Egan JJ et al. 2011. ATS/ERS/JRS/ALAT Committee on Idiopathic Pulmonary Fibrosis. An official ATS/ERS/JRS/ALAT statement: Idiopathic pulmonary fibrosis: Evidence-based guidelines for diagnosis and management. *Am J Respir Crit Care Med* 183(6):788–824.
125. Hansen JE, Wasserman K. 1996. Pathophysiology of activity limitation in patients with interstitial lung disease. *Chest* 109:1566–1576.
126. O'Donnell DE, Chau LK, Webb KA. 1998. Qualitative aspects of exertional dyspnea in patients with interstitial lung disease. *J Appl Physiol* 84(6):2000–2009.
127. Holland AE, Hill CJ, Conron M et al. 2008. Short term improvement in exercise capacity and symptoms following exercise training in interstitial lung disease. *Thorax* 63:549–554.
128. Nishiyama O, Kondoh Y, Kimura T et al. 2008. Effects of pulmonary rehabilitation in patients with idiopathic pulmonary fibrosis. *Respirology* 13:394–399.
129. Ferreira A, Garvey C, Connors GL et al. 2009. Pulmonary rehabilitation in interstitial lung disease: Benefits and predictors of response. *Chest* 135(2):442–447.
130. Ryerson CJ, Cayou C, Topp F et al. 2014. Pulmonary rehabilitation improves long-term outcomes in interstitial lung disease: A prospective cohort study. *Respir Med* 108(1):203–210.
131. Downman L, Hill CJ, Holland AE. 2014. Pulmonary rehabilitation for interstitial lung disease. *Cochrane Database Syst Rev* 10:CD006322. doi: 10.1002/14651858.CD006322.pub3.
132. Dowman L, McDonald C, Hill C et al. 2013. The benefits of exercise training in interstitial lung disease: Protocol for a multicentered randomized controlled trial. *BMC Pulm Med* 13:8.
133. Pulhan, MA, Gimeno-Santos E, Scharplatz M et al. 2011. Pulmonary rehabilitation following exacerbations of chronic obstructive pulmonary disease. *Cochrane Database Syst Rev.* (10):CD005305. doi: 10.1002/14651858.CD005305.pub3.

22 Geriatric Strokes and Brain Injuries

Jean L. Nickels and Maya Modzelewska

CONTENTS

22.1 GERIATRIC STROKE

22.1.1 EPIDEMIOLOGY

As the population continues to age, there will be a greater incidence of stroke[1] and a greater need for stroke rehabilitation. Stroke remains the third leading cause of death in the United States and the most common cause of disability.[1] It is also one of the leading diagnoses requiring inpatient rehabilitation in the older adults. Age remains one of the most significant risk factors for stroke.[2] For every year after age 55, the stroke rate more than doubles in men and women. Almost three-fourths of all strokes occur in people over the age of 65.[3] Early poststroke rehabilitation focuses on regaining as much independence as possible and improving function, while addressing and managing secondary stroke prevention and minimizing risk factors. Elderly stroke survivors are at risk of developing physical, psychological, social, and functional sequelae that further decrease their quality of life (QOL). Concern is not only for repercussions of the first stroke but also for recurrence of stroke. With an aging population and an increasing average lifespan, the prevalence of stroke survivors is also likely to increase.[1] Due to continuing improvements in public recognition of stroke warning signs and risk factors as well as imaging and interventions, more and more older adults are surviving stroke.[4]

According to World Health Organization statistics, the incidence and prevalence of stroke are 9.0 million and 30.7 million, respectively, with a higher incidence found in the Western Pacific, Europe, and Southeast Asia. Due to advances in Western healthcare, the prevalence of stroke since 1970 has decreased 42% whereas it has more than doubled in low-income to middle-income countries.[5] It is estimated that the prevalence of stroke among Americans aged 65 and older is 40/1000 persons, and 1 in 10 Americans over 75 has experienced a stroke.[6] There are about 4,500,000 stroke survivors alive today in the United States.[1] Each year, approximately 795,000 people experience a new or recurrent stroke in the United States; of these, 610,000 are first strokes and 185,000 are recurrent strokes.[6] Projections suggest that by 2030, there will be a 24.9% increase in the incidence of stroke.[7] Reports indicate that 75%–89% of strokes occur in individuals aged >65 years. Of these strokes, 50% occur in people who are aged ≥70 years and nearly 25% occur in individuals who are aged >85 years.[8] The highest prevalence and annual rate of first-ever strokes are reported in those who are 80 years or older.[9]

Stroke incidence for men is greater than that for women at younger ages, but not at older ages.[1] Stroke incidence in men is 1.25 times higher than that in women, but because women live longer than men, more women than men die from stroke each year.[1] The incidence of stroke is higher in men up to age 75, similar in the 75–84 age group, and higher in women in the age group greater than 85.[1]

The stroke incidence in African American men is 2- to 3-fold higher than that in Caucasians between the ages of 45 and 85. The incidence of stroke among African American women in this population is also higher than that in Caucasian women. The increased incidence in blacks correlates to increased risk factors, such as diabetes mellitus, hypertension, heart disease, smoking, excessive alcohol use, and sickle cell disease.[10]

Stroke accounts for roughly 1 out of every 19 deaths in the United States, and approximately 130,000 people die each year from stroke in the United States.[11]

The death rate from stroke doubles every 10 years between ages 55 and 85.[2] Stroke mortality began to decline in the 1970s and in the 1980s, likely secondary to improved detection and treatment of risk factors, particularly hypertension.[12] The rate of decline has now slowed.[13] Although stroke mortality rates have declined rapidly over the past 30 years, the decline has reached a plateau.[14] As the percentage of older individuals grows, we can expect that the magnitude of those affected by stroke is projected to increase. Pooled data from multiple studies also showed that in individuals over age 70, the 1-year mortality was 24% in Caucasian men and 27% in Caucasian women, but 25% in African American men and 22% in African American women. The mean age of stroke death was 79.6 years, but men had a younger age at stroke death than women.[1] A higher in-hospital mortality rate (16%–33% in older vs. 4%–18% in younger) has been consistently reported for octogenarians compared with younger patients. This seems due to several factors, including worse premorbid function, more severe strokes, prevalence of comorbidities, and higher rates of secondary complications.[15]

22.1.2 Risk Factors

22.1.2.1 Nonmodifiable

There are multiple risk factors for stroke that also increase with age. In fact, the single most important risk factor for stroke is advanced age.[2] In the elderly, age is also the most significant independent risk factor for stroke-associated mortality in both sexes.[16] Other factors such as previous strokes are more likely to have occurred in elderly patients.[10]

22.1.2.2 Modifiable

22.1.2.2.1 Hypertension

Hypertension is the most significant modifiable risk factor for stroke in any age group.[14] Data from 2007 to 2010 suggest that 64.1% of men aged 65–74, 71.7% men aged 75 and over, 69.3% women aged 65–74, and 81.3% women over 75 years of age suffer from hypertension.[17] Mechanisms for increased prevalence of hypertension in the elderly include stiffening of large arteries, endothelial dysfunction, cardiac remodeling, autonomic dysregulation, and renal aspects.[10] Multiple meta-analyses of randomized trials of antihypertensive medications have shown that a 10–20 mmHg reduction in systolic blood pressure and 5–6 mmHg reduction in diastolic blood pressure are associated with a 35% reduction in stroke risk in both hypertensive and normotensive patients.[10] For the geriatric population, thiazide diuretics and angiotensin-converting enzyme (ACE) inhibitors have been recommended as first-line treatment for hypertension.[18]

In older adults up to the age of 80 with systolic blood pressure over 160 mmHg, antihypertensive treatment is associated with significant reduction in stroke and cardiovascular events.[19]

22.1.2.2.2 Smoking

Data from the Framingham study have confirmed that smoking is independently associated with an increased risk in atherothrombotic stroke in men and women. The relative risk of heavy smokers (defined as >40 cigarettes/day) is twice that of light smokers (<10 cigarettes per day). Cessation of smoking reverses risk to that of nonsmokers within 5 years after quitting.[20]

22.1.2.2.3 Hypercholesterolemia

Elevated serum levels of cholesterol are common in older adults. Elevated total cholesterol and decreased high-density lipoprotein (HDL) levels predispose older adults to stroke.[21] Among persons over 65 years or more, approximately 20% of men and 40% of women have total blood cholesterol level of 240 mg/dL or higher.[22] While evidence linking hypercholesterolemia to increase stroke incidence is weak, it does strongly influence coronary artery disease and atherosclerosis and there is a link between carotid artery atherosclerosis and increased serum cholesterol levels.[10] The use of HMG-CoA reductace inhibitors can reduce the incidence of stroke as well as help to stabilize atherosclerotic plaque and reduce inflammation.[10] There are fewer studies on the effect of statins on stroke prevention in older adults. The largest trials to date suggest a beneficial effect for stroke prevention with statins in high-risk elderly subjects <82 years of age.[23] The most recent treatment guidelines suggest that the target low-density lipoprotein (LDL) for high-risk patients, including those with recent myocardial infarction (MI), cardiovascular disease with diabetes, and severe/poorly controlled risk factors of metabolic syndrome, is <70 mg/dL.[24]

22.1.2.2.4 Diabetes Mellitus

It has been established that diabetes mellitus is a major risk factor for stroke.[25] This can partially be attributed to the higher prevalence of hypertension and heart disease among people with diabetes. Even after controlling for these other risk factors, diabetes has been found to independently double the risk of stroke.[14] Other aspects of glucose metabolism, such as insulin resistance and hyperinsulinemia, may also increase stroke risk.[10] The prevalence of type 2 diabetes increases with age, with 16.5% of men and 12.8% of women 75–84 years old with type 2 diabetes.[26]

22.1.2.2.5 Heart Disease

Carotid artery stenosis plays a vital role in increasing the risk of stroke by decreasing blood flow to the brain.[10] Carotid endarterectomy is indicated in patients with 70%–99% stenosis. Outcomes are even better in the elderly than younger population. Medical management is preferred for asymptomatic elderly patients with <70% stenosis.[23] Data from the North American Symptomatic Carotid Endarterectomy Trial demonstrated a 17% absolute reduction in stroke incidence with carotid endarterectomy over a 2-year follow-up period in patients with critical stenosis of 70%–99%. This represents a relative risk reduction of 65%. The relative benefits of surgical treatment for asymptomatic carotid stenosis are marginal, suggesting that carotid endarterectomy should be reserved for patients who are otherwise medically stable, have >80% stenosis, and who are expected to live 5 years or longer. Patients with less than 50% carotid stenosis should be treated with antiplatelet medications, statins, and lifestyle modification.

Antiplatelet therapy reduces the incidence of stroke in patients at high risk for atherosclerosis and in those with known symptomatic cerebrovascular disease. For most patients with noncardioembolic stroke, use of a daily antiplatelet agent is recommended by the American Association of Chest Physicians.[24] .

22.1.2.2.6 Atrial Fibrillation

Atrial fibrillation is strongly correlated with ischemic stroke and is the most common clinically significant arrhythmia in the elderly. It is also the most treatable cardiac risk factor for stroke.[27] The incidence and prevalence of atrial fibrillation increase with age. For every 10 years above the age of 55, the incidence of atrial fibrillation doubles.[1] Persons with nonvalvular atrial fibrillation have five times greater relative risk for cardioembolic stroke, and for people with rheumatic heart disease, there is a 17-fold increase.[10] Multiple clinical trials have shown warfarin to be effective in reducing stroke risk in older adults.[28] It has been found to reduce the relative risk of stroke by 58%–86% over control subjects in the Copenhagan AFA-SAK and SPAF studies in patients with nonvalvular atrial fibrillation.[10] A second phase of the SPAF trial (SPAF II) compared warfarin with aspirin to determine which medication provided better stroke prevention for subjects over the age of 75 years with nonvalvular atrial fibrillation.[29] The study concluded that care must be taken when considering anticoagulation in patients older than 75 years, as the risk of intracranial hemorrhage is higher in elderly persons even without the use of warfarin.[10]

22.1.3 ACUTE HOSPITAL COURSE AND ROLE OF REHABILITATION

The most commonly used treatment for ischemic stroke is intravenous recombinant tissue plasminogen activator (r-tPA), a thrombolytic agent that is Food and Drug Administration (FDA)-approved for use within the first 4.5 hours of stroke onset.[10] There are well-supported data that show that if given within 3 hours of onset of stroke symptoms, it can reduce the absolute risk of death or dependency by 16%. Better outcomes have been found in patients with mild-to-moderate impairments, under the age of 75 years old, and with administration within 90 minutes of onset. It is controversial whether elderly age is a risk factor for hemorrhagic transformation in the setting of thrombolytic treatment. There is concern that aging itself incurs an inherently increased risk due to underlying changes in physiology, such as impaired clearance of medications, increased vascular frailty, and the development of age-related white matter disease and cerebral amyloid angiopathy.[15] The safety and efficacy of intravenous tPA use in the elderly population, however, have not been adequately studied because most randomized clinical trials have excluded very elderly patients (≥80 years).[15]

In addition to intravenous tPA, many centers are now using intra-arterial (IA) tPA for large-vessel occlusions of the middle cerebral artery (MCA) or basilar artery who present within 6 hours of onset. There are also endovascular techniques used to mechanically remove a thrombus from major cerebral arteries. Although IA recanalization techniques are promising for the treatment of select patients with ischemic stroke, there are few data on the outcome and efficacy of IA recanalization techniques in patients older than 80.[15]

22.1.4 STROKE-RELATED IMPAIRMENTS

Stroke-related physical disability can decrease the quality of daily living, increase burden of care on families, and increase the need for long-term institutionalization. The prognosis for functional recovery in stroke is influenced by a broad array of neurological, functional, and psychosocial factors. Many stroke survivors can regain functional independence (50%–70%); however, 15%–30% are permanently disabled and 30% require institutionalized care 3 months after onset.[1] A total of 40% of stroke patients are left with moderate functional impairments and 15%–30% with severe disability.[30] Dysphagia occurs in approximately one-third to half of all stroke survivors, increasing their risk of aspiration pneumonia, malnutrition, and dehydration.[10] Malnutrition has been found in 8%–34% of patients with stroke. Nutritional status has been found to correlate with long-term outcome after stroke and has also been linked to length of stay (LOS) and functional outcome.[10] Poor nutrition can also increase the risk of infections and pressure sores and decrease functional outcomes.[10]

Approximately one-third to half of stroke survivors experience speech and language disorders.[10] Recovery from aphasia usually occurs at a slower rate over a longer period of time than motor recovery.[10] Most aphasia recovery occurs in the first 3–6 months, up to 12 months. Patients with nonfluent aphasia have generally a less favorable prognosis than those with fluent aphasia. Language comprehension usually returns sooner and to a fuller extent. Language and visual–spatial function recovered over 12 months, whereas cognitive function improved only during the first 3 months.[10]

In general, recovery of basic activities of daily living (ADLs) has plateaued by 12.5 weeks, in 95% of stroke patients, according to the Copenhagen study on outcomes and time course of recovery in stroke.[30] Time course of recovery is strongly related to initial severity.[30] The best function in ADLs is generally reached within 8.5 weeks with mild stroke, 13 weeks in patient with moderate stroke, 17 weeks in patient with severe stroke, and 20 weeks in patients with very severe stroke.[30]

22.1.5 STROKE REHABILITATION

Stroke rehabilitation begins during the acute hospitalization, as soon as the diagnosis of stroke is established and life-threatening problems are under control.

The highest priorities during this early phase are to prevent recurrence of stroke and complications, ensure proper management of general health functions, mobilize the patient, encourage resumption of self-care activities, and provide emotional support to the patient and family.[29] Minimizing the risk of recurrent stroke and promoting secondary stroke prevention is especially applicable in the elderly population given their increased risk factors.

After the "acute" phase of stroke care, the focus of care turns to assessment and recovery of any residual physical and cognitive deficits, as well as compensation for residual impairment.[29] A growing body of evidence indicates that patients do better with a well-organized, multidisciplinary approach to postacute rehabilitation after a stroke, including physical, occupational, and speech and language therapies.[29]

22.1.6 STROKE AND REHABILITATION OUTCOMES

Outcomes following stroke can be assessed in different ways, including morbidity, mortality, level of impairment, length of hospital stay, cost of care, functional independence, discharge location, and QOL. Functional levels can be assessed as functional independence at the time of discharge, or amount of improvement from admission to discharge. Potential predictors of outcome at all ages include type and severity of the stroke, degree of physical impairment, cognitive function, communication, comorbidities, coping ability, community support, and type of rehabilitation. The strongest predictor of discharge functional ability in the general population has been found to be admission functional ability.[31]

Predicting the outcome of stroke in the geriatric population based on age and comorbidities has been difficult. It is well known that elderly patients have poorer outcomes associated with ischemic stroke and that strokes tend to be more severe. They have significantly higher in-hospital and 3-month mortality rates and are less likely to be discharged home than their younger counterparts.[15]

Even with identical severity, increased age was associated with greater disability in ADLs and mobility.[16] Patients over 85 years old were almost 10 times as likely to show a low response to rehabilitation in ADLs and almost 6 times as likely to show a low response to mobility as younger patients.[16]

There have been numerous studies that have reported associations between age and poor outcomes. The predictive value of age in the literature, however, depends on evaluation of the outcome. The negative impact of age on functional outcome is most apparent when functional status at discharge is being assessed. Conversely, when change of function is assessed, age tends not to influence outcome negatively.[32] It is difficult to distinguish between age itself and age-associated factors such as comorbidities that have a negative influence on functional outcome, including ischemic heart disease, hypertension, diabetes, and altered cognitive capacity.[32] In addition, several studies have demonstrated the definite benefits of intensive stroke rehabilitation programs in maximizing functional recovery regardless of age and without increased therapy resources.[32]

Comorbidities and age were not associated with prolonged stays at the rehabilitation center.[33] Comorbidity and age did not uniquely contribute to predicting length of hospital stay, however there is evidence that suggests that they are important factors in determining functional outcome after stroke.[10] Some studies have found that very old age (>85) was a strong predictor of poor outcome. For example, in the Auckland Stroke Study, long-term very old (≥85) stroke survivors were found to have poorer basic ADLs after 6 years when compared with age-matched control subjects.[33]

In addition to older age, other negative predictors of outcome in stroke include history of previous stroke, urinary or bowel incontinence, visuospatial deficits, cognitive impairment, speech impairment, depression, coronary artery disease, and absence of a supportive caregiver.[31]

22.1.7 Challenges to Rehabilitation of Stroke in the Elderly

At baseline, the elderly population faces increasing difficulty with mobility, ADLs, and instrumental ADLs (IADLs). All of these factors can contribute to functional decline even without the involvement of stroke deficits. Additionally, other factors related to normal aging can provide additional barriers to rehabilitation. Decreased visual acuity, presbyopia, cataracts, and macular degeneration can compound visual field cuts and neglect. Auditory changes (presbyacusis, otosclerosis) can compound difficulty with comprehension and ability to understand and carry over instructions in therapies, which can compound deficits such as aphasia. Sarcopenia is common in the elderly.[34] Along with frailty, sarcopenia can contribute to decreased mobility and ability to complete ADLs and IADLs even premorbidly. Additionally, elderly patients are at an increased risk premorbidly for malnutrition and depression, which may worsen following a stroke as a function of dysphagia and prolonged hospital stays.

Another characteristic of the rehabilitation of older adults is the prevalence of concomitant cognitive problems.[35] This adds an additional challenge with learning, remembering, and being able to apply new compensatory techniques as well as concerns for safety and problem solving. Despite the difficulties associated with the rehabilitation of older adults poststroke, even a small improvement in independence can improve QOL.

22.1.8 Challenges to Community Reentry

The presence of a supportive and involved community support system can often mean the difference between returning home to the community versus discharge to another institution. The younger population is not only more likely to have a living spouse to provide support to aid in community reentry, but also more likely to be in good health to provide more physical assistance. It is important to identify and involve social support early in order to facilitate a smoother discharge to home. This supports the need for evaluation of social situation to best determine appropriate levels of rehabilitations. At the time of discharge, home nursing visits, outpatient or home therapies, and community transportation should be set up to facilitate a successful transition to home.

22.2 GERIATRIC BRAIN INJURY

22.2.1 EPIDEMIOLOGY

22.2.1.1 Traumatic Brain Injury

The risk of traumatic brain injury (TBI) has a trimodal peak. Risk is higher in the 0–4 years, 15–19 years, and over 65 years of age groups.[36] In the United States, the rate of geriatric TBI appears to be increasing. In 1999, there were 17,657 persons 65 years and older hospitalized with TBI for an age-adjusted rate of 155.9/100,000 population.[37] Rates of TBI increased with each decade of age.[37] Persons aged 85 or older had nearly twice the rate of TBI hospitalizations or persons aged 75–84 had more than four times the rate of those aged 65–74.[37] The percentage of those with moderate TBI increased markedly with age, coinciding with a decrease in mild TBI.[37] By the 2002–2006 period, there were 141,998 TBI-related hospital-related emergency department (ED) visits/year, 81,499 TBI-related hospitalizations/year, and 14,347 TBI-related deaths/year in this age group.[36] The highest rates of TBI-related hospitalization and death rate occurred in adults aged 75 years and older (339/100,000 and 57/100,000 population, respectively).[36] The rates of TBI increased further for persons 65 and older between the 2003 and 2004 and the 2009/2010 fiscal years.[38] Rates continued to demonstrate an increased risk for each decade of age.[38]

Racial differences were also noted. Caucasians had the highest TBI-related hospitalizations in geriatric age groups,[37,39–42] with the possible exception in one study in which American Indian/Alaska Natives ranked highest in the 65–74 age group.[37]

Gender studies were inconsistent showing higher percentages of women,[40] higher percentages of men,[36,43] or no differences[39] in TBI rates in the older age groups. However, men over 80 tended to have a more severe Glasgow Coma Score (GCS) than women in the same age group.[44]

Patients over 55 were more likely to be college educated.[45] A higher proportion of younger adults have private insurance, and a higher percentage of older adults were on federally funded programs.[46]

22.2.1.2 Nontraumatic Brain Injury

Epidemiological studies regarding nontraumatic brain injury (nTBI) are very limited for the geriatric population. Those with nTBI tended to be older than those with TBI.[47] As age increased, rates of hospitalization for nTBI also increased.[38]

22.2.2 CAUSES OF BRAIN INJURY

22.2.2.1 Traumatic Brain Injury

In the majority of studies, falls are the leading cause of injury in the older adult (65 years and over) group.[36–38,40,41,45,48] Between 2002 and 2006, TBI causes for the older adult were 60.7% falls, 7.9% motor vehicle collision (MVC), 24.7% unknown, 5.7% struck by/against, 1% assault.[36]

As age increased, the percentage of falls increased and that of MVC decreased.[38] The most common causes of falls were simple fall,[49] falls on the same level, and falls on or from steps/stairs.[38] In the "old old" (over 80 years) group, falls tended to occur on staircases, icy sidewalks, getting up after a meal, getting out of bed to use the washroom, and fall off ladder.[44] Persons who fell were more likely to have three or more comorbid conditions compared with those who sustained a TBI from MVC.[37] Intracranial hemorrhage was more likely to occur following a fall than MVC.[37] Subdural hematomas (SDHs) were more common in the older adult group.[46] Intracranial hemorrhage was the most common TBI-associated diagnosis in those aged 85 and older.[37] The risk of pelvic fracture regardless of cause of TBI increased with age.[37] Falls were a more common cause in 55–74 age groups if they had a history of alcohol abuse.[50] However, the presence of alcohol in the blood was less common in older adults than younger adults.[45] Falls were more common in those with visual problems.[50] This raises the question whether identifying and treating alcoholism and visual deficits in older patients may help prevent TBI.[50]

When injury was caused by MVC, those over 65 tended to be the driver more than passenger and the passenger more than pedestrian.[37] The main secondary injuries were in the lower extremities followed by the thorax and upper limbs.[51]

However, pedestrian injury risk becomes higher for the 75 and older group compared to the 65–74 age group.[37,52] The risk of a pedestrian receiving an intracranial injury after being hit by a car increases steadily with age, and even more for elderly (over 65 years) pedestrians. In contrast, the number of fractures remains steady.[53] For the over 65 years age group, risk of intracranial injury was equal for males and females. For all age groups, men were at slightly higher risk for fractures and intracranial injury.[53] The authors propose that the increased risk of intracranial injuries may be related to the reduction of size of the brain and/or weaker neck muscles.[53]

Comorbid conditions that were similar between elderly patients with TBI included hypertension, diabetes mellitus, cardiac arrhythmias, and fluid and electrolyte imbalances.[37] Persons who fell were more likely to have chronic pulmonary disease, Alzheimer's and other dementias, and Parkinson's disease.[37] Of those older subjects who tested positive for alcohol, the cause of TBI was more likely to be a MVC than a fall.[37] In the over 85 group, MVCs were more common in those who had congestive heart failure and endocrine disorders.[50]

While assaults were a more common etiology of TBI in the middle-aged group, there is evidence that violent acts against the elderly are increasing, especially in urban areas.[54] Suicide risk is highest in adults over 65 years.[55] The most common method is by a firearm.[55,56] However, in urban settings, older adults may choose to jump from a height.[55,56] Risk factors for suicide attempts in this age group include being white and male, a history of depression, chronic pain or illness, and social isolation.[55,57]

Elderly (65 and older) had a higher rate of SDH.[58] GCS at the accident scene was higher in the elderly group.[58] But after age 80, epidural hematomas were unlikely.[44]

In gender studies, men over 80 were more likely to have hematomas and contusions than women and were more likely to have a more severe GCS.[44]

22.2.2.2 Nontraumatic Brain Injury

The most common causes of nTBI were brain tumors, anoxia, and vascular insults.[38] Other causes included encephalitis, meningitis, encephalopathy, infections, and toxins. With increasing age, the percentage of tumors decreased and the percentage due to anoxia and vascular insults increased.[38] In the oldest age group (85 and older), the percentage of women with nTBI increased compared with that of men.[38] nTBI tended to be more common in the 65–74 age group while TBI tended to be more common in the 85+ age group.[38]

22.2.3 IMAGING

Older adults had a higher risk of three or more brain lesions by computed tomography (CT), also a higher incidence of brain contusion, SDH, intracerebral hematomas, cerebral edema, and midline shift.[48,49] SDH volumes were larger in the older age group.[49] Midline shift was greater in the older age group.[44,49] Both larger SDH volume and larger midline shift correlated with poorer outcomes.[49] Older patients who have sustained falls have an increased risk of intracranial hemorrhage and, in particular, SDHs.[37,46] Pedestrians hit by motor vehicles, those who fell, and those who were assaulted had larger gray and white matter lesion volumes than with other causes of TBI.[59] Older age was associated with larger lesion volumes both in the total brain and in each brain region, but most particularly for the frontal areas.[59] However, the elderly were less likely to sustain a skull fracture or bony or metal fragments in the brain.[54]

Older age groups had a lower risk of heterotopic ossification after severe TBI.[60]

22.2.4 Acute Care

In a 1993 study, there were no significant differences between older and younger age groups with respect to field intubation and pharmacological paralysis.[48] But a 2013 study showed that fewer elderly patients were intubated at the scene.[58] Intracranial pressure and cerebral perfusion pressure were less commonly monitored in the elderly patients (65 and older).[58]

Patients over 65 years were less likely to get a CT scan within 6 hours of arriving in emergency room.[61]

A similar number of older and young adults were admitted to the intensive care unit (ICU), and treatments were similar.[40] Older patients had more preinjury medical conditions.[40]

The difference in time elapsed between treatment and surgery was not different for young versus elderly groups.[49] However, rates of transfer to neurosurgery were lower for older patients (over 65) than younger patients, independent of size of hematoma, type of intracranial hemorrhage, presence of preexisting medical conditions, other serious extracranial injuries, and measures of physiological status.[61] The presence of hypotension or hypoventilation may have prevented transfer.[61] It is not documented whether family decisions or advanced care directives played a role. For mild TBIs, the rate of neurosurgical intervention was the same between older and younger adults.[40]

Just as in younger individuals, elderly persons who experience a TBI must be monitored for elevations of intracranial pressure, which may cause further brain injury.[62] Elevated pressures should be reduced with appropriate measures such as evacuation of hematoma(s), osmotic diuresis, and/or induction of coma.[62] Mechanical ventilation is no longer routinely used because it lowers cerebral pressure by inhibiting blood flow.[62]

Early mobilization is essential to prevent pressure sores, contractures, spasticity, venous thromboembolism (VTE), cardiac (and muscular) deconditioning, atelectasis, aspiration, pneumonia, constipation, urinary retention, infection, and mood disorders.[54] Range of motion and orthotic devices or splints that are properly fitted should be initiated, and family members, nurses, and patients should be taught their use.[62] Periods of prolonged bed rest may result in orthostatic hypotension, especially in the elderly.[62] Abdominal binders, elastic pressure stocking, and adjustment of medications may help prevent drops in blood pressure.[62] Repeat imaging should be done for worsening cognitive skills, worsening gait, and incontinence to evaluate for recurrent hemorrhage or development of hydrocephalus.[62]

Speech language pathology/therapy should be involved early.[62] Communication should be assessed ,and communication boards or devices should be provided as appropriate.[62] An assessment should be made for swallowing safety, and the appropriate food and liquid consistency should be started. Nonparental methods of nutrition should be started if patient must be fed nothing by mouth (NPO) due to dysphagia.[62] A dietician or nutritionist should be involved early. Nutrition should be assessed on admission as many older adults may have premorbid nutritional deficiencies.[54] TBI may also cause anosmia or alterations in taste further decreasing the desire to eat.[54]

Medications require special consideration in the older adult group. The elderly are more likely to have more medications prior to their injury.[54] Their medication regimen should be simplified, and nonessential medications should be discontinued.[54] Delirium may be common in the older adult with TBI. Medications are more likely to cause delirium in the elderly.[54] Pain medications may contribute to delirium. Nonmedication alternatives for pain treatment should be considered, including repositioning, ice, heat, and massage.[54]

Around-the-clock acetaminophen is often preferred.[54] Nonsteroidal anti-inflammatory drugs (NSAIDs) and narcotics should be used cautiously and with consideration to side effects including acute kidney injury, delirium, peptic ulcer disease, and cardiac toxicity.[54] Negative cognitive effects may also be seen in the use of tricyclic antidepressants and gabalins (such as pregabalin or gabapentin) used for neuropathic pain treatment.[54] Safety must be closely guarded in the delirious patient to prevent falls and wandering.[54]

Sensory deprivation may occur in the elderly in the intensive care or acute care units. Older patients may have premorbid vision and hearing loss. The TBI may cause middle ear damage. Preexisting peripheral neuropathies may also impair sensation. Sensory deprivation and the TBI may lead to behavioral and psychological problems.

These may include disruptions of the sleep–wake cycle, attention deficits, agitation, and depression. Attention deficit can be treated in older adults without coronary artery disease with methylphenidate.[54,63] Amantadine, modafinil, and selective serotonin reuptake inhibitors (SSRIs) are usually safe to have a longer onset.[54] Amantadine, SSRIs, and beta-blockers may be helpful with agitation, and benzodiazepines should be avoided.[54] Agitation may be reduced by identifying and removing noxious stimuli and by avoiding overstimulation. Traditional anti-agitation antipsychotics, such a haloperidol, may slow neurological recovery.[55] Normalization of the sleep–wake cycle can be achieved with limitation of nighttime interruptions, addressing pain and a routine daytime schedule.[54] Antihistamines and benzodiazepines should be avoided. Involving family members, friends, psychological and pastoral counseling, and the use of methylphenidate or SSRIs will all help with depression.[54]

VTE prophylaxis should be initiated early. Unfractionated heparin and low-molecular-weight heparins must be used with caution in those with intracranial hemorrhages.[54] Intermittent pneumatic pressure stockings should be considered in those where heparin is contraindicated. No evidence-based consensus is present regarding the timing of VTE prophylaxis with heparins. It is probably safe to use heparin after diffuse axonal injury (DAI) within 1 week.[54]

Posttraumatic seizures may occur within the first 7 days after TBI. These typically do not recur. The use of antiepileptic drugs (AEDs) is not recommended after 7 days by the American Academy of Neurological Surgeons or the American Academy of Physical Medicine and Rehabilitation.[54] The risk of recurrent seizure is higher if seizures occur more than 7 days after TBI. A neurologist skilled in geriatrics should help to select an appropriate AED, with the least cognitive side effects. Knowledge of premorbid alcohol or benzodiazepine abuse may help prevent seizures by placing these patients on withdrawal prophylaxis.[54]

Spasticity is a velocity-dependent increase in resistance to passive stretch and may occur in patients with TBI. Goals of spasticity management are facilitating hygiene, positioning, and mobility while reducing pain.[62] Stretching, range of motion of the limbs, and proper positioning all help to decrease spasticity.[62] Several oral medications are available including diazepam, baclofen, and tizanidine. All of these medications may cause alterations in arousal and cognition in the elderly.[62] Clonidine may lower blood pressure. Intrathecal baclofen pumps, phenol blocks, and Botox injections can be considered but are generally not used in the acute hospital setting.

Patients may suffer from urinary retention or incontinence. Older patient' may have premorbid urination issues such as retention from benign prostatic hypertrophy, incontinence from pelvic relaxation after childbirth, impaired bladder capacity with aging, and decreased ability to suppress bladder contractions with aging.[54] TBI may further aggravate these issues due to loss of sensation, loss of mobility to access the toilet, loss of communication of the need to void, loss of cognition, and medication effects. An indwelling catheter may prevent retention and incontinence, while maintaining intact skin, but may lead to infections over time. After the removal of indwelling catheters, patients should receive timed toileting, intermittent straight catheterization, measurement of postvoiding residuals, and consideration for the use of condom catheters.[54] Urology may need to be involved for urodynamic studies and bladder management.

Patients may suffer from either constipation or diarrhea. Constipation may be managed with dietary fiber and probiotics, limiting the use of narcotics and limiting immobility.[54] Diarrhea may require adjustment of laxative and stool softeners, adjustments of tube feedings, and ruling out *Clostridium difficile* infection.[54]

22.2.5 Acute Care Outcomes

22.2.5.1 In-Hospital Mortality and Complication Rates

Mortality rate in the hospital was higher for the elderly (65 and over) group, dying on an average of 5–11 days after TBI, compared with 1.8–2 days out in the younger group.[37,48,49] Deaths in the younger group were due to the direct effects of the brain injury or systemic complications resulting from the brain injury, whereas more of the elderly patients died from pulmonary, cardiac, or multisystem organ failure.[48,49] Ten percent of those aged 60 or more, with GCS of 5 or less, survived to be discharged, compared with 41% of those 20–40 years old.[48] Some have proposed that this increase in mortality may be related to other effects of aging, including cerebrovascular atherosclerosis, decreased free-radical clearance, decreased intracranial pressure, increased cerebral perfusion pressure, impairment of autoregulation, and pressure reactivity, and/or the more frequent use of anticoagulants may contribute to the higher mortality rate.[55]

As age increased, mortality in the hospital also increased.[38] There was a 6%–8% increase in death risk for every additional year of age at the time of injury.[64,65] Mortality rate in the old old group (80 and over) was poorer for men than women.[44] The overall mortality rate for this old old group was 25%.[44] However, as the group reached the 85+ age group, mortality was not significantly different in the general age-matched population.[64] However, those with TBI at 85+ could expect to have their life expectancies shortened by about 0.5 years.[64] In those over 65, women had a 48% lower risk of death than men.[64] Those who were never married at the time of injury had a 48% lower risk of death than those who were married.[64] Those who suffered a fall were 1.5 times more likely to die than those involved in an MVC.[63] There was a 2% decrease in mortality for every 1 point the discharge motor functional independence measure (FIM) score increased and a 5% increase in mortality for every 1 point the disability rating score (DRS) score increased at discharge from rehab.[64] Causes of death in 65–74 year olds: aspiration pneumonia (12× increased risk), sepsis or mental disorder (9×), pneumonia (5×), and respiratory or circulatory condition (2×) than age-matched controls[64]; in those 75–85 years: fall-related injury (11×), aspiration pneumonia (7×), sepsis (6×), unintentional injury (4×), pneumonia (3×), and respiratory condition (2×) than age-matched controls[64]; and in 85+ group: aspiration pneumonia (11×) and respiratory condition (2×) than age-matched controls.[64]

For those who were injured in MVC, there was greater mortality and more severe injury in those older patients with vision problems, slower reflexes, decreased bone density, comorbid conditions, frailty, cognitive impairment, and alcohol and medication use.[55]

Prior MI correlated with increased risk of in-hospital death in patients 55 and older.[50] Although higher mortality was related to having a history of MI, duration of time since MI and cardiac function were not related to mortality.[50] Comorbidities correlated with increased ICU LOS but not acute hospital LOS.[50]

In-hospital complication rate was similar as was LOS.[40] The rate of posttraumatic epilepsy was not different between older and younger groups.[45,46] Seizures most commonly began within the first week.[46] For both younger and older adults, the most common complications were respiratory failure (39% older, 26% younger), pneumonia (26% older, 15% younger), and urinary tract infection (UTI) (48%, 20%)—only for UTI was the difference significant.[45,46]

Of the older adults with nTBI, almost one-third died in hospital, with the risk of death increasing with increasing age.[38] They were more likely to die than TBI patients.[38]

22.2.6 Disposition Following Acute Care

The average LOS was the same for older and younger adults in acute care[45]; however, for the "old old" (over 80 years), LOS was increased compared with younger patients the same degree of injury by 3–4 days.[38]

Almost 50% of the older adults with TBI were discharged home, followed by 11% to inpatient rehabilitation and 9% to long-term care (LTC)[38] (see Figure 22.1). The likelihood of discharge to

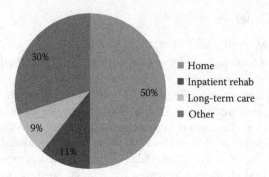

FIGURE 22.1   Disposition setting for older adults with TBI after acute care.

home declines as age groups increase, and the likelihood of admission to acute rehabilitation and other settings such as residential facilities, LTC, and continuing care centers (CCCs) for both TBI and nTBI increases.[37,38,40,47] Men were less likely than women to resume prior living situation and function.[44]

For all age groups with nTBI, 39% of those discharged home were over 65, 62.3% of those discharged to inpatient rehab were over 65, and 60.6% of those discharged to "other" were over 65[47] (see Figures 22.2 and 22.3). However, for the elderly nTBI group, the majority were discharged home followed by LTC then inpatient rehab. Like TBI patients, as age increased, discharge was less likely to home and more likely to LTC or inpatient rehab.[38]

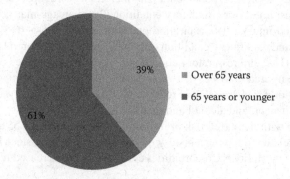

FIGURE 22.2   Percentage of discharges by age to home after acute care for nTBI.

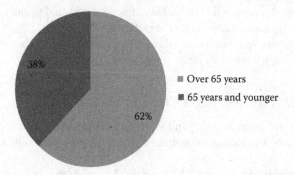

FIGURE 22.3   Percentage of discharges by age to inpatient rehab after acute care for nTBI.

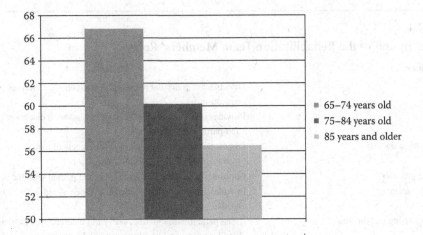

FIGURE 22.4 Percentage of home discharge by age after nTBI acute care.

For those discharged alive, the percentage of "good recovery" as measured by the Glasgow Outcome Scale (GOS) decreased with age (66.8% 65–74 year old, 60.2% 75–84 years, 56.5% of those 85 and older)[37] (see Figure 22.4).

22.2.7 REHABILITATION OPTIONS

Rehabilitation can be offered at several levels following the acute hospital stay.

A thorough understanding of the patient's preinjury physical and cognitive status, behavioral issues, chronic medical issues, and social support network will be essential to assess the potential for rehabilitation.[54] Elderly spouses may have their limitations as caregivers, and adult daughters are more likely to be involved with postacute care.[54] Consultation with the Physical Medicine and Rehabilitation team is warranted to determine the best rehabilitation approach.

At any level, the rehabilitation approach should be multidisciplinary and should include the following: patient, family/caregivers, primary care physician (internist, geriatrician, family practitioner), neurologist, neurosurgeon, physiatrist (physician specialist in Rehabilitation Medicine), nursing, physical therapist, occupational therapist, speech language pathologist, nutritionist, social worker, and neuropsychologist. It may also include pastoral care, pet or music therapist, recreational therapist, psychiatrist, palliative care specialist, wound care specialist, orthopedist or general surgeon, and/or urologist, as well as others who may be involved in the patient's care (see Table 22.1). The care should be patient/caregiver centered and directed, meaning the team should develop goals based on the needs of the patient and caregiver, rather than the goals of the medical team.

At each level of rehabilitation, the focus is on functional improvement in areas of mobility, self-care tasks, swallowing, language, and cognition. Both patients and their caregivers receive training. The patient is evaluated for and trained in the use of the appropriate adaptive equipment. Medical monitoring is available for the prevention of common complications and for the treatment of medical comorbidities.

Patients whose needs cannot be managed in the community should be referred to institutionalized or inpatient rehabilitation units or centers.

Options include the following:

1. *Acute inpatient rehabilitation:* Patients should be medically stable, require at least two therapies, be able to cognitively and physically participate in 3 hours of therapies 5–6 days a week, have a reasonable expectation to make significant functional gains, have the medical

TABLE 22.1

Brief Description of the Rehabilitation Team Members' Roles

Team Member	Role
Patient	Directs team goals and plans and participates in therapies and education
Caregiver	Provides input into discharge goals, assists with discharge planning, and participates in training
Physiatrist (rehab doctor)	Directs the rehabilitation team in all aspects of care and medical management of the rehabilitation patient
Primary care provider	Coordinates medical management of the patient with the physiatrist
Specialist physician	Provides recommendations regarding specialized areas of medical needs
Nursing and nursing technicians	Assist patient with toileting, skin care, medication, bowel and bladder needs, and positioning; provide patient and caregiver education regarding bowel and bladder programs, skin care, and medications; and provide input to the therapists regarding carryover of mobility, cognition, speech, swallow, and ADLs when not in therapy
Physical therapist	Provides therapy to improve mobility and balance
Occupational therapist	Provides therapy to improve ADLs and to improve upper extremity function, trunk control, and bed mobility
Speech language pathologist	Provides therapy to address impaired swallowing, language, and/or cognition
Nutritionist	Advises staff and educates patients and families regarding patient dietary needs
Social worker and discharge care coordinator	Assist with team, patient, and family with discharge planning and financial and coping needs
Pastoral care	Provides emotional support and assists with coping
Recreational therapist	Explores and connects patient with avocational interests and community resources
Pet/music therapist	Provides patient-directed emotional support and coping strategies
All team members	Coordinate care with other team members to maximize benefit for patient and provide patient and caregiver education

necessity for close monitoring and care by nurses and physicians trained in rehabilitation, and have a reasonable discharge plan to the community in a reasonable period of time.

2. *Subacute or skilled nursing facility (SNF) rehabilitation:* Patients should be medically stable so as not to require frequent physician monitoring, able to participate in 1.5 hours of therapy daily, and have the expectation to make functional gains, with goal of getting to community at discharge.
3. *Skilled nursing rehabilitation with restorative therapies:* This is recommended for patients for whom long-term institutionalization is likely, but for whom short-term therapies will provide an improvement in function.

If the patient's family or a caregiver can manage the patient's care at home, rehab options include the following:

1. *Home care services:* Provides community health nurse, evaluation for home health aides, and home therapy services, usually one to three times a week, for patient who lack the ability to leave home.

2. *Outpatient therapies:* Provides outpatient therapy services for patients who are no longer home bound and have access to transportation, usually provided one to three times a week.

The duration of rehabilitation is determined by functional improvement but may also be limited by insurance coverage.

At discharge, the rehabilitation team will coordinate with the family and patient to arrange for the next appropriate level of rehab and to provide the needed durable medical and adaptive equipment and the appropriate socialization opportunities. A combination of family members, visiting nursing services, and privately reimbursed companions may be necessary for home discharge.[55] Driving may not yet be appropriate and may require clearance from neurology, neurosurgery, and ophthalmology. Driving may also require cognitive and physical testing as well as on-road testing.[54] The multidisciplinary team will also need to establish return to work parameters if appropriate.

22.2.8 REHABILITATION OUTCOMES

Literature is focused predominantly on acute inpatient rehab outcomes. Studies are sparse for outcomes from other levels of rehab.

Older patients were both admitted and discharged to rehabilitation at more impaired disability ratings; however, gains made in rehabilitation were no different in younger groups.[40,45,46] Fewer older patients were discharged to the community.[45] Older patients stayed longer in acute inpatient rehabilitation units,[46] but as age increased, rehabilitation LOS decreased.[42] Older patients had higher rehabilitation charges.[45,46] Most of older adults (82%) were discharged to the community from rehab, but this was significantly less than that in the younger group (93%). Older patients were more likely to be discharged from rehabilitation with a GOS score of severe disability.[40] However, there was no difference in GOS from young to older groups at 6 months.[40]

Among those over 65, the older the age and the lower the discharge FIM motor and cognitive scores, the higher the likelihood of need for home care services.[42] Gender was not related to likelihood of discharge to home.[42] However, women needed more healthcare services at discharge from rehab than men.[42] Of older patients admitted to rehab, the average number of comorbidities was 8.[42] Nearly two-thirds were discharged home from rehab.[42] Women were more likely to be unmarried and living alone.[42] Women in the older groups had slightly higher admission and discharge motor and cognitive scores and were discharged about 1 day earlier than men.[42] Functional gain, however, was similar in men and women.[42]

Caucasian patients had higher discharge motor, cognition, and total functional scores at discharge from inpatient rehab as measured by the FIM, followed by Hispanics and African Americans.[39] Caucasian patients had the shortest LOS on acute rehab.[39] This is despite Caucasians being more likely to have three or more comorbidities.[39] Hispanics were most likely to be discharged home, followed by African Americans and then Caucasian. African Americans were the most likely to be institutionalized, with fewer being admitted to assisted living settings.[39] Male patients were less likely to be discharged home than female patients.[39] Patients who were not married were less likely to go home and more likely to be admitted to assisted living facilities.[39] Patients who were living at home prior to admission were more likely to be discharged home.[39] Overall, 30% were discharged to subacute care, skilled nursing facilities (SNFs), intermediate care units, or acute care units.[39]

22.2.9 READMISSION RATES AND CAUSES

Age is unrelated to readmission rates at 1 and 5 years after acute and inpatient rehabilitation.[65]

A higher percentage of early admissions were planned for orthopedic or reconstructive surgery or were readmitted for infections, particularly pneumonia, hardware infection, meningitis, or gastrointestinal (GI) infections.[66] By 5 years out, the rate of elective readmission declined, as did the rate of infections. At this time, the most common infections requiring readmission were pneumonia, and then hardware infection.[66] As time from discharge progressed from 1 to 5 years, the rates of readmission for psychiatric reasons or seizure are increased.[66]

22.2.10   COMMUNITY REINTEGRATION AND LONG-TERM OUTCOMES

After discharge to the community or to an institutionalized setting, elderly patients require frequent and multidisciplinary follow-up. Patients may have multiple comorbidities physically, psychologically, financially, and environmentally that must be addressed.

At 3 months after TBI, comorbidity was more common in the 65 and older age group. A total of 4% of the elderly (65 and older) group was working compared with 60% of the adult group (16–64 years).[58] Although, older patients were more likely to be unemployed or retired at injury, a greater percentage failed to return to work after being injured.[67] Older TBI patients were more likely to live dependently postinjury.[67] Adults 65 and older were more likely to report no unmet needs at discharge to home than younger adults.[68] Nevertheless, some reported one to over three unmet needs.[68]

Cognitive deficits within 3 months after TBI in patients over 50 years compared with age-matched controls included deficits in naming, fluency, memory, and executive function.[69] However, they exhibited similar learning abilities.[69] The authors report that this is a similar pattern to younger survivors. Severity of injury and coexistence of physical injuries did not correlate with return to work.[69]

The main risk factor for significant mood or anxiety symptoms was younger age (older age less likely).[70] Other factors unrelated to age included poor physical functioning, inadequate social support, being a white women, being retired or unemployed, pre-TBI psychiatric diagnosis, and history of multiple concussions.[70]

Over half of the elderly patients died within 10 years of injury, a higher rate than younger cases.[41] In mild TBI, with increasing age, mortality increased at 6 weeks, 6 months, and 10 years.[41] More recent calendar year of injury was associated with a lower risk of mortality at 6 months but not at 10 years.[41] As more older adults had more severe injury, increased mortality risk was no longer significant when corrected for severity of injury.[41] Females over 60 had a lower rate of survival at 6 months.[52] Authors propose that females have lower body weight, more predisposed to hypotension, and have lower total body blood volumes than men.[52]

One year after injury, a significantly higher proportion of older adults were rated as disabled compared with younger adults, regardless of injury severity.[43] As the age increased, the proportion of individuals rated at achieving good recovery declined.[43] At 1 year after injury, more older adults were rated with severe disability, vegetative state or dead.[43] Mortality rate was higher at 1 year for older adults.[43] Significantly, fewer older adults returned to their prior living situation, with a higher percentage now requiring a more supervised setting.[43] Employment rates were not different for older versus younger adults.[43] Older adults required a longer period of time to follow simple commands.[43] Older adults were more likely to suffer complications of cardiac arrest, ventriculitis, and sepsis.[43]

Community reintegration outcomes: QOL is rated lower in older adults with TBI.[71] Following TBI, most but not all studies indicated that older people have poorer community integration outcomes than their younger counterparts, having greater difficulty getting places, shopping, and managing money.[71] Gender studies were conflicting in regards to whether males or females had a more difficult time integrating.[71] Many integration problems arise once service utilization rates fall off after discharge, suggesting the need for longer term follow-up.[71] Long-term needs identified across studies included behavioral control, emotional/mental health support, cognitive problems, mobility barriers, support group assistance, disease process education, and financial and life planning assistance.[71] These needs should be addressed over time according to individual needs and not at one set time point.[71] Older adults were more likely to be unemployed after TBI and are more likely to retire.[71]

22.2.11 POSTREHABILITATION FOLLOW-UP CONSIDERATIONS

Patients 55 and older with TBI who needed rehab were evaluated at 2–4 years postinjury. The most frequent comorbidities were rheumatisms, neck or back pain, vision problems, cardiovascular problems, depression, and confusion.[51] Male gender, shorter acute LOS, fewer comorbid conditions, and access to home modification services were associated with long-term functional independence in self-care and in mobility.[51] Another study looked at TBI patients 1–4 years after TBI. Adults 55 years and older were more likely to have metabolic/endocrine disorders, have neurological complaints, and report orthopedic or muscular symptoms compared with younger TBI subjects or healthy age-matched subjects.[72] Younger TBI persons were more likely to complain of sleep difficulties.[72] Regardless of age, there were more symptoms reported with milder injuries.[72] Younger subjects reported more symptoms than older subjects.[72]

22.2.12 AGING WITH TBI

TBI is a risk factor for Alzheimer's dementia. The risk is increased in those individuals with apolipoprotein E4 (APOE4).[54]

Major depression and anxiety are common as those with TBI age. There is also an increased risk for suicide.[55] A small percentage of older depressed adults will present with psychotic features such as nonbizarre paranoia.[55] The most frequent anxiety disorder is posttraumatic stress disorder, followed by generalized anxiety disorder, panic disorder, and obsessive–compulsive disorder.[55] The presence of psychiatric diagnoses with TBI has a negative impact on community integration.[55] SSRIs and supportive therapy, such as cognitive behavioral therapy, are appropriate treatments, and benzodiazepines should be avoided.[55]

Sexuality may be negatively impacted by aging and by TBI. Treatment of erectile dysfunction in older men with medications such as sildenafil should be cautious and is contraindicated in those on nitrates and with coronary artery disease and hypertension.[54]

REFERENCES

1. Rosamond W, Flegal K, Friday G et al. Heart disease and stroke statistics—2007 update: A report from the American Heart Association Statistics Committee and Stroke Statistics Subcommittee. *Circulation* 115, 2007: e69–e171.
2. Sacco R, Benjamin E, Broderick JP et al. Risk factors. *Stroke* 28, 1997: 1507–1517.
3. Centers for Disease Control and Prevention. *Stroke Facts and Statistics*. Atlanta, GA: CDC, Division for Heart Disease and Stroke Prevention; 2006.
4. Barker WH, Mullooly JP. Stroke in a defined elderly population, 1967–1985: A less lethal and disabling but no less common disease. *Stroke* 28, 1997: 284–290.
5. Kim AS, Johnston SC. Global variation in the relative burden of stroke and ischemic heart disease. *Circulation* 124, 2011: 314–323.
6. Adams PF, Hendershot GE, Marano MA. Current estimates from the National Health Interview Survey, 1996. *Vital Health Stat* 10, 1999: 1–203.
7. Roger VL, Go AS, Llyod-Jones DM et al. Heart disease and stroke statistics—2007 update: A report from the American Heart Association. *Circulation* 125, 2012: e2–e220.
8. Chen RL, Balami JS, Esiri M et al. Ischemic stroke in the elderly: An overview of evidence. *Nat Rev Neurol* 6, 2010: 256–265.
9. Black-Schaffer R, Winston C. Age and functional outcome after stroke. *Top Stroke Rehabil* 11, 2004: 23–32.
10. Harvey RL, Roth EJ, Yu DT et al. Stroke syndromes. In *Physical Medicine and Rehabilitation*, Braddom RL, Chan L, Harrast MR et al. (Eds.). Philadelphia, PA: Elsevier Saunders; 2011: 1175–1222.
11. Kochanek KD, Jiaquan X, Murphy SL et al. Deaths: Final data for 2009. *Natl Vital Stat Rep* 60, 2011: 1–116.
12. Gillum RF. New considerations in analyzing stroke and heart disease mortality trends. The Year 2000 Age Standard and the International Statistical Classification of Diseases and Related Health Problems, 10th Revision. *Stroke* 33, 2002: 1717–1722.

13. Cooper R, Sempos C, Hsieh SC et al. Slowdown in the decline of stroke mortality in the United States, 1978–1986. *Stroke* 21, 1990: 1274–1279.

14. Howard G, Howard V, Katholi C et al. Decline in US stroke mortality: An analysis of temporal patterns by sex, race, and geographic region. *Stroke* 32, 2001: 2213–2220.

15. Heitsch L, Panagos PD. Treating the elderly stroke patient: Complications, controversies, and best care metrics. *Clin Geriatr Med* 29, 2013: 231–255.

16. Khaw KT, Barrett-Connor E, Suarez L et al. Predictors of stroke-associated mortality in the elderly. *Stroke* 15, 1984: 244–248.

17. Health, United States. *With a Focus on Emergency Care.* National Center for Health Statistics; 2012. Available at: www.cdc.gov/nchs/data/hus/hus12.pdf

18. Chobanian A, Bakris GL, Black HR et al. The Seventh Report of the Joint National Committee on Prevention, Detection, Evaluation, and Treatment of High Blood Pressure: The JNC 7 report. *JAMA* 289, 2003: 2560–2572.

19. Beckett N, Nunes M, Bulpitt C. Is it advantageous to lower cholesterol in the elderly hypertensive? *Cardiovasc Drugs Ther* 14, 2000: 397–405.

20. Wolf PA, D'Agostino RB, Kannel WB et al. Cigarette smoking as a risk factor for stroke: The Framingham study. *JAMA* 259, 1988: 1025–1029.

21. Sarti C, Kaarisalo M, Tuomilehto J. The relationship between cholesterol and stroke: Implications for antihyperlipidaemic therapy in older persons. *Drugs Aging* 17, 2000: 33–51.

22. Davidson MH, Kurlandsky SB, Kleinpell RM. Lipid management and the elderly. *Prev Cardiol* 6, 2003: 128–133.

23. Andrawes WF, Bussy C, Belmin J. Prevention of cardiovascular events in elderly people. *Drugs Aging* 22, 2005: 859–876.

24. Sacco RL, Adams R, Albers G et al. AHA/ASA guidelines: Guidelines for prevention of stroke in patients with ischemic stroke or transient ischemic attack. *Stroke* 37, 2006: 577–617.

25. Air EL, Kissela BM. Diabetes, the metabolic syndrome, and ischemic stroke: Epidemiology and possible mechanisms. *Diabetes Care* 30, 2007: 3131–3140.

26. Wilson PW, Kannel WB. Obesity, diabetes, and risk of cardiovascular disease in the elderly. *Am J Geriatr Cardiol* 11, 2002: 119–123, 125.

27. Go A. The epidemiology of atrial fibrillation in elderly persons: The tip of the iceberg. *Am J Geriatr Cardiol* 14, 2005: 56–61.

28. Cooper H. Trials of newer approaches to anticoagulation in atrial fibrillation. *J Interv Card Electrophysiol* 10(Suppl. 1), 2004: 27–31.

29. Jorgensen HS, Nakayama H, Raaschou HO et al. Outcome and time course of recovery in stroke. Part II: Time course of recovery. The Copenhangan Stroke Study. *Arch Phys Med Rehabil* 76, 1995: 406–412.

30. Duncan PW, Zorowitz R, Bates B et al. AHA/ASA management of adult stroke rehabilitation care: A clinical practice guideline. *Stroke* 36, 2005: e100–e143.

31. Jongbloed I. Prediction of function after stroke: A critical review. *Stroke* 17, 1986: 765–775.

32. Bagg S, Pombo AP, Hopman W. Effect of age on functional outcomes after stroke rehabilitation. *Stroke* 33, 2002: 179–185.

33. Hackett ML, Duncan JR, Anderson CS et al. Health related quality of life among long term survivors of stroke: Results from the Auckland Stroke Study, 1991–1992. *Stroke* 3, 2000: 440–447.

34. Nair K. Age related changes in muscle. *Mayo Clin Proc* 75, 2000: S14–S18.

35. Tatemichi TK, Desmond DW, Stern Y et al. Cognitive impairment after stroke: Frequency, patterns, and relationship to functional abilities. *J Neurol Neurosurg Psychiatry* 57, 1994: 202–207.

36. Faul M, Xu L, Wald MM et al. *Traumatic Brain Injury in the United States: Emergency Department Visits, Hospitalization, and Deaths, 2002–2006.* Atlanta, GA: Centers for Disease Control and Prevention; 2010. http://www.cdc.gov/traumaticbraininjury/pdf/blue_book.pdf.

37. Coronado, VG, Thomas KE, Sattin RW et al. The CDC traumatic brain injury surveillance system: Characteristics of persons aged 65 years and older hospitalized with a TBI. *J Head Trauma Rehabil* 20, 2005: 215–228.

38. Chan V, Zagorski B, Parsons D et al. Older adults with acquired brain injury: A population based study. *MBC Geriatr* 13, 2013: 97–108.

39. Chang PJ, Ostir BM, Kuo Y et al. Ethnic differences in discharge destination among older patients with traumatic brain injury. *Arch Phys Med Rehabil* 89, 2008: 231–236.

40. Mosenthal AC, Livingston DH, Lavery RF et al. The effect of age on functional outcome in mild traumatic brain injury: 6-month report of a prospective multicenter trial. *J Trauma Injury Infect Crit Care* 56, 2004: 1042–1048.

41. Testa Flaada J, Leibson CL, Mandrekar JN et al. Relative risk of mortality after traumatic brain injury: A population-based study of the role of age and injury severity. *J Neurotrauma* 24, 2007: 435–445.

42. Graham JE, Radice-Neumann DM, Reistetter TA et al. Influence of sex and age on inpatient rehabilitation outcomes among older adults with traumatic brain injury. *Arch Phys Med Rehabil* 91, 2010: 43–50.

43. Rothweiler B, Temkin NR, Dikmen SS. Aging effect on psychosocial outcome in traumatic brain injury. *Arch Phys Med Rehabil* 79, 1998: 881–887.

44. Amacher AL, Bybee DE. Toleration of head injury by the elderly. *Neurosurgery* 20, 1987: 954–958.

45. Frankel JE, Marwitz JH, Cifu DX et al. A follow-up study of older adults with traumatic brain injury: Taking into account decreasing length of stay. *Arch Phys Med Rehabil* 87, 2006: 57–62.

46. Cifu DX, Kreutzer JS, Marwitz JH et al. Functional outcomes of older adults with traumatic brain injury: A prospective, multicenter analysis. *Arch Phys Med Rehabil* 77, 1996: 883–888.

47. Chen AY, Zagorski B, Parsons D et al. Factors associated with discharge destination from acute care after acquired brain injury in Ontario, Canada. *BMC Neurol* 12, 2012: 16–24.

48. Pennings JL, Bachulis BL, Simons CT et al. Survival after severe brain injury in the aged. *Arch Surg* 128, 1993: 787–793.

49. Howard MA, Gross A, Dacey RG Jr et al. Acute subdural hematomas: An age-dependent clinical entity. *J Neurosurg* 71, 1989: 858–863.

50. Thompson HJ, Dikmen S, Temkin N. Prevalence of comorbidity and its association with traumatic brain injury and outcomes in older adults. *Res Gerontol Nurs* 5, 2012: 17–24.

51. Lecours A, Sirois MJ, Ouellet MC et al. Long-term functional outcome of older adults after a traumatic brain injury. *J Head Trauma Rehab* 27, 2012: 379–390.

52. Ponsford JL, Myles PS, Cooper DJ et al. Gender differences in outcome in patients with hypotension and severe traumatic brain injury. *Injury* 39, 2008: 67–76.

53. Richards D, Carroll J. Relationship between types of head injury and age of pedestrian. *Accid Anal Prev* 47, 2012: 16–23.

54. Englander J, Cifu DX, Trean T. The older adult. In *Brain Injury Medicine: Principles and Practice*. Zasler ND, Katz DI, Zafonte RD (Eds.). New York: Demos Medical Publishing; 2007: 315–332 (e-pages 352–369).

55. Thompson HJ, McCormick QC, Kagan SH. Traumatic brain injury in older adults: Epidemiology, outcomes, and future implications. *J Am Geriatr Soc* 54, 2006: 1590–1595.

56. Abrams RC, Marzuk PM, Tardiff K et al. Preference for fall from height as a method of suicide by elderly residents of New York City. *Am J Public Health* 95, 2005: 1000–1002.

57. Binder S. Injuries among older adults: The challenge of optimizing safety and minimizing unintended consequences. *Inj Prev* 8(Suppl. 4), 2002: IV2–IV4.

58. Rφe C, Skandsen T, Anke A et al. Severe traumatic brain injury in Norway: Impact of age on outcome. *J Rehabil Med* 45, 2013: 734–740.

59. Schönberger M, Ponsford J, Reutens D et al. The relationship between age, injury severity, and MRI findings after traumatic brain injury. *J Neurotrauma* 36, 2009: 2157–2167.

60. Simonsen LL, Sonne-Holm S, Krasheninnikoff M et al. Symptomatic heterotopic ossification after very severe traumatic brain injury in 114 patients: Incidence and risk factors. *Injury* 38, 2007: 1146–1150.

61. Munro PT, Smith RD, Parke TR. Effect of patients' age on management of acute intracranial haematoma: Prospective national study. *BMJ* 325, 2002: 1001–1005.

62. Flanagan SR, Hibbard MR, Riordan B et al. Traumatic brain injury in the elderly: Diagnostic and treatment challenges. *Clin Geriatr Med* 22, 2006: 449–468.

63. Kaelin D, Cifu DX, Matthies B. Methylphenidate effect on attention deficit in the acutely brain-injured adult. *Arch Phys Med Rehabil* 77, 1996: 6–9.

64. Harrison-Felix C, Kolalowsky-Hayner SA, Hammond FM et al. Mortality after surviving traumatic brain injury: Risks based on age groups. *J Head Trauma Rehabil* 27, 2012: E45–E56.

65. Harison-Felix CL, Whiteneck GG, Jha A et al. Mortality over four decades after traumatic brain injury rehabilitation: A retrospective cohort study. *Arch Phys Med Rehabil* 90, 2009: 1506–1513.

66. Marwitz JH, Cifu DX, Englander J et al. A multi-center analysis of rehospitalizations five years after brain injury. *J. Head Trauma Rehabil* 16, 2001: 307–317.

67. Testa JA, Malec JF, Moessner AM et al. Outcome after traumatic brain injury: Effects of aging on recovery. *Arch Phys Med Rehabil* 86, 2005: 1815–1823.

68. Pickelsimer EE, Selassie AE, Sample PL et al. Unmet service needs of persons with traumatic brain injury. *J Head Trauma Rehabil* 22, 2007: 1–13.

69. Goldstein FC, Levin HS, Presley RM et al. Neurobehavioral consequences of closed head injury in older adults. *J Neurol Neurosurg Psychiatry* 57, 1994: 961–966.

70. Horner MD, Selassie AW, Lineberry L et al. Predictors of psychological symptoms 1 year after traumatic brain injury: A population-based, epidemiological study. *J Head Trauma Rehabil* 23, 2008: 74–83.

71. Ritchie L, Wright-St Clair V, Keogh J et al. Community integration following traumatic brain injury: A systematic review of the clinic implications of measurement and service provision for older adults. *Arch Phys Med Rehabil* 95, 2014: 163–171.

72. Breed ST, Flanagan SR, Watson KR. The relationship between age and the self-report of health symptoms in persons with traumatic brain injury. *Arch Phys Med Rehabil* 85, 2004: S61–S67.

23 Cancer Rehabilitation

Susan Maltser and B. Allyn Behling-Rosa

CONTENTS

23.1 INTRODUCTION

Cancer rehabilitation is a discipline of physical medicine and rehabilitation that aims to achieve the highest level of function and quality of life for patients throughout the continuum of cancer care, including treatment and survivorship. The need for comprehensive rehabilitation services has been well studied. A landmark study by Lehman et al.[1] revealed that 50% of cancer patients have a need for rehabilitation due to deficits in ambulation and activities of daily living (ADL). They also noted that cancer patients will likely develop psychological dysfunction that will require support; comprehensive rehabilitation facilitates early identification of these impediments, allowing patients to make functional gains. This is especially true in the geriatric cancer patient who is more likely to already present with functional decline. The geriatric cancer population also has an increased need for rehabilitation services due to underlying comorbidities associated with aging such as osteoporosis, osteoarthritis, cognitive deficits, and polypharmacy. One study notes that 75% of these patients may require help with at least one ADL.[2] Rehabilitation of elderly patients with cancer has also been demonstrated to improve physical and psychological well-being; as such, rehabilitation services are a critical part of supportive care for a cancer patient.[3] Thus, a complete physiatric assessment of an elderly cancer patient should include identification and assessment of comorbid disease and psychosocial status to predict potential impairments the patient may develop from cancer and cancer treatment.

23.2 EPIDEMIOLOGY AND REHABILITATION THROUGH THE CONTINUUM

According to prevalence estimates, there were over 13.8 million cancer survivors in 2010, of which 58% were over 65 years of age; if incidence and survival rates remain stable through 2020, the number of survivors will increase by 31% to over 18 million.[4] With increased survivorship, patients will face more disability as a result of their cancer and associated cancer treatment. One study has even shown that patients have more psychological distress from living with disability incurred from cancer than the cancer diagnosis itself.[5]

In 2008, it was estimated that over 14% of the 40 million individuals admitted to U.S. hospitals were aged 75–84 years, and another 8% were over the age of 85 years.[6] In addition to being over 80 years of age, there are several other factors that predict longer hospital stay and increased cost of hospitalization, including female gender, history of delirium and/or dementia, reduced functional ability, and the likelihood of requiring an alternative living arrangement after discharge.[7]

The need for rehabilitation services after hospitalization is dependent on a cancer patient's functional impairments. Following discharge from the hospital, a patient may go home with home care rehabilitative services, as needed. However, if there is more severe functional impairment, an eligible patient may go to an inpatient facility for acute rehabilitative care. In order to qualify for acute inpatient rehabilitation, the patient must be able to tolerate 3 hours of therapy daily, require a daily physician visit, and have a qualifying diagnosis.

A study evaluating functional outcomes for inpatient cancer rehabilitation found that patients with the diagnosis of cancer made significant functional improvement, irrespective of their age.[8] Specifically, patients who received inpatient rehabilitation following the diagnosis of glioblastoma, the most common and lethal brain tumor, demonstrated significant functional improvement in mobility, ambulation, and self-care. It was determined that this population had comparable rates of discharge to the community with shorter length of stay, as to stroke and traumatic brain injury patients; additionally, they had increased quality of life following discharge.[9]

For those who do not qualify for acute inpatient rehabilitation, a skilled nursing facility or subacute rehabilitation facility may be appropriate. Unfortunately, one-third of elderly patients are admitted to a subacute rehabilitation facility in the last 6 months of life.[10] Yet subacute rehabilitation is deemed more appropriate for a patient who may have had a functional decline during hospitalization but is expected to make functional gains and return to the community. It may not be ideally suited for advanced cancer patients with end-of-life issues. Advanced cancer patients require an emphasis on symptom management and palliation. For those patients, conversations with their physician about prognosis and goals of care are crucial.[11] In these cases, admission to an inpatient hospice program or discharge to home hospice services may be more appropriate.

A patient may be eligible for hospice when facing the end stage of chronic illness, with declining health, progression of disease, and nonresponse to treatment. Any member of the healthcare team can initiate a hospice referral. Medicare benefits cover the services provided by the hospice care team, which includes a physician for oversight, hospice nurse practitioners, skilled nursing, social services, home health aides, and therapists for physical, occupational, and speech, as well as supportive and spiritual counseling for patients and families.[12]

Palliative care is a multidisciplinary specialty that works to prevent suffering and promote maximal quality of life by management of symptoms, improving function, and providing psychological support to both patient and family. It is provided to increase tolerability of treatments, decrease the need for hospitalization, and increase patient and family satisfaction at end of life. Additionally, palliative care has to be shown to reduce the amount of time end-stage cancer patients spend in the acute care settings.[13,14] One study of metastatic nonsmall cell lung cancer patients enrolled in an early palliative care program showed improvement in mood and quality of life. Despite receiving less aggressive end-of-life treatments, their median survival was longer than the patients in control group.[15] Even during the end stage of their illness, studies have demonstrated that patients continue to work toward improvements in ambulation, with participation in physical therapy successful in promoting mobility. Typical interventions provided by physical therapists include mobility and transfer training, as well as modalities such as hot packs, massage, and transcutaneous electrical nerve stimulation (TENS). Occupational therapists also promote independence with feeding, improve other ADL, provide equipment for the home, and can train caregivers on patient safety in the home.[16]

23.3 FUNCTIONAL ASSESSMENT TOOLS IN THE REHABILITATION OF CANCER PATIENTS

A reliable and valid assessment tool is vital for the rehabilitation team to evaluate the cancer patient's status before, during, and after the rehabilitative program such that practical short- and long-term goals may be devised for the patient. A patient's chronologic age does not always reflect his or her overall health status. To help predict the risk of postoperative, or postchemo- or radiotherapeutic complications in elderly patients, several assessment tools have been developed to assess physical functioning, comorbidities, polypharmacy, nutrition, cognition, and emotional status.[17,18] Studies confirm that stratification based on a comprehensive geriatric assessment predicts potential complications in elderly patients electively undergoing surgery or receiving chemotherapy for cancer.[19,20] The first of these tools to be developed was the Comprehensive Geriatric Assessment (CGA). The CGA is performed before radio- or chemotherapy to help establish a patient's baseline functional level and is used to evaluate a patient's functional status, gait, balance and risk for falls, cognitive status, affective status, nutritional status, pain, and social function.[21] In the late 1940s, Karnofsky and Buchrenal developed another clinical scale to measure functional performance in patients with cancer, especially prior to chemotherapy. The Karnofsky Performance Scale (KPS) has since become the most widely used tool for this purpose. Specifically, it evaluates cardiac function, pulmonary function, and exercise tolerance.[17,18] The KPS can also be used after treatment so as to help coordinate rehabilitative and support services.

23.4 CANCER-RELATED SYNDROMES

23.4.1 RADIATION FIBROSIS

Radiotherapy as part of a combined modality program has become an integral part of cancer treatment with the intention to cure, eliminate, or prevent cancer recurrence.[22] Unfortunately, radiation-induced side effects are a major cause of long-term disability for cancer patients. Radiation fibrosis describes the clinical symptoms that arise from progressive fibrotic tissue sclerosis. Its severity is directly related to radiation dosimetry, including total dose, fraction size, and duration of treatment.[23,24] The pathophysiology of radiation fibrosis is thought to develop from an activation of the coagulation system, complicated by inflammation and tissue remodeling. The accumulation of fibrin in the intravascular, perivascular, and extravascular compartments is thought to be responsible for the progressive tissue fibrosis.[25]

Clinical syndromes from radiation fibrosis may present acutely after treatment or may be considered early delayed (3 months after completion) or delayed (more than 3 months after completion of radiotherapy).[14,25] Neuromuscular complications of radiation fibrosis are due to the effect of the radiation on all neural structures in the radiation field and present as pain, weakness, spasticity, and/or bowel and bladder impairments. More than one structure at a time can be affected, and sometimes it is the combined damage of various neural structures that leads to neurologic deficits.[25]

The radiation field usually encompasses several muscles, such as the sternocleidomastoid, trapezius, scalenes, and cervical paraspinals that can present with weakness and painful spasm.[25] The brachial and lumbosacral plexus can also be affected, leading to pain and weakness. Neuropathic pain is thought to be caused by ectopic activity in the sensory nerves within the radiation field. Weakness can be caused by fibrosis at any level of the neuromuscular axis including the brain, nerve roots, or peripheral nerves. Radiation damage to muscles may also cause myopathy which can exacerbate pain and weakness.[14] Less commonly, radiation myelopathy is also a potential complication if the spinal cord should be within the radiation treatment field.[25]

It is well recognized that Hodgkin's lymphoma survivors' upper cervical nerve roots, plexus, and shoulder girdle musculature are significantly affected after being treated with mantle radiation.[26] These patients frequently present with weakness in their neck extensors, leading to "head drop," as well as pain in the cervical and thoracic muscles.[27] Elderly Hodgkin's lymphoma patients treated many years prior with mantle radiation may have since developed cervical spinal stenosis and radiculopathy, which now exacerbates symptoms of their concomitant radiation fibrosis. Persistent pain and being unable to maintain one's head position upright may make task-specific ADL' (such as driving) more difficult to perform and increase the risk for trauma and falls.[25] Current management of neck extensor and shoulder girdle muscle weakness includes physical therapy with focus on strength training, postural retraining, and energy conservation with neck bracing.[28]

Head-and-neck cancer patients treated with radiation therapy may also develop radiation fibrosis that presents as cervical dystonia and trismus. Cervical dystonia, also known as spasmodic torticollis, is caused by painful muscle contractions in the neck that can be confirmed by clinical and electromyographic findings; it has also presented as a dropped-head syndrome.[29] Trismus describes a limitation in mouth-opening secondary to spasm or fibrosis of the muscles of mastication, commonly presenting after radiation to the temporomandibular joint, masseter, or pterygoid muscles.[30] Normal mouth opening ranges from 35 to 45 mm, with males having slightly larger mouth opening than females. Prevalence of trismus with conventional radiation is estimated to be 25%, and increases with increasing doses of radiation, especially in excess of 60 Gy.[31,32] Patients with recurrence of oro- or nasopharyngeal cancer postradiation appear to be at higher risk of developing trismus than those receiving their first treatment; this suggests that the effects of radiation are cumulative, with trismus presenting toward the end of radiation therapy or at any time in the subsequent 24 months. Limited mouth opening frequently results in reduced nutritional status, significant weight loss, and nutritional deficits, and it can significantly affect the patient's quality of life, with deficits in expression, feeding, and performing dental hygiene.[33] The pain associated with cervical dystonia and trismus may be treated using oral neuropathic pain medications such as gabapentin, pregabalin, and duloxetine, as well as topical compounded creams for those elderly patients sensitive to side effects of medications. In addition, myofascial trigger point injections may provide adjunctive pain relief. The injection of botulinum toxin into painful muscles for cervical dystonia has been shown to relieve pain, but not improve function.[34] Moreover, physical therapy and botulinum toxin injection have demonstrated a limited role in treating trismus-associated pain and spasm; they have not significantly improved mouth opening.[27,35,36] Fortunately, various devices have recently been developed that have significantly improved the range of mouth opening and thus may likely optimize function (Therabite Jaw Motion Rehabilitation System and the Dynasplint Trismus System).[28]

23.4.2 Lymphedema

Lymphedema is a chronic progressive condition that can be debilitating while impairing function.[37] Lymphedema can be classified as primary, which is congenital in nature, or secondary, considered the most common cause of lymphedema in the United States. Secondary lymphedema is often the result of treatment for cancer.[38] While the exact prevalence is unknown, it is estimated that 3–5 million people suffer from lymphedema in the United States.[39] Moreover, as cancer patients survive and live longer, this number is anticipated to rise. In addition, as this population ages, other comorbidities common to the geriatric population, such as peripheral vascular disease and diabetes, will impact the course and treatment of lymphedema.[40]

The lymphatic system serves to absorb, filter, and transport lymphatic fluid. Surgery, trauma, and radiation can lead to a reduction in volume transport, potentially leading to lymphedema. While it is most commonly associated with breast cancer and melanoma, lymphedema can present in any body part affected by surgery and radiation, including cancers of the cervix, vulva, and prostate, as well as lower extremity sarcoma and head-and-neck cancers.[41] Lymphedema can be seen immediately following treatment or occur many years later; most will occur within 2 years.[42] Whether primary or secondary in nature, lymphedema is progressive in development. The International Society of Lymphology has endorsed a staging system (0–3) for lymphedema. Stage 0 lymphedema is considered a subclinical or latent condition where swelling is not evident, despite impaired lymphatic transport. Most patients are asymptomatic, but some report a feeling of heaviness in the limb. Stage 1 lymphedema is spontaneously reversible that is soft, pitting, and resolves after elevation. In Stage 2, the limb presents as being firmer due to fibrotic tissue and scarring. It temporarily reduces in swelling with prolonged elevation, but not to complete resolution. Stage 3 lymphedema presents as a limb that is grossly enlarged, with hardening and thickening, but without reduction with prolonged elevation.[36]

Risk factors for the development of lymphedema are multifactorial, including the location of the tumor, stage, type of surgery, radiation, and chemotherapy. The number of lymph nodes removed and the patient's BMI can also increase the risk for developing lymphedema, with overweight patients having a significantly higher risk.[43] In the elderly population, patients may present with new onset or exacerbation of lymphedema decades following the original surgery as the risk of lymphedema increases with age.[44]

Diagnosis of breast cancer-related lymphedema is highly patient dependent and may remain undiagnosed until it becomes a significant source of morbidity. Common presentation includes complaints of swelling, heaviness, achiness, and functional decline. A difference of 2 cm or greater between involved and uninvolved limbs is considered diagnostic for mild lymphedema.[45] The first step in treatment is education as patients have very little knowledge of the signs and symptoms of lymphedema prior to their diagnosis.[46] Treatment of lymphedema entails the use of multiple modalities, with complete decongestive therapy (CDT) being the mainstay of treatment. This particular therapy includes a combination of manual lymphatic drainage, compression bandaging, therapeutic exercise, and education on skin and nail care.[47] A large study of CDT demonstrated a volume reduction of 59% for the upper extremity, as well as 90% maintenance of volume reduction for those who continued a maintenance program.[48] Maintenance lymphedema therapy includes the use of compression sleeves and gloves, as well as self-massage and exercise. There is strong evidence that an exercise program including resistive exercises is also considered safe and beneficial.[46] Even in the palliative care setting, lymphedema treatment has been shown to improve the quality of life of patients.[49] Patients are educated on wearing compression garments during the day, in addition to self-massage techniques and volume measurements. Maintenance therapy is particularly challenging in geriatric patients due to reduced ability to don and doff the necessary garments, as well as poor skin integrity potentially inducing skin tears and wound care issues, which may also be complicated by comorbidities such as diabetes mellitus and peripheral vascular disease.

23.4.3 NEUROLOGICAL COMPLICATIONS

The incidence of all primary CNS tumors is 20.6 cases per 100,000 individuals, with the greatest incidence among patients aged 75–84 years increased significantly to 63.75 per 100,000 individuals.[50] Older patients make up half of the patients with high-grade gliomas, and advanced age and poor functional status at diagnosis are consistently associated with a poorer prognosis.[51] The most common diagnosis of brain cancer is metastatic; this is related to the increase in overall primary cancer survival, enhanced imaging techniques, and early detection.[52] The most common primary malignancies to metastasize to the brain are breast, lung, and melanoma.[45] Signs and symptoms of brain tumors depend on the location of the tumor, with the majority of tumors in the elderly developing in the cerebral hemispheres. Clinical presentation includes cognitive decline, gait and balance abnormalities, and has to be differentiated from normal effects of aging and other cerebrovascular disease. Half of patients with malignant gliomas have a poor performance status at the time of diagnosis, as measured by the Karnofsky performance score.[53]

The Dietz classification divides the rehabilitation intervention of brain tumors into four categories: preventative, restorative, supportive, and palliative. Most patients seen by rehabilitation specialists will fall into the supportive category—those who may have permanent residual deficit from the disease and its treatment.[54] Such patients may present with gait abnormality, hemiparesis, dysphagia, aphasia, and cognitive deficits, and it is this particular group that benefits most from inpatient rehabilitation.[55] There is also growing evidence regarding the efficacy of inpatient rehabilitation for patients with brain tumors, with functional outcomes comparable to patients with stroke and traumatic brain injury. Research has also demonstrated that a majority of patients with primary and metastatic brain tumors can achieve functional gains as measured by functional independence measurement (FIM) score and are able to return home after discharge.[56] Given the functional impairments found in these patients, inpatient rehabilitation is likely being underutilized.[57] Unique challenges with this patient population include disease status, recovery curve, prognosis, and ongoing medical challenges throughout the course of treatment.[55] Special considerations in providing rehabilitative therapy often include mitigation of side effects from radiation and chemotherapy, seizure medications, fatigue, and cognitive abnormalities. Chemotherapy is often used for patients with brain tumors, especially primary malignant tumors. An oral alkylating agent, Temozolomide (Temodar), is commonly used as adjuvant chemotherapy combined with radiation in high-grade gliomas. It can cause fatigue, headaches, nausea, thrombocytopenia, and neutropenia.[58] Many patients with brain tumors are also prescribed steroids to treat edema. Even at physiologic doses, there can be bone loss with glucocorticoid use. For patients that are taking more than 5 mg of Prednisone (or its equivalent) for 3 months, the American College of Rheumatology recommends supplementation with calcium and vitamin D, bisphosphonates, and weight-bearing exercises to prevent osteoporosis.[59]

Another important deficit in brain tumor patients is new onset of swallowing dysfunction, which occurs in about 63% of the patients.[60] Dysphagia often results in aspiration, dehydration, and malnutrition, which affects quality of life and long-term prognosis. The site of the tumor, type of surgery, chemotherapy, and radiation all contribute to the development of dysphagia.[61] In a study comparing patients with dysphagia from brain tumors versus stroke, patients presented with similar rates of dysphagia when matched for age, site of lesion, and functional status, showing comparable swallowing gains with therapy.[62,63]

Cognition affects learning and memory, arousal and attention, executive function, and language.[64] In general, cognitive dysfunction can be seen across the spectrum of brain tumors and can also be debilitating. It may result from the tumor itself, surgery, and chemo- or radiotherapy, and is considered a negative prognostic indicator.[53] It is also considered an independent prognostic factor that can signal a recurrence. Whole-brain radiotherapy used in metastatic disease has especially been associated with cognitive decline.[65] For most patients with brain metastases, controlling the tumor is the most important factor in stabilizing cognitive function. In a study of 139 patients with brain tumors, more than 90% of the patients displayed impairments in at least one area of cognition. Impairments of executive function were observed for 78% of the patients, and impairments of memory and attention were observed in more than 60% of the patients.[66] Treatment of cognitive dysfunction includes minimizing medications associated with cognitive side effects, treating concomitant depression, and implementing neurorehabilitative and cognitive therapy. Cognitive therapy includes utilizing preserved cognitive strengths as compensation for identified weaknesses. Cognitive aids such as memory books, alarms, and electronic organizers are also used.[67] In a study evaluating cognitive therapy, patients underwent a comprehensive inpatient rehabilitation program showing significant functional gains, increased independence, and productivity.[68,69] In patients with brain tumors and cognitive dysfunction, methylphenidate and donepezil have both been found to be beneficial.[55,70]

23.4.4 SPINAL CORD INJURY

Epidural spinal cord compression is one of the most feared complications of cancer and occurs in up to 5% of cancer patients (approximately 80,000 patients per year).[71,72] Cancer-related spinal cord compression has been reported to be 10%–14% of new-onset spinal cord injury cases. These patients tend to be older, female, married, and not working when compared to traumatic spinal cord injury.[73] As such, special consideration needs to be given to these patients' comorbid conditions, polypharmacy, and challenges in discharge planning. For example, in elderly patients, treatment of pain and spasticity may be challenging due to medication adverse effects of sedation. Moreover, impaired memory or dementia may interfere with carry-over during the rehabilitation process.[74]

Primary malignant tumors of the spine account for less than 5% of primary bone tumors, with the majority of bone cancer cases metastatic in nature. Multiple myeloma is particularly common in the elderly population, whereas sarcoma and plasmocytoma are more common in the general population.[75] While all tumors can metastasize to the spine, the most common to do so include breast, lung, prostate, colon, thyroid, and kidney.[76] The mechanism of metastases is largely via hematogenous spread of malignant cells to the vertebral body through the Batson plexus.[77]

Pain is the initial symptom of epidural compression, and this is usually progressive such that back pain in a patient with cancer warrants an urgent evaluation to exclude spinal cord compression.[78] Unlike degenerative joint disease, pain from spinal metastases and pathological fractures due to metastases is most commonly found in the thoracic spine.[76] The back pain commonly increases in intensity when the patient lies in a supine position, thus may be recalled as being only present at night. Pain may also be worse at night when endogenous cortisol is at its lowest level, which can subsequently increase tumor pressure. Later, other neurological findings may present such that pain is followed by weakness, sensory loss, and sphincter dysfunction.[79] Overall prognosis is determined by neurological function at diagnosis. Magnetic resonance imaging (MRI) of the entire spine with gadolinium is the imaging of choice in evaluating for spinal cord compression. In any case, one-third of patients have multiple sites of spinal cord compression at the time of diagnosis.[76]

Treatment for spinal cord compression includes high-dose corticosteroids, and this is started immediately in patients with neurologic compromise. A definitive course of therapy is decided after the patient's response to corticosteroids is noted.[63] For example, successive treatment for squamous cell carcinoma (SCC) involves radiation therapy, decompressive surgery, or both. For esophageal squamous cell carcinoma (ESCC) cases, radiotherapy alone is the most common treatment and results in decreased pain and improved function.[80] Fortunately, newer techniques of image-guided, intensity-modulated radiotherapy now permit higher doses to be precisely delivered to tumor sites with minimal spinal cord exposure, providing adequate symptom relief with minimal side effects.[81] Neurosurgical intervention prior to radiotherapy is sometimes indicated in patients with rapidly evolving neurologic deficits from vertebral bone compression.[66] There is also evidence that decompressive surgery in addition to radiation therapy improves ambulation, continence, and survival in patients with solitary compressive sites by radio-resistant tumors.[82]

Intramedullary spinal cord metastasis is much rarer, affecting less than 1% of patients who have cancer. Unlike epidural metastases, these metastases tend to affect the cervical cord and conus medullaris. In these cases, imaging of the entire cord and brain is necessary as it has been associated with brain involvement. Treatment includes corticosteroids and radiation therapy.[71]

Lastly, leptomeningeal metastases—diffuse metastases that surround the spinal cord and the brain—may induce myelopathy. Presentation can include polyradicular involvement with pain, weakness, paresthesias, and areflexia.[83] Evaluation of leptomeningeal metastasis requires contrast-enhanced brain and spine MRIs. Treatment includes steroids, radiation, and intrathecal chemotherapy, for those cancers that are responsive. While treatment is considered palliative and prognosis poor, it can help preserve neurological function for some time.[84]

Some have concerns whether a cancer patient with SCC metastases should participate in acute rehabilitation as she or he will likely have a shortened life expectancy. In reality, prognosis after ESCC is variable, with 1 year mortality estimated to be 80% and several patients surviving much longer.[14] Several studies have demonstrated that inpatient rehabilitation has indeed benefitted patients with ESCC, with one study revealing an improvement in FIM scores from 62 on admission to 84 at discharge.[69,85] Another study among traumatic spinal cord injury patients confirmed that there was no relationship between age at discharge and modified Barthel index. Instead, higher functional discharge scores were associated with paraplegia, incomplete lesions, and higher level of functional status at the time of admission. This study also revealed an increased need by the elderly for assistance in bathing, upper and lower body dressing, stair climbing, and transfers to chair, toilet, and bath—but only in patients with complete paraplegia.[86]

23.5 PARANEOPLASTIC SYNDROMES

Paraneoplastic syndromes typically present when antibodies are produced against tumors that express certain proteins. New onset of a paraneoplastic syndrome should trigger a workup for primary malignancy or a recurrence. Rapid onset of symptoms can differentiate paraneoplastic syndrome from noncancer-related etiology.[87] It has been estimated that paraneoplastic syndromes affect up to 8% of patients with cancer, and those most frequently associated with these syndromes are small cell lung cancer, breast cancer, gynecologic tumors, and hematologic malignancies. In some cases, diagnosis of paraneoplastic syndrome may predate the diagnosis of primary tumor.[88]

Paraneoplastic syndromes with neurological involvement occur in approximately 1% of cancer patients and can produce a multitude of neurological deficits that may be disabling for cancer patients.[89] Treatment includes intravenous immunoglobulin, steroids, and immunosuppressants.[90] The type of rehabilitation program initiated is determined by the type of deficits that are incurred. For example, a patient with ataxia due to paraneoplastic cerebellar degeneration would benefit from gait and balance training, and management of tremors. Secondary limbic encephalitis may be difficult to differentiate from acute psychiatric disorder but may still benefit from a brain injury rehabilitation program. Moreover, a patient with weakness in hand intrinsic muscles secondary to cerebral cortical involvement would benefit from an occupational therapy program.[14]

23.6 CHEMOTHERAPY-INDUCED PERIPHERAL NEUROPATHY

Chemotherapy-induced peripheral neuropathy (CIPN) is a common complication of cancer treatment and has the potential to cause pain in addition to disability.[76] While chemotherapy is effective in shrinking tumor size, it can have short- and long-term side effects on the peripheral nervous system, including damage to the motor, sensory, and autonomic nerves. The incidence of CIPN is extremely variable based on the agent used and has been reported to range from 30% to 40% across all chemotherapy agents.[74] Unfortunately, symptoms of CIPN are cumulative as treatment progresses. Comorbidities such as alcohol abuse and diabetes may also predispose cancer patients to develop more severe forms of peripheral neuropathy.[91] A baseline history and physical highlighting peripheral nervous system findings may be important when selecting a pretreatment chemotherapy agent (Figure 23.1).

During chemotherapy treatment, patients should also be screened for symptoms such as pain and numbness. Physical examination should include muscle strength, sensation, reflexes, gait, and functional evaluation.[92] It is anticipated that most damage will be to sensory nerves, leading to

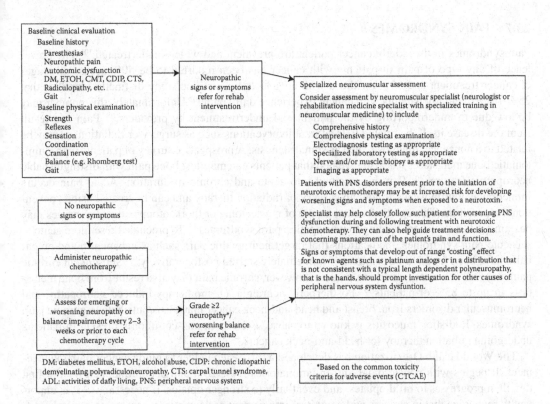

FIGURE 23.1 Neuropathy assessment algorithm used before and during administration of neurotoxic chemotherapy for breast cancer. (From Stubblefield MD, McNeely ML et al. A prospective surveillance model for physical rehabilitation of women with breast cancer: Chemotherapy-induced peripheral neuropathy. *Cancer.* 2012;118(8 Suppl):2250–2260.)

numbness and paresthesias. Painful sensations can include dysesthesias and be characterized as electric, burning, and/or lancinating. Treatment of pain from CIPN includes the use of Gabapentin, Pregabalin, Duloxetine, Amitrptyline, and opioids.[93] A review of data for the American Society of Clinical Oncology clinical practice guidelines shows Duloxetine to be the most effective for CIPN.[94] Involvement of the motor nerves, which is less common, can lead to muscle weakness, ultimately leading to difficulty with ADL and falls.[95] One assessment tool designed to identify CIPN is the Common Terminology Criteria for Adverse Events (CTCAE) scale developed by the Eastern Cooperative Oncology Group. This scale separates paresthesias, motor symptoms, and sensory symptoms by Grades 1–5.

While some studies show similar rates of CIPN in the elderly population, the elderly are seemingly more prone to long-term morbidity as a result.[96] This includes poor balance, muscle weakness, and increased risk of falls, which can increase with cumulative doses of chemotherapy.[97] Identifying those individuals at risk for falls and intervening before adverse effects occur may ultimately improve functional outcomes. Treatment includes patient education on compensatory strategy for those with decreased sensation and proprioception. Services may also include proper skin care, reminders on not to pick up hot objects with insensate hands, and utilizing other senses such as vision to compensate for poor balance. Modification of the home environment may also be necessary to prevent falls.[98] Physical and occupational therapists may also individualize therapies, including therapeutic exercises to strengthen muscles of the extremities, balance retraining, and prescription of orthotics and assistive devices.[98] Specifically, interventions for balance training have been shown to be effective in improving patients' balance among patients with diabetic peripheral neuropathy.[99,100]

23.7   PAIN SYNDROMES

Pain syndromes in the elderly cancer patient are prevalent and widely undertreated.[101] The prevalence of any type of pain in patients with cancer has been reported to be 50% across all stages of cancer treatment and 65% for those with advanced disease; one study distinctly identifies that 25%–40% of elderly patients with cancer experience daily pain.[102] Unfortunately, this number may be low due to underreporting by the patient and undertreatment by providers.[101] Pain can result from the disease itself, be related to treatment interventions such as surgery or radiation, or may be related to a noncancer diagnosis such as spinal stenosis. A prospective survey of patients with symptomatic bone metastases has also revealed that patients can manifest bone pain with distinguishable neuropathic features.[103] Pain is classified into acute and chronic in duration. Acute pain occurs immediately within weeks following surgery or radiation therapy and can be treated using conventional algorithms. Through the radical nature of mastectomy or thoracotomy surgeries, nerves may be damaged or stretched, leading to neuropathic pain syndromes.[82] To preclude these more acute to subacute pain syndromes, medications that target neuropathic pain such as gabapentin and pregabalin have been found to be effective if immediately started postoperatively.[104] Subsequent chronic pain may still originate from these injuries; however, chronic pain may also result from bone metastasis in up to 85% of patients.[102] Postherpetic neuralgia, chemotherapy-induced neuropathy, and neuromuscular disorders from breast and head-and-neck cancer may also contribute to chronic pain syndromes. Radiation mucositis is known to cause severe pain and commonly present in patients undergoing radiation therapy for head-and-neck cancers.

The World Health Organization has developed a three-step ladder to guide cancer pain management. It begins with nonsteroidal anti-inflammatories (NSAIDs) and acetaminophen for the first tier, then progresses to mild opiates, and eventually to stronger opiates, if necessary.[105] It is important to recognize that in patients with cognitive impairment or dementia, assessing pain may be difficult. Nonverbal cues such as grimacing, groaning, and confusion may lead to diagnosis of pain.[106] Advanced patient age also presents a challenge in prescribing medications such that comorbid conditions, declining cognitive function, poor nutrition, and end-organ dysfunction can substantially limit the effectiveness of treatment. Additionally, the use of polypharmacy in the elderly commonly leads to drug interactions which can increase toxicity or reduce efficacy. It is imperative to be aware of all drugs used in cancer and pain treatment that may predispose the patient to nephrotoxicity. Concomitant use of NSAIDs should be used with caution with elderly patients undergoing chemotherapy as NSAIDs may contribute to renal insufficiency, congestive heart failure, and peptic ulcer disease. For this reason, acetaminophen is the preferred drug for mild pain.[107] Opiates such as morphine, oxycodone, hydromorphone, and fentanyl are generally well tolerated, if used appropriately. Unfortunately, opiates may metabolize more slowly in older patients, making them more sensitive to the side effects, and thus should be carefully titrated for pain control.[108]

In addition to using medications, there are a number of modalities that can be used by physiatrists and therapists to benefit the geriatric cancer patient, including stretching, the use of assistive devices to offload a painful limb, bracing, and injections. The use of cryo- and heat therapies, manual medicine, and TENS unit has also been demonstrated to alleviate pain.[109]

23.7.1   Postmastectomy Pain Syndrome

Postmastectomy pain syndrome is a condition that occurs after breast procedures such as lumpectomy, axillary lymph node dissection, mastectomy, and reconstruction.[110] It is commonly seen in younger patients, with up to 40% of patients experiencing some sort of chronic pain.[111] The pathophysiology is likely neuropathic and includes damage to nerves in the axilla and the chest wall during surgery.[112] Symptoms include phantom breast sensations, dysesthesias, and intercostobrachial neuralgia.[113] Neuroma pain may also be identified by a focal point of hypersensitivity along the incision.[90] Physical examination should include assessment of the incision line for mobility and the presence of neuroma or seroma. There may also be sensory loss or dysesthesias along the dermatomal distribution of the intercostal nerves if they should be injured during surgery. Neurologic examination should focus on testing the strength of the shoulder girdle musculature, including those muscles innervated by the thoracodorsal, long thoracic, and medial and lateral pectoral nerves. Postoperative treatment includes minimizing postoperative pain with desensitization techniques.[114] Neuropathic pain medications and compounded creams are also helpful for those with pain.[115] Although not ideal, opioids may need to be used for individuals with persistent pain not responding to other treatments. Physical therapy efforts should focus on improving the mobility of the shoulder girdle muscles, including the pectoralis minor and major, and latissimus dorsi.[116]

23.7.2 POST-THOROCOTOMY PAIN SYNDROME

Post-thorocotomy pain syndrome occurs in about 50% of patients following thorocotomy.[117] It presents with persistent pain at the incision site as well as along the distribution of the intercostal nerve, for longer than 2 months in duration.[94] It is believed to result from intercostal neuralgia caused by multiple mechanisms, including poorly repositioned rib fractures, costochondral dislocation, costochondritis, intercostal neuroma, nerve entrapments, or local infections.[118] It is often described as sharp, lancinating pain accompanied by dysesthesias.[119] Altered biomechanics from the dissection of latissimus dorsi during the thoracotomy procedure also contributes to abnormal shoulder function.[95] Musculoskeletal examination should closely inspect the incision site, palpate the chest wall to exclude costochondritis, and range the shoulder so as to evaluate associated musculature with careful attention to myofascial pain and muscle atrophy.[116] Patients may benefit from postoperative pulmonary rehabilitation consisting of energy conservation and breathing techniques, aerobic conditioning following the surgery, scar mobilization, and soft tissue massage. Pain should also be treated aggressively with neuropathic pain medications, topical lidocaine, compounded creams, and intercostal nerve blockade.[98] Preemptive thoracic epidural analgesia initiated before surgical incision has previously been shown to significantly reduce the severity of acute postoperative pain but seems to have had no effect on the incidence of chronic pain 6 months after surgery.[120] Alternative pain management strategies have also involved direct manual costovertebral joint manipulation, with good effects.[121]

23.7.3 UPPER EXTREMITY PAIN DISORDERS

Complaints of pain in the upper extremity and neck are common by those treated by surgery for melanoma and cancer of the breast and lung. It is estimated that upper extremity pain is experienced in seven out of eight breast cancer patients.[122] Unfortunately, the cause of pain may be multifactorial and thus difficult to treat; the etiology may be benign, related to the malignancy, or its treatment.[116] Careful history and physical examination of the musculoskeletal and neurologic system will likely provide clues to its origin. Inspection for muscle atrophy from radiation, range of motion testing of the shoulder, examination of the chest wall and axilla, and a careful examination of incisions of postmastectomy patients may reveal a neuroma, seroma, and soft tissue changes and contractures.

23.7.4 CERVICAL RADICULOPATHY

A common cause of upper extremity pain is cervical radiculopathy, an impingement of the nerve root(s) exiting the vertebral foramen—most commonly at the C5–C6 disc, followed by C6–C7.[123] Radiculopathies in the elderly are frequently caused by degenerative disease of the spine and discs, leading to painful symptoms. Malignancy of the neural components or nerve root invasion by a tumor may cause or exacerbate radicular symptoms.[124] Furthermore, radiation to the head and neck may induce radiation fibrosis that affects nerve roots and peripheral nerves alike, leading to arm pain, sensory changes, weakness, and loss of reflexes. Physical examination should include a range of motion of the cervical spine, assessment of paraspinal musculature, and provocative testing such as Spurling's maneuver. Neurological examination should focus on muscle strength, sensory testing, and reflexes. In a patient with known malignancy and worsening neck pain, imaging should be obtained using MRI with and without gadolinium.[125] Treatment of cervical radiculopathy includes physical therapy, occupational therapy, pain medication, and interventional pain procedures. Ultimately, surgery is reserved for those with rapid-onset or severe neurological deficits, or intractable pain.[123]

23.8 BRACHIAL PLEXOPATHY

Brachial plexopathy has also been commonly associated with breast cancer treatment, as well as has been induced by radiation treatments for other malignancies occurring in proximity to the brachial plexus.[126] Radiation plexopathy presents with upper extremity weakness without pain, originating within the upper trunk of the brachial plexus. Lymphedema is often secondary in onset, with most patients developing these symptoms within 3 years of radiotherapy, although later presentations may occur.[127] Physical examination will initially reveal shoulder girdle weakness and then subsequent involvement of the entire arm as the disorder progresses.[128] Management of radiation-induced brachial plexopathy is largely supportive. Pain should be controlled, and weakness mediated with bracing.[129] Neoplastic brachial plexopathy presents with sensory loss and pain that originates in the lower trunk and progresses to the entire plexus. The presence and severity of the pain help distinguish this particular condition from radiation-induced plexopathy.[116] MRI and electrodiagnostic studies may also help differentiate between neoplastic and radiation-induced plexopathy. For instance, myokymic discharges on electromyography are suggestive of radiation plexopathy, though its presence does not rule out tumor recurrence.[130] Neoplastic brachial plexopathy is best managed by treating the underlying malignancy with radiation and chemotherapy.[116]

23.9 SHOULDER PAIN

The prevalence of shoulder pain in the elderly ranges from 21% to 27% and increases with advanced age.[131] Rotator cuff dysfunction is generally a common musculoskeletal disorder in elderly patients, often underdiagnosed and undertreated. Etiology of rotator cuff disease is multifactorial and encompasses rotator cuff impingement, tendinosis, and tears, and can lead to difficulties with ADL' and functional independence. Shoulder pain is frequently encountered in breast cancer patients, as well as those suffering from melanoma and lung cancer. A 5-year follow-up study demonstrated that the prevalence of shoulder pain among breast cancer patients is 30%–40%, with restrictions in mobility of the arm and shoulder, and associations with poor quality of life.[132] Weakness in the rotator cuff muscles following mastectomy also indirectly causes impingement of the rotator cuff.[129] Moreover, patients with premorbid C5–C6 radiculopathy or radiation-induced plexopathy may also be at higher risk for rotator cuff weakness.[116] Shoulder pain from rotator cuff dysfunction presents as a dull ache that extends over the shoulder and deltoid muscle. Overhead activities exacerbate pain which frequently worsens at night.[133] Physical examination will reveal positive findings in reduced range of motion, impingement tests, and weakness during muscle testing. Imaging with plain radiographs and MRI confirm and help delineate adhesive capsulitis from rotator cuff tendonitis as often these two conditions coexist and make diagnosis challenging.[129] Management of rotator cuff dysfunction includes pain control with local injections, topical medications, and NSAIDs. Physical therapy should be prescribed for increasing the range of motion and strengthening scapular stabilizers, and cryotherapy and ultrasound should also be provided to decrease pain and improve joint mobility.[134]

23.10 BONE METASTASES

Bone metastases are a frequent complication of advanced cancer. Cancers of the breast, prostate, lung, kidney, and thyroid account for 80% of the metastases.[135] While the true incidence of bone disease is unknown, over half of deaths have bone metastases on autopsy.[108] There are over 20,000 cases of spinal cord compression resulting from spinal metastases. These figures emphasize the importance of being able to recognize and manage this complication of advanced disease in order to maintain function. As patients live longer and survive their primary malignancy, it is important to recognize the presentation of bone metastases. Bone metastases are seen most commonly in the axial skeleton, followed by the femur, humerus, skull, ribs, and pelvis. Metastatic disease must be ruled out in patients with a known history of cancer presenting with bone pain.[136] Pain at presentation is usually functional in nature. For example, groin pain worse with active flexion may point to an impending pathologic fracture. Evaluation of suspicious bone metastases on radiographs must be reevaluated via bone scan. Generally speaking, MRI is best suited for evaluation of spinal metastases.[137] Spinal metastases typically present with pain, often leading to neurological deficit, including motor and sensory deficits, bowel and bladder abnormalities, as well as ataxia. More common complications of bone metastases include pain, hypercalcemia, spinal cord compression, and pathologic fractures. Fortunately, with recent technological and pharmaceutical advances, patients with bone metastases have increasing rates of survival (mean survival of 20 months).[138]

Predicting which metastatic lesions will lead to pathological fracture is of great interest. A common scoring system developed by Mirels accounts for the site, the size, and the type of lesion (lytic or blastic) as well as the type of pain (functional vs. nonfunctional). This algorithm allows the physician to score each potential site and better predict the possibility of fracture such that appropriate interventions may be initiated. Mirels' studies revealed that functional pain was the single best predictor of pathological fracture.[112] In another study of cancer patients with bone metastases undergoing inpatient rehabilitation, Bunting et al. found that overall, undergoing a rehabilitation program did not increase the chance of fractures, such that fractures occurred even while patients were lying in bed. One explanation for this is that pathologic fractures ultimately happen with progression of the disease, as opposed to activity.[139] Some accommodations are made for patients with metastatic lesions: prohibition of resistive exercises on the involved limb with limitations to only active range of motion, maintenance of nonweight-bearing restrictions, and bracing to the affected extremity, as well as providing education on proper transfer techniques.[183]

Medical therapy for metastatic disease includes chemotherapy, hormone therapy, bisphosphonates such as zoledronic acid, and RANK ligand inhibitors such as Denosumab. Bisphosphonates inhibit osteoclasts and bone resorption. They significantly reduce skeletal-related events (fractures, need for radiation or surgery, hypercalcemia, and spinal cord compression).[140] A Cochrane review demonstrated that bisphosphonates decrease bone pain and improve quality of life.[141] Complications of bisphosphonates use include nephrotoxicity, hypocalcemia, osteonecrosis of jaw, and atypical fractures. Adverse events related to nephrotoxicity and osteonecrosis of the jaw may also be increased in the elderly population.[116] Palliation of painful spinal metastases via radiotherapy has been demonstrated to be highly effective.[142] Surgical stabilization may also be needed for those patients that have neurologic deterioration, instability, fracture, or intractable pain. Overall, when compared with radiotherapy alone, surgery plus radiation may increase patient survival, neurologic function, continence, and ambulation.[66]

23.11 EXERCISE IN ELDERLY CANCER PATIENTS

23.11.1 INDICATIONS AND CONTRAINDICATIONS FOR EXERCISE

Physical activity has been shown to benefit the patient over the course of the cancer experience. An increasing number of studies have examined the therapeutic value of exercise during primary cancer treatment. There is strong evidence supporting exercise as not only safe and feasible during cancer treatment, but also that moderate exercise improves fatigue, mood, anxiety, depression, and self esteem. Exercise can be used to improve cardiovascular fitness, muscle strength, and body composition.[143,144] For patients with malignancies, there are few standard precautions during rehabilitation that should be followed. Unfortunately, cancer survivors have been identified as being more sedentary than desired by cancer rehabilitation team members. Observations reveal that survivors tend to decrease their physical activity levels after the diagnosis of cancer, with progressively lesser amounts and intensities of activity through the treatment period, and thereafter, rarely returning to premorbid levels of activity.[145,146]

23.12 FATIGUE

Cancer-related fatigue has also been a major detriment to the quality of life in cancer patients, defined as a "persistent, subjective sense of tiredness related to cancer or cancer treatment that interferes with usual function."[147] It can be related to radiation, chemotherapy, anemia, and depression.[148] Although there has been scarcity of evidence-based interventions to manage this type of fatigue, anemia correction and low-impact exercise have had sufficient research to support their effectiveness, while psychosocial support, energy conservation, and sleep therapy have also contributed to improvements in cancer-related fatigue.[149] One study evaluating the effects of modafinil on cancer-related fatigue among 631 patients receiving chemotherapy demonstrated that patients with severe baseline fatigue greatly benefited from the use of the drug, although patients with mild or moderate fatigue did not achieve as much improvement in symptoms.[150] There is also limited evidence that advanced cancer patients receiving methylphenidate reported less fatigue.

23.13 MODALITIES IN CANCER REHABILITATION

Physical modalities have not been well studied in cancer patients, so safety and efficacy are not certain. Caution is used for most modalities directly over tumor sites, and deep heat modalities such as ultrasound or phonophoresis are usually contraindicated over a tumor site.[151] Spinal traction is also avoided in patients with spinal bone metastasis or significant osteoporosis. Many other modalities such as cryotherapy, biofeedback, iontophoresis, TENS, and massage are generally believed to be safe.[151] Exercise can counteract the effects of inactivity and improve psychological status. Cryotherapy is usually applied as ice packs, ice compression wraps, or ice massage. It may be implemented at bedside or in the gym as adjunctive pain management options, thus decreasing the need for pain medications.[129] Heat therapies can decrease pain and muscle spasms, and decrease joint stiffness. Contraindications to use of heat therapies include not applying them to areas with sensory deficits, atrophy, acute inflammation, or those that have been exposed to radiation.[152] Biofeedback has been shown to reduce physiological arousal (EMG, pulse rate, and systolic and diastolic blood pressure) and reductions in anxiety and nausea following chemotherapy. TENS creates a therapeutic effect by causing muscle contractions and is used in those with inflammatory conditions, muscle spasms, or contusions. Via the gate mechanism of sensory feedback to the spinal cord, awareness of pain is prevented and short-term pain relief results. Myofascial therapy/massage is performed to deliberately stimulate lymph flow and perfusion, minimize muscle tightness and pain, and facilitate stretching and range of motion, in addition to fibrolytic and counterstimulatory effects. A 2013 feasibility study demonstrated that postmassage symptom scores on questionnaires showed statistically significant decreases in pain, stress/anxiety, and fatigue in Veterans Administration Medical Center patients receiving basic massage for supportive care at home.[153]

23.14 PRECAUTIONS IN CANCER REHABILITATION

Radiotherapy and chemotherapy cause different types of bone marrow injury.[154] For this reason, neutropenia and thrombocytopenia are common complications after radiotherapy that can cause treatment interruptions and increase the risks of infection or bleeding. Among National Cancer Institute-designated comprehensive cancer centers, physical therapy restrictions are in place to hold therapies for patients with platelets below 25,000 μL.[132] Chemotherapy-induced neutropenia typically occurs 3–7 days following administration of chemotherapy. Survivors with leucopenia and compromised immune function should avoid public gyms and other public places until their white blood cell counts return to safe levels. Anemia is less of a concern than thrombocytopenia, given the associated risk of intracranial hemorrhage or uncontrolled bleeding, unless it is severe.[155]

REFERENCES

1. Lehmann JF, DeLisa JA et al. Cancer rehabilitation: Assessment of need, development, and evaluation of a model of care. *Arch Phys Med Rehabil.* 1978;59(9):410–419.
2. Flood KL, Carroll MB et al. Geriatric syndromes in elderly patients admitted to an oncology-acute care for elders unit. *J Clin Oncol.* 2006;24(15):2298–2303.
3. Penedo FJ, Schneiderman N et al. Physical activity interventions in the elderly: Cancer and comorbidity. *Cancer Invest.* 2004;22(1):51–67.
4. Mariotto AB, Yabroff KR et al. Projections of the cost of cancer care in the United States: 2010–2020. *J Natl Cancer Inst.* 2011;103(2):117–128 and 103(8):699 correction.
5. Banks E, Byles JE et al. Is psychological distress in people living with cancer related to the fact of diagnosis, current treatment or level of disability? Findings from a large Australian study. *Med J Aust.* 2010;193(5 Suppl):S62–S67.
6. Agency for Healthcare Research and Quality, Rockville, MD. More than one in five hospital patients in 2008 were born in 1933 or earlier: Research activities. 2011, No. 366. http://www.ahrq.gov/news/newsletters/research-activities/feb11/0211RA34.html.
7. Lim SC, Doshi V et al. Factors causing delay in discharge of elderly patients in an acute care hospital. *Ann Acad Med Singapore.* 2006;35:27–32.
8. Roberts PS, Nuno M et al. The impact of inpatient rehabilitation on function and survival of newly diagnosed patients with glioblastoma. *PM & R.* 2014;6(6): 514–521.
9. Huang ME, Cifu DX et al. Functional outcome after brain tumor and acute stroke: A comparative analysis. *Arch Phys Med Rehabil.* 1998;79(11):1386–1390.
10. Dy SM, List DJ et al. A quality improvement initiative for improving appropriateness of referrals from a cancer center to subacute rehabilitation. *J Pain Symptom Manage.* 2014;48(1):127–131.
11. Hearn J and Higginson IJ. Do specialist palliative care teams improve outcomes for cancer patients? A systematic literature review. *Palliat Med.* 1998;12(5):317–332.
12. Centers for Medicare and Medicaid Services. Medicare hospice benefits. Official Medicare Program legal guidance is contained in the relevant statutes, regulations, and rulings. http://www.medicare.gov/pubs/pdf/02154.pdf.
13. Higginson IJ and Evans CJ. What is the evidence that palliative care teams improve outcomes for cancer patients and their families? *Cancer J.* 2010;16(5):423–435.
14. Stubblefield M and O'Dell M. (Eds.). (2009). Radiation Fibrosis Syndrome. In: *Cancer Rehabilitation: Principle and Practice.* New York: Demos Publishing. Pages 723–747.
15. Temel JS, Greer JA et al. Early palliative care for patients with metastatic non-small-cell lung cancer. *N Engl J Med.* 2010;363(8):733–742.
16. Okamura H. (Foundation for Promotion of Cancer Research). Importance of rehabilitation in cancer treatment and palliative medicine. *Jpn J Clin Oncol.* 2011;41(6):733–738.
17. O'Toole DM and Golden AM. Evaluating cancer patients for rehabilitation potential. *West J Med.* 1991;155:384–387.
18. Oken, MM, Creech, RH et al. Toxicity and response criteria of the Eastern Cooperative Oncology Group. *Am J Clin Oncol.* 1982;5:649–655.
19. Kristjansson SR, Nebakken A et al. Comprehensive geriatric assessment can predict complications in elderly patients after elective surgery for colorectal cancer: A prospective observational cohort study. *Crit Rev Oncol Hematol.* 2010;76(3):208–217.
20. Massa E, Madeddu C et al. An attempt to correlate a "Multidimensional Geriatric Assessment" (MGA), treatment assignment and clinical outcome in elderly cancer patients: Results of a phase II open study. *Crit Rev Oncol Hematol.* 2008;66:75–83.
21. Monfardini S and Balducci L. A comprehensive geriatric assessment (CGA) is necessary for the study and the management of cancer in the elderly. *Eur J Cancer.* 1999;35:1771–1772.
22. Lawrence TS, Ten Haken RK et al. Principles of Radiation Oncology. In: DeVita VT Jr., Lawrence TS, Rosenberg SA, editors. *Cancer: Principles and Practice of Oncology.* 8th ed. Philadelphia, PA: Lippincott Williams and Wilkins, 2008.

23. Stubbenfield MD. Radiation fibrosis syndrome: Neuromuscular and musculoskeletal complications in cancer survivors. *PM & R.* 2011;3(11):1041–1054.

24. Late Complications of Head and Neck Radiation. Oral Complications of Chemotherapy and Head/Neck Radiation (PDQ®). National Cancer Institute at the National Institutes of Health. http://www.cancer.gov/cancertopics/pdq/supportivecare/oralcomplications/HealthProfessional/page16.

25. Hojan K and Milecki P. Opportunities for rehabilitation of patients with radiation fibrosis syndrome. *Rep Pract Oncol Radiother.* 2014;19(1):1–6.

26. Rowin J, Cheng G et al. Late appearance of dropped head syndrome after radiotherapy for Hodgkin's disease. *Muscle Nerve.* 2006;34(5):666–669.

27. Dijkstra PU, Sterken MW et al. Exercise therapy for trismus in head and neck cancer. *Oral Oncol.* 2007;43(4):389–394.

28. Stubblefield MD, Manfield L et al. A preliminary report on the efficacy of dynamic jaw opening device (Dynasplint Trismus System) as part of multimodal treatment of trismus in patients with head and neck cancer. *Arch Phys Med Rehabil.* 2010;91(8):1278–1282.

29. Astudillo L, Hollington L et al. Cervical dystonia mimicking dropped-head syndrome after radiotherapy for laryngeal carcinoma. *Clin Neurol Neurosurg.* 2003;106(1):41–43.

30. Dijkstra PU, Kalk WW et al. Trismus in head and neck oncology: A systematic review. *Oral Oncol.* 2004;40(9):879–889.

31. Bensadoun RJ, Riesenbeck D et al. A systematic review of trismus induced by cancer therapies in head and neck cancer patients. *Support Care Cancer.* 2010;18(8):1033–1038.

32. Teguh DN, Levendag PC et al. Trismus in patients with oropharyngeal cancer: Relationship with dose in structures of mastication apparatus. *Head Neck.* 2008;30(5):622–630.

33. Hsiung CY, Huang EY et al. Intensity-modulated radiotherapy for nasopharyngeal carcinoma: The reduction of radiation-induced trismus. *Br J Radiol.* 2008;81(970):809–814.

34. Stubblefield MD, Levine A et al. The role of botulinum toxin type A in the radiation fibrosis syndrome: A preliminary report. *Arch Phys Med Rehabil.* 2008;89(3):417–421.

35. Dijkstra PU, Sterken MW et al. Trismus in head and neck oncology: A systematic review. *Oral Oncol.* 2004;40(9):879–889.

36. The International Society of Lymphology. The diagnosis and treatment of peripheral lymphedema. 2013. http://www.u.arizona.edu/~witte/ISL.htm (Accessed March 1).

37. Ahmed RL, Prizment A et al. Lymphedema and quality of life in breast cancer survivors: The Iowa Women's Health Study. *J Clin Oncol.* 2008;26(35):5689–5696.

38. Warren AG, Brorson H et al. Lymphedema: A comprehensive review. *Ann Plast Surg.* 2007;59(4):464–472.

39. Lawenda BD, Mondry TE et al. Lymphedema: A primer on the identification and management of a chronic condition in oncologic treatment. *CA Cancer J Clin.* 2009;59(1):8–24.

40. Konecne S and Perdomo M. Lymphedema in the elderly: A special needs population. *Top Geriatr Rehabil.* 2004;20(2):98–113.

41. Tiwari P, Coriddi M et al. Breast and gynecologic cancer-related extremity lymphedema: A review of diagnostic modalities and management options. *World J Surg Oncol.* 2013;11:237.

42. Norman SA, Localio SA et al. Lymphedema in breast cancer survivors: Incidence, degree, time course, treatment, and symptoms. *J Clin Oncol.* 2009;27(3):390–397.

43. Yen TW, Fan X et al. A contemporary, population-based study of lymphedema risk factors in older women with breast cancer. *Ann Surg Oncol.* 2009;16(4):979–988.

44. Ahmed, RL, Schmitz KH et al. Risk factors for lymphedema in breast cancer survivors: The Iowa Women's Health Study. *Breast Cancer Res Treat.* 2011;130(3):981–991.

45. Johnson JD and Young B. Demographics of brain metastasis. *Neurosurg Clin N Am.* 1996;7(3):337–344.

46. Kwan ML, Cohn JC et al. Exercise in patients with lymphedema: A systematic review of the contemporary literature. *J Cancer Surviv.* 2011;5(4):320–336.

47. Mondry TE, Riffenburgh RH et al. Prospective trial of complete decongestive therapy for upper extremity lymphedema after breast cancer therapy. *Cancer J.* 2004;10(1):42–48.

48. Ko DS, Lemer R et al. Effective treatment of lymphedema of the extremities. *Arch Surg.* 1998;133(4):452–458.

49. Clemens KE, Jaspers B et al. Evaluation of the clinical effectiveness of physiotherapeutic management of lymphoedema in palliative care patients. *Jpn J Clin Oncol.* 2010;40(11):1068–1072.

50. Flowers A. Brain tumors in the older person. *Cancer Control.* 2000;7(6):523–538.

51. Buckner JC. Factors influencing survival in high-grade gliomas. *Semin Oncol.* 2003;30(6 Suppl 19):10–14.

52. Eichler AF and Loeffler JS. Multidisciplinary management of brain metastases. *Oncologist.* 2007;12(7):884–898.

53. Taphoorn MJ and Klein M. Cognitive deficits in adult patients with brain tumours. *Lancet Neurol.* 2004;3(3):159–168.

54. Stubblefield M and O'Dell M. (Eds.). (2009). Rehabilitation of Patients with Brain Tumors. In: *Cancer Rehabilitation: Principle and Practice.* New York: Demos Publishing. Pages 518–521; also in *Neurosurgery.* 2000 Aug;47(2):324–333; discussion 333–334.

55. Shaw EG, Rosdhal R et al. Phase II study of donepezil in irradiated brain tumor patients: Effect on cognitive function, mood, and quality of life. *J Clin Oncol.* 2006;24(9):1415–1420.

56. Tang V, Rathbone M et al. Rehabilitation in primary and metastatic brain tumours: Impact of functional outcomes on survival. *J Neurol.* 2008;255(6):820–827.

57. O'Dell MW, Barr K et al. Functional outcome of inpatient rehabilitation in persons with brain tumors. *Arch Phys Med Rehabil.* 1998;79(12):1530–1534.

58. MacDonald DR. Temozolomide for recurrent high-grade glioma. *Semin Oncol.* 2001;28(4 Suppl 13): 3–12.

59. American College of Rheumatology Ad Hoc Committee on Glucocorticoid Induced Osteoporosis: 2001 update. *Arthritis Rheum.* 2001;44:1496–1503.

60. Vargo M. Brain tumor rehabilitation. *Am J Phys Med Rehabil.* 2011;90(5 Suppl 1):S50–S62.

61. Wesling M, Brady S et al. Dysphagia outcomes in patients with brain tumors undergoing inpatient rehabilitation. *Dysphagia.* 2003 Summer;18(3):203–210.

62. Park DH, Chun MH et al. Comparison of swallowing functions between brain tumor and stroke patients. *Ann Rehabil Med.* 2013;37(5):633–641. Epub 2013 Oct 29.

63. Jeba GR, Ramkumar G et al. Interventions for the treatment of metastatic extradural spinal cord compression in adults. *Cochrane Database Syst Rev.* 2008;(4):CD006716.

64. Tucha O, Smely C et al. Cognitive deficits before treatment among patients with brain tumors. *Neurosurgery.* 2000;47(2):324–333; discussion 333–334.

65. Tallet AV, Azria D et al. Neurocognitive function impairment after whole brain radiotherapy for brain metastases: Actual assessment. *Radiat Oncol.* 2012;7:77.

66. Patchell RA, Tibbs PA et al. Direct decompressive surgical resection in the treatment of spinal cord compression caused by metastatic cancer: A randomised trial. *Lancet.* 2005;366(9486):643–648.

67. Gehring K, Sitskoom MM et al. Cognitive rehabilitation in patients with gliomas: A randomized, controlled trial. *J Clin Oncol.* 2009;27(22):3712–3722.

68. Marciniak CM, Sliwa JA et al. Functional outcomes of persons with brain tumors after inpatient rehabilitation. *Arch Phys Med Rehabil.* 2001;82(4):457–463.

69. Parsch D, Mikut R et al. Postacute management of patients with spinal cord injury due to metastatic tumour disease: Survival and efficacy of rehabilitation. *Spinal Cord.* 2003;41(4):205–210.

70. Meyers CA, Weitzner MA et al. Methyphenidate therapy improves cognition, mood, and function of brain tumor patients. *J Clin Oncol.* 1998;16(7):2522–2527.

71. Byrne TN. Spinal cord compression from epidural metastases. *N Engl J Med.* 1992;327(9):614–619.

72. Graber JJ and Nolan CP. Myelopathies in patients with cancer. *Arch Neurol.* 2010;67(3):298–304.

73. McKinley WO, Seel RT et al. Nontraumatic spinal cord injury: Incidence, epidemiology, and functional outcome. *Arch Phys Med Rehabil.* 1999;80(6):619–623.

74. Mohile SG, Klepin HD et al. Considerations and controversies in the management of older patients with advanced cancer. *Am Soc Clin Oncol Educ Book.* 2012;32:321–328.

75. Sundaresan N, Rosen G et al. Primary malignant tumors of the spine. *Orthop Clin North Am.* 2009;40(1):21–36.

76. Hershman DL, Lacchetti C et al. Prevention and management of chemotherapy-induced peripheral neuropathy in survivors of adult cancers: American Society of Clinical Oncology. Clinical Practice Guideline. *J Clin Oncol.* 2014;32:1941–1967.

77. Arguello F. Pathogenesis of vertebral metastasis and epidural spinal cord compression. *Cancer.* 1990;65(1):98–106.

78. Helweg-Larsen S and Sørensen PS. Symptoms and signs in metastatic spinal cord compression: A study of progression from first symptom until diagnosis in 153 patients. *Eur J Cancer.* 1994;30A(3):396.

79. Stubblefield M and O'Dell M. (Eds.). (2009). Spinal Cord. In: *Cancer Rehabilitation: Principle and Practice.* New York: Demos Publishing. Pages 533–551; also in Neurosurgery. 2000 Aug;47(2):333–334.

80. Gerszten PC, Mendel E et al. Radiotherapy and radiosurgery for metastatic spine disease: What are the options, indications, and outcomes? *Spine.* 2009;34(22 Suppl):S78.

81. Yamada Y, Lovelock DM et al. A review of image-guided intensity-modulated radiotherapy for spinal tumors. *Neurosurgery.* 2007;61(2):226–235; discussion 235.

82. Braddom RL (Ed.). (2011). Cancer rehabilitation. In: *Physical Medicine and Rehabilitation.* 4th ed. Philadelphia, PA: Elsevier-Saunders. Pages 1370–1398.

83. Custodio CM. Electrodiagnosis in cancer treatment and rehabilitation. *Am J Phys Med Rehabil.* 2011;90(5 Suppl 1):S38–S49.

84. Chamberlain MC. Leptomeningeal metastasis. *Curr Opin Oncol.* 2010;22(6):627–635.

85. Murray PK. Functional outcome and survival in spinal cord injury secondary to neoplasia. *Cancer.* 1985;55(1):197–201.

86. Yarkony GM, Roth EJ et al. Spinal cord injury rehabilitation outcome: The impact of age. *J Clin Epidemiol.* 1988;41(2):173–177.

87. Braik T, Evans AT et al. A practical review: Paraneoplastic neurological syndromes: Unusual presentations of cancer. *Am J Med Sci.* 2010;340(4):301–308.

88. Pelosof LC and Gerber DE. Paraneoplastic syndromes: An approach to diagnosis and treatment. *Mayo Clin Proc.* 2010;85(9):838–854.

89. Honnorat J and Cartalat-Carel S. Advances in paraneoplastic neurological syndromes. *Curr Opin Oncol.* 2004;16(6):614–620.

90. Stubblefield M and O'Dell M. (Eds.). (2009). Upper extremity disorders in cancer. In: *Cancer Rehabilitation: Principle and Practice.* New York: Demos Publishing. Pages 693–710.

91. Wolf S, Barton D et al. Chemotherapy-induced peripheral neuropathy: Prevention and treatment strategies. *Eur J Cancer.* 2008;44(11):1507–1515.

92. Stubblefield MD, McNeely ML et al. A prospective surveillance model for physical rehabilitation of women with breast cancer: Chemotherapy-induced peripheral neuropathy. *Cancer.* 2012;118(8 Suppl):2250–2260.

93. Visovsky C, Collins M et al. Putting evidence into practice: Evidence-based interventions for chemotherapy-induced peripheral neuropathy. *Clin J Oncol Nurs.* 2007;11(6):901–913.

94. Gerner P. Post-thoracotomy pain management problems. *Anesthesiol Clin.* 2008;26(2):255–vii.

95. Li WW, Lee TW et al. Shoulder function after thoracic surgery. *Thorac Surg Clin.* 2004;14(3):331–343.

96. Argyriou AA, Polychronopoulos P et al. Is advanced age associated with increased incidence and severity of chemotherapy-induced peripheral neuropathy? *Support Care Cancer.* 2006;14(3):223–229.

97. Tofthagen C, Overcash J et al. Falls in persons with chemotherapy-induced peripheral neuropathy. *Support Care Cancer.* 2012;20(3):583–589.

98. Hughes R and Gao F. Pain control for thoracotomy. *Contin Educ Anaesth Crit Care Pain.* 2005;5(2):56–60.

99. Richardson JK, Sandman D et al. A focused exercise regimen improves clinical measures of balance in patients with peripheral neuropathy. *Arch Phys Med Rehabil.* 2001;82(2):205–209.

100. Richardson JK, Thies SB et al. Interventions improve gait regularity in patients with peripheral neuropathy while walking on an irregular surface under low light. *J Am Geriatr Soc.* 2004;52(4):510–515.

101. Bemabei R, Gambassi G et al. Management of pain in elderly patients with cancer: SAGE Study Group: Systematic assessment of geriatric drug use via epidemiology. *JAMA.* 1998;279(23):1877–1882.

102. Portenoy RK. Cancer pain: Epidemiology and syndromes. *Cancer.* 1989;63(11 Suppl):2298–2307.

103. Kerba M, Wu J et al. Neuropathic pain features in patients with bone metastases referred for palliative radiotherapy. *J Clin Oncol.* 2010;28:4892–4897.

104. Raptis E, Vadalouca A et al. Pregabalin vs. opioids for the treatment of neuropathic cancer pain: A prospective, head-to-head, randomized, open-label study. *Pain Pract.* 2014;14(1):32–42.

105. Stjemsward J. WHO cancer pain relief programme. *Cancer Surv.* 1988;7(1):195–208.

106. AGS Panel. The management of persistent pain in older persons. *J Am Geriatr Soc.* 2002;50(6 Suppl):S205–S224.

107. Stubblefield M and O'Dell M. (Eds.). (2009). Geriatric Issues in Cancer Rehabilitation. In: *Cancer Rehabilitation: Principle and Practice.* New York: Demos Publishing. Pages 869–880.

108. Bunting RW and Shea B. Bone metastasis and rehabilitation: Cancer rehabilitation in the new millennium. *Cancer Suppl.* 2001;92(4):1020–1028.

109. Menefee LA and Monti DA. Nonpharmacologic and complementary approaches to cancer pain management. *J Am Osteopath Assoc.* 2005;105(Suppl 5):S15–S20.

110. Vilholm OJ, Cold S et al. The postmastectomy pain syndrome: An epidemiological study on the prevalence of chronic pain after surgery for breast cancer. *Br J Cancer.* 2008;99(4):604–610.

111. Smith WC, Bourne D et al. A retrospective cohort study of post mastectomy pain syndrome. *Pain.* 1999;83(1):91–95.

112. Mirels H. Metastatic disease in long bones. A proposed scoring system for diagnosing impending pathologic fractures. *Clin Orthop Relat Res.* 1989;(249):256–264.

113. Carpenter JS, Andrykowski MA et al. Postmastectomy/postlumpectomy pain in breast cancer survivors. *J Clin Epidemiol.* 1998;51(12):1285–1292.

114. Katz J, Poleshuck EL et al. Risk factors for acute pain and its persistence following breast cancer surgery. *Pain.* 2005;119(1–3):16–25.

115. Dirks J, Fredensborg BB et al. A randomized study of the effects of single-dose gabapentin versus placebo on postoperative pain and morphine consumption after mastectomy. *Anesthesiology.* 2002;97(3):560–564.

116. Gridelli C. The use of bisphosphonates in elderly cancer patients. *Oncologist.* 2007;12(1):62–71.

117. Karmakar MK and Ho AM. Postthoracotomy pain syndrome. *Thorac Surg Clin.* 2004;14(3):345–352.

118. Strebel B and Ross S. Chronic post-thoractomy pain syndrome. *CMAJ.* 2007;177(9):1027, 1029.

119. Wildgaard K, Ravn J et al. Chronic post-thoracotomy pain: Critical review of pathogenic mechanisms and strategies for prevention. *Eur J Cardiothorac Surg.* 2009;36(1):170–180.

120. Bong C, Samuel M et al. Effects of pre-emptive epidural analgesia on post-thoracotomy pain. *J Cardiothorac Vasc Anaesth.* 2005;19(6):786–793.

121. Minor A. Alternative management for post-thoracotomy pain syndrome. *Can J Surg.* 1996;39:430–431.

122. Stubblefield MD and Custodio CM. Upper-extremity pain disorders in breast cancer. *Arch Phys Med Rehabil.* 2006;87(3 Suppl 1):S96–S99.

123. Rand MV. Cervical spondylosis: Recognition, differential diagnosis, and management. *Ochsner J.* 2001;3(2):78–84.

124. Shelerud RA and Paynter KS. Rarer causes of radiculopathy: Spinal tumors, infections and other unusual causes. *Phys Med Rehabil Clin N Am.* 2002;13(3):645–696.

125. Stubblefield MD and Keole N. Upper body pain and functional disorders in patients with breast cancer. *PM & R.* 2014;6(2):170–183.

126. Jaeckle KA. Neurologic manifestations of neoplastic and radiation induced plexopathies. *Semin Neurol.* 2010;30:254–262.

127. Fathers E, Thrush D et al. Radiation-induced brachial plexopathy in women treated for carcinoma of the breast. *Clin Rehabil.* 2002;16(2):160–165.

128. Kori SH, Foley KM et al. Brachial plexus lesions in patients with cancer: 100 cases. *Neurology.* 1981;31(1):45–50.

129. Management of cancer pain: Clinical practice guidelines. 1994. AHCPR Publication No. 94-0592. Rockville, MD: U.S. Department of Health and Human Services.

130. Harper CM, Thomas JE et al. Distinction between neoplastic and radiation-induced brachial plexopathy, with emphasis on the role of EMG. *Neurology.* 1989;39(4):502–506.

131. Lin JC, Weintraub N et al. Nonsurgical treatment for rotator cuff injury in the elderly. *J Am Med Dir Assoc.* 2008;9(9):626–632.

132. Nesvold IL, Reinertsen KV et al. The relation between arm/shoulder problems and quality of life in breast cancer survivors: A cross-sectional and longitudinal study. *J Cancer Surviv.* 2011;5(1):62–72.

133. Gomoll AH, Katz JN et al. Rotator cuff disorders: Recognition and management among patients with shoulder pain. *Arthritis Rheum.* 2004;50(12):3751–3761.

134. Frieman BG, Albert TJ et al. Rotator cuff disease: A review of diagnosis, pathophysiology, and current trends in treatment. *Arch Phys Med Rehabil.* 1994;75(5):604–609.

135. Buckwalter JA and Brandser EA. Metastatic disease of the skeleton. *Amer Fam Phys.* 1997;55(5):1761–1768.

136. Stubblefield M and O'Dell M. (Eds.). (2009). Bone Metastases. In: *Cancer Rehabilitation: Principle and Practice.* New York: Demos Publishing. Pages 773–785.

137. Rosenthal DI. Radiologic diagnosis of bone metastases. *Cancer.* 1997;80(8 Suppl):1595–1607.

138. Healey JH and Brown HK. Complications of bone metastases: Skeletal complications of malignancy: Surgical management. *Cancer Suppl.* 2000;88(12):2940–2951.

139. Bunting R, Lamont-Havers W et al. Pathologic fracture risk in rehabilitation of patients with bony metastases. *Clin Orthop Relat Res.* 1985;(192):222–227.

140. Saad F, Gleason D et al. Long-term efficacy of zoledronic acid for the prevention of skeletal complications in patients with metastatic hormone-refractory prostate cancer. *J Natl Cancer Inst.* 2004;96(11):879–882.

141. Wong MH, Stockler MR et al. Bisphosphonates and other bone agents for breast cancer. *Cochrane Database Syst Rev.* 2012;2:CD003474.

142. Ziellinski S. Shorter course of radiotherapy effective for palliation of painful bone metastases. *J Natl Cancer Inst.* 2005;97(11):785.

143. Courneya KS. Exercise in cancer survivors: An overview of research. *Med Sci Sports Exerc.* 2003;35:1846–1852.

144. Schmitz KH, Holtzman J et al. Controlled physical activity trials in cancer survivors: A systematic review and meta-analysis. *Cancer Epidemiol Biomarkers Prev.* 2005;14:1588–1595.

145. Irwin ML, Crumley D et al. Physical activity levels before and after a diagnosis of breast carcinoma: The health, eating, activity, and lifestyle (HEAL) study. *Cancer.* 2003;97:1746–1757.

146. Courneya KS and Friedenreich CM. Relationship between exercise during treatment and current quality of life among survivors of breast cancer. *J Psychosoc Oncol.* 1997;15:35–57.

147. Campos MP, Hassan BJ et al. Cancer-related fatigue: A practical review. *Ann Oncol.* 2011;22(6): 1273–1279.

148. Wagner LI and Cella D. Fatigue and cancer: Causes, prevalence and treatment approaches. *Br J Cancer.* 2004;91(5):822–828.

149. Mock V. Evidence-based treatment for cancer-related fatigue. *J Natl Cancer Inst Monogr.* 2004;32:112–118.

150. Jean-Pierre P, Morrow GR et al. A phase 3 randomized, placebo-controlled, double-blind, clinical trial of the effect of modafinil on cancer-related fatigue among 631 patients receiving chemotherapy: A University of Rochester Cancer Center Community Clinical Oncology Program Research base study. *Cancer.* 2010;116(14):3513–3520.

151. Stubblefield M and O'Dell M. (Eds.). Therapeutic modalities. In: *Cancer Rehabilitation: Principle and Practice.* New York: Demos Publishing. 2009; pp. 797–801.

152. DeLisa JA and Gans BM. (Eds.). (1998) Physical Agents. In: *Rehabilitation Medicine.* Philadelphia, PA: Lippincott-Raven. Pages 483–504.

153. Kozak L, Vig E et al. A feasibility study of caregiver-provided massage as supportive care for veterans with cancer at home. *J Support Oncol.* 2013;11(3):133–143.

154. MacManus M, Lamborn K et al. Radiotherapy-associated neutropenia and thrombocytopenia: Analysis of risk factors and development of a predictive model. *Blood.* 1997;89(7):2303–2310.

155. Rock CL, Doyle C et al. Nutrition and physical activity guidelines for cancer survivors. *CA Cancer J Clin.* 2012;62(4):243–274.

24 Spinal Cord Injury in Older Adults

Philippines G. Cabahug, Albert C. Recio, and Jeffrey B. Palmer

CONTENTS

24.1 INTRODUCTION

The management of individuals living with chronic spinal cord injury (SCI) presents with distinct challenges that necessitate the practitioner to have an understanding of the interaction of the complex changes following SCI with the physiology of aging. Advances in emergent, acute medical and rehabilitation management have contributed to improved survival and life expectancy rates of persons with SCI. However, a person with SCI is not exempt from medical conditions that may plague their able-bodied counterparts. It is important to recognize that these conditions may have atypical manifestations in the SCI population.

24.1.1 CHANGING FACE OF MORTALITY AND LIFE EXPECTANCY IN SPINAL CORD INJURY

It is estimated that in the United States, the annual incidence of SCI (excluding those who die at the scene of the accident) is approximately 40 cases/million or approximately 12,500 new cases each year. The average age of injury has increased from 29 years in the 1970s to 42 years in 2010. Approximately 80% of SCIs occur in males. The most common etiology of SCI is due to motor vehicle crashes, followed by falls, acts of violence (commonly gunshot wounds), and sports injuries.[1]

A study by Jain et al. assessed the trends in acute traumatic SCI incidence, etiology, and mortality using the Nationwide Inpatient Sample (NIS) databases from 1993 to 2012 which included a total of 63,109 patients. They found that the overall absolute number of cases modestly increased with the incidence rate remaining stable (53 cases/million with estimated 13,706 cases in 1993 to 54 cases/ million with estimated 16,965 cases in 2012).[2] The largest increase in incidence was observed in older patients (men aged 65–74 years from 84 cases/million or 695 cases in 1993 to 131 cases/ million 1465 cases in 2012). SCI secondary to falls increased significantly from 28% (1997–2000) to 66% (2010–2012) in those aged 65 years and older. Prior studies have noted this trend as well.[3,4]

Aside from the increasing incidence of SCI in the elderly population, more persons with SCI survive their initial insult and are living longer. More than 40% of individuals with SCI living in the United States are older than 40 years, and more than 25% of those with SCI have lived with their injury for more than 20 years.[5]

The life expectancy of individuals following SCI has increased; however, this is still significantly reduced when compared with the general population. In addition to this, life expectancy within the SCI population varies with the severity of injury and the age at injury. Those with motor incomplete injuries have longer life expectancy compared with those with complete paraplegia or tetraplegia. Life expectancy declines with increased age at the time of injury.[1,5] We thus have two different populations to consider: those who are aging with an SCI and those who have sustained their SCI late in life.

24.2   AGING AND SPINAL CORD INJURY

The term "accelerated aging" has been used to describe the altered aging trajectory seen in individuals with physical disability, such as SCI. Aging begins at about the age of 20 years, when peak capacity of the different organ systems is reached. At the peak of development, organ systems have as much as 50% excess capacity. It is postulated that the rate of normal decline is about 1% per year across organ systems. When capacity drops below 40% (at about 75 years), the organ system becomes vulnerable to adverse events (trauma, stress, infection). Genetics and lifestyle factors also play a role in the aging of organ systems. Persons with SCI do not age at a rate of 1% per year, but at a rate of about 1.5% per year, depending on the organ system. Individuals who sustain their injury before maturity may have less reserve capacity.[6]

The accelerated aging seen in SCI is therefore influenced by the combination of the physiologic changes associated with the neurologic injury and impairments leading to immediate and long-term effects on body systems.[5]

24.2.1   RESPIRATORY SYSTEM

SCI initially results in a restrictive impairment secondary to muscle paralysis. Neurologic level and completeness of injury are important factors in the acute period.[7] Individuals with complete tetraplegia are at the highest risk, followed by those with incomplete tetraplegia and paraplegia.[8] Injuries at the level of T12 and above present with impaired muscular function that results in a decline in vital capacity (VC) and ability to cough.[9] Injuries above T7 display bronchial hyperactivity, resulting in bronchoconstriction and airway obstruction.[6,10]

The early development of scoliosis, kyphosis, and increasing spasticity leads to further respiratory impairment. The reduced lung and chest wall compliance, reduced lung capacity, and inability to breathe deeply and generate an effective cough can lead to atelectasis and pneumonia.[11] This is of concern as respiratory diseases are the leading cause of mortality in the SCI population, of which pneumonia accounts for 70.1%.[12]

In addition to this, sleep disordered breathing (SDB), characterized by sleep apnea, oxygen desaturation, and snoring, is more prevalent in SCI populations and may either increase or persist with the aging process in persons with SCI.[13] Higher rate of SDB in individuals with SCI is noted within weeks of injury and continues in the following years with prevalence ranging from 25% to 53%.[14]

Older age at the time of injury is also associated with higher risk of respiratory complications.[15] Studies also show increased incidence of pneumonia and atelectasis in older SCI patients compared with younger SCI patients, regardless of the duration of injury. A British study of 834 persons with SCI of at least 20 years post injury showed that the incidence of pneumonia increased with age, from 1.6% at the <30 years age group to 5.6% in the >60 years age group.[16] Similar results were seen in the U.S. Model Systems data, with pneumonia increasing from 1.5% in the <30 years age group to 8.2% in the >76 years age group.[7] Other studies suggest that respiratory function declines with the duration of injury independent of age even in paraplegia, and smoking exacerbates the decline in forced VC.[17,18]

The combined effects of SCI and older age lead to significant respiratory dysfunction in individuals with both acute and chronic SCIs. Practitioners should include in their periodic health assessment surveillance of VC, especially in patients with tetraplegia. A sleep study (polysomnography) is necessary for diagnosing SDB, especially obstructive sleep apnea (OSA). Untreated OSA can lead to hypertension, cognitive impairment, and mood disorders. The treatment of choice for OSA is nocturnal continuous positive airway pressure (CPAP) therapy; it is safe and highly effective. In terms of personal behavioral modifications, maintenance of appropriate weight to reduce the risk of further respiratory compromise is optimal, and smoking cessation programs should be encouraged. Aggressive management of community-acquired pneumonia, including hospitalization, mobilization of pulmonary secretions using manually assisted coughing and mechanical cough assistance, and prompt administration of antibiotics is recommended.[19]

Cervical SCI commonly causes paralysis of the muscles of expiration. These muscles are essential for generating the elevated subglottal air pressure that is needed for cough. Thus, individuals with cervical SCI are unable to generate a cough that is effective in clearing the airways, making them highly vulnerable to pneumonia. Assisted cough is essential for respiratory health in these individuals.

Persons with a VC of <2 L are at the greatest risk of late-onset ventilatory failure and may benefit from oxygen supplementation and assisted ventilation during periods of respiratory compromise. Patients with higher-level SCI should be taught a preventative home program of incentive spirometry, postural drainage, assisted coughing, and breathing exercises. Regular resistive inspiratory muscle trainings in patients with chronic cervical SCI result in decreased restrictive impairment and dyspnea when performing ADLs. Smoking cessation programs should be offered to decrease incidence of mucus production and respiratory complications.[11] In addition to yearly influenza immunization, they should receive pneumococcal vaccination every 5 years.[20]

24.2.2 Cardiovascular System

When SCI results in loss of input from the sympathetic nervous system (T6 and above), bradycardia, bradyarrhythmia, and hypotension often result.[21] The combination of impaired autonomic control, decreased musculature available for exercise, sedentary lifestyle, and the resultant decreased cardiovascular fitness increases the risk of cardiovascular disease (CVD), which has emerged in recent years as a leading cause of death for those with SCI.[1,22] There is a higher prevalence of CVD in SCI in comparison to the ambulatory population. For instance, the prevalence rates of symptomatic CVD in SCI have approximated to 30%–50%[23] in comparison to 5%–10% in the able-bodied population.[24] Moreover, the prevalence of asymptomatic CVD is 60%–70% in persons with SCI.[25,26] These are alarming statistics that place significant burden upon the patient, family, and society as a whole. Patterns in causes of death following SCI have undergone substantial change. Whiteneck et al. report that CVD is the most frequent cause of death among persons with SCI more than 30 years after injury (46% of all deaths) and over 65 years old (35% of all deaths).[16]

There is ample evidence that body composition changes can play a major role in negatively affecting the individual's health. Marked physical inactivity after SCI has been associated with lower HDL cholesterol, elevated LDL cholesterol and triglycerides, increased adiposity, and abnormal glucose homeostasis. There is a consensus that low serum HDL cholesterol is common in SCI. About 10% of the able-bodied population have HDL levels <35 mg/dL versus 40% in SCI population.[26] In a study of 541 subjects with chronic SCI, lower levels of serum HDL were found in the subjects with tetraplegia than in those with paraplegia. Furthermore, those motor complete SCIs had lower HDL levels, suggesting that decreased physical activity is a contributor to lowering HDL levels. Approximately 25% of the general population is considered to have elevated levels of LDL cholesterol. Individuals with SCI have LDL levels similar to that of the general population.[26]

The loss of muscle mass is critical because insulin acts peripherally on the individual's muscle mass for metabolism of glucose. After SCI, atrophy of skeletal muscle decreases muscle mass. At 24 weeks after injury, the cross-sectional muscle mass of the leg is about 45%–80% of age-matched controls.[27] Bauman and colleagues have shown high rates of abnormal glucose tolerance and prevalence of frank diabetes in individuals with SCI compared to age-matched controls. After a 75 g oral glucose tolerance test, 22% of individuals with SCI met the criteria for diabetes versus only 6% of able-bodied subjects. Only 38% of individuals with tetraplegia and 50% of those with paraplegia had a normal response to this glucose tolerance test versus 82% of age-matched controls. In veterans with SCI, the prevalence of type II diabetes mellitus was threefold higher than that of able-bodied controls.[28] Subjects with tetraplegia have been found to have a reduction in glucose transport that is proportional to the loss of muscle mass. Glucose tolerance ensues as higher plasma levels of insulin levels are required to maintain normal blood glucose levels. Elevated serum insulin levels and other abnormalities in glucose metabolism, even if not meeting the criteria for absolute diabetes, are considered to be atherogenic conditions, increasing the risk for coronary heart disease (CHD).

Periodic assessment of risk factors such as blood lipids, glucose, weight, dietary habits, smoking, activity level, and alcohol consumption can help identify modifiable risk factors. Cigarette smokers with SCI had lower HDL regardless of gender, ethnicity, level, or completeness of lesion. Excessive alcohol intake may depress serum HDL cholesterol levels. Moderate alcohol consumption has been reported to increase serum HDL cholesterol levels. However, in obese subjects, this beneficial effect of alcohol raising serum HDL level may not occur.[29]

When adverse lipid profiles require pharmacological management, compliance with medication regimens should be encouraged. Greater emphasis on increasing HDL should be considered in persons with SCI. Exercise training is an important therapeutic intervention for reducing the risk for CVD as it appears that ordinary activities of daily living are not sufficient to maintain cardiovascular fitness in SCI. Exercise training can be an effective means of attenuating the progression of CVD and related comorbidities in persons with SCI. Research evidence shows various exercise modalities like functional electric stimulation (FES) leg cycling, arm ergometry, resistance training (RT), and body weight-supported treadmill training (BWSTT) can improve abnormalities in lipid and glucose metabolism and promote cardiovascular fitness in SCI. There is growing evidence from several trials that FES training for a minimum of 3 days per week for 2 months can improve oxidative metabolism,[30–32] exercise tolerance, and cardiovascular fitness.[31,33–36]

24.2.3 Genitourinary System

Following SCI, there is loss of volitional control over micturition and loss of coordination of detrusor and sphincter reflexes, resulting in a neurogenic bladder. Neurogenic bladder may be classified anatomically (supraspinal, suprasacral, infrasacral, peripheral autonomic, or muscular) or functionally (based on cystometric or urodynamic evaluations). Presently, a combination of both functional and anatomic classifications is used. Injuries above the sacral micturition center (above S2) result in an upper motor neuron (UMN) bladder, with detrusor hyperreflexia or detrusor–sphincter dyssynergia and elevated lower urinary tract pressure that can lead to hypertrophy of the detrusor muscle and decreased bladder compliance. Cumulatively, these may result in the development of vesicoureteral reflux (VUR) with hydronephrosis and upper urinary tract deterioration. Injuries below the sacral micturition center result in a lower motor neuron (LMN) or flaccid bladder, with failure to empty.

An indwelling Foley catheter (FC) is placed during the acute postinjury period as patients are usually in spinal shock. The bladder is acontractile and areflexic, and patients will have urinary retention generally lasting from 6 to 12 weeks. Spinal shock, however, may last anywhere from a week to a year, and its return is heralded by return of delayed plantar response, bulbocavernosus reflex, anal wink, and muscle stretch reflexes. Once medically stable, the FC may be discontinued, and clean intermittent catheterization (CIC) may be initiated. CIC is done every 4 hours with goal catheter volumes of <500 mL.[37]

Long-term management of neurogenic bladder (Table 24.1) depends on several factors: level of lesion (UMN vs. LMN bladder), completeness of injury, other comorbidities, gender, hand function, motivation, and availability of caregivers. The goals of management remain the same: obtain a "balanced bladder" with high bladder capacity and low bladder pressures; achieve urinary continence through socially acceptable methods of bladder drainage; and minimize the risk of urinary tract infections (UTIs) and risk of deterioration and/or infection of the upper urinary tract.[38]

CIC is often considered to be the best option, provided that the patient has sufficient hand function, is highly motivated and compliant, or has a willing caregiver. It is recommended that CIC is performed several times daily with goal catheterized volumes of <500 mL and a total fluid intake of approximately 2000 mL daily. Indwelling catheterization, either through an indwelling

TABLE 24.1

UMN and LMN Bladder

	UMN	LMN
Level of lesion	Above sacral micturition center (above S2)	• Involves sacral micturition center (S2–S4) or • Involves solely peripheral innervation of the bladder
Characteristics	Results from spastic bladder and/or incompetent sphincter Small, overactive, spastic bladder Failure to store	Results from flaccid bladder and/or overactive sphincter Large, areflexic, flaccid bladder Failure to empty
Examples	SCI: return of reflex arc after trauma Multiple sclerosis Stroke (subacute, detrusor hyperreflexia)	SCI: spinal shock (loss of reflex arc after initial trauma) Cauda equina, conus medullaris syndrome Stroke (acute, detrusor areflexia)
Management options	Behavioral: timed voids Intermittent catheterization Collecting devices: diaper, condom catheter, indwelling catheter Drugs to facilitate urine storage • Antimuscarinics • Oxybutynin, tolterodine well established; caution in using oxybutynin due to potential for cognitive impairment • Beta agonists (mirabegron) • Calcium channel blockers • Botulinum A injections Surgery: augmentation, continent diversion, denervation procedures	Behavioral: intermittent catheterization Collecting device: diaper, condom catheter, indwelling catheter Crede maneuver (bladder compression)[a] Valsalva maneuver (abdominal straining)[a] Drugs to induce urination • Bethanechol • Alpha blockers (for sphincter dyssynergia) Tamsulosin and other alpha blockers may cause hypotension Surgery: neurostimulation

Note: Some causes may display features of both UMN and LMN pathology at different times through the course of disease.

[a] Creates high bladder pressures; avoid in urethral pathology, hydronephrosis, or VUR or UTI.

FC or placement of a suprapubic tube (SPT), is considered in patients with poor hand skills, high fluid intake, cognitive impairments, elevated detrusor pressure, or need for temporary management of VUR. The SPT should be considered if urethral pathology is present, there is FC blockage, or catheter insertion is difficult. The advantages of using SPT include easier and less frequent catheter changes (can change even in a wheelchair), less urethral discomfort, less likely to cause autonomic dysreflexia (AD), and less likely to become blocked. It is easier to maintain hygiene in women with an SPT.

One must consider potential complications from bladder management itself. Indwelling catheters cause higher rates of bladder calculi (stones), UTIs, and bladder cancer.[39,40] CIC is considered the safest method of bladder management in terms of preventing stones, infections, and urethral erosions. However, there is an increased risk of strictures and false passages with CIC.[41]

The use of oral anticholinergics is associated with improved bladder compliance, lower leak point pressures, less hydronephrosis, and fewer febrile UTIs. Potential side effects from anticholinergic medications include dry mouth, constipation, blurry vision, sedation, and urinary retention. Oxybutynin, an anticholinergic commonly used in the treatment of UMN neurogenic bladder, is associated with cognitive deficits. Alpha blockers, which are used to relax spastic sphincter, can lead to dizziness and postural hypotension and are not well tolerated in the older adults.

UTI and its complications were formerly the leading cause of mortality in patients with SCI. With the advancements in urologic management and antibiotic treatment options, it now accounts for only 3.1%–5.4% of deaths.[1,42] UTIs are among the most frequent reasons for rehospitalizations in the years following SCI.[43,44]

Elderly individuals are at increased risk for UTIs, which may be related to a decline in immune function, postmenopausal changes, and effects of prostatism.[45] Signs and symptoms of UTI may be subtle in elderly persons with SCI, who may present with confusion or lethargy rather than common signs such as dysuria, frequency, malodorous/cloudy urine, urinary incontinence, increased spasticity, hematuria, fever, chills, and leukocytosis.[11] Diagnosis of UTI in SCI patients can be challenging as they have absent or impaired pain sensation, and bladder colonization with bacteriuria is frequent in those who use urinary catheters (indwelling or intermittent). UTI is characterized by the onset of new symptoms and not just the presence of bacteria or white blood cells (WBC) in the urine (Table 24.2). Antibiotic treatment of *asymptomatic* bacteriuria is not recommended.[46,47] Routine antibiotic

---

TABLE 24.2

Diagnosis of UTI in Neurogenic Bladder

Symptoms (two or more)	Fever >38°C
	Increased spasticity
	AD (injuries T6 and above)
	Worsening/new urinary incontinence or leakage
	Cloudy urine with increased odor
	Back pain
	Vague abdominal pain or discomfort
Urine studies	Positive urinalysis: >10 WBC/HPF on microscopy
	Positive urine culture
	1. Intermittent catheterized specimen: 10^2 CFU/mL
	2. Condom catheter specimen: >10^4 CFU/mL
	3. Indwelling and suprapubic catheter specimens: any value

Source: Jahromi, M. S., A. Mure, and C. S. Gomez. 2014. *Current Urology Reports* 15 (9): 433; McKibben, M. J. et al. 2015. *Urologic Clinics of North America.* 42 (4): 527–536; National Institute on Disability and Rehabilitation Research Consensus Statement. 1992. *The Journal of the American Paraplegia Society* 15 (3): 194–204.

prophylaxis may increase the risk of bacterial resistance and is not recommended for asymptomatic bacteriuria in patients with SCI.

Other strategies to prevent UTI in SCI include the use of hydrophilic, closed system catheters, antibiotic-coated catheters; use of introducer tip catheters that bypass the colonized distal urethra; bladder irrigation (irrigation solutions vary from saline to antibiotic irrigants such as neomycin or polymyxin); and bacterial interference with intravesical inoculation of benign organisms (*Escherichia coli* HU2117). Supplements such as cranberry and D-mannose (with mixed results) have been shown to alter bacterial biofilm load in the bladder and may help reduce the risk of UTI.[46,48]

Long-term urologic care of individuals with SCI should include education on adequate hydration (about 2 L/day) and compliance with hygienic bladder management, screening for infections, stones, upper-tract deterioration, and cancer. The incidence of bladder carcinoma in patients with SCI is reported to be between 2% and 10%, with squamous carcinoma, the most common histologic type.[49–51] Long-term indwelling catheter use is strongly associated with a fourfold risk of bladder cancer.[52] Indwelling SPT or urethral catheter for >5–10 years should undergo annual cystoscopy to screen for bladder cancer and stones. Urodynamic studies should be performed in all individuals with neurogenic bladder as soon as stable bladder function has been achieved, or if there has been a change in clinical urologic status (e.g., increased leakage in between catheterization, development of new calculi or hydronephrosis, deterioration in renal function). Annual renal ultrasound is used to assess the size and morphology of the kidneys. Renal ultrasound scanning is a sensitive modality to monitor renal function.[40,46]

Erectile dysfunction in chronic SCI may be related to the prevalence of common risk factors such as hypertension, hyperlipidemia, smoking, and diabetes. Decreased testosterone levels with longer duration of injury may be related to hypothalamic pituitary dysfunction and prolonged sitting and scrotal hyperthermia.[53] Testosterone therapy may be considered in older men after screening for prostate cancer, dyslipidemia, and other potential complications of testosterone treatment.[54]

Aside from annual lab work and imaging to monitor renal function and morphology, one should also evaluate the appropriateness of the individual's existing bladder program. The practitioner should monitor for any changes in the patient's needs and function that may affect his ability to perform (independently or with assistance) the bladder program. For example, the development of arthritis in the hands, spinal deformities, or progressive upper-limb weakness may interfere with the patient's ability to do CIC regularly.

24.2.4 GASTROINTESTINAL SYSTEM

Bowel dysmotility occurs immediately after SCI and can continue throughout the life span. There is prolonged colonic transit time, especially in left colon and rectum in patients with SCI. Depending on the level of injury, individuals may develop an UMN or LMN bowel syndrome. An LMN or areflexic bowel syndrome, common in lower lumbar and sacral SCI and cauda equina syndromes, produces segmental peristalsis, prolonged rectosigmoid transit times, and constipation, with a high risk of frequent incontinence because of a flaccid external sphincter mechanism. UMN (reflexive bowel) dysfunction results in abnormalities involving the entire colon, with markedly delayed colon and rectal transit times. This produces constipation with fecal retention behind a spastic anal sphincter.[15,55–57]

Constipation is common in patients with SCI, regardless of their age. Approximately half of the individuals with SCI report constipation, incomplete evacuation, and intermittent abdominal distention, and approximately one-third of them report gastrointestinal pain and fecal incontinence.[58,59] Constipation is more likely in older or longer duration of injury.[60] At 20 years post SCI, 42% had difficulties in constipation, 27% fecal incontinence, and 35% gastrointestinal (GI) pain.[16,61] Diarrhea alternating with constipation can develop. This is related to fecal impaction, a potentially serious complication, which may be caused by reduction in activity, diet, inadequate fluid intake, inefficient or infrequent bowel routine, stress, and side effects of medication for pain, depression, spasticity, and detrusor hyperreflexia.

A comprehensive history and physical examination of the abdomen (including rectal examination) should be done at the onset of SCI and at least annually thereafter.

Patient history should include premorbid GI function and medical conditions, current bowel program, including patient satisfaction; current GI symptoms (distention, constipation, diarrhea, unplanned evacuation, etc.); medication use; and potential effect on the bowel program. Current function including the ability to learn and direct care, arm and hand function, trunk control, tone, home accessibility, and equipment needs should also be assessed. Regardless of which type of bowel dysfunction, the goals of bowel management are to achieve predictable and effective bowel evacuation and to prevent incontinence, chronic constipation, and complications such as hemorrhoids, fissures, rectal prolapse, proctitis, and fecal impaction. The bowel program should be revised as needed throughout the continuum of care.[62]

Other GI complications include dysphagia (22.5%–30%), gastroesophageal reflux disease (up to 22% prevalence), and the formation of gallstones (17%–31%).[63–65] Diagnosis of acute abdominal emergencies in SCI may be delayed. With the loss of somatic sensation in SCI above T7, classic symptomatology may be absent, mild, or atypical in presentation. Initial laboratory findings may be unremarkable. Mortality from acute abdominal emergencies is approximately 10%–15%. It is thus important for the clinician to have a high index of suspicion and utilize appropriate radiologic investigations to facilitate early and correct diagnosis of acute abdomen.[66–68]

Nonpharmacologic therapy for reflux includes lifestyle modifications, such as decreasing caffeine intake, chocolate, peppermint, alcohol, and smoking cessation, staying upright after meals and avoiding meals immediately before bedtime. Pharmacologic therapy includes use of H2 blockers and proton pump inhibitors. Prophylactic cholecystectomy is not warranted because risk for biliary complications is not of sufficient magnitude.[11,15]

Persons with SCI are considered to be at equal risk with the general population for colorectal cancer. They should be screened according to national guidelines with an annual digital rectal examination and tested for occult blood beginning 50 years of age. Fecal occult blood may not be a reliable screening tool due to the presence of hemorrhoids or other rectal pathology. Screening periodically by sigmoidoscopy (every 5 years) or colonoscopy (every 10 years) is recommended beginning at 50 years of age.[69]

24.2.5 Nervous System

Physiologic changes of an aging nervous system include loss of vibratory sensation, muscle mass, and strength, slower reaction time, decreased fine coordination and agility, decreased deep tendon reflexes, and deteriorating balance. The histologic changes in an aging spinal cord demonstrate loss of myelinated tracts as well as loss of anterior horn cells. Significant changes may not occur until the fifth decade.[70] With the compound effects of aging and damage to the cord following injury, one may expect progressive deterioration in neurologic function beyond that imposed by the original injury.

A study of individuals aging with SCI of more than 20 years duration showed that 12% reported some sensory loss, and more than 20% reported increasing motor deficits over the years. A Canadian study found self-reported prevalence of neurologic deterioration in 11% of 633 patients with traumatic SCI. Further research is needed as it remains uncertain whether age-related loss of myelinated tracts and dropout of anterior horn cells contribute to these reported symptoms.[71,72]

Late neurologic change is not uncommon in SCI. Almost 20% of patients with chronic SCI report late-onset muscle weakness or sensory loss. Peripheral nerve dysfunction due to age-related anterior horn cell dropout, loss of myelinated tracts, median or ulnar nerve entrapment, cervical spinal stenosis, or radiculopathy can lead to progression of weakness.[73]

There is a high incidence of upper-limb neuropathies in individuals with long-term SCI. Up to 63% of people with paraplegia show evidence of these both on electrodiagnostic studies and on symptom surveys. The median nerve at the wrist is most frequently involved. Ulnar nerve entrapments at the elbow and wrist are also common. Treatment involves assessing the biomechanics and ergonomics of mobility and activities of daily living (including transfers), modification of activities, evaluation of current wheelchair and propulsion technique, relative rest with wrist or elbow splinting as appropriate, corticosteroid injection therapy, and surgical release if conservative measures fail.[74]

Neurologic deterioration in patients with chronic SCI is commonly a result of syringomyelia (this term includes progressive cystic posttraumatic myelopathy, progressive noncystic, or myelomalacic myelopathies). It is the progressive enlargement of a cystic cavity originating at the site of injury that extends in either a cephalad or a caudal direction of the spinal cord. Its incidence ranges from <1% to 7%; however, its radiologic and autopsy incidence is higher. Arachnoid membrane scarring, which interferes with spinal fluid flow and spinal cord mobility, seems to be an underlying mechanism. It is more frequently seen in complete injuries, cervical and thoracic injuries, and older age at the onset of SCI. In 5% of patients with chronic SCI, it occurs within the first 10 years of injury.[75]

Syringomyelia should be suspected when one demonstrates late-onset pain, weakness, dissociated sensory loss (especially pain/temperature sensation), loss of reflexes and changes in spasticity, increasing dysreflexia, and the development of a variable positional Horner's syndrome. It is imperative to rule out syringomyelia, which can progress to respiratory centers and brainstem. Diagnosis is based on a combination of history and physical findings and confirmed with MRI. Surgical treatment is warranted in progressive neurologic deterioration, which includes untethering of the arachnoid scar and shunting of cyst cavity fluid.[76,77]

24.2.6 INTEGUMENT

Changes in the aging skin include thinning of the epidermis; flattening of the dermal–epidermal junction; and decreased dermal vascularity, elasticity, and collagen content. These changes predispose the aging skin to injury. There are decreased tolerance to shearing forces and increased risk of epidermal detachment and blister formation. Risk of thermal injury is also increased due to diminished vascularity and sweating.[78,79]

Paralysis, spasticity, and lack of sensory protection in an individual with SCI increase the risk of skin trauma, leading to the development of pressure ulcers. Pressure ulcers are the most common long-term skin problem seen in SCI. Patients with SCI have greater susceptibility to pressure ulcers with aging as the skin loses elasticity, firmness, thickness, moisture, sensitivity, and vascularity. SCI may result in increased collagen metabolism, thus elevating susceptibility to pressure ulcers.[13]

The risk of skin injury increases with the level of injury and time. Those with complete tetraplegia have the highest risk, with 40% prevalence in pressure ulcers at the 20-year follow-up. There is a statistically significant increase in the average number of pressure ulcers from 5 to 20 years of follow-up. The incidence of pressure ulcers increases from 15% at 1 year post injury to nearly 30% at 20 years postinjury.[78,79]

The cornerstone of skin management in SCI is the primary prevention. Education of the patient and care providers should include skin protection, pressure relief, maintenance of skin hygiene, and routine skin checks. Wheelchair seating evaluation and provision of a suitable seating cushion and mattress are beneficial. Once pressure ulcers occur, basic principles of pressure relief, debridement, and asepsis are the foundation of successful conservative management. Wounds can be managed conservatively with appropriate dressings, local debridement, and electric stimulation. Vacuum-assisted wound closure may also be considered in deeper wounds. Larger and deeper wounds may require surgical intervention with myocutaneous flap closure.[80]

Chronic open sores are associated with the development of squamous carcinoma in the sore, including Marjolin's ulcer, with one study recommending biopsy of chronic ulcer more than 10 years duration.[81]

Aside from vigilant surveillance for pressure ulcers, one should check for other common skin complications such as the development of intertrigo and cellulitis. Patients who use condom catheters may develop contact dermatitis, erosions, and macerations. Sun-exposed areas should be evaluated for malignancies such as melanoma, basal cell, and squamous carcinoma.

24.2.7 IMMUNE SYSTEM

Aging in the able-bodied population is associated with a decline in immune system function and an increased risk of infection. However, one must remember that aging of the immune system is influenced by multiple factors. Exposure to pathogens throughout one's lifespan, preexisting comorbidity, depression, deterioration of support systems, pain, and the influence of medications are some factors that can influence immune function as one ages. There appears to be a cyclical association between aging and infection as aging is a major risk factor for infection, and infection may also contribute to the aging process.[82]

Individuals with SCI have impairments in ectodermal and mucosal barrier defenses. The absence of normal autonomic and sensory function to the skin increases the risk for skin breakdown and pressure ulcer formation. There is loss of normal neurologic innervations needed to maintain normal lung, bladder, and gastrointestinal mucosal barriers. For example, unopposed vagal innervation to the airway submucosal glands results in mucous hypersecretion in the lungs. Innate and acquired immunity is also affected in SCI. Acute and chronic SCIs are associated with deficits in global immune function and persistence of a chronic inflammatory state.[83,84] There are studies which suggest that the immune system after SCI is compromised at both the acute and chronic stages of injury compared with able-bodied persons, suggesting reduced reserve capacity for resisting infection.[13]

There is evidence of diminished immune function in people with SCI above T10 neurologic level, which is demonstrated by impaired bacterial phagocytosis.[85] The presence of indwelling urinary catheters and skin ulcers may be associated with an ongoing systemic inflammatory response.[86]

UTIs are known to be more prevalent in the elderly compared with younger persons; the confluence of aging and SCI results in increased risk for UTI. A longitudinal study of people with SCI more than 20 years duration showed a dramatic increase in UTIs among those aged 60 years and over, with a slight increase in frequency of infection between the 10th and 30th postinjury year.[16] This is of significance as UTI is the most common cause of infection in patients with SCI, occurring at a rate of 2.5 times per patient per year.[87] Diagnosis of UTI in this population is challenging. Patients are insensate and often lack specific urinary symptoms usually associated with UTI. Almost all patients with indwelling FCs and about two-thirds of patients who perform intermittent catheterization have bacteriuria. Thus, the clinician should take into consideration not only laboratory findings of UTI but also subtle clinical presentation (increased spasticity, worsening AD, change in voiding habits, increased bladder spasm, fever, and suprapubic or flank discomfort).

The incorporation of aggressive preventative strategies, early identification of disease process and management, is critical in this population. Appropriate immunization protocols (flu and pneumonia vaccines) should be instituted. Exercise and rehabilitation therapies are associated with improved cellular immunity in persons with SCI.[88–90]

24.2.8 MUSCULOSKELETAL SYSTEM

Normal aging of the musculoskeletal system is associated with loss of lean muscle and strength, and deterioration of articular cartilage function. Between the ages of 25 and 50 years, skeletal muscle mass declines at an average of 4% per decade. After the age of 50 years, the rate of muscle mass loss increases to 10% per decade. In aging, there is loss of type II muscle fibers with relative loss of size of the remaining type II fibers. Collagen, a building block of ligaments, tendon, and cartilage, becomes less soluble, more brittle, and easily damaged. Decreased resistive exercise, decreases in hormonal levels (growth hormone, testosterone, and thyroxine), and neuromuscular changes including structural and functional changes in the spinal cord and neuromuscular junction can contribute to loss of muscle mass.[6,91]

The cellular and hormonal changes of aging are amplified in SCI. However, there is a predominantly type I muscle fiber atrophy instead, secondary to the loss of neural influence and mechanical loading.[92] The rate of sarcopenia is 3.2% in SCI versus 1% per decade in able-bodied men. Sarcopenia and adiposity have been linked to cardiovascular deconditioning, insulin resistance, and increased risk for diabetes, which has been reported to be four times more common in men with SCI.[93] Persons with SCI have decreased lean mass and increased fat mass compared to age- and sex-matched controls. A spinal cord-injured person on average is 13% ± 1% fatter per unit body mass index (BMI) than age- and sex-matched controls. This is related to age but not to the level of SCI. With decreased lean body mass, there is decrease in protein storage and daily calorie needs, which makes increasing fat mass and obesity more likely.[91]

24.2.8.1 Shoulder Pain

In patients with SCI, the increased demand for muscles and tendons to do activities that they were not designed for with compromised biomechanics leads to increased risk for injury and cumulative trauma. Upper extremity (UE) pain is reported by more than 50% of SCI patients, with a 33%–67% prevalence rate.[74,94]

Transfer activities, wheelchair propulsion, and pressure relief maneuvers most commonly produce UE discomfort. The shoulder is the most frequently affected, followed by the wrist (Table 24.3). The prevalence and severity of UE pain generally increased with duration of injury and age. The incidence of degenerative shoulder changes after SCI may be higher in persons with advanced age (older than 30 years) who are <10 years post injury, suggesting that degenerative changes may have occurred earlier.[13]

TABLE 24.3

Causes of Upper Extremity Pain in SCI

Shoulder	Acute muscle strain
	Overuse syndromes (rotator cuff disease, subacromial impingement, tendinitis, tears, etc.)
	Acromioclavicular joint deterioration
	Anterior shoulder instability
	Osteolysis of distal clavicle
	Osteonecrosis of humeral head
	Adhesive capsulitis
Elbow	Cubital tunnel syndrome
	Olecranon bursitis
	Medial epicondylitis
	Lateral epicondylitis
Wrist	Carpal tunnel syndrome
	Ulnar nerve entrapment at the wrist
	De Quervain's tenosynovitis
	Scaphoid impaction syndrome
	Carpal instability
Other	Fractures
	Osteoarthritis
	Myofascial pain syndromes
	Cervical radiculopathy
	Referred pain (nociceptive visceral pain, e.g., cholecystitis, acute abdomen, and cardiac)

Source: Capoor, J. and A. B. Stein. 2005. *Physical Medicine and Rehabilitation Clinics of North America* 16 (1): 129–161.

Imaging modalities used in evaluation of UE pain in SCI include x-rays, arthrography, and MRI. X-rays have limited value, whereas arthrography and MRI imaging have better yield with regard to showing impingement and rotator cuff tears. Diagnostic musculoskeletal ultrasound allows for dynamic evaluation of the rotator cuff for impingement and tears; however, it is limited in visualizing the glenoid labrum.

In managing shoulder pain in this population, one should include a periodic review of daily activities and mobility mechanics, review ergonomics, environmental adaptations, assess posture, and current wheelchair, and incorporate range of motion management, activity modification, and an exercise to address the posterior shoulder girdle. Individuals with overuse syndrome often have muscular imbalance at the glenohumeral joint, with anterior musculature developed significantly more than muscles posterior to the shoulder.[74]

24.2.8.2 Osteoporosis and Pathologic Fractures

Osteoporosis is often seen as part of aging, especially in postmenopausal women (though it also occurs in aging men). However, in individuals with SCI, accelerated osteoporosis is a major risk factor for pathologic fractures.

Lower extremity osteoporosis develops rapidly in the first year post injury with a third of the original bone mass being lost by 16 months post injury.[8] In those with a complete SCI, there is a 25% loss at the hip and 37% loss at the knee within 16 months from injury. Those with complete SCI are more likely to sustain post-SCI fractures and lose bone more consistently and to a greater extent than incomplete SCI.[6] Regional bone loss may occur at rates approaching 1% of bone mineral density per week for the first several months after injury. Areas of high bone loss include the distal femur, proximal tibial, and more distal bony sites. The increased rate of bone loss continues beyond the first year of injury for at least the next 3–8 years, however, at a slower rate.[53]

Treatment of osteoporosis in individuals with SCI includes pharmacologic therapies (bisphosphonates, teriparatide), mechanical loading (weight bearing, functional electrical stimulation [FES], application of low-intensity high-frequency vibration), or combined pharmacologic and mechanical therapy.[53] Because calcium deficiency, vitamin D deprivation, and secondary hyperparathyroidism may also contribute to osteoporosis in chronic SCI, supplemental vitamin D and calcium are also recommended.

The incidence of pathologic fractures in chronic SCI is 2%–6%.[78] These may be caused by minor trauma (transfers, fall from wheelchair) or may be undetected due to impaired sensation. Paraplegics have a higher incidence of pathologic fractures as they are typically more mobile and have increased participation in physical activities. Supracondylar femoral fractures are the most common, followed by proximal tibia and tibial shaft fractures, femoral shaft and neck, and humerus. A 50% reduction in bone mineral density (BMD) at the knee appears to be the fracture breakpoint.[95]

Treatment of pathologic fractures in the aged SCI population should follow general orthopedic principles. Surgical management is indicated, even in complete injuries or nonambulatory patients, when conservative methods will not control rotational deformities or correct alignment, impaired vascular supply, impractical splinting options, or shortening/angulation of the limb will result in impaired function or cosmesis.[96]

24.3 FUNCTIONAL AND PSYCHOSOCIAL ASPECTS OF AGING WITH SCI

Aging is often associated with declining function. As one ages, decreased muscle strength, sensory loss, decreased aerobic capacity, slowed reflexes, generalized fatigue, and arthritic changes contribute to loss of independence. Data from the National Center for Health Statistics show that 61.1% of noninstitutionalized adults aged 65 years and older have some degree of activity limitation.[97]

Individuals with SCI experience accelerated functional decline with aging. Older individuals begin to experience functional decline sooner after injury compared to people who are younger at the time of injury.[98]

Compared with the general population, individuals with SCI experience increased disability and dependency at younger ages (early 40s and 50s).[6] It has been reported that the average age that additional functional assistance is first needed for those with tetraplegia or tetraparesis is 49 years and for paraplegics or paraparesis is 54 years.[99] This may be due to lower reserve capacity in the different organ systems, increased physical demands that lead to earlier cumulative wear and tear, and secondary conditions that often complicate health in patients with SCI.[6,100] Fatigue, pain, and new-onset muscle weakness are the most common symptoms that herald functional decline. Nearly 70% of people with SCI will receive some form of assistance and support from family members. Evidence suggests that SCI survivors' need for help increases as they age.[99,101] One thing to consider is that SCI caregivers are also changing and have their own age-related health issues.[15]

Methods to optimize and maintain functional independence should include modifications of activities, evaluation and use of adaptive equipment and technology, and assistance from other individuals if necessary. Access to environment is an important predictor of life satisfaction and quality of life (QOL). Long-term follow-up should include a review of perceived and real environmental barriers. Access to healthcare and supportive services are important to minimize the decline in health and function that is seen in patients with long-term SCI.

Depression is common among individuals with SCI, with an estimated mean prevalence of 22%.[102] It is greater for those who are older and who have been injured longer.[103] Individuals with SCI have a suicide rate which is two to six times greater than able-bodied persons. In a recent study by Cao et al., suicide mortality has decreased in patients with SCI; however, it still remains three times higher than that of the general population.[104] Annual screening for depression is recommended. Prescription of antidepressants (especially tricyclics) should be done with care in patients with SCI because of their anticholinergic effects.[105]

In spite of a rise in medical and functional problems, reported QOL and life satisfaction remain relatively good and stable in patients aging with SCI. Changes in functional ability, considerable psychological distress, and social disadvantage appear to be accommodated over time.[106]

24.4 REHABILITATION

The influence of age on treatment decisions and neurologic and functional recovery in patients with SCI is controversial. SCI sustained at an older age (>60 years) usually occurs secondary to low-energy trauma (e.g., fall from a standing height). They tend to have incomplete cervical lesions, often presenting as a central cord syndrome, which is generally considered to have a favorable prognosis for functional recovery.[107–109] On the other hand, individuals with nontraumatic SCI also tend to be older, with myelopathy from spinal stenosis or tumor compression as leading causes. Tetraplegia was more common in degenerative conditions, while paraplegia was more common in patients with tumor or vascular etiology of SCI.[78,110]

Elderly individuals were found to have higher mortality rates following SCI.[111] They have concurrent comorbidities and preexisting medical conditions (CVD, cerebrovascular disease, pulmonary disease, and dementia), which increase their risk of perioperative events. They are at risk for delays in transfer to specialized treatment centers and delays from acute admission to surgical intervention.[107] They are at increased risk for postoperative and medication-related adverse effects.[112,113] These factors may interfere with the rehabilitation process, preventing them from attaining maximal possible capacity levels.

However, this should not preclude elderly SCI patients from receiving aggressive rehabilitation management. Elderly SCI patients demonstrate better recovery of motor deficit (i.e., improvement in motor scores).[114] A study by Furlan et al. showed that neurologic recovery 1 year after injury as measured by motor and sensory scores in SCI patients aged ≥65 years did not differ from younger SCI patients.[111] Although neurologic recovery is demonstrated, this does not correspond to improvement in functional outcomes.[115,116] Elderly patients with traumatic SCI had less favorable functional recovery as assessed by Spinal Cord Independence Measure (SCIM) scores[114,116] and Functional

Independence Measure (FIM) scores[117] within 1 year after injury. Thus rehabilitation for older SCI patients should incorporate strategies to translate the motor recovery to improvement in function and activities of daily living (ADL).

Older age at the onset of injury and longer duration of living with an SCI are associated with more frequent and severe health conditions. The most common secondary conditions and

TABLE 24.4
Recommendations at Follow-Up

Organ System	Effects of SCI	Recommendations
Respiratory	• Injuries T12 and higher: impaired cough, decreased VC • Injuries T7 and higher: bronchial hyperactivity • Tetraplegics: impaired ventilation • Higher risk of respiratory infections SDB	• Assess lung function (VC) especially in tetraplegia • Annual influenza vaccination • ≥ 65 years old: pneumococcal vaccination (PCV13, PPSV23) • Sleep study if suspect SDB
Cardiovascular	• Decreased HDL and physical activity, insulin resistance, increased % body fat • Injuries T6 and above: autonomic dysfunction: orthostatic hypotension, AD, bradycardia, bradyarrhythmia	• Identify and address modifiable risk factors for CVD: lipid panel, glucose, weight, diet, smoking, alcohol consumption, activity level • Be aware of atypical or absent signs of CVD • Patient and family education regarding signs of AD and orthostatic hypotension and immediate management
Genitourinary	• Loss of bladder control (UMN vs. LMN) • Increased UTIs • Bladder stones • Risk for bladder cancer (indwelling catheters)	• Periodic urologic assessment of upper and lower urinary tract[a] • Caution with anticholinergics in elderly due to possible cognitive deficits
Gastrointestinal	• Loss of bowel control (UMN vs. LMN) • Gallstones • Constipation • Incontinence	• Routine colon cancer screening from 50 to 75 years of age • Fecal occult tests may be false positive • Patients may present with atypical presentation of abdominal pain or absence of GI symptoms
Skin	• Increased risk of pressure ulcers	Education on pressure relief, skin checks
Musculoskeletal	• Overuse injuries • Disuse osteoporosis and increased risk of fractures • Chronic pain (musculoskeletal, neuropathic) • Heterotopic ossification	• Assess motor, sensory, range of motion, current function • Caution with pain medications (polypharmacy, drug–drug interactions, and altered pharmacokinetics in aging)
Neurologic	• Entrapment neuropathies • Syringomyelia • Concomitant cognitive deficits in dual injuries (SCI + TBI)	• Assess biomechanics and ergonomics of mobility and ADLs • Neuropsychology evaluation
Psychosocial	• Risk for depression • Risk for suicide • Risk for social isolation	• Screen for depression • Address coping, adjustment skills

Note: VC, vital capacity; PCV13, 13-valent pneumococcal conjugate vaccine as per CDC recommendations; PPSV23, 23-valent pneumococcal polysaccharide vaccine as per CDC recommendations.

[a] Done annually for first 3 years post SCI until health is established or after major change in urologic management; may include renal ultrasound and renal perfusion scan.

symptoms include pain, problems with bowel and bladder management, muscle spasms, fatigue, heart burn, and osteoporosis.[118] These occur at a higher rate in the elderly SCI and in those with long duration of injury. The older one is at the time of injury, the more rapid his disability increases over time. In contrast, the younger the individual is, the less slowly their disability increases as they age.[119] Individuals aging with an SCI are able to maintain their QOL and participation; however, the development of secondary conditions and a decline in function over time is most likely to occur. In a study by Saunders et al., the prevalence of chronic health conditions is increased with increasing age. High cholesterol, hypertension, and diabetes were the most frequently reported chronic health conditions. Hypertension and cancer were increased in those living longer with SCI.[120]

It is imperative that rehabilitation interventions continue after discharge from acute inpatient rehabilitation. A yearly follow-up is recommended to include evaluation of the different organ systems affected by SCI, screening for secondary health conditions, screening for depression, assessment of function, equipment needs, environmental access, etc. (Table 24.4).

24.5 EXERCISE IN SCI

Exercise and therapy are essential to recovery in older people with SCI as they are in the young. The exercise prescription should be individualized and should encompass exercise mode, intensity, duration, and frequency. In addition to this, one should take into account the altered circulatory and autonomic functions following SCI.

Higher heart rate (HR) responses are usually elicited from upper-limb activities compared with lower-limb exercises. Individuals with SCI can have compromised relationships between exercise intensity (i.e., metabolic demand) and heart rate. Persons with injuries above the sympathetic outflow at T1 may experience a blunted rise of HR during exercise. Maximal heart rate may be reduced to 110–130 beats per minute.[121] Thus, heart rate may not be an accurate index of exercise intensity after SCI. Age-adjusted methods to assess exercise intensity may overestimate the true work intensity in those with SCI. An alternative to use is the Borg Rating of Perceived Exertion (RPE), which is based on patient perception of effort or the "Talk Test" wherein the patient maintains a moderate intensity of exercise at which conversation is comfortable.[122]

Various exercise modes employed for persons with SCI include exercise by neuromuscular electrical stimulation, cycling exercise, bipedal ambulation using FES, arm endurance training, and arm resistance exercise.[122] Locomotor training (LT) and RT are used to stimulate both musculoskeletal and neuromuscular adaptations after SCI. Both interventions can counteract the effect of SCI and aging on skeletal muscle atrophy. In a 10-week study by Gorgey et al., a combined program of LT and RT enhanced walking recovery in elderly persons with chronic incomplete SCI.[123] A preliminary study of underwater treadmill training in incomplete SCI showed improvements in leg strength, balance, and walking performance.[124]

There are certain precautions that should be taken into account when designing an exercise program for individuals with SCI.

AD may occur in patients with injuries at or above T6. Prompt recognition of AD, removal of the offending stimulus, and administration of a fast-acting peripheral vasodilator (such as Nitropaste 2%) are advised to prevent the life-threatening complications of AD such as stroke, seizures, myocardial infarct, and death. A comprehensive clinical practice guideline regarding recognition and management of AD was released by the Consortium of Spinal Cord Medicine.[125]

When electrical stimulation precipitates symptoms of AD, prophylaxis with slow calcium channel blockers, or alpha 1 selective adrenergic antagonist may be needed. Electrical stimulation is contraindicated in patients who develop severe spasticity or spastic response to introduction of electric current. Fractures and joint dislocation may be caused by asynergistic movement of limbs against force imposed by electrical stimulation or exercise devices.

Postexercise hypotension can occur and is associated with loss of vasomotor response after orthostatic repositioning; however, these episodes can decrease with upper-limb training.

To prevent overuse injuries of the arms and shoulders, exercise intensities should be conservative at start of the training. Assessment of the wheelchair and seating system must ensure that the wheelchair provides stability, efficiency, and safety at high repetition rates.

Persons with SCI often lack sudomotor responses below their level of injury and are challenged to maintain thermal stability, especially in those with higher levels of injury. Mean body temperature and heat content increase more rapidly in persons with SCI than in those who are neurologically intact. Pre-exercise hydration, limiting duration, and intensity of activities performed in hot or cold environments, and layering of clothes should be considered.[126]

24.6 CONCLUSION

Elderly individuals, whether they sustained their injury at an old age or are aging with an SCI, will require comprehensive medical and rehabilitative follow-up throughout their life span. Old age does not preclude them from participating and benefitting from rehabilitation interventions. As they age, clinicians should monitor for the long-term sequela of SCI and chronic health conditions as these can exacerbate functional decline and lead to loss of independence and negatively affect QOL. With proper care, older individuals with SCI can lead active, productive, and rewarding lives.

REFERENCES

1. National Spinal Cord Injury Statistical Center. Spinal Cord Injury (SCI) Facts and Figures at a Glance. University of Alabama at Birmingham, accessed March 21, 2015, https://www.nscisc.uab.edu/Public/Facts%202015.pdf.
2. Jain, N. B., G. D. Ayers, E. N. Peterson, M. B. Harris, L. Morse, K. C. O'Connor, and E. Garshick. 2015. Traumatic spinal cord injury in the United States, 1993–2012. *JAMA* 313 (22): 2236–2243.
3. Devivo, M. J. 2012. Epidemiology of traumatic spinal cord injury: Trends and future implications. *Spinal Cord* 50 (5): 365–372.
4. Van den Berg, M. E., J. M. Castellote, I. Mahillo-Fernandez, and J. de Pedro-Cuesta. 2010. Incidence of spinal cord injury worldwide: A systematic review. *Neuroepidemiology* 34 (3): 184–192.
5. Groah, S. L., S. Charlifue, D. Tate, M. P. Jensen, I. R. Molton, M. Forchheimer, J. S. Krause et al. 2012. Spinal cord injury and aging: Challenges and recommendations for future research. *American Journal of Physical Medicine and Rehabilitation/Association of Academic Physiatrists* 91 (1): 80–93.
6. Kemp, B. J., R. H. Adkins, and L. Thompson. 2004. Aging with a spinal cord injury: What recent research shows. *Topics in Spinal Cord Injury Rehabilitation* 10 (2): 175–197.
7. McKinley, W. O., A. B. Jackson, D. D. Cardenas, and M. J. DeVivo. 1999. Long-term medical complications after traumatic spinal cord injury: A regional model systems analysis. *Archives of Physical Medicine and Rehabilitation* 80 (11): 1402–1410.
8. Charlifue, S., A. Jha, and D. Lammertse. 2010. Aging with spinal cord injury. *Physical Medicine and Rehabilitation Clinics of North America* 21 (2): 383–402.
9. Sipski, M. L. and J. S. Richards. 2006. Spinal cord injury rehabilitation. *American Journal of Physical Medicine and Rehabilitation* 85 (4): 310–342.
10. Adkins, R. H. 2004. Research and interpretation perspectives on aging related physical morbidity with spinal cord injury and brief review of systems. *NeuroRehabilitation* 19 (1): 3–13.
11. Capoor, J. and A. B. Stein. 2005. Aging with spinal cord injury. *Physical Medicine and Rehabilitation Clinics of North America* 16 (1): 129–161.
12. Devivo, M. and Y. Chen. 2011. Epidemiology of traumatic spinal cord injury. In: *Spinal Cord Medicine*, edited by S. Kirshblum and D. Campagnolo. 2nd ed. Philadelphia, PA: Lippincott, Williams and Wilkins.
13. Hitzig, S. L., J. J. Eng, W. C. Miller, B. M. Sakakibara, and SCIRE Research Team. 2011. An evidence-based review of aging of the body systems following spinal cord injury. *Spinal Cord* 49 (6): 684–701.
14. Leduc, B. E., J. H. Dagher, P. Mayer, F. Bellemare, and Y. Lepage. 2007. Estimated prevalence of obstructive sleep apnea-hypopnea syndrome after cervical cord injury. *Archives of Physical Medicine and Rehabilitation* 88 (3): 333–337.

15. Jha, A. and S. Charlifue. 2011. Aging in SCI. In: *Spinal Cord Injury Medicine*, edited by S. Kirshblum and D. Campagnolo. 2nd ed. Philadelphia, PA: Lippincott, Williams and Wilkins.

16. Whiteneck, G. G., S. W. Charlifue, H. L. Frankel, M. H. Fraser, B. P. Gardner, K. A. Gerhart, K. R. Krishnan et al. 1992. Mortality, morbidity, and psychosocial outcomes of persons spinal cord injured more than 20 years ago. *Paraplegia* 30 (9): 617–630.

17. Linn, W. S., R. H. Adkins, H. Gong Jr, and R. L. Waters. 2000. Pulmonary function in chronic spinal cord injury: a cross-sectional survey of 222 Southern California adult outpatients. *Archives of Physical Medicine and Rehabilitation* 81 (6): 757–763.

18. Linn, W. S., A. M. Spungen, H. Gong Jr, R. H. Adkins, W. A. Bauman, and R. L. Waters. 2001. Forced vital capacity in two large outpatient populations with chronic spinal cord injury. *Spinal Cord* 39 (5): 263–268.

19. Burns, S. P. 2007. Acute respiratory infections in persons with spinal cord injury. *Physical Medicine and Rehabilitation Clinics of North America* 18 (2): 203–216.

20. Waites, K. B., K. C. Canupp, Y. Y. Chen, M. J. DeVivo, and M. H. Nahm. 2008. Revaccination of adults with spinal cord injury using the 23-valent pneumococcal polysaccharide vaccine. *The Journal of Spinal Cord Medicine* 31 (1): 53–59.

21. Furlan, J. C. and M. G. Fehlings. 2008. Cardiovascular complications after acute spinal cord injury: Pathophysiology, diagnosis, and management. *Neurosurgical Focus* 25 (5): E13.

22. Bauman, W. and A. Spungen. 2001. Carbohydrate and lipid metabolism in chronic spinal cord injury. *Journal of Spinal Cord Medicine* 24 (4): 266–277.

23. Groah, S. L., D. Weitzenkamp, D. Sett, B. Soni, and G. Savic. 2001. The relationship between neurological level of injury and symptomatic cardiovascular disease risk in the aging spinal injured. *Spinal Cord* 39 (6): 310–317.

24. Myers, J., M. Lee, and J. Kiratli. 2007. Cardiovascular disease in spinal cord injury: An overview of prevalence, risk, evaluation, and management. *American Journal of Physical Medicine and Rehabilitation/Association of Academic Physiatrists* 86 (2): 142–152.

25. Bauman, W. A. and A. M. Spungen. 2008. Coronary heart disease in individuals with spinal cord injury: Assessment of risk factors. *Spinal Cord* 46 (7): 466–476.

26. Bauman, W. A., A. M. Spungen, R. H. Adkins, and B. J. Kemp. 1999. Metabolic and endocrine changes in persons aging with spinal cord injury. *Assistive Technology: The Official Journal of RESNA* 11 (2): 88–96.

27. Castro, M. J., D. F. Apple Jr, E. A. Hillegass, and G. A. Dudley. 1999. Influence of complete spinal cord injury on skeletal muscle cross-sectional area within the first 6 months of injury. *European Journal of Applied Physiology and Occupational Physiology* 80 (4): 373–378.

28. Bauman, W. A. and A. M. Spungen. 2001. Carbohydrate and lipid metabolism in chronic spinal cord injury. *The Journal of Spinal Cord Medicine* 24 (4): 266–277.

29. Hagiage, M., C. Marti, D. Rigaud, C. Senault, F. Fumeron, M. Apfelbaum, and A. Girard-Globa. 1992. Effect of a moderate alcohol intake on the lipoproteins of normotriglyceridemic obese subjects compared with normoponderal controls. *Metabolism: Clinical and Experimental* 41 (8): 856–861.

30. Andersen, J. L., T. Mohr, F. Biering-Sorensen, H. Galbo, and M. Kjaer. 1996. Myosin heavy chain isoform transformation in single fibres from M. Vastus lateralis in spinal cord injured individuals: Effects of long-term functional electrical stimulation (FES). *Pflugers Archiv: European Journal of Physiology* 431 (4): 513–518.

31. Mohr, T., J. L. Andersen, F. Biering-Sorensen, H. Galbo, J. Bangsbo, A. Wagner, and M. Kjaer. 1997. Long-term adaptation to electrically induced cycle training in severe spinal cord injured individuals. *Spinal Cord* 35 (1): 1–16.

32. Crameri, R. M., P. Cooper, P. J. Sinclair, G. Bryant, and A. Weston. 2004. Effect of load during electrical stimulation training in spinal cord injury. *Muscle and Nerve* 29 (1): 104–111.

33. Pollack, S. F., K. Axen, N. Spielholz, N. Levin, F. Haas, and K. T. Ragnarsson. 1989. Aerobic training effects of electrically induced lower extremity exercises in spinal cord injured people. *Archives of Physical Medicine and Rehabilitation* 70 (3): 214–219.

34. Hooker, S. P., S. F. Figoni, M. M. Rodgers, R. M. Glaser, T. Mathews, A. G. Suryaprasad, and S. C. Gupta. 1992. Physiologic effects of electrical stimulation leg cycle exercise training in spinal cord injured persons. *Archives of Physical Medicine and Rehabilitation* 73 (5): 470–476.

35. Barstow, T. J., A. M. Scremin, D. L. Mutton, C. F. Kunkel, T. G. Cagle, and B. J. Whipp. 1996. Changes in gas exchange kinetics with training in patients with spinal cord injury. *Medicine and Science in Sports and Exercise* 28 (10): 1221–1228.

36. Thijssen, D. H., P. Heesterbeek, D. J. van Kuppevelt, J. Duysens, and M. T. Hopman. 2005. Local vascular adaptations after hybrid training in spinal cord-injured subjects. *Medicine and Science in Sports and Exercise* 37 (7): 1112–1118.

37. Samson, G. and D. D. Cardenas. 2007. Neurogenic bladder in spinal cord injury. *Physical Medicine and Rehabilitation Clinics of North America* 18 (2): 255–274.

38. Consortium for Spinal Cord Medicine. 2006. Bladder management for adults with spinal cord injury: A clinical practice guideline for health-care providers. *The Journal of Spinal Cord Medicine* 29 (5): 527–573.

39. Welk, B., F. Fuller, H. Razvi, and J. Denstedt. 2012. Renal stone disease in spinal-cord injured patients. *Journal of Endourology* 26 (08): 954–959.

40. Linsenmeyer, T. 2007. Update on bladder evaluation recommendations and bladder management guideline in patients with spinal cord injury. *Current Bladder Dysfunction Reports* 2: 134–140.

41. Weld, K. and R. Dmochowski. 2000. Effect of bladder management on urological complications in spinal cord injured patients. *The Journal of Urology* 163 (3): 768–772.

42. Garshick, E., A. Kelley, S. A. Cohen, A. Garrison, C. G. Tun, D. Gagnon, and R. Brown. 2005. A prospective assessment of mortality in chronic spinal cord injury. *Spinal Cord* 43: 408–416.

43. DeJong, G., W. Tian, C. Hsieh, C. Junn, C. Karam, P. Ballard, R. Smout et al. 2013. Rehospitalization in the first year of traumatic spinal cord injury after discharge from medical rehabilitation. *Archives of Physical Medicine and Rehabilitation* 94 (4 Suppl): S87–S89.

44. Cardenas, D., J. Hoffman, S. Kirshblum, and W. Mckinley. 2014. Etiology and incidence of rehospitalization after traumatic spinal cord injury: A multicenter analysis. *Archives of Physical Medicine and Rehabilitation* 85 (11): 1757–1763.

45. Detweiler, K., D. Mayers, and S. Fletcher. 2015. Bacteruria and urinary tract infections in the elderly. *Urologic Clinics of North America* 42: 561–568.

46. Goetz, L. L. and A. P. Klausner. 2014. Strategies for prevention of urinary tract infections in neurogenic bladder dysfunction. *Physical Medicine and Rehabilitation Clinics of North America* 25 (3): 605–618.

47. Chenoweth, C. E., C. V. Gould, and S. Saint. 2014. Diagnosis, management, and prevention of catheter-associated urinary tract infections. *Infectious Disease Clinics of North America* 28 (1): 105–119.

48. Jahromi, M. S., A. Mure, and C. S. Gomez. 2014. UTIs in patients with neurogenic bladder. *Current Urology Reports* 15 (9): 433.

49. Kalisvaart, J. F., H. K. Katsumi, L. D. Ronningen, and R. M. Hovey. 2010. Bladder cancer in spinal cord injury patients. *Spinal Cord* 48 (3): 257–261.

50. Kaufmann, J. M., B. Fam, and S. C. Jacobs. 1977. Bladder cancer and squamous metaplasia in spinal cord injury patients. *Journal of Urology* 118: 967–971.

51. Locke, J. R., D. E. Hill, and Y. Walzer. 1985. Incidence of squamous cell carcinoma in patients with long term catheter drainage. *Journal of Urology* 133: 1034–1035.

52. Groah, S. D. Weitzenkamp, D. Lammertse, G. Whiteneck, D. Lezotte, and R. Hamman. 2002. Excess risk of bladder cancer in spinal cord injury: Evidence for an association between indwelling catheter use and bladder cancer. *Archives of Physical Medicine and Rehabilitation* 83: 346–351.

53. Bauman, W. A., M. F. La Fountaine, and A. M. Spungen. 2014. Age-related prevalence of low testosterone in men with spinal cord injury. *The Journal of Spinal Cord Medicine* 37 (1): 32–39.

54. Gruenewald, D. and A. Matsumoto. 2003. Testosterone supplementation therapy for older men: Potential benefits and risks. *The Journal of the American Geriatrics Society* 51 (1): 101–115.

55. Steins, S. S., S. B. Bergman, and L. L. Goetz. 1997. Neurogenic bowel dysfunction after spinal cord injury: Clinical evaluation and rehabilitative management. *Archives of Physical Medicine and Rehabilitation* 78 (3): S86–S102.

56. Stern, M. 2006. Neurogenic bowel and bladder in the older adult. *Clinics in Geriatric Medicine* 22 (2): 311–330.

57. Lynch, A. C., A. Antony, B. R. Dobbs, and F. A. Frizelle. 2001. Bowel dysfunction following spinal cord injury. *Spinal Cord* 39: 193–203.

58. De Looze, D., M. Van Lare, M. Muynck, R. Beke, and A. Elewaut. 1998. Constipation and other chronic gastrointestinal problems in spinal cord injury patients. *Spinal Cord* 36 (1): 63–66.

59. Harari, D., M. Sarkarati, J. Gurwitz, G. McGlinchey-Berroth, and K. Minaker. 1997. Constipation related symptoms and bowel program concerning individuals with spinal cord injury. *Spinal Cord* 35 (6): 394–401.

60. Faaborg, P. M., P. Christensen, N. Finnerup, S. LAurberg, and K. Krogh. 2008. The pattern of colorectal dysfunction changes with time since spinal cord injury. *Spinal Cord* 46 (3): 234–238.

61. Menter, R. R., J. Bach, D. J. Brown, G. Gutteridge, and J. Watt. 1997. A review of the respiratory management of a patient with high level tetraplegia. *Spinal Cord* 35 (12): 805–808.

62. Consortium for Spinal Cord Medicine. 1998. Neurogenic bowel management in adults with spinal cord injury: Clinical practice guidelines. *The Journal of Spinal Cord Medicine* 21 (3): 248–293.

63. Ebert, E. 2012. Gastrointestinal involvement in spinal cord injury: A clinical perspective. *Journal of Gastrointestinal and Liver Diseases* 21 (1): 75–82.

64. Singh, G. and G. Triadafiliopouls. 2000. Gastroesophageal reflux disease in patients with spinal cord injury. *The Journal of Spinal Cord Medicine* 23 (1): 23–27.

65. Moonka, R., S. A. Stiens, W. J. Resnicj, J. M. McDonald, W. B. Eubank, J. A. Dominitz, and M. G. Stelzner. 1999. The prevalence and natural history of gallstones in spinal cord injured patients. *Journal of the American College of Surgeons* 189 (3): 274–281.

66. Sarifakioglu, B., S. I. Afsar, S. A. Yalauzdag, K. Ustaomer, and S. Ayas. 2014. Acute abdominal emergencies and spinal cord injury, our experiences: A retrospective clinical study. *Spinal Cord* 52 (9): 697–700.

67. Miller, B. J., T. Geraghty, C. Wong, D. Hall, and J. Cohen. 2001. Outcome of the acute abdomen in patients with previous spinal cord injury. *ANZ Journal of Surgery* 71 (7): 407–411.

68. Bar-On, Z. and A. Ohry. 1995. The acute abdomen in spinal cord injury individuals. *Paraplegia* 33 (12) 704–706.

69. U.S. Preventive Services Task Force. 2015. Final Update Summary: Colorectal Cancer: Screening. U.S. Preventive Services Task Force. July 2015. accessed February 28, 2016. http://www.uspreventiveservicestaskforce.org/Page/Document/UpdateSummaryFinal/colorectal-cancer-screening

70. Shaffer, S. W. and A. L. Harrison. 2007. Aging of the somatosensory system: A translational perspective. *Physical Therapy* 87 (2): 193–2007.

71. Hitzig, S. L., M. Tonack, K. A. Campbell, C. F. McGillivray, K. A. Boschen, K. Richards, and B. C. Craven. 2008. Secondary health complications in an aging canadian spinal cord injury sample. *American Journal of Physical Medicine and Rehabilitation/Association of Academic Physiatrists* 87 (7): 545–555.

72. Jha, A., S. Charlifue, and D. Lammertse. 2010. Spinal cord injury and aging. In: *Spinal Cord Medicine Principles and Practice*, edited by V. Lin. 2nd ed. New York: Demos Medical.

73. Bursell, J. P., J. W. Little, and S. A. Stiens. 1999. Electrodiagnosis in spinal cord injured persons with new weakness or sensory loss: Central and peripheral etiologies. *Archives of Physical Medicine and Rehabilitation* 80 (8): 904–909.

74. Consortium for Spinal Cord Medicine. 2005. Preservation of upper limb function following spinal cord injury: A clinical practice guideline for health-care professionals. *The Journal of Spinal Cord Medicine* 28 (5): 434–470.

75. Vannemreddy, S. S. V. P., D. W. Rowed, and N. Bharatwal. 2002. Posttraumatic syringomyelia: Predisposing factors. *British Journal of Neurosurgery* 16 (3): 276–283.

76. Edgar, R. and P. Quail. 1994. Progressive post-traumatic cystic and non-cystic myelopathy. *British Journal of Neurosurgery* 8 (1): 7–22.

77. Falci, S., A. Holtz, E. Akesson, M. Azizi, P. Ertzgaard, C. Hultling, A. Kjaeldgaard et al. 1997. Obliteration of a posttraumatic spinal cord cyst with solid human embryonic spinal cord grafts: First clinical attempt. *Journal of Neurotrauma* 14 (11): 875–884.

78. McKinley, W. O., R. T. Seel, and J. T. Hardmand. 1999. Nontraumatic spinal cord injury: Incidence, epidemiology, and functional outcome. *Archives of Physical Medicine and Rehabilitation* 80 (6): 619–623.

79. Charlifue, S., D. P. Lammertse, and R. H. Adkins. 2004. Aging with spinal cord injury: Changes in selected health indices and life satisfaction. *Archives of Physical Medicine and Rehabilitation* 85 (11): 1848–1853.

80. Consortium for Spinal Cord Medicine. 2014. *Pressure Ulcer Prevention and Treatment Following Injury: A Clinical Practice Guideline for Health-Care Providers*. 2nd ed. Paralyzed Veterans of America.

81. Eltorai, I. M., R. E. Montroy, M. Kobayashi, J. Jakowatz, and P. Guttirerez. 2002. Marjolin's ulcer in patients with spinal cord injury. *Journal of Spinal Cord Medicine* 25 (3): 191–196.

82. Gavazzi, G., Krause, K. 2002. Ageing and infection. *The Lancet Infectious Diseases* 2 (11): 659–666.

83. Frost, F. and L. Pien. 2010. Spinal cord injury and aging. In: *Spinal Cord Medicine Principles and Practice*, edited by V. Lin. 2nd ed. New York: Demos Medical.

84. Allison, D. J. and D. S. Ditor. 2015. Immune dysfunction and chronic inflammation following spinal cord injury. *Spinal Cord* 53 (1): 14–18.

85. Campagnolo, D. I., J. A. Bartlett, R. J. Chatterton, and S. E. Keller. 1999. Adrenal and pituitary hormone patterns after spinal cord injury. *American Journal of Physical Medicine and Rehabilitation* 78 (4): 361–366.

86. Frost, F., M. Roach, I. Kushner and P. Schreiber. 2005. Inflammatory C-reactive protein and cytokine kevkes in asymptomatic people with chronic spinal cord injury. *Archives of Physical Medicine and Rehabilitation* 86: 312–317.

87. Siroky, M. B. 2002. Pathogenesis of bacteriuria and infection in the spinal cord injured patient. *The American Journal of Medicine* 113 (Suppl 1A): 67S–79S.

88. Nash, M. S. 1994. Immune responses to nervous system decentralization and exercise in quadriplegia. *Medicine and Science in Sports and Exercise* 26 (2): 164–171.

89. Kliesch, W. F., J. M. Cruse, R. E. Lewis, G. R. Bishop, B. Bracking, and J. A. Lampton. 1996. Restoration of depressed immune function in spinal cord injury patients receiving rehabilitation therapy. *International Medical Society of Paraplegia* 34: 82–90.

90. Leicht, C. C., V. L. Goosey-Tolfrey, and N. C. Bishop. 2013. Spinal cord injury: Known and possible influences on the immune response to exercise. *Exercise Immunology Review* 19: 144–163.

91. Chiodo, A. 2010. Musculoskeletal aging in spinal cord injury. *Topics in Spinal Cord Injury Rehabilitation* 15 (3): 11–20.

92. Ciciliot, S., A. C. Rossi, K. A. Dyar, B. Blaauw, and S. Schiaffino. 2013. Muscle type and fiber type specificity in muscle wasting. *The International Journal of Biochemistry and Cell Biology* 45 (10): 2191–2199.

93. Bauman, W. and A. Spungen. 2001. Body composition in aging: Adverse changes in able-bodied persons and in those with spinal cord injury. *Topics in Spinal Cord Injury Rehabilitation* 6 (3): 22–36.

94. Jain, N. B., L. H. Higgins, J. N. Katz, and E. D. Garshick. 2010. Association of shoulder pain with the use of mobility devices in persons with chronic spinal cord injury. *PM&R: The Journal of Injury, Function and Rehabilitation* 2 (10): 896–900.

95. Garland, D. R., R. H. Adkins, C. A. Stewart, and R. Ashford. 2005. Fracture threshold and risk for osteoporosis and pathologic fractures in individuals with spinal cord injury. *Topics in Spinal Cord Injury Rehabilitation* 11 (1): 61–69.

96. Scleza, W. M. and T. Dyson-Hudson. Neuromusculoskeletal complications of spinal cord injury. In: *Spinal Cord Injury Medicine*, edited by S. Kirshblum and D. Campagnolo. 2nd ed. Philadelphia, PA: Lippincott, Williams and Wilkins.

97. National Center for Health Statistics. 2015. *Health, United States 2014 with Special Feature on Adults Aged 55–64*. Hyattsville, MD: U.S. Department of Health and Human Services.

98. Charlifue, S., K. Gerhart, and G. Whiteneck. 1998. Conceptualizing and quantifying functional change: An examination of aging with spinal cord injury. *Topics in Geriatric Rehabilitation* 13 (3): 35–48.

99. Gerhart, K. A., E. Bergstrom, S. W. Charlifue, R. R. Menter, and G. G. Whiteneck. 1993. Long-term spinal cord injury: Functional changes over time. *Archives of Physical Medicine and Rehabilitation* 74 (10): 1030–1034.

100. Thompson, L. 1999. Functional changes in persons aging with spinal cord injury. *Assistive Technology: The Official Journal of RESNA* 11 (2): 123–129.

101. Liem, N. R., M. A. McColl, W. King, and K. M. Smith. 2004. Aging with a spinal cord injury: Factors associated with the need for more help with activities of daily living. *Archives of Physical Medicine and Rehabilitation* 85 (10): 1567–1577.

102. Williams, R. and A. Murray. 2015. Prevalence of depression after spinal cord injury: A meta-analysis. *Archives of Physical Medicine and Rehabilitation* 96: 133–140.

103. Krause, J. J., B. Kemp, and J. Coker. 2000. Depression after spinal cord injury: Relation to gender, ethnicity, aging, and socioeconomic factors. *Archives of Physical Medicine and Rehabilitation* 81 (8): 1099–1109.

104. Cao, Y., J. F. Massaro, J. S. Karuse, Y. Chen, and M. J. Devivo. 2014. Suicide mortality after spinal cord injury in the united states: Injury cohorts analysis. *Archives of Physical Medicine and Rehabilitation* 95 (2): 230–235.

105. Consortium for Spinal Cord Medicine. 1998. *Depression Following Spinal Cord Injury: A Clinical Practice Guideline for Primary Care Physicians*. Paralyzed Veterans of America.

106. Savic, G., S. Charlifue, C. Glass, B. Soni, K. Gerhart, and A. Jamous. 2010. British ageing with SCI study: Changes in physical and psychosocial outcomes over time. *Topics in Spinal Cord Injury Rehabilitation* 15 (3): 41–53.

107. Ahn, H., C. S. Bailey, C. S. Rivers, V. K. Noonan, E. C. Tsai, D. R. Fourney, N. Attabib et al. 2015. Effect of older age on treatment decisions and outcomes among patients with traumatic spinal cord injury. *Canadian Medical Association Journal* 187 (12): 873–880.

108. Lenehan, B., J. Street, P. O'Toole, A. Siddiqui, and A. Poynton. 2009. Central cord syndrome in ireland: The effect of age on clinical outcome. *European Spine Journal* 18 (10): 1458–1463.

109. Hagen, E. M., J. A. Aarli, and M. Gronning. 2005. The clinical significance of spinal cord injuries in patients older than 60 years of age. *Acta Neurologica Scandinavica* 112 (1): 42–47.

110. New, P. W., R. K. Reeves, E. Smith, I. Eriks-Hoogland, A. Gupta et al. 2016. International retrospective comparison of inpatient rehabilitation for patients with spinal cord dysfunction: Differences according to etiology. *Archives of Physical Medicine and Rehabilitation* 97 (3): 380–385.

111. Furlan, J. C., M. B. Bracken, and M. G. Fehlings. 2010. Is age a key determinant of mortality and neurological outcome after acute traumatic spinal cord injury? *Neurobiology of Aging* 31: 434–446.

112. Street, J. T., V. K. Noonan, A. Cheung, C. G. Fisher, and M. F. Dvorak. 2015. Incidence of acute care adverse events and long term health-related quality of life in patients with TSCI. *The Spine Journal* 15 (5): 923–932.

113. Krassioukov, A. V., J. C. Fulan, and M. G. Fehlings. 2003. Medical co-morbidities, secondary complications, and mortality in elderly with acute spinal cord injury. *Journal of Neurotrauma* 20 (4): 391–399.

114. Jakob, W., M. Wirz, H. J. van Hedel, V. Dietz, and EM-SCI Study Group. 2009. Difficulty of elderly SCI subjects to translate motor recovery—"Body Function"—into daily living activities. *Journal of Neurotrauma* 26 (11): 2037–2044.

115. Furlan, J. C. and S. L. Hitzig. 2013. The influence of age on functional recovery of adults with spinal cord injury or disease after inpatient rehabilitative care: A pilot study. *Aging Clinical and Experimental Research* 25: 463–471.

116. Wirz, M., Dietz, V., and the EMSCI Network. 2015. Recovery of sensorimotor function and activities of daily living after cervical spinal cord injury: The influence of age. *Journal of Neurotrauma* 32 (3): 194–199.

117. Wilson, J. R., A. M. Davis, A. V. Kulkarni, A. Kiss, R. F. Frankowski, R. G. Grossman, M. G. Fehlings. 2014. Defining age-related differences in outcome after traumatic spinal cord injury: Analysis of a combined, multicenter dataset. *The Spine Journal* 14 (7): 1192–1198.

118. Jensen, M. P., A. R. Truitt, K. G. Schomer, K. M. Yorkston, C. Baylor, and I. R. Molton. 2013. Frequency and age effects of secondary health conditions in individuals with spinal cord injury: A scoping review. *International Spinal Cord Society* 51 (12): 882–892.

119. Rodakowski, J., E. Skidmore, S. J. Anderson, A. Begley, M. P. Jensen, O. D. Buhule, M. L. Boninger. 2014. Additive effect of age on disability for individuals with spinal cord injuries. *Archives of Physical Medicine and Rehabilitation* 95 (6): 1076–1082.

120. Saunders, L. L., A. Clarke, D. G. Tate, M. Forcheimer, and J. S. Krause. 2015. Lifetime prevalence of chronic health conditions among persons with spinal cord injury. *Archives of Physical Medicine and Rehabilitation* 96 (4): 673–679.

121. Bizzarini, E., M. Saccavini, F. Lipanje, P. Magrin, C. Malisan, and A. Zampa. 2005. Exercise prescription in subjects with spinal cord injuries. *Archives of Physical Medicine and Rehabilitation* 86: 1170–1175.

122. Nash, M. S. 2010. Spinal cord medicine principles and practice. In: *Cardiovascular Fitness and Exercise Prescription after Spinal Cord Injury*, edited by V. Lin. 2nd ed. New York: Demos Medical.

123. Gorgey, A. S., H. Poarch, J. Miller, T. Castillo, and D. R. Gater. 2010. Locomotor and resistance training restore walking in an elderly person with a chronic incomplete spinal cord injury. *NeuroRehabilitation* 26 (2): 127–133.

124. Stevens, S. L., J. L. Caputo, D. K. Fuller, and D. W. Morgan. 2015. Effects of underwater treadmill training on leg strength, balance, and walking performance in adults with incomplete spinal cord injury. *The Journal of Spinal Cord Medicine* 38 (1): 91–101.

125. Consortium for Spinal Cord Medicine. 2002. Acute management of autonomic dysreflexia: individuals with spinal cord injury presenting to health-care facilities. *The Journal of Spinal Cord Medicine* 25 (Suppl 1): S67–S88.

126. Jacobs, P. L. and M. S. Nash. 2004. Exercise recommendations for individuals with spinal cord injury. *Sports Medicine (Auckland, N.Z.)* 34 (11): 727–751.

127. McKibben, M. J., P. Seed, S. S. Ross, and K. M. Borawski. 2015. Urinary tract infection and neurogenic bladder. *Urologic Clinics of North America.* 42 (4): 527–536.

128. National Institute on Disability and Rehabilitation Research Consensus Statement. 1992. The prevention and management of urinary tract infections among people with spinal cord injuries. *The Journal of the American Paraplegia Society* 15 (3): 194–204.

25 Parkinson's Disease and Rehabilitation

Rachel A. Biemiller and Irene Hegeman Richard

CONTENTS

25.1 INTRODUCTION

Parkinson's disease (PD) is a progressive, neurodegenerative condition that was once thought to affect only motor function (hence its designation as a "movement disorder") but is now known to have widespread effects in the central and autonomic nervous systems. We now realize that it results not only tremor, slowness, stiffness, and gait disturbance but also cognitive impairment, psychiatric symptoms, and urinary and gastrointestinal dysfunction. Unfortunately, the cause and cure remain elusive. This is worrisome given the increasing numbers of people diagnosed with PD. Over the next few decades, the worldwide baby boomer population will enter its senior years, and the number of PD patients is expected to explode. One estimate states that by 2030 the number of people diagnosed with PD will double to 8.7–9.3 million people [1]. Despite the expected increase in demand, the number of neurologists is woefully low. The United States alone needs 11% more neurologists, and this need is expected to increase to 19% by 2025 [2]. This means that many other physicians and healthcare professionals will be more likely to find themselves caring for patients with PD whose management involves both medical and nonmedical approaches. This chapter is intended to serve as a PD primer for non-neurologists and will discuss the basics about the disease and its management.

25.2 PATHOPHYSIOLOGY AND EPIDEMIOLOGY: BASICS

Though the etiology is still unknown, many signs and symptoms of PD stem from a loss of dopaminergic cells mostly in the substantia nigra pars compacta (SNC). This loss prevents adequate communication with the striatum (caudate and putamen), which is imperative for proper motor control [3]. These changes lead to dysregulation of the nigrostriatal pathway and are responsible for the motor symptoms seen in PD. Besides the fading of the SNC, a hallmark pathological sign is the presence of intracellular inclusions known as Lewy bodies. They are made up of alpha-synuclein and ubiquitin proteins [4]. It remains unclear what role, if any, the Lewy bodies play in the progression of PD. Other affected systems include the noradrenergic, serotonergic, and acetyl-cholinergic [5]. This broad involvement of multiple neural pathways is the reason why PD affects far more than just the motor system. PD is primarily seen in adults over 60 years of age, though it can present earlier. Onset before the age of 40 years is less common and referred to as "early-onset" PD. Studies have shown that starting at the age of 65 years, the prevalence and incidence of PD gradually increase without any discernible decline. For example, the mean prevalence of PD in patients aged 65–69 years is 553.52/100,000 but increases to 2948.93/100,000 at ages above 85 years. It is also more commonly seen in white males, though both genders and all races can be affected [6].

Though the vast majority of PD cases are sporadic, there are several familial genes of which to be aware. The two most common forms are *LRRK2* and *PARK2*. The *LRRK2* gene is autosomal dominant and has variable penetrance. While it is responsible for only 1%–2% of all PD cases, it is much more common among individuals of Ashkenazi Jewish decent. *PARK2* causes about 1% of PD cases and is autosomal recessive. Many other genes have been described but are too rare to calculate their overall contribution to the PD population. They include autosomal dominant, recessive, and x-linked variations [7].

25.3 THE "CLASSIC" MOTOR FEATURES OF PD

As previously stated, the classic PD presentation includes three cardinal features: tremor, rigidity, and bradykinesia. However, patients rarely present with all three and frequently exhibit other symptoms as well. Patients or their families may note a tremor in a hand, a change in handwriting, a decrease in facial expression, or a general slowing down. It is also important to remember that idiopathic PD is generally asymmetric at onset.

Some patients may be diagnosed soon after the onset of motor features, while others may experience a delay in diagnosis (depending on the nature of their symptoms and to whom they initially present). PD is currently diagnosed on clinical grounds based on a history of gradual symptom onset and exam evidence of at least two of the three "cardinal" signs. However, by the time these motor features are present, the majority of the dopaminergic neurons have died. These pathologic changes in the brain have begun years prior to the onset of the hallmark PD symptoms. We now realize that there are "premotor" symptoms that may be risk factors for or, more likely, earlier manifestations of PD. These symptoms will be discussed in more detail later and may include decreased sense of smell (hyposmia), constipation, abnormal sleep activity, and depression. Some of the most disabling symptoms in PD are those which generally appear with advancing disease and do not respond well to dopaminergic therapy. These include postural instability and gait impairment, disorders of speech and swallowing, and cognitive decline [8].

25.3.1 RESTING TREMOR

An asymmetric resting tremor (which goes away with movement of the affected limb) is relatively specific for PD. However, about one-third of patients with PD do not have a tremor. PD tremor may present in the legs as well as the hands and may involve the chin. It should be noted that a subtle tremor may only be observed when the patient is concentrating on a task involving the contralateral limb or may become apparent in the hand only when the patient is ambulating. The tremor at rest is to be distinguished from that which occurs with posture or action [9,10].

25.3.2 RIGIDITY

Rigidity reflects an increase in muscle tone associated with disorders of the basal ganglia and differs from spasticity. Spasticity is generally seen in disorders of the upper motor neuron such as stroke and multiple sclerosis and creates a spastic "catch" like a clasp knife, which is noted only with increasing speed. Rigidity is constant despite the velocity with which the limb is moved. In addition, whereas rigidity is generally accompanied by bradykinesia and perhaps tremor, spasticity tends to be accompanied by hyperreflexia and weakness. Tremor superimposed on rigidity can yield a "cogwheel" sensation when the limb is passively moved by the examiner. Rigidity can range from a very slight resistance to a severe stiffness limiting full range of motion. It can be present in both axial (neck and trunk) and appendicular (extremities) muscle groups and is typically enhanced when the patient is distracted with another task involving the contralateral limb (such as drawing an imaginary circle with the opposite hand). This is particularly important in the beginning of the disease when rigidity may only be noticed when distraction techniques are employed [11].

25.3.3 BRADYKINESIA

Slowness of movement, or bradykinesia, is the last "cardinal" feature of PD. Some patients may attribute their slowing to "old age" and tend to ignore this symptom at first; however, careful questioning can reveal that this gradual process occurs much faster than expected age-related slowing. Patients may find that they are falling behind when walking with their spouses or friends when a year or two ago they could keep pace. Others may notice that it takes them longer to do things such as cook or clean the house. On examination, patients may have decreased facial expression, also known as masked facies or hypomimia. This can range from a decreased blink rate to a complete lack of facial expression. There may be a general paucity of movements with decreased spontaneous gesturing, particularly of the more affected side. One can assess for bradykinesia by having the patient perform finger taps. They should be asked to tap the index finger to the thumb at least 10 times (one side at a time) as fast as they can while keeping the excursion as wide as possible. In patients with PD, this task will be associated with reduced amplitude, speed, and rhythm. Heel tapping (raising the foot about 3 inches off of the floor) can be done to assess the lower extremities in the same way [12,13].

Rigidity and bradykinesia can result in a loss of dexterity. Tasks that require quick and nimble movements such as writing and buttoning can become cumbersome and may be the first thing a patient notices [14]. Patients may also experience shoulder pain and difficulties rolling over in bed [15]. Sometimes, this phenomenon will be reported by the patient as weakness, though examination will reveal full power on formal strength testing.

25.3.4 POSTURAL INSTABILITY AND GAIT IMPAIRMENT

While there may be subtle abnormalities of gait in early PD (such as reduced arm swing of the affected side), significant gait and balance dysfunction are generally seen with more advanced disease. Patients with PD often demonstrate reduced velocity, stride, and step length with increased truncal flexion. They may use extra steps and turn "en bloc," rather than pivoting on one foot. Postural instability is characterized by a tendency to fall backward (retropulsion). Freezing of gait (FOG) is an involuntary cessation of movement that results in the halting of gait and commonly occurs with gait initiation, turning, when approaching a target, and when navigating around obstacles or through narrow spaces [16,17]. In cross-sectional studies, 32%–54% of people with PD suffer from FOG, and the prevalence increases with disease duration and Hoehn and Yahr stage [17–20]. The presence of FOG is associated with lower quality of life [18,20] and is associated with an increased risk of falling [21,22]. Both postural instability and FOG are thought to result from widespread neuronal loss and are generally not responsive to dopaminergic therapies [23].

Early problems with gait and balance may be seen in the postural instability gait disorder ("PIGD") subtype of PD (as opposed to the "tremor predominant" subtype, which tends to have a more benign course) but should also raise suspicion for one of the Parkinson's plus conditions such as multiple system atrophy (MSA) [24].

25.4 DISORDERS OF SPEECH AND SWALLOWING

Dysarthria is a common manifestation of PD that generally worsens with disease progression. Patients with PD are often said to manifest a "hypophonic dysarthria," the characteristics of which include lack of inflection, reduced volume (hypophonia), and imprecise articulation with variations in speed (sometimes referred to as "festination" of speech) [25]. Dyskinesias involving the mouth and tongue can also affect speech, and communication may be further impaired by the lack of facial expression and spontaneous gesturing.

Dysphagia is another symptom that worsens with disease progression. Although the majority of patients have evidence of abnormal swallowing on formal testing, many are unaware of the problem, which can lead to aspiration [26]. Dysphagia in PD is characterized by abnormalities in various phases of swallowing, including abnormal bolus formation, transfer, and esophageal dysmotility [27]. Sialorrhea (drooling) in PD appears to be due to reduced swallowing and forward head posture, rather than increased saliva production [28,29].

25.5 NONMOTOR FEATURES

25.5.1 AUTONOMIC SYMPTOMS

Autonomic symptoms in PD include orthostatic hypotension (OH), urinary urgency, erectile dysfunction, delayed gastric emptying, and constipation. OH can be part of the disease itself and tends to be worsened by many of the dopaminergic medications. A patient is considered to have OH when they demonstrate a 20 or greater point drop in the systolic blood pressure upon standing. Because of the autonomic dysfunction, they generally do not demonstrate the increase in pulse as would someone who is hypovolemic. Patients may be asymptomatic or may complain of lightheadedness upon first arising from a lying or seated to a standing position. In severe cases, OH may cause syncope and is associated with a greater incidence of falls. Attempts can be made to decrease medications that may be worsening the OH. These may include dopaminergic medications (particularly agonists) as well as medications frequently used for urinary difficulties associated with benign prostatic hypertrophy. Conservative measures include elevating the head of the bed, compression stockings, increasing fluid intake, and liberalizing salt in the diet. More severe cases may require addition of a medication to raise blood pressure such as fludrocortisone or midodrine. Unfortunately, these measures may result in supine hypertension, which has its own risks [30].

Constipation, due to involvement of the autonomic nervous system responsible for bowel motility, frequently occurs in PD and may precede motor symptoms. One study followed men between 51 and 75 years of age for 24 years and documented bowel movement frequency and the development of PD in this population. It found that those patients who had less than one bowel movement per day on average were 2.7 times more likely to develop PD than those who had one bowel movement a day. This PD risk decreases with an increase in bowel movement frequency [31].

25.5.2 OLFACTORY DYSFUNCTION

Loss of sense of smell (anosmia) or decreased sense of smell (hyposmia) is associated with pathological involvement of the olfactory bulb and precedes the onset of motor symptoms on average by 4 years prior to PD diagnosis [32]. This symptom has been found equally across both genders and may affect up to 90% of patients with PD at some point in their disease course [33]. However, impaired olfaction is not specific to PD as it is also seen in other neurodegenerative diseases such as Alzheimer's.

25.5.3 REM SLEEP BEHAVIOR DISORDER

Patients with PD have a higher than normal rate of developing RBD (rapid eye movement [REM] Sleep Behavior Disorder) [34]. In RBD, there is a loss of the atonia that prevents movement in the extremities and chin during REM sleep. Movements during vivid and often violent dreams may result in injury to patients or their bed partners [35]. RBD may precede the development of PD symptoms by decades. However, it should be noted that RBD can also precede MSA and dementia with Lewy bodies (DLB) and seems to be related to the synucleopathies in general [36].

25.5.4 DEPRESSION

Depression is common in PD and may precede the development of motor symptoms. Though prevalence estimates vary, approximately half of PD patients experience clinically significant depressive symptoms. Depression in PD is thought to be part of the disease itself, rather than simply a reaction to the diagnosis or disability. Hypotheses regarding the pathophysiology include disruption of mesolimbic circuitry and abnormalities of neurotransmitter function [37]. Depression may be another "premotor" symptom of PD for some patients. One study followed over 23,000 patients and found that those with depression had a 3.24-fold greater risk of developing PD [38].

25.5.5 OTHER PSYCHIATRIC SYMPTOMS

In addition to depression, anxiety and apathy are common in PD and are thought to be related to the underlying disease process. While both anxiety and apathy may be associated with a depressive disorder, they may also occur in its absence [39,40]. Psychiatric symptoms related to the use of antiparkinsonian medications include drug-induced psychosis (visual hallucinations sometimes accompanied by paranoid delusions) and impulse control disorders (such as pathological gambling) [41].

25.5.6 Cognitive Impairment

Cognitive impairment is common in PD. It tends to be mild and circumscribed early on. Patients may note problems with attention, multitasking, and spontaneous recall. There is a great deal of heterogeneity among patients with regard to the timing and degree of cognitive impairment, but frank dementia, particularly in advanced disease, is not uncommon [42]. If, however, significant cognitive impairment occurs within the first year of motor symptom onset, a diagnosis of DLB should be considered (see discussion below). It is also possible that some patients with PD may develop a second cause of dementia, such as Alzheimer's disease. Regardless, one should evaluate for treatable causes of cognitive impairment such as vitamin B12 deficiency, hypothyroidism, anxiety, and depression [43].

25.6 DIFFERENTIAL DIAGNOSIS

25.6.1 Essential Tremor

Essential tremor (ET) is another common cause of tremor. Unlike PD, ET tends to run in families (which is why it has been referred to as benign familial tremor) with an autosomal dominant pattern of inheritance. The main difference between ET and PD is that, in ET, the tremor generally emerges with action (as the target is approached) and tends to be more symmetric. While tremor in the hands is frequent, it may also involve the head and voice. Though uncommon, tremor can be present at rest in particularly severe cases of ET in which there is a marked postural and action tremor [44]. It should be noted that PD patients may have some degree of tremor with posture or action as well.

25.6.2 Medication-Induced Parkinsonism

Medications that block postsynaptic dopamine receptors can cause parkinsonism that may be difficult to distinguish from idiopathic PD by examination alone. These include neuroleptic agents and many of the "atypical" antipsychotics, as well as some antiemetics (metoclopramide and promethazine). Most of these symptoms resolve when the medication has been stopped, so it is important to review medications carefully. It is also important to avoid using any of these medications in patients with PD [45].

25.6.3 Parkinson's Plus Syndromes

There are other neurodegenerative diseases that may have parkinsonian motor dysfunction as a prominent feature and should be considered in the differential diagnoses. As a group, these conditions are often referred to as Parkinson's plus syndromes.

MSA is a neurodegenerative disorder that affects patients of the same age as PD. There are two types of MSA: parkinsonism type (MSA-P) and cerebellar type (MSA-C). Early in the disease process, it may be difficult to tell an MSA variant from PD. Typically, MSA progresses much faster than PD, with early development of autonomic failure [46]. Also, carbidopa–levodopa (C/L), the mainstay treatment of PD, has limited efficacy in MSA [47].

Progressive supranuclear palsy (PSP) is another Parkinson's plus syndrome characterized by postural instability, axial rigidity (involving neck and trunk), eye movement abnormalities (usually starting with impaired down gaze), early cognitive impairment, and difficulty swallowing. Like MSA, PSP does not respond well to C/L and progresses at a much faster rate than PD [48].

DLB is associated with parkinsonian motor features and early cognitive impairment (within a year of onset of motor symptoms) that progresses to dementia over a relatively short time period. DLB is also associated with spontaneous visual hallucinations and waxing and waning levels of cognition and consciousness [49].

Until recently, the diagnosis of PD was purely clinical, requiring two of the three cardinal symptoms to be present to make the diagnosis. The recent use of the DaTscan, a single photon emission computer tomography (SPECT) nuclear medicine study that uses a radioactive ligand for the dopamine transporter, has enhanced the ability to separate PD from some other conditions [50]. The DaTscan will reflect decreased dopamine uptake in the basal ganglia in patients with PD. It may be helpful to distinguish between such diagnoses as ET and PD or mediation-induced parkinsonism and PD but not at separating PD from other neurodegenerative diseases such as Parkinson's plus syndromes. The bulk of the diagnosis therefore remains based on clinical judgment [51].

25.7 TREATMENTS

There is no cure for PD nor is there any intervention that has been proved to slow progression. Treatment is predominately focused on symptom management. Pharmacotherapy for the motor features related to dopaminergic deficiency is the mainstay of PD therapy. Tremor is not always easy to treat as it tends to be variably responsive to medications. In cases of severe, treatment-refractory tremor, deep brain stimulation (DBS) surgery may be considered. Bradykinesia and rigidity tend to have a more consistent response to antiparkinsonian medications. Both pharmacological and nonpharmacological approaches are used to treat the nonmotor features, including depression, anxiety, medication-induced psychosis, dementia, constipation, urinary urgency/frequency, and OH [52]. Treatment of gait and balance disorders as well as that of speech and swallowing dysfunction is largely nonpharmacologic at this time and includes physical therapy, speech therapy, and lifestyle modifications. Surgical intervention is an option, not only for those patients who have treatment-refractory tremor but also for those who had a good response to levodopa but developed motor complications (dyskinesias and wearing off of medication prior to next scheduled dosage) [53].

25.7.1 CARBIDOPA–LEVODOPA

C/L is the primary medication used in PD. Levodopa is taken up into the brain and converted to dopamine by the remaining nigral neurons. The carbidopa prevents dopa decarboxylase from converting levodopa to dopamine while still in the bloodstream. The dosage of C/L is started low and increased gradually as necessary and tolerated. The most common side effects are nausea, dizziness due to OH, psychosis, and, over time, motor fluctuations [54,55].

25.7.2 DOPAMINE AGONISTS

Dopamine agonists (DAs) stimulate the postsynaptic dopamine receptors. The two most commonly used DAs are pramipexole and ropinirole, both of which can be taken multiple times a day or taken once daily in an extended release form [56,57]. Rotigotine is another DA that comes in a 24-hour transdermal patch [58]. These medications can be useful as monotherapy early in PD or in conjunction with C/L later in the disease course. The benefit of the DA is that they are not as likely to be associated with dyskinesias or motor fluctuations. These medications, however, are more likely to cause side effects such as sedation, psychosis, light headedness, edema, and impulse control disorders [59].

Apomorphine is a fast-acting and effective agonist sometimes used as a rescue therapy. However, it is not commonly used because it can be associated with severe nausea requiring pretreatment with an antiemetic, and it is only available as an injection [60].

25.7.3 MAO-B INHIBITORS

Rasagiline and selegiline are inhibitors of monoamine oxidase B (MAO-B), an enzyme that breaks down dopamine in the brain. There is some evidence to suggest that rasagiline may slow disease progression, but questions remain regarding this issue. It is sometimes prescribed early in the disease course "just in case" it has any neuroprotective potential [61,62]. Selegiline has been used for years and is available in a generic form. It has an amphetamine metabolite, which could be helpful for daytime fatigue but may contribute to insomnia. Both medications tend to be relatively well tolerated, though they have theoretical potential for medication and dietary interactions [63]. Also, they may contribute to psychosis, OH, and dyskinesias [64].

25.7.4 AMANTADINE

An antiviral agent is not the one that most people associate with PD, but amantadine is a commonly used antiparkinsonian medication. It has multiple postulated mechanisms of action, including anticholinergic effects. It is the only PD medication currently available that may reduce levodopa-induced dyskinesias [65] in addition to helping the underlying PD motor symptoms. It can be associated with psychosis, cognitive impairment, insomnia, dry mouth, constipation, urinary retention, as well as edema and a relatively benign skin change known as livedo reticularis [66].

25.7.5 CATECHOL-O-METHYL TRANSFERASE INHIBITORS

Catechol-O-methyl transferase (COMT) inhibitors are used in conjunction with levodopa. They decrease the methylation of levodopa and prolong its effects. Entacapone is the most common COMT inhibitor with tolcapone being another alternative rarely used due to potential hepatotoxicity. Entacapone is available as a tablet to be given along with C/L tablets or as a combination pill with carbidopa and levodopa. Side effects of COMT inhibitors are basically those associated with C/L but may also be associated with diarrhea and a benign discoloration of the urine [67,68].

25.7.6 ANTICHOLINERGICS

Decreasing cholinergic tone relative to that of dopamine can improve motor function. Benztropine and trihexyphenidyl are anticholinergic agents that are sometimes used to treat PD motor symptoms. However, they tend to be used more among psychiatrists who prescribe them for antipsychotic-induced extrapyramidal symptoms. They are best limited to use in younger patients as older patients tend to be more sensitive to their side effects [69].

25.7.7 MOTOR COMPLICATIONS OF DOPAMINERGIC THERAPY

When initially treated with levodopa, patients do not notice any fluctuations in their motor response. However, with disease progression and continued dopaminergic therapy, most patients eventually develop motor complications, characterized by dyskinesias, wearing off, and fluctuations in motor state ("on" and "off") [52].

Dyskinesias are involuntary, wiggling movements involving the head, face, trunk, or extremities that, unlike tremor, are not rhythmic. They are most commonly associated with peak plasma levodopa levels and tend to occur when patients are having otherwise optimal effect from their medication (in the "on" state). Except in severe cases, where function is limited, or in people who are very self-conscious, patients themselves tend not to be bothered by the dyskinesias. It is usually those around them who are concerned [70].

"Wearing off" refers to the reemergence of parkinsonian symptoms (e.g., tremor and bradykinesia) prior to the next scheduled dose of levodopa. This is referred to as the "off" state. Dystonia (a sustained increase in tone that results in a fixed posture) can also be a manifestation of wearing off. It often occurs first thing in the morning, generally affects the foot and can be painful [71].

25.7.8 TREATMENT OF DEPRESSION

While tricyclic antidepressants have been shown to be effective for the treatment of depression in PD [37], their side effects are poorly tolerated at the effective dosages. This has limited their clinical use. Therefore, first-line treatment of depression in PD includes either a selective serotonin receptor inhibitor (SSRI) or selective norepinephrine receptor inhibitor (SNRI) antidepressant medication. A placebo-controlled, multicenter, clinical trial found both paroxetine (an SSRI) and venlafaxine extended release (an SNRI) to be more effective than placebo. Both medications were generally well tolerated, and neither worsened parkinsonian motor dysfunction. It should be noted, however, that about one-third of the subjects in each group were nonresponders [72]. If a patient does not respond to or tolerate a medication from one class, it would be reasonable to try one from the other class. Bupropion is an alternative antidepressant medication (neither an SSRI nor an SNRI) that might be considered, but there have been no clinical trials involving its use for the treatment of depression in PD. Pramipexole, a DA used to treat the motor features of PD, has been shown to have some antidepressant effects. However, the magnitude of these effects appears to be relatively small [73].

25.7.9 TREATMENT OF MEDICATION-INDUCED PSYCHOSIS

Psychosis in PD presents another treatment challenge. Frequently seen later in the disease and associated with cognitive impairment, psychosis can be induced by PD medications. In the early stages of the disease, PD medications can be decreased in an effort to improve hallucinations; however, there is a risk of worsening the motor symptoms. Unfortunately, many antipsychotic medications (even those considered "atypical") may worsen PD motor function. Clozapine has been shown to be effective for the treatment of psychosis in PD [74]. However, its potential to cause agranulocytosis makes its use difficult due to required long-term blood draws. Quetiapine has not been shown to definitively treat psychosis in PD, but due to its lower risk of extrapyramidal side effects and scant need for monitoring, it has been the primary medication used for psychosis in clinical practice. A recent study demonstrates the efficacy of pimavanserin, making it a promising treatment for the future [75,76].

25.7.10 DEEP BRAIN STIMULATION

DBS is a surgical procedure used for symptomatic treatment of dopa-responsive symptoms in PD. DBS is indicated for patients who have had a good response to levodopa but who have developed motor complications. It can also be used for treatment-refractory tremor [77]. The procedure involves placing electrodes into the brain with the target being either the subthalamic nucleus or globus pallidus. The surgery does not slow down the progression of PD, but it does provide continuous treatment, which minimizes dyskinesias and frequent motor fluctuations [78]. Though there is a risk of intracerebral hemorrhage (3.9%), infection (1.9%), and transient confusion (15.6%), the overall risk of permanent neurological damage from the surgery is roughly 2.8%. The presence of cognitive impairment and postural instability are relative contraindications for the procedure [79].

25.7.11 TREATMENT OF GAIT AND BALANCE IMPAIRMENT

The treatment of gait and balance impairment in PD has proved difficult. Very few aspects are responsive to dopaminergic medications, and patients are generally referred to physical therapy for evaluation and treatment, which should be individually tailored to the needs and abilities of the patient [80,81]. While there is some evidence to support the notion that, in general, PT may provide modest benefit for gait and balance, there is limited evidence upon which to base recommendations for the specific therapy or the optimal duration [82–84]. Research in this area has proved challenging given the significant interindividual symptom variability and differing rates of symptom progression over time [85]. More recently, PT strategies specific to PD have been developed. Lee Silverman Voice Treatment Big (LSVT BIG) is characterized by intensive exercising of high-amplitude movements to overcome bradykinesia in patients with PD [86]. There are also specific gait training approaches that incorporate cuing techniques to improve posture, to maintain stride, and to help "break" an episode of freezing [80,87–89]. There is also some evidence indicating that the initial benefit of therapy may be lost over time [90,91], suggesting the need for continuous or repeated courses of therapy.

25.7.12 TREATMENT OF SPEECH AND SWALLOWING DYSFUNCTION

For speech and swallowing difficulties, nonpharmacologic approaches have been the most beneficial. Speech therapy and, in particular, the Lee Silverman Voice Training Program (LSVT) have been proved to increase not only volume but also clarity of speech. Once the treatment has been completed, the patient must continue the exercises to maintain the effects [92,93].

Attempts to adjust medications generally have limited impact on swallowing dysfunction, despite some evidence to suggest that levodopa increases swallowing speed [94]. Speech and language pathologists can provide careful assessments and diagnosis of swallowing problems. Therapy may include education regarding swallowing techniques, exercises that can improve dysphagia, and suggestions for dietary alternatives food consistency [91,95,96]. Some patients may ultimately require placement of a feeding tube.

25.7.13 EXERCISE

There have been several animal studies suggesting that intense exercise may protect nigral neurons from the effects of toxins such as 6-OH dopa [97]. There are also a number of studies suggesting that specific forms of exercise, including Tai Chi [98], treadmill walking [99], resistance training [100], and bicycling [101], may improve function. The main limitations in these studies are their small size and short follow-up. Longer-term and larger controlled trials are still needed.

25.8 CONCLUSION

PD is and will continue to be a worldwide problem. As the population continues to age, the number of PD patients will rise, and there will be an increasing demand for neurological care. Unless the number of neurologists increases to match the demand, other providers will need to be able to recognize the common symptoms of PD and have the skills to treat them appropriately. Hopefully, this review will help future clinicians care for PD patients.

REFERENCES

1. Dorsey ER, Constantinescu R, Thompson JP, Biglan KM, Holloway RG, Kieburtz K, Marshall FJ, Ravina BM, Schifitto G, Siderowf A, Tanner CM. Projected number of people with Parkinson disease in the most populous nations, 2005 through 2030. *Neurology*. 2007; 68 (5): 384–386.
2. Dall TM, Storm, MV, Shakrabarti R, Drogan O, Keran CM, Donofrio PD, Henderson VW, Kaminski HJ, Stevens JC, Vidic TR. Supply and demand analysis of the current and future US neurology workforce. *Neurology*. 2012; 81 (5): 470–478.
3. Kish SJ, Shannak K, Hornykiewicz, O. Uneven pattern of dopaimine loss in the striatum of patients with idiopathic Parkinson's disease. *N Engl J Med*. 1998; 318 (14): 876–880.
4. Lotharius J, Brundin P. Pathogenesis of Parkinson's disease: Dopamine, vesicles and alpha synuclein. *Nat Rev Neurosci*. 2002; 3 (12): 932–942.
5. Aarsland D, Pahlhagen S, Ballard CG, Ehrt U, Svenningsson P. Depression in Parkinson disease-epidemiology, mechanisms and management. *Nat Rev Neurol*. 2011; 8 (1): 35–47.

6. Willis AW, Evanoff BA, Lian M, Criswell SR, Racette BA. Geographic and ethnic variation in Parkinson disease: A population based study of US medicare beneficiaries. *Neuroepidemiology*. 2010; 34 (3): 143–151.

7. Faralow J, Pankratz N, Wojcieszek J, Foroud T. GeneReviews [Internet]. Seattle, WA: University of Washington; c2004. Parkinson Disease Overview: Causes [2014, May 22]; [about 5 screens]. Available from: http://www.ncbi.nlm.nih.gov/books/NBK7269/#A53983.

8. Gelb DJ, Oliver E, Gilman S. Diagnostic criteria for Parkinson disease. *JAMA Neurol*. 1999; 56 (1): 33–39.

9. Deuschl G, Bain P, Brin M. Consensus statement of the Movement Disorder Society on tremor. Ad hoc scientific committee. *Mov Disord*. 1998; 13 (Suppl 3): 2–23.

10. Quinn NP, Schneider SA, Schwingenshuh P, Bhatia KP. Tremor-some controversial aspects. *Mov Disord*. 2011; 26 (1): 18–23.

11. Fung VSC, Burne JA, Morris JGL. Objective quantification of resting and activated parkinsonian rigidity: A comparison of angular impulse and work scores. *Mov Disord*. 2000; 15 (1): 48–55.

12. Hallett M. Bradykinesia: Why do Parkinson's patients have it and what trouble does it cause. *Mov Disord*. 2011; 26 (9): 1579–1581.

13. Bologna M, Fabbrini G, Marsili L, Defazio G, Thompson PD, Beraredlli A. Facial bradykinesias. *J Neurol Neurosurg Psychiatry*. 2013; 84 (6): 681–685.

14. Proud EL, Morris ME. Skilled hand dexterity in Parkinson's disease: Effects of adding a concurrent task. *Arch Phys Med Rehabil*. 2010; 91 (5): 794–799.

15. Madden MB, Hall DA. Shoulder pain in Parkinson's disease: A case-control study. *Mov Disord*. 2010; 25 (8): 1105–1106.

16. Giladi N, McDermott MP, Fahn S, Przedborski S, Jankovic J, Stern M, Tanner C, Parkinson Study Group. Freezing of gait in PD: Prospective assessment in the DATATOP cohort. *Neurology*. 2001; 56: 1712–1721.

17. Giladi N, McMahon D, Przedborski S, Flaster E, Guillory S, Kostic V, Fahn S. Motor blocks in Parkinson's disease. *Neurology*. 1992; 42: 333–339.

18. Perez-Lloret S, Negre-Pages L, Damier P, Delval A, Derkinderen P, Destée A, Meissner WG, Schelosky L, Tison F, Rascol O. Prevalence, determinants, and effect on quality of life of freezing of gait in Parkinson disease. *JAMA Neurol*. 2014; 71: 884–890.

19. Ou R, Guo X, Song W, Cao B, Yang J, Wei Q, Shao N, Shang H. Freezing of gait in Chinese patients with Parkinson disease. *J Neurol Sci*. 2014; 345: 56–60.

20. Amboni M, Stocchi F, Abbruzzese G, Morgante L, Onofrj M, Ruggieri S, Tinazzi M et al. Prevalence and associated features of self-reported freezing of gait in Parkinson disease: The DEEP FOG study. *Parkinsonism Relat Disord*. 2015; 21: 644–649.

21. Paul SS, Allen NE, Sherrington C, Heller G, Fung VS, Close JC, Lord SR, Canning CG. Risk factors for frequent falls in people with Parkinson's disease. *J Parkinsons Dis*. 2014; 4: 699–703.

22. Almedia LR, Sherrington C, Allen NE, Paul SS, Valenca GT, Oliveira-Filho J, Canning CG. Disability is an independent predictor of falls and recurrent falls in people with Parkinson's disease without a history of falls: A one-year prospective study. *J Parkinsons Dis*. 2015; 5: 855–864.

23. Schoneburg B, Mancini M, Horak F, Nutt JG. Framework for understanding balance dysfunction in Parkinson's disease. *Mov Disord*. 2013; 28 (11): 1474–1482.

24. Thenganatt MA, Jankovic J. Parkinson disease subtypes. *JAMA Neurol*. 2014; 71 (4): 499–504.

25. Stewart C, Winfield L, Hunt A, Bressman SB, Fahn S, Blitzer A, Brin MF. Speech dysfunction in early Parkinson's disease. *Mov Disord*. 1995; 10 (5): 562–565.

26. Robbins JA, Logermann JA, Kirshner HS. Swallowing and speech production in Parkinson's disease. *Ann Neurol*. 1986; 19 (3): 283–287.

27. Bushmann M, Dobmeyer SM, Leeker L, Perlmutter JS. Swallowing abnormalities and their response to treatment in Parkinson's disease. *Neurology*. 1989; 39 (10): 1309–1314.

28. Johnston BT, Li Q, Castell JA, Castell DO. Swallowing and esophageal function in Parkinson's disease. *Am J Gastroenterol*. 1995; 90 (10): 1741–1746.

29. Begheri H, Damase-Michel C, Lapeyre-Mestre M, Cismondo S, O'Connell D, Senard JM, Rascol O, Montastruc JL. A study of salivary secretion in Parkinson's disease. *Clin Neuropharmacol*. 1999; 22 (4): 213–215.

30. Sharabi Y, Goldstein DS. Mechanisms of orthostatic hypotension and supine hypertension in Parkinson disease. *J Neurol Sci*. 2011; 310 (1–2): 123–128.

31. Abbot RD, Petrovitch H, White LR, Masaki KH, Tanner CM, Curb JD, Grandinetti A, Blanchette PL, Popper JS, Ross GW. Frequency of bowel movements and the future risk of Parkinson's disease. *Neurology*. 2001; 15 (3): 456–462.

32. Ross GW, Petrovitch H, Abbott RD, Tanner CM, Popper J, Masaki K, Launer L, White LR. Association of olfactory dysfunction with risk for future Parkinson's disease. *Ann Neurol.* 2008; 63 (2): 167–173.

33. Doty RL, Deems DA, Stellar S. Olfactory dysfunction in parkinsonism: A general deficit unrelated to neurologic signs, disease stage or disease duration. *Neurology.* 1988; 38 (8): 1237–1244.

34. Schenck CS, Bundlie SR, Ettinger MG, Mahowald MW. Chronic behavioral disorders of human REM sleep: A new category of parasomnia. *Sleep.* 1986; 9 (2): 293–308.

35. Comella CL, Nardine TM, Diederich NJ, Stebbins GT. Sleep-related violence, injury and REM sleep behavior disorder in Parkinson's disease. *Neurology.* 1998; 51 (2): 526–529.

36. Claassen DO, Josephs KA, Ahlskog JE, Silber MH, Tippmann-Peikert M, Voeve BF. REM sleep behavior disorder preceding other aspects of synucleopathies by up to half a century. *Neurology.* 2010; 75 (6): 494–499.

37. Rocha F, Murad M, Sumpf B, Hara C, Cintia F. Antidepressants for depression in Parkinson's disease: Systematic review and metaanalysis. *J Psychopharmacol.* 2013; 27 (5): 417–423.

38. Shen CC, Tsai SJ, Perng CL, Kuo BIT, Yang AC. Risk of Parkinson disease after depression: A nationwide population-based study. *Neurology.* 2013; 81 (17): 1538–1544.

39. Richard IH. Anxiety disorders in Parkinson's disease. *Adv Neurol.* 2005; 96: 42–55.

40. Richard IH. Depression and apathy in Parkinson's disease. *Curr Neurol Neurosci Rep.* 2007; 7 (4): 295–301.

41. Voon V, Fernagut PO, Wickens J, Baunez C, Rodriguez M, Pavon N, Juncos JL, Obeso JA, Bezard E. Chronic dopaminergic stimulation in Parkinson's disease: From dyskinesias to impulse control disorders. *Lancet Neurol.* 2009; 8 (12): 1140–1149.

42. Muslimovic D, Post B, Speelman JD, Schmand B. Cognitive profile of patients with newly diagnosed Parkinson disease. *Neurology.* 2005; 65 (8): 1239–1245.

43. Arlt S. Non-Alzheimer's disease-related memory impairment and dementia. *Dialogues Clin Neurosci.* 2013; 15 (4): 465–473.

44. Louis ED. Essential tremor. *Lancet Neurol.* 2005; 4 (2): 100–110.

45. Bondon-Guitton E, Perez-Lloret S, Bagheri H, Brefel C, Rascol O, Montastruc JL. Drug-induced parkinsonism: A review of 17 years' experience in regional pharmacovigilance center in France. *Mov Disord.* 2011; 26 (12): 2226–2231.

46. Watanabe H, Aaito Y, Terao S, Ando T, Kachi T, Mukai E, Aiba I et al. Progression and prognosis in multiple system atrophy: An analysis of 230 Japanese patients. *Brain.* 2002; 125 (5): 1070–1083.

47. Flabeau O. Multiple system atrophy: Current and future approaches to management. *Ther Adv Neurol Disord.* 2010; 3 (4): 249–263.

48. Oaki Y, Ben-shlomo Y, Lees AJ, Daniel SE, Colosimo C, Wenning G, Quinn N. Accuracy of clinical diagnosis of progressive supranuclear palsy. *Mov Disord.* 2004; 19 (2): 181–189.

49. McKeith I, Mintzer J, Aarsland D, Burn D, Chiu H, Cohen-Mansfield J, Dickson et al. Dementia with Lewy bodies. *Lancet Neurol.* 2004; 3 (1): 19–28.

50. Bjaj N, Hauser RA, Grachev ID. Clinical utility of dopamine transporter single photon emission CT (DaT-SPECT) with (^{123}I) ioflupane in diagnosis of parkinsonian syndromes. *J Neurol Neurosurg Psychiatry.* 2013; 84 (11): 1288–1295.

51. Tolosa E, Borght TV, Moreno E. Accuracy of DaTSCAN (^{123}I-ioflupane) SPECT in diagnosis of patients with clinically uncertain parkinsonism: 2-Year follow up of an open label study. *Mov Disord.* 2007; 22 (16): 2346–2351.

52. Connolly BS, Lang AE. Pharmacological treatment of Parkinson disease: A review. *JAMA.* 2014; 311 (16): 1670–1683.

53. Munhoz RP, Cerasa A, Okun MS. Surgical treatment of dyskinesia in Parkinson's disease. *Front Neurol.* 2014; 5: 65.

54. Koller WC, Hutton JT, Tolosa E, Capilldeo R, Carbidopa/Levodopa Study group. Immediate-release and controlled release carbidopa/levodopa in PD: A 5 year randomized multicenter study. *Neurology.* 1999; 53 (5): 1012–1019.

55. Koller WC, Hubble JP. Levodopa therapy in Parkinson's disease. *Neurology.* 1990; 40 (10 Suppl 3): suppl40–47.

56. Holloway RG, Shoulson I, Fahn S, Kieburtz K, Lang A, Marek K, McDermott M et al. Pramipexole vs levodopa as initial treatment for Parkinson disease: A 4 year randomized controlled trial. *Arch Neurol.* 2004; 61 (7): 1044–1053.

57. Adler CH, Sethi KD, Hauser RA, Davis TL, Hammerstad JP, Bertoni J, Taylor RL, Sanchez-Ramos J, O'brien CF. Ropinirole for treatment of early Parkinson's disease. The Ropinirole study group. *Neurology.* 1997; 49 (2): 393–399.

58. Watts RL, Jankovic J, Waters C, Rajput A, Boroojerdi B, Rao J. Randomized, blind, controlled trial of transdermal rotigotine in early Parkinson disease. *Neurology*. 2007; 68 (4): 272–276.

59. Stowe RL, Ives NJ, Clarke C, Van Hilten J, Ferreira J, Hawker RJ, Shah L, Wheatley K, Gray R. Dopamine agonist therapy in early Parkinson's disease. *Cochrane Database Syst Rev*. 2008; (2): CD006564. doi: 10.1002/14651858.CD006564.pub2.

60. Poewe W, Wenning GK. Apomorphine: An underutilized therapy for Parkinson's disease. *Mov Disord*. 2000; 15 (5): 789–794.

61. Parkinson Study Group. A controlled trial of rasagiline in early Parkinson disease: The TEMPO study. *Arch Neurol*. 2002; 59 (12): 1937–1943.

62. Blandini F. Neuroprotection by rasagiline: A new therapeutic approach to Parkinson's disease? *CNS Drug Rev*. 2005; 11 (2): 183–194.

63. Fabbrini G, Abbruzzese G, Marconi S, Zappia M. Selegiline: A reappraisal of its role in Parkinson disease. *Clin Neuropharmacol*. 2012; 35 (3): 134–140.

64. Ives NJ, Stowe RL, Wheatley K. Monamine oxidase type B inhibitors in early Parkinson's disease: Metal-analysis of 17 randomised trials involving 3523 patients. *BMJ*. 2004; 329 (7466): 593.

65. Verhagen Metman L, Del Dotto P, van den Munckof P, Fang J, Mouradian MM, Chase TN. Amantadine as treatment for dyskinesias and motor fluctuations in Parkinson's disease. *Neurology*. 1998; 50 (5): 1323–1326.

66. Crosby N, Deane KH, Clarke CE. Amantadine in Parkinson's disease. *Cochrane Database Syst Rev*. 2003; (1): CD003468.

67. Nutt JG. Catechol-o-methyltransferase inhibitors for treatment of Parkinson's disease. *Lancet*. 1998; 351 (9111): 1221–1222.

68. Brooks DJ. Safety and tolerability of COMT inhibitors. *Neurology*. 2004; 62 (1 Suppl 1): S39–S46.

69. Katzenschlager R, Sampaio C, Costa J, Lees A. Anticholinergics for symptomatic management of Parkinson's disease. *Cochrane Database Syst Rev*. 2003; (2): CD003735.

70. Manson A, Stirpe P, Schrag A. Levodopa-induced-dyskinesias clinical features, incidence, risk factors, management and impact on quality of life. *J Parkinsons Dis*. 2012; 2 (3): 189–198.

71. Weiner WJ. Motor fluctuations in Parkinson's disease. *Rev Neurol Dis*. 2006; 3 (3): 101–108.

72. Richard IH, McDermott MP, Kurlan R, Lyness JM, Como PG, Pearson N, Factor SA et al. A randomized, double-blind, placebo-controlled trial of antidepressants in Parkinson disease. *Neurology*. 2012; 78 (16): 1229–1236.

73. Seppi K, Weintraub D, Coelho M, Perez-Lloret S, Fox SH, Katzenschlager R, Hametner EM, Poewe W, Rascol O, Goetz CG, Sampaio C. The Movement Disorders Society evidence-based medicine review, update: Treatments for the non-motor symptoms of Parkinson disease. *Mov Disord*. 2011; 26 (S3): S43–S80.

74. Parkinson's Study Group. Low-dose clozapine for the treatment of drug induced psychosis in Parkinson's disease. *N Eng J Med*. 1999; 340 (10): 757–763.

75. Aarsland D, Taylor JP, Weintraub D. Psychiatric issues in cognitive impairment. *Mov Disord*. 2014; 29 (5): 651–662.

76. Hack N, Fayad SM, Monari EH, Akbar U, Hardwick A, Rodriguez RL, Malaty IA et al. An eight-year clinic experience with clozapine use in a Parkinson's disease clinic setting. *PLoS One*. 2014; 9 (3): e91545. doi: 10.1371/journal.pone.0091545.

77. Weaver FM, Follet K, Stern M, Hur K, Harris C, Marks WJ, Rothlind J et al. Bilateral deep brain stimulation vs best medical therapy for patients with advanced Parkinson disease: A randomized controlled trial. *JAMA*. 2009; 301 (1): 63–73.

78. Rodriguez-Orzo MC, Obeso JA, Lang AE, Houeto JL, Pollak P, Rehncrona S, Kulisevsky J et al. Bilateral deep brain stimulation in Parkinson's disease: A multicenter study with 4 years follow-up. *BMJ*. 2005; 128 (10): 2240–2249.

79. Kleiner-Fisman G, Herzog J, Fiman DN, Tamma F, Lyons KE, Hawa R, Lang AE, Deuschl G. Subthalamic nucleus deep brain stimulation: Summary and meta-analysis of outcomes. *Mov Disord*. 2006; 21 (Suppl 14): S290– S304.

80. Rubinstein TC, Giladi N, Hausdorff JM. The power of cueing to circumvent dopamine deficits review of physical therapy treatment of gait disturbances in Parkinson's disease. *Mov Disord*. 2002; 17 (6): 1148–1160.

81. Abbruzzese G, Marchese R, Avanzino L, Pelosin E. Rehabilitation for Parkinson's disease: Current outlook and future challenges. *Park Relat Disord*. 2016; 22: s60–s64.

82. Tomlinson CL, Patel S, Meek C, Herd CP, Clarke CE, Stowe R, Shah L, Sackley C, Deane KHO, Wheatley K, Ives N. Physiotherapy intervention in Parkinson's disease: Systematic review and meta-analysis. *BMJ*. 2012; 345: e5004. doi: 10.1136/bmj.e5004.

83. Clarke CE, Patel S, Ives N, Rick, CE, Dowling F, Woolley R, Wheatley K et al. Physiotherapy and occupational therapy vs no therapy in mild to moderate Parkinson disease: A randomized clinical trial. *JAMA Neurol.* 2016; 73 (3): 291–299. doi 10:10.1001/jamaneurol.2015.4452.

84. Tomlinson CL, Patel S, Meek C, Heard CP, Clarke CE, Stowe R, Shah L, Sackley CM, Deane KHO, Wheatley K, Ives N. Physiotherapy versus placebo or no intervention in Parkinson's disease (review). *Cochrane Library.* 2013; (9): CD002817. doi: 10.1002/14651858.CD002817.pub4.

85. Ellis TD, Cavanaugh JT, Earhart GM, Ford MP, Foreman KB, Thackeray A, Thiese MS, Dibble LE. Identifying clinical measures that most accurately reflect the progression of disability in Parkinson disease. *Park Relat Disor.* 2016; 25: 65–71. http://dx.doi.org/10.1016/j.parkreldis.2016.02.006

86. Janssens J Malfroid K, Nyffeler T, Bohlhalter S, Vanbellingen T. Application of LSVT BIG intervention to address gait, balance, bed mobility, and dexterity in people with Parkinson disease: A case series. *Phys Ther.* 2014; 94 (7): 1014–1023. doi: 10.2522/.

87. Nieuwboer A, Kwakkel G, Rochester L, Jones D, van Wegen E, Willems AM, Chavret F, Hetherington V, Baker K, Lim I. Cueing training in the home improves gait-related mobility in Parkinson's disease: The RESCUE trial. *J Neurol Neurosurg Psychiatry.* 2007; 78: 134–140.

88. Fietzek UM, Schroeteler FE, Ziegler K, Zwosta J, Ceballos-Baumann AO. Randomized cross-over trial to investigate the efficacy of a two-week physiotherapy programme with repetitive exercises of cueing to reduce the severity of freezing of gait in patients with Parkinson's disease. *Clin Rehabil.* 2014; 28: 902–911.

89. Velik R, Hoffmann U, Zabaleta H, Marti Masso JF, Keller T. The effect of visual cues on the number and duration of freezing episodes in Parkinson's patients. *Conf Proc IEEE Eng Med Biol Soc.* 2012; 2012: 4656–4659.

90. Wade DT, Gage H, Owen C, Trend P, Grossmith C, Kaye J. Multidisciplinary rehabilitation for people with Parkinson's disease: A randomized controlled study. *J Neurol Neurosurg Psychiatry.* 2003; 74 (2): 158–162.

91. Gage H, Storey L. Rehabilitation for Parkinson's disease: A systematic review of available evidence. *Clin Rehabil.* 2004; 18: 463–482.

92. Dumer AL, Oster H, McCabe D, Rabin LA, Spielman JL, Ramig LO, Borod JC. Effects of the Lee Silverman Voice Treatment (LSVT LOUD) on hypomimia in Parkinson's disease. *J Int Neuropsychol Soc.* 2014; 20 (3): 302–312.

93. Cannito MP, Suiter DM, Beverly D, Chorna L, Wolf T, Pfeiffer RM. Sentence intelligibility before and after voice treatment in speakers with idiopathic Parkinson's disease. *J Voice.* 2012; 26 (2): 214–219.

94. Clarke CE, Gullaksen E, Macdonald S, Lowe R. Referral criteria for speech and language therapy assessment of dysphagia caused by idiopathic Parkinson's disease. *Acta Neurol Scand.* 1998; 97: 27–35.

95. Nagaya M, Kachi T, Yamada T. Effect of Swallowing training on swallowing disorders in Parkinson's disease. Scan J Rehabil Med 2000; 32: 11–15.

96. Tjaden K. Speech and swallowing in Parkinson's disease. Top Geriatr Rehabil 2008; 24: 115–126.

97. Zigmond MJ, Smeyne RJ. Exercise: Is it a neuroprotective and if so, how does it work? *Parkinsonism Relat Disord.* 2014; 20 (Suppl 1): S123–S127.

98. Li F, Harmer P, Liu Y, Eckstrom E, Fitzgeral K, Stock R, Chou LS. A randomized controlled trial of patient-reported outcomes with Tai Chi exercise in Parkinson's disease. *Mov Disord.* 2014; 29 (4): 539–545.

99. Mehrholz J, Friis R, Kugler J, Twork S, Storch A, Pohl M. Treadmill training for patients with Parkinson's disease. *Cochrane Database Syst Rev.* 2010; (1): CD007830. doi: 10. 1002/14651858.CD007830.

100. Scandalis TA, Bosak A, Berliner JC, Helman LL, Wells MR. Resistance training and gait function in patients with Parkinson's disease. *Am J Phys Med Rehabil.* 2001; 80 (1): 38–43.

101. Snijders AH, Toni I, Ruzicka E, Bloem BR. Bicycling breaks the ice for freezers of gait. *Mov Disord.* 2011; 26 (3): 367–371.

26 Aging and Intellectual/Developmental Disabilities

Kathleen M. Bishop

CONTENTS

26.1 INTRODUCTION

As a healthcare or service provider, it is likely you will have patients with intellectual/developmental disabilities (IDDs) sometime during your career. It is hoped that this chapter will help when you provide the quality care for all of your patients, including adults with IDD, so that each can return to a high quality of life.

Aging is aging regardless of the preexisting conditions such as IDDs. Each adult will age uniquely within patterns of aging with a set of experiences, unique capacities and challenges, and resources. It is important to understand that as a healthcare or service provider each adult needs to be listened to and understood from their individual baseline of functioning not compared to other adults in the general population.[1-3]

This chapter is intended to outline healthcare challenges and risk factors for older adults with IDDs so that each adult with IDD can be assured of quality of healthcare from the hospital bed to the community for the return to the home. As with any older adult, the more knowledge each provider has about healthy aging, the increased likelihood for that quality of care.[1,4]

26.2 BACKGROUND

Larger percentages of adults with IDD in the United States are living into their 70s and beyond, parallel with the extended longevity of adults in the general population.[2,4,5] It is estimated that there are approximately 650,000 adults 60 years and older with IDD and related conditions; population

519

projections further note that this number will double by 2030.[3,5] The U.S. 2010 census indicates that there are a total of 1.2 million persons (adults and children) with intellectual disabilities (IDs) and another 944,000 with other developmental disabilities such as cerebral palsy or autism. Additionally, there are another 2.4 million of older adults who report in the 2010 census that they have Alzheimer's disease (AD), senility, or dementia.[6]

An example of the rapid growth in the number of older adults with IDD is the number of older adults with Down syndrome (DS), one of the more commonly recognized IDDs, that have doubled since the 1980s.[4] Another estimate frequently used is that for every thousand people in the population, approximately four to five people will fall into the classification of IDD. It is not known how many of these are considered older adults. While it is clear that more reliable estimates are still needed, it is also increasingly likely that regardless of the human service career, especially with healthcare provision, there will likely be contact with individuals with IDD.[3,4,6,7]

It is also estimated that there are at least double the numbers of adults with IDD who have never sought assistance from an agency or a formal diagnosis and therefore are not counted in the estimated numbers. Many of these older adults live at home with their aging caregivers, who are also experiencing age-related changes and progressively need more day-to-day help.[8] As caregivers age, both families and individuals living with IDD are increasingly likely to need assistance from agencies and service providers in the community.[1,3,7,9]

IDD is characterized by significant limitations in both intellectual functioning and adaptive behavior, which covers many everyday social and practical skills. By federal definition, this disability originates before age 18 and is expected to last over the lifetime of the individual. The more commonly occurring types of disabilities include autism, Asperger syndrome, DS, and cerebral palsy. Each category of IDD has its own characteristics, challenges, and risk factors associated with aging. Some of the specific categories will be discussed below.

The term "intellectual disability" is the current terminology used and commonly accepted by advocates and in legislation, replacing the term "mental retardation" that has taken on very negative connotations. In the previous quarter of a century, the term "mental retardation" was used under the classification of developmental disabilities, which covers various disabilities beyond cognitive impairment that affect functioning and ability to live independently. The term "developmental disability" is a much broader term encompassing a variety of classifications and syndromes.[10] For the purposes of this chapter, the term "IDD" will be used so as to be inclusive of a broader group of adults.

There are very clear diagnostic categories defined federally and also by each state for service eligibility. For further information on specific diagnostic categories, please go to the website for the American Association on Intellectual and Developmental Disabilities, a national organization for advocacy and education on IDD. Adults may have been classified as having a developmental disability determining eligibility for services in one state and not be eligible for services in another.[10] For the purposes of this chapter, any one deemed to have a form of IDD regardless of classification in the state he or she currently resides is included in the discussion as it is the risk factors for early mortality, comorbidity, and reduced quality of life that are the considerations here.[2]

For you as a healthcare provider, the diagnosis can help guide you to possible risk factors as well as service eligibility for when the patient is able to be discharged from the hospital or rehabilitation facility. It is essential to remember that each patient or consumer of services needs to be treated as an individual with respect regardless of the level of disability and communication challenges.[1–3]

In the past, adults with IDD lived shorter lives with fewer adults living independently in the community. The numbers of older adults as well as the percentages of adults with IDD living in the community, that is, not under the auspices of a specific agency, have increased.[2,5] This growth in numbers and increase in independent living can be attributed to improved medical knowledge and care, better living conditions, deinstitutionalization, and the same reasons that people in the general population are living longer.[9]

People with IDD are living longer to the point where their life expectancy is nearly comparable to that of the general population. Furthermore, even those with severe/profound IDD who have more complex health issues have a life expectancy rapidly approaching 60.[11,12] The severity of the disability will affect activities of daily living, learning, socialization, and vocation, thus affecting the person's ability to live independently.[10,13,14] However, many adults with IDD live independently in the community or with their families. It is estimated that approximately 5% of adults with IDD live in residential facilities for adults with IDD, with the majority living in the community with both formal and informal supports.[9,15]

The more severe the disability, the more likely there will be an impact on the factors of aging that include physical capability, environment, lifestyle, and attitude, thus increasing the risk for a negative effect on the health and wellness of the older adult as well as on quality of life. The disabilities of DS and cerebral palsy tend to result in an earlier onset of age-related conditions such as arthritis in adults with cerebral palsy.[12]

Initial evidence indicates that older individuals with IDD have similar or even higher rates of age-related conditions than older persons without lifelong disabilities, making diagnosis of underlying conditions more challenging.[2,3] However, adults with IDD are at risk for the same age-related diseases such as cardiovascular disease, stroke, sleep disorders, thyroid disease, and vitamin B12 deficiency. The same process of differential diagnosis should be conducted as would be done for any older person who exhibits symptoms of disease or decline.[16] The major difference in treatment is that referring to the baseline functioning is even more essential than in the general population as well as the need to confer with formal or informal caregivers for information on that baseline when the baseline and historical information are available.[1-3]

From a life-course perspective, as theorized by a number of gerontologists, adults with IDD are likely to be more challenged with an accumulation of life experiences that have reduced the opportunities for relationships and interactions within the community as well as employment, access to informed healthcare, and asset attainment.[1,2,4,7] All of these are factors in the general population that can predict healthy aging and risk factors.[17] It has been well documented that having a family member with IDD increases the likelihood of poverty and reduced assets for the entire family, thus impacting the family cycle as well.[17]

26.3 HISTORY OF SERVICES AND TRENDS

During the first half of the twentieth century and well into the 1970s, adults with IDD in the United States were treated within facilities for people with IDs or institutions for people with mental illness, often moving from different institutions depending on the availability of institutions and funding for placements.[18]

Prior to this placement in the mid- to late 1700s, almshouses, workhouses, poorhouses, and hospitals were opened to house adults who were unable to live independently in the community due to lack of family or others to provide the needed supports. The United States was an agricultural and far more rural country during this time, giving jobs to people with cognitive or minor physical impairments and allowing people to be able to stay in the communities when there was viable family and friends support.[18]

No formal diagnostic procedures were used; thus, individuals with mental illness and IDD were placed together in the same settings furthering the confusion for appropriate diagnosis and treatment. As part of the Eugenics movement, the legend of the Kallikak family studied by Goddard left the impression with society that there were families with "bad blood" that should be removed from society and forcefully sterilized to prevent further reproduction.[18]

For hundreds of years, the care of individuals with varying underlying causes was provided through institutions. For example, in New York State, the care of individuals with ID and mental illness was within the same state department. Regardless of the diagnosis, rather formal or informal, individuals with either diagnosis or both were transferred back and forth to facilities.[18]

Historically, people with DS were labeled as "mongoloids" because of the facial features. The syndrome was named Down syndrome because of the research of Dr. Down who noticed the similarity in features and personality characteristics. He determined that they looked like people from Mongolia and the terminology Mongoloid stuck. In more recent years, the underlying racism has been noted with a purposeful campaign to change such racist terminology but also to put people first rather than identification by the type of underlying disability.[15,19]

This later isolation and segregation has increased the stigma of cognitive impairment or physical disability with advocates, self-advocates, and family members continuing to this day to reduce the stigma and open up access to community resources, including quality healthcare.[4,15,20]

Healthcare providers today are still dealing with the myths associated with IDD and overlapping of diagnosis along with a general lack of information on aging in adults with IDD.[4] This is in spite of the fact that the deinstitutionalization movement began in the late 1980s with a national trend to close down large institutions providing care for people with IDD. By the twenty-first century, most states had closed or were in the process of closing state-run large facilities and developing community supports to keep more people in their communities with their friends and families. But closure could not occur overnight given that many people had been permanently separated from their families, with some siblings not even knowing of the existence of their siblings with IDD.[2,15]

Family members, self-advocates, and advocates today emphasize the need to use a person-centered approach with each adult with IDD, regardless of the level of functioning and communication capacity. It cannot be stressed enough that this means providing healthcare services in a respectful manner, always including the adult and any advocates present in the process, including decision-making about appropriate healthcare interventions.[1,2,20]

26.4   LIFESTYLE AND LIVING ARRANGEMENTS

The living situation of each adult with IDD who you come in contact with is likely to vary. Understanding the living situation to which the patient will return is essential for successful interventions and follow-up care, especially for discharge planners. As much of this information should be gathered by healthcare professionals as it is pertinent to the healthy healing of adults requiring healthcare services.[2,3,15,20]

The major indicators for older people for emotional and economic well-being are marital status and the support social network available to the older adults. Adults with IDD are less likely to be married or have children and have fewer relationships than older adults in the general population.[1,4,9,15] If each adult lived at home with his or her parents, as each ages, there is increasing likelihood of difficulties remaining independent unless a sibling or other adult has replaced the parents in providing supports. After the death of the primary caregiver, it is more likely remaining family will be seeking assistance from disability service agencies. Sometimes, a health crisis will cause the family to seek this sooner.[1,3,15]

26.5   SPECIFIC IDDS

26.5.1   Down Syndrome

DS is the most easily recognized IDD and one of the most common around the world. Adults with DS who have full expression of the trisomy 21 in every cell of the body have similar facial characteristics, palm of the hand abnormalities, and personality characteristics. Because of these similarities and the known early aging into risk factors, especially for AD, this is also one of the most researched IDDs. The underlying cause for most individuals with DS is the presence of three complete copies of chromosome 21 secondary to meiotic nondisjunction. DS is the number one genetic cause of cognitive impairment as well as the most common chromosomal disorder.[2,19,21]

Research has established the underlying genetic link between trisomy 21 and AD. It has been observed and researched that by the age of 40 years, all adults with DS exhibit some measure of neuropathological defects when an autopsy is performed postmortem that are indicative of Alzheimer's type disease.[2,21]

The clinical symptoms during the lifetime, however, are variable with approximately 40%–50% by some estimates of adults with DS not exhibiting the clinical signs.[2,3,20] Others estimate that by the age of 30, individuals with DS usually develop amyloid plaques and neurofibrillary tangles, which develop into the clinical symptoms for about 70% of people with DS by the chronological age of 70.[19]

Many healthcare providers have read initial research conducted in the 1970s and 1980s on DS and AD that concluded 100% of people with DS, if they lived long enough, would develop the symptoms of AD. More recent research concludes that about 30% will not demonstrate the symptoms of AD but healthcare providers are often unfamiliar with the more recent research.[3,20] Thus, adults with DS are often diagnosed with AD much earlier in the process of diagnosis than the general population without ruling out other underlying causes for the cognitive and functioning decline or behavioral changes.[1] This topic will be discussed further in this chapter under Health Disparities and Challenges (see Section 26.6).

26.5.2 Cerebral Palsy

Cerebral palsy is a disorder of movement, muscle tone, range of motion limitations, and/or posture that is caused by damage to the brain during fetal development or shortly after birth.[22,23] The impairment to movement can include abnormal posture, involuntary movements, and spasticity in any of the limbs preventing control of the limbs and movement for mobility. Swallowing disorders and communication challenges are very common as these are functions related to movement. Secondary conditions can include epilepsy, blindness, or deafness. There is great variation in the effect of the brain damage on each individual,[22,23] making it even more essential to observe and interact with each adult and advocate to learn about the individual.[1,4]

Adults with cerebral palsy will present to the healthcare provider with symptoms that can be found in the general population but with likely higher risk factors for specific conditions and diseases. Not all adults with cerebral palsy have cognitive impairment with many adults functioning at an average or above-average intellectual level. As cerebral palsy is a motor disorder, verbal communication is often affected, resulting in possible difficulties understanding the adult with cerebral palsy.[4,22,23]

Some of the well-documented secondary conditions for adults with cerebral palsy include higher risk for respiratory and swallowing disorders, muscle–skeletal issues, pain, and early onset of loss of bone density with an increased likelihood for fractures and urinary tract infections.[2,4,23] A few of the secondary conditions will be discussed below.

Adults with cerebral palsy have been challenged over the life span by ambulation difficulties, resulting in immobility or poor postural positions creating stress on various body organs. The immobility will likely increase the risk for early onset of pain from arthritis and lowered bone density as compared to other adults of the same gender and chronological age. This can cause significant pain that may also be related to undetected bone fractures.[2,4] Respiratory problems, including bronchitis and more frequent pneumonias, as the adult grows older will also result due to the lifetime accumulation of the immobility.[4,24]

The prescribing of medications to control pain or seizures, another secondary condition of cerebral palsy, can also block the absorption of needed vitamins and minerals that support healthy bone growth. This in combination with a sedentary life style, the lack of weight-bearing exercise, and the lack of exposure to vitamin D through natural sunlight all can combine to increase the risk factor for pain, constipation, skin breakdown, and frequent bone fractures.[2,4]

The subsequent discomfort and difficulty communicating the reason for the discomfort can be exhibited as unpleasant behavior requiring behavioral plans or behavioral intervention. The symptoms and cause for the symptoms are then overlooked as a problem of underlying physical problems or disease process.[4,20,24] All of these symptoms should be attended to, and you should never assume that these are behaviors typical of people with cerebral palsy or IDD (known as diagnostic overshadowing or blaming a preexisting condition for the current symptoms). The symptoms should be noted and included for ruling out the cause for decline while treating when appropriate.[2,4,7,20]

The above accumulation of life-course challenges also increases the risk for swallowing disorders as well as gastrointestinal (GI) problems, including dysphagia, reflux, anemia, eating disorders, and aspiration.[2,4] The GI problems can also cause oral health problems, including dental erosion of existing teeth. Bowel and bladder function can be reduced causing increased infections, urinary retention, and constipation. As with any adult with IDD, a differential diagnosis should be conducted on the adult to determine possible causes for the symptoms and decline observed.[2,20]

26.5.3 DUAL OR MULTIPLE DIAGNOSIS

Adults with IDD may have multiple diagnoses, including mental health disease, or two or more diagnosis of developmental disabilities. All of the preexisting conditions should be considered in terms of the whole patient and for clues in diagnosing current underlying problems for the presenting symptoms. Each preexisting condition also adds a cadre of risk factors that should be taken into account in assessment and intervention decisions.[7,20]

For example an adult with Asperger's syndrome and another common secondary condition such as epilepsy or a mental illness, both risk factors for adults with Asperger's syndrome, would be considered to have a dual diagnosis. Asperger's syndrome is a syndrome on the Autism Spectrum with an average or above average intellectual quotient (IQ) usually challenged with sensory processing. This results in a need for structure and predictability in physical and social environment.[25] A presenting patient with this disorder may be reluctant to be touched, participate in laboratory tests, especially in closed areas, or may not be able to sit still for questioning on symptoms. While this may occur with any adult, the behavior will likely appear more obvious and make the examination more difficult. Baseline information and assistance from caregivers can help make the examination easier with an increased likelihood of positive outcomes.[25]

26.6 HEALTH DISPARITIES AND CHALLENGES

In the general population, an increase in physical and mental limitations is expected by the later part of the Third Age.[1] It is well documented that while adults with IDD are living longer there are healthcare disparities and challenges to receiving quality healthcare due to the preexisting disability. There are also increased risk factors with the onset of age-related conditions and diseases occurring earlier or with more severity in adults with IDD.[2,24]

This makes it essential that differential diagnosis is conducted to rule out and treat all causes for decline or behavioral changes. It is important that an assumption of loss and disability is not an automatic conclusion as this then increases the risk for diagnostic overshadowing.[20,24] Diagnostic overshadowing occurs when the preexisting disability is blamed for the decline or behavioral changes rather than looking for other underlying causes unrelated to the disability or existing diagnosis. The tendency for diagnostic overshadowing, even if the practitioner is not aware of this tendency, cannot be overlooked, making it essential to communicate with the advocates and the adult with disability to determine the baseline functioning and behavior.[1,7]

Adults with IDD are often at a higher risk for health problems as compared to the general population due to obesity, hypertension, epilepsy, poor dental health, and challenges with mental health.[4,7,12,24]

Adults with IDD may also experience multiple or compound assumptions related to the preexisting disability, aging itself, and other factors such as ethnicity, gender, and income status. The resulting disparities can interfere with quality of healthcare, especially when combined with the general lack of research and training on older adults with IDD for healthcare providers. Many advocates recommend that both formal and informal caregivers receive training on healthcare advocacy so that all can work together to promote positive healthcare outcomes.[1]

26.6.1 POLYPHARMACY AND ADVERSE EFFECTS OF MEDICATIONS

Unwanted adverse effects of medications are known to affect the older population in general, and adults with IDD are at an even greater risk due to a lifetime of long-term usage of prescribed medications for the secondary conditions often related to the preexisting disability. Many of the medications used on this adult population are not as commonly prescribed for the general population, causing the practitioner to know less about the possible adverse effects from the particular medications.[2,26,27] Additionally, adults with IDD are at a higher risk for multiple prescribing healthcare practitioners who may not have the full history and knowledge of other medications prescribed, especially by patients who cannot self-report.[2,27]

It is known that specific antipsychotics and pain medications as well as benzodiazepines and antihistamines have caused adverse effects in adults with IDD.[2,27] These side effects can include memory loss, lethargy, confusion, dizziness, and gait impairment that are also symptoms for other underlying diseases, including dementias such as Alzheimer's type dementia.[2,3,20,27]

26.7 HABILITATION VERSUS REHABILITATION FOR ADULTS WITH IDD

The terms "habilitation" and "rehabilitation" in reference to healthcare assessments and interventions as well as support follow-up often have different meanings for adults with IDD. By federal definition related to eligibility for funding of healthcare services through the Affordable Care Act, habilitation are healthcare services that help a person acquire, keep, or improve skills related to communication and activities of daily living.[28] These are skills intended to improve independence and the ability to participate as fully as possible in the community.[15]

Rehabilitation, also by federal definition, implies the healthcare services provided to help a person keep, restore, or improve already-developed skills and functioning capacity for daily living and communication. For an adult with IDD, the baseline may be lower than that expected for an adult in the general population for someone of that chronological age making the lines between habilitation, developing new skills, and rehabilitation, maintaining or restoring new skills very unclear to the healthcare provider. This is particularly true if the healthcare provider is unfamiliar with the adult with IDD and has little baseline information.[15,20,28]

As discussed in other sections of this chapter, it is essential for the provider to gather the information on baseline functioning and what has changed for the patient. Gathering of information will help the provider determine assessments and recommendations for interventions that can be both rehabilitative and habilitative in nature with the ultimate goal to promote healthy living and functioning as possible for each patient with IDD. This will also assist the practitioner with clues of symptoms that can be utilized for the best plan of care during and after initial treatment.[2,20,24]

26.7.1 DEMENTIA AND IDD

Dementia is diagnosed usually from an indication of general decline from the baseline functioning of each individual presenting with the symptoms of functional and cognitive decline.[2,3] For adults with IDD, determining the original baseline functioning can be complicated by numerous caregivers and advocates throughout the adult's lifetime and the lack of documentation regarding the baseline for the current caregivers. This becomes even more complex when the cognitive functioning is so varied among adults with IDs and does not usually compare with that of other patients in the general population.[2,7,20]

Evidence supports that adults with IDD are at least equal risk for AD and related dementias as the general population. For some identified groups of people with IDD, there is a higher risk than in the general population. This includes people with DS and adults with brain injury.[2,3] The number of older adults with IDD affected by dementia is growing and will continue to grow, providing a challenge to caregivers and the healthcare delivery system.[2,3]

For people with IDD, dementia is particularly challenging to assess and diagnose. As there is a lifetime of experiencing poorer health outcomes than the general population, this complexity increases in later years. There are many factors that contribute to this challenge, including lack of training, experience, or evidence-based practices available to the healthcare practitioner. It is important that this disparity, particularly in accurately identifying dementia in this population, is recognized. It is essential that a differential diagnosis be conducted to rule out possible causes for decline from the noted baseline so that an accurate intervention plan can be developed.[1,24]

26.8 RECOMMENDED HEALTHCARE INTERVENTION/PROVISION

The adult may or may not have access to caregivers on a 24 hour basis upon the return home, and this should be considered by the healthcare provider and discharge planners. There is also the possibility of different types of caregivers or advocates accompanying the adult when there is a healthcare emergency, including paid staff from a formal organization providing supports to people with IDD and family members or friends. If there is no accompanying advocate, regardless of the relationship with the adult with IDD, the assessment will be much more difficult if the adult is unable to communicate the symptoms. Symptoms for many diseases in older adults with IDD can indicate many different diseases or conditions as in the general population, challenging the practitioner to make accurate assessment and intervention decisions.[29,30]

To address the challenges with diagnosis and treatment, the National Task Group (NTG) on Dementia Care Practices and IDD, formed in 2011 to address the increasing challenges due to dementia in adults with IDD, developed practice guidelines for practitioner care, which will be discussed below. The practice guidelines were developed specifically for diagnosis of dementia but can be used in most situations as they include the process of gathering a baseline and differential diagnosis that can lead to the diagnoses of other diseases besides dementias.[2,3,20]

The steps recommended by the NTG for an accurate assessment of health and function in adults with IDD include evaluation, diagnosis, treatment, and follow-up. It is also noted that physicians and other healthcare professionals need information on how to implement the detection of cognitive impairment that is a requirement in the Medicare Annual Wellness visit under the Affordable Care Act, which is available online at http://www.medscape.com/viewarticle/776548.[2,3]

The evaluation remains the "cornerstone" for any diagnosis that should include a comprehensive history from caregivers and family members as well as the adult with IDD when possible. It should also include a gathering of medical and psychiatric history for preexisting conditions that may be the underlying cause for current reported symptoms. As in other older adults, the healthcare practitioner is looking for a history of sleep disorders, thyroid disease, head injury, cardiovascular disease, vitamin B12 deficiency, and metabolic disorders such as diabetes.[2,20]

As discussed above, the differential diagnosis should also include a baseline of functioning with the level of cognitive functioning, previous skill acquisition, ability to perform activities of daily living, and communication. All of this should be compared with the current level of functioning as the practitioner is looking for changes in those skills and behaviors. In an adult with IDD, who will likely have a different baseline of functioning than an adult in the general population, it is essential to look for each individual's baseline of functioning.[3,20,30] The practitioner should be looking for changes in fine and gross motor skills, memory loss in comparison to the original level of memory skills, changes in personality and behavior, and disorientation. All of these clues should be compared to the previous level of functioning.[2]

Conditions and diseases commonly observed in older adults with IDD are listed in Table 26.1. Each of these as well as conditions previously diagnosed in the patient as possible causes for the

TABLE 26.1

Conditions Causing Functioning and Cognitive Loss or Behavioral Changes in Older Adults with IDD

Medications	Polypharmacy, interactions with nutrients and minerals, unwanted adverse effects, self-administering or not following the prescription directions, weight loss, lifelong usage and accumulation of medications, drug-to-drug interactions.
Sensory impairments	Hearing and visual loss, loss of sense of taste and smell, vestibular and proprioceptor sensory disturbances, inability to detect sensory stimuli and respond appropriately, tactile disturbances.
Metabolic disorders	Diabetes, anemia, hypoglycemia/hyperglycemia, vitamin deficiencies, including vitamin B12, electrolyte imbalances.
Seizures	Undetected or increased seizures.
Cardiovascular	Heart disease, stroke, transient ischemic attack (TIA).
Environmental contributors	Environments not designed to meet the changing needs and challenges, sensory overload within environments, lack of meaningful sensory stimulation, lack of accessibility and usability.
Mental illness	Depression and other mood disorders, long-term grief.
Sleep problems	Sleep apnea, interrupted sleep, too much sleep during daytime causing interrupted sleep at night, environmental stimulation interfering with sleep patterns, eating and drinking too much just prior to bedtime, nighttime incontinence.
Pain	Undetected and untreated pain, lack of pain management.
Mobility problems	Arthritis, osteoporosis, undetected fractures, deconditioning in muscles, reduction in stamina.
Social challenges	Loss of significant others, including family, caregiving staff, and peers, change in routine such as loss of work or retirement, change in residence and/or program, inability to communicate verbally with others or listened to when attempting to communicate.

Source: Bishop, K. M., Robinson, L. and VanLare, S. 2013. *Journal of Psychosocial Nursing*, 5(1), 15–18.; Jokinen, N. et al. and National Task Group on Intellectual Disabilities and Dementia Practices. 2013. *Journal of Policy and Practice in Intellectual Disabilities*, 10, 1–24. doi: 10.1111/jppi.12016.; Moran, J. et al. 2013. *Mayo Clinic Proceedings*, 88(8), 831–860; Robinson, L. et al. 2012. *Journal of Gerontological Social Work*, 55, 175–190.

current symptoms should be ruled out. If they cannot be ruled out, then further evaluation and assessment should be conducted in those specific systems.[2,3,12,29]

As discussed above, medications should be carefully examined for possible causes for the changes and decline noted. Particular attention should be paid to polypharmacy and the number of multiple prescribing physicians who may not have full information of the current medications and medication history. Gait stability, urinary retention, constipation, and confusion should be noted as these can be nonspecific signs that suggest possible adverse effects.[26,27]

When available, a family history should be reviewed for detecting the history of diseases in immediate relatives. This review should include looking for cerebrovascular disease, stroke, diabetes, heart disease, rheumatoid arthritis, and dementias of the Alzheimer's type. The history can indicate risk factors for the presenting adult. The potential for multiple underlying causes should also be considered as in the general population and more typical in older adults.[1,7]

The social environment and any changes in the environment should also be noted. Aging adults with IDD, as in the general population, are at risk for family members or friends experiencing declining health, the leaving of the family home, changes in employment and functionality, and frequent turnover of caregivers. The accumulation of these life events can cause depression or other mental health problems and should be ruled out as part of the differential diagnosis.[3,15]

Psychiatric illness may look different in adults with IDD, and there is a substantial risk for diagnostic overshadowing, blaming the mental illness on behaviors related to the preexisting disability. A good resource for review of mental disorders in this population is the *Diagnostic*

Manual—Intellectual Disability (DM-ID): A Clinical Guide for Diagnosis of Mental Disorders in Persons with Intellectual Disability.[2,24,31]

The current living environment and the level of support are also important for consideration, especially in terms of discharge planning and follow-up care. All of the above information should be cross-referenced by the healthcare practitioner, considering the whole picture and possible multiple causes for the presenting changes and decline. It is important to never assume the cause of the decline until the totality of information, as much as possible, is gathered and compared as part of the differential diagnosis.[1,7,20]

26.9   HEALTHCARE ADVOCACY AND STRATEGIES FOR CARE

The challenges discussed above require advocacy by everyone involved in the process to assure quality healthcare, which is of course essential for maintaining quality of health and life in later years.[3,15,20] Nurses, other clinicians, and family can play an essential role in the identification of changes and unmet needs for people with IDD and mental health diagnoses to help prevent the misdiagnosis of symptoms when an older adult is exhibiting decline or change in behavior.[2,32]

Challenges to providing quality care requiring advocacy include—but are not limited to— lack of knowledge about aging with a complex array of preexisting diagnoses, polypharmacy, and increasing numbers of vulnerable adults in the general population and the IDD subpopulation. These factors can lead to lack of appropriate assessments or interventions, as well as diagnostic overshadowing.[20,30,32]

It is essential that the practitioner and caregivers work together to assure accuracy in the process of ruling out underlying causes for decline and behavioral changes. Listening, mutual respect for the information each has to offer, and good communication between the caregivers and diagnostician will likely result in a more accurate diagnosis and interventions. Best practices include sharing as much information between healthcare providers and caregivers/advocates as relevant and legally permissible to provide clues for diagnosis and treatment of underlying causes.[1,4,15]

Good communication of medical history and current symptoms by healthcare advocates is essential for receiving appropriate and timely treatment. The baseline cognitive functioning (prior to disease process) of an individual with IDD will determine the ability to recognize and communicate any changes to the healthcare providers. Without knowledge of baseline abilities, health, and functional status, misdiagnosis can occur, especially if the provider is comparing the adult's functioning to the general population rather than who that individual has been throughout a lifetime.[2,3,7] A misdiagnosis can result in the prescribing of inappropriate medications, overlooking significant risk factors or symptoms, and/or missed opportunities for treatment to maintain or improve overall health status.[1]

Individuals with IDD may be alone, with family members, or have staff from a service agency when they arrive in the emergency room (ER) or are hospitalized. Communication will be the key between the health provider, the patient with IDD, and any healthcare advocates accompanying the individual. Typically, if the adult is living in a residential facility, there will be staff accompanying to help provide information for assessment, treatment, and healthcare decisions made. The adult should be included in those decisions as much as possible. If the adult is not able to make decisions for himself or herself, then there are usually legal provisions made for another adult to speak on the individual's behalf and help make the best decisions possible.[3,15]

Any decisions made to release the adult back into the community should be made based on what follow-up is available when the adult returns home. If the adult lives totally independently but is currently unable to provide the personal care needed for healing and the return to baseline, then this should be considered when determining to admit or send home.[2,4,24]

Several key areas for attention by knowledgeable advocates include transitional adjustments such as moving to a new, accessible residence without input from the adult with IDD; personal losses or change in favorite staff or death of a loved family member; and physical changes due to disease process and pain. Too often providers may not look beyond the behavior, assumption of dementia in older years, or preexisting disability to identify the real underlying physical problem.[7,12,24]

26.10   WHERE TO GO FROM HERE

It should be very clear to the reader that quality healthcare provision and follow-up cannot be delivered in isolation of the individual, family, and service support staff if the best possible outcomes are to be achieved. The healthcare provider, including discharge planners, must be working with the appropriate advocates to determine the current supports available as well as recommended contacts that may be needed to assure supports once the adult with IDD is returned to home.[3,15,20]

Referrals for additional services can be obtained via a number of routes, including area agencies on aging, state developmental disabilities agencies, local ID service providers, family physicians, consulting psychologists, care coordinators, or dementia resource centers. Formal comprehensive geriatric clinic assessments are fruitful settings for such diagnostic processes.[3,15,20]

In smaller communities and rural or remote locations, consultations may need to be arranged and conducted by professionals familiar with adults with IDs via teleconference or videoconference. Development of regional teams may also improve access and assessment services for individuals and caregivers. In any formal assessment situation, persons familiar with the adult with ID and his or her history and communication style should always accompany the adult to provide reassurances to the individual as well as to serve as a knowledgeable informant and to facilitate the exchange of information.[7,15]

It is essential that partnerships in caring for adults with IDD are developed. Hospital administrators, social workers, medical associations, and AAAs can each take a lead in assuring they are working together to avoid duplication and gaps of services. To send adults with IDD to curb after treatment for any illness, symptoms, or disease without appropriate follow-up and supports is to lose the progress that may have been gained during the hospitalization or healthcare service provision.[15,20,24]

26.11   SUMMARY AND RECOMMENDATIONS

Expertise in aging and adults with IDD is paramount for the nurses, other health professionals, and family involved in their care, especially as the family caregivers become no longer available to provide day-to-day care or advocacy. The unique challenges of aging healthfully, coupled with the physical and psychiatric diagnoses this population presents, demands this expertise if we are to ensure positive outcomes in healthcare. To enhance this expertise, the author recommends the following:

1. Healthcare educators, practitioners, and advocates for older adults with IDD need to identify content experts and work closely with those experts for the inclusion of this information as mandated training in university and college courses for healthcare providers.
2. Existing advocacy groups including the NTG on Dementia Practices and IDD and Geriatric Education Centers (GEC) such as the Finger Lakes Geriatric Education Center in Rochester, New York that have partially funded the writing of this chapter are available for sharing of expertise, best practices, and guidelines on provision of healthcare. At the federal, state, and local level, the organizations should be working in collaboration to educate caregivers, healthcare providers, and advocates on the information in this chapter. Content experts should be developed within organizations and regions. Training should include the following:
    a. Topics of adverse effects of medications on older adults with IDD, common diseases and conditions causing decline in older adults with IDD, environmental and sensory barriers, and skills of healthcare advocacy

    b. Training on observation and reporting of symptoms by individuals who cannot communicate those symptoms verbally; the symptoms may be masked or mimicked by many diseases, making this a complex process

    c. Techniques for working collaboratively to determine underlying causes for decline in older adults with IDD

3. It can be difficult for the healthcare provider who does not have relevant experience with aging or IDD to consider how the older adult's system has been compromised with premature aging due to lifelong comorbidities and medications. Whenever possible, it is helpful to seek out providers who work with agencies serving adults with IDD, along with geriatricians.

4. Evidence-based research is needed for increased understanding of the challenges and diverse needs of older adults with IDD. Thorough documentation on medical, medication, and behavioral history will make this research possible in the future.

5. Providers of services for adults with IDD need to take an active leadership in talking to individual with IDD, staff, family, and caregivers to build partnerships with community healthcare providers, develop processes for healthcare advocacy with internal and external expertise developed, and long-term care planning process to address ongoing and changing needs for older adults with IDD.

6. Care coordination and systems integration are major foci for many states and local area agencies on aging (AAAs) and others. Healthcare providers and organizations providing services or advocacy for adults with IDD need to make sure that they are part of the planning process for systems changes that must include consideration for adults with IDD in the planning.

Healthcare practitioners and caregivers must realize the important role of advocating on all levels to ensure that older adults with IDD are afforded the time and effort required to arrive at the best possible outcomes. This advocacy includes assuring accurate information for healthcare providers and preventive education for caregivers and aging individuals.[7,15,20]

Appropriate assessments and interventions, as guided by advocates, can result in older adults with IDD continuing to be involved in ongoing learning, socialization, and lifelong interests, thus assuring a meaningful existence in this last stage of life. Advocacy across the life span for adults with IDD can make a difference for quality of life, health, and functioning in later years. The author hopes this chapter will help readers to make a difference for older adults to assure the best healthcare outcomes possible.

REFERENCES

1. Bishop, K. M., Robinson, L. and VanLare, S. 2013. Healthy aging for older adults with intellectual and developmental disabilities. *Journal of Psychosocial Nursing*, 5(1), 15–18.
2. Moran, J., Rafi, M., Keller, S., Singh, B. and Janicki, M. 2013. Management of dementia in adults with intellectual disabilities. *Mayo Clinic Proceedings*, 88(8), 831–860.
3. National Task Group on Intellectual Disabilities and Dementia Practice. 2012. *"My thinker's not working": A national strategy for enabling adults with intellectual disabilities affected by dementia to remain in their community and receive quality supports*. Retrieved from www.aadmd.org/ntg/thinker.
4. Service, K. P. and Hahn, J. E. 2003. Issues in aging: The role of the nurse in the care of older people with intellectual and developmental disabilities. *Nursing Clinics of North America*, 38(2), 291–312.
5. Tyler, C. and Noritz, G. 2009. Aging adults with intellectual and other developmental disabilities. *Clinical Geriatrics*, 31(1), 85–88.
6. Brault, M. 2012. Americans with disabilities: 2010. Retrieved from http://www.census.gov/prod/2012pubs/p70-131.pdf.
7. Robinson, L., Dauenhauer, J., Bishop, K. and Baxter, J. 2012. Growing health disparities for persons who are aging with intellectual and developmental disabilities: The social work linchpin. *Journal of Gerontological Social Work*, 55, 175–190.

8. Bishop, K. M. and Lucchino, R. 2010. Module II: Matching needs to services for older adults with intellectual and developmental disabilities. In *Cross Network Collaboration for Florida, ADRC Training.* Tallahassee: Florida State Department of Elder Affairs.

9. Heller, T., Janicki, M. P., Hammel, J. and Factor, A. R. 2002. *Promoting Healthy Aging, Family Support, and Age-Friendly Communities for Persons Aging with Developmental Disabilities: Report of the 2001 Invitational Research Symposium on Aging with Developmental Disabilities.* Chicago: The Rehabilitation Research and Training Center on Aging with Developmental Disabilities, Department of Disability and Human Development, University of Illinois at Chicago.

10. American Association on Intellectual and Developmental Disabilities (AAIDD). 2013. Definition of intellectual disability. Retrieved from http://aaidd.org/intellectual-disability/definition#.UsXuQe93u00.

11. Bittles, A. H., Petterson, B. A., Sullivan, S. G., Hussain, R., Glasson, E. J. and Montgomery, P. D. 2002. The influence of intellectual disability on life expectancy. *Journal of Gerontology Series A: Biological Sciences and Medical Sciences,* 57, M470–M472.

12. Evenhuis, H., Henderson, C. M., Beange, H., Lennox, N. and Chicoine, B. 2001. Healthy ageing—Adults with intellectual disabilities: Physical health issues. *Journal of Applied Research in Intellectual Disabilities,* 14, 175–194.

13. American Psychiatric Association. 2000. *Diagnostic and Statistical Manual of Mental Disorders,* Fourth Edition. Arlington, VA: American Psychiatric Association.

14. Luckasson, R., Borthwick-Duffy, S., Buntinx, W. H. E., Coulter, D. L., Craig, E. M., Schalock, R. L., Snell, M. E. et al. 2002. *Mental Retardation: Definition, Classification, and System of Supports.* Washington, DC: American Association on Mental Retardation.

15. Jokinen, N., Janicki, M. P., Keller, S. M., McCallion, P., Force, L. T. and National Task Group on Intellectual Disabilities and Dementia Practices. 2013. Guidelines for structuring community care and supports for people with intellectual disabilities affected by dementia. *Journal of Policy and Practice in Intellectual Disabilities,* 10, 1–24. doi: 10.1111/jppi.12016.

16. McKhann, G. M., Knopman, D. S., Chertkow, H., Hyman, B. T., Jack, C. R., Jr., Kawas, C. H., Klunk, W. E. et al. 2011. The diagnosis of dementia due to Alzheimer's disease: Recommendations from the National Institute on Aging and the Alzheimer's Association Workgroup. *Alzheimer's Dementia,* 7(3), 263–269.

17. Fuller-Iglesia, H., Smith, J. and Antonucci, T. 2010. Theories of aging from a life-course and life span perspective: An overview. In T. C. Antonucci and J. S. Jackson (Eds.), *Annual Review of Gerontology and Geriatrics: Life-Course Perspectives on Late-Life Health Inequalities.* New York: Springer; Vol. 29.

18. Noll, S. and Trent, J. 2004. *Mental Retardation in America: A Historical Reader.* Berkley, CA: University of California Press.

19. Ness, S., Rafii, M., Aisen, P., Krams, M., Silverman, W. and Manji, H. 2012. Down's syndrome and Alzheimer's disease: Towards secondary prevention. *Nature Reviews,* 11, 655–656.

20. Bishop, K. M., Hogan, M., Janicki, M., Keller, S., Lucchino, R., Mughal, D., Perkins, E., Singh, B., Service, K., Wolfson, S. and The Health Planning Work Group of the National Task Group on Intellectual Disabilities and Dementia Practices. 2015. Guidelines for dementia-related health advocacy for adults with intellectual disability and dementia: National task group on intellectual disabilities and dementia practices. *Intellectual and Developmental Disabilities,* 53(1), 2–29.

21. Prasher, V. 2006. Genetics, Alzheimer's disease, and Down syndrome. In *Down Syndrome and Alzheimer's Disease: Biologic Correlates.* London, UK: Radcliffe Publishing; pp. 37–57.

22. Centers for Disease Control and Prevention. 2013. Cerebral palsy homepage. Retrieved from http://www.cdc.gov/ncbddd/cp/facts.html.

23. Mayo Clinic. 2013. Diseases and conditions. Cerebral palsy. Retrieved from http://www.mayoclinic.org/diseases-conditions/cerebral-palsy/basics/definition/CON-20030502.

24. Henderson, C. M. and Davidson, P. W. 2000. Comprehensive adult and geriatric assessment. In M. P. Janicki and E. Ansello (Eds.), *Community Supports for Aging Adults with Lifelong Disabilities.* Baltimore, MD: Paul Brookes Publishing, Inc; pp. 373–386.

25. Atwood, T. 2007. *The Complete Guide to Asperger's Syndrome.* Philadelphia, PA: Jessica Kingsley Publishers.

26. Lucchino, R. 2008. *Aging and Intellectual and Developmental Disabilities.* Santa Fe, NM: New Mexico Chapter Alzheimer's Association.

27. Lucchino, R. 2012. Introduction to adverse effects and interactions of medications. Agency Webinar Series March 8, 2012 sponsored by the Program on Aging and Developmental Disabilities (PADD), Strong Center for Developmental Disabilities, Golisano Children's Hospital, Rochester, NY.

28. New York State Speech-Language-Hearing Association Inc., NYPTA and NYSOTA 2012. New York State benchmark plan recommendations. Retrieved from http://www.healthcarereform.ny.gov/timeline/2012-0802_exchange_stakeholder/docs/nys_ot_pt_speech.pdf.

29. Henderson, C. M., Robinson, L. M., Davidson, P. W., Haveman, M., Janicki, M. P. and Albertini, G. 2008. Overweight status, obesity and risk factors for coronary heart disease in adults with intellectual disability. *Journal of Policy and Practice in Intellectual Disabilities*, 5, 174–177.

30. Janicki, M. P., Davidson, P. W., Henderson, C. M., McCallion, P., Taets, J. D., Force, L. T. and Ladrigan, P. M. 2002. Health characteristics and health services utilization in older adults with intellectual disabilities living in community residences. *Journal of Intellectual Disability Research*, 46, 287–298.

31. Fletcher, R., Loschen, E., Stavrakaki, C. and First, M. (Eds.). 2007. *Diagnostic Manual—Intellectual Disability (DM-ID): A Clinical Guide for Diagnosis of Mental Disorders in Persons with Intellectual Disability*. Kingston, NY: NADD Press.

32. Jones, S., Howard, L. and Thornicroft, G. 2008. "Diagnostic overshadowing": Worse physical health care for people with mental illness. *Acta Psychiatrica Scandinavica*, 118, 169–171.

Section IV

Health Maintenance, Caregiving, and Postacute Rehabilitation

Bedside to Curbside

27 Inpatient Rehabilitation
Acute, Subacute, and in Community Settings

Deepthi S. Saxena

CONTENTS

27.1 BACKGROUND

Rehabilitation interventions in the inpatient and outpatient settings are often required in older adults, to facilitate independent living in communities. In the older adult, hospitalization is a risk for disability, leading to decreased ability to live independently at discharge from the hospital. Hospitalization-associated disability (HAD) occurs in approximately one-third of patients aged above 70 years.[1] This is a disability that is not present 2 weeks prior to hospitalization, and it could occur even after the illnesses causing the hospitalization are treated. Postacute care (PAC) in rehabilitation settings addresses this disability in the context of medical illness/disease.

Older patients are transitioned to rehabilitation settings for the management of disabilities caused by illness, injury, and/or hospitalization. A care transition is the movement of the patient from one healthcare setting to another. Older adults are at an increased risk of suboptimal care during care transitions. Rehabilitation professionals play a critical role in efficient and safe care transitions by determining the appropriate level of care based upon the intensity of services that older patients need. Medical and geriatric rehabilitation addresses the patient's current functional status and rehabilitation goals with the intent to optimize the individual's function, and facilitate independent living. The process involves addressing diseases, particularly multiple medically complex conditions in the context of disability. Based upon the intensity of services (including medical management and rehabilitation) required by the individual, the level of care setting is determined. Transitions of care may also be appropriate for older adults living independently in communities, when they require inpatient and outpatient rehabilitation.

This section focuses on the older adult population in the United States (individuals above 65 years of age), who are eligible for Medicare. Medicare is the federal health insurance program in the United States for people who are 65 years or older, certain younger people with disabilities, and people with end-stage renal disease (permanent kidney failure requiring dialysis or a transplant. Traditional fee-for-service Medicare involved significant cost sharing from beneficiaries. For that reason, more than 90% of Medicare beneficiaries maintain supplemental insurance through their employer or private insurance, which also follows regulatory trends set by the Center for Medicare and Medicaid Services (CMS).[2]

Between 2009–2010, CMS implemented a Quality Improvement Organization (QIO) initiative, which demonstrated that Medicare beneficiaries in communities in which QI initiatives were implemented to promote evidence-based care transitions, compared with Medicare patients in communities without this QI implementation, had lower all-cause 30-day re-hospitalization rates per 1000 and all-cause hospitalization rates per 1000, but no significant reductions in the rates of all-cause 30-day re-hospitalizations as a percentage of hospital discharges.[3]

In 2013, CMS incentivized ambulatory care providers to bill under new payment codes for transitional care management services to assist with transitions of care in the first 30 days of discharge from inpatient hospital settings.

On September 18, 2014, Congress passed the Improving Medicare Post-Acute Care Transformation Act of 2014 (the IMPACT Act), which requires the submission of standardized data by long-term care hospitals (LTCHs), skilled nursing facilities (SNFs), home health agencies (HHAs), and inpatient rehabilitation facilities (IRFs).[4]

On October 29, 2015, CMS released a proposed rule that would require all hospitals and HHAs to develop a written discharge plan for every inpatient and specific categories of outpatients within 24 hours of admission. This was the first step in implementing the IMPACT Act.[5]

27.2 SPEAKING THE COMMON LANGUAGE OF FUNCTION

The World Health Organization's International Classification of Functioning, Disability and Health (ICF) is a framework that acknowledges that every human being can experience a decrement in health and thereby experience some degree of disability, thus recognizing disability as a universal and mainstream human experience. The ICF shifts focus from cause to impact, placing all health conditions on an equal footing and allowing them to be compared using a common metric—the measure of health and disability. The ICF takes into account the social aspects of disability and does not see disability only as a "medical" or "biological" dysfunction. The ICF comprises of two parts, Health Conditions and Contextual Factors. Health Conditions encompasses the three domains of Body Functions and Structure, Activities, and Participation. Contextual factors consists of the two domains of environmental and personal elements, which consider the impact of the environment on the person's functioning. Therefore, the ICF is a useful conceptual model for providers, which considers the individual's function in relation to organ-specific disease in the perspective of personal and environmental factors. For this reason, ICF-based interventions designed to modify a person's impairments, limitations in activities, and participation provide a framework to develop a comprehensive rehabilitation care plan that determines the intensity of services during care transitions to appropriate rehabilitation settings.

27.3 REHABILITATION SETTINGS

IRFs are freestanding rehabilitation hospitals or acute rehabilitation units attached to an acute hospital. Subacute rehabilitation or SNFs are freestanding units attached to an acute hospital or to a long-term care nursing facility.

The following sections focus on acute and subacute inpatient rehabilitation with emphasis on regulatory criteria, and the appropriateness of admissions to the two different settings.

27.3.1 INPATIENT REHABILITATION FACILITY OR ACUTE INPATIENT REHABILITATION

Acute inpatient rehabilitation is PAC covered under Medicare's Inpatient Hospital Services, which is covered under Medicare Part A. Care transition determinations to an IRF setting are based on providing intensive rehabilitation therapy in a resource-intensive inpatient hospital environment for patients due to the complexity of their nursing, medical management, and rehabilitation needs. In order for IRF care to be considered reasonable and necessary, the documentation in the patient's medical record must demonstrate a reasonable expectation that the following criteria were met at the time of admission:

1. The patient, within reason, is expected to actively participate in and significantly benefit from active and ongoing multiple therapeutic interventions: physical and occupational therapies, and speech-language pathology.
2. The patient must generally require an intensive rehabilitation therapy program, which consists of at least 3 hours of therapy per day at least 5 days per week. In certain well-documented cases, this may consist of up to 15 hours of intensive rehabilitation therapy within a 7-consecutive-day period from the date of admission. Function is measured with the FIM (functional independence measure) assessment instrument, which is detailed below.
3. As a result of the rehabilitation treatment, the patient can reasonably be expected to make measurable improvement value; which means, improvement to their functional capacity or adaptation to impairments within a prescribed period of time. The patient is expected to achieve independence in the domain of self-care and mobility or be expected to return to his or her prior level of functioning.
4. The patient must require supervision by a rehabilitation physician, a licensed physician with specialized training and experience in inpatient rehabilitation. The patient must engage in face-to-face visits with the physician at least 3 days per week throughout the patient's stay to assess their medical and functional status, or to modify the course of treatment as needed to maximize the patient's ability to benefit from the rehabilitation process.
5. The patient must require an intensive and coordinated interdisciplinary approach to providing rehabilitation. The IRF benefit is not an alternative to completion of the full course of treatment for the patient's medical condition in the referring hospital. While completing their course of treatment, if they are not able to participate in and benefit from the intensive rehabilitation, therapy services will not be considered reasonable and necessary. Conversely, the IRF benefit is not appropriate for patients who achieve functional independence while completing their course of treatment for the medical condition. Medicare benefits are available for such patients in a less intensive setting.

27.3.1.1 IRF Rules and Regulations

The IRF Prospective Payment System (PPS) for each patient is based on information found in the IRF Patient Assessment Instrument (PAI).

IRFs are governed by

The 60 percent rule and compliance percentage
Reasonable and necessary criteria
IRF Quality Reporting Program (QRP)

27.3.1.1.1 The 60 Percent Rule and Compliance Percentage

Medicare requires determinations of whether IRF stays are reasonable and necessary based on an assessment of each beneficiary's individual care needs. One criterion specified in the Federal Register (at 42 CFR 412.29(b)) is that a minimum of 60%, called the compliance threshold, of a facility's total inpatient population must require treatment in an IRF for one or more of the following 13 medical conditions:

1. Stroke
2. Spinal cord injury
3. Congenital deformity
4. Amputation
5. Major multiple trauma
6. Fracture of femur (hip fracture)
7. Brain injury
8. Neurological disorders, including multiple sclerosis, motor neuron diseases, polyneuropathy, muscular dystrophy, and Parkinson's disease
9. *Burns*: For the three qualifying conditions listed below, the severity and complexity can vary significantly. Additional clinical criteria were established to require evidence that other less intensive treatments were attempted and failed to improve the patient's condition before admission to the IRF:
10. Active polyarticular rheumatoid arthritis, psoriatic arthritis, and seronegative arthropathies resulting in significant functional impairment of ambulation and other activities of daily living
11. Systemic vasculidities with joint inflammation resulting in significant functional impairment of ambulation and other activities of daily living
12. Severe or advanced osteoarthritis (osteoarthrosis or degenerative joint disease) involving two or more weight-bearing joints (elbow, shoulders, hips, or knees, but not counting a joint with a prosthesis) with joint deformity and substantial loss of range of motion, atrophy of muscles surrounding the joint, and significant functional impairment of ambulation and other activities of daily living
13. Knee or hip joint replacements in an individual 85 years or older or who is morbidly obese during an acute care hospitalization immediately preceding the inpatient rehabilitation stay

27.3.1.1.2 Reasonable and Necessary Criteria

IRF care is only considered by Medicare to be reasonable and necessary if the patient meets all of the requirements outlined in the Federal Register, 42 CFR §§412.622(a)(3), (4), and (5), regardless of whether the patient is treated in the IRF for one or more of the 13 medical conditions listed above (in 42 CFR §412.23(b)(2)(ii)) or not.

Therefore, acute inpatient rehabilitation/IRFs have strict documentation requirements, which include Pre-Admission Screening (PAS); the Post-Admission Physician Evaluation (PAPE); the

Overall Plan of Care, also called the Individualized Plan of Care (IPOC); and the Admission Orders.

27.3.1.1.2.1 Pre-Admission Screening A PAS is a detailed and comprehensive primary documentation by the clinical staff of the patient's status prior to admission and of the specific reasons that the admission would be reasonable and necessary. A PAS must be done in person or through a review of the patient's medical records transmitted from the referring hospital, containing the necessary assessments to make a reasonable determination in either paper or electronic format. A rehabilitation physician must document that he or she has reviewed and concurs with the findings and results of the PAS prior to the admission. The PAS is conducted within the 48 hours immediately preceding the IRF admission and includes

- The patient's prior level of function (prior to condition leading to the need for acute rehabilitation).
- The expected level of improvement and the length of stay necessary to achieve it.
- An evaluation of the risk for clinical complications from the conditions that caused the need for an IRF admission; and the anticipated discharge destination, postdischarge treatments, and other information relevant to the care needs of the patient. "Trial" IRF admissions, to assess whether the patients would benefit significantly from treatment in the IRF or other settings, are not considered reasonable and necessary.

27.3.1.1.2.2 Postadmission Physician Evaluation The PAPE is performed by a rehabilitation physician within the first 24 hours of admission. The PAPE should indicate the medical necessity, and patient's status on admission, compared to the PAS. From this, the patient's expected course of treatment will be developed. The PAPE includes a documented history and physical exam, as well as a review of the patient's prior and current medical and functional conditions and comorbidities. If the patient has a marked improvement in functional ability since the time of the PAS, or an inability to meet the demands of the intensity of the IRF rehabilitation program, the IRF begins the process of discharging the patient to another setting of care.

27.3.1.1.2.3 Individualized Overall Plan of Care The IPOC comprises documentation from all therapy disciplines and clinicians that are involved in treating the patient. Its essential elements are details on the patient's medical prognosis and the planned interventions, functional outcomes, estimated length of stay, and discharge destination. It is completed within the first 4 days of the IRF admission, and it is the responsibility of the rehabilitation physician to adequately document that the admission is reasonable and necessary.

27.3.1.1.2.4 Admission Orders At the time of admission, the physician generates admission orders for the patient's care, which includes therapy orders and the intensity of services required.

27.3.1.2 Rehabilitation Physician and Interdisciplinary Team Approach

The complexity of the patient's condition must be such that the rehabilitation goals indicated in the PAS, the PAPE, and the IPOC can only be achieved through periodic interdisciplinary team conferences. Interdisciplinary team conferences are led by a rehabilitation physician, who is responsible for making the final decisions on the patient's care based on the documented concurrence from the teams. Interdisciplinary services cannot be provided by only one discipline. Teams work within their scopes of practice to coordinate efforts through frequent, structured, and documented communication with other teams, as well as with the patient and the patient's caregivers, to establish, prioritize, and achieve treatment goals. The interdisciplinary team must document participation by professionals from each of the following disciplines, each of whom has current knowledge of the patient:

1. A rehabilitation physician with specialized training and experience in rehabilitation services
2. A registered nurse with specialized training or experience in rehabilitation
3. A social worker or a case manager (or both)
4. A licensed or certified therapist from each therapy discipline involved in treating the patient

The periodic interdisciplinary team conferences must document

1. The patient's progress toward the rehabilitation goals
2. Barriers to goals, and possible resolutions of the same
3. The reassessment of how realistic previously established goals are
4. The monitoring and revising of the treatment plan, as needed

27.3.1.3   Individualized Therapy

A primary distinction between the IRF environment and other rehabilitation settings is the high level of physician supervision, the interdisciplinary approach to monitor functional gains, and the intensity of rehabilitation therapy services. The required individualized therapy treatments must begin within 36 hours from midnight of the day of admission to the IRF. The initial therapy evaluations constitute the beginning of the required therapy services, and are used to demonstrate the intensity of therapy services that will be provided.

27.3.1.4   Brief Exceptions Policy

If an unexpected clinical event occurs during the course of an IRF stay that limits the patient's ability to participate in the intensive therapy program for a brief period not to exceed 3 consecutive days, it does not affect the determination of the medical necessity of the IRF admission if the event, which was based on reasonable conclusions from the rehabilitation physician and teams, is well documented in the patient's medical record, along with well-documented PAS, PAPE, and IPOC.

27.3.1.5   Definition of Measurable Improvement (FIM)

The patient's progress and functional improvement is measured with the FIM, which is a proprietary assessment scale, that assesses physical and cognitive disability. This scale focuses on the burden of care—that is, the level of disability indicating the burden of caring for them.

Items are scored on the level of assistance required for an individual to perform activities of daily living. The scale includes 18 items, of which 13 items are physical domains based on the Barthel Index and 5 items are cognition items. Each item is scored from 1 to 7 based on the level of independence, where 1 represents total dependence and 7 indicates complete independence. The scale can be administered by a physician, nurse, therapist, or layperson. Possible scores range from 18 to 126, with higher scores indicating more independence. Alternatively, 13 physical items could be scored separately from the five cognitive items.

27.3.1.6   Function Independence Measure

7 Complete independence: Fully independent
6 Modified independence: Requiring the use of a device but no physical help
5 Supervision: Requiring only standby assistance or verbal prompting or help with setup
4 Minimal assistance: Requiring incidental hands-on help only (subject performs >75% of the task)
3 Moderate assistance: Subject still performs 50%–75% of the task

2 Maximal assistance: Subject provides less than half of the effort (25%–49%)

1 Total assistance: Subject contributes <25% of the effort or is unable to do the task

27.3.1.7 IRF Quality Reporting Program

Under the IRF-QRP, the following are reported:

1. Urinary catheter-associated urinary tract infections (CAUTI) events on all patients
2. Percent of Medicare patients with new or worsened pressure ulcers since admission
3. Inpatient Hospital-Onset Methicillin-Resistant *Staphylococcus Aureus* Bacteremia Outcome Measure (National Quality Forum [NQF] #1716)
4. Facility-Wide Inpatient Hospital-Onset Clostridium Difficile Infection Outcome Measure (NQF #1717)
5. For FY 2016, IRFs must report quality data for influenza vaccination coverage among healthcare personnel in the IRF setting for the period October 1, 2014 (or when the vaccine becomes available) through March 31, 2015, and each October 1 through March 31 thereafter.
6. For FY 2017, IRFs must report quality data on the percent of patients who are assessed and appropriately given the seasonal influenza vaccination as well as a risk-adjusted version of the pressure ulcer measure.
7. For FY 2014 and each subsequent year thereafter, IRFs that do not report quality data are to be subjected to a 2 percentage point reduction to the applicable market basket increase factor.

27.3.2 SUBACUTE REHABILITATION

There are variations in the use of the term "subacute rehabilitation." The general consensus is that it is a niche in the continuum of care between acute-hospital care and long-term, nursing home care.[6]

According to the Joint Commission on Accreditation of Healthcare Organizations (JCAHO), subacute rehabilitation is a comprehensive inpatient care designed for someone who has had an acute illness, injury, or exacerbation of a disease process.

In subacute rehabilitation:

1. Goal-oriented treatment is provided, immediately after acute hospitalization to treat one or more specific, active, and/or complex medical conditions and to administer one or more technically complex treatments, in the context of a person's underlying long-term conditions.
2. The individual's condition does not need care heavily dependent on high-technology monitoring or complex diagnostic procedures.
3. The individual requires the coordinated services of a team of physicians, nurses, and other disciplines trained in the management of specific conditions.
4. The rehabilitation services are more intensive than traditional nursing facility care and less than acute hospital and acute rehabilitation (IRF) care.
5. The individual receives frequent recurrent assessment and review of the clinical course and a treatment plan until their condition is stabilized or the predetermined treatment course is completed.

27.3.2.1 Resource Utilization Groups

Medicare reimbursement in subacute rehabilitation is under a PPS that is adjusted according to the resources required by each patient. The resource utilization groups (RUGs) system has three tiers with eight major classification groups and one or two different types of splits (within each major group).[6]

The eight major categories are

Category I	Rehabilitation plus extensive services
Category II	Rehabilitation
Category III	Extensive services
Category IV	Special care
Category V	Clinically complex
Category VI	Impaired cognition
Category VII	Behavior problems
Category VIII	Reduced physical function

The system is hierarchical, with each resident classified into the highest tier for which he/she meets the requirements based on data from standardized resident assessments (Minimum Data Set [MDS] discussed below).

Subacute rehabilitation facilities receive per diem payments for each patient, which are case-mix-adjusted based on the classification groups. RUGs are determined through MDS under Category II, Rehabilitation. There are five RUG categories according to the number of minutes of rehabilitation that is provided:

1. *Ultra high*: Treatment minimum of 720 minutes, during which the patient receives services from at least two disciplines; one discipline at least 5-days per week and one discipline 3-days per week.
2. *Very high*: Treatment minimum of 500 minutes provided by at least one discipline 5 days per week.
3. *High*: Treatment minimum of 325 minutes from at least one discipline 5 days per week.
4. *Medium*: Treatment minimum of 150 minutes from three disciplines 5 days per week.
5. *Low*: Treatment minimum of 45 minutes weekly over at least 3 days.

27.3.2.2   Length of Stay

1. *Short stays*: 3–30 days. 75% of care is either medically complex or rehabilitative.
2. *Medium stays*: 31–90 days. 22% of care is both medical and rehabilitative.
3. *Long stays*: 91 days to less than 2 years. 3% of care is either for catastrophic illness or illnesses with a very slow rate of recovery.

27.3.2.3   Minimum Dataset

The Minimum Data Set 3.0 (MDS) is a federally mandated periodic evaluation, utilizing the Resident Assessment Instrument (RAI)-MDS[6] tool for

1. Implementing standardized assessment
2. Facilitating care management

The MDS contains information on functional, medical, cognitive, psychological, and social status. It is a patient-centered, clinically relevant, valid, and reliable tool created with the intention to decrease burden on providers, improve quality of care, and facilitate individualized care.

The average time to complete MDS 3.0 is 60 minutes. The MDS focuses on "patient reported" outcomes. Examples of the measurement tools used in MDS include Patient Health Questionnaire (PHQ 9), which takes 4 minutes, Brief Interview for Mental Status (BIMS), which takes 3.2 minutes, and the Pain items take 2.0 minutes. Since the subacute rehabilitation team involving therapy disciplines also evaluates these different sections, it is most effective and efficient to use a team meeting to gather information needed for these assessments.

Physicians as team leaders can contribute maximally by understanding medical rehabilitation aspects of these assessments and by speaking the same languages as the teams.

CMS requires that assessments in the MDS are done at periodic intervals. The facility requires that individual staff members or a team are involved in these assessments. The MDS coordinator or the resident care management director (RCMD) does timely and accurate completion of both the RAI and care management process from admission to discharge in accordance with company policies and procedures, State and Federal guidelines, and all other entities as appropriate while maintaining responsibility for coordinating information systems operations and education for the clinical department.

The Omnibus Budget Reconciliation Act (OBRA/1987) regulations require nursing homes that are Medicare and/or Medicaid certified to conduct initial and periodic assessments for all their residents.

All residents are required to have the RAI process completed regardless of age, or payer source.

Assessment reference date (ARD) refers to the last day of the observation (or "look back") period that the assessment covers for the resident. Since a day begins at 12:00 a.m. and ends at 11:59 p.m., the ARD must also cover this time period. The facility is required to set the ARD on the MDS Item Set or in the facility software within the required timeframe of the assessment type being completed. This concept of setting the ARD is used for all assessment types (OBRA and Medicare-required PPS) and varies by assessment type and facility determination. Most of the MDS 3.0 items have a 7-day look-back period. As an example, if a patient has an ARD of July 1, 2011, then all pertinent information starting at 12 a.m. on June 25 and ending on July 1 at 11:59 p.m. should be included for MDS 3.0 coding.

27.3.2.4 Frequencies of PPS Scheduled Assessments for a Medicare Part A Stay

1. *Five-day scheduled assessment*: The initial MDS to be complete is called the *entry tracking record*. The entry tracking record of the MDS form is the demographic section only and must be completed with each admission and readmission of a resident to the SNF. The entry tracking record is due within 7 days of the date of admission or readmission where day one is counted from the day that the resident enters/reenters.
2. *Fourteen-day scheduled assessment*: The next OBRA MDS is the admission assessment. The admission MDS is due within 14 days of the resident being admitted to the facility. If the patient does not remain in the facility for the 14-day duration, this assessment is not required.
3. *Thirty-day scheduled assessment*: The ARD (Item A2300) must be set on days 27 through 29 of the Part A SNF covered stay. It authorizes payment from days 31 through 60 of the stay, as long as all the coverage criteria for Part A SNF-level services continue to be met.
4. *Sixty-day scheduled assessment*: The ARD (Item A2300) must be set on days 57 through 59 of the Part A SNF covered stay. It authorizes payment from days 61 through 90 of the stay, as long as all the coverage criteria continue to be met.
5. *Ninety-day scheduled assessment*: The ARD (Item A2300) must be set on days 87 through 89 of the Part A SNF covered stay. It authorizes payment from days 91 through 100 of the stay, as long as all the coverage criteria continue to be met.
6. Readmission/return assessment
7. Other Medicare required assessment (OMRA)

27.3.2.5 Start of Therapy OMRA

Start of therapy (SOT) OMRA is completed only to classify a resident into a RUG-IV rehabilitation plus extensive services or rehabilitation group. If the RUG-IV classification does not meet a rehabilitation plus extensive services or a rehabilitation (therapy) group, the assessment will not be accepted by CMS and cannot be used for Medicare billing. The ARD must be set on days 5–7 after the start of therapy, whichever is the earliest date.

27.3.2.6 End of Therapy OMRA

End of therapy (EOT) OMRA is required when the resident is classified in a RUG-IV rehabilitation plus extensive services or rehabilitation group and continues to need Part A SNF-level services after the planned or unplanned discontinuation of all rehabilitation therapies for 3 or more consecutive days.

27.3.2.7 Change of Therapy OMRA

Change of therapy (COT) OMRA is required when the resident is receiving a sufficient level of rehabilitation therapy to qualify for an ultra high, very high, high, medium, or low rehabilitation category and when the intensity of therapy (indicated by the total reimbursable therapy minutes [RTM] delivered, and other therapy qualifiers such as number of therapy days and disciplines providing therapy), changes to such a degree that it would no longer reflect the RUG-IV classification and payment assigned for the resident based on the most recent assessment.

27.3.2.8 RAI: Sections

CMS regulates that all MDS forms must follow sections A–Z:
- Section A: Identification Information
- Section B: Hearing, Speech, and Vision
- Section C: Cognitive Patterns
- Section D: Mood
- Section E: Behavior
- Section F: Preferences for Customary Routine and Activities
- Section G: Functional Status
- Section H: Bladder and Bowel
- Section I: Active Disease Diagnosis
- Section J: Health Conditions
- Section K: Swallowing and Nutritional Conditions
- Section L: Oral and Dental Status
- Section M: Skin Conditions
- Section N: Medications
- Section O: Special Treatments and Procedures
- Section P: Restraints
- Section Q: Participation in Assessment and Goal Setting
- Section T: Therapy Supplement
- Section V: Care Area Assessment (CAA) Summary
- Section X: Correction Requested
- Section Z: Assessment Administration

Best practice model of care in subacute rehab:

- Physiatrist
- Case manager
- MDS coordinator
- Nursing
- Speech language pathologist
- Physical therapist
- Occupational therapist
- Nutritionist/dietician

- Wound nurse
- Psychology services (licensed mental health professional)
- Audiologist
- Optometrist
- Respiratory therapy
- Recreational therapy

Functional levels in MDS 3.0

- 0 = Independent
- 1 = Set up assistance
- 2 = Supervision
- 3 = Limited assistance, with weight bearing
- 4 = Extensive assistance, 1 person assist with patient performing part of the activity
- 5 = Extensive assistance, 2+ person assist with patient performing part of the activity
- 6 = Total dependence, 1 person assist with patient unable or unwilling to perform any part of the activity
- 7 = Total dependence, 2+ person assist with patient unable or unwilling to perform any part of the activity
- 8 = Activity did not occur

27.3.2.9   Basic Rules Governing Subacute Rehabilitation Facilities

1. *Three Midnight Hospital Stay Rule*[7,8]: The statutory requirement is that patients spend at least three consecutive days in a hospital as an inpatient in order to qualify for Medicare coverage of a subsequent stay in an SNF. This is different from the two-midnight standards for hospitals which are standards for physicians to apply in making inpatient admission decisions. If a physician believes a patient will require at least two midnights in the hospital, the physician should admit the patient to inpatient status; however, patients need three midnights as inpatients to qualify for Medicare coverage in an SNF.
2. The beneficiary is entitled to up to 100 days of skilled nursing coverage per spell of illness, and the beneficiary must have a daily skilled need. This does not mean that the beneficiary is guaranteed the 100 days, but that the subacute rehabilitation or skilled coverage is available for 100 days based on medical necessity. The beneficiary must have a *daily* rehabilitation and/or skilled need.

    The coverage is *per spell of illness*, and not per facility.
3. *30-Day Rule:* There is a 30-day grace period after discharge from the hospital to activate the insurance, for that spell of illness.
4. Medicare Part A does not cover long-term care. Medicaid or Veterans Administration (VA) benefits cover long-term care. However, the subacute or skilled facility can provide billable and reimbursable services to the patient under other insurance in long-term care under Medicare A if there is a new illness and a need; or if they get discharged out of Part A and go back to long-term care and have a daily need for Physical Therapy (PT), Occupational Therapy (OT), and Speech Language Pathology (SLP), and Nursing.

27.3.2.10   Reimbursement

From days 1 through 20, Medicare reimburses 100% of the RUG. From days 21 through 100, Medicare reimburses 80% of the RUG. Medicare calls the rest of the 20% a copayment and the beneficiary is responsible to pay this portion.

They may

1. Pay privately
2. Have the portion covered by Medicaid, which is state-level coverage

3. Use a supplemental plan (i.e., AARP)
4. Use a Medicare replacement insurance or Medicare replacement plan, which requires RUGs as well

27.3.3 OUTPATIENT REHABILITATION SERVICES

Outpatient rehabilitation can be provided in outpatient clinic areas.

27.3.3.1 Home Health

This is covered under Medicare Part A. In this setting, face-to-face physician visits are required within 90 days to establish medical necessity. Therapy, with PT, OT, and SLP, and skilled nursing in this setting are provided when medical necessity is determined, and if the patient is homebound only. Intermittent nursing or therapy is provided 7 days per week or 8 hours per day. Patients must have a support system to meet the needs of living at home and in the community.

27.3.3.2 Clinic, Hospital-Based, or Independent Outpatient Rehabilitation

This is covered under Medicare Part B and based on a physician's prescription of rehabilitation services to include physical therapy, occupational therapy, or speech language pathology, and conducts a periodical review of outcomes, progress, and goals. The patient must be able to get to the sites of therapy provided.

27.4 OUTCOMES BASED ON A SITE OF CARE

The effect of the site of care on rehabilitation outcomes still requires research and study, though it has been established that certain neurological conditions, particularly, stroke, are better treated in an interdisciplinary setting such as IRF, and with the multidisciplinary approach.[9] A study by the American Medical Rehabilitation Providers Association (AMRPA) concluded that IRF patients experienced an 8% lower mortality rate during the 2-year study period than SNF patients and 5% fewer emergency room visits per year, and for 5 of the 13 conditions, IRF patients experienced significantly fewer readmissions per year.[10]

REFERENCES

1. K. E. Covinsky, E. Pierluissi, and C. B. Johnston. Hospitalization-associated disability "She was probably able to ambulate, but I'm not sure". *JAMA*. 2011;306(16):1782–1793, doi:10.1001/jama.2011.1556.
2. B. Umans and K. L. Nonnemaker. Fact Sheet 149, January, 2009. AARP Public Policy Institute, Washington, DC, http://assets.aarp.org/rgcenter/health/fs149_medicare.pdf.
3. Brock J, Mitchell J, Irby K et al. Association between quality improvement for care transitions in communities and rehospitalizations among Medicare beneficiaries. *JAMA*. 2013;309(4):381–391.
4. https://www.cms.gov/Medicare/Quality-Initiatives-Patient-Assessment-Instruments/Post-Acute-Care-Quality-Initiatives/IMPACT-Act-of-2014-and-Cross-Setting-Measures.html.
5. http://www.ntocc.org/News/tabid/59/post/cms-proposes-new-discharge-planning-requirementsfor-hospitals/Default.aspx.
6. CMS's RAI Version 3.0 Manual.
7. 78 Fed. Reg. 50495, 50906-954 (August 19, 2013). CMA, Observation Status: New Final Rules from CMS Do Not Help Medicare Beneficiaries (Weekly Alert, August 29, 2013), http://www.medicareadvocacy.org/observation-status-new-final-rules-from-cms-do-not-help-medicare-beneficiaries/.
8. http://www.medicareadvocacy.org/new-cms-rules-do-not-change-requirement-for-3-day-qualifying-inpatient-hospital-stay/#_edn1.
9. P. Langhorne, J. Bernhardt, and G. Kwakkel. Stroke rehabilitation. *Lancet*. 2011;377(9778):1693–1702.
10. A. Dobson, J. E. DaVanzo, A. El-Gamil, J. W. Li, and N. Manolov. Assessment of Patient Outcomes of Rehabilitative Care Provided in Inpatient Rehabilitation Facilities (IRFs) and after Discharge. Prepared for ARA Research Institute. March 7, 2014.

28 Complementary and Alternative Medicine in Older Adults

B. Allyn Behling-Rosa

CONTENTS

28.1 BACKGROUND

This chapter is designed to review various geriatric topics within the field of rehabilitation as it pertains to the use of complementary and alternative medicine that may be helpful when optimizing function, or so as to delay neuropsychiatric or physiological degenerative processes. It is organized into issues of health and disabilities older adults face within the field of rehabilitation medicine.

Although the acronym "CAM" combines complementary and alternative medicine, distinguishing the two is important. Rossi et al. define CAM as "a wide range of pharmaceutical-type and nonpharmacological therapies that do not, on the whole, fall within the sphere of conventional medicine."[1] Complementary interventions are intended to supplement mainstream standards of care to control symptoms and bolster physical and emotional well-being throughout treatment, whereas alternative interventions are used in place of conventional ones.

It is important to note that the biologically based CAM practices and some forms of alternative medical systems are regulated under the Dietary Supplemental and Education Act of 1994, which defined dietary supplements as a product (other than tobacco) intended to supplement the diet for ingredients such as vitamins, minerals, herbs, or other botanicals, amino acids, and substances such as enzymes, organ tissues, glandulars, and metabolites.[2] This Act does not require purity, safety, or efficacy testing of supplements, nor may they claim treatment effects for specific disease processes via marketing or advertising.

In hopes to better define and regulate the above-mentioned interventions, the National Institutes of Health (NIH) set the definition of CAM as a group of diverse medical and healthcare systems, practices, and products that are not generally considered part of conventional medicine and practiced by holders of a medical doctorate and osteopathic medicine doctorate or allied health professionals, such as physical therapists, psychologists, and registered nurses. In 1998, the NIH's National Center for Complementary and Integrative Health (NCCIH, formerly the National Center for Complementary and Alternative Medicine [NCCAM]) revised its categorization of CAM therapies into the following:

- Natural products (i.e., herbal medicines, vitamins, minerals, and dietary supplements)
- Mind–body medicine (i.e., meditation, yoga, acupuncture, and Tai Chi)
- Manipulative and body-based practices (i.e., spinal manipulation and massage therapy)
- Movement therapies (i.e., Feldenkrais method, Alexander technique, and Pilates)
- Practices of traditional healers (i.e., Native American practices)
- Energy medicine (i.e., magnet therapy, light therapy, Reiki, and healing touch)
- Whole medical systems (i.e., traditional Chinese medicine, osteopathic medicine)

In 2007, Americans across all age groups spent a total of $22 billion out-of-pocket on CAM consumables (i.e., classes and products) and an additional $11.9 billion for visits to CAM practitioners. This equates to a total of 39.9 billion, or 11.2% of their out-of-pocket healthcare expenses.[3] Comprehensive studies have suggested that users of complementary and alternative therapies are primarily college-educated women, aged 35–49 years, who have annual incomes greater than $50,000 and live in the western section of the United States.[4,5] Further studies have indicated that users of CAM are characterized as having chronic health conditions and a holistic health orientation, and as being members of cultural groups that have a commitment to a personal growth psychology.[6]

As previously mentioned, most CAM research and epidemiology has been conducted in general adult populations aged 18–65 years, and there are even fewer studies focused on the safety and efficacy of these interventions in older adults. It is generally understood, however, that adjunctive therapeutic options among older persons have significantly increased over the last decade.[7] A small pilot study evaluating surveys from 60 individuals across three senior centers in 2004 reported 80% of elders using two or more complementary and/or alternative therapies. The most commonly used therapies (ranked in order of prevalence) used for staying healthy, and for pain and symptom management are acupuncture, hypnosis, yoga, homeopathy, touch therapies, and Tai Chi.[6] Another larger survey conducted in 2006 by the American Association of Retired Persons and the NCCIH reported that 54% of persons over 65 years of age had used some kind of CAM therapy or practice.[8]

Another relevant fact is that a large proportion of older adults do not consume well-balanced meals with sufficient amounts of many nutrients, and less than 50% of adults over the age of 51 meet the American Dietetic Association's estimated average requirement (EAR) for folate, vitamin E, and magnesium from food sources alone. Even after accounting for supplementation, their research notes that approximately only 80% met the EAR for vitamins A, B6, B12, C, and E; folate; iron; and zinc, but not magnesium.[9]

Many patients with chronic health conditions seek alternative and complementary therapies. The following pages summarize research studies that have positively supported the use of CAM modalities for various conditions and disease states in patients over the age of 65 years. Also noted are some noteworthy study results regarding individuals between 50 and 65 years of age. Again, this chapter is divided into sections of evidence issues common in rehabilitation of older adults.

28.2 WELLNESS AND QUALITY OF LIFE

Wellness can be defined as an overall feeling of well-being due to a healthy balance of mind, body, and spirit. How one perceives his or her well-being, or lack thereof, is called quality of life. The following section describes various evidence-based options to improve health, wellness, and components of one's quality of life.

28.2.1 NATURAL PRODUCTS

While it is true that many people cannot afford to pay more for quality food, many more of us can. Per Michael Pollan,[10] "…just in the last decade or two we've somehow found … spending more for better food is less a matter of ability than priority." Additionally, female sex, ethnicity, low income, and limited education contribute to nutritional inadequacy.[11] Furthermore, there are several other barriers to eating appropriate foods and supplements to support health and well-being: lack of sense of urgency, social and cultural symbolism, poor taste, and lack of information.[12]

28.2.1.1 Dietary Supplements and Nutritional Therapies

28.2.1.1.1 Probiotics
A double-blind randomized study of colorectal cancer survivors 56.18 ± 0.86 years old were supplemented probiotics twice daily for 12 weeks with a significant improvement in irritable bowel symptoms, fatigue- and colorectal cancer-related quality of life, and functional well-being scores.[13]

28.2.1.1.2 Eicosapentaenoic Acid
Nutritional interventions have shown increased subjective energy and less fatigue, but not improvement in quality of life or prognosis in nonsmall-cell lung cancer patients. A randomized prospective trial on supplementation with eicosapentaenoic acid (EPA) in 46 patients with advanced nonsmall-cell lung cancer on paclitaxel and cisplatin/carboplatin treatment showed that patients receiving the supplement gained lean body mass, as well as had decreases in fatigue, loss of appetite, and neuropathy.[14] However, there were no differences noted in response rate or overall survival, as compared to the control group.

28.2.1.2 Herbal Preparations

28.2.1.2.1 Ginkgo biloba
A recent study to evaluate the changes in glycemic index in older adults with type 2 diabetes mellitus using antioxidant *Ginkgo biloba* leaves dry extract, green tea dry extract, or placebo capsules after 9 and 18 months discovered that subjects perceived they suffered significantly less stress and had improved quality of life with the use of *Ginkgo biloba* extract, with no differences detected using the green tea extract or placebo.[15]

28.2.1.2.2 Cat's Claw (Uncaria tomentosa)
In 2014, a treatment regimen of a native Amazon plant that demonstrates anti-inflammatory and antitumoral properties was evaluated for symptom management in patients with advanced solid tumors. The prospective phase II study assessed the effects of a 300 mg daily dose of the extract in patients with mean age of 64 years with advanced solid tumors who had no further treatment options and a life expectancy of at least 2 months. Study results reported that although there was no tumor response detected, treatment improved the subjects overall quality of life and social functioning, and reduced fatigue.[16]

28.2.2 Mind–Body Medicine

Mind–body medicine is thought to use the power of thoughts and emotions to influence physical and mental health. The most well-known modalities of mind–body medicine are meditation, yoga, acupuncture, and Tai Chi.

28.2.2.1 Meditation

Meditation and other relaxation techniques have been shown by Shennen and colleagues in a recent study to significantly alleviate anxiety, depression, and stress, and even enhance immune function.[17]

Several years later, two meta-analyses found that various mindfulness-based stress-reduction techniques reduced depression, and alleviated anxiety and stress in breast cancer patients, which significantly improved their quality of life.[18,19]

28.2.2.2 Yoga

Originally developed in ancient India, yoga is characterized as a study of self-awareness through body poses, breath work, and meditation. In European and American cultures, yoga is practiced as a form of exercise and relaxation.[3] Although popular since the 1970s, it has recently shown promise as a beneficial therapeutic intervention targeting many lifestyle-related health conditions.

According to a community-based interventional study on menopausal women, regular practice of yoga at home for 35–40 min over 18 weeks improved physical, psychological, social, and environmental domains of quality of life after 6, 12, and 18 weeks of yoga therapy.[20]

In a study with chronic poststroke hemiparetic individuals participating in several weeks of guided yoga practice, subjects perceived significant improvements in quality of life associated with motor function and recovery, despite not having any significant improvements in objective motor function measures.[21] They also reported significant improvements in memory-related quality of life scores and clinically relevant decreases in anxiety.

28.2.2.3 Tai Chi

An ancient Chinese martial arts practice, Tai Chi is increasingly used as a form of conditioning exercise and has recently grown in popularity in the United States. It combines deep diaphragmatic breathing, relaxation, and slow, flowing movements.[22]

In 2004, a systematic review of literature demonstrated significant improvements in balance, strength, flexibility, cardiopulmonary function, mood, anxiety, self-efficacy, pain reduction, and health-related quality of life with the practice of Tai Chi.[23]

28.2.3 Manipulative and Body-Based Practices

Massage therapy is defined as the systematic manipulation of soft tissues, this is increasingly being integrated into several inpatient and outpatient management protocols.

A study by Munk et al. cited that massage is associated with self-reported fewer limitations due to physical or emotional issues, more energy, less fatigue, better social functioning, and better overall health.[24]

28.2.4 Movement Therapies

Physical function is an important predictor of health outcomes in older adults, and the ability to perform activities of daily living independently is intrinsic to their quality of life. However, it seems that exercise alone is insufficient to preserve physical function and thus maintain quality of life.[25] Although power training has been shown to be more effective than conventional resistance training for enhancing muscle power,[26] it has not been clear whether this translates into improvements in physical function that exceed those of resistance training,[27,28] which highlights the use of lengthening, or eccentric, contractions.

Prevention of physical disability among older adults has best been addressed by physical exercise, with guidelines generally recommending resistance and aerobic training.[29]

Research has also reported significant variability in the responsiveness of older adults to standardized training programs, with some regimens more effective than others when addressing specific age-related physical impairments that eventually lead to functional decline.[30]

To date, older adults' muscle strength has been shown to be preserved to a greater extent during eccentric contractions as compared to concentric muscle contractions[26]; eccentric contractions appear to allow the older person to train with greater relative intensity, and possibly greater cortical activation and thus neuromuscular adaptation.

28.2.5 ENERGY MEDICINE

28.2.5.1 Reiki

The Japanese Usui system of Reiki was developed to facilitate healing through the transfer of spiritual energy, or Qi, from the practitioner to the patient. It is often used to mitigate stress and reduce pain.

Unfortunately, a systematic review of trials in cancer patients had mixed results,[31] concluding that although Reiki seemed to improve a general sense of well-being, there was inconclusive evidence in its efficacy to relieve pain and anxiety.[32] Researchers ultimately believed that positive changes were likely due to the one-on-one support during disease interventions, regardless of whether Reiki or sham was used.[33]

28.2.6 WHOLE MEDICAL SYSTEMS

28.2.6.1 Kneipp Therapy

Considered a form of prevention and treatment and designed in 2007 by a Catholic priest nonprofessional medical practitioner Sebastian Kneipp, Kneipp therapy is a combination of hydrotherapy, herbal medicine, mind–body medicine, physical activities, and healthy eating.

A 2011 study assessed outcomes in four such German nursing homes with residents 83.2 ± 8.1 years, with caregivers indicating that residents had experienced superior health-related quality of life while receiving Kneipp therapy as part of daily routine care.[34]

28.2.6.2 Osteopathic Manipulative Medicine

Osteopathic physicians, referred to as Doctors of Osteopathic Medicine (DO), undergo the same education and residency training as allopathic physicians (MD), as well as must complete over 200 hours of additional training in manual diagnostic and treatment techniques known as Osteopathic Manipulation (OMT). OMT is specifically used to optimize, palliate, or prevent various autonomic, visceral, and neuromusculoskeletal somatic dysfunctions and conditions.

A pilot study of 21 Caucasian subjects with mean age 87 years (range 74–96 years) conducted by Snider et al. reported that twice monthly focused musculoskeletal physical examinations plus OMT or light touch protocols over 5 months reduced the number of hospitalizations and medication usage in elderly nursing home patients.[35]

Another interesting study, although not necessarily directly related to quality of life, retrospectively reviewed cost of care for over 1550 patients with acute low back pain who visited a Floridian hospital between 2002 and 2005. It reported that OMT patients had 18.5% fewer prescriptions written, 74.2% fewer radiographs, 76.9% fewer referrals, and 90% fewer magnetic resonance imaging scans.[36] Furthermore, total costs were $38.26 lower per patient, with average prescription costs $19.53 and radiologic costs $63.81 less on average.

28.3 NEUROCOGNITIVE ABNORMALITIES

Alzheimer disease and related dementia (ADRD) is the most common mental disorder diagnosed in older Americans, with over 5 million people affected in 2010.[43]

Recent data on the role of cardiovascular factors in the development of Alzheimer disease and other dementia states suggest that certain neurocognitive abnormalities may be preventable. Relative CAM interventions for neurocognitive abnormalities, which may prove beneficial, are discussed next.

28.3.1 NATURAL PRODUCTS

28.3.1.1 Diet

Neuroimaging and pathology studies have demonstrated that glucose intolerance, diabetes mellitus, hypertension, hyperlipidemia, and obesity contribute to not only vascular dementia but also to the risk of neurodegenerative dementia.[37]

28.3.1.1.1 Mediterranean Diet

This diet is characterized by a low intake of dairy products, meat, and saturated fatty acids, with regular modest intake of alcohol.

In a study of over 2200 New York older adults, the 4-year follow-up data associated the Mediterranean diet with a reduced risk of mild cognitive impairment and Alzheimer disease, such that cognitive dysfunction had a dose–response relationship to diet adherence, but not necessarily due to vascular mechanisms.[38]

These same researchers further demonstrated that adherence to the Mediterranean diet was protective against mild cognitive impairment in another long-term study of almost 1400 subjects after approximately 5 years.[39]

A third study by Feart and colleagues reported that close adherence to this diet was also associated with slower cognitive decline as measured by scores on the Mini-Mental State Examination (MMSE), although the actual incidence of Alzheimer disease was not reduced.[40]

28.3.1.1.2 Caloric Restriction

The effects of caloric restriction has been reviewed for its effects on cognitive performance over 3 months in a small study of 50 elderly individuals, specifically in those with normal or mildly overweight body habitus, as compared to control groups with unsaturated fatty acids supplementation versus a control diet.[41] The caloric restriction group exhibited not only reduced levels of fasting insulin and C-reactive protein, but also increased verbal memory scores, especially in those with the best adherence.

Attempts to replicate these results but in a younger patient population did not demonstrate any consistent patterns of changes in cognitive function.[42,43]

28.3.1.2 Dietary Supplements and Nutritional Therapies

Despite observational studies indicating that omega-3 fatty acids, antioxidants, B vitamins, and special diets may have a protective effect,[44] studies have been limited and results inconsistent, likely due to the complexity of nutritional and lifestyle-confounding variables.[45–47]

28.3.1.2.1 Melatonin

Numerous studies have shown decreased melatonin levels in the elderly as compared to subjects under age 30.[48] Moreover, chronic pain,[49] myocardial infarction,[50] and ischemic stroke[51] are also strongly associated with decreased melatonin levels. Melatonin deficiency is due to three potential factors: medications, age-related changes, and melatonin suppression from comorbid medical condition. Melatonin levels are profoundly decreased with use of beta-blockers[52] and nonsteroidal anti-inflammatories,[53] which are commonly used in the elderly.

These findings have led to multiple research studies investigating the beneficial effects of melatonin to treat several conditions. For instance, a 1998 study by Jean-Louis et al. noted improved memory recall and concentration without increased subjective fatigue, in mild cognitively impaired subjects taking melatonin 6 mg daily.[54]

28.3.1.2.2 Vitamin D

It is estimated that community-living older adults in the United States and Europe are generally malnourished, if not significantly deficient in vitamin D,[55] which has been shown to play an important role in neurogenesis, beta-amyloid clearance, and the expression of other neurotrophic factors.[56-58]

In the first prospective study on whether low levels of serum 25-hydroxyvitamin D was associated with cognitive decline, over 850 participants over the age of 65 years were followed over 6 years. It was noted that participants who were severely 25(OH)-D deficient were more likely than those sufficient to have substantial cognitive decline on the Mini Mental State Examination (MMSE).[59]

However, a systematic review conducted about the same time by Annweiler et al. found inconclusive evidence in the association between vitamin D and cognitive function.[60]

28.3.1.2.3 Vitamin E

Cognitive changes in almost 3000 subjects aged 65–102 years from the Chicago Health and Aging Project were measured at 6 months and 3 years by Morris et al. The study reported a 36% reduction in the rate of cognitive decline among persons in the highest quintile of total vitamin E intake, as compared to the lowest quintile in a model adjusted for age, race, sex, educational level, current smoking, alcohol consumption, total caloric intake, and total intakes of vitamins A and C and beta-carotene.[61]

28.3.1.3 Herbal Preparations

28.3.1.3.1 Ginkgo biloba *Leaf Extract*

A 2014 systematic review and meta-analysis of older adults with neuropsychiatric symptoms taking a daily dose of 240 mg *Gingkgo biloba* Leaf Extract revealed statistical significance in delaying decline in cognition and function, with improvements in behavior and global change. (However, the Alzheimer subgroup results were disappointing.)[62]

28.3.1.4 Japanese Medicine

Cholinesterase inhibitors are considered standard therapeutic agents for dementia, but because of limited benefits, they are often combined with other biologically active agents.

A traditional Japanese herbal medicine called Kami-Untan-To (KUT) is known to upregulate the expression of choline acetyltransferase as well as increase acetylcholine levels in mice.[63]

Between 2003 and 2005, Japanese researchers conducted an observer-blind, donepezil monotherapy controlled trial versus a combination of donepezil plus KUT for 12 weeks. Despite the small sample size and observation period, it appeared that the combination with KUT was more beneficial than donepezil alone when comparing posttreatment MMSE and Alzheimer Disease Assessment Scale-cognitive subscale scores.[64] Moreover, single-photon emission computed tomography demonstrated significant increases in regional cerebral blood flow within the KUT plus donepezil subjects.

28.3.1.5 Exercise

Several studies have provided insight into specific influences on cognitive decline, such as poor social connections with infrequent participation in social activities.[65]

Another study illustrated that a decrease in activity of more than 60 min per day over 10 years would result in a 1.8–3.5 times the 10-year cognitive decline rate than those who maintained activity.[66] This research is supportive of the fact that any activity or engagement that increases both the number of connections and the overall time spent in activity outside of a sedentary lifestyle may deter or slow the rate of cognitive decline.

28.3.1.6 Music Therapy

Music therapy has been informally used in residential care units to enhance communication, emotional, cognitive, and behavioral skills in older adults diagnosed with dementia.

A 2010 review reported that music therapy reduced levels of agitation in older people with dementia, as well as improved participants' mood and socialization skills.[67]

In another study, cognitively impaired psychiatric inpatients participated in an 8-week trial assigned to music therapy or control treatment. With MMSE used to assess cognition three times each week (prior to intervention, immediately after the intervention, and the morning following the intervention), it was discovered that the MMSE scores immediately after the intervention as well as the following day improved 2 to 3.69 points, respectively, as compared to the control group (but no subjects demonstrated retention of changes the following week).[68]

28.3.2 MANIPULATIVE AND BODY-BASED PRACTICES

Per a Cochrane Database review performed in 2006, very limited reliable evidence was available in favor of massage and touch interventions. However, hand massage was cited as a potential complement to other therapies for the management of short-term reduction of behavioral and agitation associated with dementia.[69]

A more recent study performed by Suzuki et al. in 2010 demonstrated that soft tactile massage performed 30 times over 6 weeks for 20 minutes prevented decline in "intellectual" and "emotional" function scores in elderly patients with severe dementia, as well as reduced chromogranin A (CgA, an indicator of stress) levels after 6 weeks.[70]

28.3.3 MOVEMENT THERAPIES: EXERCISE

Hamer and Chida explored the relationship between physical activity and neurodegenerative diseases in meta-analyses of prospective cohort studies published up until 2007. Results demonstrated that compared to the highest level of physical activity, subjects who had the lowest level, suffered a 72% relative risk for dementia and 55% relative risk for Alzheimer disease.[71]

28.3.4 ENERGY MEDICINE

28.3.4.1 Reiki

In 2010, a small empirical study of 24 patients by Crawford and colleagues[72] explored the efficacy of using Reiki therapy so as to improve posttest scores (prescores between 20 and 24) on the Annotated Mini-Mental State Examination (AMMSE) and Revised Memory and Behavior Problems Checklist (RMBPC) after four weekly sessions, as compared to a control group. This study was also interesting because 46% of its subjects were of American Indian descent. Results indicated statistically significant increases in mental functioning and memory and behavior problems.

However, some believe that positive changes from this aforementioned study was likely due to one-on-one support during interventions.[33]

28.3.4.2 Magnetic Therapy

A proof of concept study by Bentwich et al. utilized daily high-frequency repetitive transcranial magnetic stimulation (TMS) to six brain regions as an adjunct to cognitive training (total five sessions per week) for 6 weeks, followed by maintenance sessions twice weekly for an additional 3 months.[73] Endpoints were evaluated at 6 weeks and 4.5 months, and discovered an improvement of approximately 4 points on the Alzheimer Disease Assessment Scale-Cognitive (ADAS-cog) and 1.0 and 1.6 points, respectively, on the Clinical Global Impression of Change (CGIC).

28.4 PSYCHIATRIC ABNORMALITIES

Late-life psychiatric issues such as depression are challenging to treat due to the concern over polypharmacy, drug–drug interactions, and medication-related side effects to which the elderly are especially vulnerable. Fortunately, research conducted by Bassuk and colleagues in 1997 did not support the hypothesis that depressive symptoms were associated with the onset or the rate of cognitive decline among elderly persons.[74] Relative CAM interventions for psychiatric abnormalities, which may prove beneficial, are discussed below.

28.4.1 Dietary Supplements and Nutritional Therapies

28.4.1.1 Magnesium

A large questionnaire provided to over 5700 individuals 46–49 and 70–74 years old demonstrated a statistically significant inverse association between magnesium intake and standardized depression scores not confounded by age, gender, body habitus, or blood pressure.[75]

A smaller study in 2008 found that oral administration of 450 mg of elemental magnesium was just as efficacious as imipramine 50 mg in the treatment of newly diagnosed depression in the elderly with type 2 diabetes and hypomagnesemia.[76]

28.4.1.2 Melatonin

A large meta-analysis performed in 2004 suggested that melatonin had clinically insignificant benefit for sleep efficiency, but subjects with primary insomnia did benefit from over a 7-min improvement in sleep latency (onset). The same study also evaluated older adults with delayed sleep phase syndrome. These subjects did benefit more significantly from melatonin replacement, just over 38 min faster sleep onset.[77]

28.4.1.3 Herbal Preparations

28.4.1.3.1 St. John's Wort (Hypericum perforatum L.)

A recent meta-analysis[78] emphasized that despite generally positive evidence to support the use of St. John's wort for the treatment of depression, overall results have been mixed, especially when considering newer studies comparing the herbal therapy against serotonin-selective receptor inhibitors.[79]

28.4.2 Mind–Body Medicine

28.4.2.1 Meditation

Meditation therapy has been successfully used in prostate and breast cancer outpatients to help improve sleep.[80]

28.4.2.2 Tai Chi

Sleep disturbances are common in older adults. Li et al. evaluated whether Tai Chi would benefit individuals aged 60–92 years with moderate sleep disturbance into 1-hour thrice-weekly sessions of Tai Chi or low-impact exercise for 24 weeks. Tai Chi participants cited significant improvements in sleep quality, sleep-onset latency, sleep duration, sleep efficiency, and sleep disturbances, as well as cited improvements in general health-related quality of life and daytime sleepiness.[81]

Wang and colleagues reported significantly greater improvements in pain, physical function, depression, self-efficacy, and health status in those practicing Tai Chi as compared to control participants.[82]

28.4.2.3 Yoga

A recent trial by Taibi and Vitiello supports standardized evening yoga practice in middle-aged to older women as a potential treatment for OA-related insomnia, after participating in an 8-week yoga program, including 75-minute weekly classes and 20 minutes of nightly home practice.[83]

Another study conducted over a 6-month treatment period compared yoga (60-minute session 6 days a week, with a 15-minute evening session), Ayurvedic therapy, and a control group in 69 older adults. Participants noted a 1 hour of increased total sleep time relative to pretreatment, this improvement being significantly higher than changes in the control or Ayurveda groups.[84]

28.4.2.4 Acupressure

Acupressure is considered a noninvasive traditional Asian technique that involves stimulation of meridian or acupoints on the body via fingertips. Its objectives include stimulation of the body's immune system to self-heal, relief of muscular tension, and promotion of endorphin release. Another form of acupressure is auricular therapy, which involves pressure applied to acupoints via medicinal seeds, or magnets.[85,86]

A study performing acupressure therapy to institutionalized older adults elicited statistically significant improvements in both sleep quality and number of nocturnal awakenings relative to its two placebo arms (sham and conversation).[87]

Agitated behavior in patients with dementia has also been treated with acupressure, with one study noting reductions in several metrics of agitation within the acupressure arm relative to the control arm.[88]

Regarding auricular therapy, Suen et al. observed statistically significant improvements in sleep latency and sleep efficiency, and an overall increase of 35 minutes in total sleep time.[86] A follow-up study of the Suen et al. cohort demonstrated that insomnia symptoms remained ameliorated in the treatment group relative to the control groups.[85]

28.4.3 Manipulative and Body-Based Practices

28.4.3.1 Massage Therapy

One study examined the use of aromatherapy massage for hospice patients using self-report measures of sleep. This randomized, placebo-controlled study noted no benefits in quality of life or pain control; however, there were statistically significant improvements in sleep and depression.[89]

28.4.4 Energy Medicine

28.4.4.1 Light Therapy

Abnormal sleep patterns tend to be associated with disruption of circadian rhythms, with several reasons noted why older adults suffer an increased risk for circadian disruption: hypothalamic nuclei controlling the circadian rhythm are less active; older adults have reduced optical transmission at short wavelengths; and generally they lead more sedentary indoor lifestyles with less access to bright daylight.[90] To compound these issues, there is not always enough circadian stimulation from daylight inside residences, as light levels drop quickly just after 3–4 m away from a window, even on a sunny day.[91]

Royer et al. conducted a trial that demonstrated that the administration of hypothalamus-sensitive blue short-wavelength light to long-term-care elders for 30 minutes per day, Monday through Friday, for 4 weeks led to significant cognitive improvements compared to placebo.[90]

Evening light exposure has also been shown to be effective in consolidating awake versus sleep rhythms of those with Alzheimer dementia, and helping them to sleep better at night.[92,93]

Research conducted by Figueiro and colleagues also noted that short-wavelength blue light administered for 2 hours in the early evening was also shown to be effective in increasing sleep efficiency in older adults with Alzheimer dementia and related disorders.[94]

28.4.4.2 Magnet Therapy

Repetitive transcranial magnetic stimulation (rTMS) is a form of brain stimulation therapy that uses magnetic pulses instead of electricity to activate parts of the brain. Developed in 1985, rTMS has been studied as a possible therapy for depression, and has since been also applied for other neurological and psychological disorders.

A study with over 300 subjects by O'Reardon et al. demonstrated how daily prefrontal TMS was comparable if not superior to treatment with currently approved antidepressant medication treatments.[95] After such supportive results, the U.S. Food and Drug Association approved rTMS in 2008 as a treatment for patients with major depression who did not respond to antidepressants.

Follow-up studies by McDonald et al. in 2011 and Mantovani and colleagues in 2012 reported not only class I evidence of safety and efficacy of rTMS as drug-free monotherapy,[96] but also on the 3-month durability of TMS monotherapy antidepressant response with 58% classified as in remission and only 2% meeting criteria for relapse.[97]

The most recent research confirms that rTMS is a safe and effective adjunctive treatment to medications in elderly treatment-resistant depressed patients, as illustrated by over 58% having significant mood improvement, 50% having achieved remission, and over 41% having achieved partial response.[98]

Using a different type of magnetic therapy option, 60 participants over 60 years old who were suffering from sleep disturbances were treated with auricular therapy using magnetic pearls over 3 weeks, with significant improvements in nocturnal sleep time and sleep efficiency.[86]

Another small study on 15 older adults in Hong Kong demonstrated long-term effects of improved nocturnal sleep time and efficiency (quality and quantity) up to 6 months after 3 weeks of auricular therapy using magnetic pearls.[85]

28.5 CARDIOVASCULAR DISEASES

The frequency of CAM use by older adults with cardiovascular disease has been declining over the last decade.[99] According to one study of 235 subjects undergoing a phase 3 cardiac rehabilitation program (20% were aged 55–65 years and 76% were over 65 years), 67% admitted to taking vitamin or mineral supplements, and 38% took herbal or natural products.[100] According to this study, the most commonly used therapy was omega-3 products.

28.5.1 NATURAL PRODUCTS

28.5.1.1 Diet

28.5.1.1.1 High Fiber

Dietary fiber has been shown to reduce blood pressure, obesity, insulin resistance, and clotting factors—all independent risk factors for coronary heart disease.[101]

Additionally, an older meta-analysis of 67 controlled trials studying the cholesterol-lowering effect of four types of soluble fiber (oat, psyllium, pectin, and guar gum) reported small but significant reductions in total cholesterol and low-density lipoprotein (LDL).[102] It is thus recommended that older adults maintain a diet enriched by foods that provide a total of at least 5–10 g of soluble fiber daily.[103]

28.5.1.1.2 Low Fat

The prevalence of obesity among older adults has increased during the past 25 years. Along with the increased risk of cardiovascular disease, diabetes, and several cancers, obesity is associated with increased risk of physical and cognitive disability.[104]

Low-fat and extremely low-fat diets have been used successfully to treat established coronary artery disease[105] since the National Cholesterol Education Program issued their 2004 practice guidelines on the prevention and management of high cholesterol in adults recommending less than 7% of calories from saturated fat and less than 200 mg of dietary cholesterol daily.[106]

28.5.1.1.3 The Lyon Diet

The Lyon Diet Heart Study tested the effectiveness of a Mediterranean-type diet, modified by substitution of canola oil margarine for olive oil, with older subjects suffering 72% fewer cardiovascular events and 60% lower all-cause mortality.[107]

28.5.1.1.4 Indo-Mediterranean Diet

Findings from the Lyon Diet Study were reproduced using an Indo-Mediterranean diet, upon which older adults increased consumption of fruits, vegetables, nuts, whole grains, and mustard and soybean oils to reduce overall cardiovascular events by 45% and sudden cardiac death by 66%.[108]

28.5.1.1.5 DASH Diet

The Dietary Approaches to Stop Hypertension (DASH) study is also commonly recommended to older adults to reduce blood pressure via increased intake of fruit, vegetables, and low-fat dairy product consumption.[109]

28.5.1.2 Dietary Supplements and Nutritional Therapies

28.5.1.2.1 Stanols/Sterol Esters

Dietary modification to lower LDL-C cholesterol may be achieved by incorporating plant sterols and stanols, compounds that cannot be synthesized by humans and may only be obtained by dietary consumption.

Cater et al. performed three small studies[110] to determine whether a substantial reduction in LDL-C can be obtained in postmenopausal women with hypercholesterolemia. The results of study 1 determined that there was no difference in LDL-C concentrations among the 2, 3, and 4 g per day dosing of plant stanol ester; however, the 2 g per day dosing resulted in a 12% reduction in LDL-C. The results of study 2 showed that these esters significantly reduced LDL-C by 13%, with a 13% reduction in both non-high-density lipoprotein cholesterol (HDL-C) and apoprotein B (APO-B). Study 3 reported an additional 15% reduction in LDL-C as well as a decrease in C-reactive protein by 42%, as compared to placebo when added to men already receiving statin therapy. Thus, the National Cholesterol Expert Treatment Panel III currently recommends the consumption of 2 g of plant stanol/sterols daily to reduce LDL-C and cardiovascular risk.

28.5.1.2.1.1 *Nuts* Three of the largest studies evaluating multiple population groups, ages, races, and gender have found a consistent inverse relationship between nut consumption, especially walnuts and almonds, and coronary risk.[111–113]

28.5.1.2.1.2 *Caffeine* In the older cohort of the Rotterdam Study, an inverse association was demonstrated between tea drinking and advanced aortic atherosclerosis.[114] Data from a more recent follow-up of the Rotterdam Study highlighted a strong inverse relation between tea intake (greater than 375 mL/day) and myocardial infarction with the relation being stronger in women than in men.[115]

28.5.1.2.2   ʟ-Arginine

ʟ-Arginine is an amino acid substrate for nitric acid synthase (NOS), the enzyme that produces the vasodilator nitric oxide, which has been shown to reduce vascular stiffness.

A small study in 1997 demonstrated that ʟ-arginine improves exercise tolerance in patients with chronic stable angina by significantly increasing maximum workload in metabolic equivalent task (METs), as well as mean exercise time.[116]

Maxwell and colleagues also demonstrated that via ingestion of a nutrient bar (2 bars per day) containing 3.2 g of ʟ-arginine and a placebo bar containing 0.59 g of ʟ-arginine over 2 weeks, flow-mediated vasodilation, treadmill exercise time (20% increase over placebo), and quality of life scores improved significantly in stable class II/III angina patients.[117]

28.5.1.2.3   Beta-Carotene

A 2003 meta-analysis of eight trials evaluating beta-carotene in over 113,000 patients revealed a small but significant increase in all-cause mortality and cardiovascular death; thus supplementation is not recommended.[118]

28.5.1.2.4   Chelation

Chelation therapy has been used in the treatment of atherosclerotic cardiovascular disease consisting of a series of intravenous infusions containing disodium ethylene diamine tetraacetic acid (EDTA) in combination with vitamins.[2] Historically, EDTA has been effective in removing toxic heavy metals from the blood and is currently FDA-approved to treat heavy metal poisoning, but its application to treat coronary artery disease has not been approved.

Most evidence supporting the use of EDTA chelation therapy has not shown superiority to placebo, and is associated with considerable risks.[119]

A 5-year prospective study of subjects aged 50–72 years with a history of myocardial infarction were evaluated in regard to cardiovascular events or all-cause mortality after 40 infusions of EDTA chelation as compared to placebo. Only for the 31% of subjects that had diabetes mellitus did the EDTA infusions reduce the primary endpoints (death, reinfarction, stroke, coronary revascularization, or hospitalization for angina) 25% versus 38% placebo, with all-cause mortality also reduced 10% versus 16% placebo. The number needed to treat to reduce primary endpoint over 5 years was 6.5, with no reduction in cardiovascular events in nondiabetics, thus provides insufficient evidence to support the use of chelation therapy for the treatment of patients who have had a myocardial infarction.[120,121]

28.5.1.2.5   Coenzyme Q_{10}

Also known as ubiquinone, vitamin Q_{10}, or ubidecarenone, coenzyme Q_{10} (CoQ_{10}) acts as a free radical scavenger and membrane stabilizer.

There have been over 40 controlled trials on the clinical effects of CoQ_{10} on cardiovascular disease, a majority of which show benefit in subjective (quality of life, decrease in hospitalizations) and objective (increased left ventricular ejection fraction, stroke index) parameters.[2]

A 2008 study of 236 New York Heart Association (NYHA) class II heart failure patients with median age of 77 years demonstrated that plasma coenzyme Q_{10} levels was an independent predictor of mortality.[122]

A 2006 meta-analysis was conducted, which reported a 3.7% net improvement in ejection fraction in older patients with chronic heart failure who used CoQ_{10} supplementation versus placebo, and an even more profound improvement of 6.4% in those subjects who were not receiving angiotensin converting enzyme (ACE)-inhibitor therapy.[123]

28.5.1.2.6   Folic Acid/Folate

A meta-analysis of 14 prospective cohort studies found that elevated homocysteine levels moderately increased the risk of a first cardiovascular event, regardless of age and duration of follow-up.[124] Intake of folate, vitamin B6, and B12 are inversely related to homocysteine levels.

In 2002, the effects of folic acid supplementation on plasma homocysteine in individuals aged 65–75 years were supplemented 400 mcg or more over 6 weeks with significant lowering of homocysteine levels as compared to placebo; this study recommended that a daily folic acid intake of 926 mcg would be required to ensure that 95% of older adults population would be without cardiovascular risk from folate deficiency.[125]

A large study released in 2006 by Bonaa and colleagues of over 3700 subjects showed that although homocysteine levels were lowered by 27% in patients given 0.8 mg folic acid plus 0.4 mg vitamin B12 or 40 mg of vitamin B6, in the group given folic acid plus vitamins B12 and B6, there was actually a trend toward increased risk for recurrent myocardial infarction, stroke, and sudden death.[126]

A meta-analysis performed by Wang et al. in 2007 confirmed that folic acid supplementation can effectively reduce the risk of stroke in primary prevention via decreasing the concentration of homocysteine at least 18% over duration of more than 36 months.[127]

28.5.1.2.7   Magnesium

A recent meta-analysis of 20 randomized studies including both normotensive and hypertensive subjects detected a dose-dependent blood pressure reduction with magnesium supplementation.[128]

Another study with oral magnesium therapy (365 mg twice daily for 6 months) in 187 patients with coronary artery disease (CAD) demonstrated a 14% improvement in exercise duration combined with a decrease in exercise-induced chest pain compared to no change in the placebo group.[129]

A 2006 meta-analysis determined that magnesium supplementation for 4–16 weeks may be effective in reducing plasma fasting glucose levels and raising HDL cholesterol in adult patients with type 2 diabetes.[130]

Recent research by Barbagallo et al. reported that diabetic adults over the age of 65 years who had received over 368 mg/day of elemental magnesium had significant improvement in postischemic endothelial function.[131]

28.5.1.2.8   Melatonin

Research has demonstrated a mild reduction in blood pressure with physiologic doses of melatonin[132]; however, those subjects concomitantly taking nifedipine had a mean increase in systolic blood pressure of 6.5 mmHg and a diastolic blood pressure increase of 4.9 mmHg.[133] A larger review in 2004 confirmed these findings.[134]

28.5.1.2.9   Omega-3 Fatty Acids

The Gruppo Italiano per lo Studio della Sopravvivenza nell'Infarto Miocardico (GISSI) (Italian group for the study of the survival of Myocardial Infarction)-Prevenzione study from 1999 investigated the association of omega-3 fatty acid supplements (1 g/day) and coronary heart disease risk. The study effectively demonstrated total mortality reduction by 20% and sudden death by 45%.[135]

In 2008, the GISSI investigators further evaluated the addition of omega-3 fatty acids on atherothrombotic cardiovascular disease, including arrhythmias. More than 7000 chronic heart failure patients with NYHA class II and III were randomized to the fatty acids or placebo, while maintaining their regular traditional heart failure medications. Study findings observed modest cardiovascular benefits: 56 patients needed to be treated for a median duration of 3.9 years to avoid one death; or 44 patients to avoid one cardiac event like death, or an admission to the hospital.[136]

In the OMEGA-REMODEL study with 350 postmyocardial infarction subjects who received a daily 4 g dose of omega-3 fatty acids (Lovaza, GlaxoSmithKline) versus placebo over 6 months, MRI interpretation revealed a significant reduction in the left ventricular end systolic volume index and myocardial extracellular volume fraction (an estimation of how much fibrosis occurs following a heart attack). The study also showed a significant reduction in inflammatory biomarkers C-reactive protein, myeloperoxidase, and ST2 (marker of severity of adverse cardiac remodeling and fibrosis).[137]

28.5.1.2.10   Vitamin C

In the recent pooled analysis from the Pooling Project of Cohort Studies on Diet and Coronary Disease, those subjects with higher supplemental vitamin C intake (greater than 700 mg/day) had a 25% reduced risk of coronary heart disease.[138]

Nevertheless, the current consensus does not find a value for supplemental vitamin C in preventing heart disease.[139]

28.5.1.2.11   Vitamin E

Upon review of primary prevention trials, a lower coronary heart disease risk at higher intake of dietary vitamin E was present when adjusted for age and energy intake; however, supplemental vitamin E intake was found not to be significantly related to a reduced risk of coronary heart disease.[138]

A meta-analysis of seven randomized trials of vitamin E (50 units to 800 units) in 81,788 patients confirmed that vitamin E did not reduce mortality or decrease cardiovascular death or cerebrovascular accident.[118]

A 2009 trial that prospectively followed over 35,000 men with prostate cancer uncovered an increased risk for prostate cancer in those who consumed vitamin E,[140] with a follow-up study in 2011 confirming the same.[141]

28.5.1.3   Herbal Preparations

28.5.1.3.1   Chinese Medicine

Over a 100 patients over the age of 55 years were randomized into a standardized treatment group for coronary heart disease plus a Chinese medicine combination called Liandouqingmai Recipe, or a control group. After treatment for 14 days, physical limitation, angina stability, angina frequency, treatment satisfaction, and disease perception levels were significantly increased compared to controls.[142] Moreover, subject serum levels of IL-6, hs-C-reactive protein, and peripheral blood leukocytes were significantly lower as compared to control subjects.

28.5.1.3.2   Garlic

Garlic has recently been used by patients with hypercholesterolemia, with several studies including a meta-analysis review supporting a 5%–15% reduction in serum cholesterol, but whether this is significant is in question.[143–145] A follow-up study in 2000 by Superko et al. reported that garlic had no effect on major plasma lipoproteins and that it does not impact HDL subclasses, Lp(a), apolipoprotein B, postprandial triglycerides, or LDL subclass distribution.[146]

28.5.1.3.3   Ginkgo biloba Leaf Extract

Ginkgo leaf is obtained from the *Ginkgo biloba* tree with the mechanism of benefit unknown. *Gingko* does not appear to interact or adversely affect concomitant therapy with cardiac glycosides, and it appears to provide some benefit in the treatment of peripheral arterial disease.[2]

A study by Di Pierro in 2010 did not recommend the concomitant use of *Ginkgo* with aspirin, nonsteroidal anti-inflammatory drugs, anticoagulants, clotting factor, or platelet inhibitors due to increased antiplatelet effect and bleeding time.[147]

However, a recent meta-analysis review on over 1900 adults of which 87% had dementia, peripheral artery disease, or diabetes mellitus determined that there was no higher bleeding risk associated with standardized *Ginkgo biloba* extract.[148]

An earlier meta-analysis evaluated the safety of *Ginkgo* where several interventions for claudication remarked on modest improvements in pain-free walking distance, approximately 34 m, in study subjects taking *Ginkgo biloba* extract at doses of 120–160 mg a day over 24 weeks. Overall, this analysis showed that pain-free walking was statistically increased with *Ginkgo*, although whether these improvements are clinically significant is unclear.[149]

Garder et al. evaluated the effects of *Gingko biloba* on treadmill walking time several years later, and again noted an increase in walking time by 40% in the *Ginkgo* group and by 10% in the placebo group, without adverse effects.[150]

28.5.1.3.4   Ginseng

Ginseng has been traditionally used by Koreans to revitalize the body and mind, increase physical strength, prevent aging, and increase vigor. Ginseng is commonly used by older adults with cardiovascular risk factors such as hypertension, hypercholesterolemia, and oxidative damage.

Research on the use of ginseng has demonstrated effects of vasodilation to improve blood circulation as well as to reduce systolic blood pressure at lower doses.[151]

Ginseng has also been observed to improve arterial stiffness in subjects with hypertension via its vasomotor effects.[152,153]

Recent research on red ginseng identifies improvements in coronary flow reserve,[154] as well as inhibition of platelet aggregation and coagulation activity.[155]

28.5.1.3.5   Hawthorn Berry (Crataegus) Extract

The medicinal properties of the antioxidant hawthorn berry have been used by many cultures for several indications. Recent research has focused on the use in congestive heart failure, hypertension, and ischemic heart disease due to its inotropic effects and as a peripheral vasodilator so as to increase myocardial perfusion and stroke volume and reduce afterload.

In Germany, hawthorn can be prescribed for "mild cardiac insufficiency."[2] Despite inconsistent preparation concentrations and dosages, trials have been consistent with regard to positive outcomes.

A 2003 meta-analysis undertaken by Pittler et al. showed definite benefits in the treatment of congestive heart failure over placebo.[156] Compared to digoxin in mild heart failure, hawthorn has a wider therapeutic range, lower risk in toxicity, and less of an arrhythmogenic potential; is safer to use in renal insufficiency; and can be safely used with diuretics and laxatives.[157]

In 2004, a study by Habs noted that fewer patients in the hawthorn extract cohort required orthodox medications such as ACE inhibitors, cardiac glycosides, diuretics, and beta-blockers than in the comparative cohort.[158]

These findings were replicated by Zick et al. in 2008 with regard to the reduced need for diuretic medications in the hawthorn cohort.[159] The last study available for review was published in 2009 by Zick and colleagues who noted that hawthorn seemed to provide no symptomatic or functional benefits when given with standard medical therapy to patients with NYHA class II and III, except for a modest improvement in left ventricular ejection fraction.[160] Still, several clinical points must be considered: hawthorn can significantly enhance the activity of digoxin, and close monitoring is necessary when combining it with beta-blockers and class III antiarrhythmics.[161]

28.5.1.3.6   Horse Chestnut (Aesculus hippocastanum) Seed Extract

Also known as buckeye or Spanish chestnut, horse chestnut seed extract has traditionally been used as a remedy for hemorrhoids and to treat chronic venous insufficiency in those without renal insufficiency or hepatic impairment.[162]

The German Commission E has approved the use of horse chestnut seed extract in chronic venous insufficiency.[2]

A 1998 systematic review on over 1000 subjects demonstrated improvements in lower extremity edema at the calf and ankle secondary to chronic venous insufficiency comparable to compression stockings.[163] Symptoms such as leg pain, pruritus, fatigue, and tenseness were also reduced.

M.H. Pittler and E. Ernst identified 14 trials consisting of over 1500 patients with chronic venous insufficiency undergoing treatments with horse chestnut seed extract. As compared to placebo, administration of oral preparations was associated with improvements in edema, pruritus, and reductions in ankle and calf circumference and leg volume, as well as a significant reduction in leg pain.[164]

28.5.1.3.7 Red Yeast Rice (Monascus purpureus)

Red yeast rice is a fermentation product of a mixture of several species of *Monascus* fungi that grow on rice containing 3-hydroxyl-3-methyl-glutaryl (HMG)-CoA reductase-inhibiting compounds that is currently used to reduce cholesterol levels.

Li and colleagues demonstrated how red yeast rice extract (600 mg twice daily, lovastatin equivalent 5–6 mg/day) for 4.5 years in over 1500 subjects 60 years of age and older with hypertension and a previous heart attack reduced incidence of coronary heart disease events, nonfatal myocardial infarction, and all-cause mortality. Unfortunately, the results did not report statistically significant improvement in stroke or cardiac revascularization, as compared to placebo.[165]

A 2011 prospective study was performed in 80 adult subjects over 75 years of age that were statin-intolerant and were refusing other hypercholesterolemic agents. They were randomized to either a nutraceutical-combination pill containing berberine 500 mg, policosanol 10 mg, red yeast rice 200 mg, folic acid 0.2 mg, CoQ_{10} 2.0 mg, and astaxanthin 0.5 mg, or a placebo over 12 months of treatment. Results on the use of red yeast rice included a well-tolerated reduction of 20% of total cholesterolemia, 31% of LDL levels, and 10% of insulin resistance as compared to placebo.[166]

A year later, a systematic review of 22 randomized controlled trials (RCTs) (N = 6520), primarily conducted in China using 600–2400 mg red yeast rice extract daily (lovastatin content 5–20 mg), assessed outcomes in patients with known Coronary heart disease (CHD) and dyslipidemia and found significant reductions in coronary heart disease mortality, incidence of myocardial infarctions, and revascularization compared to placebo, but not when compared to statin therapy.[167]

28.5.2 MIND–BODY MEDICINE

Acute arousal leads to sympathetic nervous system stimulation with activation of excessive cortisol, epinephrine, and aldosterone. When arousal is maintained for long periods of time, the elevation in blood pressure remains even if the inciting stimulus is removed. At this stage, the hypertension is not sustained by increased cardiac output but by increased vascular resistance secondary to increased cardiac output and vasoconstriction.[2]

Feelings of frustration, exhaustion, and helplessness can also activate the pituitary and adrenocortical hormones. Fortunately, studies observing the effects of nonpharmacological treatments to manage stress such as meditation, acupuncture, biofeedback, and music therapy have been found to be effective in decreasing blood pressure and the development of hypertension.[168]

28.5.3 MUSIC THERAPY

In the older adults (mean age 83 years) suffering from moderate to severe dementia, systolic blood pressure measurements were significantly lower in participants of a 2-year research study of group music therapy carried out once weekly. Moreover, physical and mental states of those music therapy group participants during the 2 years were maintained better than nonmusic therapy group members.[169]

28.5.4 MOVEMENT THERAPIES

28.5.4.1 Cardiac Rehabilitation Exercise

Benefits of regular exercise for older adults are well documented and include improved cardiopulmonary function, lowered blood pressure, increased bone mineral content, increased muscle strength and energy, joint flexibility, as well as enhanced motivation and confidence in the ability to perform activities of daily living.[170] Thus, studies were performed to evaluate older coronary artery disease patients after outpatient cardiac rehabilitation.

The most significant study demonstrated statistically greater improvements in function and quality of life scores as compared to patients less than 55 years (27% vs. 20%, 20% vs. 14%, respectively), but not as much benefit in aerobic and anaerobic thresholds (32% vs. 44%, 13% vs. 18%, respectively).[171]

In a large study by the Ochner Heart and Vascular Institute, marked benefits of formal inpatient phase II cardiac rehabilitation and exercise training programs in coronary artery disease patients over 75 years of age, especially women, showed benefits on plasma lipids, obesity indices, exercise capacity, peak oxygen consumption, depression, and quality of life.[172] There has since been support by cardiologists and cardiac rehabilitation specialists to follow basic exercise prescription recommendations provided by Lavie and colleagues consisting of dynamic or aerobic exercise performed at 65%–85% of maximal heart rate intensity, for a duration of 20–30 minutes per day (40–50 minutes for obese patients) at a frequency of 3–5 exercise sessions per week.[173]

28.5.4.2 Isometric Exercise

Recent meta-analyses report that isometric or resistance exercise does not significantly lower or raise resting blood pressure, but it has been shown to improve cardiac performance during daily activities of living (which often involve isometric exercises, i.e., carrying groceries, taking the garbage out, moving a nonrolling assistive device).[173] Thus, light isometrics such as hand grips and light weight lifting has been proven safe and essential to prevent muscle mass and bone density decline in older patients, and should be recommended to hypertensive patient as part of a comprehensive treatment regimen.[174]

A large, longitudinal population study of over 142,000 subjects 35–70 years of age performed across 17 countries over 4 years referred to as the Prospective Urban–Rural Epidemiology (PURE) study illustrated that grip strength was inversely related with all-cause mortality, cardiovascular mortality, noncardiovascular mortality, myocardial infarction, and stroke. Moreover, grip strength was considered a stronger predictor of all-cause and cardiovascular mortality than systolic blood pressure.[175]

28.6 PULMONARY DISEASE

28.6.1 NATURAL PRODUCTS

Lung cancer accounts for about 27% of all cancer deaths, and is by far the leading cause of cancer death among both men and women, with two out of three people diagnosed with lung cancer over the age of 65 years.[176] Of course, it is well known that the primary cause of lung cancer is exposure to tobacco smoking, but even prior to that, smokers are subject to a higher risk of developing chronic respiratory diseases.

Chronic lower respiratory diseases have been the third leading cause of death since 2008 in the United States, with the most common condition being chronic obstructive pulmonary disease (COPD). COPD is characterized by incompletely reversible limitation in airflow. A physiological variable—the forced expiratory volume in one second (FEV1)—is often used to grade the severity of COPD. However, patients with COPD also manifest other signs and symptoms not reflected by the FEV1 endpoint. Moreover, as immune and musculoskeletal function becomes impaired with age, pulmonary endpoints are made even less reliable as markers of capacity due to concomitant chronic conditions of atelectasis, recurrent pulmonary infections, or aspiration pneumonitis.

Researchers have since recognized that in adults over the age of 70 years, the association that as COPD progresses with its dyspnea, fatigue, inactivity, deconditioning, and aging, individuals are subject to a higher mortality rate, as well as increased disability, social restriction, and depression.[177] Thus, as rehabilitation specialists, we are obligated to at least consider other potential options to optimize these patients' health and function.

28.6.1.1 Dietary Supplements and Nutritional Therapies

Patients with COPD are also at high risk of malnourishment due to weight loss, muscle and fat mass depletion, which has been associated with respiratory dysfunction, and exercise tolerance and endurance.[178]

In a study of older Chinese adults over 55 years, daily antioxidant supplementation with omega-3, vitamins A, C, and E, and dietary fish intake of at least three times weekly were individually associated with improvements in forced expiratory volume in the first second.[179] Until recently, no research has demonstrated how oral nutritional supplementation may affect readmission risk.

A retrospective study of over 10,300 hospitalizations revealed that using instrumental variables analysis, oral nutritional supplementation during hospitalization for COPD cases was associated with a 1.9 day (21.5%) decrease in length of stay, a hospitalization cost reduction of $1570 (12.5%), and a 13.1% decrease in probability of a 30-day readmission.[180]

28.6.2 Mind–Body Medicine

28.6.2.1 Meditation

According to a recent systematic review and meta-analysis by Faver-Vetergaard et al., when analyzing individual intervention types, cognitive behavioral therapy appeared to be effective for improving psychological outcomes in patients suffering from COPD, whereas for physical outcomes, only mind–body interventions such as mindfulness-based therapy, yoga, and relaxation revealed statistically significant effects.[181]

28.6.2.2 Acupuncture

Acupuncture is a traditional Chinese practice of inserting small-gauge needles superficially into the skin along "meridians" located throughout the body so as to manipulate the circulation of one's energy, or "Qi."

A 1995 meta-analysis of the use of acupuncture in bronchial asthma, chronic bronchitis, and chronic disabling breathlessness cited no significant difference between sham and acupuncture treatments on subjects, but still with significant improvements in baseline symptoms, as well as having greater response to pharmacologic interventions allowing over 90% reduction in medication dosing.[182]

There are currently several other studies being conducted and/or systematically reviewing literature on the efficacy and safety of acupuncture in patients with COPD, emphysema, and asthma, with results not yet published.[183]

28.6.2.3 Yoga

A systematic review and meta-analysis was performed in 2014 regarding the effects of yoga training in 233 patients (mean age approximately 50 years) with COPD. The limited evidence suggested that yoga training had a positive effect on improving lung function and exercise capacity, and could be used as an adjunct to pulmonary rehabilitation.[184]

28.6.3 Manipulative and Body-Based Practices

28.6.3.1 Massage Therapy

A systematic review of databases up through 2010 for manual interventions such as massage, muscle stretching, and passive range of motion revealed poor evidence for performance-based measures of pulmonary function as an adjunctive management approach for COPD patients.[185]

28.6.4 Movement Therapies

28.6.4.1 Exercise

A meta-analysis using a total of 65 randomized control trials involving 3822 participants with chronic COPD subjects found statistically significant improvement after at least 4 weeks of exercise training with or without education and/or psychological support, including functional exercise and maximal exercise capacity, Chronic Respiratory Questionnaire scores for dyspnea, fatigue, and patients' control over disease.[186]

28.6.5 WHOLE MEDICAL SYSTEMS

28.6.5.1 Osteopathic Manipulative Medicine

A small study by Noll et al. reported that elderly hospitalized patients for pneumonia had a significantly shorter duration of intravenous antibiotic treatment and a shorter hospital stay, as compared to a control group who received light touch protocol.[187]

Noll further assessed these findings in a much larger study—the Multicenter Osteopathic Pneumonia Study in the older adults (MOPSE)—which evaluated over 400 subjects over 50 years of age hospitalized with pneumonia and the effects of conventional treatment, versus light touch or OMT for 15 minutes twice daily until discharge plus conventional treatment.

Although intention-to-treat analysis found no significant differences between the groups, per protocol analysis, researchers did find a significant difference of reduce length of stay, duration of intravenous antibiotics, death, and respiratory failure rates in the OMT group versus the convention care group.[188]

Nevertheless, in a 2010 United Kingdom evidence report, Bronfort et al. concluded that there was *inconclusive evidence for the effectiveness of manual therapy in the treatment of acute pneumonia in older hospitalized patients.*[189]

28.7 GENITOURINARY SYSTEM ABNORMALITIES

Benign prostatic hyperplasia (BPH) and prostatic inflammation affect the male quality of life secondary to obstructive and irritating lower urinary tract symptoms such as urinary hesitation, frequency, and urgency. Over the years, studies have compared therapeutic drugs versus placebo, and occasionally versus other drug classes, but there have been few studies comparing various drugs with natural products. BPH has been largely an issue of older adults, and now with increased popularity in using herbal supplements for its treatment, it is now even more appropriate to conduct these comparative studies.

28.7.1 NATURAL PRODUCTS

28.7.1.1 Herbal Preparations

28.7.1.1.1 Cernilton

In 2007, a randomized multicenter clinical trial of over 900 BPH patients was conducted from September 2002 to December 2003 across seven therapeutic drug groups, including selective adrenoceptor antagonist (terazosin, doxazosin, tamsulosin, naftopidil), 5-alpha-reductase inhibitor (finasteride, epristeride), and natural product (cernilton, prepared from *Secale cereale* [rye] pollen). According to baseline, at average follow-up of 6 months, no difference in the International Prostate Symptom Score was noted across the therapeutic intervention groups. However, prostatic volume and transitional zone volume were significantly decreased in the 5-alpha-reductase inhibitor group, and more significant symptomatic improvements were noted in the cernilton, doxazosin, and naftopidil groups.[190]

Despite trials limited by several design flaws, a Cochrane systematic review in 2012 of patient use of cernilton demonstrated modest improvements in overall urologic symptoms, including nocturia, but did not improve urinary flow rates, residual volume, or prostate size compared to placebo or comparative study agents.[191]

28.7.1.1.2 Chinese Herbal Medicine

A Chinese herbal combination called Kangquan Recipe was provided to over 50 cases of older adults with BPH, versus a control group, which was given cernilton daily for 24 weeks. After the completion of the study, the International Prostate Scoring System (IPSS) in the treatment group significantly improved compared to the control group, with maximum flow rate and average flow rates also improved. Moreover, residual urine volume and total prostatic volume in the treatment group were significantly lower, as compared with the control group.[192]

28.7.1.1.3   Prostamev Plus

A comparative study between the use of saw palmetto versus a trademarked herbal preparation of Bromeline plus Nettle, in addition to antibiotic treatment with levofloxacin for prostatitis and concurrent prostatic inflammation determined that the groups treated with Prostamev Plus achieved better improvements in the IPSS, as well as urinary flow and sexual life (in relation to erectile dysfunction).[193]

28.8   GASTROINTESTINAL DISORDERS

The prevalence of chronic gastrointestinal symptoms and the irritable bowel syndrome (IBS) in the elderly was largely unknown until 1992 when Talley and colleagues[194] evaluated responses from a mail questionnaire from age- and sex-stratified Minnesota residents aged 65–93 years. Prevalence of frequent abdominal pain was 24.3%, chronic constipation 24.1%, chronic diarrhea 14.2%, fecal incontinence more than once per week 3.7%, and symptoms compatible with IBS (greater than or equal to 3 Manning criteria) 10.9%. Furthermore, only 23% had seen a physician for pain or fecal disturbances in the prior year.

Other studies have noted that the prevalence of gastroesophageal reflux disease (GERD) increases with age, with the elderly more likely to develop severe disease. However, older patients tend to complain less due to their presentation of atypical and non-specific symptoms such as dysphagia, weight loss, or extra-esophageal symptoms.[195]

28.8.1   Natural Products

28.8.1.1   Dietary Supplements and Nutritional Therapies

Increasingly, older patients suffering from functional gastrointestinal disorders are seeking alternative treatment options. Probiotics such as *Lactobacillus* and *Bifidobacterium* have demonstrated improved symptom management in IBS.[196]

28.8.1.2   Herbal Preparations

In a 1998 meta-analysis, fixed-dose peppermint oil has been shown to improve abdominal pain, abdominal distention, and flatulence in IBS.[197]

Single-herb and fixed-dose combination herbal therapies with peppermint and/or caraway seed oil have noted improved abdominal pain, abdominal distention, and flatulence in IBS and functional dyspepsia.[198]

Artichoke leaf extract has also shown potential benefits in a placebo-controlled trial for functional dyspepsia.[199]

A postmarketing study also found significant improvements in IBS-related symptoms.[200]

28.8.2   Mind–Body Medicine

28.8.2.1   Electroacupuncture

In a 2008 double-blind, crossover study in 27 functional dyspepsia subjects, electroacupuncture at points ST36 and PC6 twice weekly for 2 weeks reduced dyspepsia symptoms by 55%, with an increase in vagal activity assessed via heart rate and plasma level of neuropeptide Y.[201]

28.8.2.2   Manual Acupuncture

In a 2009 controlled study with 68 functional dyspepsia participants, Part et al. illustrated significant improvements in dyspeptic symptoms in comparison with acupuncture at nonacupoints.[202]

28.8.2.3 Psychotherapy

A systematic review of 17 studies regarding the efficacy of cognitive behavioral therapy on functional gastrointestinal disorders such as IBS has demonstrated nearly a 50% reduction in symptoms, and a number needed to treat two subjects.[203]

28.8.2.4 Hypnotherapy

There is also compelling evidence that hypnotherapy is an effective treatment for IBS, with effects that are long-lasting contributing to decreased medical consultation and medication needs in the long term.[204]

28.8.3 WHOLE MEDICAL SYSTEMS

28.8.3.1 Osteopathic Manipulative Medicine

A total of 30 osteopathic-manipulation naïve patients who met Rome II criteria for IBS and presented with IBS symptoms more than 25% of the time received two standardized 60-min sessions of OMT or sham treatment provided at a 7-day interval. Follow-up data were collected from both participant groups, and illustrated statistically significant reduction in quality of life and IBS severity scores on Day 7 for the OMT group, as compared to the control group; however, no significant differences were noted on the 28-day follow-up evaluation. Also noted were equal reductions in depression and anxiety scores for the two groups, but unchanged stool frequency and consistency.[205]

In 2010, a small nonrandomized study of six middle-aged participants with chronic constipation was evaluated after having received semistandardized osteopathic manipulative treatments six times over a 4-week period.[206] Following this period, a significant improvement in the severity of their constipation, overall symptoms and quality of life, and colonic transit times were recorded.

In 15 patients with severe dementia and dysphagia, Bautmans et al. noted significant improvement in swallowing capacity, without adverse effects, after trained physical therapists performed one session of cervical spine mobilization similar to osteopathic-style methods, versus a control group of socializing visits.[207]

28.9 DISEASES OF MUSCULOSKELETAL SYSTEM

Among the most common and disabling medical disorders experienced by adults over 65 years are musculoskeletal impairments.[208] The most common complaints involve arthritic changes and increasing incidence of muscle weakness and restricted range of motion in the hip, knee, shoulder, ankle, and limbs.[209] In 2007, older adults used CAM most often to treat back pain (17.1%), neck pain (5.9%), joint pain or stiffness (5.2%), arthritis (3.5%), and other musculoskeletal conditions (1.8%).[3]

28.9.1 NATURAL PRODUCTS

28.9.1.1 Dietary Supplements and Nutritional Therapies

28.9.1.1.1 Coenzyme Q_{10}

While data suggest serum coenzyme Q_{10} levels are reduced at moderate doses of statin, there is little evidence to suggest that muscle coenzyme Q_{10} levels are reduced. The conclusion of this review is that there is a general lack of consistency with respect to the efficacy of coenzyme Q_{10} in clinical trials and its role in statin-associated myopathy.[210]

28.9.1.1.2 Magnesium

Over 2000 Caucasian male and female adults aged 70–79 years enrolled in the Health, Aging and Body Composition Study were observed to have their increased bone mineral density significantly associated with a greater magnesium intake.[211]

28.9.1.1.3   Methylsulfonylmethane

Methylsulfonylmethane (MSM) can be synthesized commercially, and it is also naturally present in the human body as it is metabolized from ingested dimethylsulfoxide (DMSO). Many properties have been attributed to MSM, including chemopreventative properties, anti-inflammatory activities, antiatherosclerotic action, prostacyclin synthesis inhibition, and free radical scavenging activity.[212]

After reviewing data from several other supporting studies, Debbi et al. designed a small randomized study to evaluate the efficacy and safety of MSM in treating osteoarthritis of the knee at a dosage of 1.125 g three times daily for 12 weeks, versus placebo. Mean age of patients receiving the MSM were 67 ± 9.8 years. Study results concluded that there were significant improvements in physical function from baseline to 12-week endpoint, as well as a decrease in total symptoms by 20%, pain by 21%, and stiffness by 26% in the MSM group (with an increase of 14%, 9%, and 37%, respectively, in the placebo group).[212]

28.9.2   Mind–Body Medicine

28.9.2.1   Acupuncture

Acupuncture is used by approximately 1% of people with osteoarthritis, but most who seek acupuncture do not use it specifically for treating their arthritis.[213] According to acupuncture theory, one indication that acupuncture is exerting its analgesic effects is that numbness or paresthesias are induced at the needle insertion site. It is postulated that needle placement stimulates the release of several neurotransmitters, particularly endogenous opioid peptides, which are directly involved in the suppression of pain.[214] Animal studies have further implicated adenosine A1-receptor mediation of pain suppression as well.[215]

The 2011 Cochrane review of acupuncture (16 trials, 3498 participants) in osteoarthritis of the knee and hip demonstrated neither inferiority nor superiority of treatment effect in patients with osteoarthritis. The studies indicated that at 4 weeks postprocedure, pooled benefits of acupuncture against sham controls, although statistically significant, were not clinically relevant, and the studies that used nonsham controls demonstrated more significant clinical relevance. Moreover, at the 6-month follow-up visit, acupuncture demonstrated borderline statistical significance, again with clinically irrelevant improvements in osteoarthritis pain in the knee or hip, or in function, which did not improve even when acupuncture was provided as an adjuvant therapy to an exercise-based physical therapy program.[216] All in all, the Cochrane review authors determined that benefits were likely attributable to a placebo effect due to incomplete blinding.

A study published in 2014 removing design bias regarding the application of acupuncture or other complementary therapies reported that over 280 patients with chronic knee pain had clinically modest and statistically significant improvement in pain for the needle and laser acupuncture groups, as compared to the usual care group. This study also showed that those administered needle acupuncture reported significantly greater improvements in physical functioning and pain on walking and standing at 12 weeks compared to the usual care group. However, secondary analysis comparing needle and laser acupuncture versus sham techniques found no significant differences between groups in any of the outcomes at 12 weeks and at 1 year.[217]

Fewer trials have addressed the use of acupuncture in rheumatoid arthritis. In a systematic review of eight available studies in which 536 participants were treated, six studies reported a decrease in pain attributable to acupuncture compared with controls. However, despite these favorable results, evidence regarding efficacy of acupuncture for rheumatoid arthritis is overall conflicting between the currently available placebo-controlled trials.[218]

28.9.2.2   Tai Chi

In another trial with older patients with chronic symptomatic hip and knee OA, Fransen and colleagues found that both Tai Chi and hydrotherapy classes provided large and sustained improvements in physical function after 12 weeks that were sustained at 24 weeks, as compared to the control group.[219]

In a study by Brismee et al., elderly subjects with knee OA participated in a 6-week Tai Chi program followed by 6 weeks of home Tai Chi practice demonstrated significant improvement in knee pain and physical function compared with an attention control.[220]

Hartman et al. evaluated community-dwelling older adults and the participation in regular activities versus 12 weeks of Tai Chi, which reported a significant improvement in arthritis symptoms, self-efficacy, level of tension, and satisfaction with general health status.[221]

In another study, Song and colleagues reported that older women subjects with OA performing Tai Chi over 12 weeks perceived significantly less pain and stiffness than those receiving routine care; in addition, their physical functioning, balance, and abdominal muscle strength were also significantly improved.[222]

28.9.3   MANIPULATIVE AND BODY-BASED PRACTICES

28.9.3.1   Massage Therapy

In 2010, Munk and colleagues demonstrated that massage could be an effective intervention for persistent pain relief in adults over 60 years.[24]

Research by Perlman and colleagues evaluating Swedish massage in the treatment of knee OA biweekly for 4 weeks, and then for an additional 4 weeks demonstrated significant improvements in pain, stiffness, physical functional disability domains, and visual analog scale as compared to usual care.[223]

Unfortunately, 2012 survey of research in the last decade did not demonstrate significant efficacy or cost-effectiveness of massage for fibromyalgia, or osteoarthritis of the knee and other joints.[3]

On the other hand, the Ottawa Panel systematic review was able to show that, in general, massage interventions were effective in providing short-term improvements in subacute and chronic low back pain symptoms, as well as decreasing disability immediately and 2 weeks posttreatment, when combined with therapeutic exercise and education.[224]

28.9.4   ENERGY MEDICINE

28.9.4.1   Magnetic Therapy

A small study of 15 women aged 60–70 years were administered pulsed electromagnetic therapy administered at a frequency of 33 Hz and an intensity of 50 gauss for 50 minutes per session, three sessions per week over 3 months. As compared to a control group of 15 women, they demonstrated equivalent improvements in bone mineral density in the neck of the femur and the lumbar spine (L3–L5), as measured by dual-energy x-ray absorptiometry.[225]

28.9.5   WHOLE MEDICAL SYSTEMS

28.9.5.1   Osteopathic Manipulative Medicine

A high-quality trial reported significantly greater improvement in primary outcome measures (Extended Aberdeen Spine Pain Scale) when three sessions of osteopathic manipulation were performed in addition to usual care in patients with neck or back pain in primary care settings.[226] The study also demonstrated significant improvements in the SF-12 mental score at 2 and 6 months, but showed only small nonsignificant improvements in the short-form McGill Pain Questionnaire at 2 and 6 months.

A systematic review of osteopathic manipulative medicine as treatment for musculoskeletal pain was conducted by Posadzki and Ernst in 2010, which suggested that there is no clear evidence for the effectiveness of osteopathy as a treatment of various types of musculoskeletal pain.[227] However, because their efforts lacked a critical assessment of the methodology and validity of the included primary studies, there was an enormous variability in operationalization and conceptualization of musculoskeletal spine pain and its treatment. Hence, definitive judgment could not be offered other than that future research is needed to replicate past studies using accepted standards of trial design and reporting.

28.10 NEOPLASTIC DISEASES

The use of CAM interventions has also become increasingly popular among cancer patients. According to a survey of 699 patients aged 64 years and older with cancer recruited from 24 community hospitals and affiliated cancer programs, 33% were using complementary and alternative therapies.[6] Analysis of the only nationally represented telephone survey of 2055 adults demonstrated that 30% of respondents 65 years and older reported using at least one complementary and alternative therapy in the past year.[228]

A 2015 study by Ebel et al. determined that 45% of adult cancer patients used CAM, especially those who admitted to a high external locus of control, with only 60% disclosing such use to their general practitioner and 57% to their oncologist.[229] Nonetheless, a growing number of oncologists and policy makers are encouraging use of the term "integrative oncology," which focuses solely on combining mainstream and complementary care. These integrative services facilitate communication between oncologists and patients, providing an environment where patients can share their concerns and disclose any complementary interventions they already use or would like to try.

28.10.1 NATURAL PRODUCTS

28.10.1.1 Diet

28.10.1.1.1 American Cancer Society Diet

A prospective study of over 72,000 adult women over the age of 50 noted that those who consumed a diet high in red and processed meats, refined grains, and desserts had a 16% greater risk of dying from cancer and a 21% greater risk of dying from any cause compared with those who followed the American Cancer Society's dietary guidelines (a healthful diet of mostly vegetables, fruit, fish, poultry, and whole grains).[230]

28.10.1.2 Low Sugar

No randomized control trials in humans have evaluated whether sugar promotes cancer growth or avoiding sugar will shrink a tumor, despite *in vitro* studies demonstrating that tumor cells undergo apoptosis when starved of glucose.

Nonetheless, studies have consistently shown a link between excess consumption of refined sugars and greater cancer risk, as well as a strong association between being overweight or obese and an increased likelihood of developing cancer.[231,232]

28.10.1.3 Dietary Supplements and Nutritional Therapies

Dietary supplement use has become particularly prevalent among adult oncology vitamin and mineral supplements and 14%–32% of patients begin using supplements after they are diagnosed.[233]

28.10.1.3.1 Antioxidants

When researchers began examining the role that antioxidant supplementation might play in cancer prevention, the evidence was largely disappointing.

In fact, in a 2004 meta-analysis[234] as well as several other follow-up studies,[235,236] researchers compared the effects of antioxidant supplementation with a placebo on the incidence of esophageal,

gastric, colorectal, pancreatic, head and neck, and liver cancers; they found that consuming vitamins A, C, and E and beta-carotene, and selenium supplements actually increased overall mortality,
with the exception of alpha-tocopherol—a form of vitamin E—in prostate cancer.[237]

28.10.1.3.2   Curcumin

Curcumin, East-Indian spice turmeric, has been shown to exhibit improved general health as well
as potential antitumoral activity in colorectal cancer who received curcumin supplements prior to
surgery.[238]

Nevertheless, no randomized control trials have examined the anticancer effects of curcumin,
with some research highlighting that in pharmacological doses; curcumin may interact with certain
chemotherapy agents.[239]

It is also unclear whether curcumin in isolation or with turmeric provides the greatest
benefit.[240]

28.10.1.4   Herbal Preparations

28.10.1.4.1   Chinese Herbal Medicine

Chinese herbal medicine has been used for thousands of years, with a history of use in cancer
patients to reduce the occurrence of anemia and neutropenia,[241] as well as improve quality of life in
nonsmall-cell lung carcinoma.[242]

In a Chinese retrospective study with patients of mean age 60 ± 10 years undergoing treatment
with Gefitinib for nonsmall-cell lung adenocarcinoma, researchers noted median progression-free
survival over 2 months longer and median overall survival 4 months longer in patients who had been
concomitantly taking the herbal medicines.

28.10.2   Mind–Body Medicine

28.10.2.1   Meditation

High levels of stress have been demonstrated to increase inflammation, thus increasing the risk of
developing cancer, having a recurrence, or eventually dying from the disease.[243]

Nonetheless, there is no research supporting the prevention of cancer recurrence, decreased
mortality, or increased survival from practicing various mindfulness-based stress-reduction
techniques.[18,19]

28.10.2.2   Acupuncture

Cancer patients use acupuncture primarily to help relieve pain and reduce nausea and vomiting,
with one study estimating prevalence among cancer patients to be about 5%.[230]

In a 2012 systematic review, 15 studies were reviewed and reported increased efficacy of
acupuncture in reducing cancer pain in combination with analgesics, as compared to analgesics
alone.[244]

Another review performed in 2006 included 11 trials and revealed that overall acupuncture
reduced the incidence of vomiting but not the severity of nausea, except in patients who also underwent acupressure.[245]

28.10.3   Manipulative and Body-Based Practices

28.10.3.1   Massage Therapy

A 2005 review by Corbin et al. found that more than 20% of adult cancer patients receive massage
as part of their integrative oncology programs; unfortunately, they also found potential harmful
effects of massage, ranging from bruising to internal hemorrhaging, fracture, and increased pain or
infection.[246]

One meta-analysis by Ernst et al. reviewed the application of Swedish massage as compared to light touch technique in advanced cancer patients, and demonstrated a reduction in cancer-related pain, nausea, and anxiety.[247]

28.10.4 Movement Therapies

28.10.4.1 Exercise

In 2008, the American Cancer Society reiterated recommendations, providing a wealth of new evidence to support the role of exercise in cancer prevention and for promoting overall health.[231]

Furthermore, research in patients with several cancers, including nonmetastatic breast cancer and nonmetastatic colorectal cancer suggests that exercise may not only help protect people from developing cancer but also may increase survival in those already diagnosed.[248–250]

On another note, for men with prostate cancer, a prospective study of over 47,500 men in the United States over 14 years did not find an association between exercise and survival in younger men, but in those over the age of 65, regular vigorous activity did appear to slow the progression of both advanced and fatal prostate cancer.[251]

A recent prospective study followed over a thousand men over two decades, demonstrating an association between those who engaged in more frequent and vigorous exercise had the lowest risk of dying from a range of cancers, with the best survival advantage in men who burned over 3000 calories per week—equivalent to about 45–60 minutes of hiking or jogging 5 days a week (150–200 lb man-equivalent).[252]

In a Polish prospective study regarding the integration of pulmonary rehabilitation for 90 patients with average age 61.5 ± 8.2 years with inoperable nonsmall-cell lung cancer undergoing first-line chemotherapy, it was observed that subjects tolerated chemotherapy better and had less intense clinical symptoms posttreatment. The study further reported how the subset of subjects given additional supplementation with ascorbic acid had experienced even more positive effects of pulmonary rehabilitation.[253]

28.11 CENTRAL AND PERIPHERAL NERVOUS SYSTEM DISEASES

An increased frequency of CAM used among adults in the United States has also been found in patients with neurological conditions.[254] Therapies have been used successfully for several symptoms related to several neuromuscular disorders, including those affecting balance, posture, coordination, and mobility, and often observe an improvement in risk of falls. As an example, the prevalence of CAM use in Parkinson disease is reported to be between 50% and 75%, using acupuncture, massage, yoga, herbal preparations, and supplements.[255–259]

28.11.1 Natural Products

28.11.1.1 Dietary Supplements and Nutritional Therapies

28.11.1.1.1 Caffeine

Caffeine at doses of 100 mg twice daily for 3 weeks, and then 200 mg twice daily for 3 weeks was also recently found to improve daytime somnolence, severity of motor symptoms, and other features of Parkinson disease, when compared to placebo.[260]

28.11.1.1.2 Coenzyme Q_{10}

A 2011 Cochrane Database review on the use of coenzyme Q_{10} by Liu and colleagues identified several studies involving over 450 patients with Parkinson disease, and found improvements in activities of daily living and mobility at 16 months, as compared to placebo, using a well-tolerated 1200 mg/day dose of coenzyme Q_{10}.[261]

28.11.2 Mind–Body Medicine

28.11.2.1 Dance Therapy

Dance therapy allows patients to combine sensory stimulation, physical activity, and coordination to enhance cognition and motivation.

Several studies have shown improvements in gait, balance, coordination, and posture with partnered and nonpartnered dance movements over weekly 60–90 minute dance sessions.[262–265]

28.11.2.2 Music Therapy

Music therapy also allows patients to combine sensory stimulation, physical activity, and coordination to enhance cognition and motivation.

Music therapy has been practiced for stroke, multiple sclerosis, dementia, and Parkinson disease; specifically with enhancement in recall, cognitive function, reduction of stress and anxiety, and sense of rhythm so as to contribute benefits to gait and mobility.[266]

28.11.2.3 Tai Chi

One study by Wang et al. reviewed data on older patients with stroke and arthritis, finding Tai Chi to be especially beneficial for balance and physical function.[23]

A more recent study comparing Tai Chi with resistance training and stretching for 1 hour twice weekly over 24 weeks in those with Parkinson disease showed better outcome for stability, gait strength, and motor functioning, with benefits maintained for 3 months after program ended.[267]

28.11.3 Energy Medicine

28.11.3.1 Whole-Body Vibration

Whether applied horizontally, vertically, or rotationally, this modality has been demonstrated to improve physical capacity, balance and quality of life among patients with neurological diseases, other than polio.[268]

A small study in levodopa-resistant subjects reported improved balance and gait after thirty 15-minute whole-body vibration sessions (twice daily, 5 days per week) as compared to conventional physical therapy.[269]

28.11.3.2 Light Therapy

Figueiro et al. has conducted several studies proposing night lighting approaches in the senior living environment that led to improved postural control and stability, increased velocity and decreased step-length variability during walking.

28.11.4 Whole Medical Systems

28.11.4.1 Osteopathic Manipulative Medicine

Poor balance can be related to several disorders, such as neuropathies, poor vision, and vestibular dysfunction—which can contribute to falls in the elderly.

A small study by Lopez et al. evaluated the effects of seven specific techniques with an emphasis on improving vestibular function and several cranial techniques, including treatments to the head, neck, shoulders, and thoracic spine. Participants in the OMT group received 25- to 30-minute treatment sessions once per week for 4 weeks, with statistically significant improvements in anteroposterior sway at the end of 4 weeks.[270]

Case reports from the early 1900s demonstrated that frequent Osteopathic Manipulative Treatment (OMT) sessions 2–3 times weekly over several months modestly improved gait and joint range of motion in Parkinson disease patients.[271–274]

Research conducted by Wells and treatments performed by his osteopathic medical students in 1999 focused on improving joint range of motion from the cervical spine to the ankle in patients with Parkinson disease, whereas a single OMT session was discovered to have an immediate beneficial effect on gait measures. The protocol also reported significant improvement in stride length, upper limb velocity in the shoulder, and lower hip velocity relative to control groups.[275]

Lastly, a retrospective study of cranial strain patterns compared 30 patients with Parkinson disease with age-matched controls, showing that patterns differed from normal controls, and that cranial treatment could normalize these patterns.[276] However, the clinical significance of these observations was debated at this time.[277]

28.11.4.2 Chiropractic Therapy

In 2009, Hawk et al. revealed results of a practice-based clinical trial investigating the effects of two different treatment schedules compared to no treatment for a group of older patients with dizziness, balance difficulties, and spinal pain.[278] Improvements in the Berg Balance Scale at 1 month and throughout the study period were only noted in subjects receiving spinal adjustments (plus soft tissue therapy and the application of hot packs). This particular study also noted that improvements were similar whether subjects received adjustments for 8 weeks twice per week, or via 8 weekly visits followed by 10 monthly visits, for a total of 16–18 treatments. Moreover, greater improvements in the Pain Disability Index were recorded in the extended schedule care group, as compared to the other two groups.[279]

A small study by Strunk et al. related that chiropractic therapy improved gait and balance to reduce falls via nonstandardized chiropractic therapy of instrument-assisted, flexion distraction, soft-tissue therapy such as myofascial release, postisometric relation, and heat or cold twice per week for 8 weeks.[280]

Related to earlier work conducted by osteopathic researchers, Elster reported a case of Parkinson disease whom he treated similarly to an earlier osteopathic cervical manipulation regimen over 3 months, with a 43% reduction in severity of Parkinson disease symptoms, including improved cervical range of motion, improved sleep, better energy, and decreased body stiffness.[281]

28.12 CONCLUSION

Overall quality of life has benefitted from the integration of complementary and alternative medical practices and techniques, particularly the practice of several mind–body therapies.[3] In the last quarter of a century, clinical trials and observational studies have provided encouraging evidence that diet modifications, and supplemental and mind–body interventions can offer benefits to many older adults. However, more vigorously conducted prospective trials are needed to determine which conditions are best addressed, as well as integrating comparisons with currently available procedures and pharmacologic interventions with the purpose of delaying the development of degeneration and other disorders of the neuroendomusculoskeletal systems.

Given the current rate of complementary and alternative therapy use, it will become even more important that research should focus on not only how these interventions will affect a wide range of conditions, but also how the use of CAM therapies will contribute to or lend themselves to cost savings on healthcare spending. Moreover, given the low side effect profile of mind–body interventions and their appeal as treatments under patients' control, they are likely to continue to attract practitioners, as well as the interests of medical researchers and administrators.

It is most important that providers should promote mindfulness and open discussion about supportive interventions so as to appropriately address their patients' autonomy and to enhance resilience and well-being in their overall goal of health optimization. Moreover, providers need to be familiar with these therapies' adverse effect profile, although these were not specifically addressed in this chapter.

It should be noted ConsumerLab (https://www.consumerlab.com) provides independent tests, reviews, and clinical updates on supplements and products, as well as resources for conditions, drug interactions, alternative therapies, functional foods, and homeopathy.

For further information on any of the above-mentioned interventions or therapies, the NIH maintains a website under the governance of the Center for Complementary and Integrative Health (https://nccih.nih.gov/health), which is an excellent resource for simple facts and concerns related to various products and practices. It should also be noted that several of the larger health systems across the United States, Europe, and Asia have complementary, alternative, integrated, and/or supportive therapy programs designed to provide multidisciplinary approaches to optimize the care and needs of their older patients.

REFERENCES

1. Rossi P, Di Lorenzo G, Malpezzi MG et al. Prevalence, pattern and predictors of use of complementary and alternative medicine (CAM) in migraine patients attending a headache clinic in Italy. *Cephalalgia.* 2005;25:493–506.
2. Vogel JHK, Bolling SF, Olshansky B et al. Integrating complementary medicine into cardiovascular medicine: A report of the American College of Cardiology Foundation Task Force on clinical expert consensus documents. *J Am Coll Cardiol.* 2005;46(1):184–221
3. Yachoui R and Kolansinski S. Complementary and alternative medicine for Rheumatic Diseases. *Aging Health.* 2012:8(4):403–412.
4. Druss BG, Rosenheck RA. Association between use of unconventional therapies and conventional medical services. *JAMA.* 1999;282:651–656.
5. Eisenberg DM, Davis RB, Ettner SL et al. Trends in alternative medicine use in the United States, 1990–1997: Results of a follow-up national survey. *JAMA.* 1998;280:1569–1575.
6. O'Brien King M and Pettigrew AC. Complementary and alternative therapy use by older adults in three ethnically-diverse populations: A pilot study. *Geriatr Nurs.* 2004;25(1):30–37.
7. Flaherty JH and Takahashi R. The use of complementary and alternative medical therapies among older persons around the world. *Clin Geriatr Med.* 2004;20:179–200.
8. American Association of Retired Persons, National Center for Complementary and Alternative Medicine. *Complementary and Alternative Medicine: What People 50 and Over Are Using and Discussing with Their Physicians.* Washington, D.C.: AARP; 2007.
9. Sebastian RS, Cleveland LE, Goldman JD, Moshfegh AJ. Older adults who use vitamin/mineral supplements differ from nonusers in nutrient intake adequacy and dietary attitudes. *J Am Dietetic Assoc.* 2007;107:1322–1332.
10. Pollan M. In *Defense of Food: An Eater's Manifesto.* Penguin Books, United Kingdom; 1st edition. April 28, 2009. ISBN-10: 0143114964.
11. Sharkey JR, Branch LG, Zohoori N, Giuliani C, Busby-Whitehead J, Haines PS. Inadequate nutrient intakes among homebound elderly and their correlation with individual characteristics and health-related factors. *Am J Clin Nutr.* 2002;76(6):1435–1445.
12. James D. Factors influencing food choices, dietary intake, and nutrition-related attitudes among African Americans: Application of a culturally sensitive model. *Ethnicity Health.* 2004;9(4):349–367.
13. Lee JY, Chu SH, Jeon JY Lee MK, Park JH, Lee DC, Lee JW, Kim NK. Effects of 12 weeks of probiotic supplementation on quality of life in colorectal cancer survivors: A double-blind, randomized, placebo-controlled trial. *Dig Liver Dis.* 2014;46(12):1126–1132.
14. Sanchez-Lara K, Turcott JG, Juarez-Hernandez E, Nunez-Valencia C, Villanueva G, Guevara P, De la Torre-Vallejo M, Mohar A, Arrieta O. Effects of an oral nutritional supplement containing eicosapentaenoic acid on nutritional and clinical outcomes in patients with advanced non-small cell lung cancer: Randomized trial. *Clin Nutr.* 2014;33(6):1017–1023.
15. Lasaite L, Spadiene A, Savickiene N, Skesters A, Silova A. The effect of ginkgo biloba and camellia sinensis extracts on psychological state and glycemic control in patients with type 2 diabetes mellitus. *Nat Prod Commun.* 2014;9(9):1345–1350.
16. De Paula LC, Fonseca F, Perazzo F, Cruz FM, Cubero D, Trufelli DC, Martins SP, Santi PX, da Silva EA, Del Giglio A. Uncaria tomentosa (cat's claw) improved quality of life in patients with advanced solid tumours. *J Altern Complement Med.* 2015;21(1):22–30.

17. Shennan C, Payne S, Fenlon D. What is the evidence for the use of mindfulness-based interventions in cancer care? A review. *Psychooncology.* 2011;20:681–697.

18. Zainal NZ, Booth S, Huppert FA. The efficacy of mindfulness-based stress reduction on mental health of breast cancer patients: A meta-analysis. *Psychooncology.* 2013;22:1457–1465.

19. Cramer H, Lauche R, Paul A, Dobos G. Mindfulness-based stress reduction for breast cancer—A systematic review and meta-analysis. *Curr Oncol.* 2012;19:e343–e352.

20. Jayabharathi B, Judie A. Complementary health approach to quality of life in menopausal women: A community-based interventional study. *Clin Interv Aging.* 2014;9:1913–1921.

21. Immink MA, Hillier S, Petkov J. Randomized controlled trial of yoga for chronic poststroke hemiparesis: Motor function, mental health, and quality of life outcomes. *Top Stroke Rehabil.* 2014;21(3):256–271.

22. Wang C. Tai chi and rheumatic diseases. *Rheum Dis Clin N Am.* 2011;37:19–32.

23. Wang C, Collet JP, Lau J. The effect of tai chi on health outcomes in patients with chronic conditions: A systematic review. *Arch Intern Med.* 2004;164:493–501.

24. Munk N, Kruger T, Zanjani F. Massage therapy usage and reported health in older adults experiencing persistent pain. *J Altern Complement Med.* 2011;17(7):609–616.

25. Keysor JJ, Brembs A. Exercise: Necessary but not sufficient for improving function and preventing disability? *Curr Opin Rheumatol.* 2011;23(2):211–218.

26. Roig M, O'Brien K, Kirk G, Murray R, McKinnon P, Shadgan B, Reid WD. The effects of eccentric versus concentric resistance training on muscle strength and mass in healthy adults: A systematic review with meta-analysis. *Br J Sports Med.* 2009;43(8):556–568.

27. Miszko TA, Cress ME, Slade JM, Covey CJ, Agrawal SK, Doerr CE. Effect of strength and power training on physical function in community-dwelling older adults. *J Gerontol A: Biol Sci Med Sci.* 2003;58(2):171–175.

28. Henwood TR, Riek S, Taaffe DR. Strength versus muscle power-specific resistance training in community-dwelling older adults. *J Gerontol A: Biol Sci Med Sci.* 2008;63(1):83–91.

29. Nelson ME, Rejeski WJ, Blair SN, Duncan PW, Judge JO, King AC, Macera CA, Castaneda-Sceppa C, American College of Sports Medicine, American Heart Association. Physical activity and public health in older adults: Recommendation from the American College of Sports Medicine and the American Heart Association. *Circulation.* 2007;116(9):1094–1105.

30. Buford TW, Anton SD, Clark DJ, Higgins TJ, Cooke MB. Optimizing the benefits of exercise on physical function on older adults. *PMR.* 2014; 6(6):528–543.

31. Lee MS, Pittler MH, Ernst E. Effects of Reiki in clinical practice: A systematic review of randomized clinical trials. *Int J Clin Pract.* 2008;62:947–954.

32. Thrane S, Cohen SM. Effect of Reiki therapy on pain and anxiety in adults: An in-depth literature review of randomized trials with effect size calculations. *Pain Manag Nurs.* 2014;15(4):897–908. doi: 10.1016/j.pmn.2013.07.008.

33. Catlin A, Taylor-Ford RL. Investigation of standard care versus sham Reiki placebo versus actual Reiki therapy to enhance comfort and well-being in a chemotherapy infusion center. *Oncol Nurs Forum.* 2011;38:E212–E220.

34. Ortiz M, Amman ES, Gross CS et al. Complementary medicine in nursing homes—Results of mixed methods pilot study. *BMC Complement Altern Med.* 2014;14:443.

35. Snider KT, Snider EJ, Johnson JC, Hagan C, Schoenwald C. Preventative osteopathic manipulative treatment and the elderly nursing home resident: A pilot study. *J Am Osteopath Assoc.* 2012; 112(8):489–501.

36. Crow WT, Willis DR. Estimating cost of care for patients with acute low back pain: A retrospective review of patient records. *J Am Osteopath Assoc.* 2009; 109(4):229–233.

37. Knopman DS, Roberts R. Vascular risk factors: Imaging and neuropathologic correlates. *J Alzheimers Dis.* 2010;20(3):699–709.

38. Scarmeas N, Stern Y, Mayeux R, Luchsinger JA. Mediterranean diet, Alzheimer disease, and vascular mediation. *Arch Neurol.* 2006;63:1709–1717.

39. Scarmeas N, Stern Y, Mayeux R, Manly JJ, Schupf N, Luchsinger JA. Mediterranean diet and mild cognitive impairment. *Arch Neurol.* 2009;66:216–225.

40. Feart C, Samieri C, Rondeau V et al. Adherence to a Mediterranean diet, cognitive decline, and risk of dementia. *JAMA.* 2009;302:638–48.

41. Witte AV, Fobker M, Gellner R, Knecht S, Floel A. Caloric restriction improves memory in elderly humans. *Proc Natl Acad Sci USA.* 2009;106:1255–1260.

42. Martin CK, Anton SD, Han H et al. Examination of cognitive function during six months of calorie restriction: Results of a randomized controlled trial. *Rejuvenation Res.* 2007;10:179–190.

43. Halyburton AK, Brinkworth GD, Wilson CJ et al. Low- and high-carbohydrate weight-loss diets have similar effects on mood but not cognitive performance. *Am J Clin Nutr.* 2007;86:580–587.

44. Otaegui-Arrazola A, Amiano P, Elbusto A, Urdaneta E, Martinez-Lage P. Diet, cognition, and Alzheimer's disease: Food for though. *Eur J Nutr.* 2014;53(1):1–23.

45. Luchsinger J, Mayeux R. Dietary factors and Alzheimer's disease. *Lancet Neurol.* 2004;3:579–587.

46. Morris M. The role of nutrition in Alzheimer's disease: Epidemiological evidence. *Eur J Neurol.* 2009;16:1–7.

47. Yehuda S, Rabinovitz S, Mostofsky DI. Essential fatty acids and the brain: From infancy to aging. *Neurobiol Aging.* 2005;26:98–102.

48. Sharma M, Palacios-Bois J, Schwartz G et al. Circadian rhythms of melatonin and cortisol in aging. *Biol Psychiatry.* 1989;25(3):305–319.

49. Almay BG, von Knorring L, Wetterberg L. Melatonin in serum and urine in patients with idiopathic pain syndromes. *Psychiatry Res.* 1987;22(3):179–191.

50. Brugger P, Marktl W, Herold M. Impaired nocturnal secretion of melatonin in coronary heart disease. *Lancet.* 1995;345(8962):1408.

51. Fiorina P, Lattuada G, Silvestrini C, Ponari O, Dall'Aglio P. Disruption of nocturnal melatonin rhythm and immunological involvement in ischaemic stroke patients. *Scand J Immunol.* 1999; 50(2):228–231.

52. Van Den Heuvel CJ, Reid KJ, Dawson D. Effect of atenolol on nocturnal sleep and temperature in young men: Reversal by pharmacological doses of melatonin. *Physiol Behav.* 1997;61(6):795–802.

53. Murphy PJ, Myers BL, Badia P. Nonsteroidal anti-inflammatory drugs alter body temperature and suppress melatonin in humans. *Physiol Behav.* 1996;59(1):133–139.

54. Jean-Louis G, von Gizycki H, Zizi F. Melatonin effects on sleep, mood, and cognition in elderly with mild cognitive impairment. *J Pineal Res.* 1998;25(3):177–183.

55. Holick MF. Vitamin D deficiency. *N Engl J Med.* 2007;357(3):266–281.

56. Buell JS, Dawson-Hughes B. Vitamin D and neurocognitive dysfunction: Preventing "D"ecline? *Mol Aspects Med.* 2008;29(6):415–422.

57. Masoumi A, Goldenson B, Ghirmai S et al. 1-alpha,25-dihydroxyvitamin D3 interacts with curcuminoids to stimulate amyloid-beta clearance by macrophages of Alzheimer's disease patients. *J Alzheimers Dis.* 2009;17(3):703–717.

58. McCann JC and Ames BN. Is there convincing biological or behavioral evidence linking vitamin D deficiency to brain dysfunction? *FASEB J.* 2008;22(4):982–1001.

59. Llewellyn DJ, Lang IA, Langa KM, Muniz-Terrera G, Phillips CL, Cherubini M, Ferrucci L, Melzer D. Vitamin D and risk of cognitive decline in elderly persons. *Arch Intern Med.* 2010;170(13):1135–1141.

60. Annweiler C, Allali G, Allain P et al. Vitamin D and cognitive performance in adults: A systematic review. *Eur J Neurol.* 2009;16:1083–1089.

61. Morris MC, Evans DA, Bienia JL, Tangney CC, Wilson RS. Vitamin E and cognitive decline in older persons. *Arch Neurol.* 2002;59(7):1125–1132.

62. Tan MS, Yu JT, Tan CC, Wang HF, Meng XF, Wang C, Jiang T, Zhu XC, Tan L. Efficacy and adverse effects of gingko biloba for cognitive impairment and dementia: A systematic review and meta-analysis. *J Alzheimers Dis.* 2015;43(2):589–603.

63. Wang Q, Iwasaki K, Suzuki T et al. Potentiation of brain acetylcholine neurons by Kami-untan-to (KUT) in aged mice: Implications for a possible antidementia drug. Phytomedicine. 2000;7:253–258.

64. Maruyama M, Tomita N, Iwasaki K et al. Benefits of combining donepezil plus traditional Japanese herbal medicine on cognition and brain perfusion in alzheimer's disease: A 12-week observer-blind, donepezil monotherapy controlled trial. *J Am Geriatr Soc.* 2006;54(5):869–871.

65. Zunzunegui MV, Alvarado BE, Del Ser T, Otero A. Social networks, social integration, and social engagement determine cognitive decline in community-dwelling Spanish older adults. *J Gerontol B: Psychol Sci Soc Sci.* 2003;58(2):S93–S100.

66. Van Gelder BM, Tijhuis MAR, Kalmijn S, Giampaoli S, Nissinen A, Kromhout D. Physical activity in relation to cognitive decline in elderly men: The FINE study. *Neurology.* 2004;63(12):2316–2321.

67. Wall M and Duffy A. The effects of music therapy for older people with dementia. *Br J Nurs.* 2010;19:108–113.

68. Bruer RA, Spitznagel E, Cloninger CR. The temporal limits of cognitive change from music therapy in elderly persons with dementia or dementia-like cognitive impairment: A randomized controlled trial. *J Music Ther.* 2007;44:308–328.

69. Viggo L, Hansen N, Jorgensen T, Ortenblad L. Massage and touch for dementia. *Cochrane Database Syst Rev.* 2006;(4):CD004989.

70. Suzuki M, Tatsumi A, Otsuka T et al. Physical and psychological effects of 6-week tactile massage on elderly patients with severe dementia. *Am J Alzheimers Other Demen.* 2010;25(8):680–686.

71. Hamer M and Chida Y. Physical activity and risk of neurodegenerative disease: A systematic review of prospective evidence. *Psychol Med.* 2009;39(1):3–11.

72. Crawford SE, Leaver VW, Mahoney SD. Using Reiki to decrease memory and behavior problems in mild cognitive impairment and mild Alheimer's disease. *J Altern Complement Med.* 2006;12(9):911–913.

73. Bentwich J, Dobronevsky E, Aichenbaum S, Shorer R, Peretz R, Khaigrekht M, Marton RG, Rabey JM. Beneficial effect of repetitive transcranial magnetic stimulation combined with cognitive training for the treatment of Alzheimer disease: A proof of concept study. *J Neural Transm (Vienna).* 2011;118(3):463–471.

74. Bassuk SS, Berman LF, Wypij D. Depressive symptomology and incident cognitive decline in an elderly community sample. *Arch Gen Psychiary.* 1998;55(12):1073–1081.

75. Jacka FN, Overland S, Stewart R, Tell GS, Bjelland I, Mykletun A. Association between magnesium intake and depression and anxiety in community-dwelling adults: The Hordaland Health Study. *Austral New Zeal J Psych.* 2009;43:45–52.

76. Barragan-Rodriguez L, Rodriguez-Moran M, Guerrero-Romero F. Efficacy and safety of oral magnesium supplementation in the treatment of depression in the elderly with type 2 diabetes: A randomized, equivalent trial. *Magnesium Res.* 2008;21:218–223.

77. Buscemi N, Vandermeer B, Pandya R et al. *Melatonin for Treatment of Sleep Disorders, Evidence Report/Technology Assessment No. 108.* Rockville, MD: Agency for Healthcare Research and Quality; Prepared by the University of Alberta Evidence-based Practice Center, under Contract No. 290-02-0023; November 2004. AHRQ Publication No. 05-E002-2.

78. Linde K, Ramirez G, Mulrow C, Pauls A, Weidenhammer W, Mechart D. St John's wort for depression—An overview and meta-analysis of randomised clinical trials. *BMJ.* 1996;313:253.

79. Lavretsky H. Complementary and alternative medicine use for treatment and prevention of late-life mood and cognitive disorders. *Aging Health.* 2009;5:61–78.

80. Carlson LE and Garland SN. Impact of mindfulness-based stress reduction (MBSR) on sleep, mood, stress and fatigue symptoms in cancer outpatients. *Int J Behav Med.* 2005;12(4):278–285.

81. Li F, Fisher KJ, Harmer P et al. Tai chi and self-rated quality of sleep and daytime sleepiness in older adults: A randomized controlled trial. *J Am Geriatr Soc.* 2004;52:892–900.

82. Wang C, Schmid CH, Hibberd PL et al. Tai chi is effective in treating knee osteoarthritis: A randomized controlled trial. *Arthritis Rheum.* 2009;61:545–553.

83. Taibi DM and Vitiello MV. A pilot study of gentle yoga for sleep disturbance in women with osteoarthritis. *Sleep Med.* 2011;12:512–517.

84. Manjunath NK and Telles S. Influence of yoga and ayurveda on self-rated sleep in a geriatric population. *Indian J Med Res.* 2005;121(5):683–690.

85. Suen LK, Wong TK, Leung AW, Ip WC. The long-term effects of auricular therapy using magnetic pearls on elderly with insomnia. *Complement Ther Med.* 2003;11(2):85–92.

86. Suen LK, Wong TK, Leung AW. Effectiveness of auricular therapy on sleep promotion in the elderly. *Am J Chin Med.* 2002;30(4):429–449.

87. Chen ML, Lin LC, Wu SC, Lin JG. The effectiveness of acupressure in improving the quality of sleep of institutionalized residents. *J Gerontol A: Biol Sci Med Sci.* 1999;54(8):M389–M394.

88. Yang MH, Wu SC, Lin JG, Lin LC. The efficacy of acupressure for decreasing agitated behavior in dementia: A pilot study. *J Clin Nurs.* 2007;16(2):308–315.

89. Soden K, Vincent K, Craske S, Lucas C, Ashley S. A randomized controlled trial of aromatherapy massage in a hospice setting. *Palliat Med.* 2004;18(2):87–92.

90. Royer M, Ballentine NH, Eslinger PJ, Houser K, Mistrick R, Behr R, Rakos K. Light therapy for seniors in long term care. *J Am Med Dir Assoc.* 2012;13(2):100–102.

91. Hanford N and Figueiro M. Light therapy and Alzheimer's disease and related dementia: Past, present, and future. *J Alzheimers Dis.* 2013;33(4):913–922.

92. Ancoli-Israel S, Gehrman P, Martin JL, Shochat T, Marler M, Corey-Bloom J, Levi L. Increased light exposure consolidates sleep and strengthens circadian rhythms in severe Alzheimer's disease patients. *Behav Sleep Med.* 2003;1:22–36.

93. Ancoli-Israel S, Martin JL, Kripke DF, Marler M, Klauber MR. Effect of light treatment on sleep and circadian rhythms in demented nursing home patients. *J Am Geriatr Soc.* 2002;50:282–289.

94. Figueiro MG and Rea MS. LEDs: Improving the sleep quality of older adults. *Proceedings of the CIE Midterm Meeting and International Lighting Congress*; Leon, Spain. 2005.

95. O'Reardon JP, Solvason HB, Janicak PG et al. Efficacy and safety of transcranial magnetic stimulation in the acute treatment of major depression: A multisite randomized controlled trial. *Biol Psychiatry.* 2007;62:1208–1216.

96. McDonald WM, Durkalski V, Ball ER et al. Improving the antidepressant efficacy of transcranial magnetic stimulation: Maximizing the number of stimulations and treatment location in treatment-resistant depression. *Depress Anxiety.* 2011;28:973–980.

97. Mantovani A, Pavlicova M, Avery D et al. Long-term efficacy of repeated daily prefrontal transcranial magnetic stimulation (TMS) in treatment-resistant depression. *Depress Anxiety.* 2012;29:883–890.

98. Sayar GH, Ozten E, Tan O, Tarhan N. Transcranial magnetic stimulation for treating depression in elderly patients. *Neuropsychiatr Dis Treat.* 2013;9:501–504.

99. Yeh GY, Davis RB, Phillips RS. Use of complementary therapies in patients with cardiovascular disease. *Am J Cardiol.* 2006;98:673–680.

100. Nieva R, Safavynia SA, Bishop KL, Sperling L. Herbal, vitamin, and mineral supplement use in patients enrolled in a cardiac rehabilitation program. *J Cardiopulm Rehabil Prev.* 2012;32(5):270–277.

101. Anderson JW and Hanna TJ. Impact of nondigestible carbohydrates on serum lipoproteins and risk for cardiovascular disease. *J Nutr.* 1999;129:1457S–1466S.

102. Kris-Etherton PM, Krummel D, Russell ME et al. The effect of diet on plasma lipids, lipoproteins, and coronary heart disease. *J Am Diet Assoc.* 1988;88:1373–1400.

103. Executive summary of the third report of the National Cholesterol Education Program (NCEP) expert panel on detection, evaluation, and treatment of high blood cholesterol in adults (adult treatment Panel III). *JAMA.* 2001;285:2486–2497.

104. Houston DK, Nicklas BJ, Zizza CL. Weighty concerns: The growing prevalence of obesity among older adults. *J Am Dietetic Assoc.* 2009;109:1886–1895.

105. Lichtenstein AH, Van Horn L. Very low fat diets. *Circulation.* 1998;98:935–939.

106. Grundy SM, Cleeman JI, Merz CN et al. Implications of recent clinical trials for the National Cholesterol Education Program Adult Treatment Panel III Guidelines. *J Am Coll Cardiol.* 2004;44:720–732.

107. Kris-Etherton PM, Eckel RH, Howard BV, St Jeor S, Bazzarre TL. AHA science advisory: Lyon diet heart study. Benefits of a Mediterranean-style, National Cholesterol Education Program/ American Heart Association Step I dietary pattern on cardiovascular disease. *Circulation.* 2001;103: 1823–1825.

108. Singh RB, Dubnov G, Niaz MA et al. Effect of an IndoMediterranean diet on progression of coronary artery disease in high risk patients (Indo-Mediterranean Diet Heart Study): A randomised single-blind trial. *Lancet.* 2002;360:1455–1461.

109. Sacks FM, Svetkey LP, Vollmer WM et al. Effects on blood pressure of reduced dietary sodium and the Dietary Approaches to Stop Hypertension (DASH) diet. DASH-Sodium Collaborative Research Group. *N Engl J Med.* 2001;344:3–10.

110. Cater NB, Garcia-Garcia AB, Vega GL, Grundy SM. Responsiveness of plasma lipids and lipoproteins to plant stanol esters. *Am J Cardiol.* 2005;96(Suppl):23D–28D.

111. Albert CM, Gaziano JM, Willett WC, Manson JE. Nut consumption and decreased risk of sudden cardiac death in the Physicians' Health Study. *Arch Intern Med.* 2002;162:1382–1387.

112. Hu FB, Stampfer MJ, Manson JE et al. Frequent nut consumption and risk of coronary heart disease in women: Prospective cohort study. *BMJ.* 1998;317:1341–1345.

113. Fraser GE, Sabate J, Beeson WL, Strahan TM. A possible protective effect of nut consumption on risk of coronary heart disease. The Adventist Health Study. *Arch Intern Med.* 1992;152:1416–1424.

114. Geleijnse JM, Launer LJ, Hofman A, Pols HA, Witteman JC. Tea flavonoids may protect against atherosclerosis: The Rotterdam Study. *Arch Intern Med.* 1999;159:2170–2174.

115. Geleijnse JM, Launer LJ, Van der Kuip DA, Hofman A, Witteman JC. Inverse association of tea and flavonoid intakes with incident myocardial infarction: The Rotterdam Study. *Am J Clin Nutr.* 2002;75:880–886.

116. Ceremuzynski L, Chamiec T, Herbaczynska-Cedro K. Effect of supplemental oral L-arginine on exercise capacity in patients with stable exercise angina pectoris. *Am J Cardiol.* 1997;80:331–333.

117. Maxwell AJ, Zapien MP, Pearce GL, MacCallum G, Stone PH. Randomized trial of a medical food for the dietary management of chronic stable angina. *J Am Coll Cardiol.* 2002;39:37–45.

118. Vivekananthan DP, Penn MS, Sapp SK, Hsu A, Topol EJ. Use of antioxidant vitamins for the prevention of cardiovascular disease: Meta-analysis of randomised trials. *Lancet.* 2003;361:2017–2023.

119. Ernst E. Chelation therapy for peripheral arterial occlusive disease: A systematic review. *Circulation.* 1997;96:1031–1033.

120. Escolar E, Lama GA, Mar DB et al. The effect of EDTA-based chelation regimen on patients with diabetes mellitus and prior myocardial infarction in the Trial to Assess Chelation Therapy (TACT). *Circ Cardiovasc Qual Outcomes*. 2014;7:15–24.
121. Lamas GA, Goertz C, Boineau R, Mark DB, Rozema R, Nahin RL, Lindblad L, Lewis EF, Drisko J, Lee KL. TACT Investigators. Effect of disodium EDTA chelation regimen on cardiovascular events in patients with previous myocardial infarction: The TACT randomized trial. *JAMA*. 2013;309:1241–1250.
122. Molyneux SL, Florkowski CM, George PM et al. Coenzyme Q10. An independent predictor of mortality in chronic heart failure. *J Am Coll Cardiol*. 2008;52:1435–1441.
123. Sander S, Coleman CI, Patel AA, Kluger J, White CM. The impact of coenzyme Q10 on systolic function in patients with chronic heart failure. *J Card Fail*. 2006;12:464–472.
124. Bautista LE, Arenas IA, Penuela A, Martinez LX. Total plasma homocysteine level and risk of cardiovascular disease: A meta-analysis of prospective cohort studies. *J Clin Epidemiol*. 2002;55:882–887.
125. Rydlewicz A, Simpson JA, Taylor RJ, Bond CM, Golden MHN. The effect of folic acid supplementation on plasma homocysteine in an elderly population. *QJM*. 2002;95:27–35.
126. Bonaa KH, Njolstad I, Ueland PM et al. (NORVIT Trial Investigators). Homocysteine lowering and cardiovascular events after acute myocardial infarction. *N Engl J Med*. 2006;354:1578–1588.
127. Wang X, Qin X, Demirtas H et al. Efficacy of folic acid supplementation in stroke prevention: A meta-analysis. *Lancet*. 2007;369:1876–1882.
128. Jee SH, Miller ER III, Guallar E, Singh VK, Appel LJ, Klag MJ. The effect of magnesium supplementation on blood pressure: A meta-analysis of randomized clinical trials. *Am J Hypertens*. 2002;15:691–696.
129. Shechter M, Bairey Merz CN, Stuehlinger HG, Slany J, Pachinger O, Rabinowitz B. Effects of oral magnesium therapy on exercise tolerance, exercise-induced chest pain, and quality of life in patients with coronary artery disease. *Am J Cardiol*. 2003;91:517–521.
130. Song J, He K, Levitan EB, Manson JE, Liu S. Effects of oral magnesium supplementation on glycaemic control in Type 2 diabetes: A meta-analysis of randomized double-blind controlled trials. *Diabetic Med*. 2006;23:1050–1056.
131. Barbagallo M, Dominguez LJ, Galioto A, Pineo A, Belvedere M. Oral magnesium supplementation improves vascular function in elderly diabetic patients. *Magnesium Res*. 2010;23:131–137.
132. Sewerynek E. Melatonin and the cardiovascular system. *Neuro Endocrinol Lett*. 2002;23(Suppl 1):79–83.
133. Lusardi P, Piazza E, Fogari R. Cardiovascular effects of melatonin in hypertensive patients well controlled by nifedipine: A 24-hour study. *Br J Clin Pharmacol*. 2000;49(5):423–427.
134. National Academies—Committee on the Framework for Evaluating the Safety of Dietary Supplements. *Prototype Monograph on Melatonin. Dietary Supplements: A Framework for Evaluation Safety*. Washington, D.C.: The National Academies Press; 2004. pp. D1–D71.
135. Gruppo Italiano per lo Studio della Sopravvivenza nell'Infarto miocardico. Dietary supplementation with n-3 polyunsaturated fatty acids and vitamin E after myocardial infarction: Results of the GISSIPrevenzione trial. *Lancet*. 1999;354:447–455.
136. GISSI-HF Investigators. Effect of n-3 polyunsaturated fatty acids in patients with chronic heart failure (the GISI-HF trial): A randomized, double-blind, placebo-controlled trial. *Lancet*. 2008;372:1223–1230.
137. Heydari B, Abbasi S, Shah R et al. Effect of purified omega-3 fatty acids on reducing left ventricular remodeling after acute myocardial infarction (OMEGA-REMODEL study). *American College of Cardiology 2015 Scientific Sessions*, March 16, 2015, San Diego, CA. Abstract 913-08.
138. Knekt P, Ritz J, Pereira MA et al. Antioxidant vitamins and coronary heart disease risk: A pooled analysis of 9 cohorts. *Am J Clin Nutr*. 2004;80:1508–1520.
139. Kris-Etherton PM, Lichtenstein AH, Howard BV, Steinberg D, Witztum JL. Antioxidant vitamin supplements and cardiovascular disease. *Circulation*. 2004;110:637–641.
140. Lippman SM, Klein EA, Goodman PJ. Effect of selenium and vitamin E on risk of prostate cancer and other cancers: The selenium and vitamin E cancer prevention trial (SELECT). *JAMA*. 2009;301:39–51.
141. Klein EA, Thompson IM, Tangen CM, Crowley JJ, Lucia MS, Goodman PJ. Vitamin E and the risk of prostate cancer: The selenium and vitamin E cancer prevention trial (SELECT). *JAMA*. 2011;306:1549–1556.
142. Zhu H, Lu S, Su W, Gong S, Zhang Z, Li P. Effect of liandouqingmai recipe on quality of life and inflammatory reactions of patients with coronary artery disease. *J Tradit Chin Med*. 2014;34(5):539–543.
143. Neil HAW, Silagy CA, Lancaster T et al. Garlic powder in the treatment of moderate hyperlipidemia: A controlled trial and metaanalysis. *J R Coll Physicians Lond*. 1996;30:329–334.

144. Warshafsky S, Kamer RS, Sivak SL. Effect of garlic on total serum cholesterol. A meta-analysis. *Ann Intern Med.* 1993;119:599–605.

145. Stevinson C, Pittler MH, Ernst E. Garlic for treating hypercholesterolemia. *Ann Intern Med.* 2000;133:420–429.

146. Superko HR, Krauss RM. Garlic powder, effect on plasma lipids, postprandial lipemia, low-density lipoprotein particle size, high-density lipoprotein subclass distribution and lipoprotein (a). *J Am Coll Cardiol.* 2000;35:321–326.

147. Di Pierro F, Rinaldi F, Lucarelli M, Rossoni G. Interaction between ticlopidine or warfarin or cardio-aspirin with a highly standardized deterpened *Ginkgo biloba* extract (VR456) in rat and human. *Acta Biomed.* 2010;81:196–203.

148. Kellermann AJ, Kloft C. Is there a risk of bleeding associated with standardized *Ginkgo biloba* extract therapy? A systematic review and meta-analysis. *Pharmacotherapy.* 2011;31:490–502.

149. Moher D, Pham B, Ausejo M et al. Pharmacological management of intermittent claudication: A meta-analysis of randomised trials. *Drugs.* 2000;59:1057–1070.

150. Gardner CD, Taylor-Piliae RE, Kiazand A et al. Effect of Ginkgo biloba on treadmill walking time among adults with peripheral arterial disease. *J Cardiopulm Rehabil Prev.* 2008;28:258–265.

151. Vuksan V, Stavro M, Woo M, Leiter LA, Sung MK, Sievenpiper JL. Korean red ginseng (*Panax ginseng*) can lower blood pressure in individuals with hypertension: A randomized controlled trial; *Proceedings of the 9th International Ginseng Symposium*; September 25–28, 2006; Geumsan, Korea, Seoul: Korean Society of Ginseng.

152. Jovanovski E, Jenkins A, Dias AG, Peeva V, Sievenpiper J, Arnason JT, Rahelic D, Josse RG, Vuksan V. Effects of Korean red ginseng (*Panax ginseng* C.A. Mayer) and its isolated ginsenosides and polysaccharides on arterial stiffness in healthy individuals. *Am J Hypertens.* 2010;23(5):469–472.

153. Rhee MY, Kim YS, Bae JH, Nah DY, Kim YK, Lee MM, Kim HY. Effect of Korean red ginseng on arterial stiffness in subjects with hypertension. *J Altern Complement Med.* 2011;17(1):45–49.

154. Ahn CM, Hong SJ, Choi SC, Park JH, Kim JS, Lim DS. Red ginseng extract improves coronary flow reserve and increases absolute numbers of various circulating angiogenic cells in patients with first ST-segment elevation acute myocardial infarction. *Phytother Res.* 2011;25(2):239–249.

155. Lee YH, Lee BK, Choi YJ, Yoon IK, Chang BC, Gwak HS. Interaction between warfarin and Korean red ginseng in patients with cardiac valve replacement. *Int J Cardiol.* 2010;145(2):275–276.

156. Pittler MH, Schmidt K, Ernst E. Hawthorn extract for treating chronic heart failure: Meta-analysis of randomized trials. *Am J Med.* 2003;114(8):665–674.

157. Schulz V, Hansel R, Tyler V. *Rational Phytotherapy: A Physician's Guide to Herbal Medicine.* Berlin, Heidelberg: Springer-Verlag; 1998.

158. Habs M. Prospective, comparative cohort studies and their contribution to the benefit assessments of therapeutic options: Heart failure treatment with and without Hawthorn special extract WS 1442. *Forsch Komplementarmed Klass Naturheilkd.* 2004;11(Suppl 1):36–39.

159. Zick SM, Gillespie B, Aaronson KD. The effect of Crataegus oxycantha Special Extract WS 1442 on clinical progression in patients with mild to moderate symptoms of heart failure. *Eur J Heart Fail.* 2008;10(6):587–593.

160. Zick SM, Vautaw BM, Gillespie B, Aaronson KD. Hawthorn Extract Randomized Blinded Chronic Heart Failure (HERB CHF) trial. *Eur J Heart Fail.* 2009;11(10):990–999.

161. Mashour NH, Lin GI, Frishman WH. Herbal medicine for the treatment of cardiovascular disease: Clinical considerations. *Arch Intern Med.* 1998;158:2225–2234.

162. Brinker FJ. *Herb Contraindications and Drug Interactions.* 2nd edition. Sandy, OR: Eclectic Medical Publications; 1998.

163. Valli G and Giardina EG. Benefits, adverse effects, and drug-interactions of herbal therapies with cardiovascular effects. *J Am Coll Cardiol.* 2002;39:1083–1095.

164. Pittler MH and Ernst E. Horst chestnut seed extract for chronic venous insufficiency. *Cochrane Database Syst Rev.* 2006; DOI: 10.1002/14651858.CD003230.pub3.

165. Li JJ, Lu ZL, Kou WR et al. Beneficial impact of xuezhikang on cardiovascular events and mortality in elderly hypertensive patients with previous myocardial infarction from the China Coronary Secondary Prevention Study (CCSPS). *J Clin Pharmacol.* 2009;49:947–956.

166. Marazzi G, Cacciotti L, Pelliccia F, Iaia L, Volterrani M, Caminiti G, Sposato B, Massaro R, Grieco F, Rosano G. Long-term effects of nutraceuticals (berberine, red yeast rice, policosanol) in elderly hypercholesterolemic patients. *Adv Ther.* 2011;28:1105–1113.

167. Shang Q, Liu Z, Chen K et al. A systematic review of xuezhikang, an extract from red yeast rice, for coronary heart disease complicated by dyslipidemia. *Evid Based Complement Alternat Med.* 2012;2012:636547.

168. Pelletier KR. *The Best Alternative Medicine. What Works? What Does Not?* New York: Simon & Schuster; 2000.

169. Takahashi T and Matsushita H. Long-term effects of music therapy on elderly with moderate/severe dementia. *J Music Ther.* 2006;43:317–33.

170. Elward K and Larson E. Benefits of exercise for older adults: A review of existing evidence and current recommendations for the general population. *Clin Geriatr Med.* 1992;8:35–50.

171. Lavie CJ and Milani RV. Disparate effects of improving aerobic exercise capacity and quality of life after cardiac rehabilitation in young and elderly coronary patients. *J Cardiopulm Rehabil.* 2000;20(4):235–240.

172. Lavie CJ and Milani RV. Benefits of cardiac rehabilitation and exercise training programs in elderly coronary patients. *Am J Geriatr Cardiol.* 2001;10(6):323–327.

173. Lavie CJ, Milani RV, Marks P, de Gruiter H. Exercise and the heart: Risks, benefits, and recommendations for providing exercise prescriptions. *Oshsner J.* 2001;3(4):207–213.

174. Chrysant SG. Current evidence on the hemodynamic and blood pressure effects of isometric exercise in normotensive and hypertensive persons. *J Clin Hypertension.* 2010;12(9):721–726.

175. Prospective Urban Rural Epidemiology (PURE) Study Investigators. Prognostic value of grip strength: Findings from the Prospective Urban Rural Epidemiology (PURE) study. *Lancet.* 2015;386(9990):266–272.

176. http://www.cancer.org/cancer/lungcancer-non-smallcell/detailedguide/non-small-cell-lung-cancer-key-statistics. Accessed June 20, 2015.

177. Liu Y, Croft JB, Anderson LA, Wheaton AG, Presley-Cantrell LR, Ford ES. The association of chronic obstructive disease, disability, engagement in social activities, and mortality among US adults aged 70 years or older, 1994–2006. *Int J Chron Obstruct Pulmon Dis.* 2014;9:75–83.

178. Gunay E, Kaymaz D, Selcuk NT, Erqun P, Senqul F, Demir N. Effect of nutritional status in individuals with chronic obstructive pulmonary disease undergoing pulmonary rehabilitation. *Respirology.* 2013;18(8):1217–1222.

179. Nq TP, Niti M, Yap KB, Tan WC. Dietary and supplemental antioxidant and anti-inflammatory nutrient intakes and pulmonary function. *Public Health Nutr.* 2014;17(9):2081–2086.

180. Snider JT, Jena AB, Linthicum MT, Hegazi RA, Partridge JS, LaVallee C, Lakdawalla DN, Wischmeyer PE. Effect of hospital use of oral nutritional supplementation on length of stay, hospital cost, and 30-day readmissions among Medicare patients with COPD. *Chest.* 2015;147(6):1477–1484.

181. Farver-Vestergaard I, Jacobsen D, Zachariae R. Efficacy of psychosocial interventions on psychological and physical health outcomes in chronic obstructive pulmonary disease: A systematic review and meta-analysis. *Psychother Psychosom.* 2015;84(1):37–50.

182. Jobst KA. A critical analysis of acupuncture in pulmonary disease: Efficacy and safety of the acupuncture needle. *J Altern Complement Med.* 1995;1(1):57–85.

183. Choi T, Jun JH, Choi J, Kim J, Lee MS. Acupuncture for the treatment of chronic obstructive pulmonary disease: A protocol of a systematic review. *BMJ Open.* 2014;4:e004590.

184. Liu X, Pan L, Hu Q, Dong W, Yan J, Dong L. Effects of yoga training in patients with chronic obstructive pulmonary disease: A systematic review and meta-analysis. *J Thorac Dis.* 2014;6(6):795–802.

185. Heneghan NR, Adab P, Balanos GM, Jordan RE. Manual therapy for chronic obstructive airways disease: A systematic review of current evidence. *Man Ther* 2012;17(6):507–518.

186. Lacasse Y, Brosseau L, Milne S, Martin S, Wong E, Guyatt GH, Goldstein RS, White J. Pulmonary rehabilitation for chronic obstructive pulmonary disease. *Cochrane Library.* Assessed as up-to-date: March 26, 2014, DOI: 10.1002/14651858.CD003793.pub3.

187. Noll DR, Shores JH, Gamber RG, Herron KM, Swift Jr J. Benefits of osteopathic manipulative treatment for hospitalized elderly patients with pneumonia. *J Am Osteo Assoc.* 2000;100:776–782.

188. Noll DR, Degenhardt BF, Morley TF, Blais FX, Hortos KA, Hensel K, Johnson JC, Pasta DJ, Stoll ST. Efficacy of osteopathic manipulation as an adjunctive treatment for hospitalized patients with pneumonia: A randomized controlled trial. *Osteopath Med and Primary Care.* 2010;4:2.

189. Bronfort G, Haas M, Evans R, Leininger B, Triano J. Effectiveness of manual therapies: The UK evidence report. *Chiropr Osteopat.* 2010 25;18:3.

190. Li NC, Wu SL, Jin J et al. Comparison of different drugs on the treatment of benign prostate hyperplasia. *Zhonghua Wai Ke Za Zhi.* 2007;45(14):947–950.

191. Wilt T, Mac Donald R, Ishani A, Rutks I, Stark G. Cernilton for benign prostatic hyperplasia. *Cochrane Database Syst Rev.* 2000;(2):CD001042.
192. Huang YP, Wen YH, Wu GH, Hong ZF, Xu SW, Peng AX. Clinical study on Kangquan Recipe for benign prostatic hyperplasia patients: A randomized control trial. *Chin J Integr Med.* 2014;20(12): 949–954.
193. Marzano R, Dinelli N, Ales V, Bertozzi MA. Effectiveness on urinary symptoms and erectile dysfunction of Prostamev Plus vs. only extract serenoa repens. *Arch Ital Urol Androl.* 2015;87(1):25–27.
194. Talley NJ, O'Keefe EA, Zinsmeister AR, Melton LJ 3rd. Prevalence of gastrointestinal symptoms in the elderly: A population-based study. *Gastroenterology.* 1992;102(3):895–901.
195. Calabrese C, Fabbri A, Di Febo G. Long-term management of GERD in the elderly with pantoprazole. *Clin Interv Ageing.* 2007;2(1):85–92.
196. O'Mahony L, McCarthy J, Kelly P et al. Lactobacillus and bifidobacterium in irritable bowel syndrome: Symptom responses and relationship to cytokine profiles. *Gastroenterology.* 2005;128(3):541–551.
197. Pittler MH and Ernst E. Peppermint oil for irritable bowel syndrome: A critical review and metaanalysis. *Am J Gastroenterol.* 1998;93(7):1131–1135.
198. May B, Köhler S, Schneider B. Efficacy and tolerability of a fixed combination of peppermint oil and caraway oil in patients suffering from functional dyspepsia. *Aliment Pharmacol Ther.* 2000;14(12):1671–1677.
199. Holtmann G, Adam B, Haag S, Collet W, Grünewald E, Windeck T. Efficacy of artichoke leaf extract in the treatment of patients with functional dyspepsia: A six-week placebo-controlled, double-blind, multicentre trial. *Aliment Pharmacol Ther.* 2003;18(11–12):1099–1105.
200. Walker AF, Middleton RW, Petrowicz O. Artichoke leaf extract reduces symptoms of irritable bowel syndrome in a post-marketing surveillance study. *Phytother Res.* 2001;15(1):58–61.
201. Liu S, Peng S, Hou X, Ke M, Chen JD. Transcutaneous electroacupuncture improves dyspeptic symptoms and increases high frequency heart rate variability in patients with functional dyspepsia. *Neurogastroenterol Motil.* 2008;20(11):1204–1211.
202. Park YC, Kang W, Choi SM, Son CG. Evaluation of manual acupuncture at classical and nondefined points for treatment of functional dyspepsia: A randomized-controlled trial. *J Altern Complement Med.* 2009;15(8):879–884.
203. Lackner JM, Mesmer C, Morley S, Dowzer C, Hamilton S. Psychological treatments for irritable bowel syndrome: A systematic review and meta-analysis. *J Consult Clin Psychol.* 2004;72(6):1100–1113.
204. Hefner J, Rilk A, Herbert BM, Zipfel S, Enck P, Martens U. Hypnotherapy for irritable bowel syndrome—A systematic review. *Z Gastroenterol.* 2009;47(11):1153–1159.
205. King HH. Severity of irritable bowel symptoms is reduced by osteopathy. *JAOA.* 2013;113:357–358.
206. Brugman R, Fitzgerald K, Fryer G. The effect of osteopathic treatment on chronic constipation—A pilot study. *IJOM.* 2010;13(1):17–23.
207. Bautmans I, Demarteau J, Cruts B, Lemper JC, Mets T. Dysphagia in elderly nursing home residents with severe cognitive impairment can be attenuated by cervical spine mobilization. *J Rehabil Med.* 2008;40(9):755–760.
208. Foley DJ, Cornoni-Huntley JC, White LR. Physical functioning. In: Cornoni-Huntley J et al. eds. *Established Population for Epidemiologic Studies of the Elderly: Resource Data Book.* Bethesda, MD: National Institute on Aging; 1986:56–94, NIH Publication No 86-2443.
209. Atchinson JW and English WR. Manipulative techniques for geriatric patients. *Phys Med Rehabil Clin North Am.* 1996;7:825–842.
210. Marcoff L and Thompson PD. The role of coenzyme Q10 in Statin-associated myopathy. *J Am Coll Cardiol.* 2007;49:2231–2237.
211. Ryder KM, Shorr RI, Bush AJ, Kritchevsky SB, Harris T, Stone K, Cauley J, Tylavsky FA. Magnesium intake from food and supplements is associated with bone mineral density in healthy older white subjects. *J Am Geriatr Soc.* 2005;53:1875–1880.
212. Debbi EM, Agar G, Fichman G, Ziv YB, Kardosh R, Halperin N, Elbaz A, Beer Y, Debi R. Efficacy of methylsulfonylmethane supplementation on osteoarthritis of the knee: A randomized controlled study. *BMC Complement Altern Med.* 2011;11:50.
213. Quandt SA, Chen H, Grzywacz JG et al. Use of complementary and alternative medicine by persons with arthritis: Results of the national health interview survey. *Arthritis Rheum.* 2005;53:748–755.
214. Lewith GT and Kenyon JN. Physiological and psychological explanations for the mechanism of acupuncture as a treatment for chronic pain. *Soc Sci Med.* 1984;19:1367–1378.
215. Goldman N, Chen M, Fujita T et al. Adenosine A1 receptors mediate local anti-nociceptive effects of acupuncture. *Nat Neurosci.* 2010;13:883–888.

216. Manheimer E, Cheng K, Linde K et al. Acupuncture for peripheral joint osteoarthritis. *Cochrane Database Syst Rev*. 2010;1:CD001977.
217. Hinman RS, McCrory P, Pirotta M et al. Acupuncture for chronic knee pain: A randomized clinical trial. *JAMA*. 2014;312(13):1313–1322.
218. Wang C, de Pablo P, Chen X et al. Acupuncture for pain relief in patients with rheumatoid arthritis: A systematic review. *Arthritis Rheum*. 2008;59:1249–1256.
219. Fransen M, Nairn L, Winstanley J. Physical activity for osteoarthritis management: A randomized controlled clinical trial evaluating hydrotherapy or tai chi classes. *Arthritis Rheum*. 2007;57:407–414.
220. Brismee JM, Paige RL, Chyu MC. Group and home-based tai chi in elderly subjects with knee osteoarthritis: A randomized controlled trial. *Clin Rehabil*. 2007;21:99–111.
221. Hartman CA, Manos TM, Winter C et al. Effects of tai chi training on function and quality of life indicators in older adults with osteoarthritis. *J Am Geriatr Soc*. 2000;48:1553–1559.
222. Song R, Lee EO, Lam P et al. Effects of tai chi exercise on pain, balance, muscle strength, and perceived difficulties in physical functioning in older women with osteoarthritis: A randomized clinical trial. *J Rheumatol*. 2003;30:2039–2044.
223. Perlman AI, Sabina A, Williams AL et al. Massage therapy for osteoarthritis of the knee: A randomized controlled trial. *Arch Intern Med*. 2006;166:2533–2538.
224. Ottawa panel systematic review on massage: Low back pain. *J Bodywork Movement Ther*. 2012;16(4):424–455.
225. Shanb AA, Youssef EF, El-Barkouky MG, Kamal RM, Tawfick AM. The effect of magnetic therapy and active exercise on bone mineral density in elderly women with osteoporosis. *J Musculosk Res*. 2012;15(3):176–181.
226. Williams NH, Wilkinson C, Russell I, Edwards RT, Hibbs R, Linck P, Muntz R. Randomized osteopathic manipulation study (ROMANS): Pragmatic trial for spinal pain in primary care. *Fam Pract*. 2003;20(6):662–669.
227. Posadzki P and Edzard E. Osteopathy for musculoskeletal pain patients: A systematic review of randomized controlled trials. *Clin Rheumatol*. 2011;30:285–291.
228. Foster DF, Phillips RS, Hamel MB, Eisenberg DM. Alternative medicine use in older Americans. *J Am Geriatr Soc*. 2000;48:1560–1565.
229. Wyatt GK, Friedman LL, Given CW, Given BA, Beckrow KC. CAT use among older cancer patients. *Cancer Pract*. 1999;7:136–144.
230. Heidemann C, Schulze MB, Franco OH, van Dam, Mantzoros CS, Hu FB. Dietary patterns and risk of mortality from cardiovascular disease, cancer, and all-causes in a prospective cohort of women. *Circulation*. 2008;118:230–237.
231. Kushi LH, Doyle C, McCullough M, Rock CL, Demark-Wahnefried W, Bandera EV. American Cancer Society guidelines on nutrition and physical activity for cancer prevention. *CA Cancer J Clin*. 2012;62:30–67.
232. Port AM, Ruth MR, Istfan NW. Fructose consumption and cancer: Is there a connection? *Curr Opin Endocrinol Diabetes Obes*. 2012;19:367–374.
233. Velicer CM and Ulrich CM. Vitamin and mineral supplement use among US adults after cancer diagnosis: A systematic review. *J Clin Oncol*. 2008;26:665–673.
234. Bjelakovic G, Nikolova D, Simonetti RG, Gluud C. Antioxidant supplements for prevention of gastrointestinal cancers: A systematic review and meta-analysis. *Lancet*. 2004;364:1219–1228.
235. Bairati I, Meyer F, Jobin E, Gélinas M, Fortin A, Nabid A. Antioxidant vitamins supplementation and mortality: A randomized trial in head and neck cancer patients. *Int J Cancer*. 2006;119:2221–2224.
236. Karp DD, Lee SJ, Keller SM et al. Randomized, double-blind, placebo-controlled, phase III chemoprevention trial of selenium supplementation in patients with resected stage I non-small cell lung cancer: ECOG 5597. *J Clin Oncol*. 2013;31(33):4179–4187.
237. Virtamo J, Taylor PR, Kontto J, Mannisto S, Utrainen M, Weinstein SJ, Huttunen J, Albanes D. Effects of alpha-tocopherol and beta-carotene supplementation on cancer incidence and mortality: 18-year postintervention follow-up of the alfa-tocopherol, beta-carotene cancer prevention study. *Int J Cancer*. 2014;135(1):178–185.
238. He ZY, Shi CB, Wen H, Li FL, Wang BL, Wang J. Upregulation of p53 expression in patients with colorectal cancer by administration of curcumin. *Cancer Invest*. 2011;29:208–213.
239. Somasundaram S, Edmund NA, Moore DT, Small GW, Shi YY, Orlowski RZ. Dietary curcumin inhibits chemotherapy-induced apoptosis in models of human breast cancer. *Cancer Res*. 2002;62:3868–3875.
240. Aggarwal B, Prasad S, Sung B, Krishnan S, Guha S. Prevention and treatment of colorectal cancer by natural agents from mother nature. *Curr Colorectal Cancer Rep*. 2013;9:37–56.

241. Grossi F and Tisea M. Granulocyte growth factors in the treatment of non-small cell lung cancer (NSCLC). *Crit Rev Oncol/Hematol.* 2008;58(3):221–230.

242. Xu L, Li H, Xu Z et al. Multi-center randomized double-blind controlled clinical study of chemotherapy combined with or without traditional Chinese medicine on quality of life of postoperative non-small cell lung cancer patients. *BMC Complement Altern Med.* 2012;12:112.

243. Ellsworth RE, Valente AL, Shriver CD, Bittman B, Ellsworth DL. Impact of lifestyle factors on prognosis among breast cancer survivors in the USA. *Expert Rev Pharmacoeconomics Outcomes Res.* 2012;12:451–464.

244. Choi TY, Lee MS, Kim TH, Zaslawski C, Ernst E. Acupuncture for the treatment of cancer pain: A systematic review of randomised clinical trials. *Support Care Cancer.* 2012;20:1147–1158.

245. Ezzo JM, Richardson MA, Vickers A. Acupuncture-point stimulation for chemotherapy-induced nausea or vomiting. *Cochrane Database Syst Rev.* 2006;2:CD002285.

246. Corbin L. Safety and efficacy of massage therapy for patients with cancer. *Cancer Control.* 2005;12:158–164.

247. Ernst E. Massage therapy for cancer palliation and supportive care: A systematic review of randomised clinical trials. *Support Care Cancer.* 2009;17:333–337.

248. Lemanne D, Cassileth B, Gubili J. The role of physical activity in cancer prevention, treatment, recovery, and survivorship. *Oncology (Williston Park).* 2013;27:580–585.

249. Holmes MD, Chen WY, Feskanich D, Kroenke CH, Colditz GA. Physical activity and survival after breast cancer diagnosis. *JAMA.* 2005;293:2479–2486.

250. Meyerhardt JA, Giovannucci EL, Holmes MD, Chan AT, Chan JA, Colditz GA. Physical activity and survival after colorectal cancer diagnosis. *J Clin Oncol.* 2006;24:3527–3534.

251. Giovannucci EL, Liu Y, Leitzmann MF, Stampfer MJ, Willett WC. A prospective study of physical activity and incident and fatal prostate cancer. *Arch Intern Med.* 2005;165:1005–1010.

252. Lee IM, Wolin KY, Freeman SE, Sattlemair J, Sesso HD. Physical activity and survival after cancer diagnosis in men. *J Phys Act Health.* 2014;11:85–90.

253. Tokarski S, Obrebska A, Mejer A, Kowalski J. Assessment of the clinical symptoms and treatment tolerance in patients with non-small cell lung cancer (NSCLC) undergoing first-line chemotherapy and pulmonary rehabilitation. *Pol Merkur Lekarski.* 2014;36(214):245–248.

254. Wells RE, Phillips RS, Schachter SC et al. Complementary and alternative medicine use among US adults with common neurological conditions. *J Neurol.* 2010;257:1822–1831.

255. Pecci C, Rivas MJ, Moretti CM et al. Use of complementary and alternative therapies in outpatients with Parkinson's disease in Argentina. *Mov Disord.* 2010;25:2094–2098.

256. Kim JY and Jeon BS. Complementary and alternative medicine in Parkinson's disease patients in Korea. *Curr Neurol Neurosci Rep.* 2012;12:631–632.

257. Rajendran P, Thompson RE, Reich SG. The use of alternative therapies by patients with Parkinson's disease. Neurology. 2001;57:790–794.

258. Tan LC, Lau PN, Jamora RD, Chan ES. Use of complementary therapies in patients with Parkinson's disease in Singapore. *Mov Disord.* 2006;21:86–89.

259. Ferry P, Johnson M, Wallis P. Use of complementary therapies and non-prescribed medication in patients with Parkinson's disease. *Postgrad Med J.* 2002;78:612–614.

260. Postuma RB, Lang AE, Munhoz RP et al. Caffeine for the treatment of Parkinson's disease: A randomized controlled trial. *Neurology.* 2012;79:651–658.

261. Liu J, Wang L, Zhan SY, Xia Y. Coenzyme Q10 for Parkinson's disease. *Cochrane Database Syst Rev.* 2011;7:CD008150.

262. Zesiewicz TA and Evatt ML. Potential influences of complementary therapy on motor and non-motor complications in Parkinson's disease. *CNS Drugs.* 2009;23:817–835.

263. Hackney ME, Earhart GM. Effects of dance on gait and balance in Parkinson's disease: A comparison of partnered and nonpartnered dance movement. *Neurorehabil Neural Repair.* 2010;24:384–392.

264. Duncan RP and Earhart GM. Randomized controlled trial of community-based dancing to modify disease progression in Parkinson disease. *Neurorehabil Neural Repair.* 2012;26:132–143.

265. Heiberger L, Maurer C, Amtage F et al. Impact of a weekly dance class on the functional mobility and on the quality of life of individuals with Parkinson's disease. *Front Aging Neurosci.* 2011;3:14.

266. Stetka BS, Tomanaino CM. Mending the brain through music. *Medscape Neurol.* 2012. http://www.medscape.com/viewarticle/773401, Accessed October 24, 2014.

267. Li F, Harmer P, Fitzgerald K et al. Tai chi and postural stability in patients with Parkinson's disease. *N Engl J Med.* 2012;366:511–519.

268. Kapoor S. Rapidly emerging role of whole body vibration therapy in the management of neurologic diseases besides polio. *Arch Phys Med Rehabil.* 2011;92:677.

269. Ebersbach G, Edler D, Kaufhold O, Wissel J. Whole body vibration versus conventional physiotherapy to improve balance and gait in Parkinson's disease. *Arch Phys Med Rehabil.* 2008;89:399–403.

270. Lopez D, King HH, Knebl JA, Kosmopoulos V, Collins D, Patterson RM. Effects of comprehensive osteopathic manipulative treatment on balance in elderly patients: A pilot study. *J Am Osteopath Assoc.* 2011;111(6):382–388.

271. Burns L. Case 982:6225—paralysis agitans. In: Ashmore EF, ed. *Case Reports: Record of Cases Treated by Osteopathic Practitioners of California and Texas.* Chattanooga, TN: American Osteopathic Association; 1909:42. Series X.

272. Leslie JG. Case 862:6189—paralysis agitans. In: Ashmore EF, ed. *Case Reports: Record of Cases Treated by Osteopathic Practitioners of Idaho, Montana and Washington.* Auburn, NY: American Osteopathic Association; 1908:35–36. Series IX.

273. Ashmore EF. Case 365:6096—paralysis agitans. In: Ashmore EF, ed. *Case Reports: Record of Cases Treated by Osteopathic Practitioners.* Chattanooga, TN: American Osteopathic Association; 1905:26. Series IV.

274. Charles E. Case 366:6096—paralysis agitans. In: Ashmore EF, ed. *Case Reports: Record of Cases Treated by Osteopathic Practitioners.* Chattanooga, TN: American Osteopathic Association; 1905:27. Series IV.

275. Wells MR, Giantinoto S, D'Agate D et al. Standard osteopathic manipulative treatment acutely improves gait performance in patients with Parkinson's disease. *J Am Osteopath Assoc.* 1999;99(2):92–98.

276. Rivera-Martinez S, Wells MR, Capobianco JD. A retrospective study of cranial strain patterns in patients with idiopathic Parkinson's disease. *J Am Osteopath Assoc.* 2002;102(8):417–422.

277. Boehm KM, Lawner BJ, McFee RB. Study raises important issues about the potential benefit of osteopathy in the cranial field to patients with Parkinson's disease [letter]. *J Am Osteopath Assoc.* 2003;103(8):354–355.

278. Hawk C, Cambroon J. Chiropractic care for older adults: Effects on balance, dizziness, and chronic pain. *J Manipulative Physiol Ther.* 2009;32(6):431–437.

279. Hawk C, Cambroon JA, Prefer MT. Pilot study of the effect of a limited and extended course of chiropractic care on balance, chronic pain, and dizziness in older adults. *J Manipulative Physiol Ther.* 2009;32(6):438–447.

280. Strunk RG and Hawk C. Effects of chiropractic care on dizziness, neck pain, and balance: A single-group, preexperimental, feasibility study. *J Chiropr Med.* 2009;8(4):156–164.

281. Elster EL. Upper cervical chiropractic management of a patient with Parkinson's disease: A case report. *J Manipulative Physiol Ther.* 2000;23(8):573–577.

29 Assistive Technology for Older Adults

Marcia J. Scherer

CONTENTS

29.1 INTRODUCTION

For geriatric individuals with physical, sensory, communication, or cognitive disabilities, assistive technology devices (ATDs) can facilitate independence in accomplishing activities (i.e., the ability or capacity to execute tasks or actions such as reading, writing, walking/moving, dressing, and eating). ATDs enhance the performance of activities and participation by providing the means to get around independently (e.g., wheelchairs, adapted vehicles, and ramps), care for oneself (e.g., built-up handles on eating utensils), and interact with others (e.g., voice-controlled computer input, telephone dialing devices).[1] By enabling a person to perform desired tasks, assistive technologies (ATs) offer the potential to provide a sense of autonomy as well as connection to the community. By accommodating a person's weaknesses and supporting his or her strengths, ATs can reduce emotional and psychosocial as well as physical stress on individuals and their caregivers.[2–5]

ATs have been categorized by the International Organization for Standardization (ISO) based on a product's function as ISO-9999. The chapters in the fifth edition of ISO-9999 are listed below in Table 29.1.

29.2 LEGAL DEFINITION OF ASSISTIVE TECHNOLOGY DEVICES AND SERVICES

An ATD is what the person uses. How they obtain and maintain it falls under the purview of assistive technology services. In the United States, an assistive technology device was originally defined in the Technology Related Assistance for Individuals with Disabilities Act of 1988 (Pub. L.100-407).[6] This legislation, often called the Tech Act for short, was reauthorized in 1994, 1998, and 2004 as the Assistive Technology Act. The original Tech Act defined ATD, and this definition has remained the same throughout its reauthorizations:

> Any item, piece of equipment, or product system, whether acquired commercially, modified or customized, that is used to increase, maintain, or improve functional capabilities of individuals with disabilities (Title 29, Chapter 31, § 3002(a)(3)).

TABLE 29.1

ISO-9999 Assistive Products for Persons with Disability—Classification and Terminology

04 Assistive products for personal medical treatment

05 Assistive products for training in skills

06 Orthoses and prostheses

09 Assistive products for personal care and protection

12 Assistive products for personal mobility

15 Assistive products for housekeeping

18 Furnishings and adaptations to homes and other premises

22 Assistive products for communication and information

24 Assistive products for handling objects and devices

27 Assistive products for environmental improvement and assessment

28 Assistive products for employment and vocational training

30 Assistive products for recreation

Source: WHO Collaborating Centre for the FIC in the Netherlands. *Assistive Products for Persons with Disability— Classification and Terminology—ISO 9999*, fifth edition, 2011. Retrieved March 2, 2016 from http://www.rivm.nl/ who-fic/in/Chapters%20in%20ISO9999%202011.pdf.

The term "assistive technology service" is defined in the Act as

Any service that directly assists an individual with a disability in the selection, acquisition, or use, of an assistive technology device (Title 29, Chapter 31, § 3002(a)).

The law gives the following examples of AT services:

1. The evaluation of the assistive technology needs of an individual with a disability, including a functional evaluation of the impact of the provision of appropriate assistive technology and appropriate services to the individual in the customary environment of the individual.
2. A service consisting of purchasing, leasing, or otherwise providing for the acquisition of assistive technology devices by individuals with disabilities.
3. A service consisting of selecting, designing, fitting, customizing, adapting, applying, maintaining, repairing, replacing, or donating assistive technology devices.
4. Coordination and use of necessary therapies, interventions, or services with assistive technology devices, such as therapies, interventions, or services associated with education and rehabilitation plans and programs.
5. Training or technical assistance for an individual with a disability or, where appropriate, the family members, guardians, advocates, or authorized representatives of such an individual.
6. Training or technical assistance for professionals (including individuals providing education and rehabilitation services and entities that manufacture or sell assistive technology devices), employers, providers of employment and training services, or other individuals who provide services to, employ, or are otherwise substantially involved in the major life functions of individuals with disabilities.
7. A service consisting of expanding the availability of access to technology, including electronic and information technology, to individuals with disabilities.

(Pub. L. 105–394, §3, November 13, 1998, 112 Stat. 3631; Pub. L. 108–364, §2, October 25, 2004, 118 Stat. 1709).[7,8]

Under the Tech Act, each U.S. state and territory receives money to fund an Assistive Technology Act Project (ATAP) to provide services to persons with disabilities for their entire life span, as well as to their families or guardians, service providers, and agencies and other entities that are involved in providing services such as education and employment to persons with disabilities. The list of ATAPs can be found at this website: http://www.resnaprojects.org/allcontacts/statewidecontacts.html.

29.3 FINDING ASSISTIVE TECHNOLOGY DEVICES

The 2001 Survey of Assistive Technology and Information Technology Use and Need by Persons with Disabilities in the United States (AT Survey), was conducted over a 9-month period from March through December 2001.[9] Some of the key findings include

- Mobility devices constituted the bulk of AT used by persons with disabilities. Estimated rates of mobility device use from various surveys ranged from 2.6 percent to 90 percent, depending on the population that was studied, how assistive technology was defined and how use was measured.
- Older adults represented the most studied group of individuals and demonstrated the highest assistive technology use rates among disability groups. Persons over the age of 65 were more likely to use mobility devices (61.5 percent), hearing devices (68.6 percent) and vision devices (51 percent).
- Trends in assistive technology use from national surveys showed an increase in the use of assistive devices over time which can be attributed in part to an aging population.
- Assistive technology was widely used in the home, and these modifications often contributed to greater independence and increased levels of functioning.
- Along with national surveys, state and local surveys reported funding as a significant barrier to assistive technology use, contributing to many unmet needs.
- Computer use and information technology access was acknowledged in the research as important emerging issues in assistive technology (p. 11).

Data regarding ATD use in the United States, as reported by the National Center for Health Statistics, Centers for Disease Control and Prevention,[10] indicate the numbers of individuals using four categories of functional need:

- Approximately 7.4 million Americans used AT devices to accommodate mobility impairments.
- Approximately 4.6 million Americans used ATs to accommodate orthopedic impairments.
- Approximately 4.5 million Americans used ATs to accommodate hearing impairments.
- Approximately 500,000 Americans used ATs to accommodate vision impairments (exclusive of eyeglasses and contact lenses).

The number of users of assistive technology devices and services has increased significantly in each of the above categories since these data were collected in 1994, as have the number of available products, the styles and sizes they come in, and their features and accessories. The Centers for Disease Control and Prevention estimated that

- One in five Americans—about 53 million people—has a disability of some kind.
- 33 million Americans have a disability that makes it difficult for them to carry out daily activities; some have challenges with everyday activities, such as attending school or going to work, and may need help with their daily care.
- 2.2 million people in the United States depend on a wheelchair for day-to-day tasks and mobility.
- 6.5 million people use a cane, a walker, or crutches to assist with their mobility.[11]

AbleData is a website funded by the U.S. Department of Education, National Institute on Disability and Rehabilitation Research (http://www.abledata.com). In 2016, there are over 50,000 different ATDs listed in 20 different categories as shown in the screen shot in Figure 29.1. Once the relevant category is selected, then a hotlink will go to specific devices with further links to manufacturers for technical specifications, availability, cost, and so on.

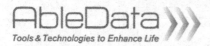

Products by Category

Aids for Daily Living (10,614)

Products to aid in activities of daily living. **Major Categories**: Bathing, Carrying, Child Care, Clothing, Dispenser Aids, Dressing, Drinking, Feeding, Grooming/Hygiene, Handle Padding, Health Care, Holding, Reaching, Time, Smoking, Toileting, Transfer.

Blind and Low Vision (6,163) Products for people with visual disabilities. **Major Categories**: Computers, Educational Aids, Health Care, Information Storage, Kitchen Aids, Labeling, Magnification, Office Equipment, Orientation and Mobility, Reading, Recreation, Sensors, Telephones, Time, Tools, Travel, Typing, Writing (Braille).

Communication (6,102) Products to help people with disabilities related to speech, writing and other methods of communication. **Major Categories**: Alternative and Augmentative Communication, Headwands, Mouthsticks, Signal Systems, Telephones, Typing, Writing.

Computers (6,208) Products to allow people with disabilities to use desktop and laptop computers and other kinds of information technology. **Major Categories**: Software, Hardware, Computer Accessories.

Controls (1,721) Products that provide people with disabilities with the ability to start, stop or adjust electric or electronic devices. **Major Categories**: Environmental Controls, Control Switches.

Deaf And Hard of Hearing (2,118) Products for people with hearing disabilities. **Major Categories**: Amplification, Driving, Hearing Aids, Recreational Electronics, Sign Language, Signal Switches, Speech Training, Telephones, Time.

Deaf Blind (177) Products for people who are both deaf and blind.

Education (3,884) Products to provide people with disabilities with access to educational materials and instruction in school and in other learning environments. **Major Categories**: Classroom, Instructional Materials.

Environmental Adaptations (3,775) Products that make the built environment more accessible. **Major Categories**: Indoor Environment, Furniture, Outdoor Environment, Vertical Accessibility, Houses, Polling Place Accessibility, Lighting, Signs.

FIGURE 29.1 Screen shot of the AbleData.com website showing 20 different categories of products.
(Continued)

Housekeeping (2,745)
Products to that assist in cooking, cleaning, and other household activities as well as adapted appliances.
Major Categories: Food Preparation, Housekeeping General, Cleaning, Ironing, Laundry, Shopping.

Orthotics (1,794)
Braces and other products to support or supplement joints or limbs.
Major categories: Head and Neck, Lower Extremity, Torso, Upper Extremity.

Prosthetics (194)
Products for amputees.
Major categories: Lower Extremity, Upper Extremity.

Recreation (5,079)
Products to assist people with disabilities with their leisure and athletic activities.
Major Categories: Crafts, Electronics, Gardening, Music, Photography, Sewing, Sports, Toys.

Safety and Security (693)
Products to protect health and home.
Major Categories: Alarm and Security Systems, Child Proof Devices, Electric Cords, Lights, Locks.

Seating (2,229)
Products that assist people to sit comfortably and safely.
Major Categories: Seating Systems, Cushions, Therapeutic Seats.

Therapeutic Aids (5,519)
Products that assist in treatment for health problems and therapy and training for certain disabilities.
Major Categories: Ambulation Training, Biofeedback, Evaluation, Exercise, Fine and Gross Motor Skills, Perceptual Motor, Positioning, Pressure/Massage Modality Equipment, Respiratory Aids, Rolls, Sensory Integration, Stimulators, Therapy Furnishings, Thermal/Water Modality Equipment, Traction.

Transportation (1,250)
Products to enable people with disabilities to drive or ride in cars, vans, trucks and buses.
Major Categories: Mass Transit Vehicles and Facilities, Vehicles, Vehicle Accessories.

Walking (2,168)
Products to aid people with disabilities who are able to walk or stand with assistance.
Major Categories: Canes, Crutches, Standing, Walkers.

Wheeled Mobility (4,101)
Products and accessories that enable people with mobility disabilities to move freely indoors and outdoors.
Major Categories: Wheelchairs (Manual, Sport, and Powered), Wheelchair Alternatives (Scooters), Wheelchair

Workplace (1,368)
Products to aid people with disabilities at work.
Major Categories: Agricultural Equipment, Office Equipment, Tools, Vocational Assessment, Vocational Training, Work Stations.

FIGURE 29.1 (Continued) Screen shot of the AbleData.com website showing 20 different categories of products.

When we see the breadth and depth of product lines available, we can appreciate just why there are over 50,000 products listed in the AbleData database. Many products and ATDs come in different sizes, styles, and with options regarding features and accessories. Providing the most appropriate AT device requires a comparison of competing products and time to trial them in actual situations of use.

A good place to begin a search is by identifying the best and most relevant category of products. A crucial point to remember, however, is that a product designed for one primary use, and eategorized in one category, may have other applications of benefit to person. For example, a vibrating and talking alarm watch is a good cognitive support technology for memory. It may, however, be listed under products for *Deaf and Hard of Hearing* and *Blind and Low Vision*.

Specialized products may exist, for example the E-pill alarm watch, but an everyday technology can often serve the same purpose, such as Google Calendar with SMS reminders sent to a cell or smartphone. Everyday wristwatches with alarms and reminding features can be just as effective for some and they can be purchased in many department stores. There are multiple models with varying numbers of alarms that can be set (daily, weekdays, or weekends) so one needs to actually see the watches in order to compare features.

The number and variety of products are large and getting larger. However, solution-seeking needs to begin with the needs and preferences of each unique individual with a disability. For example, tiny phones, small keys, and small screens are not always very useful to people with poor motor control and poor eyesight. And the demands on the user, and cognitive load, can be high.

29.4   ASSISTIVE TECHNOLOGY USE AMONG OLDER ADULTS

A research study by Mann and Tomita[12] found that older adults owned an average of 13 devices and reported using 91% of them. Overall satisfaction was 89% but this varied by device category. Hearing aids, magnifiers, canes, and wheelchairs were found to be the most problematic due to not helping with the intended task, difficulty in or security with use, product expense, discomfort, self-consciousness with use, installation and maintenance difficulties, and the need for additional assistance for use. Scherer and Cushman[13] found in their research on adults over 21 years that the four types of devices most frequently abandoned were adapted grooming aids (55% nonuse), quad canes (43%), walkers (36%), and manual wheelchairs (36%). The most frequent reason given for nonuse was that the device was no longer needed. The study also documented discrepancies in perception between therapists and consumers regarding utility and aesthetic aspects of devices.

Gitlin et al.[14] used samples of older adults discharged from hospitals or rehabilitation units to describe AT use, nonuse and perceptions of AT. While studying 86 older adults with a diverse range of diagnoses including stroke, orthopedic injury, and amputation they found that each person used an average of eight devices. Of the devices provided, 50% were used frequently, 3% were used occasionally, and 47% were seldom or never used. A smaller sample of 13 patients discharged from a rehabilitation hospital showed similar results. At one month after discharge, 45% of the devices were not being used.

In spite of the need for and availability of ATDs, approximately 30% of devices obtained overall and across ages become abandoned or discarded within a year.[15] A positive reason for this outcome may be that the person's functioning improved and the ATD is no longer needed. However, as found in the studies reported above, it remains the case that many needed ATDs are prematurely discarded by older persons. A primary reason cited for this is that there was an inadequate assessment of individualized needs and preferences and a poor match of person and technology occurred.

The Assistive Technology Device Predisposition Assessment (ATD PA)[16] emerged from research on the use and nonuse of recommended ATDs by consumers with a variety of disabilities. The ATD PA Person Form has 54 items, which have been mapped to the World Health Organization's International Classification of Functioning, Disability and Health (ICF) domains of Body Functions and Activities and Participation. The Person Form is divided into three sections: (1) A functional capabilities section which comprises of nine items and three subscales asking the participant to rate the quality of sensory/cognitive/mobility abilities on a 1–5 Likert scale; (2) a subjective well-being scale consisting of 12 items rated on a 1–5 Likert scale; (3) a personal attributes section with 33 items rated on a dichotomous scale. Subscales are affect/mood, resistance to (vs. readiness for) change, engagement in therapy (program/therapist reliance); and (4) support from others.

The ATD PA Device Form consists of 12 items addressing individuals' expectations of and readiness to use ATDs. The follow-up version assesses realization of benefit from the selected ATD.

Older adults (mean age 65) with normal hearing and comparably aged users of assistive listening devices or ALDs completed the following measures: (a) Hearing Handicap Inventory for the Elderly, (b) The Communication Profile for the Hearing Impaired (CPHI), and (c) the ATD PA. Parts of both the CPHI and the ATD PA produced significant mean differences between ALD users and nonusers, suggesting the value of assessing personality and psychosocial factors involved in technology use. Users in general attribute more value to ALDs, have higher psychological readiness for adopting technical assistance, and perceive fewer difficulties with technology use around family, friends, at work, or school than do nonusers. Then, behavioral and audiological data were obtained from 40 subjects 61–81 years of age. Group A included 20 subjects with normal audiological thresholds. Group B included 20 subjects with mild-to-moderate degrees of high-frequency hearing loss. Each subject completed a hearing loss screening survey, ATD PA, and Profile of Hearing Aid Performance (PHAP). The PHAP and hearing loss screen were adequate assessments of self-reported hearing loss, as was the subjective rating of hearing section of the ATD PA. People with high-frequency marginal hearing loss reported less satisfaction with their independence, reduced emotional well-being, and more limitation from their hearing loss than those with normal hearing. Discriminant analyses showed that the ATD PA was the best predictor of membership in Group A or Group B, correctly classifying 85% of the participants and providing psychosocial markers associated with awareness of and adaptation to hearing loss.[17,18]

The decision that a particular ATD is an appropriate and desirable support for an individual is the result of a process that is affected by unique consumer perspectives predisposing the individual to the selection of a particular ATD. To determine the adequacy of this supposition, a study was conducted to address the role of (a) consumer expectations and preferences and (b) personal characteristics on their (c) ATD predisposition or "subjective need" for an ATD as well as subsequent match of ATD and user at 6 months. 139 individuals (mean age 64.2; 54% male) were followed over time in order to gain a better understanding of the factors influencing the continued or discontinued use of mobility devices they obtained as follows: walkers (41%), straight canes (25%), wheelchair (18%), crutches (13%), and quad canes (3%). Participants were recruited at discharge from a large acute care hospital or on admission to one of two rehabilitation hospitals. Participants represented (a) 40.3% lower-extremity orthopedic conditions (traumatic injuries of the lower extremity or pelvis, e.g., hip fracture, hip replacement, femur fracture, or lower-extremity amputation), (b) 33.8% complex medical impairments (conditions not immediately life-threatening, but that posed a risk for disability and/or functional limitations, e.g., chronic obstructive pulmonary disease, various cardiovascular conditions including postmyocardial infarction and heart surgery, and postsurgical disability), and (c) 25.9% neurological (central nervous system impairments affecting mobility, e.g., cerebrovascular accident, Guillain–Barré syndrome, Parkinson's disease, multiple sclerosis, spinal cord injury, or traumatic brain injury).[19]

At 6 months, the 139 individuals had continued (47.5%), discontinued (33.1%), or substituted the use of the initial ATD (19.4%). Discriminant and general linear model (GLM) multivariate analyses showed a significant difference between the three groups according to the ATD PA baseline data.[20]

As hypothesized, respondents varied in their predispositions to ATD use according to their ATD PA Device Form total scores (weak, moderate, strong predisposition at baseline and match at 6-month follow-up). This three-group categorical dependent variable was statistically computed based on percentile score of the ATD PA Device Form total value. Only cases with complete data were used (a missing value on any variable disqualified the case from inclusion).

The more positively respondents scored their subjective well-being and personal characteristics, the more favorably predisposed they were to AT use and the better their match with the selected ATD at 6 months follow-up. For both baseline and 6-months follow-up, the overall Wilks's lambda of the discriminant function analyses was significant at the $p = .01$ level or better, indicating that the items differentiated the three groups at both baseline and 6 months follow-up. The findings gain further strength when prediction of group membership was calculated. The percent correctly predicted into one of the three groups (weak, moderate, strong ATD Match) at 6 months follow-up was 98.7%, which indicates strong accurate prediction.

The decision that a particular ATD is an appropriate and desirable support for an individual can be said to be affected by consumer personal attributes and preference as well as both subjective and objective need for the ATD. Further, these influences are associated with the subsequent match of mobility ATD and user at 6 months in terms of continued, discontinued, or substituted use of the initial ATD.

Emily Agree[21] discusses the importance and potential of "smart" technologies that integrate information technology with ATs in making possible increasingly powerful, individualized tools to assist individuals with disabilities to meet their needs. Yet, findings from 1204 individuals ranging in age from 18 to 91 years indicated that computer anxiety, fluid intelligence, and crystallized intelligence were important predictors of the use of technology.[22]

Boman et al.[23] state that everyday devices can be too complex for some persons with disabilities to master and that when new behaviors are forced upon existing routines, there is often nonuse of the device. They highlight the need for individual assessments as it is crucial to match the person with the right solution for that unique individual. Device flexibility and adaptability is also a concern with everyday technologies as cognitive tasks will vary for any given person and functioning well in one situation does not mean the individual will function as well when the setting or tasks change. Just as important is the fact that many individuals will experience progressive cognitive loss (such as those with dementia), thus requiring the device to be adaptable.

There is increasing growth in the use of information communication technologies (ICTs) such as smartphones and computers by older adults as they discover that this supports their access to information and staying current with distant friends and relatives. A study was done to test an age- appropriate needs-driven training program to promote successful use of ICTs.[24] The project used an iPad was used to provide individualized, one-on-one, home-based ICT training, which was designed to address both the instructional needs of the learner as well as the psychosocial factors influencing their receptiveness to ICTs. The project focused on anxiety and frustration reduction around about technology and learning new skills.

The breadth and frequency of ICT use, perspectives on technology, and perceived independence were recorded at baseline, during the 3-month training and at follow-up, along with an end-of-study questionnaire. Participants expressed satisfaction with both the hardware (iPad) and software (apps) in various contexts. To measure participants' changes in attitude toward ICT, the researchers used the survey of technology use (SOTU), a component of the matching person and technology (MPT) model.[16] The SOTU is a 29-item survey designed to examine an individual's predispositions to technology through his/her attitudes and experiences. It is organized into two sections: *experiences with technology* and their *personal and social characteristics*. Federici et al.[25] found these subscales to have good concurrent and discriminant validity when compared with the World Health Organization's Disability Assessment Schedule II. The SOTU is also valid across cultures when measuring attitude toward technology.

The changes in perspectives of participants toward technology as measured by the SOTU from baseline, during the ICT training, and through the 3-month follow-up revealed in positive trend in how participants viewed technology. The two items with significant change over time from a negative to a positive view were with satisfaction with technology and comfort with technology. A modest positive trend was noted in "technology adds to creativity," "technology is encouraging," "feel good around technology," and "technology raises opinion of self."

29.5   ENHANCING AT USE

It often occurs that the device that worked so well in the rehabilitation facility is not working out in the home or the workplace. For example, the power wheelchair is tearing up the carpet or the communication device is not within reach when needed.

The perspectives and expectations of others in the environments of use can be influential. Trials of equipment in actual settings of use and that involve everyone affected by the technology have proven to be cost effective in the long term because obstacles and barriers to optimal technology use are identified in time to derive solutions and alternatives.

There can be a difference between what the person can physically benefit from and what actually use (objective and subjective need for support. The *objective* need for an AT as determined by providers and measures of functional limitation may or may not match the person's or family's subjective need for that support. The predisposition to use and benefit from support can be characterized by assessing the individual's preferences and characteristics (e.g., current level of subjective quality of life, self-esteem, mood, and attitudes of and support from others).

Several researchers have emphasized the importance of understanding an individual's subjective need for an ATD as well as the functional one determined by a healthcare professional.[26-29] It is also the case that individuals with the same functional needs are apt to have very different subjective needs and vice versa. The diversity of both functional (objective) and subjective needs along with the variable interpretation of those needs by individuals and providers (i.e., the meaning the device and its use has for the person) makes it crucial to conduct a comprehensive assessment that views the patient as an equal partner in the device selection process.

Gramstad et al.[28] point out that older individuals may have ambivalent views of ATDs as being symbols of old age, weakness, and fragility, as well as instrumental in facilitating the development of enhancing independence, belonging, hope, and well-being. They caution that the frequency of ATD use as an important outcome measure may or may not correspond to the meaningfulness of the ATD as experienced by the user.

Providers must be especially cognizant of the impact of support use on individuals with new onset disability. The multiple issues that must be addressed by the individual can have an impact on that person's ability to understand the value of the support and gains that can be achieved from use of it. Given the importance of early support provision, individuals need to come to terms with living with a chronic illness or disability while trying to learn and understand treatment issues and support use. A highly positive outcome of the support decision-making process, therefore, is an individualized intervention that (a) considers the unique individual (including the nature of the disability, age at onset, and so on, as well as objective and subjective need), (b) is minimally complex, and (c) is coupled with strategies for ongoing encouragement and reinforcement of use as well as for the assessment of changing needs.

It is imperative that personal preferences are addressed as early on as possible as they are correlated with the subsequent degree of use of that support and realization of benefit from it. A comprehensive model of service delivery needs to also involve caregivers and families and match their needs to the support identified and be cognizant of any environmental barriers to use.

29.6 ENVIRONMENT EVALUATION

As noted by several researchers,[30-32] in addition to ATDs supporting physical functioning, ATDs may provide benefits such as postponement of relocation or nursing home placement, ability to access cabinets and rooms, and a return to a sense of normalcy and personal comfort. But environmental adaptations are also key to a person's healthy functioning and life quality.

Buildings for public and private use can be constructed at the outset to be accessible to persons with a variety of disabilities or, if existing, have aspects and features that have been retrofitted to meet the needs of people with all levels of capabilities. Examples of retrofitting include adding ramps or elevators so that individuals with difficulty walking can avoid the use of stairs. In addition to accessible entrances and exits, facilities and routing, this includes adequate lighting, signage, floor surfaces, and an appropriate width of corridors. The inside of public and private buildings also requires accessible washroom facilities, telephones, lifts or elevators, appliances, entries and exits, portable and stationary ramps, power-assisted doors, lever door handles, and level door thresholds. There are standards and guidelines specifying how accessibility can be achieved, one being *The Americans with Disabilities Act Accessibility Guidelines (ADAAG) Checklist for Buildings and Facilities* available at http://www.access-board.gov/adaag/checklist/a16.html. Products and technology for accessible buildings and facilities are included in ISO 9999 in the class "Assistive products for environmental improvement and assessment" and within AbleData as "Environmental Adaptations."

Many geriatric individuals live in their current home and are cared for by family members or paid personal assistants and other caregivers. Certain physical features of the home environment, however, may be safety hazards or barriers to performing routine day-to-day activities. Therefore, recommending and implementing home modifications is considered a routine part of clinical practice in home care and rehabilitation. To help in determining needed changes, Gitlin et al.[31] developed a checklist for evaluating the home environment of a person with dementia that can be applied to individuals who are aging in place or who have other disabilities. Areas assessed include the support of daily function or the performance of everyday tasks through the (1) removal of hazards, (2) physical adaptations (e.g., eliminating excess items and rearranging furniture), (3) the support of orientation through the use of visual cues, and (4) comfort enhancement.

Frisardi and Imbimbo[33] define a "smart home" as a residence equipped with technology and "smart devices" that facilitate an individual's independence and quality of life while reducing the burden on family members and other caregivers. Smart devices include sensors, actuators, and/or biomedical monitors (e.g., blood pressure and blood glucose). Advances in smart devices, mobile wireless communications, sensor networks, pervasive computing, machine learning, middleware (or software that links programs) and agent technologies, and human–computer interfaces have made workable smart homes possible.[34,35] Aldrich[36] listed five types and levels of smart homes, from least to most advanced (and intrusive):

1. Homes with intelligent objects such as talking alarms, remote controls for home appliances, a missing object finder, and adapted telephones.
2. Homes with intelligent objects that communicate. Devices include wearable monitors and sensors that detect and relay information about a person's health state. The devices are connected to a remote center, which diagnoses the situation and initiates the provision of necessary assistance (such as paramedic attention). Other examples of devices in this level include carbon monoxide detectors, smoke and fire detectors, and so on. Care delivered remotely via telecommunications technologies (telehealth, telecare, and telemedicine) are introduced in this level of smart home.
3. Connected homes have both internal and remote control of what is in the home. For example, a caregiver can check and turn off appliances from a distance.
4. Learning homes address patterns of activity in the home and the data that are recorded and accumulated are used to anticipate the resident's needs and to control the environment. For example, turning up the heat an hour before the person gets up in the morning.
5. Attentive homes continuously monitor and register the activity and location of people and items within the home and this information is used to control the devices in anticipation of the resident's needs. This is known as *context awareness*.[34]

There is a balance to be achieved between safety and security on the one hand and the loss of privacy, choice, and autonomy on the other. The more intrusive the intervention, the less privacy, choice, and autonomy exist.

29.7   SUPPORT FROM CAREGIVERS

Researchers have found that individuals who received functionally based ATs and environmental interventions showed significantly less functional decline.[12] Other forms of support come from family and paid caregivers.

According to the Family Center on Technology and Disability (FCTD), an educated and trained family is a key resource in the rehabilitation and community integration process. It is certainly the case that they have the most intimate and detailed knowledge of the person with a disability.

Paid caregivers are also a very important form of support for many persons.

Statistics from the National Alliance for Caregiving reveal that caregivers comprise 29% of the U.S. adult population, or 65.7 million adults. Of this number, half care for adult recipients and another 13% for both child and adult recipients.

There are cultural values attached to independence versus the reliance on caregivers and technologies. According to Ripat and Woodgate,[37] "although healthcare cost savings are valued in Western society, if the family culture is to provide that assistance, [assistive technology] may represent a threat to the relationship and role of the family member as care provider" (p. 92). The authors further note that while individualistic societies value independence and autonomy, collectivist society place more emphasis on community and interdependence and, thus, may not view some forms of AT favorably.

Disability is not a characteristic of an individual, but an outcome or result of a complex interrelationship among the individual's health condition, personal factors, and the external factors that represent the circumstances in which the individual lives. Disability is a situational and multidimensional phenomenon resulting from interactions within both physical and social environments. Thus, the same environment will have a varying impact on two different individuals and different environments will impact the same individual in different ways.

29.8 CONCLUDING COMMENTS

Matching an individual with the most appropriate ATD for his or her use requires an understanding of that person's personal characteristics, environments of use, and the type and degree of support from others. Rehabilitation professionals have found that the increased availability of ATD options has made the process of matching a person with the most appropriate device more complex because consumers' predisposition to, expectations for, and reactions to ATDs and their features are highly individualized and personal. These predispositions, expectations, and reactions emerge from a sense of well-being, outlook and goals for future functioning, expectations held by one's self and others, and financial and environmental support for technology use. With information from a comprehensive assessment, professionals can identify potential or existing problem areas and intervene to better ensure that the use of the technology will enhance quality of life, and the person's home and community experiences. A written summary of this information can specify what needs to be done, by whom, by when, and with what resources, thus providing professionals with appropriate questions to ask ATD providers and vendors.

REFERENCES

1. Bodine, C. 2013. *Assistive Technology and Science (The SAGE Reference Series on Disability: Key Issues and Future Directions)*. Los Angeles: Sage Publications, Inc.
2. Scherer, M.J. (Ed.). 2002. *Assistive Technology: Matching Device and Consumer for Successful Rehabilitation*. Washington, DC: APA Books.
3. Scherer, M.J. 2004. *Connecting to Learn: Educational and Assistive Technology for People with Disabilities*. Washington, DC: American Psychological Association (APA) Books.
4. Scherer, M.J. 2005. *Living in the State of Stuck: How Assistive Technology Impacts the Lives of People with Disabilities*, fourth edition. Cambridge, MA: Brookline Books.
5. Scherer M.J., Craddock G., and Mackeogh T. 2011. The relationship of personal factors and subjective well-being to the use of assistive technology devices. *Disability and Rehabilitation*, 33(10), 811–817. PMID: 20735272.
6. Assistive Technology Act of 1988, Pub. L. No. 100-407, 102 STAT. 1044. 1988. Retrieved from http://www.gpo.gov/fdsys/pkg/STATUTE-102/pdf/STATUTE-102-Pg1044.pdf.

7. Assistive Technology Act of 1998, Pub. L. No. 105-394, §§ 2 and 3. 1998.
8. Assistive Technology Act of 2004, Pub. L. No. 108-364, § 3. 2004. Retrieved from https://www.gpo.gov/fdsys/pkg/STATUTE-118/pdf/STATUTE-118-Pg1707.pdf.
9. Carlson, D. and Ehrlich, N. 2005. *Assistive Technology and Information Technology Use and Need by Persons with Disabilities in the United States*, Washington, DC: U.S. Department of Education, National Institute on Disability and Rehabilitation Research.
10. National Center for Health Statistics, Centers for Disease Control and Prevention. Number of persons using assistive technology devices. Retrieved March 7, 2016 from http://www.cdc.gov/nchs/nhis/ad292tb1.htm.
11. Eunice Kennedy Shriver National Institute of Child Health and Human Development (NICHD). How many people use assistive devices? Retrieved March 7, 2016 from https://www.nichd.nih.gov/health/topics/rehabtech/conditioninfo/pages/people.aspx.
12. Mann, W.C., Ottenbacher, K.J., Fraas, L., Tomita, M., and Granger, C.V. 1999. Effectiveness of assistive technology and environmental interventions in maintaining independence and reducing home care costs for the frail elderly: A randomized controlled trial. *Archives of Family Medicine*, 8(3), 210–217.
13. Cushman, L.A. and Scherer, M.J. 1996. Measuring the relationship of assistive technology use, functional status over time, and consumer—Therapist perceptions of ATs. *Assistive Technology*, 8(2), 103–109.
14. Gitlin, L.N., Schemm, R.L., Landsberg, L., and Burgh, D. 1996. Factors predicting assistive device use in the home by older people following rehabilitation. *Journal of Aging and Health*, 8(4), 554–575.
15. Scherer, M.J. 2014. From people-centered to person-centered services, and back again. *Disability and Rehabilitation: Assistive Technology*, 9(1), 1–2.
16. Scherer, M.J. 2005. *The Matching Person and Technology (MPT) Model Manual and Assessments*, fifth edition [CD-ROM]. Webster, NY: The Institute for Matching Person and Technology, Inc.
17. Scherer, M.J. and Frisina, D.R. 1994. Applying the matching people with technologies model to individuals with hearing loss: What people say they want—and need—from assistive technologies. *Technology and Disability: Deafness and Hearing Impairments*, 3(1), 62–68.
18. Scherer, M.J. and Frisina, D.R. 1998. Characteristics associated with marginal hearing loss and subjective well-being among a sample of older adults. *Journal of Rehabilitation Research and Development*, 35(4), 420–426.
19. Demers, L., Fuhrer, M.J., Jutai, J.W., Scherer, M.J., Pervieux, I., and DeRuyter, F. 2008. Tracking mobility-related assistive technology in an outcomes study. *Assistive Technology*, 20(2), 73–85.
20. Scherer, M.J., Jutai, J., Fuhrer, M., Demers, L., and DeRuyter, F. 2006, June. Factors impacting consumers' assistive technology device (ATD) selection. *29th Annual RESNA Conference Proceedings*. Retrieved March 10, 2016 from https://www.resna.org/sites/default/files/legacy/conference/proceedings/2006/Research/Outcomes/Scherer.html.
21. Agree, E.M. 2014. The potential for technology to enhance independence for those aging with a disability. *Disability and Health Journal*, 7, S33–S39.
22. Czaja, S.J., Charness, N., Fisk, A.D., Hertzog, C., Nair, S.N., Rogers, W.A., and Sharit, J. 2006. Factors predicting the use of technology: Findings from the center for research and education on aging and technology enhancement (create). *Psychology and Aging*, 21(2), 333–352.
23. Arthanat, S., Vroman. K.G., and Lysack C. 2014. A home-based individualized information communication technology training program for older adults: A demonstration of effectiveness and value. *Disability and Rehabilitation: Assistive Technology*. 2014 Dec 16:1–9 [Epub ahead of print].
24. Boman, I.L., Bartfai, A., Borell, L., Tham, K., and Hemmingsson, H. 2010. Support in everyday activities with a home-based electronic memory aid for persons with memory impairments. *Disability and Rehabilitation: Assistive Technology*, 5(5), 339–350.
25. Federici, S., Scherer, M., Micangeli, A., Lombardo, C., and Belardinelli, O.M. 2003. A cross-cultural analysis of relationships between disability self-evaluation and individual predisposition to use assistive technology. In Craddock, G.M., McCormack, L.P., Reilly, R.B., Knops H.T.P. (Eds.), *Assistive Technology: Shaping the Future* (pp. 941–946). Dublin, Ireland: IOS Press.
26. McCreadie, C. and Tinker, A. 2005. The acceptability of assistive technology to older people. *Ageing and Society*, 25, 91–110. doi:10.1017/S0144686X0400248X
27. Gramstad, A., Storli, S.L., and Hamran, T. 2013. "Do I need it? Do I really need it?" Elderly peoples experiences of unmet assistive technology device needs. *Disability and Rehabilitation: Assistive Technology*, 8(4), 287–293.
28. Gramstad, A., Storli, S.L., and Hamran, T. 2014. Exploring the meaning of a new assistive technology device for older individuals. *Disability and Rehabilitation: Assistive Technology*, 1–6, Posted online on May 20, 2014.

29. Scherer, M., Jutai, J., Fuhrer, M., Demers, L., and DeRuyter, F. 2007. A framework for modelling the selection of assistive technology devices (ATDs). *Disability and Rehabilitation: Assistive Technology*, 2(1), 1–8. PMID: 19263548.
30. Gitlin, L.N. 2002. Assistive technology in the home and community for older people: Psychological and social considerations. In M.J. Scherer (Ed.), *Assistive Technology: Matching Device and Consumer for Successful Rehabilitation* (pp. 109–122). Washington, DC: American Psychological Association.
31. Gitlin, L.N., Schinfeld, S., Winter, L., Corcoran, M., Boyce, A.A., and Hauck, W. 2002. Evaluating home environments of persons with dementia: Interrater reliability and validity of the Home Environmental Assessment Protocol (HEAP). *Disability and Rehabilitation*, 24(1–3), 59–71.
32. Lancioni, G.E., Perilli, V., O'Reilly, M.F., Singh, N.N., Sigafoos J., Bosco, A., Caffò, A.O., Picucci, L., Cassano, G., and Groeneweg, J. 2013. Technology-based orientation programs to support indoor travel by persons with moderate Alzheimer's disease: Impact assessment and social validation. *Research in Developmental Disabilities*, 34(1), 286–293.
33. Frisardi, V. and Imbimbo, B.P. 2011. Gerontechnology for demented patients: Smart homes for smart aging. *Journal of Alzheimer's Disease*, 23(1), 143–146.
34. Roy, N., Roy, A., and Das, S.K. 2006. Context-aware resource management in multiinhabitant smart homes: A Nash H-learning based approach. *Proceedings of the Fourth Annual IEEE International Conference on Pervasive Computing and Communications (PerCom'06)*, Pisa, Italy (pp. 148–158). http://ieeexplore.ieee.org/stamp/stamp.jsp?tp=&arnumber=1598920.
35. Schülke, A.M., Plischke, H., and Kohls, N.B. 2010. Ambient assistive technologies (AAT): Socio-technology as a powerful tool for facing the inevitable sociodemographic challenges. *Philosophy, Ethics, and Humanities in Medicine*, 5, 8. Retrieved March 10, 2016 from http://peh-med.biomedcentral.com/articles/10.1186/1747-5341-5-8.
36. Aldrich, F.K. 2003. Smart homes: Past, present and future. In R. Harper (Ed.), *Inside the Smart Home* (pp. 17–39). London, United Kingdom: Springer-Verlag.
37. Ripat, J. and Woodgate, R. 2011. The intersection of culture, disability and assistive technology. *Disability and Rehabilitation: Assistive Technology*, 6(2), 87–96.

30 Ethical Issues in Older Adults

Richard A. Demme, Bernard Sussman, and Margie Hodges Shaw

CONTENTS

30.1 INTRODUCTION

The process and activities of rehabilitation are fundamentally ethical in nature, as the preservation, restoration, and enhancement of abilities foster autonomy—living one's life as he/she sees fit, at his/her own direction. Ethical issues may become magnified in elderly patients. Despite the limited duration of benefit a procedure might have for an elderly person, the benefit may be of great consequence. The maintenance or recovery of a skill such as mobility is crucial to maintenance of independence and for quality of life. While some elderly patients may not be autonomous, the healthcare team still must consider how to maximize the benefits of treatment. Many diseases of the elderly are chronic in nature and cannot be cured. Whether or not treatments are more palliative in nature than curative, providers must be alert to the potential hazards to avoid causing harm. In this chapter, we focus on ethical issues related to medical decision-making. We review the terminology and background of ethical principles, advance directives, informed consent, capacity determination, and surrogate decision-making. We highlight important issues by the use of a representative case.

30.2 PRINCIPLES OF BIOETHICS AND BIOETHICAL DECISION-MAKING

Ethically responsible decisions incorporate respect for a person's values and preferences with her physician's professional judgment about what will best serve the patient's well-being. The frailties and limitations of the elderly, both physical and mental, may make the assessment of the patient's values and therapeutic options challenging. Each person involved in the care of the patient, and in the decision-making process, holds values and preferences that may differ significantly. Many patients and families (as well as clinicians) find communicating about the personal values and preferences that influence treatment decisions to be challenging. When ethically challenging treatment decisions arise, a thoughtful decision-making process can provide a path to a sound decision. Understanding this process requires understanding of the terminology used.

Clinical education includes instruction on the four principles of bioethics—justice, beneficence, nonmaleficence, and autonomy.[1] Physicians rely on these principles in clinical decision-making. The principle of justice requires substantive fairness and procedural fairness. Substantive fairness requires clinicians to treat similarly situated patients similarly and allocate resources fairly. The principle of justice applies to the care of every individual patient because it requires clinicians to rely on a just decision-making process. A just and fair decision-making process must include consideration of the other three principles. Beneficence is the obligation to help the patient and nonmaleficence is the obligation "to do no harm." Beneficence and nonmaleficence require clinicians to balance benefits over harms in patient care. Determining the right balance in a specific patient's care is often difficult even when the patient is a fully engaged and capable participant in the process.

Autonomy is defined as the patient's right to self-determination. The principle of autonomy, codified in the legal doctrine of informed consent, dictates the right of the adult patient with capacity to make treatment decisions. When a patient has the capacity to understand his diagnosis and prognosis and is able to express his treatment preferences, the patient's choice must be respected.

While important in clinical decision-making, the principles of bioethics neither define a fair decision-making process nor provide guidance about how to balance the principles in an individual patient's care. When, if ever, does beneficence outweigh the principle of autonomy? How does one balance beneficence and nonmaleficence? To answer these questions and prioritize the ethical principles, clinicians, whether intentionally or not, often rely on variations of the three major philosophical approaches to normative ethics. These approaches are deontology, consequentialism, and virtue ethics.

Deontological theories are rule based: obligations or duties guide actions. Deontologists tend to place a high value on the principle of beneficence and strict deontologists accept that sometimes the right action has tragic consequences. Theories of consequentialism, including utilitarianism, are concerned with outcome—consequences of actions guide actions. Consequentialists balance benefits and harms in an effort to maximize the most good among the most people and may accept an individual sacrifice, if necessary, to achieve the most good. Virtue theories focus on the character traits of the actor: good virtues guide action. The clinician who relies on virtue theory might ask, "What would the compassionate physician do?" These approaches to normative ethics include many variations and none alone provides a conclusive solution to balance the principles of bioethics in an individual patient's care. Moreover, each person caring for the patient will have her own moral tendencies. Where disagreement exists, these theories provide neither a path for decision-making nor a mechanism for conflict resolution.

Many propose the use of narrative to provide a framework for clinical decision-making.[2] Narrative theories identify the patient's stories and patient's life as unique and powerful qualitative data reflecting the patient's values and preferences. Narrative ethics allows the *patient's* moral tendencies to balance the principles of bioethics for her own care and treatment decisions. When the patient is capable of independently making treatment decisions, narrative ethics supports the patient's role as an author: autonomy outweighs the other principles. When the patient requires heightened support in making treatment decisions, the patient's right of self-determination is respected by incorporating narrative data into the decision-making process (Kohn et al.[3] provide an important discussion about the distinctions between shared decision-making and supported decision-making that go beyond the scope of this chapter).[3] The following case discussion provides an example of efforts to balance the principles of bioethics in patient care.

30.3 ADVANCE DIRECTIVES

Mr A is a 76-year-old retired college professor of literature who has been recently diagnosed with early Alzheimer's disease. Other medical problems include hypertension, type 2 diabetes, chronic kidney disease (CKD) stage 2, and osteoarthritis. He has enjoyed an intellectually stimulating life and a physically active one centered on his love of the outdoors. He takes pride and pleasure in his many interests which in addition to his life of scholarship include gardening, hiking, classical music, and amateur astronomy. He presents to the office of his primary care physician (PCP) accompanied by his wife to discuss advance directives. He has read about Alzheimer's disease and acknowledges his fear of the future. He asks for more information about what that future may be like and whether it is a good idea to draft a living will.

An advance directive refers to a written statement or document executed by an adult with the capacity to make healthcare decisions. Advance directives are designed to provide medical personnel, family members, and others information about the nature and extent of medical care to be provided in the future should a patient lose decision-making capacity.[4]

Advance directives can be procedural, substantive, or both. A procedural advance directive describes the process the medical team should follow in the event the patient loses capacity. For example, a procedural advance directive names the person who will speak on behalf of the patient. This kind of advance directive is sometimes called a "proxy." Substantive advance directives provide information about patient's wishes. Patients may request certain types of treatments or refuse others. The directions can be broad or highly specific. "Do Not Resuscitate" (DNR) and "Do Not Intubate" (DNI) orders, for example, are substantive advance directives. When the advance directive is both procedural and substantive, the proxy can use the substantive data to inform decisions.

30.3.1 SUBSTANTIVE ADVANCE DIRECTIVES

Some people use the term "living will" interchangeably with advance directive. The living will was first proposed by Luis Kutner in 1969 as an instrument to limit medical treatments for those who have lost the capacity to make medical decisions. It is called a *living* will because it expresses what types of medical treatment a person desires while he is alive, as opposed to other wills that give direction about wishes after death, such as who should receive property.[5] In 1976, California became the first state that legally sanctioned living wills. By 1992, all 50 states and the District of Columbia had passed living will legislation. The concept of the living will has spread outside the United States.[6]

A typical living will might state "In the event that my physician finds that I am in a terminal or incurable condition where death is imminent, I do not wish to receive any medical treatments or procedures that would only serve to delay my death."[4] The importance of completion of a living will that limits resuscitation for the elderly is reinforced by data demonstrating that only 18.3% of patients >65 years old survived to discharge after cardiopulmonary resuscitation (CPR) for in-hospital cardiac arrests. Older patients and those admitted from a nursing home had a poorer outcome.[7]

In an effort to encourage Americans to complete an advance directive, the United States Congress passed the Patient Self Determination Act (PSDA) in 1990. The PSDA required hospitals, nursing homes, home health agencies, hospice providers, health maintenance organizations, and other healthcare institutions to provide information about advance directives to adult patients at the time of inpatient admission or enrollment. The required information includes notice of their right to participate in and direct their own healthcare decisions, their right to accept or refuse medical or surgical treatment, and their right to prepare advance directives.

The PSDA codifies the 1990 U.S. Supreme Court ruling that "a competent person has a constitutionally protected liberty interest in refusing unwanted medical treatment" even when the treatment is life sustaining.[8] The conflict in the case (Cruzan v. Director, Missouri Department of Health) concerned the right of a surrogate decision-maker to refuse unwanted medical treatment (artificial hydration and nutrition) and the interest of the state to preserve human life. The court upheld a state's authority to set evidentiary standards and held that the state of Missouri could require "clear and convincing" evidence that a person who had lost the capacity to make medical decisions would not want to continue treatments. Justice O'Connor, in a concurring opinion, noted that similar cases could be avoided if each state recognized the authority of the patient-appointed proxy to make healthcare decisions on her behalf. "These procedures for surrogate decision making … may be a valuable additional safeguard of the patient's interest in directing his/her medical care."[9] An unambiguous, signed, and witnessed advance directive also may be a "clear and convincing" evidence of preferences.

Despite state and national efforts to encourage Americans to complete an advance directive, only a minority of people have. A Pew research survey noted a growth in the number of people who say that they have a living will from 12% in 1990% to 29% in 2006, but there has not been further growth in advance directive completion.[10] A recent mail survey designed to be representative of the nonhospitalized U.S. population reported that only 26.3% had an advance directive.[11] In hospitalized patients, the range of advance directive completion is 1%–40%.[12] Factors such as age, education, income, and culture influence the completion of advance directives. Among those in home healthcare and nursing homes, those aged 85 years and older were more than twice as likely as those under the age of 65 to have an advance directive. White nursing home residents were 3 times as likely as black residents to have living wills, and 2 times as likely as black residents to have DNR orders.[13]

It may help to consider why so few people complete advance directives. For nonhospitalized individuals, the most frequently cited reason for not having one was lack of awareness.[11] Most patients do not want to consider themselves terminally ill, and many physicians as well are reluctant to consider patients as terminally ill. The Study to Understand Prognoses and Preferences for Outcomes and Risks of Treatment (SUPPORT) showed that patients with terminal illness remained more optimistic about their prognosis than their physicians.[14] In another study, some oncology patients said that they had "full confidence in physicians" and completing an advance directive was "not important for me at the moment."[15]

Discussions about death are difficult for both patients and physicians, and are often deferred. Furthermore, there is a wide variability of both patient and physician interest, desire, and the ability to discuss end-of-life wishes. As noted above, hospitals and nursing homes are required to inform patients about their right to complete an advance directive. This is usually accomplished by the presentation of a brochure at the time of admission. One study of nursing homes found that in nearly 70% of admissions, someone other than the residents received the information about completing a directive.[16] Staff members cite residents' cognitive impairment as a reason for excluding residents from the informing process. However, even among residents who were alert and oriented, someone other than the resident received the information 47.7% of the time,[16] perhaps reflecting the reluctance to discuss end-of-life preferences.

It is also important to know that some patients do complete advance directives and to consider why. In an interview study in 1993%, 81% of patients with capacity, who were admitted to the acute medical service of a community-teaching hospital, did discuss or want to discuss advance directives in the hospital. Of these, 41% chose to forgo CPR.[17] In one study of nursing home residents, the most common reason for completing an advance directive was experience with the prolonged death of a friend or family member.[18]

Physicians should ask patients about advance planning and provide information about the purpose of advance planning, the kinds of advance directives, the logistics of how to complete one, and the costs. Patients need to know that advance directives do not require a lawyer and many templates are available for free. This general information, however, is not likely to be enough. Physicians should also consider when and under what circumstances to initiate conversations about advance planning. If these conversations are not part of hospital admissions or are routinely included in doctor–patient conversations, then, it may be difficult to decide when to introduce the subject.

In cardiac care units and oncology intensive care units, settings where patients might be greatly concerned about dying, it is curious that only a small percentage of patients have completed an advance directive or appointed a healthcare agent. In one cancer center ICU, 27% of patients had advance directives.[19] Some oncologists discuss end-of-life care with patients only after uncomfortable symptoms occur, or no further oncologic treatment is possible.[20] A survey of oncology nurses demonstrated a lack of understanding about the PSDA and advance directives and a corresponding lack of confidence in their ability to assist patients with advance directives.[21]

The American College of Cardiology/American Heart Association recommends[22] that cardiologists discuss advance directives with patients who have congestive heart failure, yet only 26% of patients in one academic medical center cardiac care unit/intensive care unit (CCU/ICU) had advance directives.[23] Perhaps, these data should not be surprising given the challenges to completing advance directives and the results of the SUPPORT study. These challenges are difficult to overcome: Use of nursing interventions to improve communication about patient end-of-life wishes did not improve the accord between patient preferences and physician recommendations regarding resuscitation.[24]

There are also problems with many completed advance directives. The language in advance directive templates is often vague and not helpful to explain wishes in specific situations. Vague language can be variably interpreted. A broad advance directive stating, "In the event my condition is hopeless, I do not wish to receive any heroic measures" does not help guide physicians to treatments a patient might actually want.[4] Physicians often do not agree when a person has an "incurable or terminal illness." There are no treatments that merely "prolong dying" that do not also "prolong living." The language also might indicate a lack of understanding of the dying process. An advance directive might document the decision to "allow natural death," but most people would not want to die in pain or short of breath, which can occur if one is allowed to die naturally.

Templates that aim for specificity have problems as well. Advance directives are available that require patients to envision a number of specific scenarios and choose a number of responses.[25] These forms can be overwhelming, and may be difficult to fill out even for someone with medical training. One cannot predict all of the clinical scenarios that might arise. An advance directive that limits treatments in a narrow set of anticipated circumstances may not apply to the predicament that the patient now faces.

A final problem that warrants discussion involves advance directives that document the desire for aggressive medical treatment regardless of the medical professionals' judgment about the benefit of such treatment. Treatment requests that extend life for patients who are not expected to recover are often frustrating for hospital staff. Such treatment may be described as "futile," but there is no medical or ethical consensus on what constitutes "futility." Courts have not overruled surrogate decisions for medical treatment even at the request of the hospital.[26] When surrogate decision-makers request aggressive treatment against medical advice, it is helpful to understand the goal of extending life and the principle of respecting the patient's wishes. Studies have shown that about 31% of people will ask for continued treatments for as long as it is possible to preserve life. "Quality of life" and "quality of death" are important for about 66% of people.[27]

Despite the problems with advance directives and concerns that the documents fall short of facilitating patients' autonomy, they may help some incapacitated patients make their preferences known. For example, a Jehovah's Witness can refuse blood transfusion. One of the author's advance directive specifies that he wants his pets to be able to visit him liberally if he is hospitalized. There are no restrictions as to what may be requested in an advance directive, but there may be hospital policy, state law, or other restrictions that limit the implementation of advance directive wishes.

In hospital settings, written advance directive guidance is often less helpful than discussions between physicians and a trusted healthcare agent. Still, the process of completing an advance directive may encourage conversation and provide the surrogate decision-maker qualitative data on the patient's wishes. The surrogate decision-maker can rely on these data to help interpret any ambiguous language. For example, if an advance directive indicates that a person would want "a trial of intubation" but would not wish to receive intensive treatments "for a prolonged time," the healthcare agent could help determine what a "prolonged time" or a reasonable "trial" would be for their loved one. High suggests that advance directive completion is most appropriate to direct care for those persons who do not have a family or other surrogates to serve as substitute decision-makers, for people who have very specific or unusual preferences, and for people who do not want their family members to make substitute healthcare decisions or who have disagreements with their family members.[28]

For the most part, simply handing out didactic information about advance directives and healthcare proxies does little to increase advance directive completion; interaction with a knowledgeable resource person and the opportunity to discuss individual concerns appears to be more effective for advance directive completion.[29] Mr A is wise to begin this conversation with his physician.

We recommend that each adult individual completes an advance directive as best as he/she can to give guidance to her healthcare agents (HCAs) and physicians. An advance directive may give physicians a better chance to provide only the desired treatment; it may lead to avoidance of non-beneficial treatments, and may lessen the burden of surrogate decision-makers.

Mr A is not sure about completing a living will. He is able to articulate that while he is uncertain about his future, he would not want to be kept alive on a machine such as a ventilator for a long time. He is confident, however, that his wife would be able to make decisions about possible treatments for him, and he would like to name her to be his healthcare agent.

30.3.2 PROCEDURAL ADVANCE DIRECTIVES: HCAs

In many of the studies cited above, patients were more likely to have named a healthcare agent than to have completed a substantive advance directive. A person chosen by the patient himself to speak for him upon losing capacity is called a proxy, or durable power of attorney for healthcare, or a Health Care Power of Attorney (HCPOA), depending on the jurisdiction. We shall refer to these chosen surrogate decision-makers as HCAs. As discussed above, it is generally more useful for healthcare providers to discuss potential treatments with living persons, than to determine whether an advance directive should apply to a specific situation that may not have been foreseen.

Choosing an HCA is simpler than filling out an advance directive and less threatening. It is easier for most people to answer the question "Is there someone you would trust to make good healthcare decisions for you if you were unable?" than to consider "what types of machines would you like us to try to keep you from dying?" A nationally representative sample of individuals living in the community, who were at least 70 years old, found that 60.8% had named HCAs.[30] Additionally, some individuals with limited capacity might still be able to pick an HCA to make decisions for them even when they themselves do not have the capacity to distinguish between the merits of complex medical treatments. However, those with the lowest quartile of global cognitive function were 76% less likely to have named an HCA than those in the highest quartile of cognitive functioning.[30]

It is still important to carefully select the best representative, discuss treatment preferences, and choose someone capable of articulating the patient's wishes. About 30% of people might not choose their spouse or emergency contact person to make their healthcare decisions.[31] Since these are the people who would most likely be contacted upon an urgent hospitalization, it is especially important for those who do not want their spouse or emergency contact to make decisions to execute an advance directive naming an HCA of their choice. A PEW study reported that 78% of people thought their closest relative should make healthcare decisions for them if they were unable to do so.[27] However, when there is family discord or disagreement, it may be best to name a friend, neighbor, coworker, or fellow parishioner as your HCA. The reasons given for choosing a particular HCA include the agent knew the patient best, was the closest relative, and was most accessible geographically.[12] When choosing a healthcare agent, an individual might consider additional factors:

Will this person respect your wishes?
Is this person the most likely to make choices that you would make?
Is this person reasonably available and willing to speak with physicians?
1. Will this person involve other loved ones to consider information about the types of treatment they think you would want?
2. Can this person determine when "enough is enough"?

Unfortunately, when individuals name an HCA, they do not always discuss treatment preferences.[32] The most crucial decision an HCA might have to make is to say when "enough is enough" and to limit further treatment to comfort measures. It may be easier for a relative to say "continue all treatments" or "add another machine" to sustain life. However, some people might not want all possible treatments. Most Americans die in hospitals, and for many patients, there is eventually an agreement to limit or discontinue certain treatments near the time of death. Some people expect that their families will make good decisions for them without explicit instruction. A commonly cited reason for not completing a living will includes a desire to "rely on the family" for making end-of-life decisions.[28] However, familial proxies' estimates of agents' preferences do not differ greatly from chance.[12] In a paired interview test, Sulmasy found that terminally ill patients and their chosen HCAs were in agreement about end-of-life choices in only 66% of the cases.[33] If a person discusses desired treatments with his/her HCA, he/she might include additional procedural direction and inform his/her agent whether he/she wants future healthcare decisions based on consideration of discussions he's/she's had with them, based on what physicians recommend, based on the style of how they lived their lives, or even what the HCA thinks is best for them.

The Terri Schiavo case illustrated the difficulties when family members could not come to a consensus about what types of treatments she would want and who should make decisions for her. Her parents wanted her to continue artificial nutrition by a tube, and her husband/guardian did not. Her parents did not accept her diagnosis of a persistent vegetative state. Her case attracted the notice of the media, the Florida state governor, and even the U.S. Congress. The resolution of her case would have been simpler if she had indicated in writing what treatments she would have wanted and/or who she would like to make decisions for her. Paula Span reported "It's not uncommon for doctors to disagree with a family about what should be done; it's not uncommon for family members to disagree—sharply and painfully—with one another." But, she notes "It's a much uglier fight if you don't have the documents."[34]

The Schiavo case is instructive in that many families learned about it through the media, and had discussions about it. In trying to elucidate the possible wishes of someone who has lost the capacity to make medical decisions, it is sometimes helpful to ask "Did your loved one indicate their own wishes about types of treatments they would wish for when the Schiavo case was in the news?"

Picking an HCA is not as easy as it might seem at first. Physicians are often faced by HCAs declaring "I know he wouldn't want that, but I can't tell you to stop." It is possible to pick more than one HCA, but they should be chosen to serve sequentially rather than simultaneously. That is, individuals should choose a primary HCA and an alternate. That way, if there is disagreement between potential HCAs about preferences, the higher-ranking agent makes the choice.

In some cases, a different approach toward advance directives may be indicated. Some people might be more concerned that the family reaches an agreement which preserves family relationships rather than name a specific agent or achieve a specific outcome. One reason cited for not filling out an advance directive is acknowledgment that a person believes his/her family will make the right decisions, without giving specific guidance. While decisions about treatments for someone without capacity need not be established in a democratic fashion, sometimes, it is useful to reach a consensus. Some people will care more about preserving relationships among their survivors than the particulars of their own death.

It is vital for healthcare providers to be sensitive to cultural differences. It is important to realize that in some cultures, it is not customary for people to make individual decisions about healthcare treatments. In a review of multiple studies in which race or ethnicity was investigated as a variable predicting treatment preferences or end-of-life decision making, nonwhites were less likely to support advance directives, African Americans were consistently found to prefer the use of life support, and Asians and Hispanics were more likely to prefer family centered decision-making than other ethnic groups.[35] In Amish communities, where health insurance is generally not carried and the community pays for member's health costs, community elders are often involved in decision-making about healthcare treatments.[36]

When someone fills out a document naming a healthcare agent, he/she should give a copy to her PCP, to other specialist physicians, and the agent. Some suggest that he/she should tape a copy to his/her refrigerator, as emergency workers are trained to look there. He/she may give her lawyer a copy, but should not lock it away or put it in a safe deposit box; it should be easy for loved ones to find. Groopman and Hartzband[37] comment that an advance directive is an "important beginning, but not the end, of understanding a patient's wishes when confronting severe illness."[37] Thorough discussion of one's wishes and values (as addressed above) should complement the advance directive document.

Upon learning more about the role of HCAs, Mr A confirms that he wants his wife to be his HCA, but if she is not available, he names his daughter as the alternate HCA.

30.4   INFORMED CONSENT

Four years later, Mr A remains at home but has become increasingly dependent on his wife for supervision. Once distinguished by his love of conversation and an ability to recite poetry by heart, his speech is now hesitant and periodically confused. He reads but he comprehends little. He is no longer able to drive because of impaired judgment and a history of becoming lost. He dresses and bathes himself but needs prompting. He appears to enjoy family gatherings with his children and grandchildren. In moments of lucidity and privacy, he confides to his wife that he hopes that soon he will not wake up. He is seen by his PCP in the emergency department of their local hospital where he has gone for symptoms of vomiting and abdominal pain. An abdominal CT scan demonstrates gallstones, acute cholecystitis, choledocholithiasis, and pancreatic inflammation. Laboratory data demonstrate elevated amylase, and white blood cell count as well as worsening renal function with a creatinine of 3.5. Mr A is admitted to the hospital for medical treatment. A surgical consultant recommends surgery. He meets with Mr A, his wife, and their daughter. He indicates that without surgery, Mr A's pancreatitis may not resolve and that even if it did there was substantial risk that it would recur. He describes the risks of surgery as significant including the possibility of worsened pancreatitis with the need for postoperative intensive care including mechanical ventilation and if his kidney function worsens dialysis on at least a temporary basis. Without surgery it is explained that he may die.

As discussed above, the legal doctrine of informed consent codifies the bioethical principle of autonomy and courts recognize the right of adult patients with the capacity to make voluntary decisions about medical treatment, including the right to refuse or withdraw life-sustaining treatment.[38] State laws govern the obligations imposed on clinicians to ensure that consent to medical treatment is informed and voluntary. While the specific statutes vary by jurisdiction and subject matter, they typically address the kind of communication required between a clinician and a patient and the information the clinician must provide for the patient to make an informed decision (e.g., information about the nature of the diagnosis and prognosis; medically indicated treatment options, including risks and benefits of each; and risks and benefits of no treatment). At the conclusion of this process, informed consent for a medical intervention is documented with the patient's signature on a form describing the intervention and information disclosed.

A focus on the legal requirements of informed consent, however, may result in a neglect of the critical features of this doctrine: "Although the informed consent doctrine has substantial foundation in law, it is essentially an ethical imperative."[39] When done well, the process of obtaining an informed consent epitomizes the best of the physician–patient relationship. The honest communication between a caring physician, who best understands the medical options, and the patient, who best understands his/her life's values and preferences, ideally leads to the medical decision that supports the patient's values and goals. However, even in the care of patients who have capacity, there are barriers to good clinical decision-making.

First, as discussed above, patients, even patients with capacity, may not want to think or talk about difficult medical decisions, especially when the decisions are significant. These are hard conversations even in the abstract. Some patients may be willing to talk about their values and preferences but do not know how to do so. Some patients may find talking with immediate family even more challenging than talking with a caring physician, nurse, social worker, or religious leader. Patients' ability to communicate with loved ones may be complicated by their relationship. A husband may not want to tell his wife that he is willing to contemplate death. He may believe that his wife does not want to have that conversation.

Second, some suggest the requirement to understand that the diagnosis and prognosis is impossible for someone without clinical knowledge and experience. The ability to repeat the information does not indicate an understanding. Others argue that even when the patient understands the biological aspects of the treatment, it is impossible to know what the future will feel like to the patient who decides to proceed. To address this concern, some identify the potential of decision aides to provide qualitative data to help inform treatment decisions. While these aides may support the patient in her decision process, they may also include a bias. For example, when clinicians want a patient to consider continuation of treatment after a life-altering trauma, they may introduce the patient to someone who is glad to have survived a similar experience. Some clinicians have created decision aides intended to be unbiased, but present data that evoke strong emotional responses.[40] Used appropriately, with nonjudgmental discussion about the information, these tools may facilitate a conversation that gives an insight into a patient's wishes. However, clinicians should carefully select decisional aides that present the information in as impartial a manner as possible and identify any bias before offering it to the patient.

Third, when decisions involve life-sustaining treatment, the discussion may be even more difficult. While it may be possible for some patients to proceed with certain aggressive treatment decisions and quickly decide that the burdens of the treatment outweigh the benefits, not all patients find this path available.

Some suggest that it is appropriate to consider important interests of the family in treatment decisions.[41] Relationships, and how one thinks about relationships, complicate the decision-making process. Patients may feel obligations to their loved ones, for example, my family is not ready for me to die so I will endure all medical interventions to prolong my life, or my healthcare costs will harm my family so I will stop this treatment. The process of informed consent should help the patient articulate his/her values and preferences, how he/she wants to make healthcare decisions, and who can support them in the process.

30.5 CAPACITY DETERMINATIONS

Whenever possible, the patient should provide consent or indicate refusal of treatment options. Assessment of the patient's capacity to make an informed decision depends upon an appraisal of the patient's understanding of the medical condition. Asking if the patients understand and have any questions is not as helpful as asking the patients to explain in their own words what they understand. The same should be done in evaluating the patient's comprehension of therapeutic options. If the patients can make, communicate, and explain the reasons for their decisions, then capacity is demonstrated. If the decision can be shown to be consistent with long-standing values and preferences, then, the evidence of capacity is further solidified.[42]

The patient's voice should be cultivated to the fullest extent possible and proposed treatment plans should be discussed in terms that are understandable to the patient when possible. Evaluating the patient's ability to make decisions requires time, patience, and clinical acumen. Conditions including hearing deficits, adverse effects of medication, illness, or hospital-related delirium may all constitute barriers to effective communication and distort the patient's capacity evaluation. Medically complicated issues and choices may require steady efforts at education and discussion to maximize the patient's ability to be self-determining. It may be necessary to conduct such an evaluation over a series of visits if the nature of the decision permits. Capacity is dynamic and may fluctuate from one evaluation to another. This process can understandably be difficult to perform effectively in the context of the demanding pace of medical practice. Nonetheless, the centrality of patient autonomy in medical ethics and the importance of finding someone capable of autonomous choice, or not, requires that all reasonable efforts be made to meet this standard of assessment.

In some instances capacity may be partial. Capacity should be evaluated on a decision-specific basis. Certain decisions may be within an individual's capabilities but not others of a more difficult nature. The existence of dementia and cognitive compromise does not, in and of itself, indicate the inability to make medical decisions. A history of getting lost in the car, or confusion about medications, does not establish the inability to evaluate medical choices. Mr A may have had the evidence of substantial memory loss when he discussed advance directives with his PCP but still had been able to identify his healthcare proxy and even indicate his preferences regarding some aspects of end-of-life care. Imagine that at that time, Mr A maintained an ability to describe experiences that would offer meaning to his life—recognition and enjoyment of time with his family, listening to music, the ability to read, enjoy food, and take pleasure being outdoors. Losing the ability to enjoy those or similar experiences would warrant a recalibration of the value of future life-sustaining medical care. As his Alzheimer's disease progresses and those sources of pleasure and meaning are lost, he might express that he would welcome a timely, peaceful death.

If a patient has limited capacity and the stakes of a medical decision entail great risk, or when refusal of recommended treatment might have life-altering consequence, it may be necessary to involve a surrogate decision-maker. As the risks involved in accepting or refusing recommended medical treatment increase, the standard of evidence of decisional capacity should correspondingly increase.[1] Imagine an elderly man with dementia and a newly diagnosed complete heart block. He expresses a desire to live and gives his consent to surgery to insert a pacemaker. The benefits of the procedure are great and the risks are limited. We would find his capacity sufficient to make this decision. Were the same patient (with the same expressed desire to live) to refuse treatment which would probably result in his death, we would, in all likelihood, find him incapable of making that decision. Whenever patients have limited or partial capacity to make medical decisions, it is best, and often mandatory, that a patient advocate be involved in medical decision-making. A patient surrogate should collaborate with the patient and physician to integrate the patient's values with the complexities of the patient's medical condition and treatment options to determine the preferred course of medical treatment.

When surgery is discussed with Mr A, his wife, and daughter, he indicates that he wants to proceed with surgery because his survival is important to him, thus providing evidence that he values his current quality of life. He has continued to enjoy time with his family, music, food, and being outdoors. Failure to proceed with surgery will lead to his death. His capacity to provide informed consent to surgery is impaired in light of his inability to gauge the complex risks and benefits of the proposed treatment. It is essential that his wife acts as his advocate and participates in the decision regarding surgery but she needs to be guided by her understanding of her husband's assessment of the value of his current life as well as her knowledge of his previously expressed preferences for medical treatment in the face of his progressive dementia.

30.6   SURROGATE DECISION-MAKING

Postoperatively (open cholecystectomy and common bile duct exploration) Mr A's medical condition deteriorates. Pancreatitis worsens, kidney function declines, large volume fluid replacement results in congestive heart failure, and diffuse fluid overload. Mr A has been intubated, sedated, and unresponsive since his surgery 1 week earlier. A family meeting is scheduled with Mr A's family, Mr A's PCP, and the ICU medical director to discuss his prognosis and what course of action is best for Mr A.

Mr A's evolving medical history illustrates the dynamic character of patient decision-making capacity. Capacity may vary over the course of time as it has for Mr A. It may vary, depending on clinical events, even within the course of several hours. It may also vary with the nature of the decision at issue.[43] In the first two scenarios Mr A demonstrates partial capacity. Following his surgery, he has lost the capacity to communicate a preference because of acute postoperative medical problems as well as the effects of sedation. In this circumstance, the responsibility for medical decisions rests entirely with his surrogates. How to incorporate information about Mr A's previously expressed wishes and values with his current critical medical condition to arrive at a consensus between surrogates and physicians regarding medical treatment is the focus of this section.

Imagine that Mr A was not intubated and sedated after surgery but still had refractory heart failure, unmitigated pancreatitis, and worsening renal function. Considering the complexities of his medical condition, the foreseeable hazards of treatment, the possible need for future mechanical ventilation and/or dialysis, as well as the uncertain but limited prospects for a positive outcome, Mr A would need the advocacy of his healthcare agent to evaluate medical decisions for him. These would not be decisions he had the capability to make in an informed manner because of his dementia, acute illness, and in view of the consequences of any choices he might make.

A determination of the global inability to make medical decisions is often an obvious clinical conclusion. The unconscious patient, the patient with advanced dementia, and the patient with expressive and receptive aphasia following a stroke are examples of individuals who are readily identified as lacking the capacity to make medical decisions. Following his surgery, Mr A is likewise clearly unable to make decisions.

In other circumstances, a determination of the loss of decision-making capacity may prove to be challenging. A determination of the inability to make informed medical decisions should rely on the same clinical criteria employed to establish decision-making capability (understanding, deliberation, explanation, and communication of decision). In many instances, a determination of compromised decision-making capacity can best be made by a physician with prior knowledge of the patient such as his PCP.[44] Instruments for assessing patient decision-making capacity may help in this process.[45] In instances where uncertainty exists regarding decisional capacity, an ethics consultation can be helpful. Enigmatic patient decisions often warrant consultative participation—for instance, a decision by a patient to forego curative, lifesaving treatment of limited risk by an apparently lucid, capable individual.[42] Where evidence of lack of capacity is related to mental health disorders, a capacity evaluation by a psychiatrist may be advisable (or in some jurisdictions legally required). Determination of lack of capacity as a consequence of intellectual or other developmental disabilities may require assessment by specifically certified healthcare personnel where they are subject to process restrictions of state law (e.g., New York).

When decision-making capability is absent, a surrogate is charged with the responsibility to make decisions that reflect the patient's previously expressed wishes whenever possible. These wishes may have been expressed in writing (advance directive) or in discussion with family or close friends. If knowledge of the patient's wishes is lacking, widely accepted bioethical guidelines suggest that substituted judgment should be used to decide on the patient's behalf. A substituted judgment is understood as the decision the patient would make if he were able to understand his current circumstances. Knowledge of the patient's values, previous conversations, prior choices regarding medical care, and the way he has lived his life are examples of the evidence that might be gathered to make a substituted judgment. The surrogate is sometimes asked to consider what the patient would tell us if able to regain capacity for 15 minutes, understand and reflect upon his medical circumstances, and then indicate his preferences. If there is insufficient knowledge of the patient to make a substituted judgment, then, clinicians and surrogate decision-makers must rely on the best interest standard. Surrogates invoking best interests make decisions that they think best serve the welfare of the patient. Best interest decisions should reflect thoughtful consideration of the potential risks and benefits of treatment in the context of the patient's overall condition. The decision should reflect the surrogate's assessment of what most individuals would choose faced with the specific decision before them.

Fulfillment of the surrogate's responsibility is often difficult. Even when there is knowledge of the patient's previously expressed wishes in an advance directive, that document may not address the situation at hand. Vague language in a living will may be vulnerable to errors of interpretation (see the discussion of advance directives above). General statements of medical preferences and personal philosophy may prove difficult to apply in actual clinical circumstances. In other cases, medical providers and family may agree that a patient's advance directive is too inflexible; its faithful execution may not be in the patient's best interest and a question may arise regarding the patient's true preferences in the current situation.[46]

In the absence of an explicit declaration of a patient's wishes that is a reliable fit for the clinical situation at hand, the use of the substituted judgment standard also can present problems. Determination of the patient's sentiments and values may be hampered by the absence of sufficient evidence. This may reflect the absence of previous discussion by the patient that is pertinent to his current medical circumstances. Alternatively the surrogate may not know the patient well enough to draw a conclusion about what he would want in his current condition. Surrogates may choose inaccurately when making a substituted judgment. As discussed above, studies have shown that in one-third of cases, surrogates are mistaken about the choice the patient would make.[47] It is also not unusual to have disagreement within a family seeking to make a group decision on behalf of the incapacitated individual. Acting in good faith, family and friends may offer differing judgments about what the patient would choose.

Using a best interest standard, surrogates may also draw conflicting conclusions about what is best for the incapacitated patient. Medical problems are often highly complex and the outcomes of clinical interventions are frequently uncertain. Intubating an elderly individual with moderate dementia for treatment of community-acquired pneumonia may provide the needed ventilator support for the initial several days of antibiotic therapy that is needed to see the patient through the acute infection. It is possible, however, that response to therapy may be meager, ventilator support prolonged, and new decisions will be needed to address treatments such as tracheostomy or artificial nutrition. Operating in conditions of uncertainty, with much at stake, divergent judgments within surrogate decision-making groups should not be surprising. Indeed, medical providers may also disagree among themselves about the best interest of the patient.

Disagreement between family and healthcare providers about how an incapacitated elderly person should be treated is a daily occurrence in modern hospitals. The drama of this conflict is often played out in the ICU where our sickest patients are treated with the most advanced medical technology and procedures. Families may be viewed as unrealistic and obstructionists by medical personnel predisposed by experience to anticipate failure of intensive therapy for the gravely ill, elderly patient. Medical teams, in turn, may be viewed as unduly pessimistic and disrespectful of the role of families advocating for the incapacitated. Both groups believe that they represent the best interest of the patient but struggle to resolve their disagreements.

Despite these problems, the role of the family surrogate is valued as a demonstration of respect for the incapacitated patient's autonomy.[48] In cases where there has been a formal designation of a healthcare proxy, the advocacy of the patient's chosen surrogate is an explicit recognition of the patient's autonomous choice. One must ask who is in the best position to know and understand an incapacitated individual's values and preferences. It seems evident that family members have a primary moral standing to advocate for the incapacitated.[48] Certainly there may be a history of estrangement or intrafamily hostility that might disqualify the family as legitimate surrogates. Customarily, however, families share a common upbringing, social and religious experiences that mold personal outlook, and ethical values. Furthermore, patients indicate that they value having family members making decisions on their behalf. Rather than favoring a strict interpretation of living wills, most patients prefer that surrogates of their choice make decisions with their physicians on the basis of existing medical conditions and knowledge of the patient's values.[49] Mr A's choice of his wife as his healthcare proxy reflects this evidence. Furthermore, his daughter's role as a support for her mother and as a participant in arriving at a surrogate decision is in keeping with what we know of how many individuals envision the family acting together to make decisions on their behalf. It is hoped that the family will successfully collaborate with medical providers in making surrogate decisions that incorporate the incapacitated individuals wishes and values with medically guided insight into the benefits and burdens of different treatment options.

Critics of the orthodox framework for a surrogate's substituted judgment have suggested alternatives to the traditional guidelines for surrogate decision-making.[50] The portrayal of a substituted judgment as an expression of the incapacitated individual's autonomous voice is thought by these critics to be misleading. A patient who has lost the capacity has lost autonomy. Formulating surrogate decisions on the basis of previously expressed advance directives is to ask the question, what did the patient choose? In the absence of a specific declaration relevant to the decision at hand, substituted judgment asks the question, what would the patient choose? This hypothetical question seeks an answer not through the exercise of the patient's autonomy but by using what we know of the patient's life to identify his preferences. This knowledge may include specific conversation about medical care in serious circumstances but is as likely to rely on what we know of the individual's choices in life, what the individual loved and made him/her happy, what he/she valued, and how that was expressed in how he/she lived. It will also be informed by knowledge of the incapacitated individual's relationships and how the effect of decisions on family and loved ones might influence the choice. As best possible, the question is answered by describing what made the individual who he/she is and what that tells us about what he/she would do. This is seen as more a matter of clarifying the authentic self as reflected in the incapacitated individual's life story.[50] We are asked to consider which decisions might honor the authenticity of that person. This approach draws from the perspective of narrative ethics which finds the evidence of moral purpose and direction in the story of our lives. This philosophical perspective does not displace the principles of bioethics but sees them given the purpose and application in the way we have lived, in the choices we have made in pursuit of happiness and meaning. Mrs A and her daughter are guided in their responsibility by an effort to make a decision on behalf of Mr A that makes sense in the story of his life. In a sense, this may amount to writing a last chapter in Mr A's life story in the way that his family thinks he would have wanted. Wrestling with probabilities of survival and the possibility of suffering associated with aggressive treatments in the ICU may be sufficient for Mr A's family to make their decision. Knowledge of how he lived his life, his active intellectual and physical engagement with the world, how he had continued to find meaning in life after his diagnosis of Alzheimer's disease, and his reflections on what he hoped the end of his life would be like give the medical information a context that may make his family's decision clearer even as they struggle. Optimally a skilled physician can help Mr A's family fulfill their responsibility as partners mutually dedicated to a decision that is best for this patient based on what is known of his authentic self and his medical prospects.

Using this alternate approach, a surrogate is asked not what her father would decide or what is in his best interest. Instead, she is asked to talk about her father's life.[51] This approach reflects respect for the incapacitated patient and initiates a partnered process of discovery that will hopefully elucidate the values, preferences, and personal commitments that indicate what decision is in keeping with the way the surrogate's father has lived his life. In the substituted interests model, the physician may recommend a course of action based upon the surrogate's account of the incapacitated person's life and values as well as an assessment of the clinical circumstances requiring choice. Surrogates are not asked to determine what is often unknowable—that is, what the patient would choose. Instead, the burden of responsibility that can seem to be overwhelming to the family is addressed in a partnered decision with members of the medical team on the basis of an assessment of the benefits and risks of treatment and what is known of the patient's values.[51]

Many geriatric medical decisions occur at the end of life. An ethical and legal consensus about decisions to withhold or withdraw life-sustaining medical treatments has existed for over 20 years.[52] All individuals with capacity are recognized to have authority to refuse any treatment, even if death is a consequence. The United States Supreme Court has recognized this right as well as the authority of patient surrogates to make any decision that a patient can (subject to process restrictions imposed by state law).[8] Both surrogates and physicians may see a significant difference in decisions to withhold a treatment as opposed to withdrawing it. Stopping the respiratory support of mechanical ventilation may be felt emotionally and ethically to be active in a way that a decision not to initiate mechanical ventilation is not. In the United States, however, no ethical or legal distinction is recognized between decisions to withhold or withdraw life-sustaining treatment. This applies to a full range of potential treatments that include mechanical ventilation, cardiac resuscitation, antibiotics, intravenous fluids, dialysis, cardiac technology (e.g., pacemakers or defibrillators), and artificial nutrition and hydration. Indeed, hesitance to withdraw life-sustaining treatments may lead to avoidance of time-limited trials of treatments such as mechanical ventilation or antibiotics for pneumonia that might prove to be effective in treating an acute life-threatening medical condition. The approach to decisions about end-of-life medical decisions for the elderly is no different than the process described above for other treatments. An evaluation of patient decision-making capacity, a conscientious informed consent process, reference to an incapacitated patient's prior wishes if relevant, and a consensus-directed deliberation with surrogates should be observed when indicated. A process that respects a patient's authentic values, while joining them with a medically guided assessment of the patient's interests, embodies familial and professional commitment to sound ethical decisions at the end of life.

REFERENCES

1. Beauchamp, T.L. and J.F. Childress. 2009. *Principles of Biomedical Ethics*, 7th ed. New York: Oxford University Press.
2. Brody, H. 1987. *Stories of Sickness*. New Haven and London: Yale University Press; Frank, A. 1995. *The Wounded Storyteller: Body, Illness and Ethics*. Chicago: Chicago University Press.
3. Kohn, N.A., J.A. Blumenthal, and A.T. Campbell. 2013. Supported decision-making: A viable alternative to guardianship? *Penn State Law Rev* 117(4): 1111–1157.
4. Basanta, W.E. 2002. Advance directives and life-sustaining treatment: A legal primer. *Hematol Oncol Clin N Am* 16: 1381–1396.
5. Haman, E.A. 2000. *How to Write Your Own Living Will*, 2nd ed. Naperville, Ill: Sphinx Publishing.
6. Hamel, C.F., L.W. Guse, P.G. Hawarnik et al. 2002. Advance directives and community dwelling older adults. *West J Nurs Res* 24(2): 143–158.
7. Silvester, W. and K. Detering. 2011. Advance directives, perioperative care, and end-of-life planning. *Best Pract Res Clin Anaesthesiol* 25: 451–460.
8. Cruzan v. Director, 1990. Missouri Department of Health, 497 U.S. 261, 278.
9. Cruzan v. Director, 1990. Missouri Department of Health, (O'Connor, J., concurring).
10. The Pew Research Center for the People and the Press. Jan 5 2006. *More Americans Discussing-and Planning-End-of-Life Treatment. Strong Public Support for Right to Die. News Release*. Washington DC.
11. Rao, J.K., L.A. Anderson, F.C. Lin et al. 2014. Completion of advance directives among U.S. consumers. *Am J Prev Med* 46(1): 65–70.
12. Miles, S.H., R. Koepp, and E.P. Weber. 1996. Advance end-of life treatment planning. *Arch Intern Med* 156: 1062–1068.
13. Jones, A.L., A.J. Moss, and L.D. Harris-Kojetin, 2011. Use of advance directives in long-term care populations. *NCHS Data Brief* 54: 1–8.
14. Teno, J., J. Lynn, N. Wenger et al. 1997. Advance directives for seriously ill hospitalized patients: Effectiveness with the patient self-determination act and the SUPPORT intervention. *J Am Geriatr Soc* 45(4): 500–507.
15. Kierner, K.A., B. Hladschik-Kermer, and H.H. Watze. 2010. Attitudes of patients with malignancies towards completion of advance directives. *Support Care Cancer* 3: 367–372.
16. Bradley, E., B. Blechner, and T. Wetle. 1997. Assessing capacity to participate in discussions of advance directives in nursing homes: Findings from a study of the Patient Self Determination Act. *J Am Geriatr Soc* 45(1): 79–83.
17. Reilly, B.M., C.R. Magnussen, J. Ross et al. 1994. Can we talk? Inpatient discussions about advance directives in a community hospital. Attending physicians' attitudes, their inpatients' wishes, and reported experience. *Arch Intern Med* 154: 2299–2308.
18. Bradley, E.H., T. Welte, and S.M. Horwitz. 1998. The patient self-determination act and advance directive completion in nursing homes. *Arch Fam Med* 7(5): 417–423.
19. Wallace, S.K., C.G. Martin, A.D. Shaw et al. 2001. Influence of an advance directive on the initiation of life support technology in critically ill cancer patients. *Crit Care Med* 29(12): 2294–2298.
20. Keating, N.L., M.B. Landrum, S.O. Rogers, Jr. et al. 2010. Physician factors associated with discussions about end-of-life care. *Cancer* 116: 998–1006.
21. Jezewski, M.A. 2005. Oncology nurses' knowledge, attitudes, and experiences regarding advance directives. *Oncol Nurs Forum* 32(2): 319–327.
22. Kumar, A., W.S. Aronow, M. Alexa et al. 2010. Prevalence of use of advance directives, health care proxy, legal guardian, and living will in 512 patients hospitalized in a cardiac care unit/intensive care unit in two community hospitals. *Arch Med Sci* 2: 188–191.
23. Kirkpatrick, J.N., C.J. Guger, M.F. Arnsdorf et al. 2007. Advance directives in the cardiac care unit. *Am Heart J* 154: 477–481.
24. Lynn, J., K.O. DeVries, H.R. Arkes et al. 2000. Ineffectiveness of the SUPPORT intervention: Review of explanations. *J Am Geriatr Soc* 48: S0206–S213.
25. Emanuel, L. and E.J. Emanuel. 1989. The Medical Directive, a new comprehensive advance care document. *J Am Med Assoc* 261: 3288–3293.
26. Miles, S.H. 1992. Interpersonal issues in the Wanglie Case. *Kennedy Inst Ethics J* 2(1): 61–72.

27. PEW Research Religion and Public Life Project. Nov 21, 2013. Views on End-of-Life Treatments. *Pew Forum* p. 1–10.
28. High, D.H. 1993. Why are elderly people not using advance directives? *J Aging Health* 5: 497–515.
29. Jezewski, M.A., M.A. Meeker, L. Sessanna et al. 2007. The effectiveness of interventions to increase advance directive completion rates. *J Aging Health* 19: 519–536.
30. McGuire, L.C., J.K. Rao, L.A. Anderson et al. 2007. Completion of a durable power of attorney for health care: What does cognition have to do with it? *Gerontologist* 47(4): 457–467.
31. Lipkin, K.M. 2006. Brief report: Identifying a proxy for health care as part of a routine medical inquiry. *J Gen Intern Med* 21: 1181–1191.
32. Cohen-Mansfield, J., J.A. Droge, and N. Billig. 1991. The utilization of the durable power of attorney for health care among hospitalized elderly patients. *J Am Geriatr Soc* 39(12): 1174–1178.
33. Sulmasy, D.P., P.B. Terry, C.S. Weisman et al. 1998. The accuracy of substituted judgments in patients with terminal diagnoses. *Ann Intern Med* 128(8): 621–629.
34. Span, P. 2009. Why do we avoid advance directives? *The New York Times.*
35. Kwak, J. and W.E. Haley. 2005. Current research findings on end-of-life decision making among racially or ethnically diverse groups. *Gerontologist* 45(5): 634–641.
36. Crawford, S.Y., A.M. Manuel, and B.D. Wood. 2009. Pharmacists considerations when serving Amish patients. *J Am Pharm Assoc* 49: 86–97.
37. Groopman, J. and P. Hartzband. 2012. Advance directives are the beginning of care, not the end. *ACP Internist.* http://www.acpinternest.org/archives/2012/07. (Accessed September 27, 2016).
38. Schloendorf v. Society of New York Hospital, 211 NY 125, 129–130, N.E. (1914)
39. President's Commission for the Study of Ethical Problems in Medicine and Biomedical and Behavioral Research. 1982. *Making Health Care Decisions: The Ethical and Legal Implications of Informed Consent in the Patient–Practitioner Relationship.* Washington, DC: U.S. Government Printing Office.
40. Volandes, A.E., M.K. Paasche-Orlow, M.J. Barry et al. 2009. Video decision support tool for advance care planning in dementia: Randomized control trial. *Brit Med J* 338: b2159.
41. Hardwig, J. 1990. What about the family? *Hasting Cent Rep* 20(2): 5–10.
42. Jonsen, A.R., M. Siegler, and W.J. Winslade. 2010. *Clinical Ethics: A Practical Approach to Ethical Decisions in Clinical Medicine. 7th ed.* New York: McGraw-Hill Medical.
43. Beauchamp, T.L. and J.F. Childress. 2001. *Principles of Biomedical Ethics. 5th ed.* New York: Oxford University Press
44. Hayley, D.C., C.K. Cassel, L. Snyder et al. 1996. Ethical and legal issues in nursing home care. *Arch Intern Med* 156(3): 249–256.
45. Sessums, L.L., H. Zembrzuska, and J.L. Jackson. 2011. Does this patient have medical decision-making capacity? *J Am Med Assoc* 306(4): 420–427.
46. Smith, A.K., B. Lo, and R. Sudore. 2013. When previously expressed wishes conflict with best interests. *JAMA Intern Med* 173(13): 1241–1245.
47. Shalowitz, D.I., E. Garrett-Mayer, and D. Wendler. 2006. The accuracy of surrogate decision makers: A systematic review. *Arch Intern Med* 166(5): 493–497.
48. Arnold, R.M. and J. Kellum. 2003. Moral justifications for surrogate decision making in the intensive care unit: Implications and limitations. *Crit Care Med* 31: S347–S353.
49. Puchalski, C.M., Z. Zhong, M.M. Jacobs et al. 2000. Patients who want their family and physician to make resuscitation decisions for them: Observations from SUPPORT and HELP. Study to understand prognoses and preferences for outcomes and risks of treatment. Hospitalized Elderly Longitudinal Project. *J Am Geriatr Soc* 48(5 Suppl): S84–S90.
50. Brudney, D. 2009. Choosing for another: Beyond autonomy and best interests. *Hastings Cent Rep* 39(2): 31–37.
51. Sulmasy, D.P. and L. Snyder. 2010. Substituted interests and best judgments: An integrated model of surrogate decision making. *J Am Med Assoc* 304(17): 1946–1947.
52. Meisel, A. 1992. The legal consensus about forgoing life-sustaining treatment: Its status and its prospects. *Kennedy Inst Ethics J* 2(4): 309–345.

31 Palliative Care and End-of-Life Issues

Rashmi Khadilkar, Hilary Yehling, and Timothy E. Quill

CONTENTS

31.1 INTRODUCTION

Public health improvements over the last century have led to significant increases in human longevity, and gains in medical science have also contributed, albeit more modestly. Many adults enjoy good health well into their later years, but eventually, most will experience one or more chronic illnesses that will impact the remainder of their lives. Advances in pharmacology, surgery, and other therapeutic modalities often allow people to live for years with such illnesses. However, these traditional modalities do not always adequately address other aspects of illness that impact quality of life, such as symptoms, emotional concerns, and care coordination needs. Palliative care is a relatively new medical specialty that aims to fill such gaps. Because the elderly bear a disproportionate amount of the burden of illness, clinicians caring for the elderly should have a solid understanding of the basic principles of palliative care, including a working knowledge of the role that rehabilitation can play in improving the quality of life.

31.2 WHAT ARE HOSPICE AND PALLIATIVE CARE?

While the primary goal of humanity's first attempts at medicine was palliation of symptoms, formalized palliative care has existed as a distinct specialty for only the past few decades. The roots of palliative care lie in the institution of hospice.

31.2.1 HOSPICE

The late nineteenth and early twentieth centuries saw the opening of facilities in the United Kingdom intended solely for the care of the dying. While working with these facilities in the 1950s and 1960s, Dame Cicely Saunders developed the modern philosophy of hospice and opened the first modern hospice home, St. Christopher's, near London. The first hospice home in the United States opened in Connecticut in 1974.

The word "hospice" comes from the Latin root "hospes," meaning "guest" or "host," and originally indicated a resting place for travelers. Today, the term has a variety of closely related meanings:

- Hospice is a *philosophy of care* that focuses on the quality of life of a terminally ill patient. Emphasis is placed on symptom management rather than disease management, as well as on the emotional and spiritual well-being of a patient and his/her family, with the goal of allowing the dying patient the greatest possible degree of comfort and dignity.
- Hospice is an *interdisciplinary team* of professionals who provide care for terminally ill patients. This team typically includes some or all of the following members: physicians, nurse practitioners, nurses, aides, social workers, chaplains, volunteers, and others. The hospice team can provide care in various settings.
- Hospice is sometimes a *place—a freestanding facility or hospital unit* that focuses solely on terminally ill patients who have elected a purely comfort-oriented approach to their care. These facilities are typically affiliated with one of the hospice *teams or agencies* in a given geographical area, and some are dependent, in addition to the hospice team, on volunteers who provide direct care and maintain the facilities. The majority of hospice care in the United States is provided in a patient's own home, whereas in England, most hospice care is facility based.
- Hospice is an *insurance benefit*—Initially, hospice services were funded through philanthropy. Over time, various major insurers began covering comfort care services for the terminally ill. In 1982, federal legislation provided for a hospice benefit through Medicare, which many other insurers now use as a model. The enactment of the Medicare benefit led to the setting of certification and licensing standards for hospice care.

Hospice should be considered when no effective medical therapies remain to treat a patient's illness or when the patient, family, and care team decide that the burdens of the available therapies outweigh the potential benefits, and that a plan of care oriented toward comfort and quality of life is appropriate. At this point, the main treating clinician may refer a patient to hospice by contacting the local hospice agency of the patient's and family's choosing. Typically, a nurse and/or social worker from the hospice agency will meet with the patient and family to determine eligibility for services and help select the best venue for hospice care. To qualify for the hospice insurance benefit, a patient must meet each of the following three conditions:

- A physician must certify that a patient is terminally ill. That is, if the patient's disease is allowed to run its natural course, the patient's life expectancy is *more likely than not* to be 6 months or less.
- The patient chooses to receive a hospice approach to treatment focusing primarily on symptoms and to forgo standard medical treatments for the terminal illness.
- The patient receives care from a hospice program that participates in the patient's insurance.

While most day-to-day hospice care is provided by nurses, aides, and family members, a physician must oversee the treatment plan and provide the necessary orders for medications, equipment, and other therapies. Hospice care may be directed by any physician—primary care provider, palliative care specialist, or other specialist—with whom the patient feels comfortable, who is willing to take on the role, and who has the skill and commitment to provide medical input into the care plan.

31.2.2 PALLIATIVE CARE

Hospice is a wonderful resource for patients who have decided to forego disease-directed therapies for a terminal illness and to focus solely on comfort and quality of life. However, many patients prefer to continue to pursue some or all disease-directed, potentially life-extending therapies which would not be covered by hospice benefits. Palliative care grew out of the limitations of hospice, which requires a patient to choose between potentially curative and life-prolonging therapies on the one hand and quality of life on the other. Like hospice, palliative care also focuses on symptom relief and on maximizing patients' quality of life. Unlike hospice, palliative care is a traditional medical consultative service and not a separate insurance benefit, and can therefore be provided concurrently with disease-directed or curative treatments. Palliative care as a medical specialty has grown tremendously over the past few decades, with many hospitals and health systems now having inpatient and (less commonly) outpatient palliative care teams to serve their patients. Palliative care prioritizes several goals that overlap with, but are in some ways distinct from, the goals of traditional medical therapy:

- Symptom management—Physical and emotional symptoms, such as pain, nausea, constipation, dyspnea, anxiety, and delirium compromise the quality of life, functional status, and dignity of patients suffering from chronic illnesses; they may also lead a patient to prematurely forego a potentially life-extending treatment due to adverse effects. Therefore, symptom relief is a primary focus of palliative care. The appropriate use of medications such as opioids, antiemetics, laxatives, and anxiolytics, as well as nonpharmacologic modalities (supportive counseling, meditation, massage, etc.), can markedly improve a patient's ability to tolerate other therapies and to derive greater enjoyment from life.
- Decision-making and goals of care—When dealing with a life-changing illness, patients face important, complicated, and time-sensitive choices. They are asked to digest information about typical disease course, prognosis, and potential benefits and burdens of treatment; they must then synthesize this information into decisions about their treatment. They may be asked to consider their goals for treatment and any limits they wish to place. They may be asked to choose a healthcare proxy to help make decisions for them in case they become incapacitated in the future. Palliative care helps patients to address this complex decision-making. This process is discussed in greater detail later in this chapter.
- Additional support—Patients with life-changing illnesses face issues that do not directly pertain to treatment. For example, they may need assistance with coordination of care and communication with their providers. They may have employment or child-care conflicts. They may need help discussing their situation with their loved ones, whose views and opinions on illness and death may differ from the patient's own. They may have difficulty confronting the possibility of distressing symptoms, functional decline, or death. Palliative care can provide social, psychological, and spiritual support alongside disease-directed treatments to meet nonmedical as well as medical challenges.
- End-of-life care—While palliative care may be delivered alongside traditional medical and geriatric care for months or even years, at some point, the major focus of treatment may shift from cure and prolongation of life more exclusively to comfort and quality of life. When this occurs, palliative care comes to the forefront of the patient's management and the patient may be offered enrollment into hospice care. The more a patient's physical, emotional, and spiritual concerns are addressed throughout the course of an illness, the more likely the transition to hospice can be made in a timely way, providing it is acceptable to the patient and family. A palliative plan of care can certainly be effectively implemented for the first time in a dying patient if it has been avoided or not needed earlier in the patient's illness.

A comparison of hospice and palliative care is shown in Table 31.1.

TABLE 31.1

Summary of the Similarities and Differences between Palliative Care and Hospice

	Palliative Care	Hospice
Who can get it?	Any patient with a serious acute or chronic illness	Any patient with a terminal illness (i.e., an illness expected to cause death within 6 months) who is willing to forgo disease-directed treatment
Time frame	Any time after diagnosis of a serious illness	When life expectancy is *more likely than not* to be 6 months or less
Insurance aspects	No specific benefit	Specific benefit covered under Medicare, Medicaid, and most commercial plans
Concurrent therapies	Any disease-directed or life-prolonging therapies permitted alongside palliative treatment	Treatment is exclusively palliative; no disease-directed or life-prolonging therapies permitted
Location	Outpatient, inpatient, or residential facility; care provided by any treating doctor (primary palliative care) or by a traditional medical consultative service (specialty palliative care)	Outpatient (home, hospice facility, and nursing home) or inpatient; care provided by a dedicated hospice team with one physician identified as the primary treating physician
Philosophy of care	Focus on comfort and quality of life with emphasis on symptom management, decision-making, and psychosocial and spiritual support, potentially alongside any and all desired disease-directed therapies	Exclusive focus on comfort and quality of life with emphasis on symptom management, decision-making, psychosocial and spiritual support, and preparation for the end of life

31.3   WHO SHOULD GET AND WHO SHOULD PROVIDE PALLIATIVE CARE?

Basic palliative care can and should be a part of the treatment plan of any patient diagnosed with a serious illness from the time of diagnosis (Figure 31.1). Initially, the treatment plan is likely to focus primarily on disease management, and, if possible, cure; but symptom management and discussion of a patient's and family's hopes, fears, and concerns are also imperative throughout the course of a patient's illness. As the disease progresses, the patient may be faced with decisions about treatments that may impose greater burdens with lower probability of success and may also contend with ongoing, perhaps worsening, symptoms and a growing risk of mortality. When this occurs, palliative care takes on an increasingly larger role in the treatment plan as symptom management and decision-making support become even more central. Eventually, medical therapies may become near-futile and/or prohibitively burdensome, and a patient may choose to transition to a purely palliative plan of care and, perhaps, hospice. Because palliative care plays a role in the care of any patient with a serious illness, all clinicians should become familiar with some general palliative care principles[1]:

- Basic pain (and other symptom) management—Pain is often a prominent symptom of a serious illness and can considerably diminish functioning and participation in treatment, including rehabilitation. Careful, adequate pain management can facilitate healing and rehabilitation and can help establish and maintain trust between the patient and care team. Various classes of medication are commonly used for pain management, including opioids, neuroadjuvants (such as gabapentin and nortriptyline), nonsteroidal anti-inflammatory drugs (NSAIDs) and acetaminophen, and corticosteroids. Many clinicians avoid opioid analgesia due to the potential risk of misuse and addiction, and under-treatment of pain is unfortunately quite common. However, in seriously ill patients, especially those without a prior personal or family history of drug or alcohol addiction, the risk of opioid misuse is relatively low. There exist useful guidelines for the initiation and titration of opioids, as well as tables for the conversion between different opioid medications. The geriatric

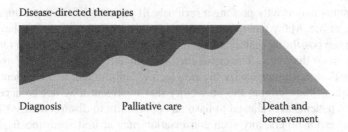

Disease-directed therapies

Diagnosis   Palliative care   Death and
                                            bereavement

FIGURE 31.1   The place of palliative care in the course of illness. (Adapted with permission from Sean Morrison.)

population is particularly sensitive to the effects of opioids. When opioids are titrated carefully ("start low and go slow"), many elders find great improvement in their pain with these medications. Some patients also benefit from interventional modalities such as nerve blocks, and still others do well with nonpharmacologic methods such as radiation therapy, massage, music therapy, or cognitive behavioral therapy. The treating clinician should be familiar with the various methods of pain management in order to incorporate them into a patient's care plan.[2] The principles of pain management outlined above can be applied to the management of other symptoms, the exploration of which is beyond the scope of this chapter.

- Decision-making and goals of care—Patients with serious illnesses face many complex decisions about treatment, and they need a context within which to make these decisions. It is usually best to begin by building a common understanding about a patient's condition and prognosis with and without treatment. Patients should be informed about the nature of their disease, including symptoms, usual course, and expected degree of morbidity. They should also be told about all reasonable therapeutic options, including the potential benefits and burdens of these options (including the possibility of withholding all disease-directed treatment). It is important to explore what patients have been told by other clinicians and to what extent that comports with the current clinician's understanding.

  Once a common understanding is established, it is then useful to explore a patient's and family's expectations, values, and short- and long-term goals with regard to illness and treatment. Does the patient expect full recovery? What tradeoff between efficacy and adverse effects would the patient be willing to accept? How would the patient (and family) handle partial or total disability and dependence as a result of the disease or of treatment? Are there cultural or spiritual factors that influence the patient's approach to illness? Is there an upcoming event in which the patient hopes to participate? What are the patient's and family's hopes and dreams for the future?

  Patients and families should have ample opportunity to ask difficult questions about the illness, proposed treatment course, and prognosis. Physicians should not shy away from offering and making recommendations based on their medical knowledge of the treatment options in light of the patient's condition and values,[3] though a patient should not be coerced into selecting a particular treatment that the clinician thinks would be best. Physicians should remember that patients' goals and values may change over time as their condition evolves and that discussions about treatment and expectations are likely to occur many times during the course of an illness.

- Setting limits on treatment—In some instances, the natural course of an illness is such that meaningful recovery is unlikely. In other cases, the available treatment options may not be consistent with a patient's value system. Therefore, it is worth discussing what, if any, limits the patient wants to place on his or her treatment, such as forgoing endotracheal intubation or cardiopulmonary resuscitation, artificial nutrition or hydration, or surgery;

these measures may briefly prolong a seriously ill patient's life without improving his or her quality of life. Many patients are reluctant to discuss these issues as they do not wish to consider the possibility that treatment may be unsuccessful and that as a result they may die sooner rather than later. The exploration of both "hoping for the best" and "preparing for the worst" can help emphasize the care team's commitment to the patient's health and wishes while acknowledging the possibility that treatment may not go according to the plan.[4] Some patients are relieved to have an opportunity to discuss their wishes and their fears, whereas for others, any such conversation may at first seem too frightening. The conversation may be difficult to start, but it is generally important for patients and families to have.

- Healthcare proxy—One of the most important decisions a patient can make when confronting a serious illness is the selection of a healthcare proxy—a person (or people) who the patient trusts to make treatment decisions in the event that the patient loses decision-making capacity in the future. Ideally, the proxy is someone close to the patient who is familiar with the patient's values and goals; the proxy's guiding principle should be to act as a surrogate for the patient and make the choices the patient would have made him- or herself if able to make and communicate a choice. In addition to choosing a proxy, the patient should be encouraged to create an advance directive, in which he or she outlines the measures (e.g., intubation, resuscitation, artificial nutrition, antibiotics, dialysis, etc.) he or she would want in the future if unable to make the decision for him- or herself. The patient should discuss his wishes directly with his family, healthcare proxy, and treating clinician once they are formulated.

Although basic palliative care should be part of the repertoire of all clinicians, whether they are general internists, geriatricians, or subspecialists, there are situations that call for referral to a palliative care specialist. Some patients may have intractable symptoms despite the treating clinician's best efforts to relieve them. There are cases in which the patient may have differing goals and expectations from his or her family or treatment team; such situations may benefit from help with conflict resolution that might be provided by a formal palliative care consultation. Sometimes, the patient's goals of care are simply not clear after reasonable efforts to ascertain, and assistance with in-depth exploration of these goals and related decision-making is desired. As the disease progresses and treatment options dwindle, patients may need to make difficult choices about the care they receive at the end of life. Because palliative care physicians frequently provide end-of-life and hospice care, they are uniquely equipped to outline the available options for such care should the primary treating clinician desire help in this process. Finally, while any physician may manage a dying patient, including in the context of hospice, it is certainly appropriate to consult a palliative care specialist for assistance with aspects of this care if needed or desired.

There is considerable overlap between the fields of palliative care and geriatrics in the management of elderly patients, such as clarifying goals of treatment, managing pain, and addressing polypharmacy. Other situations involving elderly patients call more for expertise in geriatrics rather than in palliative care. Examples include management of conditions commonly encountered in geriatrics, such as dementia and frailty. Many patients are followed by both geriatric and palliative care specialists, and a number of physicians have completed training in both fields. The specialty fields of geriatrics and palliative care have similar challenges in defining exactly who requires consultative help or referral and who can be adequately managed by nonspecialist clinicians with good general treatment skills.

31.4   HOW DOES PALLIATIVE CARE DIFFER IN THE ELDERLY?

While the basic principles of palliative care apply equally to patients of all ages, elderly patients present unique challenges to those caring for them.

31.4.1 PROGNOSTICATION

Most physicians, and especially those providing palliative care, regularly discuss information about prognosis with patients and families. This information is essential when considering one's treatment goals and the benefits and burdens of various therapies; it is also necessary when determining the optimal time for a shift in therapeutic focus and transition to hospice care. Various tools exist to aid with prognostication. The Palliative Performance Scale (PPS) considers a patient's ambulatory status, level of activity, ability for self-care, oral intake, and level of consciousness to determine an estimated survival.[5-7] The Karnofsky Performance Status (KPS) score incorporates a patient's signs and symptoms of disease (cancer), activity level, amount of assistance required, and level of medical care required; the KPS is commonly used to gauge a patient's appropriateness for chemotherapy, but is also used to estimate survival.[8,9] Disease-specific guidelines also exist, for example, the New York Heart Association class hierarchy for congestive heart failure[10] and the Model for End-Stage Liver Disease (MELD) score for liver failure.[11]

Unfortunately, while prognostication tools, along with clinical experience and judgment, provide useful information, they allow general estimations of survival that are both inaccurate and imprecise. This uncertainty is compounded in the elderly by the presence of advanced age and by comorbidities, including frailty and dementia. When discussing prognosis with a patient and family, it is important to acknowledge this uncertainty. It may be useful to state that it is impossible to predict the course of an individual patient; but that the average person with the same illness as the patient is likely to live for a certain number of days, weeks, or months; always including the proviso that a given patient's time could be longer or shorter than the general estimate.[12] Giving a general prognosis while admitting the limitations of prognostication can help patients and families plan for likely outcomes while simultaneously understanding that the decisions that they make may require reassessment if the disease does not progress as expected.

31.4.2 GOAL SETTING AND MEDICAL DECISION-MAKING

One of the main goals of geriatrics is the maintenance of function in the presence of multiple comorbid diseases. It follows that the natural course and treatment-related concerns for each of a patient's medical conditions must be considered when making decisions about a patient's overall goals of care. The therapies for one illness may worsen another illness (as in congestive heart failure and renal disease), or the therapies for a given illness may counteract those of another illness (as in drug interactions). In addition, it may be possible to successfully manage one condition that impacts longevity and quality of life (heart failure), but other conditions may remain refractory to treatment (dementia). It is not uncommon for elderly people facing multiple comorbidities to struggle with disappointment, resignation, and even depression that stems, at least in part, from their health concerns and change in quality of life.

The very concept of quality of life may differ in the elderly and infirm. Younger adults are often concerned with developing careers and with the raising of children, and they expect to enjoy many years of good health and productivity. Their goals and dreams are rooted in the future. Older adults are more likely to be retired and less likely to be responsible for children. They may therefore be less concerned with daily obligations and more concerned with spending time on relationships and enjoyable activities. They may adapt to declining mobility and independence and aim to live each day to its fullest. Their goals and values may be more rooted in the present. As such, most (but not all) may be less likely to pursue life-extending therapies that would confer additional symptomatic, financial, or logistic burdens without improving their ability to engage with life on a day-to-day basis. It is essential to recognize, of course, that many older adults, for a variety of reasons, do prefer to pursue disease-directed and life-extending therapies. In addition, some patients may choose to treat certain conditions aggressively, but not others. Ongoing discussions with patients and their families are essential to honoring their values.

31.4.3 THE ROLE OF FAMILIES AND CAREGIVERS

Patients make medical decisions within the context of their family systems. Often, families and loved ones provide encouragement and assistance; this support might be material, financial, logistical, and, of course, emotional. Sometimes, families are a source of uncertainty, conflict, and stress. Older adults may have to consider the needs and desires of spouses or siblings who are themselves infirm. They often have adult children whose opinions they also consider when making choices for themselves, especially if the older adult is increasingly reliant on his or her children for various types of assistance. Indeed, an older adult with a serious illness is likely to experience functional decline and, perhaps, cognitive decline. In some cases, an older adult lacks the ability to care for him- or herself and/or lacks the capacity to make medical decisions pertaining to his or her own treatment. In these cases, the family or caregiver must take on an expanded role in decision-making, and the consequences of any choices will greatly impact the family as well as the patient. Ideally, then, families and caregivers should be involved in the decision-making process as early as a patient will allow.

31.4.4 SPECIAL MEDICAL MANAGEMENT CONSIDERATIONS

Several factors make the provision of direct medical care more challenging in older adults.

- Symptom assessment—The assessment of symptoms such as pain, dyspnea, nausea, and anxiety can be difficult in some older adults. Some people are reluctant to reveal discomfort. They may have been trained from a young age to remain stoic. They may wish to minimize their own concerns to not burden their families and caregivers. They may fear that their independence will be curtailed if they admit to any weakness. Those with moderate dementia may not recognize their discomfort or understand what it means. Other patients, such as those with advanced dementia, are unable to clearly express their needs. For example, they may moan or become agitated with any type of discomfort, whether it is physical or emotional. Well-validated tools, such as the Pain Assessment in Advanced Dementia (PAINAD),[13] can help with the assessment of pain and can guide the appropriate selection and titration of treatment modalities; palliative care specialists and geriatricians may also be good resources.
- Medication concerns—Older adults are more likely to exhibit sensitivity to medications because of advancing age, comorbidities, impaired renal and hepatic function, and changes in body habitus. In addition, because they often take multiple medications, they are at risk for a wider range of adverse effects, additive side effects, and medication interactions. The very need to take a large number of pills, sometimes several times a day, poses a considerable burden to many people. If at all possible, the number of medications a patient takes should be minimized; combination and long-acting products should be considered when appropriate to decrease pill burden. All medications should be assessed regularly for indication, efficacy, and intolerability, and any medications that do not meet the patient's goals of care might be discontinued. Geriatric consultation may benefit any older patients and caregivers struggling with medication concerns.
- Under-treatment of pain—At the same time that unnecessary medications are stopped, some symptoms, pain in particular, are sometimes best addressed with pharmacologic measures. Patients' reluctance to take pain medication, the presence of adverse effects, and clinicians' concerns about misuse and side effects may all lead to the under treatment of pain. These are valid concerns, but adequate analgesia is essential to recovery from injury, participation in rehabilitation, and overall sense of well-being. Assistance from a palliative care specialist can be valuable in cases of inadequately treated pain.
- Agitation and delirium—Transient disturbances in consciousness and awareness are common in older adults, especially those with dementia, infection, metabolic insults, or

polypharmacy. Nonpharmacologic techniques such as reorientation to surroundings, inviting the presence of loved ones, reassurance, and music often help calm an agitated patient. Medications such as haloperidol, quetiapine, and risperidone can also be useful when used in low doses. Benzodiazepines such as lorazepam benefit some patients (especially those with coexisting anxiety disorders), but they should be used with caution as elderly patients sometimes have a paradoxical response causing more, rather than less, agitation and confusion. Physical restraints should be avoided if at all possible as they can worsen symptoms and increase the risk of injury. Tethers such as catheters or IV drips and poles should also be removed when possible. Both palliative care and geriatric specialists can help determine the optimal treatment regimen for a given patient's agitation and delirium.

31.5 REHABILITATION AND PALLIATIVE CARE IN GERIATRIC PATIENTS

It is not uncommon for older adults to participate in rehabilitation following a variety of medical conditions, such as arthritis exacerbations and joint replacement surgery, cardio- and cerebrovascular events, and deconditioning secondary to acute illness. For most of these patients, the goal of rehabilitation (to maintain functional capacity at the highest possible level in the face of physical impairment) complements that of palliative care (to maximize comfort and quality of life). When patients are terminally ill or dying, however, the aims of the two fields may diverge. Therapies that seek to improve function become inconsistent or impossible to apply in the face of terminal illness-related progressive functional decline. For dying patients, communication among themselves, their families, and their palliative and rehabilitation care providers is vital to bridge the gap between the possible and the inevitable. In many cases, a patient's short-term goals of care allow for limited-duration rehabilitation with specific outcomes and clear measures of progress. For example, a patient may wish to maintain enough strength to transfer from bed to commode with minimal assistance, or to sit upright in a bed or a chair to hold a grandchild. A family may wish to learn how to carefully feed a patient to maximize oral intake while minimizing aspiration risk. Such gains may be relatively small or short lived, but the sense of dignity and control they impart to a patient can substantially improve the patient's quality of life during his or her final weeks to months.

Conflicts between rehabilitation and palliative care also sometimes occur because of differing goals and expectations among the various parties involved in a patient's care. A patient and/or family might refuse to accept a prognosis of terminal illness and insist on intensive rehabilitation despite the physical impossibility and futility of such therapy. Conversely, some patients and families might underestimate the prognosis and potential for improvement and decline rehabilitation efforts despite a high likelihood of success. Sometimes, the source of conflict is entirely outside the scope of both patients' and care teams' control. The reimbursement scheme used in the United States often pays for treatments that improve function, but not those that promote comfort and dignity without promoting major gains in function. This can cause a great deal of frustration among those involved in a patient's care. In many cases, negotiation principles similar to those outlined above can lead to resolution; these include discussion, careful documentation, and trials of goal-directed, limited-duration rehabilitation with clear outcome measures.

31.6 THE INTERPLAY OF PALLIATIVE CARE AND REHABILITATION IN SELECTED GERIATRIC CONDITIONS

31.6.1 DEMENTIA

An 88-year-old woman has had Alzheimer's dementia for 6 years. Over the past 16 months, her functional status has declined to the point that she can no longer carry out any of her activities of daily living (ADL). She has intermittent urinary, but not fecal, incontinence. She had a urinary tract infection that required hospitalization 2 months ago. She now spends most of her time in bed.

Her son, who is her healthcare proxy, wonders whether she would be a candidate for physical therapy to improve her strength and allow her to ambulate around the house with a walker, under supervision.

Dementia is a progressive, terminal illness. It may coexist for years with other medical conditions; if one of a patient's coexisting conditions does not cause death, complications of dementia, such as aspiration pneumonia, eventually will. Dementia can be classified in various ways. It may be staged as mild (difficulties with instrumental ADL, such as bill paying), moderate (difficulties with physical household tasks), or severe (marked difficulties with self-care). The Functional Assessment Staging (FAST) score stages patients using more specific functional increments.[14]

Patients with mild and moderate dementia can and do participate in rehabilitation with the goal of improving function. Patients with more severe dementia are unlikely to make any gains in function and may not benefit from even short-term, specific goal-directed therapy. However, rehabilitation specialists might work with the caregivers of patients with severe dementia, focusing on things such as hand feeding to reduce the risk of aspiration, careful toileting to reduce the risk of infection, and prevention of pressure ulcers.

For patients with severe dementia, palliative care focuses on the management of symptoms such as pain and delirium, as well as refocusing the family on achievable goals of treatment. Because these patients lack the capacity for decision-making, their surrogates are educated about the terminal nature of dementia and the complications that often ultimately lead to death, such as urinary sepsis, aspiration pneumonia, and malnutrition. They are asked to consider and then guided through decisions such as cardiopulmonary resuscitation, endotracheal intubation, artificial nutrition and hydration, and hospitalization. Ideally, patients have in place advance directives, completed prior to their cognitive decline, to guide their decision makers. If there are no advance directives (more often than not the case), surrogates are asked to make the decisions they feel that patients would have made if able to speak for themselves ("substituted judgment"). For patients with dementia, goals of care discussions often occur after a sentinel event, such as an aspiration, infection, or hip fracture. Advanced dementia is an appropriate hospice diagnosis, although a patient must have a minimum FAST score to qualify in terms of prognosis. Hospice services can be provided in the home or, commonly, in a skilled nursing facility.

The patient in the case has severe dementia and has had a recent urinary tract infection. She is unlikely to make any functional gains with traditional rehabilitation, but she and her caregivers may benefit from additional training in toileting and positioning to prevent further infections. If not already done, her son should be educated about dementia, and discussions regarding goals of care should be held to ensure that the patient receives only the therapies consistent with her values as they are known for this clinical context. If her son agrees, a hospice referral may be considered as her advanced dementia and recent severe infection may suggest a limited prognosis of less than 6 months.

31.6.2 FAILURE TO THRIVE

An 87-year-old man is admitted to the hospital with a 6-week history of abdominal pain, nausea without vomiting, and decreased oral intake. He has lost 12 pounds over the past 3 months. Abdominal imaging reveals bladder wall thickening and retroperitoneal lymphadenopathy, but no clear cause for his symptoms. His wife of 66 years died earlier in the year after a brief illness. While saddened by the loss of his wife and by his own recent physical decline, the patient denies depression and states that he would like to live for as long as possible. He would like to participate in rehabilitation to increase his strength and activity, which he hopes will stimulate his appetite. His family asks about the placement of a feeding tube if he does not start eating soon.

Failure to thrive is defined as a greater than 5% weight loss accompanied by decreased appetite and impaired nutrition.[15] It is fairly common in older adults and can be associated with various medical conditions, including malignancy, renal disease, heart failure, and hepatic failure, as well as with depression. Treatment measures include elucidation and management of any underlying causes, as well as nutritional support in the form of favorite foods, supplements, and, in some cases, artificial nutrition.

Some patients with failure to thrive may benefit from physical therapy to address deconditioning, with the goal of increasing strength and endurance to allow greater participation in desired activities. However, others may make no gains even with aggressive therapy. The latter are patients in whom it may be appropriate to define concrete measures of progress, such as the ability to ambulate a certain distance within a given time frame, and to discontinue further therapy and reconsider the goals of care if these measures are not achieved.

The role of palliative care in failure to thrive usually comprises symptom management and goals of care discussions. Symptoms such as nausea, anorexia, fatigue, and depression can be distressing for patients and their families, but may respond to antiemetics, appetite stimulants, general stimulants, and antidepressants. Some medications impact multiple symptoms; mirtazapine, for example, can address depression and anorexia, while methylphenidate can improve fatigue, depression, and anorexia. Pain management is also important in failure to thrive, as pain, if present and undertreated, can impact both appetite and mood.

The families of patients with failure to thrive often inquire about artificial nutrition. Discussions about artificial nutrition must accompany consideration of goals of care. For patients pursuing comfort-oriented measures, artificial nutrition is unlikely to provide benefit. Patients and families may express worry about starvation in the absence of good oral intake. However, as patients near the end of life, both their nutritional needs and desire to eat decrease, and they typically experience no discomfort as a result of decreased oral intake. They should be allowed, but not forced, to eat small amounts of their favorite foods if they wish. For patients continuing with disease-directed or life-extending therapies, particularly those with mechanical swallowing obstructions or dysphagia following acute stroke, tube feeds might sometimes be appropriate, especially as a time-limited trial with predefined endpoints.

In failure to thrive, artificial nutrition is unlikely to have a long-term impact on nutritional status and still poses substantial additional risks. Feeding tubes expose patients to the possibility of surgical risk, worsening aspiration, injury from pulling on uncomfortable tubes, and physical restraints. Parenteral nutrition poses the risks of infection, thrombosis, and liver disease. In patients with declining renal or cardiac function, both tube feeds and parenteral nutrition can cause fluid overload, edema, and dyspnea. For these reasons, artificial nutrition should not be initiated without a thorough discussion of the potential burdens as well as benefits and the extent to which the nutrition will meet the patient's goals of care.

The patient in this case should receive symptomatic treatment for his nausea and, perhaps, anorexia. He should be evaluated for depression and treated if appropriate. Given his desire to live as long as possible, consideration should be given to working up his radiographic findings. The presence of malignancy would impact his prognosis, and an informed decision about how to approach the malignancy would probably guide other treatment decisions. Even if a primarily palliative approach to his malignancy were selected, a time-limited, goal-directed trial of rehabilitation may still be appropriate to try to improve his function. However, artificial nutrition is probably not appropriate as the patient continues to have some oral intake and is unlikely to benefit long-term from such an intervention. Regardless of the treatment approach chosen and the patient's long-term outlook, he should be encouraged to select a healthcare proxy, to discuss his wishes about cardiopulmonary resuscitation and his goals for ongoing care with his proxy and family, and to update his family and care team if his wishes change.

31.6.3 Cancer

A 90-year-old woman with a 7-year history of mild-to-moderately aggressive lymphoma previously treated with chemotherapy and radiation presents to the hospital with several weeks of increasing weakness, fatigue, and confusion. Workup reveals no cause for these symptoms, although it is felt that her underlying cancer may be contributing. No further treatment is available for her malignancy. During hospitalization, she lacks decision-making capacity, but is pleasant and able to converse and follow instructions. Her oral intake is poor, and she is unable to get out of bed. Her prognosis is felt to be a few weeks to a few months based on her current trajectory. Her family agrees, based on her previously expressed wishes, that she would prefer to be at home on hospice. However, they think that it would be much easier to care for her if she were stronger and able to transfer more easily and are requesting rehab admission for this reason.

In this case, the goals of rehabilitation and palliative care are similar—to improve functioning and quality of life. However, significant improvement in her functional status is unlikely. It is reasonable to have a frank discussion with the family about the potential outcomes of rehabilitation. She may improve modestly and have greater ability to transfer, giving her greater quality of life at home. On the other hand, she could remain unchanged or even continue to deteriorate. For this patient, should the family desire, a geriatric and/or rehabilitation consultation to see if a very limited-duration trial of rehabilitation (e.g., 5 days) with very concrete goals would be appropriate, with a discharge plan set up in advance for home hospice. Alternatively, the patient could get a one-time rehabilitation consultation where family and treating staff could learn safer transfer techniques. Her palliative care needs would be of paramount importance so that her quality of life could be maximized for the time remaining. These basic palliative care needs might be addressed by her primary care clinician, geriatrician, or oncologist—whichever clinician knows her best and is willing to take on that role—with formal palliative care consultation only if some aspect of her care were difficult to manage.

31.6.4 Chronic Obstructive Pulmonary Disease

An 88-year-old man with severe chronic obstructive pulmonary disease (COPD) presents for the third time in 6 months with impending respiratory failure. He went to pulmonary rehabilitation after his first hospitalization and learned some techniques to improve his breathing. Four months later, during his next hospitalization, he was intubated for 1 week; he then decided that he did not want this again, so do-not-intubate (DNI) and do-not-resuscitate (DNR) orders were instituted, with no other limitations. Two months later, when he again presented with impending respiratory failure, he was offered bilevel positive airway pressure (BiPAP) in the emergency department and was admitted to the intensive care unit. Attempts to wean him off of BiPAP were unsuccessful, as he became very short of breath and panicky after only a few minutes. A palliative care consultation was obtained.

Patients with advanced respiratory and cardiac disease face a daunting array of choices toward the end of life. While mechanical ventilation may allow patients to survive potentially reversible exacerbations of their illness, they also have the potential to prolong the very terminal phase of illnesses that are not going to reverse and for which there are no good or easy alternatives. BiPAP can help patients with advanced pulmonary disease avoid unwanted intubation and mechanical ventilation, but it can also create dilemmas in which patients who are DNR/DNI must now make an additional "life or death" decision because they cannot live without the BiPAP and are unprepared to die (especially as the result of an explicit decision).

In this circumstance, the palliative care team learned that the pulmonary team thought the odds of the patient leaving the hospital off BiPAP were very low. The patient found the BiPAP very uncomfortable and required steady doses of opioids and benzodiazepines to tolerate the mask. Because of the sedation, the patient was incapacitated to make decisions, and he had no healthcare proxy. His family felt that the patient would not want his life indefinitely sustained on the BiPAP, which they had not anticipated using in the first place. The palliative care team recommended removing the patient from the BiPAP with the expectation that he would not survive long, and they promised to do their best to keep him comfortable during the dying process. The family agreed to moving the patient to the palliative care unit and giving family members 24 hours to visit with the patient and say good-bye with the BiPAP still on. Prior to removal of the BiPAP, the doses of opioids and benzodiazepines were increased by 30% and then adjusted as per the hospital's ventilator withdrawal policy. The patient was taken off of the BiPAP and put on nasal oxygen. Medication was adjusted to keep his level of dyspnea and anxiety well controlled. He died 36 hours later with family in attendance.

31.7 CONCLUSION

With the aging of the "baby boomer" cohort in the United States, the number of older adults will skyrocket in the coming decades. This group statistically bears the brunt of acute and chronic illness. Although palliative care and geriatric care are compatible with any and all traditional medical treatments, as patients age and become more impaired, the focus of medical care for many will shift away from primarily disease-directed and potentially life-prolonging treatments more toward comfort- and quality of life-oriented treatments. Therefore, clinicians who treat older adults, whether as primary care providers or specialists, should become familiar with various principles of palliative care, including symptom management, goal setting and decision-making, and end-of-life considerations. The application of these principles throughout the course of patients' treatment will allow them to live the remainder of their lives, however long or short that might be, with the utmost comfort, fulfillment, and dignity.

REFERENCES

1. Quill, T. and Abernethy, A. 2013. Generalist plus specialist palliative care—Creating a more sustainable model. *N Engl J Med* 368:1173–1175.
2. Bial, A. and Levine, S. 2008. UNIPAC three: Assessment and treatment of physical pain associated with life-limiting illness. In *Hospice and Palliative Care Training for Physicians: A Self-Study Program [UNIPAC]*, eds. C. Storey, S. Levine, and J. Shega. Glenview, IL: American Academy of Hospice and Palliative Medicine.
3. Quill, T. and Brody, H. 1996. Physician recommendations and patient autonomy: Finding a balance between physician power and patient choice. *Ann Intern Med* 125(9):763–769.
4. Back, A., Arnold, R., and Quill, T. 2003. Hope for the best, and prepare for the worst. *Ann Intern Med* 138(5):439–443.
5. Lau, F., Downing, M., Lesperance, M. et al. 2009. Using the palliative performance scale to provide meaningful survival estimates. *J Pain Symptom Manage* 38(1):134–144.
6. Downing, M., Lau, F., Lesperance, M. et al. 2007. Meta-analysis of survival prediction with palliative performance scale. *J Palliat Care* 23(4):245–252; discussion 252–254.
7. Ho, F., Lau, F., Downing, M. et al. 2008. A reliability and validity study of the palliative performance scale. *BMC Palliat Care* 4:7–10.
8. Evans, C. and McCarthy, M. 1985. Uncertainty in terminal care: Can the Karnofsky index help? *Lancet* 25;1(8439):1204–1206.
9. Maltoni, M., Nanni, O., Scarpi, E. et al. 1994. Clinical prediction of survival is more accurate than the Karnofsky performance status in estimating life span of terminally ill cancer patients. *Eur J Cancer* 30A(6):764–766.
10. Heart Failure Society of America. NYHA Classification: The stages of heart failure. http://www.abouthf.org/questions_stages.htm (accessed February 14, 2014).
11. Kamath, P. and Kim, W. 2007. The model for end-stage liver disease (MELD). *Hepatology* 45:797–805.
12. Lamont, E. and Christakis, N. 2003. Complexities in prognostication in advanced cancer: "To help them live their lives the way they want to." *J Am Med Assoc* 290:98–104.
13. Warden, V., Hurley, A., and Volicer, L. 2003. Development and psychometric evaluation of the pain assessment in advanced dementia (PAINAD) scale. *J Am Med Dir Assoc* 4(1):9–15.
14. Tsai, S. and Arnold, R. 2006. Prognostication in dementia. http://www.mypcnow.org/blank-txv87. (accessed September 26, 2016).
15. Robertson, R. and Montagnini, M. 2004. Geriatric failure to thrive. *Am Fam Physician* 70(2):343–350.

32 Economics of Geriatric Rehabilitation

K. Rao Poduri

CONTENTS

Caring for geriatric patients is a skill and a challenge at the same time. Post-acute care is becoming more of a bigger challenge as a result of its economic impact. Throughout the world, healthcare costs for caring the growing number of older adults are reaching astronomical levels.

The growth of aging population is a global phenomenon which affects every part of the world.

By the year 2050, the world's population of 4 billion will consist of 21% each of people under 15 years and over 60 years of age.[1,2]

In Europe, there were more people over 60 years of age than under 15 years at the turn of the century and this trend will be followed by North America by 2030 and in Asia and Latin America by 2040. The current number of 89 million of the people in the world over the age of 80 will increase to 379 million by 2050; 12% of the European population will be older than 80 years of age.

Throughout the world, almost two-thirds of the childbearing rates have fallen below replacement levels due to the falling fertility rates.[3] In the later part of the twentieth century, there was a decline in fertility rates along with an average increase of life span of individuals by 20 years. In the last two decades, there is an increase in the fertility rates in many countries and the life span of individuals across the world is projected to increase by another 10 years by 2050.[4]

This trend of the aging population poses a demand on medical and social services. Chronic disease that affects the older adults more frequently causes disability and decline in function resulting in decreased quality of life and increased long-term care costs.[5]

Chronic diseases cause severe disability. Severe arthritis alone is a leading cause of disability affecting 59% of older adults in the United States.[6]

In Europe, the population over 65 is growing rapidly. It is estimated that by 2060, this group of older adults will become 29.5% of the total population of the world, an increase from 17.4% in 2010. Among the European countries, the highest number of people over 65 are found in Germany and Italy, and their numbers have doubled in less than 60 years. These two countries are facing challenges in the fields of medicine and healthcare costs.[7,8]

Increase in the prevalence of chronic diseases is one major consequence of aging of the population. In addition to cancer and diabetes, chronic respiratory and cardiovascular diseases are the main causes of death in the world.[9]

The global prevalence of the leading chronic diseases is on the rise with most of it occurring in the developing countries. Cardiovascular disease is reported as the leading cause of death in these countries and is expected to increase to 120% in females and 137% in males by 2020.[10]

The affordability of healthcare during 2005–2010 for the aging population was compared for the high-income countries: Canada, United States, and United Kingdom.[4] In all the three countries, increase in healthcare costs was attributed to the growth of the aging population. The perception in the United States is that healthcare resources of the older people are diverting the resources away from younger people but aging population is not responsible for the increase in the overall healthcare spending. However, in Canada and the United Kingdom, the steady increase in health-care costs is attributed to the aging population.

U.S. economy is the biggest and represents 20% of all global economic activity in the world. The gross domestic product (GDP) of the United States is 15-trillion dollars. The percentage of this GDP spent for healthcare costs is higher than in any other nation in the world. These healthcare costs in the United States will continue to rise at a rate of 4%–7% per annum.[2] They increased from 27.1 billion to 2.6 trillion in the last 60 years. If this trend is not controlled, healthcare spending as a percentage of GDP will reach 30% in 2035 and will become an economic burden.

The main factors for these disproportionate increases in healthcare costs are unsustainable with the GDP lagging behind. The unavoidable aging of the population is attributed to this disproportionate healthcare expenditure. Rich and Adams[2] mention that healthcare spending, relief of suffering, prolongation of life, quality of health, and resource allocation are all related to the development of technological advances. However, well-being, quality, and cost are not directly related. Besides aging of the population, other factors that influence the costs are technology, health insurance, malpractice, and overhead and administrative expenditures. Along those lines, the high per capita income and the higher standards of living in the United States compared to the rest of the world are factors attributed to the high cost of healthcare. Health care expenditures increased for each 10% increase in real income.[11] The growing group of older adults who have chronic diseases and multiple comorbidities[12,13] that sustain hip fractures, strokes, trauma, and other disabling conditions are seen by the physicians more often and they are hospitalized frequently requiring rehabilitation services adding to the healthcare costs. The prevalence of chronic diseases that bring disability and dependence in this ever-increasing older adult population has a toll on the quality of life of the individuals and society and escalates healthcare costs. Prevalence of one or more chronic conditions in older adults was found to be 82% higher compared to those without those conditions. Sixty-two percent of the 82% had multiple chronic conditions. Wolff et al.[14] reported that patients with a number of chronic conditions had more inpatient admissions and hospitalizations with preventable complications. People older than 65 years with four or more chronic conditions were 99 times more likely to have an admission than those without any chronic conditions. The cost increased with the number and types of chronic conditions. For an individual, it was $211 without a chronic condition and $13,973 with four or more types of chronic conditions. Hoffman et al.[15] reported that 88% of the population older than 65 years had one or more chronic conditions compared to 45% in the general population. The risk of an avoidable inpatient admission or a preventable complication in an inpatient setting increases dramatically with the number of chronic conditions. Better primary care, especially coordination of care, could reduce avoidable hospitalization rates, especially for individuals with multiple chronic conditions.

The effects of multimorbidity and its implications are well studied. Multimorbidity is the presence of two or more chronic disorders.[16] In Switzerland, they found that multimorbidity was associated with higher cost of care and higher healthcare utilization in the older population.[17] It is observed that older adults had multiple comorbidities and chronic diseases, which affect them disproportionately. Multimorbidity is also associated with socioeconomic factors. Low-income groups have higher multimorbidity and incur higher costs of care.[18] In the United States, 75% of the healthcare costs account for the management of chronic diseases.[19,20] The healthcare resources are not equally distributed among the populations. In 2008 and 2009, half the healthcare expenditure in the United States was spent for the 5% of the sickest population. Forty-two percent of the costs were for the older adults comprising of 13.2% of the population. Chronic diseases in older adults resulted in these increased expenses. A systematic review of 35 studies by Lehnert et al.[21] identified that there is a curvilinear and near-exponential relationship between healthcare costs and multiple chronic conditions and costs increase with each additional condition. Chronic conditions seem to cluster in individuals, and people with any one condition are prone to have other additional conditions.[14] The leading causes of disability and death in the older adults are due to chronic diseases and are attributed to obesity and smoking.[22] The economic burden in this case is cumulative. In the United States, 80% of the older adults have at least one chronic condition and 50% have at least two and the treatment costs twice as much as compared to people with no chronic diseases. Similarly, treating patients with multiple comorbidities costs 7 times more than treating people with one comorbidity.[23,24]

Additionally, the process of aging is associated with disability from sarcopenia, which is prevalent in 45% of people in the United States over the age of 65. Sarcopenia is the progressive loss of muscle mass and causes functional decline and disability. The economic impact of sarcopenia is estimated to be $18.5 billion when the cost of disability is multiplied by the number of older adults.[24]

Older adults in the United States have the highest rate of obesity in the world.[22] Obesity and its resultant comorbidities such as coronary heart disease, stroke, diabetes, and cancer further increase the healthcare expenses. The rate of obesity in adults has risen threefold since the 1960s. Finkelstein et al.[25] pointed out in 2006 that the cost of caring for the obese is 42% higher than treating the nonobese.[23] By 2008, the prevalence of obesity combined with the 21% for healthcare spending adds up to $147 billion each year.[26] As the rate of obesity increases, the related healthcare costs are expected to rise exponentially.

In addition, elective and nonelective surgeries in older adults are reported to have higher morbidity and mortality.[27] Their perioperative and postoperative care usually occurs in intensive care units. They account for 50% of all ICU admissions[28] and they are responsible for 20%–30% of overall healthcare costs in the United States. Twenty percent of these adults die within 3 months[29] and 70% of all the hospital deaths are of the older adults. The cost of the hospitalizations resulting in deaths is 2.7 times higher than when patients are discharged alive.

Functional disability and aging: Each year, up to 10% of the nondisabled adults who are 75 years and older living in the community lose independence for basic activities of daily living (ADL).[30] Hence, assessment and interventions are crucial to prevent further disease, injuries, and dependence. Higher incidence of hospitalizations and associated costs are described in a study by Ferrucci et al.[31] and resource consumption by Wolinksy et al.[32] Subsequent risk of being placed in a long-term care or nursing homes and even death with functional dependence is imminent in this population.[33,34]

A study by Fried et al.[35] in 2001 described that patients with progressive decline in functional status required more services and increased healthcare costs. Almost half of the total expenditure was accounted for 19.6% of the community-dwelling individuals who were 72 years or older and had stable dependence but declined further. This is a burden on the government-funded short- and long-term care services. There is a definite effect of healthcare spending on age. There are differences in functional decline and disability for different age groups in different countries for mobility and IADLs. Levels of disability were found to be lower in Eastern Europe followed by England, Southern Europe, and lowest in Northern and Western Europe. High levels of disability with small age-related changes between 50 and 85 were found in the United States. Age-related increases in disability were noted to be higher in Eastern and Southern Europe than in the United States.[36] IADL dependence was noted in 70 years and older age groups. In the United States and England, poor socioeconomic groups had higher dependency and age-related functional deficits with advanced age. Compared to the United States, age-related functional decline was high at 75–85 years of age in Eastern and Southern Europe. Despite the variations in disability and functional decline, the healthcare costs per capita are higher for persons who are 65 years and older. For an individual in the United States, the expenditure in 2000s was $12,100 compared to $6800 in Canada and $3600 in the United Kingdom.[37]

The differences in the expenditures in developed and developing countries are the availability of acute care and long- term care in institutional services in the developed countries. As mentioned earlier, the utilization of medical services and the cost of care are higher for the older adults. These differences may be attributed to income growth and medical and technological advances. Very little is known about the medical care and its cost in the developing world. The World Health Organization (WHO), National Institution on Aging, and National Institute of Health[38] report that the cost of care for heart disease, stroke, and cancer are the main reasons for the disease burden of care in the developed countries. The analysis in this report indicates that diabetes, heart disease and stroke, and their impact on economic loss in 2006 to be $20–30 million in Vietnam and Ethiopia and almost one billion dollars both in China and India. These losses are expected to double in the near future. Between 2006 and 2015, the estimated disease-related economic loss in 23 nations is $84 billion. As regards cancer, due to the increase in the aging population, there were 13-million cases in 2009 costing $286 billion. It is projected that there will be 17 million new cases by 2020 and 27 million by 2030 and half of these cases are expected to be seen in Asia.[38] As older individuals are surviving longer, in order to prolong life, majority of the healthcare costs are spent during the years close to death. Across the world, the medical treatment for the very old is questionable based on the attitudes such as ageism. However, in the United States, the healthcare expenditures toward the end of life are not on the rise compared to healthcare spending in general.[39] In the decades to come, aging population will clearly influence patterns of healthcare spending and sustainability of provision of care. As people age with accompanying functional dependence, the healthcare demands for long-term care increase with a strain on personal family and governmental resources. Between 1990 and 2001, in the United States, the costs for nursing home and home care were $132 billion[40] in the United States; patients and families were responsible for 25% and 57% was paid by the federal government. Currently, these figures are already surpassing the projected 20%–21% for 2020. The increasing trends of the growing older adults and less taxpaying population (due to the increasing number of older adults) will deplete the resources further.[41] Additionally, older adults will have difficulty with the availability of family and friends to provide care.

Another study was conducted in Netherlands by Blom et al.[42] on the effectiveness and cost-effectiveness of a proactive, goal-oriented, integrated care model in general practice for older people. They concluded that using this model of care plans for older people with complex problems can be a valuable tool in general practice, but no direct beneficial effect was found for older persons. They explained that older patients with complex problems were already satisfied with the care offered by their general practitioners and the change in satisfaction was not significant with this model. Nevertheless, no significant improvement was found in quality of life or functional status of the older adults after 1-year follow-up.

Since cardiovascular diseases, cancer, diabetes, and stroke are the leading causes of morbidity and mortality, providing healthcare addressing these conditions in the older adults with quality and safety is paramount. Patient and family education for the preventive measures is critical.

The topics on cancer, diabetes, and stroke are covered in the previous chapters. Health care should be provided in an integrated care model that focuses on the ability of the older adults than their disability. The Geriatric Resources for Assessment and Care of Elders (GRACE) program, developed at the Indianapolis-based Wishard Health Services is one such model to address the healthcare needs of the vulnerable older adults by an interdisciplinary geriatrics team. Care plans are developed by a team of nurse practitioner and social worker in conjunction with the primary care physicians to address ambulation, urinary continence, nutrition, pain, vision, hearing, medications, health maintenance, advance care planning, dementia, depression, and caregiver burden. Hong et al.[43] compared 18 successful complex care management programs and found that effective programs customize their approach to care their patients with care coordination and utilize technology to boost their efforts. These programs aim at treating "high-need, high-cost" patients who suffer from multiple complex medical conditions. Care coordination will optimize care of the older adults and can potentially improve outcomes and reduce costs. Positive outcomes were especially noted in high-risk and medically complex populations that require expensive treatments and repeated hospitalizations.[44] The care coordination will optimize care of the older adults and can also potentially improve outcomes and reduce costs. Positive outcomes were especially noted in high-risk and medically complex populations that require expensive treatments and repeated hospitalizations (Stefanacci RG). An interdisciplinary care team that provides care in the continuum is regarded as the current "Best Practice." Care coordination model can provide higher quality of care with lower costs for the patients as well as for the healthcare systems. According to the American

College of Physicians, uncoordinated care results in more costs to the patients and the systems, due to the duplication of services and increase in preventable hospital admissions. It is estimated that patients receiving uncoordinated care pay 75% more for their healthcare than those who obtain coordinated care.[45] Marek et al.[46] have shown that with coordinated care approach, older adults improved their ADL skills and decreased pain. They incorporated home visits and comprehensive needs assessments of patients into their model. Care coordination can be provided in many settings in the continuum of care, that is, hospitals, nursing homes, outpatient settings, and in the patient homes in the community. Since primary care physicians provide care in the outpatient setting, the best site for care coordination should reside in their offices. The next site of care coordination is in the patient's home and it is ideal to have a combination of home care and office-based care.

Care coordination is especially crucial during care transitions from one site to another in the continuum. Coleman[47] and his team have addressed patient safety during care transitions by identifying "The Four Pillars" across many settings of care from the hospitals to physician offices to patient homes. These pillars are (1) medication management consisting of medication reconciliation, (2) use of dynamic patient-centered record, (3) primary care and specialists follow-up, and (4) patient awareness of red flags.

Geriatricians and healthcare providers should embrace this concept of care coordination model of care and provide high quality of care which is cost effective and has proven to be successful.

The experiences among high-need older adult patients in Australia, Canada, France, Germany Netherlands, Norway, Sweden, Switzerland, and the United States were compared.[44] It was reported that the "high-need patients" have three or more comorbidities and use more healthcare services and face more financial barriers and coordination of care problems compared with other older adults. These issues were more pronounced in the United States. The comparative success of other countries is a reflection of the policies of their healthcare agencies which particularly target high-need patients. To improve the health status of the older adults and reduce the costs of care, the United States needs to adopt similar models of care.

The WHO[45] reports in 2015 that healthcare expenditure per person actually fell after the age of around 75 in high-income countries, while expenditures have increased for providing long-term care. Health care costs increase with age and peak at 65–74 years, and they begin to fall for acute and elective admissions to hospital and outpatient care. The report also mentions that older people in low-income countries use health services considerably less frequently than the younger adults. Poorer older adults with greater healthcare needs use health services less often than their richer counterparts in high-income countries.

The current health of the older adults is not keeping pace with the longevity that medical advances and technology bestowed on this population.[17] The older adults face physical and psychological barriers in accessing healthcare, further compromising their health.[46] Cost appears to be one of the major factors associated with the lack of access to care.[50] Out-of-pocket expenses are a financial burden for people over 65 years when insurances do not cover their medical needs.

According to the WHO,[49] older adults are not a financial burden to the healthcare.[47,51] The challenges and the impacts of aging population and its healthcare needs should prepare the younger generation of healthcare professionals with proper training in geriatrics and gerontology.[48,52]

REFERENCES

1. Harper S. Economic and social implications of aging societies. *Science*. 2014 Oct 31; 346(6209):587–591.
2. Rich PB, Adams SD. Health care: Economic impact of caring for geriatric patients. *Surg Clin North Am*. 2015 Feb; 95(1):11–21.
3. United Nations. *World Population Prospects: The 2012 Revision* (medium variant), 2013, http://esa.un.org/wpp.
4. Gusmano MK, Allin S. Framing the issue of ageing and health care spending in Canada, the United Kingdom and the United States. *Health Econ Policy Law*. 2014 Jul; 9(3):313–328.

5. Trends in aging—United States and worldwide. *Centers for Disease Control and Prevention (CDC) MMWR Morb Mortal Wkly Rep.* 2003 Feb 14; 52(6):101–104, 106.

6. CDC. Prevalence of self-reported arthritis or chronic joint symptoms among adults—United States, 2001. *MMWR* 2002; 51:948–950.

7. European Commission. Active ageing. [Cited Jul 28 2015]. Available from: http://ec.europa.eu/social/main.jsp?catId=1062.

8. United Nations. *World Population Ageing 2013.* New York: UN, 2013. [Cited Jul 28 2015]. Available from: http://www.un.org/en/development/desa/population/publications/pdf/ageing/World PopulationAgeingReport2013.pdf.

9. Yach D, Hawkes C, Gould CL, Hofman KJ. The global burden of chronic diseases: Overcoming impediments to prevention and control: Special Communication | June 2, 2004. *J Am Med Assoc.* 2004; 291(21):2616–2622.

10. Leeder S, Raymond S, Greenberg H, Liu H, Esson K. *A Race against Time: The Challenge of Cardiovascular Disease in Developing Economies.* New York: Columbia University, 2004.

11. Liu S, Chollet D. Price and income elasticity of the demand for health insurance and health care services: A critical review of the literature. *Math Policy Res.* 2006 Mar 24; 1–50.

12. Barnett K, Mercer SW, Norbury M, Watt G, Wyke SB. Epidemiology of multimorbidity and implications for health care, research, and medical education: A cross-sectional study. *Lancet.* 2012 Jul 7; 380(9836):37–43.

13. Framing the issue of ageing and health care... *Health Econ Policy Law.* 2014 Jul; 9(3):313–328. (Epub Apr 23 2014.) http://www.ncbi.nlm.nih.gov/pubmed/24759155.

14. Wolff JL, Starfield B, Anderson G. Prevalence, expenditures, and complications of multiple chronic conditions in the elderly. *Arch Intern Med.* 2002 Nov 11; 162(20):2269–2276.

15. Hoffman C, Rice D, Sung HY. Persons with chronic conditions: Their prevalence and costs. *J Am Med Assoc.* 1996; 276(18):1473–1479.

16. Koller D, Schon G, Schafer I, Glaeske G, Van den Bussche H, Hansen H. Multimorbidity and long-term care dependency—A five-year follow-up. *BMC Geriatr.* 2014; 14:70.

17. Bähler C, Huber CA, Brüngger B, Reich O. Multimorbidity, health care utilization and costs in an elderly community-dwelling population: A claims data based observational study. *BMC Health Serv Res.* 2015 Jan 22; 15:23.

18. Kuo RN, Lai MS. The influence of socio-economic status and multimorbidity patterns on healthcare costs: A six-year follow-up under a universal healthcare system. *Int J Equity Health.* 2013 Aug 20; 12:69.

19. Cohen SB, Yu W. Agency for Healthcare Research and Quality (AHRQ) Statistical Brief. The concentration and persistence in the level of health expenditures over time: Estimates for the U.S. population, 2008–2009. 2012. Available at: http://meps.ahrq.gov/data_files/publications/st354/stat354.pdf.

20. Centers for Disease Control and Prevention (CDC). Public health and aging: Trends in aging—United States and worldwide. *MMWR Morb Mortal Wkly Rep.* 2003; 52:101–106.

21. Lehnert T, Heider D, Leicht H, Heinrich S, Corrieri S, Luppa M, Riedel-Heller S, König HH. Review: Health care utilization and costs of elderly persons with multiple chronic conditions. *Med Care Res Rev.* 2011 Aug; 68(4):387–420.

22. Ehrlich E, Kofke-Egger H, Udow-Phillips M. *Health Care Cost Drivers: Chronic Disease, Comorbidity, and Health Risk Factors in the US and Michigan.* Ann Arbor (MI): Center for Healthcare Research and Transformation, 2010.

23. Stanton MW, Rutherford MK. *The High Concentration of US Health Care Expenditures.* Rockville (MD): Agency for Healthcare Research and Quality (AHRQ), 2005.

24. Janssen I, Shepard DS, Katzmarzyk PT et al. The healthcare costs of sarcopenia in the United States. *J Am Geriatr Soc.* 2004; 52:80–85.

25. Finkelstein EA, Trogdon JG, Cohen JW et al. Annual medical spending attributable to obesity: Payer- and service-specific estimates. *Health Aff.* 2009; 28:w822–w831.

26. Cawley J, Meyerhoefer C. The medical care costs of obesity: An instrumental variables approach. *J Health Econ.* 2012; 31:219–230.

27. Ingraham AM, Cohen ME, Raval MV. Variation in quality of care after emergency general surgery procedures in the elderly. *J Am Coll Surg.* 2011; 212:1039–1048.

28. Menaker J, Scalea TM. Geriatric care in the surgical intensive care unit. *Crit Care Med.* 2010; 38:S452–S459.

29. Yu W, Ash AS, Levinsky NG et al. Intensive care unit use and mortality in the elderly. *J Gen Intern Med.* 2000; 15:97–102.

30. Gill TM, Williams CS, Tinetti ME. Assessing risk for the onset of functional dependence among older adults: The role of physical performance. *J Am Geriatr Soc*. 1995; 43:603–609.
31. Ferrucci L, Guralnick JM, Pahor M, Corti MC, Havlik RJ. Hospital diagnoses, medicare charges, and nursing home admissions in the year when older persons become severely disabled. *J Am Med Assoc*. 1997; 277:728–734.
32. Wolinsky FD, Culler SD, Callahan C, Johnson RJ. Hospital resource consumption among older adults: A prospective analysis of episodes, length of stay, and charges over a seven-year period. *J Gerontol*. 1994; 49:S240–S252.
33. Foley DJ, Ostfeld AM, Branch LG, Wallace RB, McGloin J, Cornoni-Huntley JC. The risk of nursing home admission in three communities. *J Aging Health*. 1992 May; 4(2):155–173.
34. Wolinksy FD, Callahan CM, Fitzgerald JF et al. The risk of nursing home placement and subsequent death among older adults. *J Gerontol*. 1992; 47:S173–S182.
35. Fried TR, Bradley EH, Williams CS, Tinetti ME. Functional disability and health care expenditures for older persons. *Arch Intern Med*. 2001; 161(21):2602–2607.
36. Wahrendorf M, Reinhardt JD, Siegrist J. Relationships of disability with age among adults aged 50 to 85: Evidence from the United States, England and Continental Europe. *PLoS ONE*. 2013; 8(8):e71893. doi: 10.1371/journal.pone.0071893.
37. Anderson GF, Hussey PS. Population aging: A comparison among industrialized countries. *Health Aff*. 2000; 19:191–203.
38. World Health Organization. National Institute on Aging, National Institute of Health: NIH publication no. 11-7737, October 2011.
39. Kinsella K, Wan H. U.S. Census Bureau, International Population Reports, p95/09-1, *An Aging World: 2008*, U.S. Government Printing Office, Washington, DC, 2009.
40. Levit K, Smith C, Cowan C, Lazenby H, Sensenig A, Catlin A. Trends in U.S. health care spending, 2001. *Health Aff*. 2003; 22:154–164.
41. Kinsella K, Velkoff V. *U.S. Census Bureau. An Aging World: 2001*. Washington, DC: U.S. Government Printing Office, 2001; series P95/01-1.
42. Blom J, den Elzen W, van Houwelingen AH, Heijmans M, Stijnen T, Van den Hout W, Gussekloo J. Effectiveness and cost-effectiveness of a proactive, goal-oriented, integrated care model in general practice for older people. A cluster randomized controlled trial: Integrated Systematic Care for Older People—The ISCOPE study. *Age Ageing*. 2016 Jan; 45(1):30–41.
43. Hong CS, Siegel AL, Ferris TG. Caring for high-need, high-cost patients: What makes for a successful care management program? *Issue Brief (Commonw Fund)*. 2014 Aug; 19:1–19. www.commonwealthfund.org.
44. Stefanacci RG. Care coordination today: What, why, who, where, and how? *Clin Geriatr*. 2013 Mar; 21(3):12–16.
45. The Value of Nursing Care Coordination. A white paper of the American Nurses Association, n.d., Retrieved April 19, 2016, from http://www.nursingworld.org/carecoordinationwhitepaper.
46. Marek KD, Adams SJ, Stetzer F, Popejoy L, Rantz M. The relationship of community-based nurse care coordination to costs in the Medicare and Medicaid programs. *Res Nurs Health*. 2010 Jun; 33(3):235–242. doi: 10.1002/nur.20378.
47. Coleman EA, Parry C, Chalmers S, Min S. The care transitions intervention: Results of a randomized controlled trial. *Arch Intern Med*. 2006; 166(17):1822–1828. doi: 10.1001/archinte.166.17.1822.
48. Sarnak DO, Ryan J. How high-need patients experiences the health care system in nine countries. *Issue Brief (Commonw Fund)*. 2016 Jan; 1:1–14.
49. World Health Organization Report on Aging and Health: www.who.int/entity/ageing/publications/world-report-2015/en/-32k.
50. Fitzpatrick AL, Powe NR, Cooper LS, Ives DG, Robbins JA. Barriers to health care access among the elderly and who perceives them. *Am J Public Health*. 2004 Oct; 94(10):1788–1794.
51. Gulland A. Older people are not a burden, says WHO. *Brit Med J*. 2015; 351:h5272.
52. Mateos-Nozal J, Beard JR. Global approaches to geriatrics in medical education. *Eur Geriatr Med*. 2011; 2(2):87–92. World Report on Ageing and Health.

33 Aging Gracefully
A Global Perspective

Brian Tucker and K. Rao Poduri

CONTENTS

33.1 INTRODUCTION

Age, generally refers to the "length of life," or "existence" or to the "later part of life." In short, aging also is referred to as "Growing old." By all statistics, the world's population is getting older and people over 65 are going to outnumber their counterparts by 2050. People are living longer due to improvements in healthcare, nutrition, and technology. This shift in population provides great possibilities, but not without challenges.

In the United States, the term older adults is used for people over 65 years. In other parts of the world, such as New Guinea, anyone 50 years and older is considered *lapun,* or an old man. The people of Greek island of Ikaria, a small Mediterranean island, are 4 times more likely than their American counterparts to live to 90, and are noted to live on an average 8–10 years longer with cancer or heart disease. And this island's longevity is attributed to relaxed life style and dietary habits. It is said that the perception of aging varies from one society to another, and it changes over time within any given society.

The United Nations (UN) calls people 60 years and older as elderly and has a policy to support aging populations around the world. The United Nations General Assembly voted on December 14, 1990 to establish October 1 as the International Day of Older Persons to recognize and acknowledge the contributions made by this population to the world. The holiday was observed on October 1, 1991 for the first time. The purpose of this celebration is to raise awareness about issues affecting the elderly, such as senescence and elder abuse.

The American Geriatric Society prefers to use the term older adults as opposed to elderly as it is associated with frailty. Surprisingly, when asked how they feel, the older adults often remark that they often feel younger than their years or say that the best years are yet to come for them. In January 2014, the Pew Research Center on Global Attitudes and Trends published the attitudes about aging and the global perspectives describing the problems of aging. For instance, nine-in-ten Japanese, eight-in-ten South Koreans and seven-in-ten Chinese, and more than 50% of people in Europe, Germany, and Spain are concerned about aging as a major problem for their countries. However, in the United States, only one-in-four are concerned about aging despite the economic burden described in the previous chapter. The aging population raises concerns in many aspects, and it is projected that population in the United States will grow more rapidly than in Europe, East Asia, and Latin America.

There is an increase in the growth of the aging world population due to declines in mortality and fertility rates. Life expectancy is at all-time high and it puts a strain on the health of individuals. The twentieth century was known for population growth and the twenty-first century will be known for aging. There is an escalation of age and age-related diseases causing a burden not only on individuals and families but also on social, economic, and healthcare systems. The major concerns with advancing age are health of the population and healthcare expenditures. The last few decades were marked with significant contributions to the development of new drugs, clinical interventions for Alzheimer's disease, cancer, type II diabetes, cardiovascular diseases, and understanding of age and age-related diseases and their treatments. The research and the impact of the discoveries have led to this explosion of the aging population. Now, it is not the cure of the disease with medical and technological advances that becomes relevant to this population but it is the quality of life of the older adults that is meaningful with or without the disease.

In the prehistoric societies, the physical and mental health of older people and the society's economy dictated the view of older adults.[1]

33.2   PHYSICAL AND MENTAL HEALTH OF THE OLDER ADULTS

Age-related physical conditions include hypertension, heart disease, diabetes, osteoporosis, arthritis, hearing loss, and impairment of vision in addition to the physiological changes described in Chapter 1. Cognitive decline and speed of information processing may decrease resulting in memory loss. Functional decline due to the above conditions results in dependence for everyday activities that increases with age. It is reported that 9% of those between ages 65 and 69 and up to 50% of older Americans over 85 are dependent on caregivers for activities of daily living (ADL) and mobility. In addition, depression, dementia, and anxiety disorders are also found in older adults that may impact quality of life and may require institutionalization. There is a difference in the way older adults exhibit cognitive deficits, some showing significant deficits while others performing as well as young adults.[2] This phenomenon is well described in a study by Cabeza et al.[3] in which the differences are explained on neural basis. The high-performing older adults were noted in that study to counteract age-related neural decline by reorganizing brain functions with similar neural network as young adults. They concluded that low-performing young adults utilize their brain function inefficiently.

33.3   AGING GRACEFULLY

Older women outnumbered older men in the United States. Lunenfeld and Stratton[4] argue that in order for the women to age gracefully and continue to maintain functional independence, the healthcare system needs to address preventive strategies to reduce or minimize frailty, cancer, cardiac, and metabolic diseases and prevent the resulting disabilities. Balance between life expectancy and maintenance of health are the main goals to achieve graceful aging.

Socioeconomic status clearly has an impact on morbidity and mortality of various diseases. Racial and ethnic backgrounds, poverty, education, and marital status were described as predictors of health expectancy, morbidity, and mortality. Thirty seven key indicators were reported to have an influence on health status and behaviors of older adults in 2012 by the Federal Interagency Forum on Aging-Related Statistics.[5] The important factors are as follows: 1. *Population*: the number of older Americans, racial and ethnic composition, marital status educational attainment, living arrangements, and older veterans. 2. *Economic factors:* poverty, income, sources of income, net worth, participation in labor force, total expenditures, and housing problems. 3. *Health status*: life expectancy, mortality, chronic health conditions, sensory impairments and oral health, respondent-assessed health status, depressive symptoms, and functional limitations. 4. *Health risks and behaviors*: vaccinations, mammography, diet quality, physical activity, obesity, cigarette smoking, air quality, and use of time. 5. *Healthcare*: use of healthcare services, healthcare expenditures, prescription drugs, sources of health insurance, out-of-pocket healthcare expenditures, sources of payment for healthcare services, veterans' healthcare, residential services, and personal assistance and equipment. There is a need to collect more data for residential care, elder abuse, informal care, functioning and disability, mental and cognitive functioning, pension measures, and end-of-life issues addressing the type of care received (hospice and intensive care unit/coronary care units) and place of death in the days to months preceding death. There are health risks and behaviors that can be modified to promote aging as an enjoyable and graceful experience.

Lunenfeld[6] in his editorial emphasizes that the promotion of healthy aging and the prevention, or drastic reduction, of morbidity and disability among the elderly must assume a central role in the formulation of health and social policies. It must emphasize an all-encompassing, lifelong approach to the aging process beginning with pre-conceptual events and focus on appropriate interventions at all stages of life. Environmental, economical, behavioral, and other factors determine aging and life expectancy. He went on to discuss the following specific measures for the promotion of healthy aging:

1. The promotion of a safe environment
2. Healthy lifestyle including proper nutrition
3. Appropriate exercise
4. Avoidance of smoking
5. Avoidance of drug and alcohol abuse
6. Social interactions to maintain good mental health
7. Preventive medical strategies to delay, decrease, or prevent frailty and disabilities
8. Medical healthcare including the control of chronic illnesses

All the above measures when applied to the older adults' life styles will accomplish the goal of aging gracefully. Some of these factors were emphasized in the previous chapters.

In general, older adults receive healthcare in primary care settings, but it is not clear that whether they receive the standard of care for chronic disease management, geriatric syndromes, and recommended preventive services. The Geriatric Resources for Assessment and Care of Elders (GRACE) model of primary care[7] was developed for low-income geriatric population to optimize health and functional status, decrease healthcare, utilization, and avoid institutionalization into long-term care facilities. Other investigators have studied various interventions for improving care of the older adults such as outpatient geriatric evaluation and management.[8] Counsell et al.[9] studied a multi-component interventional approach of care for hospitalized older people in a community-teaching hospital and showed that it is possible to prevent ADL decline and/or nursing home placement at discharge without adverse effects or increased costs.

The effect of preventive home visits on functional status, nursing home admission, and mortality were studied through a meta-regression analysis.[10] In this study, functional decline in the elderly and potential for nursing home admissions were assessed via home visits by implementing primary, secondary, and tertiary prevention measures. They were found to be effective if the assessments were based on multidimensional geriatric interventions linked with several follow-up visits. Survival was more effective for the young–old rather than the old–old population.

Semi-structured interviews by 17 experts in preventive elderly care and three group interviews with volunteer elderly advisors were conducted in Netherlands.[11] Qualitative analysis revealed that the needs of the frail older adults are not sufficiently addressed in spite of a number of initiatives being available for preventive care.

Japan has the longest life expectancy compared to the rest of the countries in the world. They created promotion systems[12] toward improving the care of the older adults and their participation in social activities. There are several initiatives in all aspects of life spanning from building geriatric medical centers in each area, home-based multidisciplinary care to educational reforms in undergraduate and postgraduate, and lifelong education and promotion of gerontology to name a few. With the above measures, Japan is expected to be a role model and sets an example to the rest of the countries. Japan is the "front-runner of super-aged societies"[13] and believes that conventional medical care must be upgraded to meet the needs of the aging society and move ahead from "cure-seeking medical care" to "cure and support-seeking medical care" with a goal of improving the quality of life of its aging population. True to the title of this book *Geriatric Rehabilitation from Bed Side to Curbside*, Japan embraces the concept of "hospital-centered medical care" to "community-oriented medical care" to promote and maximize function and independence and improves graceful aging of older adults.

In conclusion, information technology revolution in the recent years has an impact, in that older adults feel left out. The people in their 20s and 30s are at the center of the information age and the effect of the information age on the older adults also may dictate the view on how they perceive themselves. To combat the various deficits such as mobility difficulties, social isolation, and loneliness that accompany older adults, Technologies for Aging Gracefully lab (TAGlab) was formed in 2009[14] and their mission is to enable full participation in society by individuals with special needs. As the older adults outnumber the youth, they face several challenges that may include maintaining self-esteem, coping with vulnerability,[15] and preparing for retirement. Socioemotional selectivity theory says that older adults invest greater resources in emotionally meaningful activities and focus on positivity than negativity. These attitudes in turn may help to cope with age-related social and health issues and aim toward aging gracefully.

REFERENCES

1. Sokolovsky J. *The Cultural Context of Aging: Worldwide Perspectives*, 3rd edition. Connecticut: Praeger. December 30, 2008.
2. Christensen H, Mackinnon AJ, Korten AE, Jorm AF, Henderson AS, Jacomb P, Rodgers B. An analysis of diversity in the cognitive performance of elderly community dwellers: Individual differences in change scores as a function of age. *Psychol Aging* 1999; 14: 365–379.
3. Cabeza R, Anderson ND, Locantore JK, McIntosh AR. Aging gracefully: Compensatory brain activity in high-performing older adults. *Neuroimage* 2002; 17(3): 1394–1402.
4. Lunenfeld B, Stratton P. The clinical consequences of an ageing world and preventive strategies. *Best Pract Res Clin Obstet Gynaecol* 2013; 27(5): 643–659. E pub Mar 28 2013.
5. Older Americans 2012: Key indicators of well-being available on line http://www.agingstats.gov (Federal Interagency Forum on Aging Related Statistics).
6. Lunenfeld B. An aging world—Demographics and challenges. *Editorial Gynecol Endocrinol* 2008; 24(1): 1–3.
7. Counsell SR, Callahan CM, Buttar AB, Clark DO, Frank KI. Geriatric resources for assessment and care of elders (GRACE): A new model of primary care for low-income seniors. *J Am Geriatr Soc* 2006; 54(7): 1136–1141.
8. Boult C, Boult LB, Morishita L et al. A randomized clinical trial of outpatient geriatric evaluation and management. *J Am Geriatr Soc* 2001; 49: 351–359.
9. Counsell SR, Holder CM, Liebenauer LL et al. Effects of a multicomponent intervention on functional outcomes and process of care in hospitalized older patients: A randomized controlled trial of acute care for elders (ACE) in a community hospital. *J Am Geriatr Soc* 2000; 48: 1572–1581.
10. Stuck AE, Egger M, Hammer A et al. Home visits to prevent nursing home admission and functional decline in elderly people: Systematic review and meta-regression analysis. *J Am Med Assoc* 2002; 287: 1022–1028.
11. Lette M, Baan CA, van den Berg M, de Bruin SR. Initiatives on early detection and intervention to proactively identify health and social problems in older people: Experiences from the Netherlands. *BMC Geriatr* 2015; 15: 143.
12. Arai H, Ouchi Y, Yokode M et al. Members of subcommittee for aging. Toward the realization of a better aged society: Messages from gerontology and geriatrics. *Geriatr Gerontol Int.* 2012; 12(1): 16–22.
13. Arai H, Ouchi Y, Toba K et al. Japan as the front-runner of super-aged societies: Perspectives from medicine and medical care in Japan. *Geriatr Gerontol Int.* 2015; 15 (6): 673–687.
14. Baecker RM, Moffatt K, Massimi M. Technologies for aging gracefully. *Mag Interact* 2012; 19(3): 32–36.
15. Perry VG, Wolburg JM. Aging gracefully: Emerging issues for public policy and consumer welfare. *J Consum Aff Spec Issue: Aging Consum* 2011; 45(3): 365–371.

Index

Printed in the United States
by Baker & Taylor Publisher Services